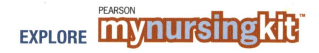 

EXPLORE **mynursingkit**™

PEARSON

D0076798

STEP 1: Register

All you need to get started is a valid email address and the access code below. To register, simply:

1. Go to **www.mynursingkit.com**. Click on the appropriate book cover.
2. In the "First-Time User" column, click "**Register**."
3. Read the **License Agreement** and **Privacy Policy**. If you accept, click "**I Accept**."
4. Under "**Do you have a Pearson account**?" select:
   - "**Yes**" if you have a Pearson account and know your Login Name and Password.
   - "**Not Sure**" if you do not know if you already have an account or do not recall your Login Name and Password.
   - "**No**" if you are sure you do not have a Pearson account.
5. Using a coin, scratch off the silver coating below to reveal your access code. Do not use a knife or other sharp object, which can damage the code.
6. Enter your access code in lowercase or uppercase, without the dashes, then click "**Next**."
7. Follow the on-screen instructions to complete registration.

After completing registration, you will be sent a confirmation email that contains your Login Name and Password. Be sure to save this email for future reference.

Your Access Code is:

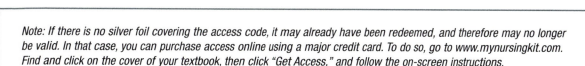

Note: If there is no silver foil covering the access code, it may already have been redeemed, and therefore may no longer be valid. In that case, you can purchase access online using a major credit card. To do so, go to www.mynursingkit.com. Find and click on the cover of your textbook, then click "Get Access," and follow the on-screen instructions.

STEP 2: Log in

1. Go to **www.mynursingkit.com**.
2. Find and click on the appropriate book cover. Cover must match the textbook edition used for your class.
3. Enter the Login Name and Password that you created during registration. If unsure of this information, refer to your registration confirmation email.
4. Click "**Login**."

Got technical questions?

Customer Technical Support: To obtain support, please visit us online anytime at http://247pearsoned.custhelp.com where you can search our knowledgebase for common solutions, view product alerts, and review all options for additional assistance.

SITE REQUIREMENTS

For the latest updates on Site Requirements, go to www.mynursingkit.com. Find and click on the cover of the book you are using. Click on "**Needs help?**" link at bottom of page. Under "**Technical Problems**" select the link "**What do I need on my computer to use this site?**"

Important: Please read the Subscription and End-User License agreement, accessible from the book website's login page, before using the *mynursingkit* website. By using the website, you indicate that you have read, understood, and accepted the terms of this agreement.

Classroom

- Detailed lecture notes organized by learning outcome
- Suggestions for classroom activities
- Guide to relevant additional resources
- Comprehensive PowerPoint™ presentations integrating lecture, images, animations, and videos
- Classroom Response questions
- Image Gallery
- Video and Animation Gallery
- Online course management systems complete with instructor tools and student activities available in a variety of formats

PEARSON mynursinglab

- Saves instructors time by providing quality feedback, ongoing formative assessments and customized remediation for students.
- Provides easy, one-stop access to a wealth of teaching resources, such as test item files, PowerPoint™ slides, and video suggestions.
- A built-in electronic gradebook tracks students' progress on assessment and remediation activities.

Clinical

- Suggestions for Clinical Activities and other clinical resources organized by learning outcome

Real Nursing Simulations Facilitator's Guide: Institutional Edition

- 25 simulation scenarios that span the nursing curriculum
- Consistent format includes learning objectives, case flow, instructions for set up, student debriefing questions and more!
- Companion online course cartridge with student exercises, activities, videos, skill checklists, and reflective questions also available for adoption

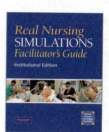

NCLEX-RN®

- Test Item Files with NCLEX®-style questions and complete rationales for correct and incorrect answers mapped to learning outcomes. *Available in TestGen, Par Test, and MS Word*

Instructor Resources

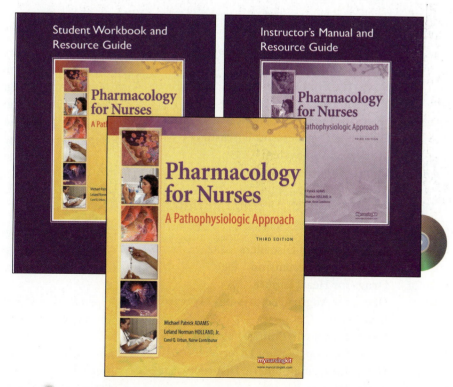

Student Workbook and Resource Guide

Instructor's Manual and Resource Guide

Pharmacology for Nurses
A Pathophysiologic Approach
THIRD EDITION

Michael Patrick ADAMS
Leland Norman HOLLAND, Jr.
Carol Q. Urban, Nurse Contributor

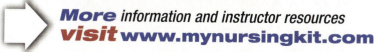

More information and instructor resources
visit www.mynursingkit.com

Brief Contents

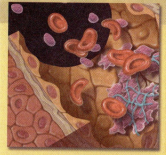

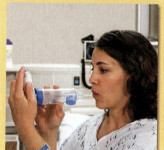

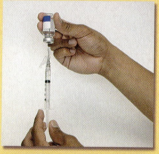

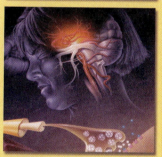

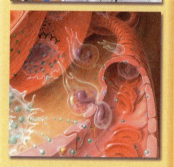

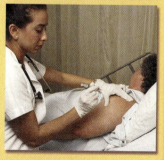

Pharmacology for Nurses

A Pathophysiologic Approach

THIRD EDITION

Michael Patrick Adams
Professor, Biological Sciences
Formerly Dean, Health Occupations
Pasco-Hernando Community College

Leland Norman Holland, Jr.
Instructor
Hillsborough Community College, Southshore Center

Carol Q. Urban, Nurse Contributor
Assistant Dean, Undergraduate Nursing
Assistant Professor
George Mason University

Pearson

Boston   Columbus   Indianapolis   New York   San Francisco   Upper Saddle River

Amsterdam   Cape Town   Dubai   London   Madrid   Milan   Munich   Paris   Montreal   Toronto

Delhi   Mexico City   São Paulo   Sydney   Hong Kong   Seoul   Singapore   Taipei   Tokyo

Library of Congress Cataloging-in-Publication Data

Adams, Michael
  Pharmacology for nurses : a pathophysiologic approach / Michael Patrick Adams, Leland Norman Holland Jr.—3rd ed.
    p. ; cm.
  Includes bibliographical references and index.
  ISBN-978-0-13-508981-1
  1. Pharmacology. 2. Nursing. I. Holland, Leland Norman. II. Title.
  [DNLM: 1. Drug Therapy—nursing. 2. Pharmacology—Nurses' Instruction. WB 330 A215p 2011]
  RM301.A32 2011
  615'.1—dc22

2009053910

Publisher: Julie Levin Alexander
Assistant to Publisher: Regina Bruno
Editor-in-Chief: Maura Connor
Assistant to the Editor-in-Chief: Marion Gottlieb
Executive Acquisitions Editor: Kelly Trakalo
Editorial Assistant: Lauren Sweeney
Development Editor: Michael Giacobbe
Media Product Manager: Travis Moses-Westphal
Director of Marketing: David Gesell
Marketing Specialist: Michael Sirinides
Marketing Assistant: Crystal Gonzalez
Managing Editor, Production: Patrick Walsh
Production Editor: Barb Tucker, S4Carlisle Publishing Services
Production Liaison: Anne Garcia
Media Project Manager: Rachel Collett
Manufacturing Manager: Ilene Sanford
Art Director: Christopher Weigand
Interior/Cover Design: Christine Cantera
Manager, Image Rights and Permissions: Zina Arabia
Manager, Visual Research: Beth Brenzel
Manager, Cover Visual Research & Permissions: Karen Sanatar
Image Permission Coordinator: Vicki Menanteaux
Composition: S4Carlisle Publishing Services
Printer/Binder: Quebecor World Color/Versailles
Cover Printer: Lehigh-Phoenix Color/Hagerstown

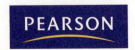

www.pearsonhighered.com

10 9 8 7 6 5 4 3 2 1
ISBN-13: 978-0-13-508981-1
ISBN-10:   0-13-508981-6

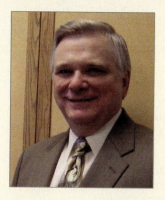

Michael Patrick Adams, PhD, is an accomplished educator, author, and national speaker. The National Institute for Staff and Organizational Development in Austin, Texas, named Dr. Adams a Master Teacher. He has published two other textbooks with Pearson Publishing: *Core Concepts in Pharmacology* and *Pharmacology: Connections to Nursing Practice.*

Dr. Adams obtained his Master's degree in Pharmacology from Michigan State University and his Doctorate in Education at the University of South Florida. Dr. Adams was on the faculty of Lansing Community College and St. Petersburg College, and was Dean of Health Programs at Pasco-Hernando Community College for 15 years. He is currently Professor of Biological Sciences at Pasco-Hernando Community College.

I dedicate this book to nursing educators, who contribute every day to making the world a better and more caring place.

—MPA

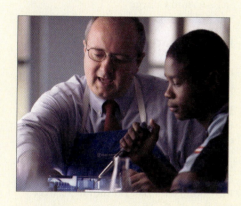

Leland Norman Holland, Jr., PhD (Norm) over 20 years ago started out like many scientists, planning for a career in basic science research. He was quickly drawn to the field of teaching in higher medical education, where he has spent most of his career since then. Among the areas where he has been particularly effective are preparatory programs in nursing, medicine, dentistry, pharmacy, and allied health. Dr. Holland is both an affiliate and supporter of nursing education nationwide. He brings to the profession a depth of knowledge in biology, chemistry, and medically related subjects such as microbiology, biological chemistry, and pharmacology. Dr. Holland's doctoral degree is in medical pharmacology. He is very much dedicated to the success of students and their preparation for work–life readiness. He continues to motivate students in the lifelong pursuit of learning.

I would like to thank the willful encouragement of Farrell and Norma Jean Stalcup. I dedicate this book to my beloved wife, Karen, and my three wonderful children, Alexandria Noelle, my double-deuce daughter, Caleb James, my number-one son, and Joshua Nathaniel, my number three "O."

—LNH

NURSE CONTRIBUTOR

Carol Quam Urban, PhD, RN is the Assistant Dean for Undergraduate Nursing and an Assistant Professor in the School of Nursing, College of Health and Human Services at George Mason University where she teaches undergraduate courses in pharmacology and pathophysiology. Her current research interests focus on improving learning for students at-risk for academic difficulties, outcomes-based education, effective educational models using computer-based learning, and service-based learning. She has also published articles on the ethical needs of at-risk students.

She is a member of Sigma Theta Tau - Epsilon Zeta chapter, Alpha Chi, the National Association for Developmental Education, National College Learning Center Association, and the College Reading and Learning Association. At George Mason University, she serves on the General Education Committee and the Distance Education Council.

To my daughter, Joy, an extraordinary, resilient young woman. And in memory of my son, Keith, the bravest and happiest soul I know.

—CQU

Thank You

The authors wish to convey their special thanks to the many nurse contributors and reviewers who provided their unique knowledge and expertise to this project. Their insights, suggestions, eye for detail, and dedication to quality nursing education were evident and enabled us to prepare an accurate, relevant, and useful pharmacology textbook.

SUPPLEMENT CONTRIBUTORS

Rosemary Bakasa, RN, MSN, PhD
Bryant and Stratton College—
Eastlake Campus
Eastlake, Ohio
Instructor's Resource Manual
PowerPoints

Marge Gingrich, RN, MSN
Harrisburg Area Community College
Harrisburg, Pennsylvania
MyNursingLab

Sandra L. Gustafson, RN, MA
Hibbing Community College
Hibbing, Minnesota
MyNursingLab

Frank Lyerla, PhD, RN
Southern Illinois University Edwardsville
Edwardsville, Illinois
Test Bank

Barbara Maxwell, RN, MS, LNC
State University of NY at Ulster
Stone Ridge, New York
Instructor's Resource Manual

Pamela Newland, PhD, BSN, MSN
Southern Illinois University Edwardsville
Edwardsville, Illinois
Test Bank
MyNursingLab

Janine Ray, BA, BSN, MSN, RN, CRRN
Cisco College
Cisco, Texas
MyNursingLab

REVIEWERS

Joy Ache-Reed, RN, MSN
Indiana Wesleyan University
Marion, Indiana

Exzelia O. Alfred, RN, BSN, MA, MEd
Kent State University, Tuscarawas
New Philadelphia, Ohio

Rosemary Bakasa, RN, MSN, PhD
Bryant and Stratton College—
Eastlake Campus
Eastlake, Ohio

Kathy Black, MSN
Iowa Western Community College
Council Bluffs, Iowa

Ilene Borze, RN, MS
Gateway Community College
Phoenix, Arizona

Donna L. Bumpus, RN, MSN
Lamar University
Beaumont, Texas

Darlene Clark, RN, MSN
Pennsylvania State University
University Park, Pennsylvania

Lucille Dirk, RN, MSN
ATS Institute of Technology
Highland Heights, Ohio

MaryAnn Edelman, RN, MS, CNS
Kingsborough Community College
Brooklyn, New York

Jacqueline Frock, RN, MSN
Oklahoma City Community College
Oklahoma City, Oklahoma

Mēki Jacobs Graham, RN, MSN
University of North Carolina
at Pembroke
Pembroke, North Carolina

Sandra L. Gustafson, RN, MA
Hibbing Community College
Hibbing, Minnesota

Lorrie S. Jones, ARNP-C
Polk State College
Winter Haven, Florida

Kathleen Krov, RN, MSN, CNM, CNE
Raritan Valley Community College
Somerville, New Jersey

Lora J. Leonard, RN, MSN
Kent State University, Ashtabula Regional Campus
Ashtabula, Ohio

Barbara Maxwell, RN, MSN, LNC
State University of NY at Ulster
Stone Ridge, New York

Lora McGuire, RN, MS
Joliet Junior College
Joliet, Illinois

Cydney King Mullen, RN, PhD
Sandhills Community College
Pinehurst, North Carolina

Christina Carol Olson, RN, MSN
San Antonio College
San Antonio, Texas

Janice Ramirez, RN, MSN, BC, CRRN, CNE
North Idaho College
Coeur d'Alene, Idaho

Laurie Simmons, BSN, MSN, MEd
Kirkwood Community College
Cedar Rapids, Iowa

Ann Underwood Smith, RN, MSN, FNP, CNOR
Piedmont Virginia Community College
Charlottesville, Virginia

Marianne F. Swihart, RN, BSN, MEd, MSN, CRNI, WCON, PCCN
Pasco-Hernando Community College
New Port Richey, Florida

Annie Thomas, RN, PhD
Marcella Niehoff School of Nursing
Chicago, Illinois

Kathy Trummer, RN, MS, CNS
Front Range Community College—
Westminster Campus
Westminster, Colorado

Keith T. Veltri, BS, PH, PharmD
Adelphi School of Nursing
Garden City, New York

Daryle Wane, PhD, ARNP, FNP-BC
Pasco-Hernando Community College
New Port Richey, Florida

Nancy Lynn Whitehead, MS, FNP-C, CSN, CLNC
Milwaukee Area Technical College
Milwaukee, Wisconsin

When students are asked which subject in their nursing program is the most challenging, pharmacology always appears near the top of the list. The study of pharmacology demands that students apply knowledge from a wide variety of the natural and applied sciences. Successfully predicting drug action requires a thorough knowledge of anatomy, physiology, chemistry, and pathology as well as the social sciences of psychology and sociology. Not properly applying pharmacology can result in immediate and direct harm to the patient; thus, the stakes in learning the subject are high.

Pharmacology cannot be made easy, but it can be made understandable, if the proper connections are made to knowledge learned in these other disciplines. The vast majority of drugs in clinical practice are prescribed for specific diseases, yet many pharmacology textbooks fail to recognize the complex interrelationships between pharmacology and pathophysiology. When drugs are learned in isolation from their associated diseases or conditions, students have difficulty connecting pharmacotherapy to therapeutic goals and patient wellness. The pathophysiology approach of this textbook gives the student a clearer picture of the importance of pharmacology to disease, and, ultimately, to patient care. The approach and rationale of this textbook focus on a holistic perspective to patient care, which clearly shows the benefits and limitations of pharmacotherapy in curing or preventing illness. Although difficult and challenging, the study of pharmacology is truly a fascinating, lifelong journey.

ORGANIZATION AND STRUCTURE— A BODY SYSTEM AND DISEASE APPROACH

Pharmacology for Nurses: A Pathophysiologic Approach is organized according to body systems (units) and diseases (chapters). Each chapter provides the complete information on the drug classifications used to treat the disease(s) classes. Specially designed numbered headings describe key concepts and cue students to each drug classification discussion.

The pathophysiology approach clearly places the drugs in context with how they are used therapeutically. The student is able to locate easily all relevant anatomy, physiology, pathology, and pharmacology in the same chapter in which the drugs are discussed. This approach provides the student with a clear view of the connection between pharmacology, pathophysiology, and the nursing care learned in other clinical courses.

The vast number of drugs available in clinical practice is staggering. To facilitate learning, we use prototypes where the one or two most representative drugs in each classification are introduced in detail in the chapter. Students are less intimidated when they can focus their learning on one representative drug in each class.

New to This Edition

The third edition of *Pharmacology for Nurses: A Pathophysiologic Approach* has been thoroughly updated to reflect current pharmacologic drugs and processes.

- NEW! Research boxes provide evidence-based practice as it is applicable to pharmacology.

- EXPANDED! Complementary and Alternative boxes now include 20 of the top natural therapies.

- EXPANDED! Pharmacotherapy Illustrated diagrams to help students visualize the connection between pharmacology and the patient.

- NEW! Pharmacologic and therapeutic drug classes have been added to all prototype drug boxes.

- NEW! Lifespan boxes discuss specific considerations for specific population groups.

- NEW! Treating the Diverse Patient features discuss the nursing considerations of a diverse population.

- Updated! Nursing Process Focus Charts

- Enhanced and Revised! End of chapter NCLEX questions now include alternative format items and complete rationales.

- NEW! Appendix on the ISMP's List of High-Alert Medications has been added.

- NEW! Information on weight-loss drugs and obesity has been added.

A Note About Terminology

The term "health care provider" is used to denote the physician, nurse practitioner, and any other health professional who is legally authorized to prescribe drugs.

ACKNOWLEDGMENTS

When authoring a textbook such as this, a huge number of dedicated and talented professionals are needed to bring the initial vision to reality. Kelly Trakalo, Senior Acquisitions Editor, and Maura Connor, Editor-in-Chief, are responsible for helping us sculpt the vision for the text. Our Developmental Editor, Michael Giacobbe, supplied the expert guidance and leadership to keep everyone on task and to be certain it reached its fruition on time. Providing the necessary expertise for our comprehensive supplement package was Lauren Sweeney, Editorial Assistant.

The design staff at Pearson, especially Chris Weigand, created magnificent text and cover designs. Overseeing the production process with finesse was Anne Garcia, Production Liaison. Barb Tucker and the staff at S4Carlisle provided expert and professional guidance in all aspects of the art and production process.

Although difficult and challenging, the study of pharmacology is truly a fascinating, lifelong journey. We hope that we have written a textbook that helps make that study easier and more understandable so that nursing students will be able to provide safe, effective nursing care to patients undergoing drug therapy. We hope students and faculty will share with us their experiences using this textbook and all its resources.

Learning Pharmacology in Context

25.2 Pathogenesis of Angina Pectoris

The classic presentation of angina pectoris is steady, intense pain in the anterior chest, sometimes accompanied by a crushing or constricting sensation. The discomfort may radiate to the left shoulder and proceed down the left arm and it may extend posterior to the thoracic spine or move upward to the jaw. In some patients, the pain is experienced in the midepigastrium or abdominal area. Recent studies indicate that women do not always present with the classic symptoms

◄ **The organization by body systems (units) and diseases** (chapters) clearly places the drugs in context with how they are used therapeutically. You can easily locate all relevant anatomy, physiology, pathophysiology, and pharmacology in the same chapter in which we present complete information for the drug classifications used to treat the disease(s) in each chapter. This organization builds the connection between pharmacology, pathophysiology, and the nursing care you learn in your clinical nursing courses.

Drugs at a Glance presents a quick way for you to see the classifications and prototypes that are covered in the chapter, organized by disorder drug class. ▶

DRUGS AT A GLANCE

ORGANIC NITRATES *page 341*
- *nitroglycerin (Nitrostat, Nitro-Bid, Nitro-Dur, others)* *page 344*

BETA-ADRENERGIC BLOCKERS (ANTAGONISTS) *page 343*
- *atenolol (Tenormin)* *page 347*

CALCIUM CHANNEL BLOCKERS *page 343*
- *diltiazem (Cardizem, Cartia XT, Dilacor XR, Taztia XT, Tiazac)* *page 348*

THROMBOLYTICS *page 348*
- *reteplase (Retavase)* *page 351*

ADJUNCT DRUGS FOR MYOCARDIAL INFARCTION *page 349*

PHARMFACTS

Angina Pectoris
- Over 9 million Americans have angina pectoris; 500,000 new cases occur each year.
- 20% of the deaths due to cardiovascular disease are attributed to smoking.

Myocardial Infarction
- More than 1.1 million Americans experience a new or recurrent MI each year.
- About one third of the patients experiencing MIs will die from them.
- About 60% of the patients who died suddenly of MI had no previous symptoms of the disease.

◄ **PharmFacts** present pertinent facts and statistics related to the disease, providing you with a social and economic perspective of the disease.

Prototype Approach and Prototype Drug boxes clearly ▶ summarize important medications. They include:

- Actions and Uses
- Administration Alerts
- Pharmacokinetics, including onset of action, duration, half-life, and peak effect, when known
- Adverse Effects and Contraindications
- Interactions with drugs, herbs, and food
- Treatment of overdose and antidotes, where applicable

Pr Prototype Drug | Escitalopram Oxalate *(Lexapro)*

Therapeutic Class: Antidepressant; anxiolytic   **Pharmacologic Class:** Selective serotonin reuptake inhibitor (SSRI)

ACTIONS AND USES

Escitalopram is a selective serotonin reuptake inhibitor (SSRI) that increases the availability of serotonin at specific postsynaptic receptor sites located within the CNS. Selective inhibition of serotonin reuptake results in antidepressant activity without production of symptoms of sympathomimetic or anticholinergic activity. This medication is indicated for conditions of generalized anxiety and depression. Unlabeled uses include the treatment of panic disorders.

ADMINISTRATION ALERTS

- This medication should not be started until 14 days have elapsed after discontinuing any MAOI drugs.
- In cases of renal or hepatic impairment or in older adults, reduced doses are advised.
- Dose increments should be separated by at least 1 week.
- Pregnancy category C.

PHARMACOKINETICS
Onset: With once-daily dosing, steady-state plasma concentrations can be reached within 1 wk
Peak: 5 h
Half-life: 25–35 h
Duration: Variable

ADVERSE EFFECTS

Serious reactions include dizziness, nausea, insomnia, somnolennce, confusion, and seizures if taken in overdose.

Contraindications: This drug should not be used in patients who are breast-feeding or within 14 days of MAOI therapy.

INTERACTIONS

Drug–Drug: MAOIs should be avoided due to serotonin syndrome, marked by autonomic hyperactivity, hyperthermia, rigidity, diaphoresis, and neuroleptic malignant syndrome. Combination with MAOIs could result in hypertensive crisis, hyperthermia, and autonomic instability.
Escitalopram will increase plasma levels of metoprolol and cimetidine. Concurrent use of alcohol and other CNS depressants may enhance CNS depressant effects; patients should avoid alcohol when taking this drug.

Lab Tests: Unknown

Herbal/Food: Use caution with herbal supplements such as St. John's wort, which may cause serotonin syndrome and increase the effects of escitalopram.

Treatment of Overdose: There is no specific treatment for overdose. Treat symptoms, as indicated, including dizziness, confusion, nausea, vomiting, tremor, sweating, tachycardia, and seizures.

Refer to MyNursingKit for a Nursing Process Focus specific to this drug.

See Chapter 16, page 191, for Nursing Process Focus: Patients Receiving Antidepressant Therapy ∞ .

Teaching Through Visuals

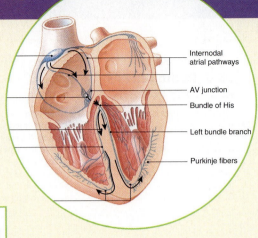

Vivid and colorful illustrations help you review specific anatomy, physiology, and pathophysiology for a body system to help you better understand the impact of disease on that system. ▶

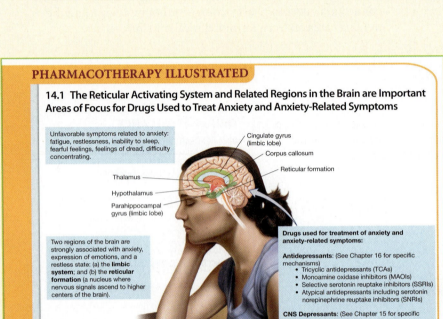

PHARMACOTHERAPY ILLUSTRATED

14.1 The Reticular Activating System and Related Regions in the Brain are Important Areas of Focus for Drugs Used to Treat Anxiety and Anxiety-Related Symptoms

Unfavorable symptoms related to anxiety: fatigue, restlessness, inability to sleep, fearful feelings, feelings of dread, difficulty concentrating.

Cingulate gyrus (limbic lobe)
Corpus callosum
Reticular formation
Thalamus
Hypothalamus
Parahippocampal gyrus (limbic lobe)

Two regions of the brain are strongly associated with anxiety, expression of emotions, and a restless state: (a) the **limbic system**; and (b) the **reticular formation** (a nucleus where nervous signals ascend to higher centers of the brain).

Drugs used for treatment of anxiety and anxiety-related symptoms:

Antidepressants: (See Chapter 16 for specific mechanisms)
• Tricyclic antidepressants (TCAs)
• Monoamine oxidase inhibitors (MAOIs)
• Selective serotonin reuptake inhibitors (SSRIs)
• Atypical antidepressants including serotonin norepinephrine reuptake inhibitors (SNRIs)

CNS Depressants: (See Chapter 15 for specific mechanisms)
• Benzodiazepines
• Barbiturates
• Other drugs

◀ **Pharmacotherapy Illustrated** boxes visually illustrate the drug therapy process and its impact on the disease, showing you specifically how the drug acts to counteract the effects of disease on the body.

Mechanism of Action animated tutorials featured in **MyNurskingKit** clearly show drug action at the molecular, tissue, organ, and system levels. ▼

MECHANISM OF ACTION ANIMATIONS

Drug	Chapter	Drug	Chapter	Drug	Chapter	Drug	Chapter
Acetaminophen	Ch. 33	Doxazosin	Ch. 23	Lidocaine	Ch. 19	Ranitidine	Ch. 40
Acyclovir	Ch. 36	Epinephrine	Ch. 29	Lisinopril	Ch. 24	Reteplase	Ch. 25
Amiodarone	Ch. 26	Epoietin alfa	Ch. 28	Methotrexate	Ch. 37	Salmeterol	Ch. 39
Atorvastatin	Ch. 22	Escitalopram	Ch. 14	Methylphenidate	Ch. 16	Saquinavir	Ch. 36
Calcitriol	Ch. 47	Estradiol	Ch. 45	Morphine	Ch. 18	Sildenafil	Ch. 46
Ciprofloxacin	Ch. 34	Fluconazole	Ch. 35	Naproxen	Ch. 33	Spironolactone	Ch. 30
Cyclobenzaprine	Ch. 21	Fluoxetine	Ch. 16	Nifedipine	Ch. 23	Tegaserod	Ch. 41
Cyclophosphamide	Ch. 37	Furosemide	Ch. 24	Omeprazole	Ch. 40	Valproic acid	Ch. 15
Diazepam	Ch. 15	Glipizide	Ch. 44	Oxycodone	Ch. 18	Venlafaxine	Ch. 16
Digoxin	Ch. 24	Heparin	Ch. 27	Penicillin	Ch. 34	Warfarin	Ch. 27
Diphenhydramine	Ch. 38	Interferon alfa	Ch. 32	Pilocarpine	Ch. 49	Zidovudine	Ch. 36
Dopamine	Ch. 29	Levadopa	Ch. 20	Propranolol	Ch. 26	Zolpidem	Ch. 14

Providing a Nursing Focus

Once you understand how a drug works on the body—i.e., its actions, therapeutic effects, potential side effects and interactions, and more—you begin to understand the "why" of the interventions you will take as the nurse. Each chapter guides you to the content that is essential for you to provide safe, effective drug therapy.

Nursing Process Focus charts present need-to-know nursing actions presented in a way that helps the student or new practitioner think like a nurse about medications—from assessment, nursing diagnoses, planning, implementation with interventions and rationales, through evaluation—and including patient teaching and discharge planning.

Additional **Nursing Process Focus** charts are available on **MyNursingKit**.

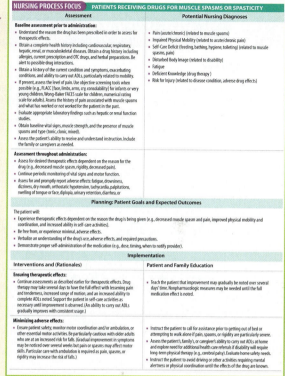

RESEARCH SHOWS

The Question: Are there areas of patient drug therapy where adverse drug events have consistently contributed to serious injury, disability, or death?
The Study: Researchers recently completed a review of all adverse drug events reported to the FDA since 2006. In looking at medications for a range of disorders, including heart failure, asthma, coagulation defects, bipolar disorder, depression, epilepsy, and pain treatments, clinicians found 10 potentially fatal drugs: dioxin, bandronate, clonazepam, heparin, capecitabine, methadone, ritonavir, isotretinoin, fentanyl, and interferon beta. In some instances, drug fatalities were associated with

◀ **NEW! Research Boxes** have been added throughout to provide evidence-based practice as it is applicable to pharmacology.

AVOIDING MEDICATION ERRORS

The FDA and the American Hospital Association track drug errors that occur in health care settings. The five most common causes of medication errors are:
- Incomplete patient information (e.g., not knowing about patients' allergies, other medicines they are taking, previous diagnoses, or lab results)
- Unavailable drug information (e.g., current warnings issued by the FDA)
- Miscommunication of drug orders (e.g., illegible handwritten orders, confusion between drugs with similar names, misuse of zeroes and decimal points, unclear abbreviations)

◀ **Avoiding Medication Errors** are brief patient-based scenarios that illustrate potential pitfalls that nurses encounter and can lead to medication errors. Each scenario ends with a question asking you to identify what went wrong, enabling you to watch for similar situations and deliver medications safely.

COMPLEMENTARY AND ALTERNATIVE THERAPIES

Cayenne for Muscular Pain and Tension
Cayenne (*Capsicum annum*), also known as chili pepper, paprika, or red pepper, has been used as a remedy for minor muscle pain or tension. Capsaicin, the active ingredient in cayenne, diminishes the chemical messengers that travel through the sensory nerves, thereby decreasing the sensation of pain (Nelson, Ragan, Bell, Ichiyama, & Iwamoto, 2004). Capsaicin cream (0.025% to 0.075%) may be applied directly to the affected area up to four times a day. Its effect accumulates over time, so creams containing capsaicin need to be applied regu-

◀ **NEW! Complementary and Alternative Therapies** boxes present popular herbal or dietary supplements patients may use along with conventional drugs. As a nurse, you need to assess clients to see if they are using any natural remedies that may have interactions with medications they are taking.

Lifespan Considerations boxes present a variety of special issues related to age, gender, and psychosocial concerns that nurses must consider during drug therapy. ▼

NEW! Treating the Diverse Patient boxes provide additional coverage related to culture and ethnicity. ▶

TREATING THE DIVERSE PATIENT

Non–English-Speaking and Culturally Diverse Patients
Nurses should know, in advance, what translation services and interpreters are available in their health care facility to assist with communication. The nurse should use interpreter's services when available, validating with the interpreter that he or she is able to understand the patient. Many dialects are similar but not the same, and knowing another language is not the same as understanding the culture. Can the interpreter understand the patient's language and cultural expressions or nuances well enough for effective communication to occur? If a family member is interpreting, especially if a child is interpreting for a parent or

LIFESPAN CONSIDERATIONS

The New Fountain of Youth?
Seen as the new fountain of youth, botulinum toxin type A (Botox Cosmetic) injections were approved by the FDA for the temporary improvement in the appearance of moderate to severe frown lines (vertical lines between the brows) in adult patients aged 65 years or younger. It works to relax frown muscles by blocking nerve impulses that trigger wrinkle-causing muscle contractions, creating a smooth appearance between the brows. Administered in a few tiny injections of purified protein, this minimally invasive treatment is simple and quick, and delivers dramatic results with minimal discomfort. Re

Home & Community Considerations alert you to concerns and teaching implications for care settings outside the hospital. ▶

HOME & COMMUNITY CONSIDERATIONS

Caring for Loved Ones With Alzheimer's Disease
The diagnosis of Alzheimer's disease is devastating to the patient and family members alike. Family members must deal with many unexpected changes. The personality of the patient with Alzheimer's disease slowly changes and may include paranoia, anger, and frustration. Many families attempt to care for their loved one at home for as long as possible. A frightening aspect of Alzheimer's disease is the tendency for the patient to wander away. The patient easily becomes lost after leaving the familiarity of the home environment. This tendency to wander is believed to be linked to anxiety on the part of the AD

Putting It All Together

The tools at the end of each chapter and on the accompanying media resources help you test your understanding of the drugs and nursing care presented in that chapter. Using these tools will help you succeed in your pharmacology course, in the clinical setting, on the NCLEX-RN®, and ultimately in professional nursing practice.

Chapter REVIEW

KEY CONCEPTS

The numbered key concepts provide a succinct summary of the important points from the corresponding numbered section within the chapter. If any of these points are not clear, refer to the numbered section within the chapter for review.

13.1 The peripheral nervous system is divided into a somatic portion, which is under voluntary control, and an autonomic portion, which is involuntary and controls smooth muscle, cardiac muscle, and glandular secretions.

13.2 Stimulation of the sympathetic division of the autonomic nervous system causes symptoms of the fight-or-flight response, whereas stimulation of the parasympathetic branch induces rest-and-digest responses.

13.3 Drugs can affect nervous transmission across a synapse by preventing the synthesis, storage, or release of the neurotransmitter; by preventing the destruction of the neurotransmitter; or by binding neurotransmitters to the receptors.

13.4 Norepinephrine is the primary neurotransmitter released at adrenergic receptors, which are divided into alpha and beta subtypes. Acetylcholine is the other primary neurotransmitter of the autonomic nervous system.

13.5 Acetylcholine is the primary neurotransmitter released at cholinergic receptors (nicotinic and muscarinic) in both the sympathetic and parasympathetic nervous systems. It is also the neurotransmitter at nicotinic receptors in skeletal muscle.

13.6 Autonomic drugs are classified by the receptors they stimulate or block: Sympathomimetics stimulate target tissue innervated by sympathetic nerves, and parasympathomimetics stimulate target tissue innervated by parasympathetic nerves; adrenergic antagonists inhibit functionality of the sympathetic division, whereas anticholinergics inhibit functionality of the parasympathetic branch.

13.7 Sympathomimetics act by directly activating adrenergic receptors, or indirectly by increasing the release of norepinephrine from nerve terminals. They are used primarily for their effects on the heart, bronchial tree, and nasal

13.8 Adrenergic antagonists are used primarily for h sion and are the most widely prescribed class nomic drugs.

13.9 Parasympathomimetics act directly by sti cholinergic receptors or indirectly by inhibiti cholinesterase. They have few therapeutic uses of their numerous side effects.

13.10 Anticholinergics act by blocking the effects o choline at muscarinic receptors, and are used to cretions, treat asthma, and prevent motion sick

◀ **Key Concept Summary** provides expanded summaries of concepts that correlate to sections within the chapter. You can use this succinct summary to ensure that you understand the concepts before moving on to the next chapter. The numbering of these concepts helps you easily locate that section within the chapter if you need further review.

NCLEX-RN® REVIEW QUESTIONS

1 Following administration of an adrenergic (sympathomimetic) drug, the nurse would assess for which adverse drug effects?
   1. Insomnia, nervousness, and hypertension
   2. Nausea, vomiting, and hypotension
   3. Nervousness, drowsiness, and dyspnea
   4. Bronchial dilation, hypotension, and bradycardia

2 Therapeutic uses for anticholinergics include: (Select all that apply.)
   1. peptic ulcer disease.
   2. bradycardia.
   3. decreased sexual function.
   4. irritable bowel syndrome.

NCLEX-RN® Review Questions prepare you for course exams on the chapter content using all NCLEX® formats. Appendix D provides answers and rationales. ▶

CRITICAL THINKING QUESTIONS

1. A 24-year-old patient (gravida 3, para 1) is admitted to the labor and delivery unit and states that she is having contractions. She is at 32 weeks gestation. The obstetrician initially begins tocolysis with magnesium sulfate and then switches the patient to terbutaline (Brethine), 5 mg PO every 4 hours around the clock. The nurse recognizes terbutaline as a beta₂-adrenergic agent. What nursing assessments should be made with a patient receiving terbutaline therapy? What education does the patient require in relation to terbutaline therapy? How will the nurse evalu

3. A 42-year-old male patient was diagnosed with Parkinson's disease 4 years ago. He is being treated with a regimen of amantadine (Symmetrel), an indirect-acting dopaminergic agent, and benztropine mesylate (Cogentin). The nurse recognizes Cogentin as an anticholinergic agent. What should the nurse assess this patient for? Discuss the potential side effects of benztropine that the nurse should assess for in this patient.

See Appendix D for answers and rationales for all activities.

◀ **Critical Thinking Questions** help you apply the essential components of nursing care through case-based scenarios. Appendix D provides answers.

MyNursingKit Each chapter ▶ provides a reminder to visit MyNursingKit™ (www.mynursingkit.com) for additional chapter review and resources.

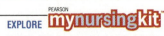

EXPLORE mynursingkit™

MyNursingKit is your one stop for online chapter review materials and resources. Prepare for success with additional NCLEX®-style practice questions, interactive assignments and activities, web links, animations and videos, and more!

Register your access code from the front of your book at
www.mynursingkit.com.

Contents

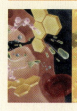

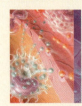

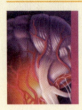

UNIT 4 THE CARDIOVASCULAR AND URINARY SYSTEMS   281

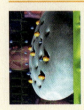

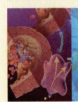

UNIT 6 THE RESPIRATORY SYSTEM   571

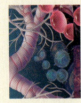

Chapter 38 Drugs for Allergic Rhinitis and the Common Cold   572

Chapter 39 Drugs for Asthma and Other Pulmonary Disorders   589

UNIT 7 THE GASTROINTESTINAL SYSTEM   605

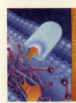

Chapter 40 Drugs for Peptic Ulcer Disease   606

UNIT 9   THE INTEGUMENTARY SYSTEM AND EYES/EARS   729

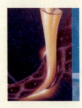

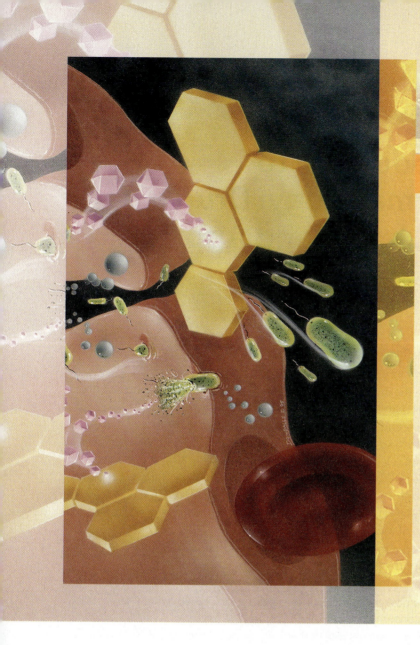

Core Concepts in Pharmacology

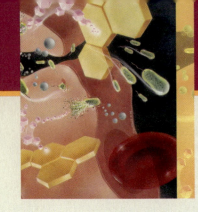

Chapter 1

Introduction to Pharmacology: Drug Regulation and Approval

LEARNING OUTCOMES

After reading this chapter, the student should be able to:

1. Identify key events in the history of pharmacology.
2. Explain the interdisciplinary nature of pharmacology, giving examples of subject areas needed to learn the discipline well.
3. Compare and contrast therapeutics and pharmacology.
4. Compare and contrast traditional drugs, biologics, and alternative therapies.
5. Identify the advantages and disadvantages of prescription and over-the-counter (OTC) drugs.
6. Identify key U.S. drug regulations that have ensured the safety and efficacy of medications.
7. Discuss the role of the U.S. Food and Drug Administration (FDA) in the drug approval process.
8. Explain the four stages of approval for therapeutic and biologic drugs.
9. Discuss how the FDA has increased the speed with which new drugs reach consumers.
10. Identify the nurse's role in the drug approval process.

KEY TERMS

biologics *page 4*
clinical investigation *page 6*
clinical phase trials *page 6*
complementary and alternative therapies *page 4*
drug *page 4*
Food and Drug Administration (FDA) *page 5*

FDA's Critical Path Initiative *page 6*
formulary *page 4*
Investigational New Drug Application (IND) *page 7*
medication *page 4*
NDA review *page 7*

pharmacology *page 3*
pharmacopoeia *page 4*
pharmacotherapy *page 4*
postmarketing surveillance *page 7*
preclinical investigation *page 6*
therapeutics *page 4*

More drugs are being administered to patients than ever before. More than 3 billion prescriptions are dispensed each year in the United States. About one half of all Americans take one prescription drug regularly, and one out of six persons takes at least three prescription drugs. The purpose of this chapter is to introduce the subject of pharmacology and to emphasize the role of government in ensuring that drugs, herbals, and other natural alternatives are safe and effective for public use.

1.1 History of Pharmacology

The story of pharmacology is rich and exciting, filled with accidental discoveries and landmark events. Its history likely began when humans first used plants to relieve symptoms of disease. One of the oldest forms of health care, herbal medicine has been practiced in virtually every culture dating to antiquity. The Babylonians recorded the earliest surviving "prescriptions" on clay tablets in 3000 B.C. At about the same time, the Chinese recorded the *Pen Tsao* (Great Herbal), a 40-volume compendium of plant remedies dating to 2700 B.C. The Egyptians followed in 1500 B.C. by archiving their remedies on a document known as the *Eber's Papyrus*.

Little is known about pharmacology during the Dark Ages. Although it is likely that herbal medicine continued to be practiced, few historical events related to this topic were recorded. Pharmacology, and indeed medicine, could not advance until the discipline of science was eventually viewed as legitimate by the religious doctrines of the era.

The first recorded reference to the word *pharmacology* was found in a text entitled "Pharmacologia sen Manductio and Materiam Medicum," by Samuel Dale, in 1693. Before this date, the study of herbal remedies was called "Materia Medica," a term that persisted into the early 20th century.

Although the exact starting date is obscure, modern pharmacology is thought to have begun in the early 1800s. At that time, chemists were making remarkable progress in isolating specific substances from complex mixtures. This enabled scientists to isolate the active agents morphine, colchicine, curare, cocaine, and other early pharmacologic agents from their natural products. Using standardized amounts, pharmacologists could then study their effects in animals more precisely. Indeed, some of the early researchers used themselves as test subjects. Frederich Serturner, who first isolated morphine from opium in 1805, injected himself and three friends with a huge dose (100 mg) of his new product. He and his colleagues suffered acute morphine intoxication for several days afterward.

Pharmacology as a distinct discipline was officially recognized when the first department of pharmacology was established in Estonia in 1847. John Jacob Abel, who is considered the father of American pharmacology owing to his many contributions to the field, founded the first pharmacology department in the United States at the University of Michigan in 1890.

In the 20th century, the pace of change in all areas of medicine continued exponentially. Pharmacologists no longer needed to rely on the slow, laborious process of isolating active agents from scarce natural products; they could synthesize drugs in the laboratory. Hundreds of new drugs could be synthesized and tested in a relatively short time. More importantly, it became possible to understand how drugs produced their effects, down to their molecular mechanism of action.

The current practice of pharmacology is extremely complex and far advanced compared with its early, primitive history. Nurses who consult with pharmacists in the use of pharmacologic substances and other health professionals who practice it must never forget its early roots: the application of products to relieve human suffering. Whether a substance is extracted from the Pacific yew tree, isolated from a fungus, or created totally in a laboratory, the central purpose of pharmacology is to focus on the patient and to improve the quality of life.

1.2 Pharmacology: The Study of Medicines

The word **pharmacology** is derived from two Greek words, *pharmakon,* which means "medicine," and *logos,* which means "study." Thus, pharmacology is most simply defined as the study of medicine. Pharmacology is an expansive subject ranging from understanding how drugs are administered, to where they travel in the body, to the actual responses produced. To learn the discipline well, nursing students need a thorough understanding of concepts from various foundation areas such as anatomy and physiology, chemistry, microbiology, and pathophysiology.

More than 10,000 brand-name drugs, generic drugs, and combination drugs are currently available. Each has its own characteristic set of therapeutic applications, interactions, side effects, and mechanisms of action. Many drugs are prescribed for more than one disease, and most produce multiple effects on the body. The study of pharmacology is further complicated by knowing that drugs may elicit different responses depending on individual patient factors such as age, sex, body mass, health status, and genetics. Indeed, learning the applications of existing medications and staying current with new drugs introduced every year is an enormous challenge for the nurse. The task, however, is a critical one for both the patient and the health care practitioner. If applied properly, drugs can dramatically improve the quality of life. If applied improperly, drugs can produce devastating consequences.

1.3 Pharmacology and Therapeutics

It is obvious that a thorough study of pharmacology is important to health care providers who prescribe drugs on a daily basis. Nurses are most often the health care providers directly involved with patient care and are active in educating, managing, and monitoring the proper use of drugs. This applies not only to nurses in clinics, hospitals, and home health care settings but also to nurses who teach and

MyNursingKit Old-Fashioned Remedies

to new students entering the nursing profession. In all these cases, it is necessary that individuals have a thorough knowledge of pharmacology to perform their duties. As nursing students progress toward their chosen specialty, pharmacology is at the core of patient care and is integrated into every step of the nursing process. Learning pharmacology is a gradual, continuous process that does not end with graduation. One never completely masters every facet of drug action and application. That is one of the motivating challenges of the nursing profession.

Another important area of study for the nurse, sometimes challenging to distinguish from pharmacology, is the study of therapeutics. Therapeutics is slightly different from the field of pharmacology, although the disciplines are closely connected. **Therapeutics** is the branch of medicine concerned with the prevention of disease and treatment of suffering. **Pharmacotherapy,** or *pharmacotherapeutics,* is the application of drugs for the purpose of disease prevention and the treatment of suffering. Drugs are just one of many tools available to the nurse for these purposes.

1.4 Classification of Therapeutic Agents as Drugs, Biologics, and Alternative Therapies

Substances applied for therapeutic purposes fall into one of the following three general categories:

• Drugs or medications
• Biologics
• Alternative therapies

A **drug** is a chemical agent capable of producing biologic responses within the body. These responses may be desirable (therapeutic) or undesirable (adverse). After a drug is administered, it is called a **medication.** From a larger perspective, drugs and medications may be considered a part of the body's normal activities, from the essential gases that we breathe to the foods that we eat. Because drugs are defined so broadly, it is necessary to clearly distinguish them from other substances such as foods, household products, and cosmetics. Many agents such as antiperspirants, sunscreens, toothpaste, and shampoos might alter the body's normal activities, but they are not necessarily considered medically therapeutic, as are drugs.

Although most modern drugs are synthesized in a laboratory, **biologics** are agents naturally produced in animal cells, by microorganisms, or by the body itself. Examples of biologics include hormones, monoclonal antibodies, natural blood products and components, interferons, and vaccines. Biologics are used to treat a wide variety of illnesses and conditions.

Other therapeutic approaches include **complementary and alternative therapies.** These involve natural plant extracts, herbs, vitamins, minerals, dietary supplements, and many techniques considered by some to be unconventional. Such therapies include acupuncture, hypnosis, biofeedback, and massage. Because of their great popularity, herbal and alter-

native therapies are featured throughout this text wherever they show promise in treating a disease or condition. Herbal therapies are presented in chapter 10∞.

1.5 Prescription and Over-the-Counter Drugs

Legal drugs are obtained either by a prescription or over the counter (OTC). There are major differences between the two methods of dispensing drugs. To obtain prescription drugs, the person must receive a written order from a person with the legal authority to write such a prescription. The advantages to requiring an authorization are numerous. The physician or nurse practitioner has an opportunity to examine the patient and determine a specific diagnosis. The practitioner can maximize therapy by ordering the proper drug for the patient's condition, and by conveying the amount and frequency of drug to be dispensed. In addition, the health care provider has an opportunity to teach the patient the proper use of the drug and what side effects to expect. In a few instances, a high margin of safety observed over many years can prompt a change in the status of a drug from prescription to OTC.

In contrast to prescription drugs, OTC drugs do not require a physician's order. In most cases, patients may treat themselves safely if they carefully follow instructions included with the medication. If patients do not follow these guidelines, OTC drugs can have serious adverse effects.

Patients prefer to take OTC drugs for many reasons. They are obtained more easily than prescription drugs. No appointment with a physician is required, thus saving time and money. Without the assistance of a health care provider, however, choosing the proper drug for a specific problem can be challenging for a patient. OTC drugs may react with foods, herbal products, prescription medications, or other OTC drugs. Patients may not be aware that some OTC drugs can impair their ability to function safely. Self-treatment is sometimes ineffectual, and the potential for harm may increase if the disease is allowed to progress.

1.6 Drug Regulations and Standards

Until the 19th century, there were few standards or guidelines in place to protect the public from drug misuse. The archives of drug regulatory agencies are filled with examples of early medicines, including rattlesnake oil for rheumatism; epilepsy treatment for spasms, hysteria, and alcoholism; and fat reducers for a slender, healthy figure. Many of these early concoctions proved ineffective, though harmless. At their worst, some contained hazardous levels of dangerous or addictive substances. It became quite clear that drug regulations were needed to protect the public.

The first standard commonly used by pharmacists was the **formulary,** or list of drugs and drug recipes. In the United States, the first comprehensive publication of drug standards, called the *U.S. Pharmacopoeia* (*USP*), was established in 1820. A **pharmacopoeia** is a medical reference summarizing standards of drug purity, strength, and directions for synthesis. In 1852, a national professional society of pharmacists called the American Pharmaceutical Association

(APhA) was founded. From 1852 to 1975, two major compendia maintained drug standards in the United States, the *U.S. Pharmacopoeia* and the *National Formulary* (*NF*) established by the APhA. All drug products were covered in the *USP*; pharmaceutical ingredients were covered in the *NF*. In 1975, the two entities merged into a single publication, the *U.S. Pharmacopoeia–National Formulary* (*USP-NF*). The current document of about 2,400 pages contains 3,777 drug monographs in 164 chapters. Official monographs and interim revision announcements for the *USP-NF* are published regularly, with the full bound version printed every 5 years. Today, the USP label can be found on many medications verifying the purity and exact amounts of ingredients found within the container. Sample labels are illustrated in ➤ Figure 1.1.

In the early 1900s, the United States began to develop and enforce tougher drug legislation to protect the public. In 1902, the Biologics Control Act helped to standardize the quality of serums and other blood-related products. The Pure Food and Drug Act of 1906 gave the government power to control the labeling of medicines. In 1912, the Sherley Amendment prohibited the sale of drugs labeled with false therapeutic claims that were intended to defraud the consumer. In 1938, Congress passed the Food, Drug, and Cosmetic Act. This was the first law preventing the sale of drugs that had not been thoroughly tested before marketing. Later amendments to this law required drug companies to prove the safety and efficacy of any drug before it could be sold within the United States. In reaction to the rising popularity of dietary supplements, Congress passed the Dietary Supplement Health and Education Act of 1994 in an attempt to control misleading industry claims. A brief timeline of major events in U.S. drug regulation is shown in ➤ Figure 1.2.

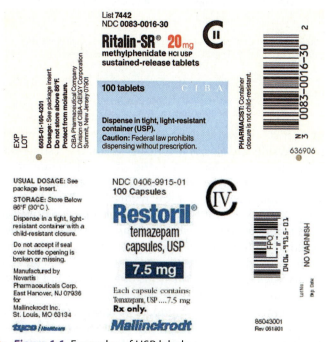

➤ **Figure 1.1** Examples of USP labels
Source: Courtesy of Novartis Pharmaceuticals Corporation and Mallinckrodt Pharmaceuticals.

1.7 The Role of the Food and Drug Administration

Much has changed in the regulation of drugs in the past 100 years. In 1988, the **Food and Drug Administration (FDA)** was officially established as an agency of the U.S. Department of Health and Human Services. The Center for Drug Evaluation and Research (CDER), a branch of the FDA, exercises control over whether prescription drugs and OTC drugs may be used for therapy. The CDER states its mission as facilitating the availability of safe, effective drugs; keeping unsafe or ineffective drugs off the market; improving the health of Americans; and providing clear, easily understandable drug information for safe and effective use. Any pharmaceutical laboratory, whether private, public, or academic, must solicit FDA approval before marketing a drug.

Another branch of the FDA, the Center for Biologics Evaluation and Research (CBER), regulates the use of biologics including serums, vaccines, and blood products. One historical achievement involving biologics was the 1986 Childhood Vaccine Act. This act authorized the FDA to acquire information about patients taking vaccines, to recall biologics, and to recommend civil penalties if guidelines regarding biologics were not followed.

The FDA also oversees administration of herbal products and dietary supplements through the Center for Food Safety and Applied Nutrition (CFSAN). Herbal products and dietary supplements are regulated by the Dietary Supplement Health and Education Act of 1994. This act does not provide the same degree of protection for consumers as the Food, Drug, and Cosmetic Act of 1938. For example, herbal and dietary supplements can be marketed without prior approval from the FDA. This act is discussed in more detail in chapter 10∞.

1.8 Stages of Approval for Therapeutic and Biologic Drugs

The amount of time spent by the FDA in the review and approval process for a particular drug depends on several checkpoints along a well-developed and organized plan.

TIMELINE	REGULATORY ACTS, STANDARDS, AND ORGANIZATIONS
1820	A group of physicians established the first comprehensive publication of drug standards called the **U.S. Pharmacopeia (USP)**.
1852	A group of pharmacists founded a national professional society called the **American Pharmaceutical Association (APhA)**. The APhA then established the **National Formulary (NF)**, a standardized publication focusing on pharmaceutical ingredients. The *USP* continued to catalogue all drug related substances and products.
1862	This was the beginning of the **Federal Bureau of Chemistry**, established under the administration of President Lincoln. Over the years and with added duties, it gradually became the Food and Drug Administration (FDA).
1902	Congress passed the **Biologics Control Act** to control the quality of serums and other blood-related products.
1906	**The Pure Food and Drug Act** gave the government power to control the labeling of medicines.
1912	**The Sherley Amendment** made medicines safer by prohibiting the sale of drugs labeled with false therapeutic claims.
1938	Congress passed the **Food, Drug, and Cosmetic Act**. It was the first law preventing the marketing of drugs not thoroughly tested. This law now provides for the requirement that drug companies must submit a New Drug Application (NDA) to the FDA prior to marketing a new drug.
1944	Congress passed the **Public Health Service Act**, covering many health issues including biological products and the control of communicable diseases.
1975	The *U.S. Pharmacopeia* and *National Formulary* announced their union. The **USP-NF** became a single standardized publication.
1986	Congress passed the **Childhood Vaccine Act**. It authorized the FDA to acquire information about patients taking vaccines, to recall biologics, and to recommend civil penalties if guidelines regarding biologic use were not followed.
1988	The **FDA** was officially established as an agency of the **U.S. Department of Health and Human Services**.
1992	Congress passed the **Prescription Drug User Fee Act**. It required that nongeneric drug and biologic manufacturers pay fees to be used for improvements in the drug review process.
1994	Congress passed the **Dietary Supplement Health and Education Act** that requires clear labeling of dietary supplements. This act gives the FDA the power to remove supplements that cause a significant risk to the public.
1997	The **FDA Modernization Act** reauthorized the Prescription Drug User Fee Act. This act represented the largest reform effort of the drug review process since 1938.
2002	The **Bioterrorism Act** implemented guidelines for registration of selected toxins that could pose a threat to human, animal, or plant safety and health.
2007	The **FDA Amendments Act** reviewed, expanded, and reaffirmed legislation to allow for additional comprehensive reviews of new drugs and medical products. This extended the reforms imposed from 1997. The **FDA's Critical Path Initiative** was a part of this reform.

➤ *Figure 1.2* A historical timeline of regulatory acts, standards, and organizations

Therapeutic drugs and biologics are reviewed in four phases. These phases, summarized in ➤ Figure 1.3, are as follows:

1. Preclinical investigation
2. Clinical investigation
3. Review of the New Drug Application (NDA)
4. Postmarketing surveillance

Preclinical investigation involves extensive laboratory research. Scientists perform many tests on human and microbial cells cultured in the laboratory. Studies are performed in several species of animals to examine the drug's effectiveness at different doses, and to look for adverse effects. Extensive testing on cultured cells and in animals is essential because it allows the pharmacologist to predict whether the drug will cause harm to humans. Because laboratory tests do not al-ways reflect the way a human responds, preclinical investigation results are always inconclusive. Animal testing may overestimate or underestimate the actual risk to humans.

In January 2007, the FDA restated its concern that a number of innovative and critical medical products had decreased since the 1990s. The **FDA's Critical Path Initiative** was an effort to modernize the sciences to enhance the use of bioinformation to improve the "safety, effectiveness, and manufacturability of candidate medical products." Listed areas of improvement have been the fields of genomics and proteonomics, imaging, and bioinformatics.

Clinical investigation, the second stage of drug testing, takes place in three different stages termed **clinical phase trials**. Clinical phase trials are the longest part of the drug approval process. Clinical pharmacologists first perform tests on healthy volunteers to determine proper dosage and to as-

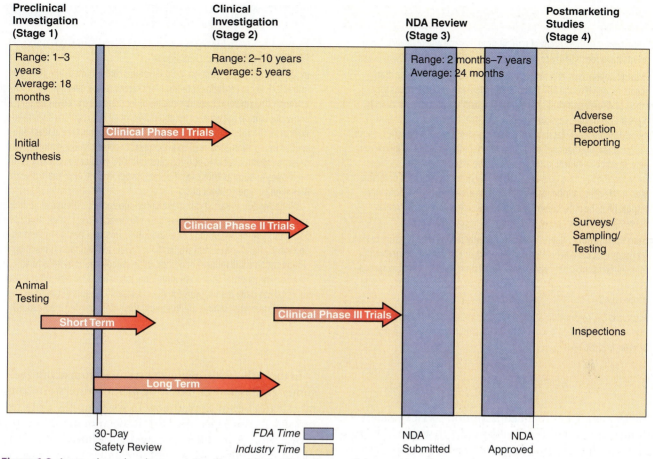

> *Figure 1.3* A new drug development timeline, with the four phases of drug approval

sess for adverse effects. Large groups of selected patients with the particular disease are then given the medication. Clinical investigators from different medical specialties address concerns such as whether the drug is effective, worsens other medical conditions, interacts unsafely with existing medications, or affects one type of patient more than others.

Clinical phase trials are an essential component of drug evaluations due to the variability of responses among patients. If a drug appears to be effective and without serious side effects, approval for marketing may be accelerated, or the drug may be used immediately in special cases with careful monitoring. If the drug shows promise but precautions are noted, the process is delayed until the pharmaceutical company remedies the concerns. In any case, a New Drug Application (NDA) must be submitted before a drug is allowed to proceed to the next stage of the approval process. An **Investigational New Drug Application (IND)** may be submitted for Phase I clinical trials when it is determined there are significant therapeutic benefits, and the product is reasonably safe for initial use in humans (e.g., HIV-positive patients). Companies usually begin developing a brand name for drugs during Phase I of the IND process.

The **NDA review** is the third stage of the drug approval process. During this stage, the drug's brand name is finalized. Clinical phase III trials and animal testing may continue depending on the results obtained from preclinical

testing. By law, the FDA is permitted 6 months to initially review an NDA. If the NDA is approved, the process continues to the final stage. If the NDA is rejected, the process is suspended until noted concerns are addressed by the pharmaceutical company. The average NDA review time for new drugs is approximately 17–24 months.

Postmarketing surveillance, the final stage of the drug approval process, begins after clinical trials and the NDA review have been completed. The purpose of this stage is to survey for harmful drug effects in a larger population. Some adverse effects take longer to appear and are not identified until a drug is circulated to large numbers of people. One example is the diabetes drug troglitazone (Rezulin), which was placed on the market in 1997. In 1998, Britain banned its use after discovering at least one death and several cases of liver failure in diabetic patients taking the medication. The FDA became aware of a number of cases in the United States in which Rezulin was linked with liver failure and heart failure. Rezulin was recalled in March 2000 after health care providers asked the FDA to reconsider its therapeutic benefits versus its identified risks. The FDA withdrew 11 prescription drugs from the market between 1997 and 2000. Drug recalls continue to occur.

The FDA holds public meetings annually to receive feedback from patients and professional and pharmaceutical organizations regarding the effectiveness and safety of new drug therapies. If the FDA discovers a serious problem, it will mandate that the drug be withdrawn from the market.

The Question: Are there areas of patient drug therapy where adverse drug events have consistently contributed to serious injury, disability, or death?

The Study: Researchers recently completed a review of all adverse drug events reported to the FDA since 2006. In looking at medications for a range of disorders, including heart failure, asthma, coagulation defects, bipolar disorder, depression, epilepsy, and pain treatments, clinicians found 10 potentially fatal drugs: dioxin, bandronate, clonazepam, heparin, capecitabine, methadone, ritonavir, isotretinoin, fentanyl, and interferon beta. In some instances, drug fatalities were associated with complications of drug delivery, such as overstrength tablets or defective medical devices. In other cases, potentially adverse drug reactions were responsible. The most common reactions were cardiac dysrhythmias, depression with self-injury, and severe cutaneous reactions.

Nursing Implications: Nurses should constantly review the literature to look for drugs that have been reported, recalled, or considered dangerous due to manufacturing safety issues. In areas of drug therapy where common or repetitive adverse reactions have been noted, special cautions should be exercised.

Source: Moore, T. J., Cohen, M. R., & Furberg, C. D. QuarterWatch 2008 Quarter 2. Institute for Safe Medication Practices. January 15, 2009. http://www.ismp.org/QuarterWatch/200901.pdf

Prescription Drug Costs and the "Doughnut Hole" for Senior Citizens

In January 2006, prescription drug coverage through Medicare Part D went into effect, in part to help protect senior citizens (those over age 65) from catastrophic drug expenditures. Americans older than age 65 constitute only 13% of the population but account for about 34% of all prescriptions dispensed and 40% of all OTC medications. More than 80% of all seniors take at least one prescribed medication each day. The average older person is taking more than four prescription medications at once, plus two OTC medications. Many of these medicines—such as those for diabetes, hypertension, and heart disease—are taken on a permanent basis.

While Medicare Part D did make some substantial differences in helping seniors pay for their medications, a gap in coverage occurs when drug spending totals are between $2,250 and $5,100. This gap has been termed the "doughnut hole" and current studies have suggested that seniors reaching that doughnut hole will reduce spending on their medications by 14% to 40%, depending on whether they have additional insurance coverage. With most seniors taking daily medications for chronic conditions, this decrease in spending may mean that seniors are foregoing their most needed medications.

The FDA has a free e-mail subscription service to alert the consumer regarding drugs and products withdrawn from the market. Special committees also address important issues such as potential prescription errors and the screening of drug names. Proprietary drug names may be changed if considered a significant safety risk. The naming of drugs is discussed more thoroughly in chapter 2∞.

1.9 Recent Changes to the Drug Approval Process

The process of isolating or synthesizing a new drug and testing it in cells, experimental animals, and humans can take many years. The NDA can include dozens of volumes of experimental and clinical data that must be examined in the drug review process. Some NDAs contain more than 100,000 pages. Even after all experiments have been concluded and clinical data have been gathered, the FDA review process can take several years.

Expenses associated with development of a new drug can cost pharmaceutical manufacturers millions of dollars. A recent study estimated the cost to bring a new drug to market at $802 million. These companies are often critical of the regulatory process and are anxious to get the drug marketed to recoup their research and development expenses. The public is also anxious to receive new drugs, particularly for diseases that have a high mortality rate. Although the criticisms of manufacturers and the public are certainly understandable—and sometimes justified—the fundamental priority of the FDA is to ensure that drugs are safe. Without an exhaustive review of scientific data, the public could be exposed to dangerous medications, or those that are ineffective in treating disease.

In the early 1990s, owing to pressures from organized consumer groups and various drug manufacturers, governmental officials began to plan how to speed up the drug review process. Reasons identified for the delay in the FDA drug approval process included outdated guidelines, poor communication, and insufficient staff to handle the workload.

In 1992, FDA officials, members of Congress, and representatives from pharmaceutical companies negotiated the Prescription Drug User Fee Act on a 5-year trial basis. This act required drug and biologic manufacturers to provide yearly product user fees. This added income allowed the FDA to hire more employees and to restructure its organization to more efficiently handle the processing of a greater number of drug applications. The result of restructuring was a resounding success. From 1992 to 1996, the FDA approved double the number of drugs while cutting some review times by as much as half. In 1997, the FDA Modernization Act reauthorized the Prescription Drug User Fee Act. Nearly 700 employees were added to the FDA's drug and biologics program, and more

Time Length for New Drug Approvals

- It takes about 11 years of research and development before a drug is submitted to the FDA for review.
- Phase I clinical trials take about 1 year and involve 20 to 80 normal, healthy volunteers.
- Phase II clinical trials last about 2 years and involve 100 to 300 volunteer patients with the disease.
- Phase III clinical trials take about 3 years and involve 1,000 to 3,000 patients in hospitals and clinic agencies.
- For every 5,000 chemicals that enter preclinical testing, only 5 make it to human testing. Of these 5 potential drugs, only 1 is finally approved.

TABLE 1.1	Steps of Approval for Drugs Marketed Within Canada
Step 1	Preclinical studies or experiments in culture, living tissue, and small animals are performed, followed by extensive clinical trials or testing done in humans.
Step 2	A drug company completes a drug submission to Health Canada. This report details important safety and effectiveness information including testing data, how the drug product will be produced and packaged, and expected therapeutic benefits and adverse reactions.
Step 3	A committee of drug experts including medical and drug scientists reviews the drug submission to identify potential benefits and drug risks.
Step 4	Health Canada reviews information about the drug product and passes on important details to health practitioners and consumers.
Step 5	Health Canada issues a Notice of Compliance (NOC) and Drug Identification Number (DIN). Both permit the manufacturer to market the drug product.
Step 6	Health Canada monitors the effectiveness of the drug and any concerns after it has been marketed. This is done by regular inspection, notices, newsletters, and feedback from consumers and health care practitioners.

Therapeutic Products Directorate (TPD) authorizes marketing of a pharmaceutical drug or medical device, once a manufacturer presents sufficient scientific evidence of the product's safety, efficacy, and quality as required by the Canadian Food and Drugs Act and Regulations. The Biologics and Genetic Therapies Directorate (BGTD) regulates biologic drugs (drugs derived from living sources) and radiopharmaceuticals. Products regulated by the BGTD include blood products, vaccines, tissues, organs, and gene therapy products. The Natural Health Products Directorate (NHPD) is the regulating authority for natural health products for sale in Canada.

The Canadian Food and Drugs Act is an important regulatory document specifying that drugs cannot be marketed without a Notice of Compliance (NOC) and Drug Identification Number (DIN) from Health Canada. Foods, drugs, cosmetics, and therapeutic devices must follow established guidelines for approval. Any drug that does not comply with standards established by recognized pharmacopoeias and formularies in the United States, Europe, Britain, or France cannot be labeled, packaged, sold, or advertised in Canada.

1.11 Nurses and the Drug Approval Process

In nursing, it is during the postmarketing surveillance period of Phase IV (Step 6 in Canada) that nurses have the most frequent opportunities to participate in the drug approval process. While nurses working at larger, urban medical centers may participate in administering medications during Phase II and III trials, *all* nurses administering medications monitor for therapeutic effects and adverse reactions from the drugs they give to their patients. Whenever a possible drug reaction is noted, nurses are responsible for reporting the reaction to the prescriber and appropriate health care agency personnel (e.g., risk management, pharmacist). By monitoring for and reporting adverse effects, nurses can ensure that better postmarketing surveillance is achieved. The role and responsibilities of the nurse in drug administration are discussed in more depth in chapter 3∞.

than $300 million was collected in user fees. The FDA Amendments Act expanded the reform effort in 2007 by allowing more U.S. resources to be used for comprehensive reviews of new drugs. In 2008, the target base revenue for new drugs was over $392 million.

1.10 Canadian Drug Standards

The drug approval process in Canada is illustrated in Table 1.1. In Canada as in the United States, drug testing and risk assessment is a major priority. Health Canada is the federal department working in partnership with provincial and territorial governments. The Health Products and Food Branch (HPFB) of Health Canada is responsible for ensuring that health products and foods approved for sale to Canadians are safe and of high quality. The HPFB regulates the use of therapeutic products through directorates. The

 Chapter REVIEW

KEY CONCEPTS

The numbered key concepts provide a succinct summary of the important points from the corresponding numbered section within the chapter. If any of these points are not clear, refer to the numbered section within the chapter for review.

1.1 The history of pharmacology began thousands of years ago with the use of plant products to treat disease.

1.2 Pharmacology is the study of medicines. It includes the study of how drugs are administered and how the body responds.

1.3 The fields of pharmacology and therapeutics are closely connected. Pharmacotherapy is the application of drugs to prevent disease and ease suffering.

1.4 Therapeutic agents may be classified as traditional drugs, biologics, or alternative therapies.

1.5 Drugs are available by prescription or over the counter (OTC). Prescription drugs require an order from a health care provider.

1.6 Drug regulations were created to protect the public from drug misuse, and to assume continuous evaluation of safety and effectiveness.

1.7 The regulatory agency responsible for ensuring that drugs and medical devices are safe and effective is the Food and Drug Administration (FDA).

1.8 There are four stages of approval for therapeutic and biologic drugs. These progress from cellular and animal testing to use of the experimental drug in patients with the disease.

1.9 Once criticized for being too slow, the FDA has streamlined the process to get new drugs to market more quickly.

1.10 Drug standards also ensure the effectiveness and safety of drugs for Canadian consumers.

1.11 Nurses may participate in several phases of the drug approval process but will have the most frequent opportunities during Phase IV, postmarketing surveillance.

CRITICAL THINKING QUESTIONS

1. Explain why a patient might seek treatment from an OTC drug instead of a more effective prescription drug.

2. How does the FDA ensure the safety and effectiveness of drugs? How has this process changed in recent years?

3. In many respects, the role of the FDA continues long after the initial drug approval. Explain the continued involvement of the FDA.

4. Identify opportunities that nurses have in educating, administering, and monitoring the proper use of drugs.

See Appendix D for answers and rationales for all activities.

EXPLORE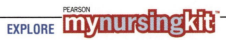

MyNursingKit is your one stop for online chapter review materials and resources. Prepare for success with additional NCLEX®-style practice questions, interactive assignments and activities, web links, animations and videos, and more!

Register your access code from the front of your book at
www.mynursingkit.com.

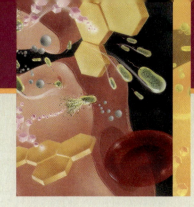

Chapter 2

Drug Classes and Schedules

LEARNING OUTCOMES

After reading this chapter, the student should be able to:

1. Explain the basis for placing drugs into therapeutic and pharmacologic classes.
2. Discuss the prototype approach to drug classification.
3. Describe what is meant by a drug's mechanism of action.
4. Distinguish between a drug's chemical name, generic name, and trade name.
5. Explain why generic drug names are preferred to trade name drugs.
6. Discuss why drugs are sometimes placed on a restrictive list, and the controversy surrounding this issue.
7. Explain the meaning of a controlled substance.
8. Explain the U.S. Controlled Substance Act of 1970 and the role of the U.S. Drug Enforcement Agency in controlling drug abuse and misuse.
9. Identify the five drug schedules and give examples of drugs at each level.

KEY TERMS

bioavailability *page 14*
chemical name *page 12*
combination drug *page 13*
controlled substance *page 14*
dependence *page 14*

generic name *page 13*
mechanism of action *page 12*
pharmacologic classification *page 12*
prototype drug *page 12*

scheduled drugs *page 14*
therapeutic classification *page 12*
trade name *page 13*
withdrawal *page 14*

The student beginning the study of pharmacology is quickly confronted with hundreds of drugs having specific dosages, side effects, and mechanisms of action. Without a means of grouping or organizing this information, most students would be overwhelmed by the vast amounts of new data. Drugs can be classified by a number of different methods that provide logical systems for identifying drugs and determining the limitations of their use. This chapter presents methods of grouping drugs: by therapeutic or pharmacologic classification, and by drug schedules.

2.1 Therapeutic and Pharmacologic Classification of Drugs

One useful method of organizing drugs is based on their therapeutic usefulness in treating particular diseases. This is referred to as a **therapeutic classification.** Drugs may also be organized by **pharmacologic classification.** A drug's pharmacologic classification refers to the way an agent works at the molecular, tissue, and body system level. Both types of classification are widely used in categorizing the thousands of available drugs.

Table 2.1 shows the method of therapeutic classification, using cardiac care as an example. Many different types of drugs affect cardiovascular function. Some drugs influence blood clotting, whereas others lower blood cholesterol or prevent the onset of stroke. Drugs may be used to treat elevated blood pressure, heart failure, abnormal rhythm, chest pain, heart attack, or circulatory shock. Thus, drugs that treat cardiac disorders may be placed in several types of therapeutic classes, for example, anticoagulants, antihyperlipidemics, and antihypertensives.

A therapeutic classification need not be complicated. For example, it is appropriate to simply classify a medication as a "drug used for stroke" or a "drug used for shock." The key to therapeutic classification is to clearly state what a particular drug does clinically. Other examples of therapeutic classifications include antidepressants, antipsychotics, drugs for erectile dysfunction, and antineoplastics.

The pharmacologic classification addresses a drug's **mechanism of action,** or *how* a drug produces its effect in the

body. Table 2.2 shows a variety of pharmacologic classifications using hypertension as an example. A diuretic treats hypertension by lowering plasma volume. Calcium channel blockers treat this disorder by decreasing cardiac contractility. Other drugs block intermediates of the renin–angiotensin pathway. Notice that each example describes *how* hypertension might be controlled. A drug's pharmacologic classification is more specific than a therapeutic classification and requires an understanding of biochemistry and physiology. In addition, pharmacologic classifications may be described with varying degrees of complexity, sometimes taking into account drugs' chemical names.

When classifying drugs, it is common practice to select a single drug from a class and compare all other medications with this representative drug. A **prototype drug** is the well-understood drug model with which other drugs in its representative class are compared. By learning the characteristics of the prototype drug, students may predict the actions and adverse effects of other drugs in the same class. For example, by knowing the effects of penicillin V, students can extend this knowledge to the other drugs in the penicillin class of antibiotics. The original drug prototype is not always the most widely used drug in its class. Newer drugs in the same class may be more effective, have a more favorable safety profile, or have a longer duration of action. These factors may sway health care providers from using the original prototype drug. In addition, health care providers and pharmacology textbooks sometimes differ as to which drug should be the prototype. In any case, becoming familiar with the drug prototypes and keeping up with newer and more popular drugs is an essential part of mastering drugs and drug classes.

2.2 Chemical, Generic, and Trade Names for Drugs

A major challenge in studying pharmacology is learning the thousands of drug names. Adding to this difficulty is the fact that most drugs have multiple names. The three basic types of drug names are chemical, generic, and trade names.

A **chemical name** is assigned using standard nomenclature established by the International Union of Pure and Applied Chemistry (IUPAC). A drug has only one chemical name,

TABLE 2.2 Organizing Drug Information by Pharmacologic Classification

FOCUSING ON HOW A THERAPY IS APPLIED: PHARMACOTHERAPY FOR HYPERTENSION MAY BE ACHIEVED BY:

Mechanism of Action	Pharmacologic Classification
lowers plasma volume	diuretic
blocks heart calcium channels	calcium channel blocker
blocks hormonal activity	angiotensin-converting enzyme inhibitor
blocks physiologic reactions to stress	adrenergic antagonist
dilates peripheral blood vessels	vasodilator

TABLE 2.1 Organizing Drug Information by Therapeutic Classification

THERAPEUTIC FOCUS: CARDIAC CARE / DRUGS AFFECTING CARDIOVASCULAR FUNCTION

Therapeutic Usefulness	Therapeutic Classification
influence blood clotting	anticoagulants
lower blood cholesterol	antihyperlipidemics
lower blood pressure	antihypertensives
restore normal cardiac rhythm	antidysrhythmics
treat angina	antianginals

which is sometimes helpful in predicting a substance's physical and chemical properties. Although chemical names convey a clear and concise meaning about the nature of a drug, they are often complicated and difficult to remember or pronounce. For example, few nurses know the chemical name for diazepam: 7-chloro-1,3-dihydro-1-methyl-5-phenyl-2H-1,4-benzodiazepin-2-one. In only a few cases, usually when the name is brief and easily remembered, will nurses use chemical names. Examples of useful chemical names include lithium carbonate, calcium gluconate, and sodium chloride.

More practically, drugs are sometimes classified by a *portion* of their chemical structure, known as the chemical group name. Examples are antibiotics such as the fluoroquinolones and cephalosporins. Other common examples include the phenothiazines, thiazides, and benzodiazepines. Although chemical group names may seem complicated when first encountered, knowing them will become invaluable as the nursing student begins to learn and understand major drug actions and adverse side effects.

The **generic name** of a drug is assigned by the U.S. Adopted Name Council. With few exceptions, generic names are less complicated and easier to remember than chemical names. Many organizations, including the Food and Drug Administration (FDA), the U.S. Pharmacopoeia, and the World Health Organization (WHO), routinely describe a medication by its generic name. Because there is only one generic name for each drug, health care providers often use this name, and students generally must memorize it.

A drug's **trade name** is assigned by the company marketing the drug. The name is usually selected to be short and easy to remember. The trade name is sometimes called the proprietary or product or brand name. The term *proprietary* suggests ownership. In the United States, a drug developer is given exclusive rights to name and market a drug for 17 years after a new drug application is submitted to the FDA. Because it takes several years for a drug to be approved, the amount of time spent in approval is usually subtracted from the 17 years. For example, if it takes 7 years for a drug to be approved, competing companies will not be allowed to market a generic equivalent drug for another 10 years. The rationale is that the developing company should be allowed sufficient time to recoup the millions of dollars in research and development costs in designing the new drug. After 17 years, competing companies may sell a generic equivalent drug, sometimes using a different name, which the FDA must approve.

Trade names may be a challenge for students to learn because of the dozens of product names containing similar ingredients. A **combination drug** contains more than one active generic ingredient. This poses a problem in trying to match one generic name with one product name. As an example, Table 2.3 considers the drug diphenhydramine (generic name), also called Benadryl (one of many trade names). Diphenhydramine is an antihistamine. Low doses of diphenhydramine may be purchased over the counter (OTC); higher doses require a prescription. When looking for diphenhydramine, the nurse may find it listed under

TABLE 2.3	Examples of Brand-Name Products Containing Popular Generic Substances
Generic Substance	**Brand Names**
aspirin	Acuprin, Anacin, Aspergum, Bayer, Bufferin, Ecotrin, Empirin, Excedrin, Maprin, Norgesic, Salatin, Salocol, Salsprin, Supac, Talwin, Triaphen-10, Vanquish, Verin, ZORprin
diphenhydramine	Allerdryl, Benadryl, Benahist, Bendylate, Caladryl, Compoz, Diahist, Diphenadril, Eldadryl, Fenylhist, Fynex, Hydramine, Hydril, Insomnal, Noradryl, Nordryl, Nytol, Tusstat, Wehdryl
ibuprofen	Advil, Amersol, Apsifen, Brufen, Haltran, Medipren, Midol 200, Motrin, Neuvil, Novoprofen, Nuprin, Pamprin-IB, Rufen, Trendar

many trade names, such as Allerdryl and Compoz, provided alone or in combination with other active ingredients. Ibuprofen and aspirin are additional drug examples with different trade names. The rule of thumb is that the active ingredients in a drug are described by their generic name. The generic name of a drug is usually lowercased, whereas the trade name is capitalized.

2.3 Differences Between Brand-Name Drugs and Their Generic Equivalents

During its 17 years of exclusive rights to a new drug, the pharmaceutical company determines the price of the medication. Because there is no competition, the price is generally quite high. The developing company sometimes uses legal tactics to extend its exclusive rights, since this can mean hundreds of millions of dollars per year in profits for a popular medicine. Once the exclusive rights end, competing companies market the generic drug for less money, and consumer savings may be considerable. In some states, pharmacists may routinely substitute a generic drug when the prescription calls for a brand name. In other states, the pharmacist must dispense drugs directly as written by a health care provider or obtain approval before providing a generic substitute. Drugs not approved are placed on a restrictive list.

The companies marketing brand-name drugs often lobby aggressively against laws that might restrict the routine use of their brand-name products. The lobbyists claim that significant differences exist between a trade-name drug and its generic equivalent, and that switching to the generic drug may be harmful for the patient. Consumer advocates, on the other hand, argue that generic substitutions should always be permitted because of the cost savings to patients.

Are there really differences between a brand-name drug and its generic equivalent? The answer is unclear. Despite the fact that the dosages may be identical, drug formulations are not always the same. The two drugs may have different

---

PHARMFACTS

Marketing and Promotional Spending

- When generic versions of paclitaxel (Taxol) became available, various legal tactics by Bristol-Myers Squibb delayed their entry to market. The estimated additional cost to consumers for 2 more years of patent extension was more than $1 billion.

- Promotional spending on prescription drugs rose to over $28 billion in 2008, up from $16.6 billion in 2000 and $9.2 billion in 1996.

- Spending on consumer drug advertisements on television and in print media increased to over $4.1 billion in 2008, up from $2.5 billion in 2000 and $791 million in 1996.

- Consumer advocates claim that promotional advertisements drive up demand for the newer, more expensive drugs over the older, less costly drugs that might be equally effective.

---

inert ingredients. For example, if the drug is in tablet form, the active ingredients may be more tightly compressed in one of the preparations.

The key to comparing brand-name drugs and their generic equivalents lies in measuring the bioavailability of the two preparations. **Bioavailability** is the physiologic ability of the drug to reach its target cells and produce its effect. Bioavailability may indeed be affected by inert ingredients and tablet compression. Anything that affects absorption of a drug, or its distribution to the target cells, can certainly affect drug action. Measuring how long a drug takes to exert its effect gives pharmacologists a crude measure of bioavailability. For example, if a patient is in circulatory shock and it takes the generic-equivalent drug 5 minutes longer to produce its effect, that is indeed significant; however, if a generic medication for arthritis pain relief takes 45 minutes to act, compared with the brand-name drug, which takes 40 minutes, it probably does not matter which drug is prescribed.

To address this issue, some states (Florida, Kentucky, Minnesota, and Missouri, for example) have compiled a negative formulary list. A *negative formulary list* is a list of trade-name drugs that pharmacists may *not* dispense as generic drugs. These drugs must be dispensed exactly as written on the prescription, using the trade-name drug the physician prescribed. In some cases, pharmacists must inform or notify patients of substitutions. Pharmaceutical companies and some health care practitioners have supported this action, claiming that generic drugs—even those that have small differences in bioavailability and bioequivalence—could adversely affect patient outcomes in those with critical conditions or illnesses. However, laws frequently change, and in many instances, the efforts of consumer advocacy groups have led to changes in or elimination of negative formulary lists.

2.4 Controlled Substances and Drug Schedules

Some drugs are frequently abused or have a high potential for addiction. Technically, *addiction* refers to the overwhelming feeling that drives someone to use a drug repeatedly.

Dependence is a related term, often defined as a physiologic or psychologic need for a substance. *Physical dependence* refers to an altered physical condition caused by the adaptation of the nervous system to repeated drug use. In this case, when the drug is no longer available, the individual expresses physical signs of discomfort known as **withdrawal.** In contrast, when an individual is *psychologically dependent*, there are few signs of physical discomfort when the drug is withdrawn; however, the individual feels an intense compelling desire to continue drug use. These concepts are discussed in detail in chapter 11∞ .

According to law, drugs that have a significant potential for abuse are placed into five categories called schedules. These **scheduled drugs** are classified according to their potential for abuse: Schedule I drugs have the highest potential for abuse, and Schedule V drugs have the lowest potential for abuse. Drugs with the highest potential for abuse (Schedule I) are restricted for use in situations of medical necessity, if at all allowed. They have little or no therapeutic value or are intended for research purposes only. Drugs in the other four schedules may be dispensed only in cases in which therapeutic value has been determined. Schedule V is the only category in which some drugs may be dispensed without a prescription because the quantities of the controlled drug are so low that the possibility of causing dependence is extremely remote. Table 2.4 gives the five drug schedules with examples. Not all drugs with an abuse potential are regulated or placed into schedules. Tobacco, alcohol, and caffeine are significant examples.

In the United States, a **controlled substance** is a drug whose use is restricted by the Controlled Substances Act of 1970 and later revisions. The Controlled Substances Act is also called the Comprehensive Drug Abuse Prevention and Control Act. Hospitals and pharmacies must register with the Drug Enforcement Administration (DEA) and then use their assigned registration numbers to purchase scheduled drugs. Hospitals and pharmacies must maintain complete records of all quantities purchased and sold. Physicians,

---

PHARMFACTS

Extent of Drug Abuse

- In 2008, more than 11.5 million people reported driving under the influence of illegal drugs during the previous year.

- In 2008, over 29.8% of the U.S. population 12 and older (70.8 million people) had smoked cigarettes during the past month. This figure includes 3.6 million young people aged 12 to 17. Although it is illegal in the United States to sell tobacco to underage youths, in most cases they are able to purchase them personally.

- From 1994 to 2008, emergency department records of abused substances such as gamma hydroxybutyric acid (GHB; street name *Fantasy*), ketamine (street names *jet, super acid, Special K,* among others), and MDMA (chemical name 3,4-methylenedioxymethamphetamine; street name *Ecstasy*) rose more than 2,000%.

- In 2008, more than 18 million Americans abused or were dependent on either alcohol or illicit drugs.

TABLE 2.4	U.S. Drug Schedules and Examples				
Drug Schedule	Abuse Potential	Potential for Physical Dependency	Potential for Psychologic Dependency	Examples	Therapeutic Use
I	highest	high	high	heroin, lysergic acid diethylamide (LSD), marijuana, and methaqualone	Limited or no therapeutic use
II	high	high	high	morphine, phencyclidine (PCP), cocaine, methadone, and methamphetamine	Used therapeutically with prescription; some drugs no longer used
III	moderate	moderate	high	anabolic steroids, codeine and hydrocodone with aspirin or Tylenol, and some barbiturates	
IV	lower	lower	lower	dextropropoxyphene, pentazocine, meprobamate, diazepam, alprazolam	
V	lowest	lowest	lowest	OTC cough medicines with codeine, diphenoxylate with atropine	Used therapeutically without prescription

nurse practitioners, and others with prescriptive authority must also register with the DEA and receive an assigned number before prescribing these drugs. Drugs with higher abuse potential have more restrictions. For example, a special order form must be used to obtain Schedule II drugs, and orders must be written and signed by the health care provider. Telephone orders to a pharmacy are not permitted. Refills for Schedule II drugs are not permitted; patients must visit their health care provider first. Those convicted of unlawful manufacturing, distributing, or dispensing of controlled substances face severe penalties.

2.5 Canadian Regulations Restricting Drugs of Abuse

In Canada, until 1996 controlled substances were those drugs subject to guidelines outlined in Part III, Schedule G, of the Canadian Food and Drugs Act. According to these guidelines, a health care provider dispensed these medications only to patients suffering from specific diseases or illnesses. Regulated drugs included amphetamines, barbiturates, methaqualone, and anabolic steroids. Controlled drugs were labeled clearly with the letter *C* on the outside of the container.

Restricted drugs not intended for human use were covered in Part IV, Schedule H, of the Canadian Food and Drugs Act. These were drugs used in the course of a chemical or analytical procedure for medical, laboratory, industrial, educational, or research purposes. They included hallucinogens such as lysergic acid diethylamide (LSD), MDMA, and 2,5-dimethoxy-4-methylamphetamine (DOM; street name *STP*). Schedule F drugs were those drugs requiring a prescription for their sale. Examples were methylphenidate (Ritalin), diazepam (Valium), and chlordiazepoxide (Librium). Drugs such as morphine, heroin, cocaine, and cannabis were covered under the Canadian Narcotic Control Act and amended schedules. According to Canadian law, narcotic drugs were labeled clearly with the letter *N* on the outside of the container.

Today Canada's federal drug control statute is the Controlled Drugs and Substances Act. It repeals the Narcotic

Control Act and Parts III and IV of the Food and Drug Act. It further establishes eight schedules of controlled substances; two classes of precursors are covered in one schedule. For a complete listing of drugs, see http://laws.justice .gc.ca/en/C-38.8/. The Controlled Drugs and Substances Act provides broad latitude to the Governor in Council to amend schedules as determined to be in the best interest of Canada's citizens. Drugs and substances covered in the Controlled Drugs and Substances Act correlate with agents named in three United Nations treaties: the Single Convention on Narcotic Drugs, the Convention on Psychotropic Substances, and the United Nations Convention Against Illicit Traffic in Narcotic Drugs and Psychotropic Substances.

Throughout Canada, both prescription and nonprescription drugs must meet specific criteria for public distribution and use. Nonprescription drugs are provided according to guidelines and acts established by the respective Canadian provinces. One recent system establishes three general drug schedules (Table 2.5). Pharmacies must monitor those drugs used specifically to treat self-limiting discomforts such as cold, flu, and mild gastrointestinal or other symptoms. Other nonprescription drugs may be sold without monitoring.

TABLE 2.5	Three-Schedule System for Drugs Sold in Canada
Drug Schedule	Drug Type
I	All prescription drugs
	Drugs with no potential for abuse
	Controlled drugs
	Narcotic drugs
II	All nonprescription drugs monitored for sale by pharmacists
III	All nonprescription drugs not monitored for sale by pharmacists

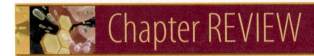

Chapter REVIEW

KEY CONCEPTS

The numbered key concepts provide a succinct summary of the important points from the corresponding numbered section within the chapter. If any of these points are not clear, refer to the numbered section within the chapter for review.

2.1 Drugs may be organized by their therapeutic or pharmacologic classification.

2.2 Drugs have chemical, generic, and trade names. A drug has only one chemical or generic name but may have multiple trade names.

2.3 Generic drugs are less expensive than brand-name drugs, but they may differ in their bioavailability; that is, the ability of the drug to reach its target tissue and produce its action.

2.4 Drugs with a potential for abuse are restricted by the Controlled Substances Act and are categorized into schedules. Schedule I drugs are the most tightly controlled; Schedule V drugs have less potential for addiction and are less tightly controlled.

2.5 Canadian regulations restrict drugs as covered in its federal drug control statute: the Canadian Controlled Drugs and Substances Act.

CRITICAL THINKING QUESTIONS

1. What is the difference between therapeutic and pharmacologic classifications? Identify the following classifications as therapeutic or pharmacologic: beta-adrenergic blocker, oral contraceptive, laxative, folic acid antagonist, and antianginal agent.

2. What is a prototype drug, and how does it differ from other drugs in the same class?

3. A pharmacist decides to switch from a trade-name drug that was ordered by the physician to a generic-equivalent drug. What advantages does this substitution have for the patient? What disadvantages might be caused by the switch?

4. Why are certain drugs placed in schedules? What extra precautions are health care providers required to take when prescribing scheduled drugs?

5. A nurse is preparing to give a patient medications and notes that a drug to be given is marked as a Schedule III drug. What does this information tell the nurse about this medication?

See Appendix D for answers and rationales for all activities.

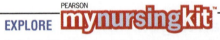

EXPLORE   PEARSON **mynursingkit™**

MyNursingKit is your one stop for online chapter review materials and resources. Prepare for success with additional NCLEX®-style practice questions, interactive assignments and activities, web links, animations and videos, and more!

Register your access code from the front of your book at
www.mynursingkit.com.

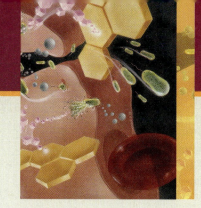

Chapter 3

Principles of Drug Administration

LEARNING OUTCOMES

After reading this chapter, the student should be able to:

1. Discuss drug administration as a component of safe, effective nursing care, utilizing the nursing process.
2. Describe the roles and responsibilities of the nurse regarding drug administration.
3. Explain how the five rights of drug administration affect patient safety.
4. Give specific examples of how the nurse can increase patient compliance in taking medications.
5. Interpret drug orders that contain abbreviations.
6. Compare and contrast the three systems of measurement used in pharmacology.
7. Explain the proper methods of administering enteral, topical, and parenteral drugs.
8. Compare and contrast the advantages and disadvantages of each route of drug administration.

KEY TERMS

The primary role of the nurse in drug administration is to ensure that prescribed medications are delivered in a safe manner. Drug administration is an important component of providing comprehensive nursing care that incorporates all aspects of the nursing process. In the course of drug administration, nurses will collaborate closely with physicians, pharmacists, and, of course, their patients. The purpose of this chapter is to introduce the roles and responsibilities of the nurse in delivering medications safely and effectively.

3.1 Medication Knowledge, Understanding, and Responsibilities of the Nurse

Whether administering drugs or supervising the use of drugs by their patients, the nurse is expected to understand the pharmacotherapeutic principles for all medications given to each patient. Given the large number of different drugs and the potential consequences of medication errors, this is indeed an enormous task. The nurse's responsibilities include knowledge and understanding of the following:

- What drug is ordered
  - Name (generic and trade) and drug classification
  - Intended or proposed use
  - Effects on the body
  - Contraindications
  - Special considerations (e.g., how age, weight, body fat distribution, and individual pathophysiologic states affect pharmacotherapeutic response)
  - Side effects
- Why the medication has been prescribed for this particular patient
- How the medication is supplied by the pharmacy
- How the medication is to be administered, including dosage ranges
- What nursing process considerations related to the medication apply to this patient

Before any drug is administered, the nurse must obtain and process pertinent information regarding the patient's medical history, physical assessment, disease processes, and learning needs and capabilities. Growth and developmental factors must always be considered. It is important to remember that a large number of variables influence a patient's response to medications. Having a firm understanding of these variables can increase the success of pharmacotherapy.

A major goal of studying pharmacology is to limit the number and severity of adverse drug events. Many adverse effects are preventable. Professional nurses can routinely avoid many serious adverse drug effects in their patients by applying their experience and knowledge of pharmacotherapeutics to clinical practice. Some adverse effects, however, are not preventable. It is vital that the nurse be prepared

PharmFacts

Potentially Fatal Drug Reactions
Toxic Epidermal Necrolysis (TEN)

- Severe and deadly drug-induced allergic reaction
- Characterized by widespread epidermal sloughing, caused by massive disintegration of keratinocytes
- Severe epidermal detachment involving the top layer of the skin and mucous membranes
- Multisystem organ involvement and death if the reaction is not recognized and diagnosed
- Occurs when the liver fails to properly break down a drug, which then cannot be excreted normally
- Associated with use of some anticonvulsants (phenytoin [Dilantin], carbamazepine [Tegretol]), the antibiotic trimethoprim/sulfamethoxazole (Bactrim, Septra), and other drugs, but can occur with the use of any prescription or OTC preparation, including ibuprofen (Advil, Motrin)
- Risk of death decreases if the offending drug is quickly withdrawn and supportive care is maintained
- Skin sloughing of 30% or more of the body

Stevens–Johnson Syndrome (SJS)

- Usually prompted by the same or similar drugs as TEN
- Begins within 1 to 14 days of pharmacotherapy
- Start of SJS usually signaled by nonspecific upper respiratory infection (URI) with chills, fever, and malaise
- Generalized blisterlike lesions follow within a few days
- Skin sloughing of 10% of the body

to recognize and respond to potential adverse effects of medications.

Allergic and anaphylactic reactions are particularly serious effects that must be carefully monitored and prevented, when possible. An **allergic reaction** is an acquired hyperresponse of body defenses to a foreign substance (allergen). Signs of allergic reactions vary in severity and include skin rash with or without itching, edema, runny nose, or reddened eyes with tearing. On discovering that the patient is allergic to a product, it is the nurse's responsibility to alert all personnel by documenting the allergy in the medical record and by appropriately labeling patient records and the medication administration record (MAR). An appropriate, agency-approved bracelet should be placed on the patient to alert all caregivers to the specific drug allergy. Information related to drug allergy must be communicated to the physician and pharmacist so the medication regimen can be evaluated for cross-sensitivity among various pharmacologic products.

Anaphylaxis is a severe type of allergic reaction that involves the massive, systemic release of histamine and other chemical mediators of inflammation that can lead to life-threatening shock. Symptoms such as acute dyspnea and the sudden appearance of hypotension or tachycardia following drug administration are indicative of anaphylaxis, which must receive immediate treatment. The pharmacotherapy of allergic reactions and anaphylaxis is covered in chapters 38 and 29∞, respectively.

3.2 The Rights of Drug Administration

The traditional **five rights of drug administration** form the operational basis for the safe delivery of medications. The five rights offer simple and practical guidance for nurses to use during drug preparation, delivery, and administration, and focus on individual performance. The five rights are as follows:

1. Right patient
2. Right medication
3. Right dose
4. Right route of administration
5. Right time of delivery

Additional rights have been added over the years, depending on particular academic curricula or agency policies. Additions to the original five rights include considerations such as the right to refuse medication, the right to receive drug education, the right preparation, and the right documentation. Ethical and legal considerations regarding the five rights are discussed in chapter 9∞.

The **three checks of drug administration** that nurses use in conjunction with the five rights help to ensure patient safety and drug effectiveness. Traditionally these checks incorporate the following:

1. Checking the drug with the MAR or the medication information system when removing it from the medication drawer, refrigerator, or controlled substance locker
2. Checking the drug when preparing it, pouring it, taking it out of the unit-dose container, or connecting the IV tubing to the bag
3. Checking the drug before administering it to the patient

Despite all attempts to provide safe drug delivery, errors continue to occur, some of which are fatal. Although the nurse is held accountable for preparing and administering medications, safe drug practices are a result of multidisciplinary endeavors. Responsibility for accurate drug administration lies with multiple individuals, including physicians, pharmacists, and other health care practitioners. It should be noted that computerized scanning systems of medication administration do not relieve the health care provider of the responsibility to continue the three checks and the use of the five rights. Scanning a bar code does not replace these checks and could result in serious medication errors. Factors contributing to medication errors are presented in chapter 9∞.

3.3 Patient Compliance and Successful Pharmacotherapy

Compliance or adherence to drug regimen is a major factor affecting pharmacotherapeutic success. As it relates to pharmacology, **compliance** is taking a medication in the manner prescribed by the health care provider, or in the case of OTC

AVOIDING MEDICATION ERRORS

The FDA and the American Hospital Association track drug errors that occur in health care settings. The five most common causes of medication errors are:

- Incomplete patient information (e.g., not knowing about patients' allergies, other medicines they are taking, previous diagnoses, or lab results)
- Unavailable drug information (e.g., current warnings issued by the FDA)
- Miscommunication of drug orders (e.g., illegible handwritten orders, confusion between drugs with similar names, misuse of zeroes and decimal points, unclear abbreviations)
- Lack of appropriate labeling when a drug is prepared and repackaged into smaller units
- Environmental factors (e.g., noise or interruptions that distract the nurse as he or she prepares to administer the medications)

Because the nurse is often the final health care provider in the chain of medication administration, extra caution must be taken to avoid these key sources of error.

drugs, following the instructions on the label. Patient noncompliance ranges from not taking the medication at all to taking it at the wrong time or in the wrong manner.

Although the nurse may be extremely conscientious in applying all the principles of effective drug administration, these strategies are of little value unless the patient agrees that the prescribed drug regimen is personally worthwhile. Before administering the drug, the nurse should use the nursing process to formulate a personalized care plan that will best enable the patient to become an active participant in his or her care (chapter 6∞). This allows the patient to accept or reject the pharmacologic course of therapy, based on accurate information that is presented in a manner that addresses individual learning styles. It is imperative to remember that a responsible, well-informed adult always has the legal option to refuse to take any medication.

In the plan of care, it is important to address essential information that the patient must know regarding the prescribed medications. This includes factors such as the name of the drug, why it has been ordered, expected drug actions,

LIFESPAN CONSIDERATIONS

The Challenges of Pediatric Drug Administration

Administering medication to infants and young children requires special knowledge and techniques. The nurse must have knowledge of growth and development patterns. When possible, the child should be given a choice regarding the use of a spoon, dropper, or syringe. A matter-of-fact attitude should be presented in giving a child medications: Using threats or dishonesty is unacceptable. Oral medications that must be crushed for the child to swallow can be mixed with flavored syrup, jelly, or fruit puree to avoid unpleasant tastes. Medications should not be mixed with certain dietary products, such as potatoes, milk, or fruit juices to mask the taste, because the child may develop an unpleasant association with these items and refuse to consume them in the future. To prevent nausea, medications can be preceded and followed with sips of a carbonated beverage that is poured over crushed ice.

associated side effects, and potential interactions with other medications, foods, herbal supplements, or alcohol. Patients need to be reminded that they share an active role in ensuring their own medication effectiveness and safety.

Many factors can influence whether patients comply with pharmacotherapy. The drug may be too expensive or may not be approved by the patient's health insurance plan. Patients sometimes forget doses of medications, especially when they must be taken three or four times per day. Patients often discontinue the use of drugs that have annoying side effects or those that impair major lifestyle choices. Adverse effects that often prompt noncompliance are headache, dizziness, nausea, diarrhea, or impotence.

Patients often take medications in an unexpected manner, sometimes self-adjusting their doses. Some patients believe that if one tablet is good, two must be better. Others believe they will become dependent on the medication if it is taken as prescribed; thus, they take only half the required dose. Patients are usually reluctant to admit or report noncompliance to the nurse for fear of being reprimanded or feeling embarrassed. Because the reasons for noncompliance are many and varied, the nurse must be vigilant in questioning patients about their medications. When pharmacotherapy fails to produce the expected outcomes, noncompliance should be considered a possible explanation.

3.4 Drug Orders and Time Schedules

Health care providers use accepted abbreviations to communicate the directions and times for drug administration. Table 3.1 lists common abbreviations that relate to universally scheduled times.

A **STAT order** refers to any medication that is needed immediately, and is to be given only once. It is often associated with emergency medications that are needed for life-threatening situations. The term *STAT* comes from *statim*, the Latin word meaning "immediately." The physician normally notifies the nurse of any STAT order so it

TABLE 3.1   Drug Administration Abbreviations

Abbreviation	Meaning
ac	before meals
ad lib	as desired/as directed
AM	morning
bid	twice per day
cap	capsule
gtt	drop
h or hr	hour
IM	intramuscular
IV	intravenous
no	number
pc	after meals; after eating
PO	by mouth
PM	afternoon
PRN	when needed/necessary
qid	four times per day
q2h	every 2 hours (even or when first given)
q4h	every 4 hours (even)
q6h	every 6 hours (even)
q8h	every 8 hours (even)
q12h	every 12 hours
Rx	take
STAT	immediately; at once
tab	tablet
tid	three times per day

The Institute for Safe Medical Practices recommends that the following abbreviations be avoided because they can lead to medication errors: q: instead use "every"; qh: instead use "hourly" or "every hour"; qd: instead use "daily" or "every day"; qhs: instead use "nightly"; qod: instead use "every other day." For other recommendations, see the official Joint Commission "Do Not Use List."

PharmFacts

Grapefruit Juice and Drug Interactions

- Grapefruit juice may not be safe for people who take certain medications.
- Chemicals (most likely flavonoids) in grapefruit juice lower the activity of specific enzymes in the intestinal tract that normally break down medications. This allows a larger amount of medication to reach the bloodstream, resulting in increased drug activity.
- Drugs that may be affected by grapefruit juice include midazolam (Versed); cyclosporine (Sandimmune, Neoral); antihyperlipidemics such as lovastatin (Mevacor) and simvastatin (Zocor); certain antihistamines such as astemizole (Hismanal); certain antibiotics such as erythromycin; and certain antifungals such as itraconazole (Sporanox), ketoconazole (Nizoral), and mibefradil (Posicor).
- Grapefruit juice should be consumed at least 2 hours before or 5 hours after taking a medication that may interact with it.
- Some drinks that are flavored with fruit juice could contain grapefruit juice, even if grapefruit is not part of the name of the drink. Check the ingredients label.

can be obtained from the pharmacy and administered immediately. The time between writing the order and administering the drug should be 5 minutes or less. Although not as urgent, an **ASAP order** (as soon as possible) should be available for administration to the patient within 30 minutes of the written order.

The **single order** is for a drug that is to be given only once, and at a specific time, such as a preoperative order. A **PRN order** (Latin: *pro re nata*) is administered *as required* by the patient's condition. The nurse makes the judgment, based on patient assessment, as to when such a medication is to be administered. Orders not written as STAT, ASAP, NOW, or PRN are called **routine orders**. These are usually carried out within 2 hours of the time the order is written by the physician. A **standing order** is written in advance of a situation that is to be carried out under specific circumstances. An example of a standing order is a set of postoperative PRN prescriptions that are written for all patients who have undergone a specific surgical procedure. A common standing order for patients who have had a tonsillectomy is "Tylenol elixir 325 mg PO every 6 hours PRN sore throat." Because of the legal implications of putting all patients into a single treatment category, standing orders are no longer permitted in some facilities.

Agency policies dictate that drug orders be reviewed by the attending physician within specific time frames, usually at least every 7 days. Prescriptions for narcotics and other scheduled drugs are often automatically discontinued after 72 hours, unless specifically reordered by the physician. Automatic stop orders do not generally apply when the number of doses or an exact period of time is specified.

Some medications must be taken at specific times. If a drug causes stomach upset, it is usually administered *with* meals to prevent epigastric pain, nausea, or vomiting. Other medications should be administered *between* meals because food interferes with absorption. Some central nervous system drugs and antihypertensives are best administered *at bedtime*, because they may cause drowsiness. Sildenafil (Viagra) is unique in that it should be taken 30 to 60 minutes prior to expected sexual intercourse, to achieve an effective erection. (Note: Sildenafil is also prescribed to hospitalized patients for pulmonary hypertension.) The nurse must pay careful attention to educating patients about the timing of their medications, to enhance compliance and to increase the potential for therapeutic success.

Once medications are administered, the nurse must correctly document that they have been given to the patient and this documentation is completed only *after* the medications have been given, not when they are prepared. It is necessary to include the drug name, dosage, time administered, any assessments, and the nurse's signature. If a medication is refused or omitted, this fact must be recorded on the appropriate form within the medical record. It is customary to document the reason, when possible. Should the patient voice any concerns or complaints about the medication, these should also be included.

3.5 Systems of Measurement

Dosages are labeled and dispensed according to their weight or volume. Three systems of measurement are used in pharmacology: metric, apothecary, and household.

The most common system of drug measurement uses the **metric system of measurement.** The volume of a drug is expressed in terms of liters (L) or milliliters (mL). The cubic centimeter (cc) is a measurement of volume that is equivalent to 1 mL of fluid, but the *cc* abbreviation is no longer used because it can be mistaken for the abbreviation for unit (u) and cause medication errors. The metric weight of a drug is stated in kilograms (kg), grams (g), milligrams (mg), or micrograms (mcg). Note that the abbreviation μg should not be used for microgram, because it too can be confused with other abbreviations and cause a medication error.

The **apothecary** and **household systems** are older systems of measurement. Although most physicians and pharmacies use the metric system, these older systems are still encountered. In 2005, the Joint Commission (JCAHO), the accrediting organization for health care agencies, added "apothecary units" to its official "Do Not Use" list. But because not all health care agencies are accredited by JCAHO and until the metric system totally replaces the other systems, the nurse must recognize dosages based on all three systems of measurement. Approximate equivalents between metric, apothecary, and household units of volume and weight are listed in Table 3.2.

Because Americans are very familiar with the teaspoon, tablespoon, and cup, it is important for the nurse to be able to convert between the household and metric systems of measurement. In the hospital, a glass of fluid is measured in milliliters—an 8-oz glass of water is recorded as 240 mL. If a patient being discharged is ordered to drink 2,400 mL of fluid per day, the nurse may instruct the patient to drink 10, 8-oz glasses or 10 cups of fluid per day. Likewise, when a child is to be given a drug that is administered in elixir form, the nurse should explain that 5 mL of the drug is approximately the same as 1 teaspoon. The nurse should encourage the use of accurate medical dosing devices at home, such as oral dosing syringes, oral droppers, cylindrical spoons, and medication cups. These are preferred over the traditional household measuring spoon because they are more accurate. Eating utensils that are commonly referred to as teaspoons or tablespoons often do not hold the volume that their names imply. Because of the differences in volumes between standard teaspoons, dessert spoons, tablespoons, and "salt spoons," it is recommended that a measuring spoon used for cooking be used rather than

TABLE 3.2	Metric, Apothecary, and Household Approximate Measurement Equivalents		
Metric	**Apothecary**	**Household**
1 mL	15–16 minims	15–16 drops
4–5 mL	1 fluid dram	1 teaspoon or 60 drops
15–16 mL	4 fluid drams	1 tablespoon or 3–4 teaspoons
30–32 mL	8 fluid drams or 1 fluid ounce	2 tablespoons
240–250 mL	8 fluid ounces (1/2 pint)	1 glass or cup
500 mL	1 pint	2 glasses or 2 cups
1 L	32 fluid ounces or 1 quart	4 glasses or 4 cups or 1 quart
1 mg	1/60 grain	———
60–64 mg	1 grain	———
300–325 mg	5 grains	———
1 g	15–16 grains	———
1 kg	———	2.2 pounds

To convert grains to grams: Divide grains by 15 or 16. To convert grams to grains: Multiply grams by 15 or 16. To convert minims to milliliters: Divide minims by 15 or 16.

household eating utensils if a more accurate dosing device is not available. Many OTC liquid medications now come with a pre-packaged medication cup to avoid under- or over-dosage problems.

ROUTES OF DRUG ADMINISTRATION

The three broad categories of routes of drug administration are enteral, topical, and parenteral, and there are subsets within each of these. Each route has both advantages and disadvantages. Whereas some drugs are formulated to be given by several routes, others are specific to only one route. Pharmacokinetic considerations, such as how the route of administration affects drug absorption and distribution, are discussed in chapter 4 ∞.

Certain protocols and techniques are common to all methods of drug administration. The student should review the drug administration guidelines in the following list before proceeding to subsequent sections that discuss specific routes of administration:

- Review the medication order and check for drug allergies.
- Wash your hands and apply gloves, if indicated.
- Use aseptic technique when preparing and administering parenteral medications.
- In all cases of drug administration, identify the patient by asking the person to state his or her full name (or by asking the parent or guardian), checking the identification band, and comparing this information with the MAR or scanner and computer.
- Ask the patient about known allergies.
- Inform the patient of the drug's name and method of administration.
- Position the patient for the appropriate route of administration.
- For enteral drugs, assist the patient to a sitting position.
- If the drug is prepackaged (unit dose), remove it from the packaging at the bedside when possible.
- Unless specifically instructed to do so in the orders, do not leave drugs at the bedside.
- Document the medication administration and any pertinent patient responses on the MAR.

3.6 Enteral Drug Administration

The enteral route includes drugs given orally and those administered through nasogastric or gastrostomy tubes. Oral drug administration is the most common, most convenient, and usually the least costly of all routes. It is also considered the safest route because the skin barrier is not compromised. In cases of overdose, medications remaining in the stomach can be retrieved by inducing vomiting. Oral preparations are available in tablet, capsule, and liquid forms. Medica-

tions administered by the enteral route take advantage of the vast absorptive surfaces of the oral mucosa, stomach, or small intestine.

TABLETS AND CAPSULES

Tablets and capsules are the most common forms of drugs. Patients prefer tablets or capsules over other routes and forms because of their ease of use. In some cases, tablets may be scored for more individualized dosing.

Some patients, particularly children, have difficulty swallowing tablets and capsules. Crushing tablets or opening capsules and sprinkling the drug over food or mixing it with juice will make it more palatable and easier to swallow. However, the nurse should not crush tablets or open capsules unless the manufacturer specifically states this is permissible. Some drugs are inactivated by crushing or opening, whereas others severely irritate the stomach mucosa and cause nausea or vomiting. Occasionally, drugs should not be crushed because they irritate the oral mucosa, are extremely bitter, or contain dyes that stain the teeth. Most drug guides provide lists of drugs that may not be crushed. Guidelines for administering tablets or capsules are given in Table 3.3 (section A).

The strongly acidic contents within the stomach can present a destructive obstacle to the absorption of some medications. To overcome this barrier, tablets may have a hard, waxy coating that enables them to resist the acidity. These **enteric-coated** tablets are designed to dissolve in the alkaline environment of the small intestine. It is important that the nurse not crush enteric-coated tablets because the medication would then be directly exposed to the stomach environment.

Studies have clearly demonstrated that compliance declines as the number of doses per day increases. With this in mind, pharmacologists have attempted to design new drugs that may be administered only once or twice daily. **Sustained-release** tablets or capsules are designed to dissolve very slowly. This releases the medication over an extended time and results in a longer duration of action for the medication. Also called extended-release (XR), long-acting (LA), or slow-release (SR) medications, these forms allow for the convenience of once- or twice-a-day dosing. Extended-release medications must not be crushed or opened.

Giving medications by the oral route has certain disadvantages. The patient must be conscious and able to swallow properly. Certain types of drugs, including proteins, are inactivated by digestive enzymes in the stomach and small intestine. Medications absorbed from the stomach and small intestine first travel to the liver, where they may be inactivated before they ever reach their target organs. This process, called *first-pass metabolism,* is discussed in chapter 4 ∞. The significant variation in the motility of the GI tract and in its ability to absorb medications can create differences in bioavailability. In addition, children and some adults have an aversion to swallowing large tablets and capsules, or to taking oral medications that are distasteful.

TABLE 3.3	Enteral Drug Administration
Drug Form	**Administration Guidelines**
A. tablet, capsule, or liquid	1. Assess that patient is alert and has ability to swallow. 2. Place tablets or capsules into medication cup. 3. If liquid, shake the bottle to mix the agent, and measure the dose into the cup at eye level. 4. Hand the patient the medication cup. 5. Offer a glass of water to facilitate swallowing the medication. Milk or juice may be offered if not contraindicated. 6. Remain with patient until all medication is swallowed.
B. sublingual	1. Assess that patient is alert and has ability to hold medication under tongue. 2. Place sublingual tablet under tongue. 3. Instruct patient not to chew or swallow the tablet, or move the tablet around with tongue. 4. Instruct patient to allow tablet to dissolve completely before swallowing saliva. 5. Remain with patient to determine that all the medication has dissolved. 6. Offer a glass of water, if patient desires.
C. buccal	1. Assess that patient is alert and has ability to hold medication between the gums and the cheek. 2. Place buccal tablet between the gum line and the cheek. 3. Instruct patient not to chew or swallow the tablet, or move the tablet around with tongue. 4. Instruct patient to allow tablet to dissolve completely before swallowing saliva. 5. Remain with patient to determine that all of the medication has dissolved. 6. Offer a glass of water, if patient desires.
D. nasogastric and gastrostomy	1. Administer liquid forms when possible to avoid clogging the tube. 2. If solid, crush finely into powder and mix thoroughly with at least 30 mL of warm water until dissolved. 3. Assess and verify tube placement. 4. Turn off feeding, if applicable to patient. 5. Aspirate stomach contents and measure the residual volume. If greater than 100 mL for an adult, check agency policy. 6. Return residual via gravity and flush with water. 7. Pour medication into syringe barrel and allow to flow into the tube by gravity. Give each medication separately, flushing between with water. 8. Keep head of bed elevated for 1 hour to prevent aspiration. 9. Reestablish continual feeding, as scheduled. Keep head of bed elevated 45° to prevent aspiration.

SUBLINGUAL AND BUCCAL DRUG ADMINISTRATION

For sublingual and buccal administration, the tablet is not swallowed but kept in the mouth. The mucosa of the oral cavity contains a rich blood supply that provides an excellent absorptive surface for certain drugs. Medications given by this route are not subjected to destructive digestive enzymes, nor do they undergo hepatic first-pass metabolism.

For the **sublingual route**, the medication is placed under the tongue and allowed to dissolve slowly. Because of the rich blood supply in this region, the sublingual route results in a rapid onset of action. Sublingual dosage forms are most often formulated as rapidly disintegrating tablets or as soft gelatin capsules filled with liquid drug.

When multiple drugs have been ordered, the sublingual preparations should be administered after oral medications have been swallowed. The patient should be instructed not to move the drug with the tongue, nor to eat or drink anything until the medication has completely dissolved. The sublingual mucosa is not suitable for extended-release formulations because it is a relatively small area and is constantly being bathed by a substantial amount of saliva. Table 3.3 (section B) and ➤ Figure 3.1a present important points regarding sublingual drug administration.

To administer by the **buccal route**, the tablet or capsule is placed in the oral cavity between the gum and the cheek. The patient must be instructed not to manipulate the medication with the tongue; otherwise, it could get displaced to the sublingual area, where it would be more rapidly absorbed, or to the back of the throat, where it could be swallowed. The buccal mucosa is less permeable to most medications than the sublingual area, providing for slower absorption. The buccal route is preferred over the sublingual route for sustained-release delivery because of the greater mucosal surface area of the former. Drugs formulated for buccal administration

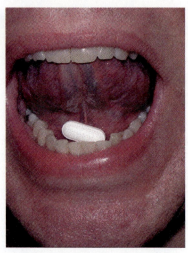

(a)

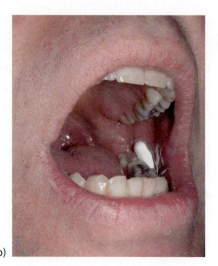

(b)

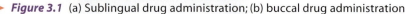

➤ *Figure 3.1* (a) Sublingual drug administration; (b) buccal drug administration

generally do not cause irritation and are small enough to not cause discomfort to the patient. As with the sublingual route, drugs administered by the buccal route avoid first-pass metabolism by the liver and the enzymatic processes of the stomach and small intestine. Table 3.3 (section C) and ➤ Figure 3.1b provide important guidelines for buccal drug administration.

NASOGASTRIC AND GASTROSTOMY DRUG ADMINISTRATION

Patients with a nasogastric tube or enteral feeding mechanism such as a gastrostomy tube may have their medications administered through these devices. A nasogastric (NG) tube is a soft, flexible tube inserted by way of the nasopharynx with the tip lying in the stomach. A gastrostomy (G) tube is surgically placed directly into the patient's stomach. Generally, the NG tube is used for short-term treatment, whereas the G tube is inserted for patients requiring long-term care. Drugs administered through these tubes are usually in liquid form. Although solid drugs can be crushed or dissolved, they tend to cause clogging within the tubes. Sustained-release drugs should not be crushed and administered through NG or G tubes. Drugs administered by this route are exposed to the same physiologic processes as those given orally. Table 3.3 (section D) gives important guidelines for administering drugs through NG or G tubes.

3.7 Topical Drug Administration

Topical drugs are those applied locally to the skin or the membranous linings of the eye, ear, nose, respiratory tract, urinary tract, vagina, and rectum. These applications include the following:

- *Dermatologic preparations:* Drugs applied to the skin, the topical route most commonly used. Formulations include creams, lotions, gels, powders, and sprays.
- *Instillations and irrigations:* Drugs applied into body cavities or orifices. These include the eyes, ears, nose, urinary bladder, rectum, and vagina.

- *Inhalations:* Drugs applied to the respiratory tract by inhalers, nebulizers, or positive-pressure breathing apparatuses. The most common indication for inhaled drugs is bronchoconstriction due to bronchitis or asthma; however, a number of illegal, abused drugs are taken by this route because it provides a very rapid onset of drug action (see chapter 11∞). Additional details on inhalation drug administration can be found in chapter 39∞.

Many drugs are applied topically to produce a *local* effect. For example, antibiotics may be applied to the skin to treat skin infections. Antineoplastic agents may be instilled into the urinary bladder via catheter to treat tumors of the bladder mucosa. Corticosteroids are sprayed into the nostrils to reduce inflammation of the nasal mucosa due to allergic rhinitis. Local, topical delivery produces fewer side effects compared with oral or parenteral administration of the same drug. This is because topically applied drugs are ab-

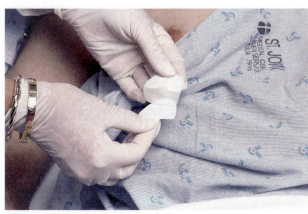

(a)

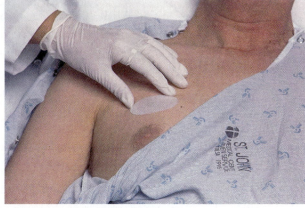

(b)

➤ *Figure 3.2* Transdermal patch administration: (a) protective coating removed from patch; (b) patch immediately applied to clean, dry, hairless skin and labeled with date, time, and initials
Source: Pearson Education/PH College.

sorbed very slowly, and amounts reaching the general circulation are minimal.

Some drugs are given topically to provide for slow release and absorption of the drug in the general circulation. These agents are administered for their *systemic* effects. For example, a nitroglycerin patch is applied to the skin not to treat a local skin condition but to treat a systemic condition, coronary artery disease. Likewise, prochlorperazine (Compazine) suppositories are inserted rectally not to treat a disease of the rectum but to alleviate nausea.

The distinction between topical drugs given for local effects and those given for systemic effects is an important one for the nurse. In the case of local drugs, absorption is undesirable and may cause side effects. For systemic drugs, absorption is essential for the therapeutic action of the drug. With either type of topical agent, drugs should not be applied to abraded or denuded skin, unless directed to do so.

TRANSDERMAL DELIVERY SYSTEM

The use of transdermal patches provides an effective means of delivering certain medications. Examples include nitroglycerin for angina pectoris and scopolamine (Transderm-Scop) for motion sickness. Although transdermal patches contain a specific amount of drug, the rate of delivery and the actual dose received may be variable. Patches are changed on a regular basis, using a site rotation routine, which should be documented in the MAR. Before applying a transdermal patch, the nurse should verify that the previous patch has been removed and disposed of appropriately. Drugs to be administered by this route avoid the first-pass effect in the liver and bypass digestive enzymes. Table 3.4 (section A) and ➤ Figure 3.2 illustrate the major points of transdermal drug delivery.

OPHTHALMIC ADMINISTRATION

The ophthalmic route is used to treat local conditions of the eye and surrounding structures. Common indications include excessive dryness, infections, glaucoma, and dilation of the pupil during eye examinations. Ophthalmic drugs are available in the form of eye irrigations, drops, ointments, and medicated disks. ➤ Figure 3.3 (a) and (b) and Table 3.4 (sec-

tion B) give guidelines for adult administration. Although the procedure is the same with a child, it is advisable to enlist the help of an adult caregiver. In some cases, the infant or toddler may need to be immobilized with arms wrapped to prevent accidental injury to the eye during administration. For the young child, demonstrating the procedure using a doll facilitates cooperation and decreases anxiety.

OTIC ADMINISTRATION

The otic route is used to treat local conditions of the ear, including infections and soft blockages of the auditory canal. Otic medications include eardrops and irrigations, which are usually ordered for cleaning purposes. Administration to infants and young children must be performed carefully to avoid injury to sensitive structures of the ear. ➤ Figure 3.4 and Table 3.4 (section C) present key points in administering otic medications.

NASAL ADMINISTRATION

The nasal route is used for both local and systemic drug administration. The nasal mucosa provides an excellent absorptive surface for certain medications. Advantages of this route include ease of use and avoidance of the first-pass effect and digestive enzymes. Nasal spray formulations of corticosteroids have revolutionized the treatment of allergic rhinitis owing to their high safety margin when administered by this route.

Although the nasal mucosa provides an excellent surface for drug delivery, there is the potential for damage to the cilia within the nasal cavity, and mucosal irritation is common. In addition, unpredictable mucus secretion among some individuals may affect drug absorption from this site.

Drops or sprays are often used for their local **astringent effect;** that is, they shrink swollen mucous membranes or loosen secretions and facilitate drainage. This brings immediate relief from the nasal congestion caused by the common cold. The nose also provides the route to reach the nasal sinuses and the eustachian tube. Proper positioning of the patient prior to instilling nose drops for sinus disorders depends on which sinuses are being treated. The same holds true for treatment of

TABLE 3.4	**Topical Drug Administration**
Drug Form	**Administration Guidelines**
A. transdermal	1. Obtain transdermal patch, and read manufacturer's guidelines. Application site and frequency of changing differ according to medication. 2. Apply gloves before handling, to avoid absorption of the agent by the nurse. 3. Remove previous medication or patch, and cleanse area. 4. If using a transdermal ointment, apply the ordered amount of medication in an even line directly on the premeasured paper that accompanies the medication tube. 5. Press patch or apply medicated paper to clean, dry, and hairless skin. 6. Rotate sites to prevent skin irritation. 7. Label patch with date, time, and initials.
B. ophthalmic	1. Instruct patient to lie supine or sit with head slightly tilted back. 2. With nondominant hand, pull lower lid down gently to expose the conjunctival sac, creating a pocket. 3. Ask patient to look upward. 4. Hold eyedropper 1/4–1/8 inch above the conjunctival sac. Do not hold dropper over eye, as this may stimulate the blink reflex. 5. Instill prescribed number of drops into the center of the pocket. Avoid touching eye or conjunctival sac with tip of eyedropper. 6. If applying ointment, apply a thin line of ointment evenly along inner edge of lower lid margin, from inner to outer canthus. 7. Instruct the patient to close eye gently. Apply gentle pressure with finger to the nasolacrimal duct at the inner canthus for 1–2 minutes, to avoid overflow drainage into nose and throat, thus minimizing risk of absorption into the systemic circulation. 8. With tissue, remove excess medication around eye. 9. Replace dropper. Do not rinse eyedropper.
C. otic	1. Instruct patient to lie on side or to sit with head tilted so that affected ear is facing up. 2. If necessary, clean the pinna of the ear and the meatus with a clean washcloth to prevent any discharge from being washed into the ear canal during the instillation of the drops. 3. Hold dropper 1/4 inch above ear canal, and instill prescribed number of drops into the side of the ear canal, allowing the drops to flow downward. Avoid placing drops directly on the tympanic membrane. 4. Gently apply intermittent pressure to the tragus of the ear three or four times. 5. Instruct patient to remain on side for up to 10 minutes to prevent loss of medication. 6. If cotton ball is ordered, presoak with medication and insert it into the outermost part of ear canal. 7. Wipe any solution that may have dripped from the ear canal with a tissue.
D. nasal drops	1. Ask the patient to blow the nose to clear nasal passages. 2. Draw up the correct volume of drug into dropper. 3. Instruct the patient to open and breathe through the mouth. 4. Hold the tip of the dropper just above the nostril, and without touching the nose with the dropper, direct the solution laterally toward the midline of the superior concha of the ethmoid bone—not the base of the nasal cavity, where it will run down the throat and into the eustachian tube. 5. Ask the patient to remain in position for 5 minutes. 6. Discard any remaining solution that is in the dropper.
E. vaginal	1. Instruct the patient to assume a supine position with knees bent and separated. 2. Place water-soluble lubricant into medicine cup. 3. Apply gloves; open suppository and lubricate the rounded end. 4. Expose the vaginal orifice by separating the labia with nondominant hand. 5. Insert the rounded end of the suppository about 8–10 cm along the posterior wall of the vagina, or as far as it will pass. 6. If using a cream, jelly, or foam, gently insert applicator 5 cm along the posterior vaginal wall and slowly push the plunger until empty. Remove the applicator and place on a paper towel. 7. Ask the patient to lower legs and remain lying in the supine or side-lying position for 5–10 minutes following insertion.

TABLE 3.4	**Topical Drug Administration** *(Continued)*
Drug Form	**Administration Guidelines**
F. rectal suppositories	1. Instruct the patient to lie on left side (Sims' position).
	2. Apply gloves; open suppository and lubricate the blunt end. Suppositories are designed for the rounded end to be facing out, to exert less pressure on the internal anal sphincter, thereby decreasing the patient's urge to push it out.
	3. Lubricate the gloved forefinger of the dominant hand with water-soluble lubricant.
	4. Inform the patient when the suppository is to be inserted; instruct the patient to take slow, deep breaths and deeply exhale during insertion, to relax the anal sphincter.
	5. Gently insert the lubricated end of suppository into the rectum, beyond the anal–rectal ridge to ensure retention.
	6. Instruct the patient to remain in the Sims' position or lie supine to prevent expulsion of the suppository.
	7. Instruct the patient to retain the suppository for at least 30 minutes to allow absorption to occur, unless the suppository is administered to stimulate defecation.

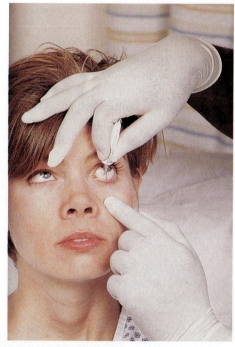

(a)

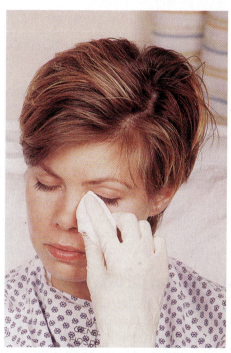

(b)

➤ *Figure 3.3* (a) Instilling an eye ointment into the lower conjunctival sac; (b) pressing on the nasolacrimal duct
Source: © Jenny Thomas Photography.

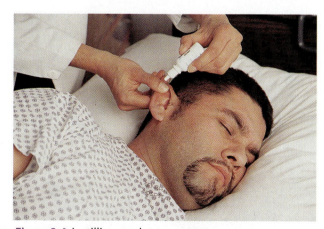

➤ *Figure 3.4* Instilling eardrops
Source: © Elena Dorfman.

the eustachian tube. Table 3.4 (section D) and ➤ Figure 3.5 illustrate important facts related to nasal drug administration.

VAGINAL ADMINISTRATION

The vaginal route is used to deliver medications for treating local infections and to relieve vaginal pain and itching. Vaginal medications are inserted as suppositories, creams, jellies, or foams. It is important that the nurse explain the purpose of treatment and provide for privacy and patient dignity. Before inserting vaginal drugs, the nurse should instruct the patient to empty her bladder, to lessen both the discomfort during treatment and the possibility of irritating or injuring the vaginal lining. The patient should be offered a perineal pad following administration. Table 3.4 (section E) and ➤ Figure 3.6 (a) and (b) provide guidelines regarding vaginal drug administration.

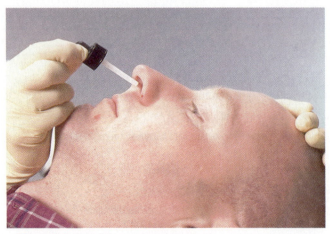

> *Figure 3.5* Nasal drug administration
Source: Pearson Education/PH College.

RECTAL ADMINISTRATION

The rectal route may be used for either local or systemic drug administration. It is a safe and effective means of delivering drugs to patients who are comatose or who are experiencing nausea and vomiting. Rectal drugs are normally in suppository form, although a few laxatives and diagnostic agents are given via enema. Although absorption is slower than by other routes, it is steady and reliable provided the medication can be retained by the patient. Venous blood from the lower rectum is not transported by way of the liver; thus, the first-pass effect is avoided, as are the digestive enzymes of the upper GI tract. Table 3.4 (section F) gives selected details regarding rectal drug administration.

3.8 Parenteral Drug Administration

Parenteral administration refers to the dispensing of medications by routes other than oral or topical. The **parenteral route** delivers drugs via a needle into the skin layers, subcutaneous tissue, muscles, or veins. More advanced parenteral delivery includes administration into arteries, body cavities

(such as intrathecal), and organs (such as intracardiac). Parenteral drug administration is much more invasive than topical or enteral. Because of the potential for introducing pathogenic microbes directly into the blood or body tissues, aseptic techniques must be strictly applied. The nurse is expected to identify and use appropriate materials for parenteral drug delivery, including specialized equipment and techniques involved in the preparation and administration of injectable products. The nurse must know the correct anatomical locations for parenteral administration, and safety procedures regarding hazardous equipment disposal.

INTRADERMAL AND SUBCUTANEOUS ADMINISTRATION

Injection into the skin delivers drugs to the blood vessels that supply the various layers of the skin. Drugs may be injected either intradermally or subcutaneously. The major difference between these methods is the depth of injection. An advantage of both methods is that they offer a means of administering drugs to patients who are unable to take them orally. Drugs administered by these routes avoid the hepatic first-pass effect and digestive enzymes. Disadvantages are that only small volumes can be administered, and injections can cause pain and swelling at the injection site.

An **intradermal (ID)** injection is administered into the dermis layer of the skin. Because the dermis contains more blood vessels than the deeper subcutaneous layer, drugs are more easily absorbed. Intradermal injection is usually employed for allergy and disease screening or for local anesthetic delivery prior to venous cannulation. Intradermal injections are limited to very small volumes of drug, usually only 0.1 to 0.2 mL. The usual sites for ID injections are the nonhairy skin surfaces of the upper back, over the scapulae, the high upper chest, and the inner forearm. Guidelines for intradermal injections are given in Table 3.5 (section A) (page 30) and ➤ Figure 3.7.

A **subcutaneous** injection is delivered to the deepest layers of the skin. Insulin, heparin, vitamins, some vaccines, and other medications are given in this area because the sites are

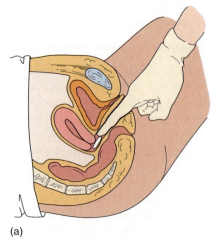

(a)

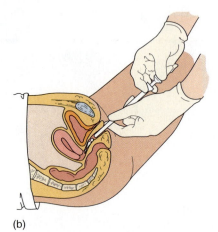

(b)

> *Figure 3.6* Vaginal drug administration: (a) instilling a vaginal suppository; (b) using an applicator to instill a vaginal cream
Source: Pearson Education/PH College.

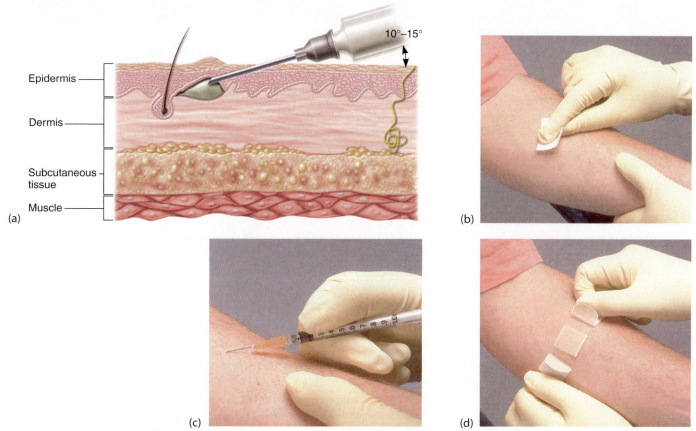

> *Figure 3.7* Intradermal drug administration: (a) cross section of skin showing depth of needle insertion; (b) the administration site is prepped; (c) the needle is inserted, bevel up at 10–15°; (d) the needle is removed and the puncture site is covered with an adhesive bandage
Source: Pearson Education/PH College.

easily accessible and provide rapid absorption. Body sites that are ideal for subcutaneous injections include the following:

- Outer aspect of the upper arms, in the area above the triceps muscle
- Middle two thirds of the anterior thigh area
- Subscapular areas of the upper back
- Upper dorsogluteal and ventrogluteal areas
- Abdominal areas, above the iliac crest and below the diaphragm, 1.5 to 2 inches out from the umbilicus

Subcutaneous doses are small in volume, usually ranging from 0.5 to 1 mL. The needle size varies with the patient's quantity of body fat. The length is usually half the size of a pinched/bunched skinfold that can be grasped between the thumb and forefinger. It is important to rotate injection sites in an orderly and documented manner to promote absorption, minimize tissue damage, and alleviate discomfort. For insulin, however, rotation should be within an anatomical area to promote reliable absorption and maintain consistent blood glucose levels. When performing subcutaneous injections, it is usually not necessary to aspirate prior to the injection. It depends upon what is being injected, and the patient's anatomy. Aspiration might prevent inadvertent ad-

ministration into a vein or artery in a thin person. If the medication should not be administered directly into a vessel, aspiration is recommended. For example, long-acting insulins should not be given IV; therefore, aspiration is justified. Heparin, on the other hand, can be safely administered IV, and so aspiration is not required. Note that tuberculin syringes and insulin syringes are not interchangeable, so the nurse should not substitute one for the other. Table 3.5 (section B) and ➤ Figure 3.8 include important information regarding subcutaneous drug administration.

INTRAMUSCULAR ADMINISTRATION

An **intramuscular (IM)** injection delivers medication into specific muscles. Because muscle tissue has a rich blood supply, medication moves quickly into blood vessels to produce a more rapid onset of action than with oral, ID, or subcutaneous administration. The anatomical structure of muscle permits this tissue to receive a larger volume of medication than the subcutaneous region. An adult with well-developed muscles can safely tolerate up to 3 mL of medication in a large muscle, although only 2 mL is recommended. The deltoid and triceps muscles should receive a maximum of 1 mL.

A major consideration for the nurse regarding IM drug administration is the selection of an appropriate injection site. Injection sites must be located away from bone, large

TABLE 3.5	Parenteral Drug Administration
Drug Form	**Administration Guidelines**
A. intradermal route	1. Prepare medication in a tuberculin or 1-mL syringe with a preattached 26- to 27-gauge, 3/8- to 5/8-inch needle.
	2. Apply gloves and cleanse injection site with antiseptic swab in a circular motion. Allow to air dry.
	3. With thumb and index finger of nondominant hand, spread skin taut.
	4. Insert needle, with bevel facing upward, at angle of 10–15°.
	5. Advance needle until entire bevel is under skin; do not aspirate.
	6. Slowly inject medication to form small wheal or bleb.
	7. Withdraw needle quickly, and pat site gently with sterile 2 × 2 gauze pad. Do not massage area.
	8. Instruct the patient not to rub or scratch the area.
	9. Draw circle around perimeter of injection site. Read in 48 to 72 hours.
B. subcutaneous route	1. Prepare medication in a 1- to 3-mL syringe using a 23- to 25-gauge, 1/2- to 5/8-inch needle. For heparin, the recommended needle is 3/8 inch and 25–26 gauge.
	2. Choose site, avoiding areas of bony prominence, major nerves, and blood vessels. For heparin, check with agency policy for the preferred injection sites.
	3. Check previous rotation sites and select a new area for injection.
	4. Apply gloves and cleanse injection site with antiseptic swab in a circular motion.
	5. Allow to air dry.
	6. Bunch the skin between thumb and index finger of nondominant hand or spread taut if there is substantial subcutaneous tissue.
	7. Insert needle at 45° or 90° angle depending on body size: 90° if obese; 45° if average weight. If the patient is very thin, gather skin at area of needle insertion and administer at 90° angle.
	8. For nonheparin injections, aspirate by pulling back on plunger. If blood appears, withdraw the needle, discard the syringe, and prepare a new injection. For heparin, do not aspirate, as this can damage surrounding tissues and cause bruising.
	9. Inject medication slowly.
	10. Remove needle quickly, and gently massage site with antiseptic swab. For heparin, do not massage the site, as this may cause bruising or bleeding.
C. intramuscular route: ventrogluteal (different administration guidelines would apply to the dorsogluteal, vastus lateralis, and deltoid muscle sites)	1. Prepare medication using a 20- to 23-gauge, 1- to 1.5-inch needle.
	2. Apply gloves and cleanse ventrogluteal injection site with antiseptic swab in a circular motion. Allow to air dry.
	3. Locate site by placing the hand with heel on the greater trochanter and thumb toward umbilicus. Point to the anterior iliac spine with the index finger, spreading the middle finger to point toward the iliac crest (forming a V). Inject medication within the V-shaped area of the index and third finger. (Note: This is how to locate the ventrogluteal site.)
	4. Insert needle with smooth, dartlike movement at a 90° angle within V-shaped area.
	5. Aspirate, and observe for blood. If blood appears, withdraw the needle, discard the syringe, and prepare a new injection.
	6. Inject medication slowly and with smooth, even pressure on the plunger.
	7. Remove needle quickly.
	8. Apply pressure to site with a dry, sterile 2 × 2 gauze and massage vigorously to create warmth and promote absorption of the medication into the muscle.

D. intravenous route	1. To add drug to an IV fluid container:
	  a. Verify order and compatibility of drug with IV fluid.
	  b. Prepare medication in a 5- to 20-mL syringe using a 1- to 1.5-inch, 19- to 21-gauge needle. (Typically in an adult, a 22-gauge needle is used for fluid administration, but the size may vary with the patient's body size and the reason for IV administration.)
	  c. Apply gloves and assess injection site for signs and symptoms of inflammation or extravasation.
	  d. Locate medication port on IV fluid container and cleanse with antiseptic swab.
	  e. Carefully insert needle or access device into port and inject medication.
	  f. Withdraw needle and mix solution by rotating container end to end.
	  g. Hang container and check infusion rate.

TABLE 3.5	**Parenteral Drug Administration** *(Continued)*
Drug Form	**Administration Guidelines**
	2. To add drug to an IV bolus (IV push) using existing IV line or IV lock (reseal):
	a. Verify order and compatibility of drug with IV fluid.
	b. Determine the correct rate of infusion.
	c. Determine if IV fluids are infusing at proper rate (IV line) and that IV site is adequate.
	d. Prepare drug in a syringe.
	e. Apply gloves and assess injection site for signs and symptoms of inflammation or extravasation.
	f. Select injection port, on tubing, closest to insertion site (IV line).
	g. Cleanse tubing or lock port with antiseptic swab and insert needle into port.
	h. If administering medication through an existing IV line, occlude tubing by pinching just above the injection port.
	i. Slowly inject medication over designated time; usually not faster than 1 mL/min, unless specified.
	j. Withdraw syringe. Release tubing and ensure proper IV infusion if using an existing IV line.
	k. If using an IV lock, check agency policy for use of saline flush before and after injecting medications.

blood vessels, and nerves. The size and length of needle are determined by body size and muscle mass, the type of drug to be administered, the amount of adipose tissue overlying the muscle, and the age of the patient. Information regarding IM injections is given in Table 3.5 and ➤ Figure 3.9. The four common sites for intramuscular injections are as follows:

1. *Ventrogluteal site:* This is the preferred site for IM injections. This area provides the greatest thickness of gluteal muscles, contains no large blood vessels or nerves, is sealed off by bone, and contains less fat than the buttock area, thus eliminating the need to determine the depth of subcutaneous fat. It is a suitable site for children and infants over 7 months of age.

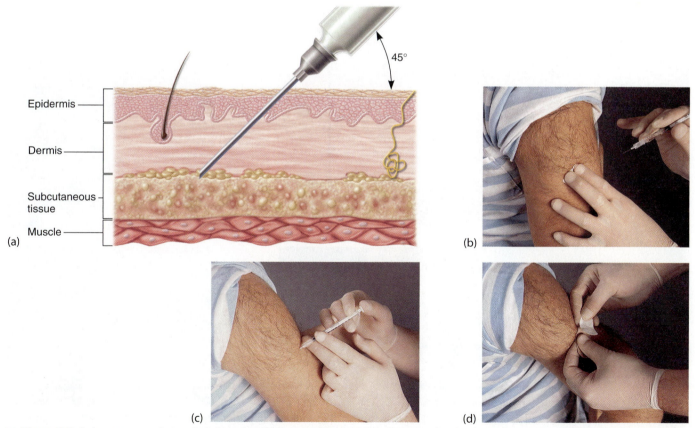

➤ *Figure 3.8* Subcutaneous drug administration: (a) cross section of skin showing depth of needle insertion; (b) the administration site is prepped; (c) the needle is inserted at a 45° angle; (d) the needle is removed and the puncture site is covered with an adhesive bandage

Source: Pearson Education/PH College.

2. *Deltoid site:* This site is used in well-developed teens and adults for volumes of medication not to exceed 1 mL. Because the radial nerve lies in close proximity, the deltoid is not generally used, except for small-volume vaccines, such as for hepatitis B in adults.

3. *Dorsogluteal site:* This site is used for adults and for children who have been walking for at least 6 months. The site is safe as long as the nurse appropriately locates the injection landmarks to avoid puncture or irritation of the sciatic nerve and blood vessels.

4. *Vastus lateralis site:* The vastus lateralis is usually thick and well developed in both adults and children. The middle third of the muscle is the site for IM injections.

INTRAVENOUS ADMINISTRATION

Intravenous (IV) medications and fluids are administered directly into the bloodstream and are immediately available for use by the body. The IV route is used when a very rapid onset of action is desired. So with other parenteral routes, IV medications bypass the enzymatic process of the digestive system and the first-pass effect of the liver. The three basic types of IV administration are as follows:

1. *Large-volume infusion:* This type of IV administration is for fluid maintenance, replacement, or supplementation. Compatible drugs may be mixed into a large-volume IV container with fluids such as normal saline or Ringer's lactate. Table 3.5 (section D) and ➤ Figure 3.10 illustrate this technique.

2. *Intermittent infusion:* This is a small amount of IV solution that is arranged tandem with or piggybacked to the primary large-volume infusion. Used to instill adjunct medications, such as antibiotics or analgesics, over a short time period. ➤ Figure 3.11 shows a Baxter infusion pump.

3. *IV bolus (push) administration:* This is a concentrated dose delivered directly to the circulation via syringe to administer single-dose medications. Bolus injections may be given through an intermittent injection port or by direct IV push. Details on the bolus administration technique are given in Table 3.5 (section D) and ➤ Figure 3.12.

Although the IV route offers the fastest onset of drug action, it is also the most dangerous. Once injected, the medication cannot be retrieved. If the drug solution or the needle is contaminated, pathogens have a direct route to the bloodstream and body tissues. Patients who are receiving IV injections must be closely monitored for adverse reactions. Some adverse reactions occur immediately after injection;

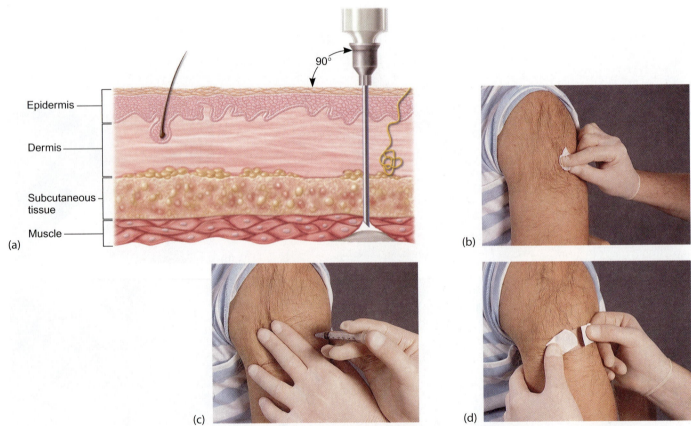

➤ **Figure 3.9** Intramuscular drug administration: (a) cross section of skin showing depth of needle insertion; (b) the administration site is prepped; (c) the needle is inserted at a 90° angle; (d) the needle is removed and the puncture site is covered with an adhesive bandage

Source: Pearson Education/PH College.

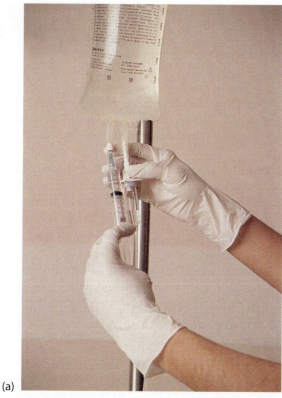

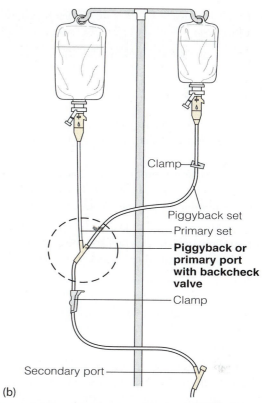

(a)   (b)

➤ **Figure 3.10** Secondary intravenous lines: (a) a tandem intravenous alignment; (b) an intravenous piggyback (IVPB) alignment

others may take hours or days to appear. Antidotes for drugs that can cause potentially dangerous or fatal reactions must always be readily available.

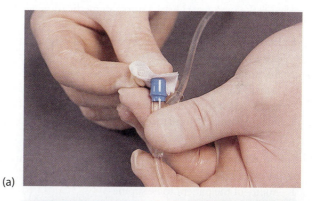

(a)

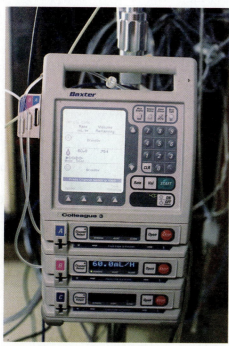

➤ **Figure 3.11** A Baxter infusion pump

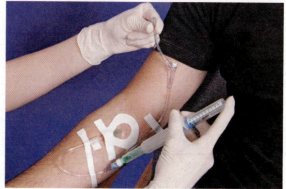

(b)

➤ **Figure 3.12** IV bolus administration. (a) The part is cleaned; (b) the drug is administered through the port using a needleless syringe

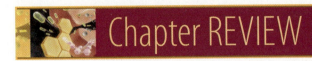

Chapter REVIEW

KEY CONCEPTS

The numbered key concepts provide a succinct summary of the important points from the corresponding numbered section within the chapter. If any of these points are not clear, refer to the numbered section within the chapter for review.

3.1   The nurse must have a comprehensive knowledge of the actions and side effects of drugs before they are administered to limit the number and severity of adverse drug events.

3.2   The five rights and three checks are guidelines for safe drug administration, which is a collaborative effort among nurses, physicians, and other health care professionals.

3.3   For pharmacologic compliance, the patient must understand and personally accept the value associated with the prescribed drug regimen. Understanding the reasons for noncompliance can help the nurse increase the success of pharmacotherapy.

3.4   There are established orders and time schedules by which medications are routinely administered. Documentation of drug administration and reporting of side effects are important responsibilities of the nurse.

3.5   Systems of measurement used in pharmacology include the metric, apothecary, and household systems. Although the metric system is most commonly used, the nurse must be able to convert dosages among the three systems of measurement.

3.6   The enteral route includes drugs given orally and those administered through nasogastric or gastrostomy tubes. This is the most common route of drug administration.

3.7   Topical drugs are applied locally to the skin or membranous linings of the eye, ear, nose, respiratory tract, urinary tract, vagina, and rectum.

3.8   Parenteral administration is the dispensing of medications via a needle, usually into the skin layers (ID), subcutaneous tissue, muscles (IM), or veins (IV).

NCLEX-RN® REVIEW QUESTIONS

1   What is the primary role of a nurse in medication administration?
1. Ensure medications are administered and delivered in a safe manner.
2. Be certain that physician orders are accurate.
3. Inform the patient that prescribed medications need be taken only if the patient agrees with the treatment plan.
4. Ensure patient compliance by watching the patient swallow all prescribed medications.

2   Before administering drugs by the enteral route, the nurse should evaluate which of the following?
1. Ability of the patient to lie supine
2. Compatibility of the drug with IV fluid
3. Ability of the patient to swallow
4. Patency of the injection port

3   Which of the following is the highest nursing priority when a patient has an allergic reaction to a newly prescribed medication?
1. Instruct the patient to remain calm.
2. Document the allergy in the medical record.
3. Notify the physician of the allergic reaction.
4. Place an allergy bracelet on the patient.

4   The order reads, "Lasix 40 mg IV STAT." Which of the following actions should the nurse take?
1. Administer the medication within 30 minutes of the order.
2. Administer the medication within 5 minutes of the order.
3. Administer the medication as required by the patient's condition.
4. Assess the patient's urinary output prior to administration and hold medication if output is less than 30 mL/h.

5   Which of the following medications would not be administered through a nasogastric tube? (Select all that apply.)
1. Liquids
2. Enteric-coated tablets
3. Sustained-release tablets
4. Finely crushed tablets
5. IV medications

6   A diabetic patient has been NPO since midnight for surgery in the morning. He usually takes an oral hypoglycemic drug to control his diabetes. What would be the best action for the nurse to take concerning the administration of his medication?
1. Hold all medications as ordered.
2. Give him the medication with a sip of water.
3. Give him half the original dose.
4. Contact the physician for further orders.

CRITICAL THINKING QUESTIONS

1. Why do errors continue to occur despite the fact that the nurse follows the five rights and three checks of drug administration?

2. What strategies can the nurse employ to ensure drug compliance for a patient who is refusing to take his or her medication?

3. Compare the oral, topical, IM, subcutaneous, and IV routes. Which has the fastest onset of drug action? Which routes avoid the hepatic first-pass effect? Which require strict aseptic technique?

4. What are the advantages of the metric system of measurement over the household or apothecary systems?

See Appendix D for answers and rationales for all activities.

PEARSON
EXPLORE   mynursingkit™

MyNursingKit is your one stop for online chapter review materials and resources. Prepare for success with additional NCLEX®-style practice questions, interactive assignments and activities, web links, animations and videos, and more!

Register your access code from the front of your book at
www.mynursingkit.com.

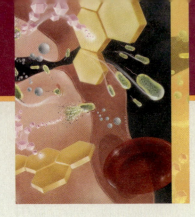

Chapter 4

Pharmacokinetics

LEARNING OUTCOMES

After reading this chapter, the student should be able to:

1. Explain the applications of pharmacokinetics to clinical practice.
2. Identify the four components of pharmacokinetics.
3. Explain how substances travel across plasma membranes.
4. Discuss factors affecting drug absorption.
5. Explain the metabolism of drugs and its applications to pharmacotherapy.
6. Discuss how drugs are distributed throughout the body.
7. Describe how plasma proteins affect drug distribution.
8. Identify major processes by which drugs are excreted.
9. Explain how enterohepatic recirculation might affect drug activity.
10. Explain the applications of a drug's plasma half-life ($t_{1/2}$) to pharmacotherapy.
11. Explain how a drug reaches and maintains its therapeutic range in the plasma.
12. Differentiate between loading and maintenance doses.

KEY TERMS

Medications are given to achieve a desirable effect. To produce this effect, the drug must reach its target cells. For some medications, such as topical agents used to treat superficial skin conditions, this is a relatively simple task. For others, however, the process of reaching target cells in sufficient quantities to produce a physiologic change may be challenging. Drugs are exposed to a myriad of different barriers and destructive processes after they enter the body. The purpose of this chapter is to examine factors that act on the drug as it travels to reach its target cells.

4.1 Pharmacokinetics: How the Body Handles Medications

The term **pharmacokinetics** is derived from the root words *pharmaco,* which means "medicine" and *kinetics,* which means "movement or motion." Pharmacokinetics is thus the study of drug movement throughout the body. In practical terms, it describes how the body deals with the medications. Pharmacokinetics is a core subject in pharmacology, and a firm grasp of this topic allows nurses to better understand and predict the actions and side effects of medications in their patients.

Drugs face numerous obstacles in reaching their target cells. For most medications, the greatest barrier is crossing the many membranes that separate the drug from its target cells. A drug taken by mouth, for example, must cross the plasma membranes of the mucosal cells of the gastrointestinal tract and the capillary endothelial cells to enter the bloodstream. To leave the bloodstream, the drug must again cross capillary cells, travel through the interstitial fluid, and depending on the mechanism of action, the drug may also need to enter target cells and cellular organelles such as the nucleus, which are surrounded by additional membranes. These are examples of just some of the barriers that a drug must successfully penetrate before it can produce a response.

While moving toward target cells and passing through the various membranes, drugs are subjected to numerous physiologic processes. For medications given by the enteral route, stomach acid and digestive enzymes often act to break down the drug molecules. Enzymes in the liver and other organs may chemically change the drug molecule to make it less active. If the drug is seen as foreign by the body, phagocytes may attempt to remove it, or an immune response may be triggered. The kidneys, large intestine, and other organs attempt to excrete the medication from the body.

These examples illustrate pharmacokinetic processes: *how the body handles medications.* The many processes of pharmacokinetics are grouped into four categories: absorption, distribution, metabolism, and excretion, as illustrated in ➤ Figure 4.1.

4.2 The Passage of Drugs Through Plasma Membranes

Pharmacokinetic variables depend on the ability of a drug to cross plasma membranes. With few exceptions, drugs must penetrate these membranes to produce their effects. Like other chemicals, drugs primarily use two processes to cross body membranes:

1. *Active transport:* This is movement of a chemical against a concentration or electrochemical gradient; *cotransport* involves the movement of two or more chemicals across the membrane.

2. *Diffusion or passive transport:* This is movement of a chemical from an area of higher concentration to an area of lower concentration.

Plasma membranes consist of a lipid bilayer, with proteins and other molecules interspersed in the membrane. This lipophilic membrane is relatively impermeable to large molecules, ions, and polar molecules. These physical characteristics have direct application to pharmacokinetics. For example, drug molecules that are small, nonionized, and lipid soluble will usually pass through plasma membranes by simple diffusion and more easily reach their target cells. Small water-soluble agents such as urea, alcohol, and water can enter through pores in the plasma membrane. Large molecules, ionized drugs, and water-soluble agents, however, will have more difficulty crossing plasma membranes. These agents may use other means to gain entry, such as protein carriers or active transport. Drugs may not need to enter the cell to produce their effects. Once bound to receptors, located on the plasma membrane, some drugs activate a second messenger within the cell, which produces the physiologic change (chapter 5 ∞).

4.3 Absorption of Medications

Absorption is a process involving the movement of a substance from its site of administration, across body membranes, to circulating fluids. Drugs may be absorbed across the skin and associated mucous membranes, or they may move across membranes that line the GI or respiratory tract. Most drugs, with the exception of a few topical medications, intestinal anti-infectives, and some radiologic contrast agents, must be absorbed to produce an effect.

Absorption is the primary pharmacokinetic factor determining the length of time it takes a drug to produce its effect. In general, the more rapid the absorption, the faster the onset of drug action. Drugs that are used in critical care are designed to be absorbed within seconds or minutes. At the other extreme are drugs such as the contraceptive Mirena (levonorgestrel–releasing intrauterine system), which is a polyethylene tube placed in the uterus. The drug is absorbed slowly and can provide contraceptive protection for up to 5 years.

Absorption is conditional on many factors. Drugs in elixir or syrup formulations are absorbed faster than tablets or

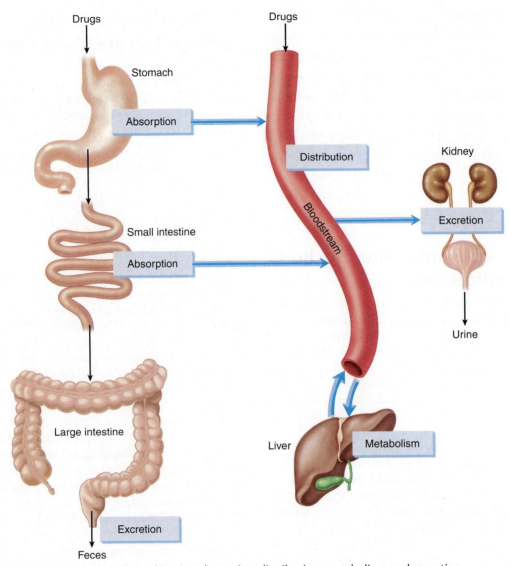

➤ *Figure 4.1* The four processes of pharmacokinetics: absorption, distribution, metabolism, and excretion

capsules. Drugs administered in high doses are generally absorbed more quickly and have a more rapid onset of action than those given in low concentrations. The speed of digestive motility, exposure to enzymes in the digestive tract, and blood flow to the site of drug administration also affect absorption. Due to the fact that drugs administered IV directly enter the bloodstream, absorption to the tissues after the infusion is very rapid. IM medications take longer to absorb.

The degree of ionization of a drug also affects its absorption. A drug's ability to become ionized depends on the surrounding pH. Aspirin provides an excellent example of the effects of ionization on absorption, as depicted in ➤ Figure 4.2. In the acid environment of the stomach, aspirin is in its *nonionized* form and thus readily absorbed and distributed by the bloodstream. As aspirin enters the alkaline environment of the small intestine, however, it becomes *ionized*. In its ionized form, aspirin is not as likely to be absorbed and distributed to target cells. Unlike acidic drugs, medications that are weakly basic are in their nonionized form in an alkaline environment; therefore, basic

drugs are absorbed and distributed better in alkaline environments such as in the small intestine. The pH of the local environment directly influences drug absorption through its ability to ionize the drug. In simplest terms, it may help the nurse to remember that acids are absorbed in acids, and bases are absorbed in bases.

Drug–drug or food–drug interactions may influence absorption. Many examples of these interactions have been discovered. For example, administering tetracyclines with food or drugs containing calcium, iron, or magnesium can significantly delay absorption of the antibiotic. High-fat meals can slow stomach motility significantly and delay the absorption of oral medications taken with the meal. Dietary supplements may also affect absorption. Common ingredients in herbal weight-loss products such as aloe leaf, guar gum, senna, and yellow dock exert a laxative effect that may decrease intestinal transit time and reduce drug absorption (Scott & Elmer, 2002). The nurse must be aware of drug interactions and advise patients to avoid known combinations of foods and medications that significantly affect drug action.

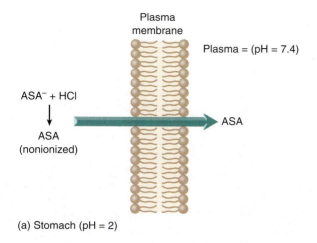

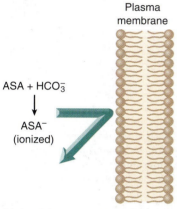

> **Figure 4.2** Effect of pH on drug absorption: (a) a weak acid such as aspirin (ASA) is in a nonionized form in an acidic environment and absorption occurs; (b) in a basic environment, aspirin is mostly in an ionized form and absorption is prevented

4.4 Distribution of Medications

Distribution involves the transport of pharmacologic agents throughout the body. The simplest factor determining distribution is the amount of blood flow to body tissues. The heart, liver, kidneys, and brain receive the most blood supply. Skin, bone, and adipose tissue receive a lower blood supply; therefore, it is more difficult to deliver high concentrations of drugs to these areas.

The physical properties of the drug greatly influence how it moves throughout the body after administration. Lipid solubility is an important characteristic, because it determines how quickly a drug is absorbed, mixes within the bloodstream, crosses membranes, and becomes localized in body tissues. Lipid-soluble agents are not limited by the barriers that normally stop water-soluble drugs; thus, they are more completely distributed to body tissues.

Some tissues have the ability to accumulate and store drugs after absorption. The bone marrow, teeth, eyes, and adipose tissue have an especially high **affinity,** or attraction, for certain medications. Examples of agents that are attracted to adipose tissue are thiopental (Pentothal), diazepam (Valium), and lipid-soluble vitamins. Tetracycline binds to cal-

cium salts and accumulates in the bones and teeth. Once stored in tissues, drugs may remain in the body for many months and are released very slowly back to the circulation.

Not all drug molecules in the plasma will reach their target cells, because many drugs bind reversibly to plasma proteins, particularly albumin, to form **drug–protein complexes.** Drug–protein complexes are too large to cross capillary membranes; thus, the drug is not available for distribution to body tissues. Drugs bound to proteins circulate in the plasma until they are released or displaced from the drug–protein complex. Only unbound (free) drugs can reach their target cells or be excreted by the kidneys. This concept is illustrated in ➤ Figure 4.3. Some drugs, such as the anticoagulant warfarin (Coumadin) are highly bound; 99% of the drug in the plasma is bound in drug–protein complexes and is unavailable to reach target cells.

Drugs and other chemicals compete with one another for plasma protein–binding sites, and some agents have a greater affinity for these binding sites than other agents. Drug–drug and drug–food interactions may occur when one drug displaces another from plasma proteins. The displaced medication can immediately reach high levels in the bloodstream and produce adverse effects. Drugs such as aspirin or valproates for example, displace Coumadin from the drug–protein complex, thus raising blood levels of free Coumadin and dramatically enhancing the risk of hemorrhage. Most drug guides give the percentage of medication bound to plasma proteins; when giving multiple drugs that are highly bound, the nurse should monitor the patient closely for adverse effects.

The brain and placenta possess special anatomic barriers that prevent many chemicals and medications from entering. These barriers are referred to as the **blood–brain barrier** and **fetal–placental barrier.** Some medications such as sedatives, antianxiety agents, and anticonvulsants readily cross the

MyNursingKit | Cytochrome Animation

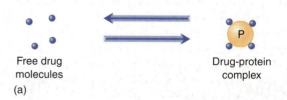

(a)

Free drug molecules

Drug-protein complex

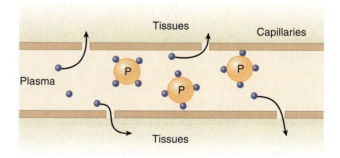

(b)

> **Figure 4.3** Plasma protein binding and drug availability: (a) drug exists in a free state or bound to plasma protein; (b) drug–protein complexes are too large to cross membranes

blood–brain barrier to produce actions in the central nervous system. In contrast, most antitumor medications do not easily cross this barrier, making brain cancers difficult to treat.

The fetal–placental barrier serves an important protective function, because it prevents potentially harmful substances from passing from the mother's bloodstream to the fetus. Substances such as alcohol, cocaine, caffeine, and certain prescription medications, however, easily cross the placental barrier and can potentially harm the fetus. Consequently, no prescription medication, OTC drug, or herbal therapy should be taken by a patient who is pregnant without first consulting with a health care provider. The health care provider should always question female patients in the childbearing years regarding their pregnancy status before prescribing a drug. Chapter 7 ∞ presents a list of drug pregnancy categories for assessing fetal risk.

4.5 Metabolism of Medications

Metabolism, also called *biotransformation*, is the process of chemically converting a drug to a form that is usually more easily removed from the body. Metabolism involves complex biochemical pathways and reactions that alter drugs, nutrients, vitamins, and minerals. The liver is the primary site of drug metabolism, although the kidneys and cells of the intestinal tract also have high metabolic rates.

Medications undergo many types of biochemical reactions as they pass through the liver, including hydrolysis, oxidation, and reduction. During metabolism, the addition of side chains, known as **conjugates**, makes drugs more water soluble and more easily excreted by the kidneys.

Most metabolism in the liver is accomplished by the **hepatic microsomal enzyme system**. This enzyme complex is sometimes called the P-450 system, named after cytochrome P-450, which is a key component of the system. As they relate to pharmacotherapy, the primary actions of the hepatic microsomal enzymes are to inactivate drugs and accelerate their excretion. In some cases, however, metabolism can produce a chemical alteration that makes the resulting molecule *more* active than the original. For example, the narcotic analgesic codeine undergoes biotransformation to morphine, which has significantly greater ability to relieve pain. In fact, some agents, known as **prodrugs**, have no pharmacologic activity unless they are first metabolized to their active form by the body. Examples of prodrugs include benazepril (Lotensin) and losartan (Cozaar).

Changes in the function of the hepatic microsomal enzymes can significantly affect drug metabolism. A few drugs have the ability to increase metabolic activity in the liver, a process called **enzyme induction**. For example, phenobarbital causes the liver to synthesize more microsomal enzymes. By doing so, phenobarbital increases the rate of its own metabolism, as well as that of other drugs metabolized in the liver. In these patients, higher doses of medication may be required to achieve the optimum therapeutic effect.

Certain patients have decreased hepatic metabolic activity, which may alter drug action. Hepatic enzyme activity is

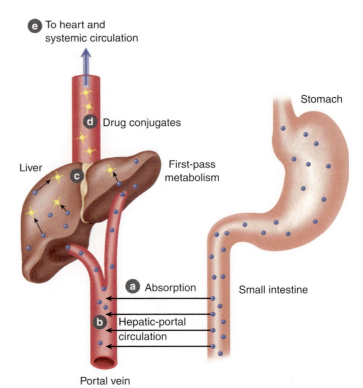

> *Figure 4.4* First-pass effect: (a) drugs are absorbed; (b) drugs enter hepatic portal circulation and go directly to liver; (c) hepatic microsomal enzymes metabolize drugs to inactive forms; (d) drug conjugates, leaving liver; (e) drug is distributed to general circulation

generally reduced in infants and elderly patients; therefore, pediatric and geriatric patients are more sensitive to drug therapy than middle-age patients. Patients with severe liver damage, such as that caused by cirrhosis, will require reductions in drug dosage because of the decreased metabolic activity. Certain genetic disorders have been recognized in which patients lack specific metabolic enzymes; drug dosages in these patients must be adjusted accordingly. The nurse should pay careful attention to laboratory values that may indicate liver disease so that doses may be adjusted.

Metabolism has a number of additional therapeutic consequences. As illustrated in ➤ Figure 4.4, drugs absorbed after oral administration cross directly into the hepatic portal circulation, which carries blood to the liver before it is distributed to other body tissues. Thus, as blood passes through the liver circulation, some drugs can be completely metabolized to an inactive form before they ever reach the general circulation. This **first-pass effect** is an important mechanism, since a large number of oral drugs are rendered inactive by hepatic metabolic reactions. Alternative routes of delivery that bypass the first-pass effect (e.g., sublingual, rectal, or parenteral routes) may need consideration for these drugs.

4.6 Excretion of Medications

Drugs are removed from the body by the process of **excretion**. The rate at which medications are excreted determines their concentration in the bloodstream and tissues. This is important because the concentration of drugs in the bloodstream determines their duration of action. Pathologic states, such as liver disease or renal failure, often increase the duration of drug action in the body because they interfere with natural excretion mechanisms. Dosing regimens must be carefully adjusted in these patients.

Although drugs are removed from the body by numerous organs and tissues, the primary site of excretion is the kidney. In an average-size person, approximately 180 L of blood is filtered by the kidneys each day. Free drugs, water-soluble agents, electrolytes, and small molecules are easily filtered at the glomerulus. Proteins, blood cells, conjugates, and drug–protein complexes are not filtered because of their large size.

After filtration at the renal corpuscle, chemicals and drugs are subjected to the process of reabsorption in the renal tubule. Mechanisms of reabsorption are the same as absorption elsewhere in the body. Nonionized and lipid-soluble drugs cross renal tubular membranes easily and return to the circulation; ionized and water-soluble drugs generally remain in the filtrate for excretion.

Drug–protein complexes and substances too large to be filtered at the glomerulus are sometimes secreted into the distal tubule of the nephron. For example, only 10% of a dose of penicillin G is filtered at the glomerulus; 90% is secreted into the renal tubule. As with metabolic enzyme activity, secretion mechanisms are less active in infants and older adults.

Certain drugs may be excreted more quickly if the pH of the filtrate changes. Weak acids such as aspirin are excreted faster when the filtrate is slightly alkaline, because aspirin is ionized in an alkaline environment, and the drug will remain in the filtrate and be excreted in the urine. Weakly basic drugs such as diazepam (Valium) are excreted faster with a slightly acidic filtrate, because they are ionized in this environment. This relationship between pH and drug excretion can be used to advantage in critical care situations. To speed the renal excretion of acidic drugs such as aspirin in an overdosed patient, an order may be written to administer sodium bicarbonate. Sodium bicarbonate will make the urine more basic, which ionizes more aspirin, causing it to be excreted more readily. The excretion of diazepam, on the other hand, can be enhanced by giving ammonium chloride. This will acidify the filtrate and increase the excretion of diazepam.

Impairment of kidney function can dramatically affect pharmacokinetics. Patients with renal failure will have diminished ability to excrete medications and may retain drugs for an extended time. Doses for these patients must be reduced, to avoid drug toxicity. Because small to moderate changes in renal status can cause rapid increases in serum drug levels, the nurse must constantly monitor kidney function in patients receiving drugs that may be nephrotoxic (low margin of safety). The pharmacotherapy of renal failure is presented in chapter 30∞.

Drugs that can easily be changed into a gaseous form are especially suited for excretion by the respiratory system. The rate of respiratory excretion is dependent on factors that affect gas exchange, including diffusion, gas solubility, and pulmonary blood flow. The elimination of volatile anesthetics following surgery is primarily dependent on respiratory activity. The faster the breathing rate, the greater the excretion. Conversely, the respiratory removal of water-soluble agents such as alcohol is more dependent on blood flow to the lungs. The greater the blood flow into lung capillaries, the greater the excretion. In contrast with other methods of excretion, the lungs excrete most drugs in their original unmetabolized form.

Glandular activity is another elimination mechanism. Water-soluble drugs may be secreted into the saliva, sweat, or breast milk. The odd taste that patients sometimes experience when given IV drugs is an example of the secretion of agents into the saliva. Another example of glandular excretion is the garlic smell that can be detected when standing next to a perspiring person who has recently eaten garlic. Excretion into breast milk is of considerable importance for basic drugs such as morphine or codeine, as these can achieve high concentrations and potentially affect the nursing infant. Nursing mothers should always check with their health care provider before taking any prescription medication, OTC drug, or herbal supplement. Pharmacology of the pregnant or breast-feeding patient is discussed in chapter 7∞.

Some drugs are secreted in the bile, a process known as *biliary excretion.* In many cases, drugs secreted into bile will enter the duodenum and eventually leave the body in the feces. However, most bile is circulated back to the liver by **enterohepatic recirculation,** as illustrated in ➤ Figure 4.5. A percentage of the drug may be recirculated numerous times with the bile. Biliary reabsorption is extremely influential in prolonging the activity of cardiac glycosides, some antibiotics, and phenothiazines. Recirculated drugs are ultimately metabolized by the liver and excreted by the kidneys. Recirculation and elimination of drugs through biliary excretion may continue for several weeks after therapy has been discontinued.

4.7 Drug Plasma Concentration and Therapeutic Response

The therapeutic response of most drugs is directly related to their level in the plasma. Although the concentration of the medication at its *target tissue* is more predictive of drug

---

LIFESPAN CONSIDERATIONS

Adverse Drug Effects and Older Adults

Adverse drug effects are more commonly recorded in older adults than in young adults or middle-age patients, because the older adult population takes more drugs simultaneously (an average of seven) than other age groups and because of normal declines in hepatic and renal function. Chronic diseases that affect pharmacokinetics are also present more often in older adults. In addition, older adults may not reliably report adverse drug effects or may consider them signs of aging or of their disease condition. One study (Lampela et al., 2007) found that when comparing adverse effects reported by patients age 75 or older with adverse effects noted by a health care provider, adverse effects were reported by only 11.4% of the patients compared to effects observed by the health care provider in 24% of the patients. The study authors recommend that health care providers inquire about possible drug-related problems even though older adults may not complain of or self-report such problems.

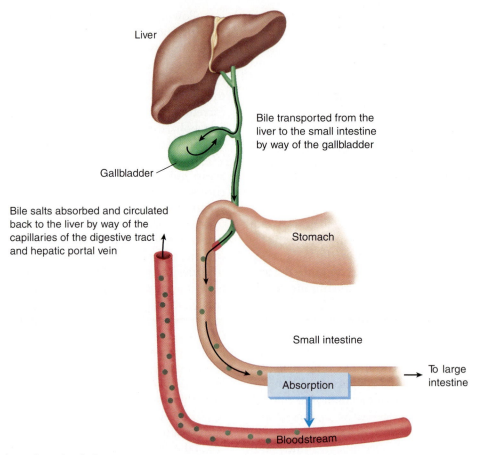

Liver

Bile transported from the liver to the small intestine by way of the gallbladder

Gallbladder

Bile salts absorbed and circulated back to the liver by way of the capillaries of the digestive tract and hepatic portal vein

Stomach

Small intestine

Absorption

To large intestine

Bloodstream

> *Figure 4.5* Enterohepatic recirculation

action, this quantity is impossible to measure in most cases. For example, it is possible to conduct a laboratory test that measures the serum level of the drug lithium carbonate (Eskalith) by taking a blood sample; it is a far different matter to measure the quantity of this drug in neurons within the CNS. Indeed, it is common practice for nurses to monitor the plasma levels of certain drugs that have a low safety profile.

Several important pharmacokinetic principles can be illustrated by measuring the serum level of a drug following a single-dose administration. These pharmacokinetic values are shown graphically in ➤ Figure 4.6. This figure demonstrates two plasma drug levels. First is the **minimum effective concentration**, the amount of drug required to produce a therapeutic effect. Second is the **toxic concentration**, the level of drug that will result in serious adverse effects. The plasma drug concentration *between* the minimum effective concentration and the toxic concentration is called the **therapeutic range** of the drug. These values have great clinical significance. For example, if the patient has a severe headache and is given half of an aspirin tablet, the plasma level will remain below the minimum effective concentration, and the patient will not experience pain relief. Two or three tablets will increase the plasma level of aspirin into the therapeutic range, and the pain will subside. Taking six or more tablets may result in adverse effects, such as GI bleeding or tinnitus. For each drug administered, the nurse's goal is to keep its plasma concentration in the therapeutic range. For some drugs, the therapeutic range is quite wide; for other medications, the difference between a minimum effective dose and a toxic dose may be dangerously narrow.

4.8 Plasma Half-Life and Duration of Drug Action

The most common description of a drug's duration of action is its **plasma half-life ($t_{1/2}$)**, defined as the length of time required for the plasma concentration of a medication to decrease by one-half after administration. Some drugs have a half-life of only a few minutes, whereas others have a half-life of several hours or days. The greater the half-life, the longer it takes a medication to be excreted. For example, a drug with a $t_{1/2}$ of 10 hours would take longer to be excreted and thus produce a longer effect in the body than a drug with a $t_{1/2}$ of 5 hours.

The plasma half-life of a drug is an essential pharmacokinetic variable with important clinical applications. Drugs with relatively short half-lives, such as aspirin ($t_{1/2}$ = 15 to 20 minutes) must be given every 3 to 4 hours. Drugs with longer half-lives, such as felodipine (Plendil) ($t_{1/2}$ = 10 hours), need be given only once a day. If a patient has extensive renal or hepatic disease, the plasma half-life of a drug will increase, and the drug concentration may reach toxic levels. In these patients, medications must be given less frequently, or the dosages must be reduced.

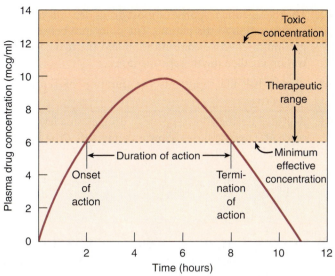

➤ **Figure 4.6** Single-dose drug administration: pharmacokinetic values for this drug are as follows: onset of action = 2 hours; duration of action = 6 hours; termination of action = 8 hours after administration; peak plasma concentration = 10 mcg/mL; time to peak drug effect = 5 hours; $t^{1/2}$ = 4 hours

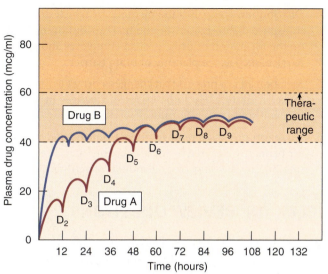

➤ **Figure 4.7** Multiple-dose drug administration: drug A and drug B are administered every 12 hours; drug B reaches the therapeutic range faster, because the first dose is a loading dose

4.9 Loading Doses and Maintenance Doses

Few drugs are administered as a single dose. Repeated doses result in an accumulation of drug in the bloodstream, as shown in ➤ Figure 4.7. Eventually, a plateau will be reached where the level of drug in the plasma is maintained continuously within the therapeutic range. At this level, the amount administered has reached equilibrium with the amount of drug being eliminated, resulting in the distribution of a continuous therapeutic level of drug to body tissues. Theoretically, it takes approximately four half-lives to reach this equilibrium. If the medication is given as a continuous infusion, the plateau can be reached quickly and be maintained with little or no fluctuation in drug plasma levels.

The plateau may be reached faster by administration of loading doses followed by regular maintenance doses. A **loading dose** is a higher amount of drug, often given only once or twice to "prime" the bloodstream with a sufficient level of drug. Before plasma levels can drop back toward zero, intermittent **maintenance doses** are given to keep the plasma drug concentration in the therapeutic range. Although blood levels of the drug fluctuate with this approach, the equilibrium state can be reached almost as rapidly as with a continuous infusion. Loading doses are particularly important for drugs with prolonged half-lives and for situations in which it is critical to raise drug plasma levels quickly, as might be the case when administering an antibiotic for a severe infection. In Figure 4.7, notice that it takes almost five doses (48 hours) before a therapeutic level is reached using a routine dosing schedule. With a loading dose, a therapeutic level is reached within 12 hours.

Chapter REVIEW

KEY CONCEPTS

The numbered key concepts provide a succinct summary of the important points from the corresponding numbered section within the chapter. If any of these points are not clear, refer to the numbered section within the chapter for review.

4.1   Pharmacokinetics focuses on the movement of drugs throughout the body after they are administered.

4.2   The physiologic properties of plasma membranes determine movement of drugs throughout the body. The four components of pharmacokinetics are absorption, metabolism, distribution, and excretion.

4.3   Absorption is the process by which a drug moves from the site of administration to the bloodstream. Absorption depends on the size of the drug molecule, its lipid solubility, its degree of ionization, and interactions with food or other medications.

4.4 Distribution comprises the methods by which drugs are transported throughout the body. Distribution depends on the formation of drug–protein complexes and special barriers such as the placenta or brain barriers.

4.5 Metabolism is a process that changes a drug's activity and makes it more likely to be excreted. Changes in hepatic metabolism can significantly affect drug action.

4.6 Excretion processes remove drugs from the body. Drugs are primarily excreted by the kidneys but may be excreted into bile, by the lung, or by glandular secretions.

4.7 The therapeutic response of most drugs depends on their concentration in the plasma. The difference between the minimum effective concentration and the toxic concentration is called the therapeutic range.

4.8 Plasma half-life represents the duration of action for most drugs.

4.9 Repeated dosing allows a plateau drug plasma level to be reached. Loading doses allow a therapeutic drug level to be reached rapidly.

NCLEX-RN® REVIEW QUESTIONS

1 A patient has an order for a tetracycline antibiotic and has been instructed to avoid taking the medication with foods, beverages, or drugs that contain calcium, iron, or magnesium. What stage of the pharmacokinetic processes is behind the rationale for this instruction?
1. Absorption
2. Distribution
3. Metabolism
4. Excretion

2 The patient has a malignant brain tumor. What property of pharmacokinetics may cause difficulty in treating her tumor?
1. Blood–brain barrier
2. Drug–protein complexes
3. Affinity for neoplasms
4. Lack of active transport

3 A patient with cirrhosis of the liver exhibits decreased metabolic activity. This will require what possible change in her drug regimen?
1. A reduction in the dosage of drugs
2. A change in the timing of medication administration
3. An increased dose of prescribed drugs
4. All prescribed drugs must be given by intramuscular injection.

4 Some drugs may be completely metabolized by the liver circulation before ever reaching the general circulation. This effect is known as what?
1. Conjugation of drugs
2. Hepatic microsomal enzyme system
3. Blood–brain barrier
4. First-pass effect

5 A patient who is in renal failure may have a diminished capacity to excrete medications. It is imperative that this patient be assessed for what development?
1. Increased creatinine levels
2. Increased levels of blood urea nitrogen
3. Drug toxicity
4. Increased levels of potassium

6 The nurse understands that with glandular activity, water-soluble drugs may be secreted into (select all that apply):
1. saliva.
2. sweat.
3. breast milk.
4. bile.
5. feces.

CRITICAL THINKING QUESTIONS

1. Describe the types of obstacles drugs face from the time they are administered until they reach their target cells.

2. Why is the drug's plasma half-life important to the nurse?

3. How does the ionization of a drug affect its distribution in the body?

4. Explain why drugs metabolized through the first-pass effect might need to be administered by the parenteral route.

See Appendix D for answers and rationales for all activities.

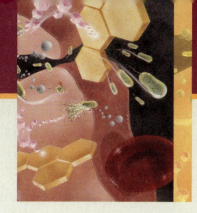

Chapter 5

Pharmacodynamics

LEARNING OUTCOMES

After reading this chapter, the student should be able to:

1. Apply principles of pharmacodynamics to clinical practice.

2. Discuss how frequency response curves may be used to explain how patients respond differently to medications.

3. Explain the importance of the median effective dose (ED_{50}) to clinical practice.

4. Compare and contrast median lethal dose (LD_{50}) and median toxicity dose (TD_{50}).

5. Discuss how a drug's therapeutic index is related to its margin of safety.

6. Identify the significance of the graded dose–response relationship to clinical practice.

7. Compare and contrast the terms *potency* and *efficacy*.

8. Distinguish between an agonist, a partial agonist, and an antagonist.

9. Explain the relationship between receptors and drug action.

10. Explain possible future developments in the field of pharmacogenetics.

KEY TERMS

In clinical practice, nurses quickly learn that medications do not affect all patients in the same way: A dose that produces a dramatic response in one patient may have no effect on another. In some cases, the differences among patients are predictable, based on the pharmacokinetic principles discussed in chapter 4 ⬤. In other cases, the differences in response are not easily explained. Despite this patient variability, health care providers must choose optimal doses while avoiding unnecessary adverse effects. This is not an easy task given the wide variation of patient responses within a population. This chapter examines the mechanisms by which drugs affect patients, and how the nurse can apply these principles to clinical practice.

5.1 Pharmacodynamics and Interpatient Variability

The term **pharmacodynamics** comes from the root words *pharmaco*, which means "medicine," and *dynamics*, which means "change." In simplest terms, pharmacodynamics refers to how a medicine *changes* the body. A more complete definition explains pharmacodynamics as the branch of pharmacology concerned with the mechanisms of drug action and the relationships between drug concentration and responses in the body.

Pharmacodynamics has important clinical applications. Health care providers must be able to predict whether a drug will produce a significant change in patients. Although clinicians often begin therapy with average doses taken from a drug guide, intuitive experience often becomes the practical method for determining which doses of medications will be effective in a given patient. Knowledge of therapeutic indexes, dose–response relationships, and drug–receptor interactions will help the nurse provide safe and effective treatment.

Interpatient variability in responses to drugs can best be understood by examining a frequency distribution curve. A **frequency distribution curve**, shown in ▶ Figure 5.1, is a graphical representation of the number of patients responding to a drug action at different doses. Notice the wide range in doses that produced the patient responses shown on the curve. A few patients responded to the drug at very low doses. As the dose was increased, more and more patients responded. Some patients required very high doses to elicit the desired response. The peak of the curve indicates the largest number of patients responding to the drug. The curve does not show the *magnitude* of response, only whether a measurable response occurred among the patients. As an example, think of the given response to an antihypertensive drug as being a reduction of 20 mmHg in systolic blood pressure. A few patients experienced the desired 20-mm reduction at a dose of only 10 mg of drug. A 50-mg dose gave the largest number of patients a 20-mm reduction in blood pressure; however, a few patients needed as much as 90 mg of drug to produce the same 20-mm reduction.

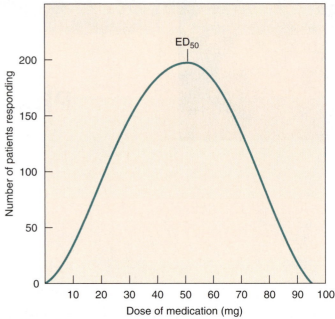

▶ **Figure 5.1** Frequency distribution curve: interpatient variability in drug response

The dose in the middle of the frequency distribution curve represents the drug's **median effective dose (ED$_{50}$)**. The ED$_{50}$ is the dose required to produce a specific therapeutic response in 50% of a group of patients. Drug guides sometimes report the ED$_{50}$ as the average or standard dose.

The interpatient variability shown in Figure 5.1 has important clinical implications. First, the nurse should realize that the standard or average dose predicts a satisfactory therapeutic response for only *half* the population. In other words, many patients will require more or less than the average dose for optimum pharmacotherapy. Using the systolic blood pressure example, assume that a large group of patients is given the average dose of 50 mg. Some of these patients will experience toxicity at this level because they needed only 10 mg to achieve blood pressure reduction. Other patients in this group will probably have no reduction in blood pressure. By observing the patient, taking vital signs, and monitoring associated laboratory data, the nurse uses skills that are critical in determining whether the average dose is effective for the patient. It is not enough to simply memorize an average dose for a drug; the nurse must know when and how to adjust this dose to obtain the optimum therapeutic response.

5.2 Therapeutic Index and Drug Safety

Administering a dose that produces an optimum therapeutic response for each individual patient is only one component of effective pharmacotherapy. The nurse must also be able to predict whether the dose is safe for the patient.

Frequency distribution curves can also be used to represent the safety of a drug. For example, the **median lethal dose (LD$_{50}$)** is often determined in preclinical trials, as part of the drug development process discussed in chapter 1 ⬤. The

LD_{50} is the dose of drug that will be lethal in 50% of a group of animals. As with ED_{50}, a group of animals will exhibit considerable variability in lethal dose; what may be a non-toxic dose for one animal may be lethal for another.

To examine the safety of a particular drug, the LD_{50} can be compared with the ED_{50}, as shown in ➤ Figure 5.2a. In this example, 10 mg of drug X is the average *effective* dose, and 40 mg is the average *lethal* dose. The ED_{50} and LD_{50} are used to calculate an important value in pharmacology, a drug's **therapeutic index,** the ratio of a drug's LD_{50} to its ED_{50}.

$$\text{Therapeutic index} = \frac{\text{median lethal dose } LD_{50}}{\text{median effective dose } ED_{50}}$$

The larger the difference between the two doses, the greater the therapeutic index. In Figure 5.2a, the therapeutic index is 4 (40 mg ÷ 10 mg). Essentially, this means that it would take an error in magnitude of *approximately* 4 times the average dose to be lethal to a patient. Thus, the therapeutic index is a measure of a drug's safety margin: The higher the value, the safer the medication.

As another example, the therapeutic index of a second drug is shown in ➤ Figure 5.2b. Drug Z has the same ED_{50} as drug X but shows a different LD_{50}. The therapeutic index for drug Z is only 2 (20 mg ÷ 10 mg). The difference between an effective dose and a lethal dose is very small for drug Z; thus, the drug has a narrow safety margin. The therapeutic index offers the nurse practical information on the safety of a drug, and a means to compare one drug with another.

Because the LD_{50} cannot be experimentally determined in humans, the **median toxicity dose (TD_{50})** is a more practical value in a clinical setting. The TD_{50} is the dose that will produce a given toxicity in 50% of a group of patients. The TD_{50} value may be extrapolated from animal data or based on adverse effects recorded in patient clinical trials.

5.3 The Graded Dose–Response Relationship and Therapeutic Response

In the previous examples, frequency distribution curves were used to graphically visualize patient differences in responses to medications in a *population*. It is also useful to visualize the variability in responses observed within a *single patient*.

The **graded dose–response** relationship is a fundamental concept in pharmacology. The graphical representation of this relationship is called a dose–response curve, as illustrated in ➤ Figure 5.3. By observing and measuring the patient's response obtained at different doses of the drug, one can explain several important clinical relationships.

The three distinct phases of a dose–response curve indicate essential pharmacodynamic principles that have relevance to clinical practice. Phase 1 occurs at the lowest doses. The flatness of this portion of the curve indicates that few target cells have yet been affected by the drug. Phase 2 is the straight-line portion of the curve. This portion often shows a linear

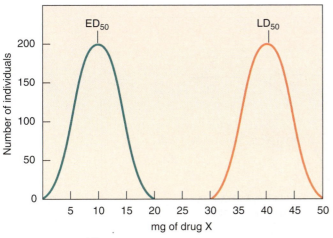

(a) Drug X : TI = $\dfrac{LD_{50}}{ED_{50}}$ = $\dfrac{40}{10}$ = 4

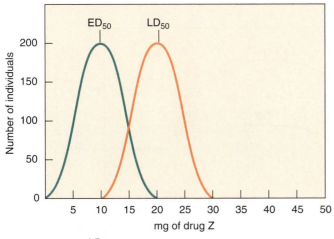

(b) Drug Z : TI = $\dfrac{LD_{50}}{ED_{50}}$ = $\dfrac{20}{10}$ = 2

➤ *Figure 5.2* Therapeutic index: (a) drug X has a therapeutic index of 4; (b) drug Z has a therapeutic index of 2

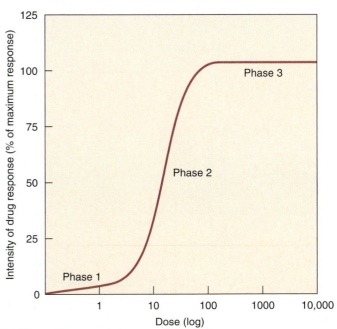

➤ *Figure 5.3* Dose–response relationship

relationship between the amount of drug administered and the degree of response obtained from the patient. For example, if the dose is doubled, twice as much response is obtained. This is the most desirable range of doses for pharmacotherapeutics, since giving more drug results in proportionately more effect; a lower drug dose gives less effect. In phase 3, a plateau is reached in which increasing the drug dose produces no additional therapeutic response. This may occur for a number of reasons. One explanation is that all the receptors for the drug are occupied. Practically it means that the drug has brought 100% relief, such as when a migraine headache has been terminated; giving higher doses produces no additional relief. In phase 3, although increasing the dose does not result in more therapeutic effect, the nurse should be mindful that increasing the dose may produce adverse effects.

5.4 Potency and Efficacy

Within a pharmacologic class, not all drugs are equally effective at treating a disorder. For example, some antineoplastic drugs kill more cancer cells than others; some

antihypertensive agents lower blood pressure to a greater degree than others; and some analgesics are more effective at relieving severe pain than others in the same class. Furthermore, drugs in the same class are effective at different doses; one antibiotic may be effective at a dose of 1 mg/kg, whereas another is most effective at 100 mg/kg. Nurses need a method to compare one drug with another so that they can administer treatment effectively.

There are two fundamental ways to compare medications within therapeutic and pharmacologic classes. First is the concept of **potency.** A drug that is more potent will produce a therapeutic effect at a lower dose, compared with another drug in the same class. Consider two agents, drug X and drug Y, that both produce a 20-mm drop in blood pressure. If drug X produces this effect at a dose of 10 mg, and drug X at 60 mg, then drug X is said to be more potent. Thus, potency is a way to compare the doses of two independently administered drugs in terms of how much is needed to produce a particular response. A useful way to visualize the concept of potency is by examining dose–response curves. Compare the two drugs shown in ➤ Figure 5.4a. In this ex-

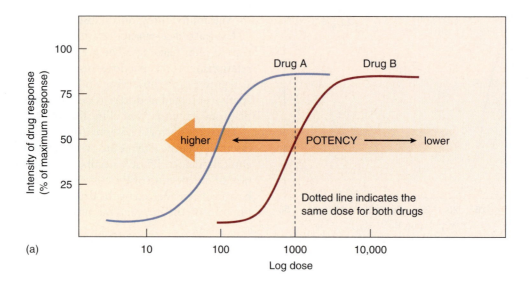

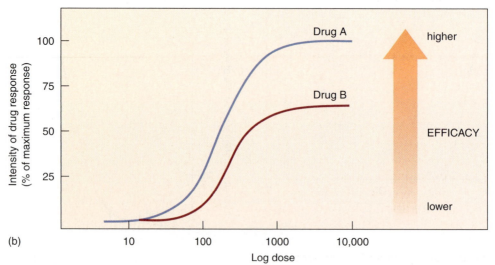

➤ **Figure 5.4** Potency and efficacy: (a) drug A has a higher potency than drug B; (b) drug A has a higher efficacy than drug B

ample, drug A is more potent because it requires a lower dose to produce the same response.

The second method used to compare drugs is called **efficacy,** which is the magnitude of maximal response that can be produced from a particular drug. In the example in ➤ Figure 5.4b, drug A is more efficacious because it produces a higher maximal response.

Which is more important to the success of pharmacotherapy, potency or efficacy? Perhaps the best way to understand these concepts is to use the specific example of headache pain. Two common OTC analgesics are ibuprofen (200 mg) and aspirin (650 mg). The fact that ibuprofen relieves pain at a lower dose indicates that this agent is *more potent* than aspirin. At recommended doses, however, both are equally effective at relieving headache pain; thus, they have the *same efficacy*. If the patient is experiencing severe pain, however, neither aspirin nor ibuprofen has sufficient efficacy to bring relief. Narcotic analgesics such as morphine have a greater efficacy than aspirin or ibuprofen and can effectively treat this type of pain. From a pharmacotherapeutic perspective, efficacy is almost always more important than potency. In the previous example, the average dose is unimportant to the patient, but headache relief is essential. As another comparison, the patient with cancer is much more concerned about how many cancer cells have been killed (efficacy) than what dose the nurse administered (potency). Although the nurse will often hear claims that one drug is more potent than another, a more compelling concern is whether the drug is more efficacious.

5.5 Cellular Receptors and Drug Action

Drugs act by modulating or changing existing physiologic and biochemical processes. To exert such changes requires that drugs interact with specific molecules and chemicals normally found in the body. A cellular macromolecule to which a medication binds in order to initiate its effects is called a **receptor.** The concept that a drug binds to a receptor to cause a change in body chemistry or physiology is a fundamental theory in pharmacology. *Receptor theory* explains the mechanisms by which most drugs produce their effects. It is important to understand, however, that these receptors do not exist in the body solely to bind drugs. Their normal function is to bind endogenous molecules such as hormones, neurotransmitters, and growth factors.

Although a drug receptor can be any type of macromolecule, the vast majority are proteins. As shown in ➤ Figure 5.5, a receptor is depicted as a three-dimensional protein associated with the cellular plasma membrane. The extracellular structural component of the receptor usually consists of several protein subunits arranged around a central canal or channel. Other receptors consist of many membrane-spanning segments inserted into the plasma membrane.

A drug attaches to its receptor in a specific manner, much like a lock and key. Small changes to the structure of a drug, or its receptor, may weaken or even eliminate binding between the two molecules. Once bound, drugs may trigger a series of **second messenger** events within the cell, such as the conversion of adenosine triphosphate (ATP) to cyclic

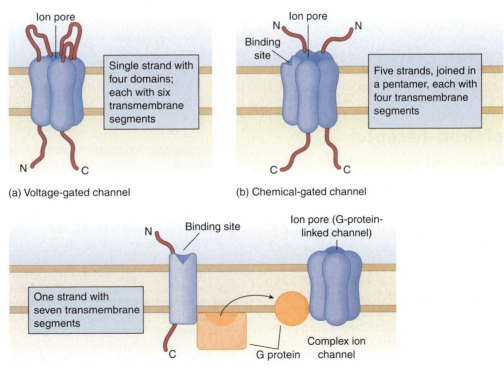

(a) Voltage-gated channel

Ion pore

Single strand with four domains; each with six transmembrane segments

(b) Chemical-gated channel

Ion pore

Binding site

Five strands, joined in a pentamer, each with four transmembrane segments

(c) G-protein-linked channel

One strand with seven transmembrane segments

Binding site

Ion pore (G-protein-linked channel)

G protein

Complex ion channel

➤ *Figure 5.5* Cellular receptors

adenosine monophosphate (cyclic AMP), the release of intracellular calcium, or the activation of specific G proteins and associated enzymes. These biochemical cascades initiate the drug's action by either stimulating or inhibiting normal activity of the cell.

Not all receptors are bound to plasma membranes; some are intracellular molecules such as DNA or enzymes in the cytoplasm. By interacting with these types of receptors, medications are able to inhibit protein synthesis or regulate cellular events such as replication and metabolism. Examples of agents that bind intracellular components include steroid medications, vitamins, and hormones.

Receptors and their associated drug mechanisms are extremely important in therapeutics. Receptor *subtypes* are being discovered and new medications are being developed at a faster rate than at any other time in history. These subtypes permit the "fine-tuning" of pharmacology. For example, the first medications affecting the autonomic nervous system affected all autonomic receptors. It was discovered that two basic receptor types existed in the body, *alpha* and *beta,* and drugs were then developed that affected only one type. The result was more specific drug action, with fewer adverse effects. Still later, several subtypes of alpha and beta receptors, including alpha$_1$, alpha$_2$, *beta*$_1$, and *beta*$_2$, were discovered that allowed even more specificity in pharmacotherapy. In recent years, researchers have further divided and refined these subtypes. It is likely that receptor research will continue to result in the development of new medications that activate very specific receptors and thus direct drug action that avoids unnecessary adverse effects.

Some drugs act independently of cellular receptors. These agents are associated with other mechanisms, such as changing the permeability of cellular membranes, depressing membrane excitability, or altering the activity of cellular pumps. Actions such as these are described as **nonspecific cellular responses.** Ethyl alcohol, general anesthetics, and osmotic diuretics are examples of agents that act by nonspecific mechanisms.

5.6 Types of Drug–Receptor Interactions

When a drug binds to a receptor, several therapeutic consequences can result. In simplest terms, a specific activity of the cell is either enhanced or inhibited. The actual biochemical mechanism underlying the therapeutic effect, however, may be extremely complex. In some cases, the mechanism of action is not known.

When a drug binds to its receptor, it may produce a response that *mimics* the effect of the endogenous regulatory molecule. For example, when the drug bethanechol (Urecholine) is administered, it binds to acetylcholine receptors in the autonomic nervous system and produces the same actions as acetylcholine. A drug that produces the same type of response as the endogenous substance is called an **agonist.** Agonists sometimes produce a greater maximal response

than the endogenous chemical. The term **partial agonist** describes a medication that produces a weaker, or less efficacious, response than an agonist.

A second possibility is that a drug will occupy a receptor and *prevent* the endogenous chemical from acting. This drug is called an **antagonist.** Antagonists often compete with agonists for the receptor binding sites. For example, the drug atropine competes with acetylcholine for specific receptors associated with the autonomic nervous system. If the dose is high enough, atropine will inhibit the effects of acetylcholine, because acetylcholine cannot bind to its receptors.

Not all antagonism is associated with receptors. *Functional* antagonists inhibit the effects of an agonist not by competing for a receptor but by changing pharmacokinetic factors. For example, antagonists may slow the absorption of a drug. By speeding up metabolism or excretion, an antagonist can enhance the removal of a drug from the body. The relationships that occur between agonists and antagonists explain many of the drug–drug and drug–food interactions that occur in the body.

5.7 Pharmacology of the Future: Customizing Drug Therapy

Until recently, it was thought that single drugs should provide safe and effective treatment to every patient in the same way. Unfortunately, a significant portion of the population either develops unacceptable side effects to certain drugs or is unresponsive to them. Many scientists and clinicians are now discarding the one-size-fits-all approach to drug therapy, which was designed to treat an entire population without addressing important interpatient variation.

With the advent of the Human Genome Project and other advances in medicine, pharmacologists are hopeful that future drugs can be customized for patients with specific genetic similarities. In the past, unpredictable and unexplained drug reactions were labeled **idiosyncratic responses.** It is hoped that performing a DNA test before administering a drug may someday address idiosyncratic differences.

TREATING THE DIVERSE PATIENT

Enzyme Deficiency in Certain Ethnic Populations

Pharmacogenetics has identified a number of people who are deficient in the enzyme glucose-6-phosphate dehydrogenase (G6PD). This enzyme is essential in carbohydrate metabolism. Males of Mediterranean and African descent are more likely to express this deficiency. It is estimated to affect 400 million people worldwide. The disorder is caused by mutations in the DNA structure that encode for G6PD, resulting in one or more amino acid changes in the protein molecule. Following administration of certain drugs, such as primaquine, sulfonamides, or nitrofurantoin, an acute hemolysis of red blood cells occurs due to the breaking of chemical bonds in the hemoglobin molecule. Up to 50% of the circulating RBCs may be destroyed. Genetic typing does not always predict toxicity; thus, the nurse must observe patients carefully following the administration of these medications. Fortunately, there are good alternative choices for these medications.

Pharmacogenetics is the area of pharmacology that examines the role of heredity in drug response. The greatest advances in pharmacogenetics have been the identification of subtle genetic differences in drug-metabolizing enzymes. Genetic differences in these enzymes are responsible for a significant portion of drug-induced toxicity. It is hoped that the use of pharmacogenetic information may someday allow for customized drug therapy. Although therapies based on a patient's genetically based response may not be cost effective at this time, pharmacogenetics may radically change the way pharmacotherapy will be practiced in the future.

 Chapter REVIEW

KEY CONCEPTS

The numbered key concepts provide a succinct summary of the important points from the corresponding numbered section within the chapter. If any of these points are not clear, refer to the numbered section within the chapter for review.

5.1 Pharmacodynamics is the area of pharmacology concerned with how drugs produce *change* in patients, and the differences in patient responses to medications.

5.2 The therapeutic index, expressed mathematically as $TD_{50} \div ED_{50}$, is a value representing the margin of safety of a drug. The higher the therapeutic index, the safer the drug.

5.3 The graded dose–response relationship describes how the therapeutic response to a drug changes as the medication dose is increased.

5.4 Potency, the dose of medication required to produce a particular response, and efficacy, the magnitude of maximal response to a drug, are means of comparing medications.

5.5 Drug–receptor theory is used to explain the mechanism of action of many medications.

5.6 Agonists, partial agonists, and antagonists are substances that compete with drugs for receptor binding and can cause drug–drug and drug–food interactions.

5.7 In the future, pharmacotherapy will likely be customized to match the genetic makeup of each patient.

NCLEX-RN® REVIEW QUESTIONS

1 What is the term for unpredictable and unexplained drug reactions?
1. Adverse reactions
2. Idiosyncratic reactions
3. Enzyme-specific reactions
4. Unaltered reactions

2 A drug that occupies a receptor site and prevents endogenous chemicals from acting is called a/an:
1. antagonist.
2. partial agonist.
3. agonist.
4. protagonist.

3 In considering the pharmacotherapeutic perspective, which property is considered to be of most importance?
1. Potency
2. Efficacy
3. Toxicity
4. Interaction with other drugs

4 The term used to describe the magnitude of maximal response that can be produced from a particular drug is:
1. efficacious.
2. toxic.
3. potent.
4. comparable.

5 Morphine has a greater efficacy than either of the OTC drugs, aspirin or acetaminophen. Based on what the nurse knows about efficacy, what patient condition might require a dose of morphine rather than either aspirin or acetaminophen?
1. A patient who is in mild pain but does not like to take aspirin or acetaminophen
2. A patient who routinely uses acetaminophen at home for pain relief
3. A patient who quickly develops allergies to multiple medications
4. A patient in moderate to severe pain after the other drugs have been ineffective for pain relief

6 A nurse reads that the drug to be given to the patient has a "narrow therapeutic index." This means that the drug:
1. has a narrow range of effectiveness and may not give this patient the desired therapeutic results.
2. has a narrow safety margin and even a small increase in dose may produce adverse or toxic effects.
3. has a narrow range of conditions or diseases that the drug will be expected to treat successfully.
4. has a narrow segment of the population for whom the drug will work as desired.

CRITICAL THINKING QUESTIONS

1. If the ED_{50} is the dose required to produce an effective response in 50% of a group of patients, what happens in the "other" 50% of the patients after a dose has been administered?

2. Two drugs are competing for a receptor on a mast cell that will cause the release of histamine when activated. Compare the effects of an agonist versus an antagonist on this receptor. Which would likely be called an antihistamine, the agonist or the antagonist?

See Appendix D for answers and rationales for all activities.

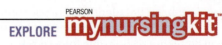

EXPLORE

MyNursingKit is your one stop for online chapter review materials and resources. Prepare for success with additional NCLEX®-style practice questions, interactive assignments and activities, web links, animations and videos, and more!

Register your access code from the front of your book at
www.mynursingkit.com.

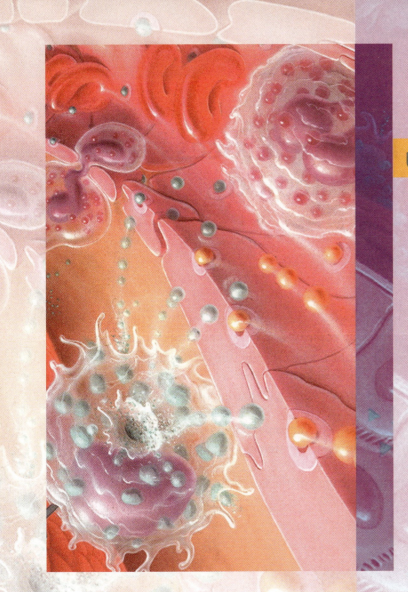

Pharmacology and the Nurse–Patient Relationship

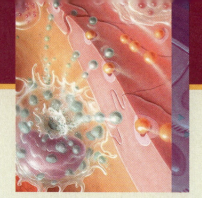

Chapter 6

The Nursing Process
in Pharmacology

LEARNING OUTCOMES

After reading this chapter, the student should be able to:

1. Compare and contrast the different steps of the nursing process.
2. Identify assessment data that is pertinent to medication administration.
3. Develop appropriate nursing diagnoses for patients receiving medications.
4. Plan realistic goals and outcomes for patients receiving medications.
5. Discuss key intervention strategies to be implemented for patients receiving medications.
6. Evaluate the outcomes of medication administration.

KEY TERMS

The **nursing process** is a systematic method of problem solving that forms the foundation of nursing practice. The use of the nursing process is particularly important for patients receiving medications. By using the steps of the nursing process, nurses can ensure that the interdisciplinary practice of pharmacology results in safe, effective, and individualized medication administration and outcomes for patients under their care. These steps are illustrated in ➤ Figure 6.1.

Most nursing students enter a pharmacology course after taking a course on the fundamentals of nursing, during which the steps of the nursing process are discussed in detail. This chapter focuses on how the steps of the nursing process can be applied to pharmacotherapy. Students who are unfamiliar with the nursing process are encouraged to consult one of the many excellent fundamentals of nursing textbooks for a more detailed explanation.

6.1 Assessment of the Patient

The **assessment phase** of the nursing process is the systematic collection, organization, validation, and documentation of patient data. Assessment is an ongoing process that begins with the nurse's initial contact with the patient and continues with every interaction thereafter.

A health history and physical assessment are completed during the initial meeting between a nurse and patient.

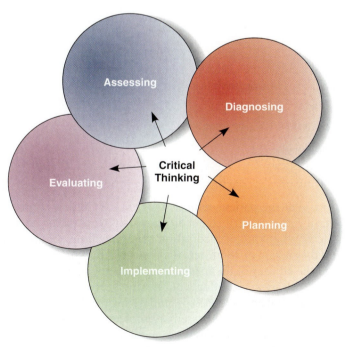

➤ *Figure 6.1* The five overlapping phases of the nursing process. Each phase depends on the accuracy of the other phases.

Baseline data are gathered on the patient that will be compared to information obtained from later interactions, during and following treatment. Assessment consists of gathering **subjective data,** which include what the patient says or perceives, and **objective data** gathered through physical assessment, laboratory tests, and other diagnostic sources.

The initial health history is tailored to the patient's clinical condition. A complete history is the most detailed, but the nurse must consider the appropriateness of this history given the patient's condition. Often the nurse takes a problem-focused or "chief complaint" history that focuses on the symptoms that led the patient to seek care. In any history, the nurse must assess key components that could potentially affect the outcomes of drug administration. Essential questions to ask in the initial history relate to history of drug allergy; past medical history; medications currently used; personal and social history including the use of alcohol, tobacco, or caffeine; health risks such as the use of street drugs or illicit substances; and reproductive health questions such as the pregnancy status of women of childbearing age. Assessment should always include the use of over-the-counter (OTC) drugs, dietary supplements, and herbal products because these agents have the potential to affect drug therapy. Table 6.1 provides pertinent questions that the nurse may ask during an initial health history that provide baseline data before medications are administered. Nurses must remember that what is *not* being said may be as important as what *is* being said. For instance, a patient may deny symptoms of pain while grimacing or guarding a certain area from being touched. Nurses must use their observation skills during the history to gather such critical data.

Along with the health history, a physical assessment is completed to gather objective data on the patient's condition. The nurse may obtain vital signs, height and weight, a head-to-toe physical assessment, and laboratory specimens. These provide the baseline data to compare with future assessments and guide the health care provider in deciding which medications to prescribe. Because many medications can affect the heart rate and blood pressure, the nurse should carefully document chronic conditions of the cardiovascular system. Baseline electrolyte values are important parameters to obtain, because many medications affect electrolyte balance. Renal and hepatic function tests are essential for many patients, particularly older adults and those who are critically ill, because kidney and liver disease often requires adjustment in drug dosages (chapter 6∞).

Once pharmacotherapy is initiated, ongoing assessments are conducted to determine the effectiveness of the medications. Assessment should first focus on determining whether the patient is experiencing the expected therapeutic benefits from the medications. For example, if a drug is given for symptoms of pain, has the pain subsided? If an antibiotic is given for an infection, have the signs of that infection improved over time? If a patient is not experiencing the therapeutic effects of the medication, then the nurse must conduct further assessment to determine possible reasons. Dosages are reviewed, and serum drug levels may be obtained.

TABLE 6.1	Health History Assessment Questions Pertinent to Drug Administration
Health History Component Areas	**Pertinent Questions**
Chief complaint	■ How do you feel? (Describe) ■ Are you having any pain? (Describe) ■ Are you experiencing other symptoms? (Especially pertinent to medications are nausea, vomiting, headache, itching, dizziness, shortness of breath, nervousness or anxiousness, palpitations or heart "fluttering," and weakness or fatigue.)
Allergies	■ Are you allergic to any medications? ■ Are you allergic to any foods, environmental substances (e.g., pollen or "seasonal" allergies), tape, soaps, or cleansers? ■ What specifically happens when you experience an allergy?
Past medical history	■ Do you have a history of diabetes, heart or vascular conditions, respiratory conditions, or neurologic conditions? ■ Do you have any dermatologic conditions? ■ How were these treated in the past? Currently?
Family history	■ Has anyone in your family experienced difficulties with any medications? (Describe) ■ Does anyone in your family have any significant medical problems?
Drug history	■ What prescription medications are you currently taking? (List drug name, dosage, and frequency of administration.) ■ What nonprescription/OTC medications are you taking? (List name, dosage, and frequency.) ■ What drugs, prescription or OTC, have you taken within the past month or two? ■ Have you ever experienced any side effects or unusual symptoms with any medications? (Describe) ■ What do you know, or what were you taught, about these medications? ■ Do you use any herbal or homeopathic remedies? Any nutritional substances or vitamins?
Health management	■ Identify all the health care providers you have seen for health issues. ■ When was the last time you saw a health care provider? For what reason did you see this provider? ■ What is your normal diet? ■ Do you have any trouble sleeping?
Reproductive history	■ Is there any possibility you are pregnant? (Ask *every* woman of childbearing age.) ■ Are you breast-feeding?
Personal–social history	■ Do you smoke? ■ What is your normal alcohol intake? ■ What is your normal caffeine intake? ■ Do you have any religious or cultural beliefs or practices concerning medications or your health that we should know about? ■ What is your occupation? What hours do you work? ■ Do you have any concerns regarding insurance or the ability to afford medications?
Health risk history	■ Do you have any history of depression or other mental illness? ■ Do you use any street drugs or illicit substances?

Assessment during pharmacotherapy should also identify any adverse effects experienced by the patient. Assessment should include the patient's perceptions of the adverse effects, as well as follow-up vital signs and laboratory reports. Here again, baseline data are compared with the current assessment to determine what changes have occurred since the initiation of pharmacotherapy. The Nursing Process Focus flowcharts provided in chapters 13 through 49∞ illustrate key assessment data that the nurse should gather that are associated with specific medications or classes of drugs.

Finally, it is important to assess the ability of the patient to assume responsibility for self-administration of medica-

tion. Will the patient require assistance obtaining or purchasing the prescribed medications, or with taking them safely? What kind of medication storage facilities exists and are they adequate to protect the patient, others in the home, and the efficacy of the medication? Does the patient understand the uses and effects of this medication and how it should be taken? Do assessment data suggest that the use of this medication might present a problem, such as difficulty swallowing large capsules or an inability to administer parenteral medications at home, when necessary?

After analyzing the assessment data, the nurse determines patient-specific nursing diagnoses appropriate for the drugs prescribed. These diagnoses will form the basis for the remaining steps of the Nursing Process.

MEDICATION ERRORS AND DIETARY SUPPLEMENTS

Herbal and vitamin supplements can have powerful effects on the body that can influence the success of prescription drug therapy. In some cases, over-the-counter supplements can enhance the effects of prescription drugs, whereas in other instances supplements may cancel the therapeutic effects of a medication. For example, many patients with heart disease take garlic supplements in addition to warfarin (Coumadin) to prevent clots from forming. Because garlic and warfarin are both anticoagulants, taking them together could result in abnormal bleeding. As another example, high doses of calcium supplements can cancel the beneficial antihypertensive effects of drugs such as nifedipine (Procardia), a calcium channel blocker.

Few controlled studies have examined how concurrent use of natural supplements affects the therapeutic effects of prescription drugs. Patients should be encouraged to report use of all over-the-counter dietary supplements to the health care provider.

6.2 Nursing Diagnoses

Nursing diagnoses are clinical judgments of a patient's actual or potential health problem that is within the nurse's scope of practice to address. Nursing diagnoses provide the basis for establishing goals and outcomes, planning interventions, and evaluating the effectiveness of the care given. Unlike medical diagnoses that focus on a disease or condition, nursing diagnoses focus on a patient's response to actual or potential health and life processes. The North American Nursing Diagnosis Association (NANDA) defines nursing diagnoses as:

A clinical judgment about individual, family, or community responses to actual or potential health/life processes. Per NANDA, nursing diagnoses provide the basis for selection of nursing interventions to achieve outcomes for which the nurse is accountable.

Nursing diagnoses are often the most challenging part of the nursing process. Sometimes the nurse identifies what is believed to be the patient's problem, only to discover from further assessment that the planned goals, outcomes, and interventions have not "solved" the problem. A key point to remember is that nursing diagnoses focus on the *patient's* needs, not the nurse's needs. A primary nursing role is to enable patients to become active participants in their own care. By including the patient in identifying needs, the nurse encourages the patient to take a more active role in working toward meeting the identified goals.

When applied to pharmacotherapy, the diagnosis phase of the nursing process addresses three main areas of concern.

- Promoting therapeutic drug effects
- Minimizing adverse drug effects and toxicity

- Maximizing the ability of the patient for self-care, including the knowledge, skills, and resources necessary for safe and effective drug administration

Nursing diagnoses that focus on drug administration may address actual problems, such as the treatment of pain; focus on potential problems such as a risk for deficient fluid volume; or concentrate on maintaining the patient's current level of wellness. The diagnosis is written as a one-, two-, or three-part statement depending on whether the nurse has identified a wellness, risk, or actual problem. Actual and risk problems include the diagnostic statement and a related factor, or inferred cause. Actual diagnoses also contain a third part, the evidence gathered to support the chosen statement. There are many diagnoses appropriate to medication administration. Some are nursing specific that the nurse can manage independently, whereas other problems are multidisciplinary and require collaboration with other members of the health care team.

Two of the most common nursing diagnoses for medication administration are *Deficient Knowledge* and *Noncompliance.* Knowledge deficit may occur when the patient was given a new prescription and has no previous experience with the medication. This diagnosis may also be applicable when a patient has not received adequate education about the drugs being prescribed. When obtaining a medication history, the nurse should assess the patient's knowledge regarding the drugs currently being taken and evaluate whether the drug education was adequate. Noncompliance, also called nonadherence, assumes that the patient was properly educated about the medication but has made the decision not to take it. It is vital that the nurse assess possible factors leading to the noncompliance *before* establishing this diagnosis. Does the patient understand why the medication was prescribed? Was dosing and scheduling information explained? Are adverse effects causing the patient to refuse the medication? Are cultural, religious, or social issues impacting the decision not to take the medication? Is the noncompliance related to inadequate financial resources?

Table 6.2 provides an abbreviated list of some of the common nursing diagnoses appropriate to drug administration. Although the list contains actual nursing diagnoses, these may also be identified as risk diagnoses. This is not an exhaustive list of all NANDA-approved diagnoses, and the establishment of new diagnoses is ongoing. The nurse is encouraged to consult books on nursing diagnoses for more information on establishing, writing, and researching other nursing diagnoses that may apply to drug administration.

6.3 Planning: Establishing Goals and Outcomes

The **planning phase** of the nursing process prioritizes diagnoses, formulates desired outcomes, and selects nursing interventions that can assist the patient to return to establish an optimum level of wellness. Short- or long-term **goals** are established that focus on what the patient will be able to do or achieve, not what the nurse will do. The objective

TABLE 6.2	Common Nursing Diagnoses Applicable to Drug Administration
NANDA-Approved Nursing Diagnoses	
Activity Intolerance	Risk for Injury
Ineffective Airway Clearance	Deficient Knowledge
Anxiety	Risk for Impaired Liver Function
Risk for Aspiration	Impaired Physical Mobility
Ineffective Breathing Pattern	Nausea
Decreased Cardiac Output	Noncompliance
Readiness for Enhanced Comfort	Imbalanced Nutrition
Impaired Verbal Communication	Impaired Oral Mucous Membrane
Constipation	Pain
Risk for Contamination	Risk for Poisoning
Ineffective Coping	Self-Care Deficit
Diarrhea	Disturbed Sensory Perception
Moral Distress	Sexual Dysfunction
Risk for Falls	Impaired Skin Integrity
Fatigue	Disturbed Sleep Pattern
Deficient Fluid Volume	Stress Overload
Excess Fluid Volume	Risk for Suicide
Impaired Gas Exchange	Impaired Swallowing
Ineffective Health Maintenance	Ineffective Therapeutic Regimen Management
Risk for Compromised Human Dignity	
Hyperthermia	Impaired Thermoregulation
Hypothermia	Disturbed Thought Processes
Incontinence	Ineffective Tissue Perfusion
Risk for Infection	Urinary Retention

Source: Adapted from North American Nursing Diagnosis Association, 2007–2008.

measures of those goals, or **outcomes**, specifically define what the patient will do, under what circumstances, and within a specified time frame. The nurse also discusses goals and outcomes with the patient or caregiver, and these are prioritized to address immediate needs first. Planning links the strategies, or interventions, to the established goals and outcomes.

Before administering medications, nurses should establish clear, realistic goals and outcomes so that planned interventions ensure safe and effective use of these agents. The nurse establishes priorities based on the assessment data and nursing diagnoses, with high-priority needs addressed before low-priority needs.

With respect to pharmacotherapy, the planning phase involves two main components: drug administration and patient teaching. The overall goal of the nursing plan of care is the safe and effective administration of medication. The nurse may focus goals related to pharmacotherapy for the short term or long term, depending on the setting and situation. For a patient with a thrombus in the lower extremity who was placed on anticoagulant therapy, a short-term goal may be that the patient will not experience an increase in clot size, as evidenced by improving circulation to the lower extremity distal to the clot. A long-term goal might focus on teaching the patient to effectively administer parenteral anticoagulant therapy at home.

Like assessment data, pharmacotherapeutic goals should focus first on the therapeutic outcomes of medications, then on the prevention or treatment of adverse effects. For the patient on pain medication, relief of pain is a priority established before treatment of the nausea, vomiting, or dizziness caused by the medication. The nurse should remember, however, that planning for the prevention or treatment of expected adverse effects is an integral step of the planning phase.

Outcomes are the specific criteria used to measure attainment of the selected goals. They are written to include the subject (usually the patient), the actions required by that subject, under what circumstances, the expected performance, and the specific time frame in which the subject will accomplish that performance. In the example of the patient who will be taught to self-administer anticoagulant therapy at home, an outcome may be written as: "Patient will demonstrate the injection of enoxaparin (Lovenox) using the preloaded syringe provided, given subcutaneously into the anterior abdominal areas, in 2 days (1 day prior to discharge)." This outcome includes the subject (patient), actions (demonstrate injection), circumstances (using a preloaded syringe), performance (SC injection into the abdomen), and time frame (2 days from now—1 day before discharge home). Writing specific outcomes also gives the nurse a concrete time frame to work toward assisting the patient to meet the goals. In the case of children or the mentally impaired, the pharmacotherapeutic outcomes include the caregiver responsible for administering the medication in the home setting.

After goals and outcomes are identified based on the nursing diagnoses, a plan of care is written. Each agency determines whether this plan will be communicated as either nursing centered, interdisciplinary, or both. All plans should be patient focused and include the patient or caregiver in their development. The goals and outcomes identified in the plan of care will assist the nurse, and other health care providers, in implementing interventions and evaluating the effectiveness of that care.

6.4 Implementing Specific Nursing Actions

The **implementation phase** is when the nurse applies the knowledge, skills, and principles of nursing care to help move the patient toward the desired goal and optimal wellness. Implementation involves *action* on the part of the nurse or patient: administering a drug, providing patient teaching, and initiating other specific actions identified by the plan of care. When applied to pharmacotherapy, the implementation phase involves administering the medication, continuing to assess the patient and monitoring drug effects, and carrying out the interventions developed in the planning phase to maximize the therapeutic response and prevent adverse events.

Non–English-Speaking and Culturally Diverse Patients

Nurses should know, in advance, what translation services and interpreters are available in their health care facility to assist with communication. The nurse should use interpreter's services when available, validating with the interpreter that he or she is able to understand the patient. Many dialects are similar but not the same, and knowing another language is not the same as understanding the culture. Can the interpreter understand the patient's language and cultural expressions or nuances well enough for effective communication to occur? If a family member is interpreting, especially if a child is interpreting for a parent or relative, be sure that the interpreter first understands and repeats the information back to the nurse before explaining it in the patient's own language. This is especially important if the translation is a summary of what was said rather than a line-by-line translation. Before an interpreter is available, or if one is unavailable, use pictures, simple drawings, nonverbal cues, and body language to communicate with the patient. Be aware of culturally based nonverbal communication behaviors (e.g., use of personal space, eye contact, or lack of eye contact). Gender sensitivities related to culture (e.g., male nurse or physician for female patients) and the use of touch are often sensitive issues. In the United States, an informal and personal style is often the norm. When working with patients of other cultures, adopting a more formal style may be more appropriate.

Monitoring drug effects is a primary intervention that nurses perform. A thorough knowledge of the actions of each medication is necessary to carry out this monitoring process. The nurse should first monitor for the identified therapeutic effect. A lack of sufficient therapeutic effect suggests the need to reassess pharmacotherapy. Monitoring may require a reassessment of the patient's physical condition, vital signs, body weight, lab values, and/or serum drug levels. The patient's statements about pain relief, as well as objective data, such as a change in blood pressure, are used to monitor the therapeutic outcomes of pharmacotherapy. The nurse also monitors for side and adverse effects and attempts to prevent or limit these effects when possible.

The intervention phase includes appropriate documentation of the administration of the medication, as well as any adverse effects observed or reported by the patient. The nurse may include additional objective assessment data, such as vital signs, in the documentation to provide more details about the specific drug effects. Statements from the patient can provide subjective detail to the documentation. Each health care facility determines where, when, and how to document the administration of medications and any follow-up assessment data that the nurse has gathered.

Patient teaching is a vital component of the nurse's interventions for a patient receiving medications. Knowledge deficit, and even noncompliance, is directly related to the type and quality of medication education that a patient receives. State nurse practice acts and regulating bodies such as the Joint Commission on Accreditation of Healthcare Organizations (JCAHO) consider teaching to be a primary role for nurses, giving it the weight of law and key importance in accreditation standards. Because the goals of pharmacotherapy are the safe administration of medications, with the best therapeutic outcomes possible, teaching is aimed at provid-

ing the patient with the information necessary to ensure this occurs. Every nurse–patient interaction can present an opportunity for teaching. Small portions of education given over time are often more effective than large amounts of information given on only one occasion. Discussing medications each time they are administered is an effective way to increase the amount of education accomplished. Table 6.3 summarizes key areas of teaching and provides sample questions the nurse might ask, or observations that the nurse can make, to verify that teaching was effective. The Nursing Process Focus flowcharts in chapters 13 through 49 also supply information on specific drugs and drug classes that is important to include in patient teaching.

Providing written material assists the patient to retain the information and review it later. Some medications come with a self-contained teaching program that includes videotapes. The nurse must always assess whether the patient is able to read and understand the material provided. Patient educational materials are ineffective if the reading level is above what the patient can understand, or is in a language unfamiliar to the patient. The nurse may have the patient summarize key points after providing the teaching to verify that the patient has understood the information.

Pediatric patients often present special challenges to patient teaching. Specialized pediatric teaching materials may assist the nurse in teaching these patients. Parents of children must be included in the medication administration process. The nurse must base medication administration in pediatric patients on safe pediatric dosages and limiting potential adverse drug reactions. Medication research often does not include children, so data are often unclear on safe pediatric doses and potential adverse drug reactions in this population. There is also a greater risk for serious medication errors, since drug administration in children often requires drug calculations using smaller doses. The nurse must be vigilant to ensure the dosage is correct because small errors in drug doses have the potential to cause serious adverse effects in infants and children.

The elderly population also presents the nurse with additional nursing considerations. Age-appropriate teaching materials that are repeated slowly and provided in small increments may assist the nurse in teaching these patients. It is often necessary to co-teach the patient's caregiver. Elderly patients often have chronic illnesses and age-related changes that may cause medication effects to be unpredictable. Because of chronic diseases, elderly patients often take multiple drugs that may cause many drug–drug interactions.

6.5 Evaluating the Effects of Medications

The **evaluation phase** compares the patient's current health status with the desired outcome. This step is important to determine if the plan of care is appropriate, if it was met, or if it needs revision. If it was met, the plan of care was appropriate, and the problem or risk was resolved. The nurse and patients can then address the next highest priority health

TABLE 6.3	Important Areas of Teaching for a Patient Receiving Medications
Area of Teaching	**Important Questions and Observations**
Therapeutic use and outcomes	▪ Can you tell me the name of your medication and what it is used for?
	▪ What will you look for to know that the medication is effective? (How will you know that the medicine is working?)
Monitoring side and adverse effects	▪ Which side effects can you handle by yourself? (e.g., simple nausea, diarrhea)
	▪ Which side effects should you report to your health care provider? (e.g., extreme cases of nausea or vomiting, extreme dizziness, bleeding)
Medication administration	▪ Can you tell me how much of the medication you should take? (milligrams, number of tablets, milliliters of liquid, etc.)
	▪ Can you tell me how often you should take it?
	▪ What special requirements are necessary when you take this medication? (e.g., take with a full glass of water, take on an empty stomach, and remain upright for 30 minutes)
	▪ Is there a specific order in which you should take your medications? (e.g., using a bronchodilator before using a corticosteroid inhaler)
	▪ Can you show me how you will give yourself the medication? (e.g., eye drops, subcutaneous injections)
	▪ What special monitoring is required before you take this medication? (e.g., pulse rate) Can you demonstrate this for me? Based on that monitoring, when should you *not* take the medication?
	▪ Do you know how, or where, to store this medication?
	▪ What should you do if you miss a dose?
Other monitoring and special requirements	▪ Are there any special tests you should have related to this medication? (e.g., finger-stick glucose levels, therapeutic drug levels)
	▪ How often should these tests be done?
	▪ What other medications should you *not* take with this medication?
	▪ Are there any foods or beverages you must not have while taking this medication?

need. If the goal was partially met, the patient is moving toward the goal, but the nurse may need to continue interventions for a longer time, or somehow modify interventions to completely resolve the problem. The nursing process comes full circle as the nurse reassesses the patient, reviews the nursing diagnoses, makes necessary changes, reviews and rewrites goals and outcomes, and carries out further interventions to meet the stated goals and outcomes.

As it relates to pharmacotherapy, evaluation is used to determine whether the therapeutic effects of the drug were achieved, as well as whether adverse effects were prevented or kept to acceptable levels. If the evaluation data show no improvement over the baseline data, the interventions may require revision. The drug dose may need to be increased, more time may be needed to achieve therapeutic drug levels, or a different or additional drug may be needed. The nurse also evaluates the effectiveness of teaching provided and notes areas where further drug education is needed.

Evaluation is not the end of the process but the beginning of another cycle as the nurse continues to work to ensure safe and effective medication use and active patient involvement in his or her care. It is a checkpoint where the nurse considers the overall goal of safe and effective administration of medications and takes the steps necessary to maximize the success of pharmacotherapy. The nursing process acts as the overall framework for working toward this success.

Chapter REVIEW

KEY CONCEPTS

The numbered key concepts provide a succinct summary of the important points from the corresponding numbered section within the chapter. If any of these points are not clear, refer to the numbered section within the chapter for review.

6.1 Assessment is the systematic collection of patient data. Assessment of the patient receiving medications includes health history information, physical assessment data, lab values and other measurable data, and an assessment of medication effects, including both therapeutic and side effects.

6.2 Nursing diagnoses are written to address the patient's responses related to drug administration. They are developed after an analysis of the assessment data, are focused on the patient's problems, and are verified with the patient or caregiver.

6.3 Goals and outcomes, which are developed from the nursing diagnoses, direct the interventions required by the plan of care. Goals focus on what the patient should be able to achieve, and outcomes provide the specific, measurable criteria that will be used to measure goal attainment.

6.4 The implementation phase involves administering the drug, and carrying out interventions to promote a therapeutic response and minimize adverse effects of the drug. Key interventions required of the nurse include monitoring drug effects, documenting medications, and patient teaching.

6.5 The evaluation phase of the nursing process compares the patient's current health status with the desired outcome. This step is important to determine if the plan of care is appropriate, if it was met, or if it needs revision. Nursing diagnoses are reviewed or rewritten, goals and outcomes are refined, and new interventions are carried out.

NCLEX-RN® REVIEW QUESTIONS

1 Which of the following is an incorrect statement regarding nursing diagnosis?
 1. It identifies the medical problem experienced by the patient.
 2. It is a clinical judgment made by the nurse.
 3. It identifies the patient's response to actual or potential health and life processes.
 4. It determines nursing interventions for which the nurse is accountable.

2 An appropriately stated goal for a patient with type 1 diabetes mellitus is:
 1. the nurse will teach the patient to recognize and respond to the signs and symptoms of hypoglycemia prior to discharge.
 2. the patient will demonstrate self-injection of insulin, using a preloaded syringe, into the subcutaneous tissue of the thigh prior to discharge.
 3. the nurse will teach the patient to accurately draw up the insulin dose in a syringe.
 4. the patient will be able to self-manage his diabetic diet and medications.

3 A 15-year-old adolescent with a history of type 1 diabetes presents to the emergency department in diabetic ketoacidosis. She has successfully self-managed her diet and insulin therapy for the past 2 years. She confides in the nurse that she deliberately skipped some of her insulin doses because she did not want to gain weight, and she is afraid of needle marks. Which of the following nursing diagnoses is most appropriate in this situation? (Select all that apply.)
 1. Deficient Knowledge
 2. Self-Care Deficit
 3. Noncompliance
 4. Ineffective Coping
 5. Disbelief

4 Which factor is most important for the nurse to assess when evaluating the effectiveness of a patient's drug therapy?
 1. Patient's promise to comply with drug therapy
 2. Patient's satisfaction with the drug
 3. Cost of the medication
 4. Evidence of therapeutic benefit

5 Which of the following part of the nursing process is where the nurse assesses the effectiveness of the medication?
 1. Assessment
 2. Implementation
 3. Diagnosis
 4. Evaluation

6 During the evaluation phase of drug administration, the nurse completes which responsibilities?
 1. Prepares and administers drugs correctly
 2. Establishes goals and outcome criteria related to drug therapy
 3. Monitors the patient for therapeutic and adverse effects
 4. Gathers data in a drug and dietary history

CRITICAL THINKING QUESTIONS

1. A 13-year-old patient from a rural community who is a cheerleader was diagnosed with type 1 diabetes. She is supported by a single mother who is frustrated with her daughter's eating habits. The patient has lost weight since beginning her insulin regimen. The nurse notes that the patient and her mother, who is very well dressed, are both extremely thin. Identify additional assessment data that the nurse would need to obtain before making the nursing diagnosis *Noncompliance*.

2. The drug regimen of the patient in question 1 is evaluated, and the health care provider suggests a subcutaneous insulin pump to help control the patient's fluctuating blood glucose levels. Write three nursing diagnoses related to this new therapy.

3. A nursing student is assigned to a licensed preceptor who is administering oral medications. The student notes that the preceptor administers the drugs safely but routinely fails to offer the patient information about the drug being administered. Identify the information that the nurse should teach the patient during medication administration.

See Appendix D for answers and rationales for all activities.

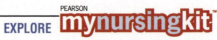

EXPLORE **mynursingkit**

MyNursingKit is your one stop for online chapter review materials and resources. Prepare for success with additional NCLEX®-style practice questions, interactive assignments and activities, web links, animations and videos, and more!

Register your access code from the front of your book at
www.mynursingkit.com.

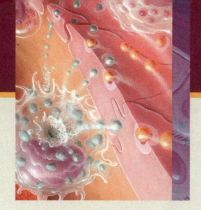

Chapter 7

Drug Administration Throughout the Life Span

LEARNING OUTCOMES

After reading this chapter, the student should be able to:

1. Describe physiological changes during pregnancy that may affect the absorption, distribution, metabolism, and excretion of drugs.
2. Describe the placental transfer of drugs from mother to infant.
3. Match the five FDA pregnancy risk categories with their definitions.
4. Identify factors that influence the transfer of drugs into breast milk.
5. Identify techniques that the breast-feeding mother can use to reduce drug exposure to the newborn.
6. Explain how differences in pharmacokinetic variables can impact drug response in pediatric patients.
7. Discuss the nursing and pharmacologic implications associated with each pediatric developmental age group.
8. Describe physiological and biochemical changes that occur in the older adult, and how these affect pharmacotherapy.
9. Develop nursing interventions that maximize pharmacotherapeutic outcomes in the older adult.

KEY TERMS

Beginning with conception, and continuing throughout the life span, organs and body systems undergo predictable physiological changes that influence the absorption, metabolism, distribution, and elimination of medications. Nurses must recognize such changes to ensure that drugs are delivered in a safe and effective manner to patients of all ages. This chapter examines how principles of developmental physiology and life span psychology apply to drug administration.

7.1 Pharmacotherapy Across the Life Span

Growth is a term that characterizes the progressive increase in *physical* size. *Development* is a related term that refers to the *functional* changes in the physical, psychomotor, and cognitive capabilities of a person. Stages of growth and physical development usually go hand in hand, in a predictable sequence, whereas psychomotor and cognitive development have a tendency to be more variable.

To provide optimum care, nurses must understand *normal* growth and developmental patterns that occur throughout the life span. It is from this benchmark that *deviations* from the norm can be recognized, so that health-pattern impairments can be appropriately addressed. For pharmacotherapy to achieve its desired outcomes, such knowledge is essential.

The development of a person is a complex process that links the biophysical with the psychosocial, ethnocultural, and spiritual components to make each individual a unique human being. This whole-person view is essential to holistic care. The very nature of pharmacology requires that the nurse consider the individuality of each patient and the specifics of age, growth, and development in relation to pharmacokinetics and pharmacodynamics.

DRUG ADMINISTRATION DURING PREGNANCY AND LACTATION

Health care providers exercise great caution when initiating pharmacotherapy during pregnancy or lactation (➤ Figure 1.2). When possible, drug therapy is postponed until after pregnancy and lactation, or nonpharmacologic alternatives are implemented. There are some serious conditions, however, that may require pharmacotherapy in such patients. For example, if the patient has epilepsy, hypertension, or a psychiatric disorder *prior to* the pregnancy, it would be unwise to discontinue therapy during pregnancy or lactation. Conditions such as gestational diabetes and gestational hypertension occur *during* pregnancy and must be treated for the safety of the growing fetus. Antibiotics may be necessary to treat infections during pregnancy; acute urinary tract infections and sexually transmitted infections are relatively common and can harm the fetus. In all cases, health care

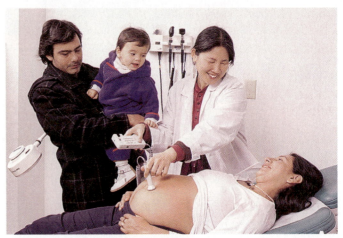

➤ *Figure 7.1* Treating the pregnant patient
Source: © Jenny Thomas Photography.

practitioners must weigh the therapeutic benefits of a given medication against its potential adverse effects.

7.2 Pharmacotherapy of the Pregnant Patient

Drug therapy in a pregnant patient requires that the nurse consider the effects of the drug on both the mother as well as on the growing fetus. The placenta is a semipermeable membrane: Some substances readily pass from mother to fetus, whereas the transport of other substances is blocked. The fetal membranes contain enzymes that detoxify certain substances as they cross the membrane. For example, insulin from the mother is inactivated by placental enzymes during the early stages of pregnancy, preventing it from reaching the fetus. In general, drugs that are water soluble, ionized, or bound to plasma proteins are less likely to cross the placenta.

PHYSIOLOGICAL CHANGES DURING PREGNANCY THAT IMPACT PHARMACOTHERAPY

During pregnancy, major physiological and anatomic changes occur in the endocrine, gastrointestinal (GI), cardiovascular, circulatory, and renal systems of women. Some of these changes alter drug pharmacokinetics and pharmacodynamics and may affect the success of therapy.

ABSORPTION Hormonal changes as well as the pressure of the expanding uterus on the blood supply to abdominal organs may affect the absorption of drugs. Gastric emptying is delayed, and transit time for food and drugs in the GI tract is slowed by progesterone, which allows a longer time for absorption of oral drugs. Gastric acidity is also decreased, which can affect the absorption of some drugs. Changes in the respiratory system during pregnancy—increased tidal volume and pulmonary vasodilation—may cause inhaled drugs to be absorbed to a greater extent.

DISTRIBUTION AND METABOLISM Hemodynamic changes in the pregnant patient increase cardiac output, increase plasma volume, and change regional blood flow. The increased blood volume in the mother causes dilution of drugs and decreases plasma protein concentrations, affecting drug distribution. Blood flow to the uterus, kidneys, and skin is increased, whereas flow to the skeletal muscles is diminished. Alterations in lipid levels may alter drug transport and distribution, especially during the third trimester. Drug metabolism increases for certain drugs, most notably anticonvulsants such as carbamazepine, phenytoin, and valproic acid, which may require higher doses during pregnancy. Fat-soluble drugs are distributed into the lipid-rich breast milk and are ultimately passed to the lactating infant.

EXCRETION By the third trimester of pregnancy, blood flow through the mother's kidneys increases 40% to 50%. This increase has a direct effect on renal plasma flow, glomerular filtration rate, and renal tubular absorption. Thus, drug excretion rates may be increased, affecting dosage timing and onset of action.

GESTATIONAL AGE AND DRUG THERAPY

A **teratogen** is a substance, organism, or physical agent to which an embryo or fetus is exposed that produces a permanent abnormality in structure or function, causes growth retardation, or causes death. The baseline incidence of teratogenic events is approximately 3% of all pregnancies. Potential fetal consequences include intrauterine fetal death, physical malformations, growth impairment, behavioral abnormalities, and neonatal toxicity.

There are no "absolute" teratogens. Whether or not a drug produces a teratogenic effect depends upon multiple, complex factors. Like other effects of drugs, there is a dose–response relationship, with risk increasing with higher doses. The timing of drug therapy and the stage of fetal development critically affect the risk for possible fetal consequences. Because of the constant changes that occur during fetal development, the specific risk is dependent on when during gestation the drug is administered. A well-known example is the drug thalidomide, which causes fetal defects during pregnancy if it is administered day 35 to 48 after the last menstrual period. The specific malformation is linked to the time of exposure to the drug: 35 to 37 days, no ears; 39 to 41 days, no arms; 41 to 43 days, no uterus; 45 to 47 days, no tibia; and 47 to 49 days, triphalangeal thumbs.

Preimplantation period: Weeks 1 to 2 of the first trimester are known as the **preimplantation period.** Before implantation, the developing embryo has not yet established a blood supply with the mother. This is sometimes called the "all-or-none" period because exposure to a teratogen either causes death of the embryo or has no effect. Drugs are less likely to cause congenital malformations during this period because the baby's organ systems have not yet begun to form. Drugs such as nicotine, however, can create a negative *environment* for the embryo and potentially cause intrauterine growth retardation.

Embryonic period: During the embryonic period, from 3 to 8 weeks postconception, there is rapid development of internal structures. This is the period of maximum sensitivity to teratogens. Teratogenic agents taken during this phase can lead to structural malformation and spontaneous abortion. The specific abnormality depends upon which organ is forming at the time of exposure.

Fetal period: The fetal phase is from 9 to 40 weeks postconception or until birth. During this time, there is continued growth and maturation of the baby's organ systems. Blood flow to the placenta increases and placental vascular membranes become thinner. Such alterations maximize the transfer of substances from the maternal circulation to the fetal blood. As a result, the fetus may receive larger doses of medications and other substances taken by the mother. Because the fetus lacks mature metabolic enzymes and efficient excretion mechanisms, medications will have a prolonged duration of action within the unborn child. Exposure to teratogens during the fetal period is more likely to produce slowed growth or impaired organ function, rather than gross structural malformations.

PREGNANCY DRUG CATEGORIES AND REGISTRIES

Fortunately, the number of prescription drugs that are strongly suspected or known to be teratogenic is small. In addition, for most clinical conditions, there are alternative drugs that can be given with relative safety. New or infrequently used drugs for which there is inadequate safety information should not be given to pregnant women unless the benefits of drug therapy clearly outweigh any theoretical risks.

The FDA has developed drug pregnancy categories that classify medications according to their risks during pregnancy. Table 7.1 lists the five pregnancy categories, which guide the health care team and the patient in selecting drugs that are least hazardous for the fetus. Examples of prescription drugs that are associated with teratogenic effects are shown in the table. In addition to prescription medications, alcohol, nicotine, and illicit drugs such as cocaine will affect the unborn child.

Testing drugs in human subjects to determine their teratogenicity is unethical and prohibited by law. Although drugs are tested in pregnant laboratory animals, the structure of the human placenta is unique. This is problematic because laboratory animals have different physiological, metabolic, and genetic characteristics. Most information about fetal malformations and abnormalities is extrapolated from these animal data and may only be crude approximations of the risk to a human fetus. The actual risk to a human fetus may be much less, or magnitudes greater, than that predicted from animal data. In a few cases, human data are available to show pregnancy risks. The following statement bears repeating: *No prescription drug, over-the-counter (OTC) medication, herbal product, or dietary supplement should be taken during pregnancy unless the physician verifies that the therapeutic benefits to the mother clearly outweigh the potential risks for the unborn.*

The current A, B, C, D, and X pregnancy labeling system is simplistic and gives no *specific* clinical information to help guide nurses or their patients about a medication's true safety. The system does not indicate how the dose should be adjusted during pregnancy or lactation. Most drugs are category C

TABLE 7.1	Current FDA Pregnancy Category Ratings with Examples	
Risk Category	Interpretation	Drugs
A	Adequate, well-controlled studies in pregnant women have not shown an increased risk of fetal abnormalities to the fetus in any trimester of pregnancy.	Prenatal multivitamins, insulin, thyroxine, folic acid
B	Animal studies have revealed no evidence of harm to the fetus; however, there are no adequate and well-controlled studies in pregnant women. OR Animal studies have shown an adverse effect, but adequate and well-controlled studies in pregnant women have failed to demonstrate risk to the fetus in any trimester.	Penicillins, cephalosporins, azithromycin, acetaminophen, ibuprofen in the first and second trimesters
C	Animal studies have shown an adverse effect and there are no adequate and well-controlled studies in pregnant women. OR No animal studies have been conducted and there are no adequate and well-controlled studies in pregnant women.	Most prescription medicines; antimicrobials such as clarithromycin, fluoroquinolones, and Bactrim; selective serotonin reuptake inhibitors (SSRIs); corticosteroids; and most antihypertensives
D	Adequate well-controlled or observational studies in pregnant women have demonstrated a risk to the fetus. However, the benefits of therapy may outweigh the potential risk. For example, the drug may be acceptable if needed in a life-threatening situation or serious disease for which safer drugs cannot be used or are ineffective.	ACE inhibitors, angiotensin receptor blockers (ARBs) in the second and third trimesters, gentamicin, ibuprofen in the third trimester, tetracyclines, Premarin, alcohol, and nicotine
X	Adequate well-controlled or observational studies in animals or pregnant women have demonstrated positive evidence of fetal abnormalities or risks. The use of the product is contraindicated in women who are or may become pregnant. There is no indication for use in pregnancy.	Accutane, misoprostol, and thalidomide

because very high doses in laboratory animals often produce teratogenic effects. All category D and X drugs should be avoided during pregnancy due to their potential for causing serious birth defects. Because a woman may obtain a prescription before she knows she is pregnant, it is crucial that the nurse ask *all* women of child-bearing age if there is the possibility of pregnancy as part of the routine teaching that accompanies giving a patient their prescription.

PREGNANCY REGISTRIES

Pregnancy registries help identify medications that are safe to be taken during pregnancy. These registries gather information from women who took medications during pregnancy. Information on babies born to women not taking the medication is then compared with data on babies born while medication was taken during pregnancy. The effects of the medication taken during pregnancy are then evaluated. Registries may be maintained by drug companies, governmental agencies, or special-interest groups. Examples of pregnancy registries include the following:

- Antipsychotic medicines: http://www.motherisk.org/women/index.jsp
- Antiretroviral medicines: http://www.apregistry.com/who.htm
- Asthma medications: http://otispregnancy.org/
- Epilepsy medications: http://www2.massgeneral.org/aed/
- Autoimmune disease medications: http://www.otispregnancy.org/hm/inside.php?sid=7&id=40

7.3 Pharmacotherapy of the Lactating Patient

A large number of drugs are secreted into breast milk. Fortunately, there are relatively few instances where drugs secreted into breast milk have been found to cause injury to infants. For the few drugs that are absolutely contraindicated during lactation, equally effective, safer alternatives are usually available. Although most medications probably cause no harm to the breast-feeding baby, their effects have not been fully studied.

As with the placenta, drugs that are ionized, water soluble, or bound to plasma proteins are less likely to enter breast milk. Central nervous system (CNS) medications are very lipid soluble and thus are more likely to be present in higher concentrations in milk and can be expected to have a greater effect on an infant. Although concentrations of CNS drugs in breast milk are found in higher amounts, they often remain at subclinical levels. Regarding the role of protein binding, drugs that remain in the maternal plasma bound to albumin are not able to penetrate the mother's milk supply. For example, warfarin is strongly bound to plasma proteins and thus has a reduced milk level because it is unable to transfer into the maternal milk.

The American Academy of Pediatrics (AAP) Committee on Drugs provides guidance on which drugs should be avoided during breast-feeding to protect the child's safety. Medications that pass into breast milk are indicated in drug guides. Nurses working with pregnant or breast-feeding women should give careful attention to this information.

TABLE 7.2	Selected Drugs Associated with Adverse Effects During Breast-Feeding	
Drug	**Reported Effect or Reasons for Concern**
acebutolol (Sectral)	Hypotension; bradycardia; tachypnea
amiodarone (Cordarone)	Hypothyroidism
amphetamine	Irritability, poor sleeping pattern
aspirin and other salicylates	Metabolic acidosis
atenolol (Tenormin)	Cyanosis; bradycardia
bromocriptine (Parlodel)	Suppresses lactation; may be hazardous to the mother
cocaine	Cocaine intoxication: irritability, vomiting, diarrhea, tremulousness, seizures
ergotamine (Ergostat)	Vomiting, diarrhea, convulsions (doses used in migraine medications)
fluoxetine (Prozac)	Feeding and sleeping disorders, reduced weight gain, colic
haloperidol (Haldol)	Decline in developmental scores
lithium (Eskalith)	One-third to one-half therapeutic blood concentration in infants
phenindione	Anticoagulant: increased prothrombin and partial thromboplastin time
phenobarbital (Luminal)	Sedation; infantile spasms after weaning from milk containing phenobarbital, methemoglobinemia
primidone (Mysoline)	Sedation, feeding problems
sulfasalazine (Azulfidine)	Bloody diarrhea

Source: From "The Transfer of Drugs and Other Chemicals into Human Breast Milk" by American Academy of Pediatrics, Committee on Drugs, 2001, *Pediatrics, 3*, pp. 776–782. Reprinted with permission.

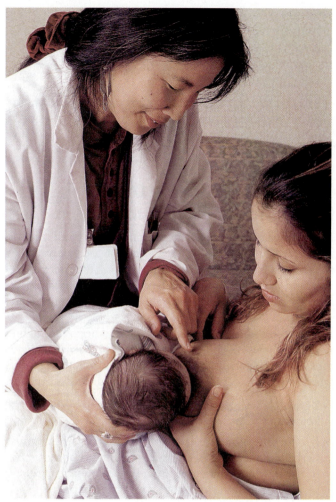

➤ *Figure 7.2* Treating the breast-feeding mother
Source: © Jenny Thomas Photography.

Selected drugs that enter the breast milk and have been shown to produce adverse effects are listed in Table 7.2.

It is important to understand factors that influence the amount of drug secreted into breast milk. This allows the nurse to aid the patient in making responsible choices regarding lactation and in reducing exposure of her newborn to potentially harmful substances (➤ Figure 7.2). The same guidelines for drug use apply during the breast-feeding period as during pregnancy—drugs should be taken only if the benefits to the mother clearly outweigh the potential risks to the infant. The nurse should explore the possibility of postponing pharmacotherapy until the baby is weaned, or perhaps selecting a safer, nonpharmacologic therapy. If a drug is indicated, it is sometimes useful to administer it immediately after breast-feeding, or when the infant will be sleeping for an extended period, so that time elapses before the next feeding. This will usually reduce the concentration of active drug in the mother's milk when she later breast-feeds her infant. The nurse can assist the mother in protecting the child's safety by teaching her to avoid illicit drugs, alcohol, and tobacco products during lactation.

When considering the effects of drugs on the breast-feeding infant, the *amount* of drug that actually reaches the infant's tissues must be considered. Some medications produce no adverse effects because they are destroyed in the infant's GI system, or are unable to be absorbed across the GI tract. Thus, although many drugs are secreted in breast milk, some are present in such small amounts that they cause no noticeable harm.

The last key factor in the effect of drugs during lactation relates to the infant's ability to metabolize small amounts of drugs. Premature, neonatal, and seriously ill infants may be at greater risk for adverse effects because they lack drug metabolizing enzymes.

Some recommendations regarding medications given during lactation are as follows (Hale, 2004):

• Drugs with a shorter half-life are preferable. Peak levels are rapidly reached and the drug is quickly cleared from the maternal plasma, which reduces the amount of drug exposure to the infant. The mother should not breast-feed while the drug is at its peak level.

• Drugs that have long half-lives (or active metabolites) should be avoided because they can accumulate in the infant's plasma. Examples include barbiturates, benzodiazepines, meperidine, and fluoxetine.

- Whenever possible, drugs with high protein-binding ability should be selected because they are not secreted as readily to the milk.

- All OTC herbal products and dietary supplements should be avoided during lactation, unless specifically prescribed by the health care provider because the safety of most of these products to the infant has not been determined.

7.4 Patient Teaching During Pregnancy and Lactation

Patient education during pregnancy and lactation is critical to the success of pharmacotherapy and to the safety of the mother and baby. The nurse should perform an in-depth history and prenatal assessment to eliminate potentially hazardous substances, substitute alternative drugs, or adjust medication dosages. The patient needs to be thoroughly informed about the risks to both herself and her unborn child related to the use of drugs, alcohol, tobacco, alternative therapies, and OTC medications. Include the following points when teaching patients about drug therapy during pregnancy:

- Keep all scheduled physician appointments and laboratory visits for testing.

- Do not take other prescription drugs, OTC medications, herbal remedies, or dietary supplements without notifying your health care provider. Your health care provider may need to change a prescribed drug to another similar drug or change the drug dosage.

- Take iron, folic acid, and multivitamin supplements as prescribed during pregnancy.

- Eliminate alcohol and tobacco use.

PharmFacts

Fetal Effects Caused by Specific Drug Use During Pregnancy

- Marijuana: low-birth-weight babies, risk of premature delivery, withdrawal symptoms (crying and trembling)
- Cocaine: increased risk of miscarriage, premature delivery, malformations of fetal limbs and kidneys, behavioral disturbances (jittery, irritable, crying)
- Heroin: increased risk of miscarriage, low-birth-weight babies, withdrawal symptoms, diarrhea, fever, sneezing, yawning, tremors, seizures, irregular breathing, and irritability, increased risk of sudden infant death syndrome (SIDS)
- Tobacco: increased risk of stillbirths, premature delivery, low-birth-weight babies, increased risk of sudden infant death syndrome (SIDS)
- Alcohol: alcohol-related birth defects ranging from miscarriage and stillbirth to fetal alcohol syndrome (small stature; joint problems; and problems with attention, memory, intelligence, coordination, and problem solving)

Source: March of Dimes, accessed at www.marchofdimes.com on November 1, 2009.

- Join a pregnancy registry if you are taking prescription drugs.

- Understand that the adverse effects of drug treatment may be confused with common discomforts of pregnancy because they may be similar. These common discomforts include nausea, vomiting, heartburn, constipation, hypotension, heart palpitations, and fatigue.

- Use nonpharmacologic alternatives such as massage for pain or calming music for anxiety, whenever possible, to minimize the need for drug therapy.

DRUG ADMINISTRATION DURING CHILDHOOD

As a child develops, physical growth and physiological changes mandate adjustments in the administration of medications. Although children may sometimes receive similar drugs via the same routes as adults, the nursing management for children is very different from that for adults. Normal physiologic changes during growth and development can markedly affect pharmacokinetics and pharmacodynamics. Factors for the nurse to consider include physiological variations, maturity of body systems, and greater fluid distribution in children. Drug dosages are vastly different in children.

For the purposes of medication administration, the pediatric patient is defined as being any age from birth to 16 years and weighing less than 50 kg. Additionally, children may be classified as neonates, infants, toddlers, preschool, school age, and adolescent.

7.5 Pharmacotherapy of Infants

Infancy is the period from birth to 12 months of age (➤ Figure 7.2). The first 28 days of life are referred to as the neonatal period. During this time, nursing care and pharmacotherapy are directed toward safety of the infant, proper dosing of prescribed drugs, and teaching parents how to administer medications properly. A primary goal is to have the child ingest the entire dose of medication without spitting it out because it is difficult to estimate the amount lost. If the child vomits immediately after taking the drug, the dose may be reordered. The following nursing interventions and parental teaching points are important for this age group:

- The infant should be held and cuddled while administering medications, and offered a pacifier if the infant is on fluid restrictions caused by vomiting or diarrhea.

- Medications are often administered to infants via droppers into the eyes, ears, nose, or mouth. Oral medications should be directed to the inner cheek and the child given time to swallow the drug to avoid aspiration. If rectal suppositories are administered, the buttocks

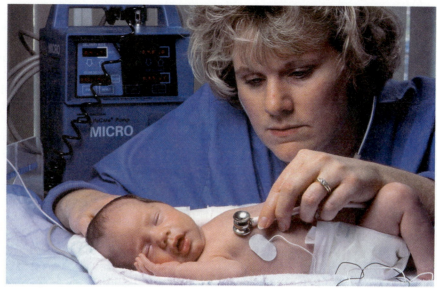

➤ *Figure 7.3* Treating the infant
Source: Pearson Education/PH College.

should be held together for 5 to 10 minutes to prevent expulsion of the drug before absorption has occurred.

- In very young infants, the medication may be given via a nipple. Some believe this is controversial since the infant may associate the nipple with medication and refuse feedings.

- Special considerations must be observed when administering intramuscular (IM) or intravenous (IV) injections to infants. Unlike adults, infants lack well-developed muscle masses, so the smallest needle appropriate for the drug should be used. For volumes less than 1 mL, a tuberculin syringe is appropriate. The vastus lateralis is a preferred site for IM injections, because it has few nerves and is relatively well developed in infants. The gluteal site is usually contraindicated because of potential damage to the sciatic nerve, injury to which may result in permanent disability.

- Because of the lack of choices for injection sites, the nurse must rotate injection sites from one leg to the next to avoid overuse and to prevent inflammation and excessive pain.

- For IV sites, the feet and scalp veins may provide more easily accessible and preferred venous access sites.

7.6 Pharmacotherapy of Toddlers

Toddlerhood is the age period from 1 to 3 years. During this time, a toddler begins to explore, wants to try new things, and tends to place everything in the mouth. This becomes a major concern for medication and household product safety. The nurse must be instrumental in teaching parents that poisons come in all shapes, sizes, and forms and include medicines, cosmetics, cleaning supplies, arts and crafts materials, plants, and food products that are improperly stored. Parents should be instructed to request child-resistant con-

tainers from the pharmacist and to stow all medications in secure cabinets.

Toddlers can swallow liquids and may be able to chew solid medications. When prescription drugs are supplied as flavored elixirs, it is important to stress that the child not be given access to the medications. Drugs must never be left at the bedside or within easy reach of the child. A child who has access to a bottle of cherry-flavored acetaminophen (Tylenol) may ingest a fatal overdose of the tasty liquid. Nurses should educate parents about the following means of protecting their children from poisoning:

- Read and carefully follow directions on the label before using drugs and OTC products.
- Store all drugs and harmful agents out of the reach of children and in locked cabinets.
- Keep all household products and drugs in their original containers. Never put chemicals in empty food or drink containers.
- Always ask the pharmacist to place the medications for everyone in the household in child-resistant containers.
- Never tell children that medicine is candy.
- Keep the Poison Control Center number near phones, and call immediately if poisoning is suspected.
- Never leave medication unattended in a child's room or in areas where the child plays.

Administration of medications to toddlers can be challenging. At this stage, the child is rapidly developing increased motor ability and learning to assert independence, but has extremely limited ability to reason or understand the relationship of medicines to health. Giving long, detailed explanations to the toddler will prolong the procedure and create additional anxiety. Short, concrete explanations followed by immediate drug administration are best for this age group. Physical comfort in the form of touching, hugging, or verbal praise following drug administration is important.

Oral medications that taste bad should be mixed with a vehicle such as jam, syrup, or fruit puree, if possible. Encourage parents to mix the medication in the smallest amount possible to ensure that the toddler receives all of it. The medication may be followed with a carbonated beverage or mint-flavored candy. Nurses should teach parents to avoid placing medicine in milk, orange juice, or cereals, because the child may associate these healthful foods with bad-tasting medications. Pharmaceutical companies often formulate pediatric medicines in sweet syrups to increase the ease of drug administration.

IM injections for toddlers should be given into the vastus lateralis muscle. IV injections may use scalp or feet veins; additional peripheral site options become available in late toddlerhood. The toddler presents additional safety issues to the nurse who is administering IV medications. The nurse must firmly secure the IV and then educate the parents about the dangers of the toddler trying to pull away too quickly from the IV pump. It is often helpful to put longer tubing on a toddler's IV to give the child more play room. Suppositories may be difficult to administer because of the child's resistance. For any of these invasive administration procedures, having a parent in close proximity will usually reduce the toddler's anxiety and increase cooperation, but ask the parent prior to the procedure if he or she would like to assist. The nurse should take at least one helper into the room for assistance in restraining the toddler if necessary.

7.7 Pharmacotherapy of Preschoolers and School-Age Children

The **preschool child** ranges in age from 3 to 5 years. During this period, the child begins to refine gross and fine motor skills and develop language abilities. The child initiates new activities and becomes more socially involved with other children.

Preschoolers can sometimes comprehend the difference between health and illness and that medications are administered to help them feel better. Nonetheless, medications and other potentially dangerous products must still be safely stowed out of the child's reach.

In general, principles of medication administration that pertain to the toddler also apply to this age group. Preschoolers cooperate in taking oral medications if they are crushed or mixed with food or flavored beverages. After a child has walked for about a year, the ventrogluteal site may be used for IM injections, because it causes less pain than the vastus lateralis site. The scalp veins can no longer be used for IV access; peripheral veins are used for IV injections.

Like toddlers, preschoolers often physically resist medication administration, and a long, detailed explanation of the procedure will likely promote anxiety. A brief explanation followed quickly by medication administration is usually the best method. Uncooperative children may need to be restrained, and patients older than 4 years may require two adults to administer the medication. Before and after medication procedures, the child may benefit from opportunities to play-act troubling experiences with dolls. When the child plays the role of doctor or nurse by giving a "sick" doll a pill or injection, comforting the doll, and explaining that the doll will now feel better, the little actor feels safer and more in control of the situation.

The **school-age child** is between 6 and 12 years of age. Some refer to this period as the *middle childhood* years. This is the time in a child's life when rapid physical, mental, and social development occur, and early ethical–moral development begins to take shape. Thinking processes become progressively more logical and consistent.

During this time, most children remain relatively healthy. Respiratory infections and GI upset are the most common complaints. Because the child feels well most of the time, there is little concept of illness or the risks involved with ingesting a harmful substance offered to the child by a peer or older person.

The nurse is usually able to gain considerable cooperation from school-age children. More detailed explanations may be of value, because the child has developed some reasoning ability and can understand the relationship between the medicine and feeling better. When children are old enough to welcome choices, they can be offered limited dosing alternatives to provide a sense of control and to encourage cooperation. The option of taking one medication before another or the chance to choose which drink will follow a chewable tablet helps distract children from the issue of whether they will take the medication at all. It also makes an otherwise strange or unpleasant experience a little more enjoyable. Making children feel that they are willing participants in medication administration, rather than victims, is an important foundation for compliance. Praise for cooperation is appropriate for any pediatric patient and sets the

---

LIFESPAN CONSIDERATIONS

Iron Poisoning

One of the leading causes of poisonings in children under the age of 6 is iron poisoning. Iron is often found in vitamins of all kinds: prenatal, pediatric, and adult vitamins. Pediatric vitamins may be particularly tempting and may have the taste and appearance of candy that the child is familiar with. Prenatal vitamins may hold a particular danger due to the increased amounts of iron and other components. And vitamins are not always considered "medicine" or locked away with other prescription medications. Older children may open the bottle, a young child may outwit a "child-resistant" top, or a bottle is left within the child's reach. Depending on the age of the child, as few as five iron-containing tablets are known to cause iron poisoning.

Symptoms of iron poisoning include nausea, vomiting, diarrhea, gastrointestinal bleeding, and can progress to coma and death. Even if iron poisoning is only suspected, the child should be taken for medical evaluation because symptoms may be delayed. Parents should be encouraged to be certain *all* medication, including OTC drugs such as vitamins, are locked away and medicine bottle tops are secured. And when visiting another home or having a visitor within the home, be sure all medication is out of a child's reach and availability, even vitamins.

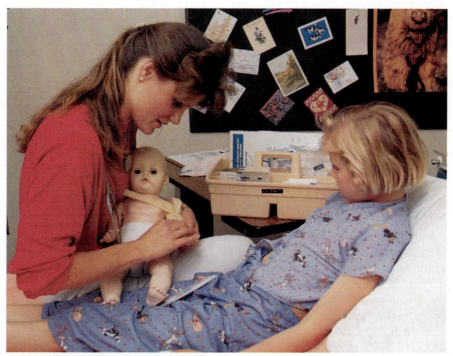

➤ *Figure 7.4* Treating the younger school-age child
Source: Pearson Education/PH College.

stage for successful medication administration in the future (➤ Figure 7.4).

School-age children can safely take chewable tablets and may even be able to swallow tablets or capsules. Because many still resist injections, it is best to have help available for these procedures. The child should never be told that he or she is "too old" to cry and resist. The ventrogluteal site is preferred for IM injections, although the muscles of older children are developed enough for the nurse to use other sites.

7.8 Pharmacotherapy of Adolescents

Adolescence occurs between ages 13 and 16 years. Rapid physical growth and psychologic maturation have a great impact on personality development. The adolescent strongly relates to peers, wanting and needing their support, approval, and presence. The strong sense of independence leads teens to self-medicate, either with or without their parent's knowledge. Treatment objectives for the nurse should include teaching parents to keep their medications safely stowed out of sight from inquisitive, experiment-minded adolescents. Parents should also be taught the signs and symptoms of drugs commonly abused by teens such as marijuana, inhalents, and methamphetamine.

The most common needs for the pharmacotherapy of teens are for skin problems, headaches, menstrual symptoms, eating disorders, contraception, alcohol and tobacco use, and sports-related injuries.

- Of primary concern to the adolescent is the initiation of sexual intercourse and the avoidance of pregnancy and sexually transmitted infections. The nurse must be prepared to address a variety of topics related to sexuality, including the importance of responsible sexual practices, condom use, and other contraceptive methods.

- Eating disorders commonly occur in this population; therefore, the nurse should carefully question adolescents about their eating habits and their use of OTC appetite suppressants or laxatives that may be contributing to bulimia or anorexia.

- Alcohol, tobacco use, and other illicit drug experimentation are common in this population. Teenage athletes may use amphetamines to delay the onset of fatigue, as well as anabolic steroids to enhance performance. The nurse assumes a key role in educating adolescent patients about the hazards of tobacco use and illicit drugs.

- The adolescent has a need for privacy and control in drug administration. The nurse should communicate with the teen more in the manner of an adult, than as a child. Teens usually appreciate thorough explanations of their treatment, and ample time should be allowed for them to ask questions.

- Despite the adolescent's need for confidentiality and privacy, confidentiality laws differ from state to state. Nurses working with the adolescent population need to be familiar with their state laws affecting confidentiality and informed consent.

- Despite their need to have independence and the desire to self-medicate, teens have a very poor understanding of medication information (Buck, 2007). Adolescents are reluctant to admit their lack of knowledge, so the nurse should carefully explain important information regarding their medications and expected side effects, even if the patient claims to understand.

DRUG ADMINISTRATION DURING ADULTHOOD

When considering adult health, it is customary to divide this period of life into three stages: **young adulthood** (18 to 40 years of age), **middle adulthood** (40 to 65 years of age), and **older adulthood** (over 65 years of age). Within each of these divisions are similar biophysical, psychosocial, and spiritual characteristics that affect nursing and pharmacotherapy.

7.9 Pharmacotherapy of Young and Middle-Aged Adults

The health status of younger adults is generally good; absorption, metabolic, and excretion mechanisms are at their peaks. There is minimal need for prescription drugs unless chronic diseases such as diabetes or immune-related conditions exist. The use of vitamins, minerals, and herbal remedies is prevalent in young adulthood. Prescription drugs are usually related to contraception or agents needed during pregnancy and delivery. Medication compliance is positive within this age range, because there is clear comprehension of benefit in terms of longevity and feeling well.

Substance abuse is a cause for concern in the 18 to 24 age group, with alcohol, tobacco products, amphetamines, and illicit drugs a problem. For young adults who are sexually active, with multiple partners, prescription medications for the treatment of herpes, gonorrhea, syphilis, and HIV infections may be necessary.

The physical status of the middle-aged adult is on a par with that of the young adult until about 45 years of age. During this period of life, numerous transitions occur that often result in excessive stress. Middle-aged adults are sometimes referred to

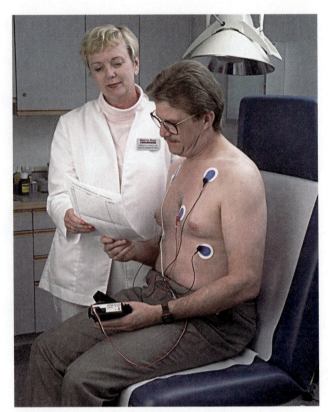

> **Figure 7.5** Treating the middle-aged adult
Source: Pearson Education/PH College.

as the "sandwich generation" because they are often caring for aging parents as well as children and grandchildren. Because of the pressures of work and family, middle-aged adults often take medication to control health alterations that could best be treated with positive lifestyle modifications. The nurse must emphasize the importance of overall health of lifestyle choices, such as limiting lipid intake, maintaining optimum weight, and exercising (➤ Figure 7.5).

Health impairments related to cardiovascular disease, hypertension, obesity, arthritis, cancer, and anxiety begin to surface in late middle age. The use of drugs to treat hypertension, hyperlipidemia, digestive disorders, erectile dysfunction, and arthritis are common. Respiratory disorders related to lifelong tobacco use or exposure to secondhand smoke and environmental toxins may develop that require drug therapies. Adult-onset diabetes mellitus often emerges during this time of life. The use of antidepressants and antianxiety agents is prominent in the population older than 50.

7.10 Pharmacotherapy of Older Adults

During the 20th century, an improved quality of life and the ability to effectively treat many chronic diseases contributed to increased longevity. The age-related changes in older adults, however, can influence the patient's response to drugs, altering both the therapeutic and adverse effects, and creating special needs and risks. As a consequence of aging,

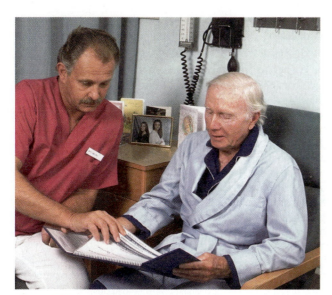

➤ *Figure 7.6* Treating the older adult
Source: Pearson Education/PH College.

patients experience an increasing number of chronic health disorders, and more drugs are prescribed to treat them.

The taking of multiple drugs concurrently, known as **polypharmacy,** has become commonplace among older adults. Patients who visit multiple physicians and use different pharmacies may experience polypharmacy because each doctor or pharmacist may not be aware of all the drugs ordered by other practitioners. Polypharmacy dramatically increases the risk for drug interactions and side effects. Nurses should urge the patient to report all prescription and OTC products on each office visit and teach the patient to use one pharmacy for their prescription needs.

Although predictable physiological and psychosocial changes occur with aging, significant variability exists among patients. For example, although cognitive decline and memory loss certainly occur along the aging continuum, there is a great variation in geriatric patients. Some older individuals do not experience cognitive impairment at all. The nurse should avoid preconceived notions that elderly patients will have physical or cognitive impairment simply because they have reached a certain age. Careful assessment is always necessary (➤ Figure 7.6).

When administering medications to older adults, the nurse should offer the patient the same degree of independence and dignity that would be afforded middle-aged adults, unless otherwise indicated. Like their younger counterparts, older patients have a need to understand why they are receiving a drug and what outcomes are expected. Accommodations must be made for older adults who have certain impairments. Visual and auditory changes make it important for the nurse to provide drug instructions in large type and to obtain patient feedback to be certain that medication instructions are understood. Elderly patients with cognitive decline and memory loss can benefit from aids such as alarmed pill containers, medicine management boxes, and

clearly written instructions. During assessment, the nurse should determine if the patient is capable of self-administering medications in a consistent, safe, and effective manner. As long as small children are not present in the household, older patients with arthritis should be encouraged to ask the pharmacist for regular screw-cap medication bottles for ease of opening.

Geriatric patients experience more adverse effects from drug therapy than other age groups. Although some of these effects are due to polypharmacy, many of the adverse events are predictable, based on normal physiological processes that occur during aging. The principal complications of drug therapy in the older adult population are due to degeneration of organ systems, multiple and severe illness, polypharmacy, and unreliable compliance. By understanding these changes, the nurse can avoid many adverse drug effects in older patients.

In geriatric patients, the functioning ability of all major organ systems progressively declines. For this reason, all phases of pharmacokinetics are affected, and appropriate adjustments in therapy need to be implemented. Although most of the pharmacokinetic changes are due to reduced hepatic and renal drug elimination, other systems may also initiate a variety of changes. For example, immune system function diminishes with aging, so autoimmune diseases and infections occur more frequently in elderly patients. Thus, there is an increased need for influenza and pneumonia vaccinations. Normal physiological changes that affect pharmacotherapy of the older adult are summarized as follows:

Absorption: In general, absorption of drugs is slower in the older adult due to diminished gastric motility and decreased blood flow to digestive organs. Because of increased gastric pH, oral tablets and capsules that require high levels of acid for absorption may take longer to dissolve, and, therefore take longer to become available to the tissues.

Distribution: Increased body fat in the geriatric patient provides a larger storage compartment for lipid-soluble drugs and vitamins. Plasma levels are reduced, and the therapeutic response is diminished. Older adults have less body water, making the effects of dehydration more dramatic and increasing the risk for drug toxicity. For example, elderly patients who have reduced body fluid experience more orthostatic hypotension. The decline in lean body mass and total body water leads to an increased concentration of water-soluble drugs, because the drug is distributed in a smaller volume of water. The aging liver produces less albumin, resulting in decreased plasma protein-binding ability and increased levels of free drug in the bloodstream, thereby increasing the potential for drug–drug interactions. The aging cardiovascular system has decreased cardiac output and less efficient blood circulation, which slow drug distribution. This makes it important to initiate pharmacotherapy with smaller dosages and slowly increase the amount to a safe, effective level.

Metabolism: Enzyme production in the liver decreases and the visceral blood flow is diminished, resulting in reduced hepatic drug metabolism. This change leads to an increase in the half-life of many drugs, which prolongs and intensifies drug response. The decline in hepatic function reduces first-pass metabolism. (Recall that first-pass metabolism relates to the amount of a drug that is removed from the bloodstream during the first circulation through the liver after the drug is absorbed by the intestinal tract.) Thus, plasma levels are elevated, and tissue concentrations are increased for the particular drug. This change alters the standard dosage, the interval between doses, and the duration of side effects.

Excretion: Older adults have reduced renal blood flow, glomerular filtration rate, active tubular secretion, and nephron function. This decreases drug excretion for drugs that are eliminated by the kidneys. When excretion is reduced, serum drug levels and the potential for toxicity markedly increase. Administration schedules and dosage amounts may need to be altered in many older adults due to these changes in kidney function. Keep in mind that the most common etiology of adverse drug reactions in older adults is caused by the accumulation of toxic amounts of drugs secondary to impaired renal excretion.

TREATING THE DIVERSE PATIENT

Patients with Speaking, Visual, or Hearing Impairments

Verbal communication disorders may make obtaining responses from the patient difficult. Communication may be facilitated by having the patient write or draw responses. Clarify by paraphrasing the response back to the patient. Use gestures, body language, and yes/no questions if writing or drawing is difficult. Allow adequate time for responses. Be especially aware of nonverbal clues, such as grimacing, when performing interventions that may cause discomfort or pain.

Provide adequate lighting for patients with visual impairments and be aware of how the phrasing of verbal communication affects the message conveyed. Remember that the nonverbal cues involved in communication may be missed by the patient. Paraphrase responses back to patients to be sure they understood the message in the absence of nonverbal cues. Explain interventions in detail before implementing procedures or activities with the patient.

Patients with hearing impairments benefit from communication that is spoken clearly and slowly in a low-pitched voice. Sit near the patient and avoid speaking loudly or shouting, especially if hearing devices are used. Limit the amount of background noise when possible. Write or draw to clarify verbal communication, and use nonverbal gestures and body language to aid communication. Allow adequate time for communication and responses. Alert other members of the health care team that the patient has a hearing impairment and may not hear a verbal answer to the nurse's call light given over an intercom system.

 # Chapter REVIEW

KEY CONCEPTS

The numbered key concepts provide a succinct summary of the important points from the corresponding numbered section within the chapter. If any of these points are not clear, refer to the numbered section within the chapter for review.

7.1 To contribute to safe and effective pharmacotherapy, it is essential for the nurse to understand and apply fundamental concepts of growth and development.

7.2 The effects of drugs on a growing embryo or fetus depends on gestational stage and the amount of drug received. Pharmacotherapy during pregnancy should be conducted only when the benefits to the mother outweigh the potential risks to the unborn child. Pregnancy categories guide the health care provider in prescribing drugs for these patients.

7.3 Breast-feeding women must be aware that many drugs and other substances can appear in milk and cause adverse effects to the infant.

7.4 Patient education is especially critical during pregnancy and lactation for the safety of the mother and baby and to ensure successful pharmacologic outcomes.

7.5 During infancy, pharmacotherapy is directed toward the safety of the child and teaching the parents how to properly administer medications and care for the infant.

7.6 Drug administration to toddlers can be challenging; short, concrete explanations followed by immediate drug administration are usually best for the toddler.

7.7 Preschool and younger school-age children can begin to assist with medication administration.

7.8 Pharmacologic compliance in the adolescent is dependent on an understanding of and respect for the uniqueness of the person in this stage of growth and development.

7.9 Young adults constitute the healthiest age group and generally need few prescription medications. Middle-aged adults begin to suffer from stress-related illness such as hypertension.

7.10 Older adults take more medications and experience more adverse drug events than any other age group. For drug therapy to be successful, the nurse must make accommodations for age-related changes in physiological and biochemical functions.

NCLEX-RN® REVIEW QUESTIONS

1 A 16-year-old adolescent is 6 weeks pregnant. The pregnancy has exacerbated her acne. She asks the nurse if she can resume taking her isotretinoin (Accutane) prescription, a category X drug. The best response by the nurse is:
1. "Since you have a prescription for Accutane, it is safe to resume using it."
2. "You should check with your physician at your next visit."
3. "Accutane is known to cause birth defects and should never be taken during pregnancy."
4. "You should reduce the Accutane dosage by half during pregnancy."

2 To reduce the effect of a prescribed medication on the infant of a breast-feeding mother, the nurse should plan to administer the medication:
1. at night.
2. immediately before the next feeding.
3. in divided doses at regular intervals around the clock.
4. immediately after breast-feeding.

3 A patient has arthritis in her hands. She takes several prescription drugs. Which statement by this patient requires follow-up by the nurse?
1. "My pharmacist puts my pills in screw-top bottles to make it easier for me to take them."
2. "I fill my prescriptions once per month."
3. "I care for my 2-year-old grandson twice a week."
4. "My arthritis medicine helps my stiff hands."

4 A nurse is administering a liquid medication to a 15-month-old child. The most appropriate approach by the nurse is to:
1. tell the child the medication is candy.
2. mix the medication in 8 oz of orange juice.
3. ask the child if she would like to take her medication now.
4. sit the child up, hold the medicine cup to her lips, and kindly instruct her to drink.

5 The nurse is preparing to give an injection to an infant. Using the image provided, select the preferred site for injections for newborns and infants.

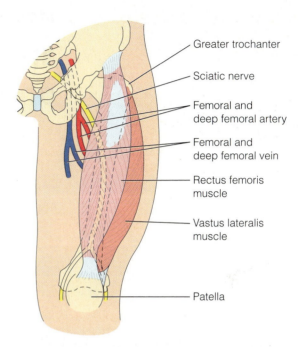

Greater trochanter

Sciatic nerve

Femoral and deep femoral artery

Femoral and deep femoral vein

Rectus femoris muscle

Vastus lateralis muscle

Patella

6 To reduce the chance of polypharmacy in the older adult, the nurse should:
1. call in all prescriptions to the patient's pharmacies rather than relying on paper copies of prescriptions.
2. give all prescriptions to the patient's family member.
3. take an OTC, prescription, and "pharmacy" history with each patient visit.
4. work with the patient's health care provider to limit the number of prescriptions.

CRITICAL THINKING QUESTIONS

1. A 22-year-old pregnant patient is diagnosed with pyelonephritis, and an antibiotic is prescribed. What information does the nurse need to safely administer the drug?

2. An 86-year-old male patient is confused and anxious. His daughter wonders if "a small dose" of diazepam (Valium) might help her father to be less anxious. Prior to responding to the daughter or consulting the prescribing authority, the nurse should review age-related concerns. What are the nurse's concerns?

3. An 8-month-old child is prescribed acetaminophen (Tylenol) elixir for management of fever. She is recovering from gastroenteritis and is still having several loose stools each day. The child spits some of the elixir on her shirt.

Does the nurse repeat the dose? What are the implications of this child's age and physical condition for oral drug administration?

See Appendix D for answers and rationales for all activities.

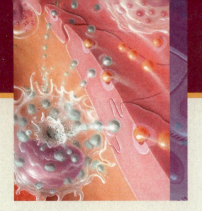

Chapter 8

Psychosocial, Gender, and Cultural Influences on Pharmacotherapy

LEARNING OUTCOMES

After reading this chapter, the student should be able to:

1. Describe fundamental concepts underlying a holistic approach to patient care and their importance to pharmacotherapy.
2. Describe the components of the human integration pyramid model.
3. Identify psychosocial and spiritual factors that can affect pharmacotherapeutics.
4. Explain how ethnicity can affect pharmacotherapeutic outcomes.
5. Identify examples of how cultural values and beliefs can influence pharmacotherapeutic outcomes.
6. Explain how community and environmental factors can affect health care outcomes.
7. Convey how genetic polymorphisms can influence pharmacotherapy.
8. Relate the implications of gender to the actions of certain drugs.

KEY TERMS

cultural competence *page 78*
culture *page 78*
ethnicity *page 78*

genetic polymorphism *page 80*
holistic *page 77*
human integration pyramid *page 77*

pharmacogenetics *page 80*
psychosocial *page 77*
spirituality *page 77*

It is convenient for a nurse to memorize an average drug dose, administer the medication, and expect all patients to achieve the same outcomes. Unfortunately, this is rarely the case. For pharmacotherapy to be successful, the nurse must assess and evaluate the needs of each individual patient. In chapter 4∞, variables such as absorption, metabolism, plasma protein binding, and excretion mechanisms were examined to help explain how these modify patient responses to drugs. In chapter 5∞, variability among patient responses was explained in terms of differences in drug–receptor interactions. Chapter 7∞ examined how pharmacokinetic and pharmacodynamic factors change patient responses to drugs throughout the life span. This chapter examines additional psychological, social, and biologic variables that must be considered to achieve optimum outcomes from pharmacotherapy.

8.1 The Concept of Holistic Pharmacotherapy

To deliver the highest quality of care, the nurse must fully recognize the individuality and totality of the patient. Each person must be viewed as an integrated biologic, psychosocial, cultural, communicating whole, existing and functioning within the communal environment. Simply stated, the recipient of care must be regarded in a **holistic** context to better understand how established risk factors such as age, genetics, biologic characteristics, personal habits, lifestyle, and environment increase a person's likelihood of acquiring specific diseases. Pharmacology has taken the study of these characteristics one step further—to examine and explain how they influence pharmacotherapeutic outcomes.

The **human integration pyramid,** shown in ➤ Figure 8.1, serves as a conceptual framework in dealing with patients in a holistic manner. This model provides a useful approach to addressing the nursing and pharmacologic needs of patients within the health care delivery system. All levels of the pyramid are interconnected and interdependent. Thus, when considering a patient's pharmacologic treatment plan, all levels of the pyramid are considered. For example, when giving a medication for the treatment of hypertension, an elderly man may experience greater effects from the medication than a younger man (age corollaries) or a woman in young adulthood (age and gender). Furthermore, patients may have different treatment outcomes related to cultural/ethnic differences because they may metabolize drugs to a different extent. By considering the levels of the human integration pyramid, the nurse can help ensure that the pharmacotherapy is not only treating symptoms, but is addressing issues related to the total patient.

By its very nature, modern (Western) medicine as it is practiced in the United States is seemingly incompatible with holistic medicine. Western medicine focuses on specific diseases, their causes, and treatments. Disease is viewed as a malfunction of a specific organ or system. Sometimes, the disease is viewed even more specifically, and categorized as a change in DNA structure or a malfunction of one enzyme. Sophisticated technology is used to identify, image, and classify the specific structural or functional abnormality. Somehow, the total patient is lost in this focus of categorizing disease. Too often, it does not matter how or why the patient developed cancer, diabetes, or hypertension, or how he or she feels about it; the psychosocial and cultural dimensions are lost. Yet, these dimensions can have a profound impact on the success of pharmacotherapy. The nurse must consciously direct care toward a *holistic* treatment of each individual patient, in his or her psychosocial, spiritual, and communal context.

8.2 Psychosocial Influences on Pharmacotherapy

The term **psychosocial** is often used in health care to describe one's psychological development in the context of one's social environment. This involves both the social and psychological aspects of a person's life. **Spirituality** incorporates the capacity to love, to convey compassion and empathy, to give and forgive, to enjoy life, and to find peace of mind and fulfillment in living. The spiritual life overlaps with components of the emotional, mental, physical, and social aspects of living.

From a health care perspective, every human being should be considered as an integrated psychosocial, spiritual being. Health impairments related to an individual's psychosocial situation often require a blending of individualized nursing care and therapeutic drugs, in conjunction with psychotherapeutic counseling. The term *psycho-social-spiritual* is appearing more frequently in nursing literature. It is now acknowledged that when patients have strong spiritual or religious beliefs, these may greatly influence their perceptions of illness and even affect the outcomes of pharmacotherapy. When illness imposes threats to health, the patient commonly presents with psychological, social, and

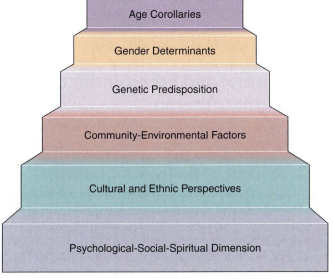

➤ *Figure 8.1* The human integration pyramid care model

spiritual issues along with physical symptoms. Patients face concerns related to ill health, suffering, loneliness, despair, and death, and at the same time look for meaning, value, and hope in their situation. Such issues can have a great impact on wellness and preferred methods of medical treatment, nursing care, and pharmacotherapy.

The psychosocial history of the patient is an essential component of the initial interview and assessment. This history delves into the personal life of the patient, with inquiries directed toward lifestyle preferences, religious beliefs, sexual practices, alcohol intake, and tobacco and nonprescription drug use. The nurse must demonstrate sensitivity when gathering these types of data. If a trusting nurse–patient relationship is not quickly established, the patient will be reluctant to share important personal data that could affect nursing care.

The psychological dimension can exert a strong influence on pharmacotherapy. Patients who are convinced that their treatment is important and beneficial to their well-being will demonstrate better compliance with drug therapy. The nurse must ascertain the patient's goals in seeking treatment, and determine whether drug therapy is compatible with those goals. Past experiences with health care may lead a patient to distrust medications. Drugs may not be acceptable for the social environment of the patient. For example, having to take drugs at school or in the workplace may cause embarrassment; patients may fear that they will be viewed as weak, unhealthy, or dependent. Some patients may believe that certain medications, such as antidepressants or antiseizure medications carry a social stigma, and therefore they will resist using them.

Patients who display positive attitudes toward their personal health and have high expectations regarding the results of their pharmacotherapy are more likely to achieve positive outcomes. The nurse plays a pivotal role in encouraging the patient's positive expectations. The nurse must always be forthright in explaining drug actions and potential side effects. Trivializing the limitations of pharmacotherapy or minimizing potential adverse effects can cause the patient to have unrealistic expectations regarding treatment. The nurse–patient relationship may be jeopardized, and the patient may acquire an attitude of distrust. As discussed in chapter 9∞, the patient has an ethical and legal right to receive accurate information regarding the benefits and effects of drug therapy.

8.3 Cultural and Ethnic Influences on Pharmacotherapy

Although often used interchangeably, the definitions of culture and ethnicity are somewhat different. An ethnic group is a community of people that share a common ancestry and similar genetic heritage. **Ethnicity** implies that people have biologic and genetic similarities. **Culture** is a set of beliefs, values, and norms that provide meaning for an individual or group. People within a culture have common rituals, religious beliefs, language, and certain expectations of behavior. Cultural and ethnic variables are important aspects of patient care that directly relate to pharmacotherapy. Both have a profound influence on patient outcomes and the oc-

---

TREATING THE DIVERSE PATIENT

Medication Adherence

Poor adherence to a prescribed medication is becoming known as America's "other drug problem" but one that has health and financial consequences even greater than substance abuse. It is estimated that approximately 50% of the 2 billion prescriptions filled each year are taken incorrectly; while one third of patients take all of their medication, one third take some, and one third do not take any at all or never fill the prescription. Approximately 23% of nursing home admissions may be due to poor medication adherence and as many as 10% of all hospital admissions. The medically underserved population, Americans of all ethnic backgrounds who are poor, lack health insurance, or have inadequate access to health care, are one of the groups most at risk.

Nurses serve a vital role in increasing medication adherence, both because of the trustful relationship nurses establish with their patients, and because they are often the main source of medication education for the patient and their families. Providing simple drug information to help the patient understand why a medication is required, when and how it should be taken, and when to call the health care provider is vital information to help increase medication adherence. With each successive health care visit, the nurse can go over the medication history, asking questions about prescribed medications, being alert to reports that the patient is not taking, or is not taking correctly, the prescribed drugs. As economic conditions sometimes result in difficult decisions between obtaining medications and other required necessities, nurses are among the health care providers in the forefront of providing medication education and follow-up that will result in positive outcomes to health and preventing negative health effects, and even larger expenditures, as a result of poor medication adherence.

---

currence of specific drug effects as perceived and interpreted by the user.

Although non-Caucasians comprise more than 25% of the U.S. population, modern clinical pharmacology has been based largely on research and clinical experiences with Caucasians. Some research now suggests that variations in metabolic processes among various ethnic groups can significantly impact drug therapy. Through technologic advancement, researchers have identified specific regions on various chromosomes that influence hepatic metabolism. Certain antidysrhythmics, antidepressants, and opioids may be metabolized differently in individuals of African, Native American, and Asian descent. As technology advances, nurses will likely begin to see variations in the prescribed amounts and forms of medication based upon the ethnicity of the patient.

Although it is impossible to have complete knowledge about the many cultural variations among patients, the nurse can strive to understand the significance of the cultural traditions and their potential impact on the patient's care. People hold cultural beliefs (religious or ideologic) that may challenge or conflict with what the health care provider believes to be in the best interests of the patient. How illness is defined can be based on the cultural beliefs of an individual. One example that illustrates this point is the difference in belief systems between age groups—each with its own unique culture.

Cultural competence in health care is the ability of practitioners to provide care to people with diverse values, beliefs, and behaviors, including the ability to adapt delivery of care to meet the needs of these patients. Cultural competence requires knowledge of this diversity, as well as an attitude of openness and sensitivity. Understanding and respecting the beliefs of the patient are keys to establishing and maintaining positive therapeutic relationships in culturally sensitive nursing care. Therapeutic communication mandates that all health care providers bear in mind the cultural, racial, and social factors that comprise each person, and how these affect behavior. Nurses can instill trust by attentiveness to individual patient beliefs and support patients' desires to seek adequate medical care when it is needed.

The nurse must keep in mind the following variables when treating patients from different ethnic groups.

- *Dietary considerations:* Cultures vary in their dietary preferences and practices. Diets that include (or exclude) certain foods have the potential to increase or decrease the effectiveness of a medication. Certain spices and herbs important to a patient's culture may affect pharmacotherapy. For example, some cultures include a diet with abundant amounts of cheese, pickled fish, or wine that can interact with medications. Certain herbs can affect antidepressants, anticoagulants, and beta blockers. Assessing the primary foods of a patient's culture is an important component of the patient's psychosocial history.

- *Alternative therapies:* Various cultural groups believe in using alternative therapies, such as vitamins, herbs, or acupuncture, either along with or in place of modern medicines. Some folk remedies and traditional treatments have existed for thousands of years and helped form the foundation for modern medical practice. For example, Chinese patients may consult with herbalists to treat diseases whereas Native Americans may collect, store, and use herbs to treat and prevent disease. Certain Hispanic cultures use spices and herbs to maintain a balance of hot and cold to promote wellness. The nurse can assess the treatments used and interpret the effect of these herbal and alternative therapies on the prescribed medications to maximize positive outcomes. The nurse can explain that certain herbs or supplements may cause potential health risks when combined with prescribed drugs.

- *Beliefs about health and disease:* Cultures view health and illness in different ways. Individuals may seek assistance from people in their own community who they believe have healing powers. Native Americans may consult with a tribal medicine man while Hispanics seek a folk healer. African Americans sometimes practice healing through the gift of laying-on-of-hands. The nurse's understanding of the patient's trust in alternative healers is important. The more nurses know about cultural beliefs, the better they can provide support and guidance to patients.

8.4 Community and Environmental Influences on Pharmacotherapy

A number of community and environmental factors have been identified that influence disease and its subsequent treatment. Population growth, complex technologic ad-

PHARMFACTS

Minority Statistics and Health Care

- In 2000, the majority ethnic group in the United States was non-Hispanic Whites, at 71%.

- By 2025, the population of non-Hispanic Whites is expected to decrease to 62%, and then fall to 55% by 2045.

- Sometime between 2050 and 2060, non-Hispanic White persons will themselves become a "minority," shrinking to less than half of all Americans.

- The infant death rate among African Americans is more than double that of whites. Heart disease death rates are more than 40% higher for African Americans than for whites. The death rate for all cancers is 30% higher for African Americans than for whites; for prostate cancer, it is more than double that for whites.

- Hispanics living in the United States are almost twice as likely to die from diabetes as are non-Hispanic whites. Hispanics also have higher rates of high blood pressure and obesity than non-Hispanic whites.

- Native Americans have an infant death rate almost double that for whites. The rate of diabetes for this population group is more than twice that for whites.

Source: "About Minority Health," Centers for Disease Control. Retrieved May 21, 2009, from http://www.cdc.gov/omhd/AMH/AMH.htm

vances, and evolving globalization patterns have all affected health care. Communities vary significantly in regard to population density, age distributions, socioeconomic levels, occupational patterns, and industrial growth. In much of the world, people live in areas lacking adequate sanitation and potable water supplies. All these community and environmental factors have the potential to affect health and access to pharmacotherapy.

Access to health care is perhaps the most obvious community-related influence on pharmacotherapy. There are many potential barriers to obtaining appropriate health care. Without an adequate health insurance plan, some people are reluctant to seek health care for fear of bankrupting the family unit. Older adults fear losing their retirement savings or being placed in a nursing home for the remainder of their lives. Families living in rural areas may have to travel great distances to obtain necessary treatment. Once treatment is rendered, the cost of prescription drugs may be far too high for patients on limited incomes. The nurse must be aware of these variables and have knowledge of social agencies in the local community that can assist in improving health care access.

Literacy is another community-related variable that can affect health care. Up to 48% of English-speaking patients do not have functional literacy—a basic ability to read, understand, and act on health information (Andrus & Roth, 2002). The functional illiteracy rate is even higher in certain populations, particularly non–English-speaking individuals and older patients. The nurse must be aware that these patients may not be able to read drug labels, understand written treatment instructions, or read brochures describing their disease or therapy. Functional illiteracy can result in a lack of understanding about the importance of

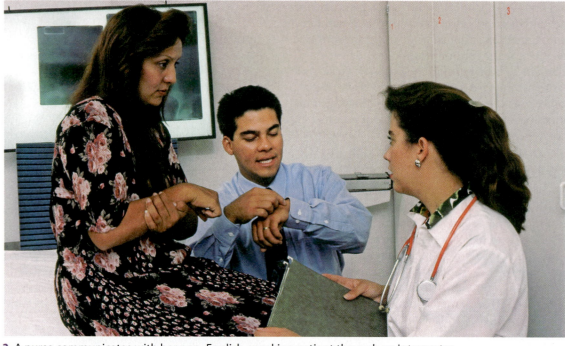

➤ *Figure 8.2* A nurse communicates with her non–English-speaking patient through an interpreter
Source: Pearson Education/PH College.

pharmacotherapy and can lead to poor compliance. The nurse must attempt to identify these patients and provide them with brochures, instructions, and educational materials that can be understood. For non–English-speaking patients or those for whom English is their second language, the nurse should have proper materials in the patient's primary language, or provide an interpreter who can help with accurate translations (➤ Figure 8.2). The nurse should ask the patient to repeat important instructions, to ensure comprehension. The use of graphic-rich materials is appropriate for certain therapies.

8.5 Genetic Influences on Pharmacotherapy

Although 99.8% of human DNA sequences are alike, the remaining 0.2% may result in significant differences in patients' ability to handle certain medications. Some of these differences are created when a mutation occurs in the portion of DNA responsible for encoding a certain metabolic enzyme. A single base mutation in DNA may result in an amino acid change in the enzyme, which alters its function. This creates a **genetic polymorphism**—two or more versions of the same enzyme. The best characterized genetic polymorphisms have been discovered in enzymes that metabolize drugs, and in proteins that serve as receptors for drugs. **Pharmacogenetics** is the study of genetic variations that give rise to differences in the way patients handle medications.

Genetic polymorphisms are most often identified in specific ethnic groups, because people in an ethnic group have been located in the same geographic area and have married

PHARMFACTS

Community Health Statistics in the United States

- Americans who live in the suburbs fare significantly better in many key health measures than those who live in the most rural and the most urban areas.

- Those who live in the suburbs of large metropolitan areas have the lowest infant mortality rates and are more likely to have health insurance and healthy lifestyles.

- Death rates for working-age adults are higher in the most rural and most urban areas.

- The highest death rates for children and young adults are in the most rural counties.

- Homicide rates are highest in the central counties of large metropolitan areas.

- Suburban residents are more likely to exercise during leisure time and more likely to have health insurance. Suburban women are the least likely to be obese.

- Both the most rural and most urban areas have a similarly high percentage of residents without health insurance.

- Teenagers and adults in rural counties are the most likely to smoke.

- Residents of the most rural communities have the fewest visits for dental care.

Source: www.cdc.gov/nchs

others within the same group for hundreds of generations. Although genetic polymorphisms are generally rare in the overall population, specific ethnic groups can sometimes express a very high incidence of these defects.

TABLE 8.1	Enzyme Polymorphisms of Importance to Pharmacotherapy	
Enzyme	Result of Polymorphism	Drugs Using This Metabolic Enzyme/Pathway
Acetyltransferase	Slow acetylation in Scandinavians, Jews, North African Caucasians; fast acetylation in Japanese	caffeine, hydralazine, isoniazid, procainamide
Debrisoquin hydroxylase	Poorly metabolized in Asians and African Americans	amitriptyline, imipramine, perphenazine, haloperidol, propranolol, metoprolol, codeine, morphine
Mephenytoin hydroxylase	Poorly metabolized in Asians and African Americans	diazepam, imipramine, barbiturates, warfarin

The relationship between genetic make-up and drug response has been documented for decades. The first polymorphism was discovered in acetyltransferase, an enzyme that metabolizes isoniazid (INH), a drug prescribed for tuberculosis. The metabolic process, known as *acetylation*, occurs abnormally slowly in certain Caucasians. The reduced hepatic metabolism and subsequent clearance by the kidney can cause the drug to build to toxic levels in these patients, who are known as *slow acetylators*. The opposite effect, fast acetylation, is found in many patients of Japanese descent.

In recent years, several other enzyme polymorphisms have been identified. Asian Americans are less able to metabolize codeine to morphine due to a genetic absence of the enzyme debrisoquin, a defect that interferes with the analgesic properties of codeine. Some persons of African American descent have decreased effects from beta-adrenergic antagonist drugs such as propranolol (Inderal), because of genetic variances in plasma renin levels. Another set of oxidation enzyme polymorphisms have been found that alter the response to warfarin (Coumadin) and diazepam (Valium). Table 8.1 summarizes the three most common polymorphisms. Expanding knowledge about the physiological impact of heredity on pharmacotherapy may someday allow for personalization of the treatment process.

8.6 Gender Influences on Pharmacotherapy

There are well-established differences in the patterns of disease between males and females. For example, women tend to pay more attention to changes in health patterns and seek health care earlier than their male counterparts. However, many women do not seek medical attention for potential cardiac problems, because heart disease has traditionally been considered to be a "man's disease." Alzheimer's disease affects both men and women, but studies in various populations have shown that between 1.5 and 3 times as many women suffer from the disease. Alzheimer's disease is becoming recognized as a major "women's health issue," along with osteoporosis, breast cancer, and fertility disorders.

Adherence with the prescribed medication regimen may be influenced by gender because the side effects are specific to either males or females. A common example is certain antihypertensive agents that have the potential to cause or worsen male impotence. Several different drugs can cause gynecomastia, an increase in breast size, which can be embarrassing for males. Similarly, certain drugs can cause masculine side effects such as increased hair growth, which can be a cause of nonadherence in women taking these medications. Also in females, the estrogen contained in oral contraceptives causes an elevated risk of thromboembolic disorders. With effective communication, gender-specific concerns regarding drug adverse effects can be brought into the open so alternative drug therapies can be considered. As with so many areas of health care, appropriate patient teaching by the nurse is a key aspect in preventing or alleviating drug-related health problems.

Local and systemic responses to some medications can differ between genders. These response differences may be based on differences in body composition such as the fat-to-muscle ratio. In addition, cerebral blood flow variances between males and females may alter the response to certain analgesics. An example is the benzodiazepines given for anxiety; women experience slower elimination rates and this difference becomes more significant if the woman is taking oral contraceptives.

In the past, the majority of drug research studies were conducted using only male subjects. It was wrongly assumed that the conclusions of these studies applied in the same manner to women. Since 1993, the FDA has formalized policies that require the inclusion of subjects of both genders during drug development. This includes analyses of clinical data by gender, assessment of potential pharmacokinetic and pharmacodynamic differences between genders, and, when appropriate, conducting additional studies specific to women's health.

Also of concern is gender inequity regarding prescription drug coverage. A common example is employer health plans that exclude women's contraceptive medications. It was not until a federal district court ruling in June 2001 that exclusion of prescription of female contraceptives by an employer's health care provider was deemed sex discrimination.

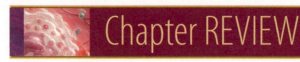

Chapter REVIEW

KEY CONCEPTS

The numbered key concepts provide a succinct summary of the important points from the corresponding numbered section within the chapter. If any of these points are not clear, refer to the numbered section within the chapter for review.

8.1 To deliver effective treatment, the nurse must consider the total patient in a holistic context.

8.2 The psychosocial domain must be considered when delivering holistic care. Positive attitudes and high expectations toward therapeutic outcomes in the patient may influence the success of pharmacotherapy.

8.3 Culture and ethnicity are two interconnected perspectives that can affect nursing care and pharmacotherapy. Differences in diet, use of alternative therapies, perceptions of wellness, and genetic makeup can influence patient drug response.

8.4 Community and environmental factors affect health and the public's access to health care and pharmacotherapy. Inadequate access to health care resources and an inability to read or understand instructions may compromise treatment outcomes.

8.5 Genetic differences in metabolic enzymes that occur among different ethnic groups must be considered for effective pharmacotherapy. Small differences in the structure of enzymes can result in profound changes in drug response.

8.6 Gender can influence many aspects of health maintenance, promotion, and treatment, as well as medication response.

NCLEX-RN® REVIEW QUESTIONS

1 The patient informs the nurse that he will use herbal compounds given by a family member to treat his hypertension. The appropriate action by the nurse is to:
1. inform the patient that the herbal treatments will be ineffective.
2. obtain more information and determine whether the herbs are compatible with medications prescribed.
3. notify the physician immediately.
4. inform the patient that the physician will not treat him if he does not accept the use of traditional medicine only.

2 The nurse provides teaching about a drug to an elderly couple. To ensure that the instructions are understood, the nurse should: (Select all that apply.)
1. provide detailed written material about the drug.
2. provide labels and instructions in large print.
3. assess the reading levels and have patients repeat instructions to determine understanding.
4. provide instructions only when family members are present.

3 The nurse must understand gender issues related to drug therapy. Important considerations include which of the following facts?
1. Men seek health care earlier than women.
2. Women suffer from Alzheimer's disease in greater numbers than men.
3. Women are more likely to stop taking medications because of side effects.
4. All drug trials are conducted on male subjects.

4 The patient informs the nurse that she will decide whether she will accept treatment after she prays with her family and minister. The nurse recognizes the role of spirituality in drug therapy as:
1. irrelevant because medications act on scientific principles.
2. important to the patient's acceptance of medical treatment and response to treatment.
3. harmless if it makes the patient feel better.
4. harmful, especially if treatment is delayed.

5 The nurse knows that patients characterized as slow acetylators:
1. are more prone to drug toxicity.
2. require more time to absorb enteral medications.
3. must be given liquid medications only.
4. should be advised to decrease protein intake.

6 A patient undergoing treatment for cancer complains about nausea and fatigue. In approaching this patient problem holistically, the nurse would:
1. give an antinausea drug as ordered and place the patient on bedrest.
2. observe for specific instances of nausea or fatigue and report them to the oncologist.
3. take a medication history on the patient, noting specific medication or food triggers.
4. talk to the patient about the symptoms, the impact they have on daily activities, and techniques that have helped lessen the problem.

CRITICAL THINKING QUESTIONS

1. A 72-year-old African American heart patient who has been treated for atrial flutter is taking warfarin (Coumadin) 2.5 mg PO once a day. He comes to the clinic for his routine international normalized ratio (INR), which is no longer in the therapeutic range. The patient lives in a rural area and has a large vegetable garden. What questions would a nurse need to ask to evaluate the cause of the decreased drug effectiveness?

2. An 82-year-old female patient is admitted to the emergency department. She has been taking furosemide (Lasix) 40 mg PO daily as part of a regimen for congestive heart failure. She is confused, dehydrated, and has lost 12 pounds this week. What gender-related considerations should the nurse make when assessing this patient?

3. A 19-year-old male patient of Mexican descent presents to a health clinic for migrant farm workers. In broken English, he describes severe pain in his lower jaw. An assessment reveals two abscessed molars and other oral health problems. Discuss the probable reasons for this patient's condition.

See Appendix D for answers and rationales for all activities.

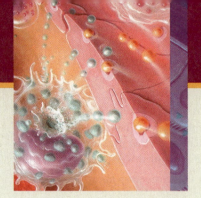

Chapter 9

Medication Errors and Risk Reduction

LEARNING OUTCOMES

After reading this chapter, the student should be able to:

1. Define medication error.
2. Identify factors that contribute to medication errors.
3. Describe specific categories of medication errors.
4. Explain the impact of medication errors on all aspects of a health care agency.
5. Describe methods of documenting medication errors and occurrences.
6. Describe strategies that the nurse can implement to reduce medication errors and incidents.
7. Identify patient teaching information that can be used to reduce medication errors and incidents.
8. Identify efforts recommended by the FDA to monitor medication errors and incidents and provide information to health care providers.
9. Explain strategies used by health care organizations to reduce the number of medication errors and incidents.

KEY TERMS

In their clinical practice, nurses maximize patient safety by striving to be 100% accurate when administering medications. Drug administration, however, requires multiple complex steps by physicians, pharmacists, nurses, and patients and can never be 100% error free. Occasionally medication errors are made that can significantly impact treatment outcomes. The purpose of this chapter is to examine the reasons for medication errors and explore strategies the nurse may use to prevent them.

9.1 Defining Medication Errors

According to the National Coordinating Council for Medication Error Reporting and Prevention (NCC MERP), a **medication error** is "any preventable event that may cause or lead to inappropriate medication use or patient harm while the medication is in the control of the health care professional, patient, or consumer." NCC MERP also classifies medication errors and has developed the **medication error index.** This index categorizes medication errors by evaluating the extent of the harm an error can cause (➤ Figure 9.1).

Stated simply, a medication error is any error that occurs in the medication administration process whether or not it harms the patient. These errors may be related to misinterpretations, miscalculations, misadministrations, handwriting misinterpretation, and misunderstanding of verbal or phone orders.

9.2 Factors Contributing to Medication Errors

To be successful, proper medication administration involves a partnership between the health care provider and the patient. This relationship is dependent on the competence of the health care provider, as well as the patient's full adherence with the drug therapy regimen. This dual responsibility provides a simple, though useful, way to conceptualize medication errors as resulting from health care provider error or patient error. Clearly, the purpose of classifying and studying these errors is not to assess individual blame but to prevent future errors.

Factors contributing to medication errors by *health care providers* include, but are not limited to, the following:

- Omitting one of the rights of drug administration (chapter 4 ∞). Common errors include giving an incorrect dose, not giving an ordered dose, and giving the wrong drug.
- Failing to perform an agency system check. Both pharmacists and nurses must collaborate on checking the accuracy and appropriateness of drug orders prior to administering drugs to patients.
- Failing to account for patient variables such as age, body size, and impairment in renal or hepatic function. Nurses should always review recent laboratory data and

other information in the patient's chart before administering medications, especially for those drugs that have a narrow margin of safety.

- Giving medications based on verbal orders or phone orders, which may be misinterpreted or go undocumented. Nurses should remind the prescriber that medication orders must be in writing before the drug can be administered.
- Giving medications based on an incomplete order or an illegible order, when the nurse is unsure of the correct drug, dosage, or administration method. Incomplete orders should be clarified with the prescriber before the medication is administered. Written orders should avoid certain abbreviations that are frequent sources of medication errors, as listed in Table 9.1.
- Practicing under stressful work conditions. Studies have correlated an increased number of errors with the stress level of nurses. Studies have also indicated that the rate of medication errors may increase when individual nurses are assigned to patients who are the most acutely ill.

Patients, or their home caregivers, may also contribute to medication errors by:

- Taking drugs prescribed by several practitioners without informing each of their health care providers about all prescribed medications.
- Getting their prescriptions filled at more than one pharmacy.
- Not filling or refilling their prescriptions.
- Taking medications incorrectly.
- Taking medications that may have been left over from a previous illness or prescribed for something else.

9.3 The Impact of Medication Errors

Medication errors are the most common cause of morbidity and preventable death within hospitals. When a medication error occurs, the repercussions can be emotionally devastating for the nurse and extend beyond the particular nurse and patient involved. A medication error can lengthen the patient's stay in the hospital, which increases costs and the time that a patient is separated from his or her family. The nurse or physician making the medication error may suffer from self-doubt and embarrassment. If a high error rate occurs within a particular unit, the nursing unit may develop a poor reputation within the facility. If frequent medication errors or serious errors are publicized, the reputation of the facility may suffer, because it may be perceived as unsafe. Administrative personnel may also be penalized because of errors within their departments or the hospital as a whole.

There are no acceptable incidence rates for medication errors. The goal of every health care organization should be to improve medication administration systems to prevent harm to patients due to medication errors. All errors, whether or not they harm the patient, should be investigated

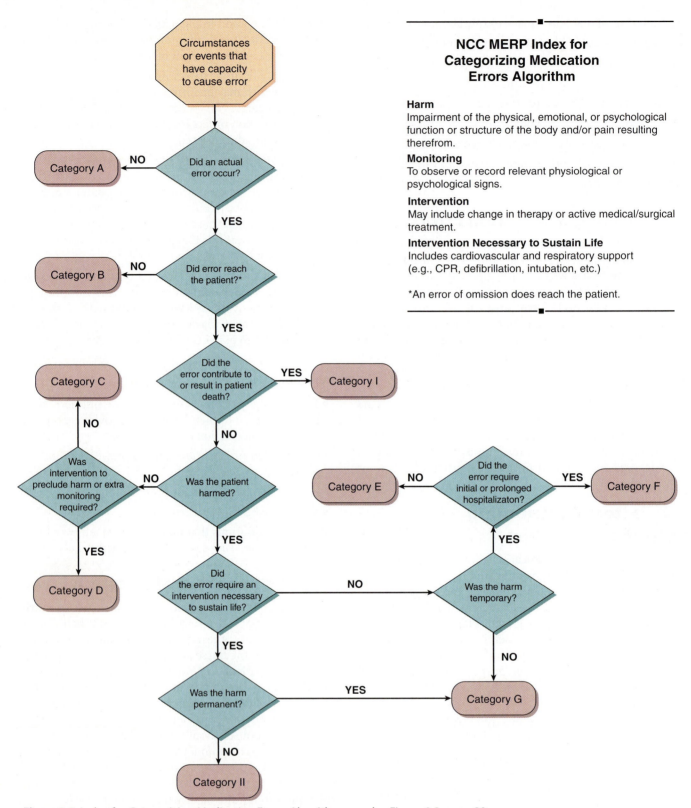

NCC MERP Index for Categorizing Medication Errors Algorithm

Harm
Impairment of the physical, emotional, or psychological function or structure of the body and/or pain resulting therefrom.

Monitoring
To observe or record relevant physiological or psychological signs.

Intervention
May include change in therapy or active medical/surgical treatment.

Intervention Necessary to Sustain Life
Includes cardiovascular and respiratory support (e.g., CPR, defibrillation, intubation, etc.)

*An error of omission does reach the patient.

➤ *Figure 9.1* Index for Categorizing Medication Errors Algorithm; see also Figure 9.2, page 89
Source: © 2001 National Coordinating Council for Medication Error Reporting and Prevention. All rights reserved.

with the goal of identifying ways to improve the medication administration process to prevent future errors. The investigation should occur in a nonpunitive manner that will encourage staff to report errors, thereby building a culture of safety within an organization. Analysis of error patterns can alert nurses and health care administrators that a new policy or procedure needs to be implemented to reduce or eliminate medication errors.

TABLE 9.1	Abbreviations to Avoid in Medication Administration	
Abbreviation	**Intended Meaning**	**Common Error**
U	Units	Mistaken as a zero or a four (4) resulting in overdose. Also mistaken for "cc" (cubic centimeters) when poorly written.
μg	Micrograms	Mistaken for "mg" (milligrams) resulting in an overdose.
q.d.	Latin abbreviation for every day	The period after the "Q" has sometimes been mistaken for an "I," and the drug has been given "QID" (four times daily) rather than daily.
q.o.d.	Latin abbreviation for every other day	Misinterpreted as "QD" (daily) or "QID" (four times daily). If the "O" is poorly written, it looks like a period or "I."
SC or SQ	Subcutaneous	Mistaken as "SL" (sublingual) when poorly written.
t i w	Three times a week	Misinterpreted as "three times a day" or "twice a week."
D/C	Discharge; also discontinue	Patient's medications have been prematurely discontinued when D/C, (intended to mean "discharge") was misinterpreted as "discontinue," because it was followed by a list of drugs.
hs	Half strength	Misinterpreted as the Latin abbreviation "HS" (hour of sleep).
cc	Cubic centimeters	Mistaken as "U" (units) when poorly written.
AU, AS, AD	Latin abbreviation for both ears, left ear, right ear	Misinterpreted as the Latin abbreviation "OU" (both eyes); "OS" (left eye); "OD" (right eye).
IU	International unit	Mistaken as IV (intravenous) or 10 (ten).
MS, MSO4, MgSO4	Confused for one another	Can mean morphine sulfate or magnesium sulfate.

Note: From the National Coordinating Council for Medication Error Reporting and Prevention, © 1998–2006. All Rights Reserved.

HOME & COMMUNITY CONSIDERATIONS

Preventing Medication Errors in the Home

The U.S. Pharmacopeia's Safe Medication Use Expert Committee (Santell & Cousins, 2004) reports that medication errors occurring in the home are the result of communication problems (21%), knowledge deficit (19%), and inadequate or lacking monitoring (4%). Ten percent of errors are caused by lack of access to information. Warfarin is the drug most frequently (9%) associated with medication errors in the home; next in frequency are insulin (7%), morphine (4%), and vancomycin (4%). At the top of the list of error type are improper dose (36%) and omission errors (28%). In this study, the patient, family, or caregiver is reported to be at fault in 39% of errors, the nurse in 36%, and the physician or pharmacist in 11%. This study points out the need for better patient education, a role in which the nurse plays a large part.

9.4 Reporting and Documenting Medication Errors

When a health care provider commits or observes an error, effects can be lasting and widespread. Although some errors go unreported, it is always the nurse's legal and ethical responsibility to report all occurrences. In severe cases, adverse reactions caused by medication errors may require the initiation of lifesaving interventions for the patient. After such an incident, the patient may require follow-up supervision and medical treatments.

The Food and Drug Administration (FDA) has coordinated the reporting of medication errors at the federal level. The FDA Safety Information and Adverse Event Reporting Program, known as MedWatch, provides important and timely clinical information about safety issues involving medical products, including prescription and over-the-counter (OTC) drugs, biologics, medical and radiation-emitting devices, and special nutritional products. The FDA encourages nurses and other health care providers to report medication errors for its database, which is used to assist other professionals in avoiding similar mistakes. Medication errors, or situations that can lead to errors, may be reported anonymously directly to the FDA by telephone or online. Since 1992, the FDA has received over 30,000 reports of medication errors. The number of actual errors may be much higher.

A second organization that has been established to provide assistance with medication errors is the National Coordinating Council for Medication Error Reporting and Prevention (NCC MERP). This organization was formed during the Pharmacopoeia Convention in 1995 to help standardize the medication error reporting system, examine interdisciplinary causes of medication errors, and promote medication safety. NCC MERP coordinates information on medication errors and provides medication error prevention education.

DOCUMENTING IN THE PATIENT'S MEDICAL RECORD

All facilities should have clear policies and procedures that provide guidance on reporting medication errors. Documentation of the error should occur in a factual manner: The nurse should avoid blaming or making judgments. Documentation does not simply record that a medical error occurred. Documentation in the medical record must include specific nursing interventions that were implemented following the error to protect patient safety, such as monitoring vital signs and assessing the patient for possible complications. Failure to report nursing actions implies either negligence (i.e., no interventions were taken) or lack of acknowledgement that the incident occurred. The nurse should also document all individuals who were notified of the error. The **medication administration record (MAR)** is another source that should contain information about what medication was given or omitted.

REPORTING THE ERROR   In addition to documenting in the patient's medical record, the nurse making or observing the medication error should complete a written report of the error. Depending on the health care agency, these reports may be called "Incident Reports," "Occurrence Reports," or similar titles. The specific details of the error should be recorded in a factual and objective manner. The report allows the nurse an opportunity to identify factors that contributed to the medication error and assists in identifying any specific performance improvement strategies that may need to be implemented. The written report is not included in the patient's medical record but is used by the agency's risk management personnel for quality improvement and assurance and may be used by nursing administration and education to identify common error occurrences and the need for performance improvement or educational intervention.

Accurate documentation in the medical record and in the error report is essential for legal reasons. These documents verify that the patient's safety was protected and serve as a tool to improve medication administration processes. Legal issues may worsen if there is an attempt to hide a mistake or delay corrective action, or if the nurse forgets to document interventions in the patient's chart.

Hospitals and health care agencies monitor medication errors through quality and performance improvement programs. The results of quality improvement programs alert staff and administrative personnel about trends within particular units and may serve as indicators of quality patient care. Through data collection, specific solutions can be created to reduce the number of medication errors. Root cause analysis, or RCA, is being implemented in many health care organizations as a method to prevent future mistakes. By answering three basic questions: What happened, why did it happen, and what can be done to prevent it from happening again?, RCA seeks to prevent another occurrence. Many agencies also continue RCA with the question, has the risk of recurrence actually been reduced?, by analyzing data postoccurrence. The overall goal of reporting medication errors and conducting follow-up assessments such as RCA, is safe and effective patient care and patient medication administration.

SENTINEL EVENTS   The Joint Commission, which accredits health care agencies, recognizes a particular form of event termed "sentinel events." Sentinel events are defined as "unexpected occurrences involving death or serious physical or psychological injury, or risk thereof" (Joint Commission, 2009). Not all errors are sentinel events and not all sentinel events occur because of an error. But because of the grave nature of the event, sentinel events are *always* investigated

and interventions put in place to ensure that the event does not recur. Root cause analysis is utilized to identify the causes and required intervention to prevent a recurrence.

9.5 Strategies for Reducing Medication Errors

What can the nurse do in the clinical setting to avoid medication errors and promote safe administration? The nurse can begin by following the steps of the nursing process:

1. *Assessment:*   Ask the patient about allergies to food or medications, current health concerns, and use of OTC medications and herbal supplements. For all medications taken prior to assessment, ensure that the patient has been receiving the right dose, at the right time, and by the right route. Assess kidney, liver, and other body system functions to determine if impairments are present that could affect pharmacotherapy. Identify areas of needed patient education with regard to medications.

2. *Planning:*   Minimize factors that contribute to medication errors: Avoid using abbreviations that can be misunderstood, question unclear orders, do not accept verbal orders, and follow specific facility policies and procedures related to medication administration. Have the patient restate dosing directions, including the correct dose of medication and the right time to take it. Ask the patient to demonstrate an understanding of the goals of therapy.

3. *Implementation:*   Be aware of and eliminate potential distractions during medication administration that could result in an error. When engaged in a medication-related task, focus entirely on the task. Noise, other events, and talking coworkers can distract the nurses' attention and result in a medication error. Practice the rights of medication administration: right patient, right time and frequency of administration, right dose, right route of administration, and right drug. Keep the following steps in mind as well:
   - Positively verify the identity of each patient using two means (e.g., name and birthdate) before administering the medication according to facility policy and procedures.
   - Use the correct procedures and techniques for all routes of administration. Use sterile materials and aseptic techniques when administering parenteral or eye medication.
   - Calculate medication doses correctly and measure liquid drugs carefully. Some medications, such as heparin, have a narrow safety margin. When giving these medications, ask a colleague or a pharmacist to check the calculations to make certain the dosage is correct. Always double-check pediatric calculations prior to administration.
   - Open medications immediately prior to administering the medication and in the presence of the patient.

- Record the medication on the MAR immediately after administration.
- Always confirm that the patient has swallowed the medication. Never leave the medication at the bedside unless there is a specific order that they may be left there.
- Be alert for long-acting oral dosage forms with indicators such as *LA*, *XL*, and *XR*. These tablets or capsules must remain intact for the extended-release feature to remain effective. Instruct the patient not to crush, chew, or break the medication in half, because doing so could cause an overdose.

4. *Evaluation:* Assess the patient for expected outcomes and determine if any adverse effects have occurred.

Nurses should know the most frequent types of drug errors and the severities of different categories of errors (➤ Figure 9.2). The FDA (Meadows, 2003) evaluated reports of fatal medication errors that it received from 1993 to 1998. The most common types of errors reported involved administering an improper dose (41%), giving the wrong drug (16%), and using the wrong route of administration (16%). Almost half of the fatal medication errors

occurred in patients older than 60 years. There is an increase in the risk for errors in the elderly population because they often take numerous medications, have multiple health care providers, and are experiencing normal age-related changes in physiology. Children are another vulnerable population because they receive medication dosages based on weight (which increases the possibility of dosage miscalculations), and the therapeutic dosages are much smaller.

Nurses must be vigilant in keeping up to date on pharmacotherapeutics and should never administer a medication until they are familiar with its uses and side effects. There are many venues by which the nurse can obtain updated medication knowledge. Each nursing unit should have current drug references available. Nurses can also call the pharmacy to obtain information about the drug or, if available, look it up on the Internet using reliable sources. Many nurses are now relying on personal digital assistants (PDAs) to provide current information. These devices can be updated daily or weekly by downloading information so that the information is current. Nurses need to familiarize themselves with research on preventing medical errors to maintain evidence-based practice skills.

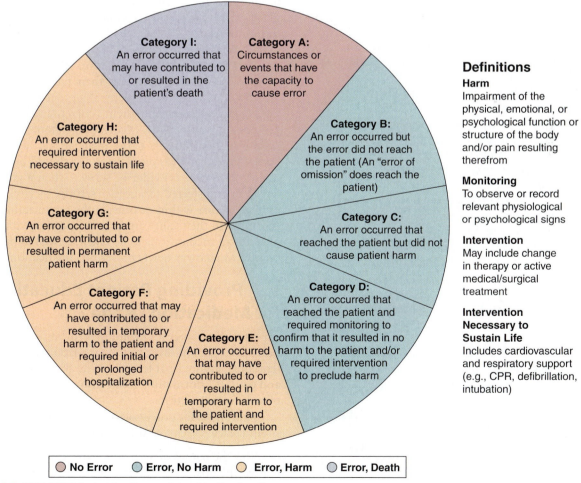

Definitions

Harm
Impairment of the physical, emotional, or psychological function or structure of the body and/or pain resulting therefrom

Monitoring
To observe or record relevant physiological or psychological signs

Intervention
May include change in therapy or active medical/surgical treatment

Intervention Necessary to Sustain Life
Includes cardiovascular and respiratory support (e.g., CPR, defibrillation, intubation)

Category I: An error occurred that may have contributed to or resulted in the patient's death

Category A: Circumstances or events that have the capacity to cause error

Category B: An error occurred but the error did not reach the patient (An "error of omission" does reach the patient)

Category H: An error occurred that required intervention necessary to sustain life

Category C: An error occurred that reached the patient but did not cause patient harm

Category G: An error occurred that may have contributed to or resulted in permanent patient harm

Category D: An error occurred that reached the patient and required monitoring to confirm that it resulted in no harm to the patient and/or required intervention to preclude harm

Category F: An error occurred that may have contributed to or resulted in temporary harm to the patient and required initial or prolonged hospitalization

Category E: An error occurred that may have contributed to or resulted in temporary harm to the patient and required intervention

○ No Error   ○ Error, No Harm   ○ Error, Harm   ○ Error, Death

➤ *Figure 9.2* NCC MERP Index for Categorizing Medication Errors
Source: © 2001 National Coordinating Council for Medication Error Reporting and Prevention. All rights reserved.

LIFESPAN CONSIDERATIONS

Age-Related Issues in Drug Administration

The Pediatric Population

- Always double-check calculations with another nurse for pediatric drug administration.
- Medications may need to be crushed or administered in a liquid form.
- Ask parents or caregivers how the child has taken medications in the past and for techniques that have been successful in administering medications. Some children will readily take medications and the drug may not need to be disguised.
- Consider the developmental stage of the patient and involve the child to the extent possible. For example, for children under 5, give simple choices and short explanations (e.g., "I have some medicine for you to drink. Would you like to hold the cup?")
- Before mixing medication into a food, beverage, or condiment, be sure that the medication does not react with that substance (e.g., acidic food sources such as orange juice may interact with penicillin). Use sugarless foods and beverages for patients who are diabetic or on ketogenic diets.
- Avoid mixing medications into any required foods such as cereal or milk because the child may refuse the food later.
- When a method of medication administration has been successful, document the technique in the child's care plan to relay the information to other caregivers.
- Remember that medications may have idiosyncratic effects on pediatric patients. Any unusual reaction should be investigated and a possible drug effect considered.

The Elderly Population

- Remember that the frequency of adverse effects of medications is increased in elderly patients because of their decreased ability to absorb and metabolize medications.
- Assess elderly patients for ability to swallow prior to administration of oral medications.
- Patients may refuse medications for many reasons: cost, size of the pill or tablet, and real or perceived adverse effects. Explore reasons for refusal and take appropriate action to ensure the issue is resolved (e.g., switch from a large, difficult to swallow pill to a smaller formulation) and that patient autonomy is respected.
- Explore the patient's normal activity and usual sleeping and waking hours. Schedule medications around these times when possible. Follow as simple a dosing schedule as possible.
- Review all medications with the patient on every health care visit. Note any complaints related to specific drugs for follow-up intervention.
- Visual changes may make medication labels difficult to read. For home administration, provide large-print instructions, make sure eyeglasses are used if needed, and recommend discussing all medications with the pharmacist each time a prescription is filled for shape, color, and size of the medication.
- For at-home care, if separate pill containers are used other than the original prescription bottle (e.g., pill containers divided by days of the week), be sure the patient, family, or caregiver retains original bottles as well as notes the color of each pill. Should a reaction occur, or should a visiting young child access the container, a more precise record of what drugs were potentially consumed will aid in treating the patient.
- Provide specific instructions for all medications (e.g., how frequently "as needed" medications can be taken). Ensure that the patient knows what to do if a medication is forgotten.

9.6 Medication Reconciliation

Many geriatric patients have several chronic medical disorders, each of which may be treated by individual specialists. It is common for these patients to receive multiple prescriptions, sometimes for the same condition, that have conflicting pharmacologic actions, a condition termed **polypharmacy.** Although not unique to older adults, polypharmacy is most often seen in this age group. Keeping track of multiple medications, their doses, indications, routes, and frequency of administration is a major challenge for both patients and health care providers. Failure to properly record medication information, and communicate that information to health care providers, is a potential cause of medication errors.

Medication reconciliation is the process of "keeping track" of a patient's medications as they proceed from one health care provider to another. Reconciliation accurately lists all medications a patient is taking in an attempt to reduce duplication, omissions, dosing errors, or drug interactions. For example, when a patient is admitted to care, the nurse records all medications the patient has been taking at home, including their dose, route, and frequency. This list is checked against admission orders and is transferred to other practitioners whenever the patient is moved to different units within the hospital. It is also checked at discharge. These "interfaces of care" are the most likely places that medication reconciliation errors have been found to occur.

In 2004, JCAHO identified hundreds of serious medication errors attributed to medication reconciliation and developed recommendations for their prevention. Hospitals are now encouraged to implement a process for documenting a complete list of the patient's current medications upon the patient's admission. Medications should include prescription medications, OTC medications, vitamins, and herbal products. This medication list should be communicated to the next provider of service when a patient is referred or transferred to another setting, service, physician, or level of care within or outside the organization. On discharge from the facility, provide the patient with the complete list of medications to be taken, as well as instructions on how to take any newly prescribed medications.

9.7 Providing Patient Education for Medication Usage

An essential strategy for avoiding medication errors is to educate the patient by providing written age-appropriate handouts, audiovisual teaching aids about the medication, and contact information about whom to notify in the event of an adverse reaction.

To minimize the potential for medication errors, the nurse should teach patients or their home caregivers the following:

- Know the names of all medications they are taking, the uses, the doses, and when and how they should be taken.
- Know what side effects need to be reported immediately.

OTC Drugs and Medication Errors

Patient use of OTC drugs and natural therapies is a common reason for adverse reactions and medication errors. For example, taking antibiotics can lower the effectiveness of oral contraceptives. OTC antihistamines can interact adversely with alcohol, sedatives, antidepressants, and antihypertensives. Encourage patients to:

- Carry a list of all medications, including OTC drugs, dietary supplements, and medicinal herbs.
- Be sure family and various health care providers have a copy of this list. Include vitamins, laxatives, sleeping pills, and birth control pills.
- If possible, use one pharmacy for all prescriptions, because the pharmacist is an excellent resource for providing information about drug–drug and herbal/food interactions.

- Read the label prior to each drug administration and use the medication device that comes with liquid medications rather than household measuring spoons.
- Carry a list of all medications, including OTC drugs, as well as herbal and dietary supplements that are being taken. If possible, use one pharmacy for all prescriptions.
- Ask questions. Health care providers want to be partners in maintaining safe medication principles.

9.8 How Health Care Facilities Are Reducing Medication Errors

There is a trend for health care agencies to use automated, computerized, locked cabinets for medication storage on patient-care units. Each nurse on the unit has a code for accessing the cabinet and removing a medication dose. These automated systems also maintain an inventory of drug supplies.

Larger health care agencies often have **risk-management** departments to examine risks and minimize the number of medication errors. Risk-management personnel investigate incidents, track data, identify problems, and provide recommendations for improvement. Nurses collaborate with the risk-management committees to seek means of reducing medication errors by modifying policies and procedures within the institution. Examples of policies and procedures include:

- Correctly storing medication (light and temperature control).
- Reading the drug label to avoid using time-expired medications.

- Avoiding the transfer of doses from one container to another.
- Avoiding overstocking of medications to prevent the expiration of medications.
- Monitoring compliance with prohibited prescription abbreviations.
- Removing outdated reference books.

9.9 Governmental and Other Agencies That Track Medication Errors

Both governmental and private agencies track medication errors and provide updated reporting for consumers and health care providers:

- The FDA's safety information and adverse-event reporting program is MedWatch. Its toll-free number is 1-800-332-1088, and its website is www.fda.gov/medwatch/how.htm.
- The Institute for Safe Medication Practices (ISMP) accepts reports from consumers and health care professionals related to medication safety. It publishes *Safe Medicine*, a consumer newsletter about medication errors.
- MEDMARX is the U.S. Pharmacopeia's anonymous medication error reporting program used by hospitals.

RESEARCH SHOWS

The Question: What are the most common types of medication errors occurring in pediatric patients?

The Study: A review of the literature going back to 1969 found only 32 relevant papers in the scientific literature that examined the incidence and nature of medication errors in children. The most common type of error was delivering an incorrect dose. In some cases, this involved administering 10 times the normal dose. The most frequent drug associated with the errors were antibiotics and sedatives. The actual error rate was not possible to calculate due to the small number of studies.

Nursing Implications: The authors offer a number of common-sense suggestions to avoid medication errors in this population, including double-checking the doses, verifying any medications or doses that appear unusual, checking for allergies before administering the drug, confirming the patient's weight is correct, and providing adequate inservices for agency personnel.

Source: Ghaleb, M. A., Barber, N., Franklin, B. D., Yeung, V., Khaki, Z. F., & Wong, I. (2006). Systematic review of medication errors in pediatric patients: Suggestions to prevent medication errors in children. The Annals of Pharmacotherapy, 40(10): 1766–1776.

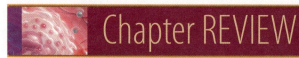

Chapter REVIEW

KEY CONCEPTS

The numbered key concepts provide a succinct summary of the important points from the corresponding numbered section within the chapter. If any of these points are not clear, refer to the numbered section within the chapter for review.

9.1 A medication error may be related to misinterpretations, miscalculations, misadministrations, handwriting misinterpretation, and misunderstanding of verbal or phone orders. Whether the patient is injured or not, it is still a medication error.

9.2 Numerous factors contribute to medication errors, including mistakes in the five rights of drug administration, failing to follow agency procedures or consider patient variables, giving medications based on verbal orders, not confirming orders that are illegible or incomplete, and working under stressful conditions. Patients also contribute to errors by using more than one pharmacy, not informing health care providers of all medications they are taking, or not following instructions.

9.3 Nurse practice acts define professional nursing, including safe medication delivery. Standards of care are defined by nurse practice acts and the rule of reasonable and prudent action.

9.4 Nurses are legally and ethically responsible for reporting medication errors—whether or not they cause harm to a patient—in the patient's medical record and on an incident report. The FDA and NCC MERP are two agencies that track medication errors and provide data to help institute procedures to prevent them.

9.5 Nurses can reduce medication errors by adhering to the four steps of the nursing process—assessment, planning, implementation, and evaluation. Keeping up to date on pharmacotherapeutics and knowing common error types are instrumental to safe medication administration.

9.6 Medication reconciliation is an important means of reducing medication errors. Medication reconciliation is a process of "keeping track" of a patient's medications as they proceed from one health care provider to another.

9.7 Patient teaching includes providing age-appropriate medication handouts, and encouraging patients to keep a list of all prescribed medications, OTC drugs, herbal therapies, and vitamins they are taking and to report them to all health care providers.

9.8 Facilities use risk-management departments and agency policies and procedures to decrease the incidence of medication errors. Automated, computerized, locked cabinets for medication storage are a means of safekeeping of medications and keeping track of inventory at the unit level.

9.9 The FDA (MedWatch), the Institute of Safe Medication Practices (ISMP), and the U.S. Pharmacopeia (MEDMARX) are three agencies that track medication errors and provide databases of error incidence, error types, and levels of harm for health care professionals and/or consumers.

NCLEX-RN® REVIEW QUESTIONS

1 Each nurse is responsible for becoming familiar with the nurse practice acts of the state in which he or she practices because these acts:
1. protect the nurse from malpractice suits.
2. contain national standards and responsibilities.
3. contain job descriptions for all nurses.
4. define nursing practice and standards of care for the nurse practicing in a specific state.

2 The nurse administers a medication to the wrong patient. The appropriate nursing action is to:
1. monitor the patient for adverse reaction before reporting the incident.
2. document the error if the patient has an adverse reaction.
3. report the error to the physician, document the medication in the patient record, and complete a report of the error for further follow-up and analysis.

4. notify the physician and document the error in a report only.

3 The patient with liver dysfunction experiences toxicity to a drug following administration of several doses. This adverse reaction may have been prevented if the nurse had followed which phase of the nursing process?
1. Assessment
2. Planning
3. Implementation
4. Evaluation

4 Nurses have a legal and moral responsibility to report medication errors. The steps of reporting these errors include:
1. punishing the nurse who committed the error.
2. monitoring unsafe medication orders.
3. identifying potential unsafe medication facilities.
4. examining interdisciplinary causes of errors and assisting professionals in ways to avoid mistakes.

5 The nurse has administered a medication to the wrong patient. Which of the following is a correct action the nurse must take? (Select all that apply.)
   1. Notify the physician.
   2. Document that a medication error occurred in the nurse's notes.
   3. Assess vital signs.
   4. Document medication on the medication administration record (MAR).
   5. Complete a facility report of the error.

6 When the nurse enters the patient's room with a medication, the patient states "I'm on the phone, just leave my pill on the table there." What would be the <u>best</u> response by the nurse?
   1. Leave the pill at the bedside as requested.
   2. Ask the patient to let the nurse know when the phone call is completed so that the nurse can return with the medication.
   3. Instruct the patient to either take the medication or refuse it.
   4. Chart the medication as "unable to give" and skip the dose.

CRITICAL THINKING QUESTIONS

1. A registered nurse is assigned to a team of eight patients. Six of these patients have medications scheduled for once-a-day dosing at 10:00 a.m. Explain how the nurse will be able to administer these drugs to the patients at the "right time."

2. A health care provider writes an order for Tylenol 3 PO q3–4 for mild pain. The nurse evaluates this order and is concerned that it is incomplete. Identify the probable concern and describe what the nurse should do prior to administering this medication.

3. A new nurse does not check an antibiotic dosage ordered by a health care provider for a pediatric patient. The nurse subsequently overdoses a 2-year-old patient, and an experienced nurse notices the error during the evening shift change. Identify each person who is responsible for the error and how each is responsible.

See Appendix D for answers and rationales for all activities.

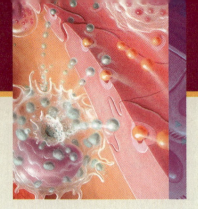

Chapter 10

Herbal and Alternative Therapies

LEARNING OUTCOMES

After reading this chapter, the student should be able to:

1. Explain the role of complementary and alternative medicine in promoting patient wellness.
2. Analyze reasons why herbal and dietary supplements have increased in popularity.
3. Identify the parts of an herb that may contain active ingredients and the types of formulations made from these parts.
4. Analyze the strengths and weaknesses of the Dietary Supplement Health and Education Act (DSHEA) of 1994.
5. Describe adverse effects that may be caused by herbal and dietary supplements.
6. Discuss the role of the nurse in teaching patients about complementary and alternative therapies.
7. Identify common drug–herbal interactions.
8. Explain how some herbal products are standardized based on specific active ingredients.

KEY TERMS

botanical   *page 95*

complementary and alternative medicine (CAM)
   page 95

dietary supplement   *page 98*

Dietary Supplement and Nonprescription Drug
   Consumer Protection Act   *page 99*

Dietary Supplement Health and Education Act
   (DSHEA) of 1994   *page 98*

herb   *page 95*

specialty supplement   *page 99*

Herbal supplements and alternative therapies represent a multibillion-dollar industry. Sales of dietary supplements alone exceed $17 billion annually, with more than 158 million consumers using them. Despite the fact that these therapies have not been subjected to the same scientific scrutiny as prescription medications, consumers turn to these treatments for a variety of reasons. Many people have the impression that natural substances have more healing power than synthetic medications. The ready availability of herbal supplements at a reasonable cost, combined with effective marketing strategies, has convinced many consumers to try them. This chapter examines the role of complementary and alternative therapies in the prevention and treatment of disease.

10.1 Alternative Therapies

Complementary and alternative medicine (CAM) comprises an extremely diverse set of therapies and healing systems that are considered to be outside mainstream health care. Although diverse, the major CAM systems have common characteristics.

- Focus on treating each person as an individual.
- Considers the health of the whole person.
- Emphasizes the integration of mind and body.
- Promotes disease prevention, self-care, and self-healing.
- Recognizes the role of spirituality in health and healing.

Because of the popularity of CAM, considerable attention has recently focused on determining its effectiveness, or lack of effectiveness. Although research into these alternative systems is underway, few CAM therapies have been subjected to rigorous clinical and scientific study. It is likely that some of these therapies will be found ineffective, whereas others will become mainstream treatments. The line between what is defined as an alternative therapy and what is considered mainstream is constantly changing. Increasing numbers of health care providers are now accepting CAM therapies and recommending them to their patients. Table 10.1 lists some of these therapies.

Nurses have long known the value of CAM in preventing and treating disease. For example, prayer, meditation, massage, and yoga have been used for centuries to treat both body and mind. From a pharmacology perspective, much of the value of CAM therapies lies in their ability to reduce the need for medications. For instance, if a patient can find anxiety relief through herbal products, massage, or biofeedback therapy, then the use of antianxiety drugs may be reduced or eliminated. Reduction of drug dose leads to fewer adverse effects and improved adherence with the therapeutic regimen.

The nurse should be sensitive to the patient's need for alternative treatment and not be judgmental. Both advantages

TABLE 10.1	Complementary and Alternative Therapies	
Healing Method	**Examples**
Alternative health care systems	Naturopathy
	Homeopathy
	Chiropractic
	Native American medicine (e.g., sweat lodges, medicine wheel)
	Chinese traditional medicine (e.g., acupuncture, Chinese herbs)
Biologic-based therapies	Herbal therapies
	Nutritional supplements
	Special diets
Manual healing	Massage
	Pressure-point therapies
	Hand-mediated biofield therapies
Mind–body interventions	Yoga
	Meditation
	Hypnotherapy
	Guided imagery
	Biofeedback
	Movement-oriented therapies (e.g., music, dance)
Spiritual	Shamans
	Faith and prayer
Others	Bioelectromagnetics
	Detoxifying therapies
	Animal-assisted therapy

and limitations must be presented to patients so they may make rational and informed decisions about their treatment. Pharmacotherapy and alternative therapies can serve complementary and essential roles in the healing of the total patient.

10.2 Brief History of Therapeutic Natural Products

An **herb** is technically a **botanical** without any woody tissue such as stems or bark. Over time, the terms *botanical* and *herb* have come to be used interchangeably to refer to any plant product with some useful application either as a food enhancer, such as flavoring, or as a medicine.

The use of botanicals has been documented for thousands of years. One of the earliest recorded uses of plant products was a prescription for garlic in 3000 B.C. Eastern and Western medicine have recorded thousands of herbs and herb combinations reputed to have therapeutic value. The most popular current herbal supplements and their claimed applications are listed in Table 10.2.

TABLE 10.4	Liquid Formulations of Herbal Products
Product	Description
Decoction	Fresh or dried herbs are boiled in water for 30–60 minutes until much of the liquid has boiled off; very concentrated
Extract	Active ingredients are extracted using organic solvents to form a highly concentrated liquid or solid form; solvent may be removed or be part of the final product
Infusion	Fresh or dried herbs are soaked in hot water for long periods, at least 15 minutes; stronger than teas
Tea	Fresh or dried herbs are soaked in hot water for 5–10 minutes before ingestion; convenient
Tincture	Active ingredients are extracted using alcohol by soaking the herb; alcohol remains as part of the liquid

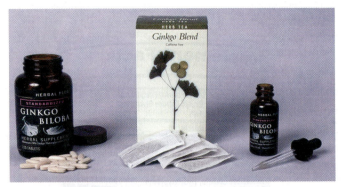

➤ *Figure 10.2* Three different ginkgo formulations: tablets, tea bags, and liquid extract

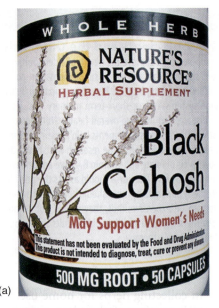

(a)

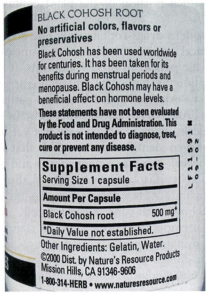

(b)

➤ *Figure 10.3* Labeling of black cohosh: (a) front label with general health claim and (b) back label with more health claims and FDA disclaimer

10.4 Regulation of Herbal Products and Dietary Supplements

Since the passage of the Food, Drug, and Cosmetic Act in 1936, Americans have come to expect that all approved prescription and OTC drugs have passed rigid standards of safety prior to being marketed. Furthermore, it is expected that these drugs have been tested for efficacy and that they truly provide the medical benefits claimed by the manufacturer. Americans cannot and should not expect the same quality standards for herbal products. These products are regulated by a far less rigorous law, the **Dietary Supplement Health and Education Act (DSHEA) of 1994.**

According to the DSHEA, "dietary supplements" are specifically exempted from the Food, Drug, and Cosmetic Act. **Dietary supplements** are defined as products intended to enhance or supplement the diet, such as botanicals, vitamins, minerals, or other extracts or metabolites that are not already approved as drugs by the FDA. A major strength of the legislation is that it gives the FDA the power to remove from the market any product that poses a "significant or unreasonable" risk to the public. It also requires these products to be clearly labeled by the manufacturer as "dietary supplements." An example of an herbal label for black cohosh is shown in ➤ Figure 10.3.

Unfortunately, the DSHEA has several significant flaws that have led to a lack of standardization in the dietary supplement industry, and to less protection for the consumer.

- Effectiveness does not have to be demonstrated by the manufacturer prior to marketing.
- The manufacturer does not have to prove the safety of the dietary supplement. To be removed from the market, the government has to provide the burden of proof to show that the supplement is unsafe.
- Dietary supplement labels must state that the product is not intended to diagnose, treat, cure, or prevent any disease; however, the label may make claims about the product's effect on body structure and function, such as the following:
  - Helps promote healthy immune systems.
  - Reduces anxiety and stress.

- Helps maintain cardiovascular function.
- May reduce pain and inflammation.
- The DSHEA does not regulate the accuracy of the label; the product may or may not contain the product listed, in the amounts claimed.

Several steps have been taken to address the lack of purity and mislabeling of herbal and dietary supplements. In an attempt to protect consumers, Congress passed the **Dietary Supplement and Nonprescription Drug Consumer Protection Act,** which took effect in 2007. Companies marketing herbal and dietary supplements are now required to include contact information (address and phone number) on the product labels for consumers to use in reporting adverse events. Companies must notify the FDA of any serious adverse event reports within 15 days of receiving such reports. Under this Act, a "serious adverse event" is defined as any adverse reaction resulting in death, a life-threatening experience, inpatient hospitalization, a persistent or significant disability or incapacity, or a congenital anomaly or birth defect, as well as any event requiring a medical or surgical intervention to prevent one of these conditions, based on reasonable medical judgment. Companies must keep records of such events for at least 6 years, and the records are subject to inspection by the FDA.

Also in 2007, the FDA announced a final rule that requires the manufacturers of dietary supplements to evaluate the identity, purity, potency, and composition of their products. The labels must accurately reflect what is in the product, which must be free of contaminants such as pesticides, toxins, glass, or heavy metals.

10.5 The Pharmacologic Actions and Safety of Herbal Products

A key concept to remember when dealing with alternative therapies is that "natural" does not always mean "better" or "safe." There is no question that some botanicals contain active chemicals as powerful as, and perhaps more effective than, some currently approved medications. Thousands of years of experience, combined with current scientific research, have shown that some herbal remedies have therapeutic actions. Because a substance comes from a natural product, however, does not make it safe or effective. For example, poison ivy is natural, but it certainly is not safe or therapeutic. Natural products may not offer an improvement over conventional therapy in treating certain disorders and, indeed, may be of no value whatsoever. Furthermore, a patient who substitutes an unproven alternative therapy for an established, effective medical treatment may delay healing, suffer harmful effects, and endanger health.

Because some herbal products contain ingredients that interact with prescription drugs, nurses should include questions on dietary supplements when obtaining medical histories. Patients taking medications with potentially serious adverse effects such as insulin, warfarin (Coumadin), or digoxin (Lanoxin) should be warned never to take any herbal product or dietary supplement without first discussing their needs with a physician. In addition, pregnant or lactating women should never take these products without approval of their health care provider. The nurse should also remember that the potential for any drug interaction increases in older adults, especially those with hepatic or renal impairment. Drug interactions with selected herbs are listed in Table 10.5. Herbal–drug interactions are noted, where applicable, in the prototype drug features throughout this text.

Another warning that must be heeded with natural products is to beware of allergic reactions. Most herbal products contain a mixture of ingredients, and it is not unusual to find dozens of different chemicals in teas and infusions made from the flowers, leaves, or roots of a plant. Patients who have known allergies to certain foods or medicines should seek medical advice before taking a new herbal product. It is always wise to take the smallest amount possible when starting herbal therapy, even less than the recommended dose, to see if allergies or other adverse effects occur.

Nurses have an obligation to seek the latest medical information on herbal products because there is a good possibility that their patients are using them to supplement traditional medicines. Patients should be advised to be skeptical of claims on the labels of dietary supplements and to seek health information from reputable sources. Nurses should never condemn a patient's use of alternative medicines, but instead should be supportive and seek to understand the patient's goals for taking the supplements. The health care provider will often need to educate patients on the role of CAM therapies in the treatment of their disorders and discuss which treatment or combination of treatments will best meet their health goals.

10.6 Specialty Supplements

Specialty supplements are nonherbal dietary products used to enhance a wide variety of body functions. These supplements form a diverse group of substances obtained from plant and animal sources. They are more specific in their action than herbal products and are generally targeted for one or a smaller number of conditions. The most popular specialty supplements are listed in Table 10.6.

In general, specialty supplements have a legitimate rationale for their use. For example, chondroitin and glucosamine are natural substances in the body necessary for cartilage growth and maintenance. Amino acids are natural building blocks of muscle protein. Flaxseed and fish oils contain omega fatty acids that have been shown to reduce the risk of heart disease in certain patients.

As with herbal products, the link between most specialty supplements and their claimed benefits is unclear. In many cases, a normal diet supplies sufficient quantities of the substance and taking additional amounts may provide no benefit. In other cases, the product is marketed for conditions for which the supplement has no proved effect. The good news is that these substances are generally not harmful, unless taken in large amounts. The bad news, however, is that they can give patients false hopes of an easy cure for chronic conditions such as heart disease or the pain of arthritis. As with herbal products, the nurse should advise patients to be skeptical about the health claims regarding the use of these supplements.

TABLE 10.5	Documented Herb–Drug Interactions	
Common (*Scientific*) Name	Interacts with	Comments
Echinacea (*Echinacea purpurea*)	Amiodarone, anabolic steroids, ketoconazole, methotrexate	Possible increased hepatotoxicity
Feverfew (*Tanacetum parthenium*)	Aspirin and other NSAIDs, heparin, warfarin (Coumadin)	Increased bleeding risk
Garlic (*Allium sativum*)	Aspirin and other NSAIDs, warfarin	Increased bleeding risk
	Insulin, oral hypoglycemic agents	Additive hypoglycemic effects
Ginger (*Zingiber officinale*)	Aspirin and other NSAIDs, heparin, warfarin	Increased bleeding risk
Ginkgo (*Ginkgo biloba*)	Anticonvulsants	Possible decreased anticonvulsant effectiveness
	Aspirin and NSAIDs	Increased bleeding potential
	Heparin and warfarin	
	Tricyclic antidepressants	Possible decreased seizure threshold
Ginseng (*Panax quinquefolius/Eleutherococcus senticosus*)	CNS depressants	Increased sedation
	Digoxin (Lanoxin)	Increased toxicity
	Diuretics	Possible attenuated diuretic effects
	Insulin and oral hypoglycemic agents	Increased hypoglycemic effects
	Warfarin	Decreased anticoagulant effects
Goldenseal (*Hydrastis canadensis*)	Diuretics	May decrease diuretic effects
St. John's wort (*Hypericum perforatum*)	CNS depressants and opioid analgesics	Increased sedation
	Cyclosporine (Sandimmune)	May decrease cyclosporine levels
	Efavirenz, indinavir	Decreased antiretroviral activity
	Protease inhibitors	Decreased antiretroviral activity of indinavir
	Selective serotonin reuptake inhibitors, tricyclic antidepressants	Possible serotonin syndrome*
	Warfarin	Decreased anticoagulant effects
Valerian (*Valeriana officinalis*)	Barbiturates, benzodiazepines and other CNS depressants	Potentiate sedation

*Serotonin syndrome: headache, dizziness, sweating, agitation
Note: Data modified from www.prenhall.com/drugguides

TABLE 10.6	Selected Specialty Supplements	
Name	Primary Uses	Supplement Feature (Chapter)
Amino acids	Build protein, muscle strength, and endurance	–
Carnitine	Enhance energy and sports performance, heart health, memory, immune function, and male fertility	24
Coenzyme Q10	Prevent heart disease, provide antioxidant therapy	22
DHEA	Boost immune functions and memory	–
Fish oil	Reduce cholesterol levels, enhance brain function, increase visual acuity (due to presence of omega-3 fatty acids)	33
Flaxseed oil	Reduce cholesterol levels, enhance brain function, increase visual acuity (due to presence of omega-3 fatty acids)	–
Glucosamine and chondroitin	Alleviate arthritis and other joint problems	47
Lactobacillus acidophilus	Maintain intestinal health	41
Selenium	Reduce the risk of certain types of cancer	
Vitamin C	Prevention of colds	

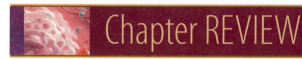

Chapter REVIEW

KEY CONCEPTS

The numbered key concepts provide a succinct summary of the important points from the corresponding numbered section within the chapter. If any of these points are not clear, refer to the numbered section within the chapter for review.

10.1 Complementary and alternative medicine is a set of diverse therapies and healing systems used by many people for disease prevention and self-healing.

10.2 Natural products obtained from plants have been used as medicines for thousands of years. Recent years have seen resurgence in the popularity of these products.

10.3 Herbal products are available in a variety of formulations; some contain standardized extracts, and others contain whole herbs.

10.4 Herbal products and dietary supplements are regulated by the Dietary Supplement Health and Education Act of 1994, which does not require safety or efficacy testing prior to marketing. Recent laws have been passed to safeguard consumer safety regarding dietary supplements.

10.5 Natural products may have pharmacologic actions and result in adverse effects, including significant interactions with prescription medications.

10.6 Specialty supplements are nonherbal dietary products used to enhance a wide variety of body functions. Like herbal products, most have not been subjected to controlled, scientific testing.

NCLEX-RN® REVIEW QUESTIONS

1 The nurse obtains information during the admission interview that the patient is taking herbal supplements. What implications does this information have for the patient's treatment?
1. This is not important, because herbal products are natural and pose no risk to the patient.
2. These products are a welcome adjunct to conventional treatment.
3. The nurse must observe the patient for allergic reactions.
4. The herbal products may interact with prescribed medications and affect drug action.

2 Appropriate teaching to provide safety for a patient who is planning to use herbal products should include which of the following?
1. Take the smallest amount possible when starting herbal therapy, even less than the recommended dose, to see if allergies or other adverse effects occur.
2. Read the labels to determine composition of the product.
3. Research the clinical trials before using the products.
4. Read the labels to determine which diseases or disorders the product has been proven to treat or cure.

3 The patient states he has been using the herbal product saw palmetto. The nurse recognizes that this supplement is often used to treat:
1. insomnia.
2. urinary problems associated with prostate enlargement.
3. symptoms of menopause.
4. urinary tract infection.

4 A patient receiving warfarin (Coumadin) therapy reports use of the herb feverfew. The nurse observes the patient for evidence of:
1. liver toxicity.
2. increased coagulation.
3. renal dysfunction.
4. increased bleeding potential.

5 The patient has been taking sertraline (Zoloft), but just added St. John's wort for his depression. He now presents to the emergency department. The nurse recognizes the signs and symptoms of serotonin syndrome as: (Select all that apply.)
1. headache.
2. dizziness.
3. agitation.
4. weight loss.
5. sweating.

6 What is the difference between an herbal product and a specialty supplement?
1. An herbal product is safer to use than a specialty supplement.
2. A specialty supplement tends to be more expensive than an herbal product.
3. A specialty supplement is a nonherbal dietary product used to enhance a variety of body functions.
4. There are less adverse effects or risk of allergy with specialty supplements than there are with herbal products.

CRITICAL THINKING QUESTIONS

1. A 44-year-old breast cancer survivor is placed on tamoxifen (Nolvadex) 20 mg PO daily. Since receiving chemotherapy, the patient has not had a menstrual cycle. She is concerned about being menopausal and wonders about the possibility of using a soy-based product as a form of natural hormone replacement. How should the nurse advise the patient?

2. A 62-year-old male patient is recuperating from a myocardial infarction. He is on the anticoagulant warfarin (Coumadin) and antidysrhythmic digoxin (Lanoxin). He talks to his wife about starting garlic to help lower his blood lipid levels, and ginseng because he has heard it helps in coronary artery disease. Discuss the potential concerns about the use of garlic and ginseng by this patient.

3. The patient has been taking St. John's wort for symptoms of depression. He is now scheduled for an elective surgery. What important preoperative teaching should be included?

See Appendix D for answers and rationales for all activities.

EXPLORE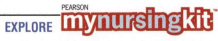

MyNursingKit is your one stop for online chapter review materials and resources. Prepare for success with additional NCLEX®-style practice questions, interactive assignments and activities, web links, animations and videos, and more!

Register your access code from the front of your book at
www.mynursingkit.com.

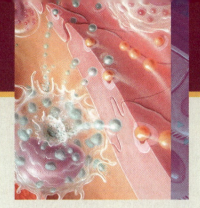

Chapter 11

Substance Abuse

LEARNING OUTCOMES

After reading this chapter, the student should be able to:

1. Explain underlying causes of addiction.
2. Compare and contrast psychologic and physical dependence.
3. Compare withdrawal syndromes for the various substance abuse classes.
4. Discuss how nurses can recognize drug tolerance in patients.
5. In the following drug classes, explain the major characteristics of abuse, dependence, and tolerance: alcohol, nicotine, marijuana, hallucinogens, CNS stimulants, sedatives, and opioids.
6. Describe the role of the nurse in delivering care to individuals who have substance abuse issues.

KEY TERMS

Throughout history, individuals have consumed both natural substances and prescription drugs to increase performance, assist with relaxation, alter psychologic state, and to enhance social interaction. Substance abuse has a tremendous societal, economic, and health impact. Although the terms *drug abuse* and *substance abuse* have been used interchangeably, *substance abuse* is often considered more inclusive because of the involved legal and illegal agents, misused household items, and drugs available for medication purposes. By definition, **substance abuse** in this chapter will be considered *the self-administration of a drug in a manner that does not conform to the norms within the patient's own culture and society.*

11.1 Overview of Substance Abuse

Abused substances belong to many diverse chemical classes. Drugs have few structural similarities, but they all have in common the ability to impact the brain and central nervous system. Some substances—such as opium, marijuana, cocaine, nicotine, caffeine, and alcohol—are obtained from natural sources. Others are synthetic or **designer drugs,** created in illegal laboratories for the purpose of profiting from illicit drug trafficking.

Abused or misused substances are not always illegal drugs. Alcohol and nicotine are two of the most commonly abused drugs. Abused legal CNS-influencing drugs include prescription medications such as methylphenidate (Ritalin) and meperidine (Demerol). Legal substances without prescription involve agents such as volatile inhalants. Ketamine and gamma hydroxybutyrate (GHB) are examples of misused legal anesthetics. Athletes often abuse legal anabolic steroids. Frequently abused illegal substances include marijuana, heroin (opioids), and hallucinogens such as lysergic acid diethylamide (LSD) and methamphetamines. Phencyclidine hydrochloride (PCP) is a hallucinogen with a history of abuse but not so much presently. Huffing of organic, household, or industrial chemical products is not uncommon. Aerosols and paint thinners are inhalants obtained without prescription.

Several drugs once used therapeutically are now illegal due to their high potential for abuse. Cocaine was once widely used as a local anesthetic, but today nearly all the cocaine acquired by users is obtained illegally. LSD is now illegal, although in the 1940s and 1950s, LSD was used in psychotherapy. Phencyclidine was popular in the early 1960s as an anesthetic, but was withdrawn from the market in 1965, because patients reported hallucinations, delusions, and anxiety after recovering from anesthesia. Many amphetamines once used for bronchodilation were discontinued in the 1980s after unpleasant psychotic episodes were reported. The sum of this information relates to the diversity of substances within our culture, which patients can either misuse or abuse.

11.2 Neurobiologic and Psychosocial Components of Substance Abuse

Addiction is an overwhelming compulsion that drives someone to take drugs repetitively, despite serious health and social consequences. It is impossible to accurately predict whether a person will become a substance abuser. Attempts to predict a person's addictive tendency using psychologic profiles or genetic markers have largely been unsuccessful. Substance abuse depends on multiple, complex, interacting variables such as described in the following categories:

- *User-related factors:* Genetic factors (e.g., metabolic enzymes, innate tolerance), personality for risk-taking behavior, prior experiences with drugs, disorders that may require a scheduled drug
- *Environmental factors:* Societal and community norms, role models, peer influences, educational opportunities

---

PharmFacts

Substance Abuse in the United States

- Twenty-eight million Americans have used illicit drugs at least once.
- Nurses and other health care providers are at increased risk for substance abuse problems especially with benzodiazepines, opioids, and alcohol. It is estimated that 6% to 8% of health professionals have a substance abuse problem.
- 25% of high school students use an illegal drug monthly.
- An estimated 2.4 million Americans have used heroin during their lives.
- About one in five Americans has lived with an alcoholic while growing up. Children of alcoholic parents are four times more likely to become alcoholics than children of nonalcoholic parents.
- Alcohol is an important factor in 68% of manslaughters, 54% of murders, 48% of robberies, and 44% of burglaries.
- Among youth between the ages of 12 and 17, 7.2 million have drunk alcohol at least once. Girls were as likely as boys to drink alcohol.
- Barbiturate overdose is a factor in almost one third of all drug-related deaths.
- 36% of 10th-grade students and 46% of 12th-grade students have reported using marijuana and hashish.
- Almost 8% of high school seniors have reported using cocaine.
- 2 million Americans have used cocaine on a monthly basis; about 567,000 have used crack cocaine.
- Approximately 70% of the cocaine entering the United States comes from Colombia and passes through south Florida.
- 16% of 8th graders and 11% of 12th graders have reported using volatile inhalants.
- 30% of all Americans are cigarette smokers, including 25% who are between the ages of 12 and 25.
- 43% of 10th-grade students and 54% of 12th-grade students have reported smoking cigarettes. 8% of 12th-grade students consume more than half a pack or more each day.
- 8% of 12th-grade students have reported using Ecstasy (MDMA).
- LSD is one of the most potent drugs known, with only 25–150 mcg constituting a dose. Almost 9% of 12th-grade students have reported using LSD.

• *Factors related to the agent or drug:* Cost, availability, dose, mode of administration (e.g., oral, IV, inhalation), speed of onset/termination, and length of drug use

In the case of legal prescription drugs, addiction may begin with a legitimate need for pharmacotherapy. For example, narcotic analgesics may be indicated for pain relief, or sedatives may be taken for a sleep disorder. These drugs may result in such a favorable experience, or for whatever reason patients determine to repeat the experience after the prescription has expired.

There is often the concern that the therapeutic use of scheduled drugs creates large numbers of addicted patients. Because of this, medications having a potential for abuse have been prescribed at the lowest effective dose and for the shortest time necessary to treat the medical problem. Prescription drugs in fact rarely cause addiction when used as prescribed and according to accepted medical protocols. As mentioned in chapters 1 and 2∞, numerous laws have been passed in an attempt to limit substance abuse and addiction. The risk of addiction caused by prescription medications is primarily a function of dose and duration of drug therapy. Nurses should be able to administer medications for the relief of patient symptoms, without unnecessary fear of producing dependency.

RESEARCH SHOWS

The Question: Are there connections between a sedentary lifestyle, stress-related disorders, and drug addiction?

The Study: Scientists are beginning to believe that exercise may help prevent addiction to alcohol and drugs, and this may apply to various chemical substances as well. Evidence suggests that exercising teens are 50% less likely to smoke than their inactive counterparts. Forty percent are less likely to experiment with marijuana. Adults who engage in some type of regular physical activity are less likely to abuse alcohol than those who sporadically exercise. Aerobic exercise tends to reduce the likelihood that members of the general population will seek out the rewarding effects of some illicit drugs such as cocaine. While studies are preliminary, many believe there is a connection between positive psychosocial activity and the natural release of brain dopamine. While it has long been established that exercise promotes positive cardiovascular and pulmonary health, focused physical activity seems to decrease the prevalence of certain stress-related disorders such as anxiety, depression, and hyperactivity in children.

Nursing Implications: When considered beneficial to patients, nurses should encourage regular physical exercise. Physical activity not only promotes positive general health but also positive mental health. Exercise may help mitigate tendencies for drug abuse.

Source: Can Physical Activity and Exercise Prevent Drug Abuse? Promoting a Full Range of Science to Inform Prevention. *Meeting of the National Institute of Drug Abuse (NIDA), National Institutes of Health (NIH), Bethesda, MD, June 5–6, 2008.*

11.3 Physical and Psychologic Dependence

Whether a substance is addictive is related to how easily an individual can stop taking the agent on a repetitive basis. When a person has an overwhelming desire to take a drug and cannot stop, this condition is referred to as *substance dependence*. Substance dependence is classified into two categories, physical dependence and psychologic dependence.

Physical dependence refers to an altered physical condition caused by the adaptation of the nervous system to repeated substance use. Over time, the body's cells become accustomed to the presence of the unnatural substance. With physical dependence, uncomfortable symptoms known as *withdrawal* result when the agent is discontinued. Repeated doses of opioids, such as morphine and heroin, may produce physical dependence rather quickly, particularly when the drugs are taken intravenously. Alcohol, sedatives, nicotine, and CNS stimulants are additional examples of substances that with extended use may easily cause physical dependence.

In contrast, **psychologic dependence** refers to a condition where no obvious physical signs of discomfort are observed after the agent is discontinued. The user, however, will have an overwhelming desire to continue drug-seeking behavior despite obvious negative economic, physical, or social consequences. Any associated intense craving may be connected with the patient's home or social environment. Strong psychologic craving may continue for months or even years and can be responsible for relapses during therapy. For psychologic dependence to occur, relatively high doses of drugs are usually taken for a prolonged period of time. Examples include marijuana and antianxiety drugs. On the other hand, psychologic dependence may develop quickly after only one use, as with crack cocaine, a potent, rather inexpensive, form of the drug.

11.4 Withdrawal Syndrome

Once a person becomes physically dependent and the substance is discontinued, **withdrawal syndrome** may occur. Prescription drugs are often used to reduce the severity of withdrawal symptoms. For example, alcohol withdrawal might be treated with the short-acting benzodiazepine, oxazepam (Serax); opioid withdrawal might be treated with methadone. Symptoms of nicotine withdrawal might be relieved with replacement therapy in the form of nicotine patches or chewing gum. For withdrawal from CNS stimulants, hallucinogens, marijuana, or inhalants, specific pharmacologic intervention might not be indicated.

Symptoms of withdrawal may be particularly severe for those who are dependent on alcohol or sedatives. Because of the severity of the symptoms, the process of withdrawal from these agents is probably best accomplished in a substance abuse treatment facility. Examples of drugs and associated withdrawal symptoms and characteristics are shown in Table 11.1.

With chronic substance abuse, people will often associate use of the substance with their conditions and surroundings, including social contacts with other users who are also taking the drug. Users tend to revert to drug-seeking behavior when they return to the company of other substance abusers. Counselors often encourage users to refrain from associating with past social contacts or having relationships with other substance abusers to lessen the possibility for relapse. The

TABLE 11.1	Selected Drugs of Abuse, Withdrawal Symptoms, and Characteristics	
Drug	**Physiologic and Psychologic Effects**	**Signs of Toxicity**
Alcohol	Tremors, fatigue, anxiety, abdominal cramping, hallucinations, confusion, seizures, delirium	Extreme somnolence, severe CNS depression, diminished reflexes, respiratory depression
Barbiturates	Insomnia, anxiety, weakness, abdominal cramps, tremor, anorexia, seizures, skin hypersensitivity reactions, hallucinations, delirium	Severe CNS depression, tremor, diaphoresis, vomiting, cyanosis, tachycardia, Cheyne–Stokes respirations
Benzodiazepines	Insomnia, restlessness, abdominal pain, nausea, sensitivity to light and sound, headache, fatigue, muscle twitches	Somnolence, confusion, diminished reflexes, coma
Cocaine and amphetamines	Mental depression, anxiety, extreme fatigue, hunger	Dysrhythmias, lethargy, skin pallor, psychosis
Hallucinogens	Rarely observed; dependent on specific drug	Panic reactions, confusion, blurred vision, increase in blood pressure, psychotic-like state
Marijuana	Irritability, restlessness, insomnia, tremor, chills, weight loss	Euphoria, paranoia, panic reactions, hallucinations, psychotic-like state
Nicotine	Irritability, anxiety, restlessness, headaches, increased appetite, insomnia, inability to concentrate, decrease in heart rate and blood pressure	Heart palpitations, tachyarrhythmias, confusion, depression, seizures
Opioids	Excessive sweating, restlessness, dilated pupils, agitation, goosebumps, tremor, violent yawning, increased heart rate and blood pressure, nausea/vomiting, abdominal cramps and pain, muscle spasms with kicking movements, weight loss	Respiratory depression, cyanosis, extreme somnolence, coma

formation of new social contacts as a result of association with self-help groups such as Alcoholics Anonymous helps some people transition to a drug-free lifestyle. Residential secondary treatment or "step down" from primary care may be required for some patients who are not ready to return to the community after detoxification.

11.5 Tolerance

Tolerance is a biologic condition that occurs when the body adapts to a substance after repeated administration. Over time, higher doses of the agent are required to produce the same initial effect. For example, at the start of pharmacotherapy, a patient may find that 2 mg of a sedative is effective for inducing sleep. After taking the medication for several months, the patient notices that it takes 4 mg or perhaps 6 mg to fall asleep. Development of drug tolerance is common for substances that affect the nervous system. Tolerance should be thought of as a natural consequence of continued drug use and not be considered evidence of addiction or substance abuse.

Tolerance does not develop at the same rate for all actions of a drug. For example, patients usually develop tolerance to the nausea and vomiting produced by narcotic analgesics after only a few doses. Tolerance to the mood-altering effects of these drugs and to their ability to reduce pain develops more slowly but eventually may be complete. On the other hand, tolerance never develops to the drug's ability to constrict the pupils. Patients will often endure annoying side effects of drugs, such as the sedation caused by antihistamines, if they know that tolerance to these effects will quickly develop.

Once tolerance develops to a substance, it often extends to closely related drugs. This phenomenon is known as **cross-tolerance**. For example, a heroin addict will become tolerant to the analgesic effects of other opioids such as morphine or meperidine. Patients who have developed tolerance to alcohol will show tolerance to other CNS depressants such as barbiturates, benzodiazepines, and some general anesthetics. This has important clinical implications for the nurse, because doses of these related medications will need to be adjusted accordingly to obtain maximum therapeutic benefit.

LIFESPAN CONSIDERATIONS

Abuse of Volatile Inhalants by Children and Adolescents

Many parents are concerned that their children will smoke tobacco or marijuana or become addicted to crack or amphetamines. Yet few parents consider that the most common sources of abused substances are readily available in their own homes. Inhaling volatile chemicals, known as *huffing*, is most prevalent in the 10- to 12-year-old age group and declines with age; one in five children has done this by the eighth grade. Virtually any organic compound can be huffed, including nail polish remover, spray paint, household glue, correction fluid, propane, gasoline, and even whipped cream propellants. These agents are available in the home, in stores, and in the workplace. They are inexpensive, legal, and can be used anytime and anywhere. Children can die after a single exposure or suffer brain damage, which may be manifested as slurred or slow speech, tremor, memory loss, or personality changes. Nurses who work with pediatric patients should be aware of the widespread nature of this type of abuse, and advise parents to keep a close watch on volatile substances.

The terms *immunity* and *resistance* are often confused with tolerance. These terms more correctly refer to the immune system and infections and should not be used interchangeably with tolerance. For example, microorganisms become resistant to the effects of an antibiotic: They do not become tolerant. Patients become tolerant to the effects of pain relievers: They do not become resistant or immune.

11.6 CNS Depressants

CNS depressants are a group of drugs that cause patients to feel sedated or relaxed. Drugs in this group include barbiturates, nonbarbiturate sedative–hypnotics, benzodiazepines, alcohol, and opioids. Although the majority of these are legal substances, they are controlled due to their abuse potential.

SEDATIVES AND SEDATIVE–HYPNOTICS

Sedatives, also known as *tranquilizers,* are prescribed for sleep disorders and certain forms of epilepsy. The two primary classes of sedatives are the barbiturates and the nonbarbiturate sedative–hypnotics. Their actions, indications, safety profiles, and addictive potential are roughly equivalent. Physical dependence, psychologic dependence, and tolerance develop when these agents are taken for extended periods at high doses (chapter 2∞). Patients sometimes abuse these drugs by faking prescriptions or by sharing their medication with friends. Sedatives are commonly combined with other drugs of abuse, such as CNS stimulants or alcohol. Addicts often alternate between amphetamines, which keep them awake for several days, and barbiturates, which are needed to help them relax and fall sleep.

Many sedatives have a long duration of action: Effects may last an entire day, depending on the specific drug. Users may appear dull or apathetic. Higher doses resemble alcohol intoxication, with slurred speech and motor incoordination. Four commonly abused barbiturates are pentobarbital (Nembutal), amobarbital (Amytal), secobarbital (Seconal), and a combination of secobarbital and amobarbital (Tuinal). The medical use of barbiturates and nonbarbiturate sedative–hypnotics has declined markedly over the past 20 years. The use of barbiturates in treating sleep disorders is discussed in chapter 14∞, and their use for epilepsy treatment is presented in chapter 15∞.

Overdoses of barbiturates and nonbarbiturate sedative–hypnotics are extremely dangerous. These drugs suppress the respiratory centers in the brain, and the user may stop breathing or lapse into a coma. Death may result from barbiturate overdose. Withdrawal symptoms from these drugs resemble those of alcohol withdrawal and may be life threatening.

Benzodiazepines are another group of CNS depressants that have a potential for abuse. They are one of the most widely prescribed classes of drugs, and have largely replaced the barbiturates for certain disorders. Their primary indication is anxiety (chapter 14∞), although they are also used to prevent seizures (chapter 15∞) and for muscle relaxation (chapter 21∞). Popular benzodiazepines include alprazo-lam (Xanax), diazepam (Valium), temazepam (Restoril), triazolam (Halcion), and midazolam (Versed).

Although they are a frequently prescribed drug class, benzodiazepine abuse is not uncommon. Individuals abusing benzodiazepines may appear carefree, detached, sleepy, or disoriented. Death due to overdose is rare, even with high doses. Users may combine these agents with alcohol, cocaine, or heroin to augment their drug experience. If combined with other agents, overdose may be lethal. The benzodiazepine withdrawal syndrome is less severe than that of barbiturates or alcohol. Due to the longer half-life of benzodiazepines, however, drug levels remain high for several weeks. This makes abuse of benzodiazepines very dangerous.

OPIOIDS

Opioids, also known as *narcotic analgesics,* are prescribed for severe pain, persistent cough, and diarrhea. The opioid class includes natural substances obtained from the unripe seeds of the poppy plant such as opium, morphine, and codeine. Synthetic drug examples are propoxyphene (Darvon), meperidine (Demerol), oxycodone (OxyContin), fentanyl (Duragesic, Sublimaze), methadone (Dolophine), and heroin. The therapeutic effects of the opioids are discussed in more detail in chapter 18∞.

The effects of *oral* opioids begin within 30 minutes and may last over a day. *Parenteral* forms produce immediate effects, including the brief, intense rush of euphoria sought by heroin addicts. Individuals experience a range of CNS effects from extreme pleasure to slowed body activities and profound sedation. Signs include constricted pupils, an increase in the pain threshold, and respiratory depression. Overdose of opioids is extremely dangerous and fatal. The pharmacotherapy of opioid blocking drugs is covered in chapter 18∞.

Addiction to opioids can occur rapidly, and withdrawal can produce intense symptoms. Although extremely unpleasant, withdrawal from opioids is not life threatening, compared to barbiturate withdrawal. Methadone is a narcotic sometimes used to treat opioid addiction. Although methadone has addictive properties of its own, it does not produce the same degree of euphoria as other opioids, and its effects are longer lasting. Heroin addicts are switched to methadone to prevent unpleasant withdrawal symptoms. Since methadone is taken orally, patients are no longer exposed to serious risks associated with intravenous drug use, such as hepatitis and AIDS. Patients sometimes remain on methadone maintenance for a lifetime. Withdrawal from methadone is more prolonged than with heroin or morphine, but the symptoms are less intense.

ETHYL ALCOHOL

Ethyl alcohol, commonly known as *alcohol,* is one of the most commonly abused drugs. Alcohol is a legal substance for adults, and it is readily available as beer, wine, and liquor. The economic, social, and health consequences of alcohol abuse are staggering. Despite the enormous negative consequences associated with long-term use, small quantities of alcohol consumed on a daily basis have been found to reduce the risk of stroke and heart attack.

Alcohol is classified as a CNS depressant because it slows the region of the brain responsible for alertness and wakefulness. Alcohol easily crosses the blood–brain barrier, so its effects are observed within 5 to 30 minutes after consumption. Effects of alcohol are directly proportional to the amount consumed, and include relaxation, sedation, memory impairment, loss of motor coordination, reduced judgment, and decreased inhibition. Alcohol also imparts a characteristic odor to the breath and increases blood flow in certain areas of the skin, causing a flushed face, pink cheeks, or red nose. Although these symptoms are easily recognized, the nurse must be aware that other substances and disorders may cause similar effects. For example, many antianxiety agents, sedatives, and antidepressants can cause drowsiness, memory difficulties, and loss of motor coordination. Certain mouthwashes contain alcohol and cause the breath to smell like alcohol. During assessment, the skilled nurse must consider these factors before confirming alcohol use.

The presence of food in the stomach slows the absorption of alcohol, thus delaying the onset of drug action. *Metabolism,* or detoxification of alcohol by the liver, occurs at a slow, constant rate, which is not affected by the presence of food. The average rate is about 15 mL per hour—the practical equivalent of one alcoholic beverage per hour. If consumed at a higher rate, alcohol will accumulate in the blood and produce greater depressant effects on the brain. Acute overdoses of alcohol produce vomiting, severe hypotension, respiratory failure, and coma. Death due to alcohol poisoning is not uncommon. The nurse should teach patients to never combine alcohol consumption with other CNS depressants because their effects are cumulative, and profound sedation or coma may result.

With acute alcohol withdrawal, benzodiazepines are the preferred drug class for treatment (Valium or Librium therapy). While the use of benzodiazepines is more guarded for longer-term therapy of alcoholism, the reality is that many alcoholics continue to receive benzodiazepines for anxiety disorders and insomnia secondary to alcohol dependence. Seizures are also a risk to the patient, even after weeks of cessation from alcohol consumption; hence, benzodiazepine step-down therapy is often beneficial.

Chronic alcohol consumption produces both psychologic and physiologic dependence and results in a large number of adverse health effects. The organ most affected by chronic alcohol abuse is the liver. Alcoholism is a common cause of *cirrhosis,* a debilitating and often fatal failure of the liver to perform its vital functions. Liver impairment causes abnormalities in blood clotting and nutritional deficiencies. It also sensitizes the patient to the effects of all medications metabolized by the liver. For alcoholic patients, the nurse should begin therapy with reduced medication doses until the adverse effects of pharmacotherapy can be assessed.

Delirium tremens (DT) may occur in individuals who have constantly consumed alcohol for a longer period of time. Symptoms are hallucinations, confusion, disorientation, and

COMPLEMENTARY AND ALTERNATIVE THERAPIES

Milk Thistle for Alcohol Liver Damage

Milk thistle is a plant found growing in North America, from Mexico to Canada, that has been used as an herbal medicine for centuries. The active ingredient in the milk thistle plant (*Silybum marianum*), silymarin, has been confirmed to exhibit hepatoprotective qualities (Rambaldi, Jacobs, Iaquinto, & Gluud, 2007). Studies have shown that silymarin is able to neutralize the effects of alcohol, and actually stimulate liver regeneration. It acts as an antioxidant and free-radical scavenger. It is typically taken for liver cirrhosis, chronic hepatitis, and gallbladder disorders. The herb has few side effects, other than mild diarrhea, bloating, and upset stomach.

Anti-inflammatory and anticarcinogenic properties have also been documented (Song et al., 2006). Milk thistle has been claimed to reduce the growth of cancer cells. Most claims regarding milk thistle have not been verified through controlled studies.

agitation. Many patients experience anxiety, panic, paranoia, and sensations of something crawling on the skin.

Alcohol withdrawal syndrome is severe and may be life threatening. Antiseizure medications may be used in the treatment of alcohol withdrawal (chapter 15∞). Long-term treatment for alcohol abuse includes behavioral counseling and self-help groups such as Alcoholics Anonymous. Disulfiram (Antabuse) may be given to discourage relapses. Disulfiram inhibits acetaldehyde dehydrogenase, the enzyme that metabolizes alcohol. If a patient consumes alcohol while taking disulfiram, he or she becomes violently ill within 5 to 10 minutes, with headache, shortness of breath, nausea/vomiting, and other unpleasant symptoms. Disulfiram is effective only in highly motivated patients, since the success of pharmacotherapy is entirely dependent on patient compliance. Alcohol sensitivity continues for up to 2 weeks after disulfiram has been discontinued. As a pregnancy category X drug, disulfiram should never be taken during pregnancy.

In addition to disulfiram, acamprosate calcium (Campral, Forest) is an FDA-approved drug for maintaining alcohol abstinence in patients with alcohol dependence. Studies comparing the therapeutic benefit of disulfiram with acamprosate have not been fully demonstrated. The drug may benefit patients who are not candidates for naltrexone therapy. (Patients receiving naltrexone therapy or patients receiving methadone treatment are subject to withdrawal symptoms.) Acamprosate's mechanism of action involves the restoration of neuronal excitation—the alteration of gamma-aminobutyrate and glutamate activity in the CNS—and does not appear to have other central nervous system actions. Adverse reactions to acamprosate include diarrhea, flatulence, and nausea. The drug is contraindicated in patients with severe renal impairment but may be used in patients at increased risk for hepatotoxicity.

11.7 Cannabinoids

Cannabinoids are substances obtained from the hemp plant *Cannabis sativa,* which thrives in tropical climates. Cannabinoid agents are usually smoked and include marijuana, hashish, and hash oil. Although more than 61 cannabinoid chemicals have been identified, the ingredient responsible for most of the psychoactive properties is **delta-9-tetrahydrocannabinol (THC).**

MARIJUANA

Marijuana, also known as *grass, pot, weed, reefer,* or *dope,* is a natural product obtained from *C. sativa.* It is the most commonly used illicit drug in the United States. Use of marijuana slows motor activity, decreases coordination, and causes disconnected thoughts, feelings of paranoia, and euphoria. It increases thirst and craving for food, particularly chocolate and other candies. One hallmark symptom of marijuana use is red or bloodshot eyes, caused by dilation of blood vessels. THC accumulates in the gonads.

When inhaled, marijuana produces effects that occur within minutes and last up to 24 hours. Because marijuana smoke is inhaled more deeply and held within the lungs for a longer time than cigarette smoke, marijuana smoke introduces four times more particulates (tar) into the lungs than tobacco smoke. Smoking marijuana on a daily basis may increase the risk of lung cancer and other respiratory disorders. Chronic use is associated with a lack of motivation in achieving or pursuing life goals.

Unlike many abused substances, marijuana produces little physical dependence or tolerance. Withdrawal symptoms are mild, if they are experienced at all. Metabolites of THC, however, remain in the body for months to years, allowing laboratory specialists to easily determine whether someone has taken marijuana. For several days after use, THC can also be detected in the urine. Despite numerous attempts to demonstrate therapeutic applications for marijuana, results have been controversial and the medical value of the drug remains to be proved.

11.8 Hallucinogens

Hallucinogens consist of a diverse class of chemicals that have in common the ability to produce an altered, dreamlike state of consciousness. The prototype substance for this class, sometimes called **psychedelics,** is LSD. All hallucinogens are Schedule I drugs: They have no medical use.

LSD

For nearly all drugs of abuse, predictable symptoms occur in every user. Effects from hallucinogens, however, are highly variable and dependent on the mood and expectations of the user and the surrounding environment in which the substance is used. Two people taking the same agent will report completely different symptoms, and the same person may report different symptoms with each use. Users who take LSD and psilocybin (magic mushrooms, or "shrooms") (➤ Figure 11.1) may experience symptoms such as laughter, visions, religious revelations, or deep personal insights. Common occurrences are hallucinations and afterimages projected onto people as they move. Users also report unusually bright lights and vivid colors. Some users hear voices; others report smells. Many experience a profound sense of truth and deep-directed thoughts. Unpleasant experiences can be terrifying and may include anxiety, panic attacks, confusion, severe depression, and paranoia.

MyNursingKit | The History of LSD

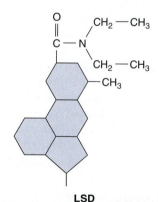

Psilocybin
(4-phosphoryl-DMT)

LSD

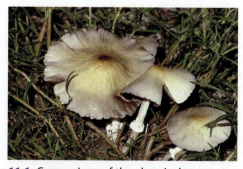

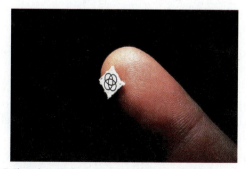

➤ *Figure 11.1* Comparison of the chemical structures of psilocybin and LSD. Psilocybin (left) is derived from a mushroom
Source: James Beveridge/Visuals Unlimited.

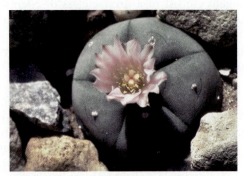

Mescaline

➤ **Figure 11.2** The chemical structure of mescaline, derived from the peyote cactus
Source: Pearson Education/PH College.

LSD, also called *acid, the beast, blotter acid,* and *California sunshine,* is derived from a fungus that grows on rye and other grains. LSD is nearly always administered orally and can be manufactured in capsule, tablet, or liquid form. A common and inexpensive method for distributing LSD is to place drops of the drug on paper, often containing the images of cartoon characters or graphics related to drug culture. The paper is dried; users then ingest the paper containing the LSD to produce the drug's effects.

LSD is distributed throughout the body immediately after use. Effects are experienced within an hour, and may last from 6 to 12 hours. LSD affects the central and autonomic nervous systems, increasing blood pressure, elevating body temperature, dilating pupils, and increasing the heart rate. Repeated use may cause impaired memory and inability to reason. In extreme cases, patients may develop psychoses. One unusual adverse effect is flashbacks, in which the user experiences the effects of the drug again, sometimes weeks, months, or years after the drug was initially taken. Although tolerance is observed, little or no dependence occurs with the hallucinogens.

OTHER HALLUCINOGENS

In addition to LSD, other abused hallucinogens include the following:

- *Mescaline:* Found in the peyote cactus of Mexico and Central America (➤ Figure 11.2)
- *MDMA (3,4-methylenedioxymethamphetamine; XTC or Ecstasy):* An amphetamine originally synthesized for research purposes that has since become extremely popular among teens and young adults
- *DOM (2,5 dimethoxy-4-methylamphetamine):* A recreational drug often linked with rave parties as a drug of choice having the name STP

- *MDA (3,4-methylenedioxyamphetamine):* Called the love drug because it is believed to enhance sexual desires
- *Phenylcyclohexylpiperidine (PCP; angel dust or phencyclidine):* Produces a trancelike state that may last for days and results in severe brain damage
- *Ketamine (date rape drug or special coke):* produces unconsciousness and amnesia; primary legal use is as an anesthetic

11.9 CNS Stimulants

Stimulants include a diverse family of drugs known for their ability to increase the activity of the CNS. Some are available by prescription for the treatment of narcolepsy, obesity, and attention deficit/hyperactivity disorder (ADHD). As drugs of abuse, CNS stimulants are taken to produce a sense of exhilaration, improve mental and physical performance, reduce appetite, prolong wakefulness, or simply "get high." Stimulants include the amphetamines, cocaine, methylphenidate, and caffeine.

AMPHETAMINES AND METHYLPHENIDATE

CNS stimulants have effects similar to those of the neurotransmitter norepinephrine (chapter 13∞). Norepinephrine affects awareness and wakefulness by activating neurons in a part of the brain called the **reticular formation.** High doses of amphetamines give the user a feeling of self-confidence, euphoria, alertness, and empowerment; but just as short-term use induces favorable feelings, long-term use often results in feelings of restlessness, anxiety, and fits of rage, especially when the user is coming down from a "high" induced by the drug.

Most CNS stimulants affect cardiovascular and respiratory activity, resulting in increased blood pressure and increased respiration rate. Other symptoms include dilated pupils, sweating, and tremors. Overdoses of some stimulants lead to seizures and cardiac arrest.

Amphetamines and dextroamphetamines were once widely prescribed for depression, obesity, drowsiness, and congestion. In the 1960s, it became recognized that the medical uses of amphetamines did not outweigh their risk for misuse. Due to the development of safer medications, the current therapeutic uses of these drugs are extremely limited. Most substance abusers obtain these agents from illegal laboratories, which can easily produce amphetamines and make tremendous profits.

Dextroamphetamine (Dexedrine) may be prescribed for short-term weight loss when all other attempts to reduce weight have been exhausted, and to treat narcolepsy. Methamphetamine, commonly called *ice,* is often used as a recreational drug by users who like the rush that it gives them. It usually is administered in powder or crystal form, but it may also be smoked. Methamphetamine is a Schedule II drug marketed under the trade name Desoxyn, although most abusers obtain it from illegal methamphetamine (*meth*) laboratories. A structural analogue of methamphetamine, methcathinone (street name, *Cat*) is made illegally and snorted, taken orally, or injected IV. Methcathinone is a Schedule I agent.

Methylphenidate (Ritalin) is a CNS stimulant widely prescribed for children diagnosed with **attention deficit/ hyperactivity disorder (ADHD)**. Ritalin has a calming effect in children who are inattentive or hyperactive. By stimulating the alertness center in the brain, the child is able to focus on tasks for longer periods. This explains the paradoxical calming effects that this stimulant has on children, which is usually the opposite of that on adults. The therapeutic applications of methylphenidate are discussed in chapter 16∞.

Ritalin is a Schedule II drug that has many of the same effects as cocaine and amphetamines. It is sometimes abused by adolescents and adults seeking euphoria. Tablets are crushed and used intranasally or dissolved in liquid and injected IV. Ritalin is sometimes mixed with heroin, a combination called a *speedball*.

COCAINE

Cocaine is a natural substance obtained from leaves of the coca plant, which grows in the Andes Mountains region of South America. Documentation suggests that the plant has been used by Andean cultures since 2500 B.C. Natives in this region chew the coca leaves, or make teas of the dried leaves. Because coca is taken orally, absorption is slow, and the leaves contain only 1% cocaine, so users do not suffer the ill effects caused by chemically pure extracts from the plant. In the Andean culture, use of coca leaves is not considered substance abuse because it is part of the social norms of that society.

Cocaine is a Schedule II drug that produces actions similar to those of the amphetamines, although its effects are usually more rapid and intense. It is the second most commonly abused illicit drug in the United States. Routes of administration include snorting, smoking, and injecting. In small doses, cocaine produces feelings of intense euphoria, a decrease in hunger, analgesia, illusions of physical strength, and increased sensory perception. Larger doses will magnify these effects and also cause rapid heartbeat, sweating, dilation of the pupils, and an elevated body temperature. After the feelings of euphoria diminish, the user is left with a sense of irritability, insomnia, depression, and extreme distrust. Some users report the sensation that insects are crawling under the skin. Users who snort cocaine develop a chronic runny nose, a crusty redness around the nostrils, and deterioration of the nasal cartilage. Overdose can result in dysrhythmias, convulsions, stroke, or death due to respiratory arrest. The withdrawal syndrome for amphetamines and cocaine is much less intense than from alcohol or barbiturate abuse.

CAFFEINE

Caffeine is a natural substance found in the seeds, leaves, or fruits of more than 63 plant species throughout the world. Significant amounts of caffeine are consumed in chocolate, coffee, tea, soft drinks, and ice cream. Caffeine is sometimes added to OTC pain relievers because it has been shown to increase the effectiveness of these medications. Caffeine travels to almost all parts of the body after ingestion, and several hours are needed for the body to metabolize and eliminate the drug. Caffeine has a pronounced diuretic effect.

Caffeine is considered a CNS stimulant because it produces increased mental alertness, restlessness, nervousness, irritability, and insomnia. The physical effects of caffeine include bronchodilation, increased blood pressure, increased production of stomach acid, and changes in blood glucose levels. Repeated use of caffeine may result in physical dependence and tolerance. Withdrawal symptoms include headaches, fatigue, depression, and impaired performance of daily activities.

11.10 Nicotine

Nicotine is sometimes considered a CNS stimulant, and although it does increase alertness, its actions and long-term consequences place it in a class by itself. Nicotine is unique among abused substances in that it is legal, strongly addictive, and highly carcinogenic. Furthermore, use of tobacco can cause harmful effects to those in the immediate area who breathe secondhand smoke. Patients often do not consider tobacco use as substance abuse.

TOBACCO USE AND NICOTINE

The most common method by which nicotine enters the body is through the inhalation of cigarette, pipe, or cigar smoke. Tobacco smoke contains more than 1,000 chemicals, a significant number of which are carcinogens. The primary addictive substance present in cigarette smoke is nicotine. Effects of inhaled nicotine may last from 30 minutes to several hours.

Nicotine affects many body systems including the nervous, cardiovascular, and endocrine systems. Nicotine stimulates the CNS directly, causing increased alertness and ability to focus, feelings of relaxation, and light-headedness. The cardiovascular effects of nicotine include an accelerated heart rate and increased blood pressure, caused by activation of nicotinic receptors located throughout the autonomic nervous system (chapter 13∞). These cardiovascular effects can be particularly serious in patients taking oral contraceptives: The risk of a fatal heart attack is five times greater in smokers than in nonsmokers. Muscular tremors may occur with moderate doses of nicotine, and convulsions may result from very high doses. Nicotine affects the endocrine system by increasing the basal metabolic rate, leading to weight loss. Nicotine also reduces appetite. Chronic smoking leads to bronchitis, emphysema, and lung cancer.

Both psychologic and physical dependence occur relatively quickly with nicotine. Once started on tobacco, patients tend to continue their drug use for many years, despite overwhelming medical evidence that the quality of life will be adversely affected and their life span shortened. Discontinuation results in agitation, weight gain, anxiety, headache, and an extreme craving for the drug. Although nicotine replacement patches and gum assist patients in dealing with the unpleasant withdrawal symptoms, only 25% of patients who attempt to stop smoking remain tobacco-free a year later.

11.11 The Nurse's Role in Substance Abuse

The nurse serves a key role in the prevention, diagnosis, and treatment of substance abuse. A thorough medical history must include questions about substance abuse. In the case of IV drug users, the nurse must consider the possibility of HIV infection, hepatitis, tuberculosis, and associated diagnoses. Patients are often reluctant to report their drug use, for fear of embarrassment or being arrested. The nurse must be knowledgeable about the signs of substance abuse and withdrawal symptoms, and develop a keen sense of perception during the assessment stage. A trusting nurse–patient relationship is essential to helping patients deal with their dependence. By using therapeutic communication skills and by demonstrating a nonjudgmental, empathetic attitude, the nurse can build a trusting relationship with patients.

It is often difficult for a health care provider not to condemn or stigmatize a patient for his or her substance abuse. Nurses, especially those in large cities, are all too familiar with the devastating medical, economic, and social consequences of heroin and cocaine abuse. The nurse must be firm in disapproving of substance abuse, yet compassionate in trying to help the patient receive treatment. A list of social agencies dealing with dependency should be readily available to provide patients. When possible, the nurse should attempt to involve family members and other close contacts in the treatment regimen. Educating the patient and family members about the long-term consequences of substance abuse is essential. Substance abuse also affects members of the health care community. Nurses should be aware of the ramifications of drug abuse and the impact this would have on the nursing license.

Chapter REVIEW

KEY CONCEPTS

The numbered key concepts provide a succinct summary of the important points from the corresponding numbered section within the chapter. If any of these points are not clear, refer to the numbered section within the chapter for review.

11.1 A wide variety of substances may be abused by individuals. All of these substances share the common characteristic of altering brain physiology and/or perception.

11.2 Addiction is an overwhelming compulsion to continue repeated drug use that has both neurobiologic and psychosocial components.

11.3 Certain substances can cause both physical and psychologic dependence, which result in continued drug-seeking behavior despite negative health and social consequences.

11.4 The withdrawal syndrome is a set of uncomfortable symptoms that occur when an abused substance is no longer available. The severity of the withdrawal syndrome varies among the different drug classes.

11.5 Tolerance is a biologic condition that occurs with repeated use of certain substances, and results in the necessity for higher doses to achieve the same initial response. Cross-tolerance occurs between closely related drugs.

11.6 CNS depressants, which include sedatives, opioids, and ethyl alcohol, decrease the activity of the brain, causing drowsiness, slowed speech, and diminished motor coordination.

11.7 Cannabinoids, which include marijuana, are the most frequently abused class of illegal substances. They cause less physical dependence and tolerance than the CNS depressants.

11.8 Hallucinogens, including LSD, cause an altered state of thought and perception similar to dreams. Their effects are extremely variable and unpredictable.

11.9 CNS stimulants—including amphetamines, methylphenidate, caffeine, and cocaine—increase the activity of the CNS and produce increased wakefulness.

11.10 Nicotine is a powerful and highly addictive cardiovascular and CNS stimulant that has serious adverse effects with chronic use.

11.11 The nurse serves an important role in educating patients about the consequences of drug abuse and in recommending appropriate treatment.

NCLEX-RN® REVIEW QUESTIONS

1 Following a surgical procedure, the patient states he does not want to take narcotic analgesics for pain because he is afraid he will become addicted to the drug. Response by the nurse is based on the knowledge that:
1. dependence on narcotics is common among postoperative patients.
2. addiction to prescription drugs is rare when used according to protocol.
3. female patients are more likely to become addicted.
4. addiction is rare if the patient has a high pain threshold.

2 The patient states she has been increasing the amount and frequency of the antianxiety drug she is using. The nurse understands that the patient has most likely developed to the drug.
1. immunity
2. tolerance
3. resistance
4. addiction

3 A 13-year-old boy has been showing signs of paranoia and anxiety and, according to his parents, has been "acting very oddly," including recently being reclusive and locking himself in his room. On occasion, the young man has shown loss of coordination and an apparent distorted sense of time. The parents are very concerned, since they have been notified by the school nurse that their son has been implicated in drug activity. In the nurse's office, the young man asks if he can have a drink of water for "dry mouth." The nurse observes that his face is flushed and his eyes reddened. Which substance has the young man most likely used?
1. Heroin
2. Crack
3. Barbiturates
4. Marijuana

4 The patient with a history of alcohol abuse is admitted to the hospital. The nursing care plan includes assessment of the patient for which of the following symptoms indicative of alcohol withdrawal?
1. Mental depression, headaches, and hunger
2. Insomnia, nausea, and bradycardia
3. Tremors, hallucinations, and delirium
4. Weakness, hypotension, and violent yawning

5 The patient states that she is going to quit smoking "cold turkey." The nurse teaches the patient to expect which of the following symptoms during withdrawal from nicotine? (Select all that apply.)
1. Headaches and insomnia
2. Increased appetite
3. Tremors
4. Insomnia
5. Increased heart rate and blood pressure

6 What is the difference between physical and psychologic dependence?
1. Physical dependence is the adaptation of the body to a substance over time such that when the substance is withdrawn, withdrawal symptoms will result. Psychologic dependence is the overwhelming desire to continue using a substance after it is stopped or withdrawn, but without physical withdrawal symptoms occurring.
2. Physical and psychologic dependence are terms that are used interchangeably. In both cases, physical withdrawal symptoms will result if the substance is withdrawn from use.
3. They occur together: psychologic dependence is the first type of dependence to occur with a substance, followed by physical dependence.
4. Psychologic dependence develops when the brain adapts over time to the use of the substance. Physical dependence is the active seeking of a substance associated with a desire to continue using the substance.

CRITICAL THINKING QUESTIONS

1. A 16-year-old female patient is hospitalized in the ICU following the ingestion of a high dose of MDMA (Ecstasy) at a street dance. Her mother cannot understand why her daughter could have such serious renal and cardiovascular complications after "just one dose." The nurse is concerned that the mother lacks sufficient knowledge to be helpful. What teaching does the nurse conduct?

2. The wife of a 24-year-old professional football player is admitted to the emergency room after being beaten and verbally abused by her husband. She says that he is under a great deal of stress and has been working hard to maintain peak athletic fitness. She says she has noticed that her husband becomes irritable easily. What assessments and interventions should the nurse perform?

3. A 44-year-old businessman travels weekly for his company and has had difficulty sleeping in "one hotel after another." He consulted his health care provider and has been taking secobarbital (Seconal) nightly to help him sleep. The patient has called the nurse at the health care provider's office and has said, "I have just got to have something stronger." What does the nurse consider as part of the assessment?

See Appendix D for answers and rationales for all activities.

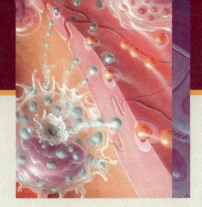

Chapter 12

Emergency Preparedness and Poisonings

LEARNING OUTCOMES

After reading this chapter, the student should be able to:

1. Explain why drugs are important in the context of emergency preparedness.
2. Discuss the role of the nurse in preparing for and responding to a bioterrorist act.
3. Identify the purpose and components of the Strategic National Stockpile (SNS).
4. Explain the threat of anthrax contamination and how it is transmitted.
5. Discuss the clinical manifestations and treatment of anthrax exposure.
6. Identify specific viruses that would most likely be used in a bioterrorist act.
7. Explain the advantages and disadvantages of vaccination as a means of preventing illness due to bioterrorist attacks.
8. Provide examples of chemical agents that might be used in a bioterrorism incident, and their treatments.
9. Describe the symptoms of acute radiation exposure and the role of potassium iodide (KI) in preventing thyroid cancer.
10. List top substances that represent human poison exposures.
11. Explain fundamental elements of toxicity treatment provided by the nurse.
12. Describe specific antidotes used to treat common overdosed substances and toxins.

KEY TERMS

activated charcoal *page 122*
acute radiation syndrome *page 120*
anthrax *page 118*
basic supportive care *page 121*
bioterrorism *page 116*

gastric lavage and aspiration *page 122*
ionizing radiation *page 120*
nerve agents *page 120*
specific antidotes *page 122*
Strategic National Stockpile (SNS) *page 118*

Syrup of Ipecac *page 122*
vaccine *page 119*
vendor-managed inventory (VMI) *page 118*
whole-bowel irrigation *page 122*

It is important that nurses understand the role that drugs play in preventing or controlling global disease and toxic outbreaks. Drugs are the most powerful tools available to the medical community for countering worldwide epidemics and bioterrorist threats. If medical personnel could not identify, isolate, or treat the causes of global diseases, a major incident could easily overwhelm health care resources and produce a catastrophic loss of life. Drugs are a major component of emergency preparedness plans. Drugs are also a component of poison removal protocols, and some drugs serve as antidotes to counteract the effects of specific poisons. This chapter discusses the role of pharmacology in the prevention and treatment of diseases or conditions that might develop in the context of a biologic, chemical, or nuclear attack and the general management of poisonings in a clinical setting.

12.1 The Nature of Bioterrorism

Prior to the September 11, 2001 terrorist attacks on the United States, the attention of health care providers regarding disease outbreaks was focused mainly on the spread of traditional infectious diseases. These included possible epidemics caused by influenza, tuberculosis, cholera, and HIV. Table 12.1 lists the 10 most dangerous infectious diseases ranked according to which disorders caused the most deaths worldwide in the year 2000. Other infectious diseases such as food poisoning and sexually transmitted diseases were also common though considered less important, because they produced fewer fatalities.

The aftermath of the September 11, 2001 attacks prompted the health care community to expand its awareness of outbreaks and treatments to include bioterrorism and the health effects of biologic and chemical weapons. **Bioterrorism** may be defined as the intentional use of infectious biologic agents, chemical substances, or radiation to cause widespread harm or illness. The public has become more aware of the threat of bioterrorism because such federal agencies as the Centers for Disease Control and Prevention (CDC) and the U.S. Department of Defense have stepped up efforts to inform, educate, and prepare the public for disease outbreaks of a less traditional nature.

The goals of a bioterrorist are to create widespread public panic and to cause as many casualties as possible. There is no shortage of agents that can be used for this purpose. Indeed, some of these agents are easily obtainable and require little

PHARMFACTS

Potential Chemical and Biologic Agents for Terrorist Attacks

- Robert Stevens, the 63-year-old employee of American Media who died in Florida on October 5, 2001, was the first person to die from anthrax in the United States in 25 years.
- In 1979, accidental release of anthrax from a research lab in the Soviet Union killed 68 people. The problem was traced to a faulty air filter.
- The Ebola virus causes death by hemorrhagic fever in up to 90% of the patients who show clinical symptoms of infection.
- Ebola viruses are found in central Africa. Although the source of the viruses in nature remains unknown, monkeys (like humans) appear to be susceptible to infection and serve as sources of the virus if infected.
- Widespread public smallpox vaccinations ceased in the United States in 1972.
- It is estimated that 7 million to 8 million doses of smallpox vaccine are in storage at the CDC. This stock cannot be easily replenished, since all vaccine production facilities were dismantled after 1980, and new vaccine production requires 24 to 36 months.
- Most nerve agents were originally produced in a search for insecticides, but because of their toxicity, they were evaluated for military use.
- Chemicals used in bioterrorist acts need not be sophisticated or difficult to obtain: Toxic industrial chemicals such as chlorine, phosgene, and hydrogen cyanide are used in commercial manufacturing and are readily available.

TABLE 12.1	The 10 Most Dangerous Infectious Diseases in the World, 2000		
Disease	Causative Agent	Target	Deaths per Year (millions)
Influenza	*Haemophilus influenzae*	Respiratory system	3.7
Tuberculosis	*Mycobacterium tuberculosis*	Lungs	2.9
Cholera	*Vibrio cholerae*	Digestive tract	2.5
AIDS	Human immunodeficiency virus	Immune response	2.3
Malaria	*Plasmodium falciparum*	Blood disorder	1.5
Measles	Rubeola virus	Lungs and meninges	0.96
Hepatitis B	Hepatitis B virus (HBV)	Liver	0.605
Whooping cough	*Bordetella pertussis*	Respiratory system	0.41
Tetanus	*Clostridium tetani*	Entire body (infections)	0.275
Dengue fever	Flavivirus	Entire body (fever)	0.14

Source: July 2001 report by the WHO/Industry Drug Development Working Group—World Health Organization: http://www.who.int/en/

or no specialized knowledge to disseminate. Areas of greatest concern include acutely infectious diseases such as anthrax, smallpox, plague, and hemorrhagic viruses; incapacitating chemicals such as nerve gas, cyanide, and chlorinated agents; and nuclear and radiation emergencies. The CDC has categorized the biologic threats, based on their potential impact on public health, as shown in Table 12.2.

12.2 Role of the Nurse in Emergency Preparedness

Emergency preparedness is not a new concept. For more than 30 years, the Joint Commission on Accreditation of Healthcare Organizations (JCAHO) has required accredited hospitals to develop disaster plans and to conduct periodic emergency drills to determine readiness. Prior to the late 1990s, disaster plans and training focused on natural disasters such as tornadoes, hurricanes and floods, or accidents such as explosions that could cause multiple casualties. In the late 1990s, the JCAHO standards added the possibility of bioterrorism and virulent infectious organisms as rare, though possible, scenarios in disaster preparedness.

In 2001 JCAHO issued new standards that shifted the focus from disaster preparedness to emergency management. The newer standards included more than just responding to the immediate casualties caused by a disaster, they also considered how an agency's health care delivery system might change during a crisis, and how it might return to normal operations following the incident. The expanded focus also included how the individual health care agency would coordinate its efforts with community resources, such as other hospitals and public health agencies. State and federal agencies revised their emergency preparedness guidelines in an attempt to plan more rationally for a range of disasters including possible bioterrorist acts.

Planning for bioterrorist acts requires close cooperation among all the different health care professionals. Nurses are central to the effort. Because a bioterrorist incident may occur in any community without warning, nurses must be prepared to respond immediately. The following elements underscore the key roles of nurses in meeting the challenges of a potential bioterrorist event:

- *Education:* Nurses should maintain a current knowledge and understanding of emergency management relating to

TABLE 12.2	Categories of Infectious Agents	
Category	Description	Examples
A	Agents that: can easily be disseminated or transmitted person to person; cause high mortality, with potential for major public health impact; might cause public panic and social disruption; or require special action for public health preparedness	*Bacillus anthracis* (anthrax) *Clostridium botulinum* toxin (botulism) *Francisella tularensis* (tularemia) Variola major (smallpox) Viral hemorrhagic fevers such as Marburg and Ebola *Yersinia pestis* (plague)
B	Agents that: are moderately easy to disseminate; cause moderate morbidity and low mortality; or require specific enhancements of CDC's diagnostic capacity and enhanced disease surveillance	*Brucella* species (brucellosis) *Burkholderia mallei* (glanders) *Burkholderia pseudomallei* (melioidosis) *Chlamydia psittaci* (psittacosis) *Coxiella burnetii* (Q fever) Epsilon toxin of *Clostridium perfringens* Food safety threats such as *Salmonella* and *E. coli* Ricin toxin from *Ricinus communis* *Staphylococcus* enterotoxin B Viral encephalitis Water safety threats such as *Vibrio cholerae* and *Cryptosporidium parvum*
C	Emerging pathogens that could be engineered for mass dissemination because of their availability, ease of production and dissemination, and potential for high morbidity and mortality rates and major health impacts	Hantaviruses Multidrug-resistant tuberculosis Nipah virus (NiV) Tick-borne encephalitis viruses Yellow fever

Source: http://www.bt.cdc.gov/agent/agentlist-category.asp

bioterrorist activities. Nurses can assist the public by providing current and accurate information about potential or real threats to public health and correcting misinformation about these topics.

- *Resources:* Nurses should maintain a current listing of health and law enforcement contacts and resources in their local communities who would assist in the event of bioterrorist activity. When appropriate, nurses may participate in local, hospital-related, or regional first-responder teams as a resource to their community.

- *Diagnosis and treatment:* Nurses should be aware of the early signs and symptoms of chemical and biologic agents, and their immediate treatment, and report the findings to the appropriate authorities.

- *Planning:* Nurses should be involved in developing emergency management plans for their own families, assisting neighbors and their communities to develop such plans, and participating through their health care agencies in disaster preparedness drills.

12.3 Strategic National Stockpile

Should a chemical or biologic attack occur, it would likely be rapid and unexpected, and would produce multiple casualties. Although planning for such an event is an important part of disaster preparedness, individual health care agencies and local communities could easily be overwhelmed by such a crisis. Shortages of needed drugs, medical equipment, and supplies would be expected.

The **Strategic National Stockpile (SNS),** formerly called the National Pharmaceutical Stockpile, is a program designed to ensure the immediate deployment of essential medical materials to a community in the event of a large-scale chemical or biologic attack. Managed by the CDC, the stockpile consists of the following materials:

- Antibiotics
- Vaccines
- Medical, surgical, and patient support supplies such as bandages, airway supplies, and IV equipment

The SNS has two components. The first is called a *push package,* which consists of a preassembled set of supplies and pharmaceuticals designed to meet the needs of an unknown biologic or chemical threat. There are eight fully stocked 50-ton push packages stored in climate-controlled warehouses throughout the United States. They are in locations where they can reach any community in the United States within 12 hours after an attack. The decision to deploy the push package is based on an assessment of the situation by federal government officials.

The second SNS component consists of a **vendor-managed inventory (VMI)** package. VMI packages are shipped, if necessary, after the chemical or biologic threat has more clearly been identified. The materials consist of supplies and pharmaceuticals more specific to the chemical or biologic agent used in the attack. VMI packages are designed to arrive within 24 to 36 hours.

The stockpiling of antibiotics and vaccines by local hospitals, clinics, or individuals for the purpose of preparing for a bioterrorist act is not recommended. Pharmaceuticals have a finite expiration date, and keeping large stores of drugs can be costly. Furthermore, stockpiling could cause drug shortages and prevent the delivery of these pharmaceuticals to communities where they may be needed most.

AGENTS USED IN BIOTERRORISM ACTS

Bioterrorists could potentially use any biologic, chemical, or physical agent to cause widespread panic and serious illness. Knowing which agents are most likely to be used in an incident helps nurses plan and implement emergency preparedness policies.

12.4 Anthrax

One of the first threats following the terrorist attacks on the World Trade Center was **anthrax.** In the fall of 2001, five people died as a result of exposure to anthrax, presumably due to purposeful, bioterrorist actions. At least 13 U.S. citizens were infected, several governmental employees were threatened, and the U.S. Postal Service was interrupted for several weeks. There was initial concern that anthrax outbreaks might disrupt many other essential operations throughout the country.

Anthrax is caused by the bacterium *Bacillus anthracis,* which normally affects domestic and wild animals. A wide variety of hoofed animals are affected by the disease, including cattle, sheep, goats, horses, donkeys, pigs, American bison, antelopes, elephants, and lions. If transmitted to humans by exposure to an open wound, through contaminated food, or by inhalation, *B. anthracis* can cause serious damage to body tissues. Symptoms of anthrax infection usually appear 1 to 6 days after exposure. Depending on how the bacterium is transmitted, specific types of anthrax "poisoning" may be observed, each characterized by hallmark symptoms. Clinical manifestations of anthrax are summarized in Table 12.3.

B. anthracis causes disease by the emission of two types of toxins, *edema toxin* and *lethal toxin.* These toxins cause necrosis and accumulation of exudate, which produces pain, swelling, and restriction of activity, the general symptoms associated with almost every form of anthrax. Another component, the *anthrax binding receptor,* allows the bacterium to bind to human cells and act as a "doorway" for both types of toxins to enter.

Further ensuring its chance for spreading, *B. anthracis* is spore forming. Anthrax spores can remain viable in soil for hundreds, and perhaps thousands, of years. Anthrax spores are resistant to drying, heat, and some harsh chemicals. These spores are the main cause for public health concern, because they are responsible for producing inhalation anthrax, the most dangerous form of the disease. After entry into the lungs, *B. anthracis* spores are ingested by macrophages and carried to lymphoid tissue, resulting in tissue necrosis, swelling, and hemorrhage. One of the main body areas affected is the mediastinum, which is a potential

TABLE 12.3	**Clinical Manifestations of Anthrax**	
Type	Description	Symptoms
Cutaneous anthrax	Most common but least complicated form of anthrax; almost always curable if treated within the first few weeks of exposure; results from direct contact of contaminated products with an open wound or cut	Small skin lesions develop and turn into black scabs; inoculation takes less than 1 week; cannot be spread by person-to-person contact
Gastrointestinal anthrax	Rare form of anthrax; without treatment, can be lethal in up to 50% of cases; results from eating anthrax-contaminated food, usually meat	Sore throat, difficulty swallowing, cramping diarrhea, and abdominal swelling
Inhalation anthrax	Least common but the most dangerous form of anthrax; can be successfully treated if identified within the first few days after exposure; results from inhaling anthrax spores	Initially, fatigue, and fever for several days, followed by persistent cough and shortness of breath; without treatment, death can result within 4–6 days

site for tissue injury and fluid accumulation. Meningitis is also a common pathology. If treatment is delayed, inhalation anthrax is lethal in almost every case.

B. anthracis is found in contaminated animal products such as wool, hair, dander, and bonemeal, but it can also be packaged in other forms, making it transmissible through the air or by direct contact. Terrorists have delivered it in the form of a fine powder, making it less obvious to detect. The powder can be inconspicuously spread on virtually any surface, making it a serious concern for public safety.

The antibiotic ciprofloxacin (Cipro) has traditionally been used for anthrax prophylaxis and treatment. For prophylaxis, the usual dosage is 500 mg PO (by mouth), every 12 hours for 60 days. If exposure has been confirmed, ciprofloxacin should immediately be administered at a usual dose of 400 mg IV (intravenously), every 12 hours. Other antibiotics are also effective against anthrax, including penicillin, vancomycin, ampicillin, erythromycin, tetracycline, and doxycycline. In the case of inhalation anthrax, the FDA has approved the use of ciprofloxacin and doxycycline in combination for treatment.

Many members of the public have become intensely concerned about bioterrorism threats and have asked their health care provider to provide them with ciprofloxacin. The public should be discouraged from seeking the prophylactic use of antibiotics in cases where anthrax exposure has not been confirmed. Indiscriminate, unnecessary use of antibiotics can be expensive, can cause significant side effects, and can promote the appearance of resistant bacterial strains. The student should refer to chapter 34∞ to review the precautions and guidelines regarding the appropriate use of antibiotics.

Although anthrax immunization (vaccination) has been licensed by the FDA for 30 years, it has not been widely used because of the extremely low incidence of this disease in the United States prior to September 2001. The **vaccine** has been prepared from proteins from the anthrax bacteria, dubbed "protective antigens." Anthrax vaccine works the same way as other vaccines: by causing the body to make protective antibodies and thus preventing the onset of disease and symptoms. Immunization for anthrax consists of three subcutaneous injections given 2 weeks apart, followed by three additional subcutaneous injections given at 6, 12, and 18 months. Annual booster injections of the vaccine are recommended. At this time, the CDC recommends vaccination for only select populations: laboratory personnel who work

with anthrax, military personnel deployed to high-risk areas, and those who deal with animal products imported from areas with a high incidence of the disease.

There is an ongoing controversy regarding the safety of the anthrax vaccine and whether it is truly effective in preventing the disease. Until these issues are resolved, the use of anthrax immunization will likely remain limited to select groups. Vaccines and the immune response are discussed in more detail in chapter 32∞.

12.5 Viruses

In 2002, the public was astounded as researchers announced that they had "built" a poliovirus, a threat that U.S. health officials thought had essentially been eradicated in 1994. Although virtually eliminated in the Western Hemisphere, polio was reported in at least 27 countries as late as 1998. The infection persists among infants and children in areas with contaminated drinking water or food, mainly in underdeveloped regions of India, Pakistan, Afghanistan, western and central Africa, and the Dominican Republic. In the United States, polio remains a potential threat in 1 of 300,000 to 500,000 patients who are vaccinated with the oral poliovirus vaccine.

The current concern is that bioterrorists will culture the poliovirus and release it into regions where people have not been vaccinated. An even more dangerous threat is that a mutated strain, for which there is no effective vaccine, might be developed. Because the genetic code of the poliovirus is small (around 7,500 base pairs), it can be manufactured in a relatively simple laboratory. Once the virus is isolated, hundreds of different mutant strains could be produced in a very short time.

In addition to polio, smallpox is considered a potential biohazard. Once thought to have been eradicated from the planet in the 1970s, the variola virus that causes this disease has been harbored in research labs in several countries. Much of its genetic code (200,000 base pairs) has been sequenced and is public information. The disease is spread person to person as an aerosol or droplets or by contact with contaminated objects such as clothing or bedding. Only a few viral particles are needed to cause infection. If the virus is released into an unvaccinated population, as many as one in three people could die.

There are no effective therapies for treating patients infected by most types of viruses that could be used in a bioterrorist attack. For some viruses, however, it is possible to create a vaccine that could stimulate the body's immune system in a manner that could be remembered at a later date. In the case of smallpox, a stockpile of the vaccine exists in enough quantity to administer to every person in the United States. The variola vaccine provides a high level of protection if given prior to exposure, or up to 3 days later. Protection may last from 3 to 5 years. The following are contraindications to receiving the smallpox vaccine, unless the individual has confirmed face-to-face contact with an infected patient:

- Persons with (or a history of) atopic dermatitis or eczema
- Persons with acute, active, or exfoliative skin conditions
- Persons with altered immune states (e.g., HIV, AIDS, leukemia, lymphoma, immunosuppressive drugs)
- Pregnant and breast-feeding women
- Children younger than 1 year
- Persons who have a serious allergy to any component of the vaccine

It has been suggested that multiple vaccines be created, mass produced, and stockpiled to meet the challenges of a terrorist attack. Another suggestion has called for mass vaccination of the public, or at least those health care providers and law enforcement employees who might be exposed to infected patients.

Vaccines have side effects, some of which are quite serious. In the case of smallpox vaccination, for example, it is estimated that there might be as many as 250 deaths for every million people inoculated. If the smallpox vaccine was given to every person in the United States (approximately 300 million), possible deaths from vaccination could exceed 75,000. In addition, terrorists having some knowledge of genetic structure could create a modified strain of the virus that renders existing vaccines totally ineffective. It appears, then, that mass vaccination is not an appropriate solution until research can produce safer and more effective vaccines.

12.6 Toxic Chemicals

Although chemical warfare agents have been available since World War I, medicine has produced few drug antidotes. Many treatments provide minimal help other than to relieve some symptoms and provide comfort following exposure. Most chemical agents used in warfare were created to cause mass casualties; others were designed to cause so much discomfort that soldiers would be too weak to continue fighting. Potential chemicals that could be used in a terrorist act include nerve gases, blood agents, choking and vomiting agents, and those that cause severe blistering. Table 12.4 provides a summary of selected chemical agents and known antidotes for chemical warfare and first-aid treatments.

The chemical category of main pharmacologic significance is **nerve agents.** Exposure to these acutely toxic chemicals can cause convulsions and loss of consciousness within seconds, and respiratory failure within minutes. Almost all

signs of exposure to nerve gas agents relate to overstimulation by the neurotransmitter acetylcholine (Ach) at both central and peripheral sites located throughout the body.

Acetylcholine is normally degraded by the enzyme acetylcholinesterase (AchE) in the synaptic space. Nerve agents block AchE, increasing the action of acetylcholine in the synaptic space; therefore, all symptoms of nerve gas exposure such as salivation, increased sweating, muscle twitching, involuntary urination and defecation, confusion, convulsions, and death are the direct result of Ach overstimulation. To remedy this condition, nerve agent antidote and Mark I injector kits that contain the anticholinergic drug atropine or a related medication are available in cases where nerve agent release is expected. Atropine blocks the attachment of Ach to receptor sites and prevents the overstimulation caused by the nerve agent. Neurotransmitters, synapses, and autonomic receptors are discussed in detail in chapter 13∞.

12.7 Ionizing Radiation

In addition to releasing biologic and chemical weapons, it is possible that bioterrorists could develop nuclear bombs capable of mass destruction. In such a scenario, the greatest number of casualties would be due to the physical blast itself. Survivors, however, could be exposed to high levels of **ionizing radiation** from hundreds of different radioisotopes created by the nuclear explosion. Some of these radioisotopes emit large amounts of radiation and persist in the environment for years. As was the case in the 1986 Chernobyl nuclear accident in Ukraine, the resulting radioisotopes could travel through wind currents, to land thousands of miles away from the initial explosion. Smaller scale radiation exposure could occur through terrorist attacks on nuclear power plants or by the release of solid or liquid radioactive materials into public areas.

The acute effects of ionizing radiation have been well documented and depend primarily on the dose of radiation that the patient receives. **Acute radiation syndrome,** sometimes called *radiation sickness,* can occur within hours or days after extreme doses. Immediate symptoms are nausea, vomiting, and diarrhea. Later symptoms include weight loss, anorexia, fatigue, and bone marrow suppression. Patients who survive the acute exposure are at high risk for developing various cancers, particularly leukemia.

Symptoms of nuclear and radiation exposure remain some of the most difficult to treat pharmacologically. Apart from the symptomatic treatment of radiation sickness, taking potassium iodide (KI) tablets after an incident or an attack is one of the few recognized approaches specifically designed to treat nuclear radiation exposure. Antidotes are available to treat exposure to radioactive plutonium, americium, curium, and cesium-137, but these are more likely to result from internal rather than external radiation exposure (Table 20.6∞). One of the main radioisotopes produced by a nuclear explosion is iodine-131. Because iodine is naturally concentrated in the thyroid gland, I-131 will immediately enter the thyroid and damage thyroid cells. For example, following the Chernobyl nuclear disaster, the incidence of thyroid cancer in Ukraine jumped from 4 to 6 cases

TABLE 12.4	Chemical Warfare Agents and Treatments	
Category	Signs of Discomfort/Fatality	Antidotes/First Aid
NERVE AGENTS		
GA—Tabun (liquid) GB—Sarin (gaseous liquid) GD—Soman (liquid) VX (gaseous liquid)	Depending on the nerve agent, symptoms may be slower to appear and cumulative depending on exposure time: miosis, runny nose, difficulty breathing, excessive salivation, nausea, vomiting, cramping, involuntary urination and defecation, twitching and jerking of muscles, headaches, confusion, convulsion, coma, death.	Nerve agent antidote and Mark I injector kits with atropine are available. Flush eyes immediately with water. Apply sodium bicarbonate or 5% liquid bleach solution to the skin. Do not induce vomiting.
BLOOD AGENTS		
Hydrogen cyanide (liquid)	Red eyes, flushing of the skin, nausea, headaches, weakness, hypoxic convulsions, death	Flush eyes and wash skin with water. For inhalation of mist, oxygen and amyl nitrate may be given. For ingestion of cyanide liquid, 1% sodium thiosulfate may be given to induce vomiting.
Cyanogen chloride (gas)	Loss of appetite, irritation of the respiratory tract, pulmonary edema, death	Oxygen and amyl nitrate may be given. Give patient milk or water. Do not induce vomiting.
CHOKING/VOMITING AGENTS		
Phosgene (gas)	Dizziness, burning eyes, thirst, throat irritation, chills, respiratory and circulatory failure, cyanosis, frostbite-type lesions	Provide fresh air. Administer oxygen. Flush eyes with normal saline or water. Keep patient warm and calm.
Adamsite—DM (crystalline dispensed in aerosol)	Irritation of the eyes and respiratory tract, tightness of the chest, nausea, and vomiting	Rinse nose and throat with saline, water, 10% solution of sodium bicarbonate. Treat the skin with borated talcum powder.
BLISTER/VESICANT AGENTS		
Phosgene oxime (crystalline or liquid) Mustard—lewisite Mixture—HL Nitrogen mustard—HN-1, HN-2, HN-3 Sulfur mustard agents	Destruction of mucous membranes, eye tissue, and skin (subcutaneous edema), followed by scab formation; irritation of the eyes, nasal membranes, and lungs; nausea and vomiting; formation of blisters on the skin; cytotoxic reactions in hematopoietic tissues including bone marrow, lymph nodes, spleen, and endocrine glands	Flush affected area with copious quantities of water. If ingested, do not induce vomiting. Flush affected area with water. Treat the skin with 5% solution of sodium hypochlorite or household bleach. Give milk to drink. Do not induce vomiting. Skin contact with lewisite may be treated with 10% solution of sodium carbonate.

Source: Chemical Fact Sheets at the U.S. Army Center for Health Promotion and Preventive Medicine website: http://chppm-www.apgea.army.mil/dts/dtchemfs.htm

per million people to 45 cases per million. If taken prior to, or immediately following, a nuclear incident, KI can prevent up to 100% of the radioactive iodine from entering the thyroid gland. It is effective even if taken 3 to 4 hours after radiation exposure. Generally, a single 130-mg dose is necessary.

Unfortunately, KI protects only the thyroid gland from I-131. It has no protective effects on other body tissues, and it offers no protection against the dozens of other harmful radioisotopes generated by a nuclear blast. As with vaccines and antibiotics, the stockpiling of KI by local health care agencies or individuals is not recommended. Interestingly, I-131 is also a medication used to shrink the size of an overactive thyroid gland. Thyroid medications are presented in chapter 43∞.

12.8 Poisonings and Fundamentals of Toxicity Treatment

In 2006, according to the American Association of Poison Control Centers, there were 2,403,539 human poison exposures in the United States. Of these exposures, both pharmaceutic and nonpharmaceutic agents were responsible for over 1,200 fatalities (Bronstein et al, 2007). Table 12.5 shows the top 25 substances involved. Among the substances, analgesics, sedative–hypnotics, antipsychotics, cold and cough preparations, antidepressants, opioids, and cardiovascular drugs were at the top of the list.

When poisonings occur, nurses must be familiar with basic elements of toxicity treatment. Measures must be taken to prevent further injury or fatality to the patient and to make a proper diagnosis. When taken properly, most pharmacologic agents do not have extremely adverse characteristics. Most pharmacologic agents approach toxicity when their doses exceed recommended ranges (chapter 4∞). Recall that medications having a lower therapeutic index are more likely to be toxic (chapter 5∞).

Substances enter the body by a variety of methods—either by inhalation, ingestion, injection, or absorption through the skin (chapter 3∞). Some poisonings are intentional; most are accidental. Sometimes the identity and doses of a poison are not known. Often, laboratory methods are necessary to identify contents of the stomach, bloodstream, and urine.

Basic supportive care is one of the first elements of toxicity treatment. Fundamental to the patient's survival is maintaining the patient's airway, breathing, and circulation. In addition, it is important to make sure that proper blood glucose levels are

TABLE 12.5	2006 Data: Top 25 Substances Involved in Human Exposures	
Substance	Number	Percentage
Analgesics	284,906	11.9
Cosmetics/personal care products	214,780	8.9
Cleaning substances (household)	214,091	8.9
Sedative–hypnotics/antipsychotics	141,150	5.9
Foreign bodies/toys/miscellaneous	120,752	5.0
Cold and cough preparations	114,559	4.8
Topical preparations	108,308	4.5
Pesticides	96,811	4.0
Antidepressants	95,327	4.0
Bites and envenomations	82,133	3.4
Cardiovascular drugs	80,426	3.3
Alcohols	76,531	3.2
Antihistamines	75,070	3.1
Food products/food poisoning	66,115	2.8
Antimicrobials	6,017	2.7
Plants	64,236	2.7
Vitamins	63,331	2.6
Hormones and hormone antagonists	51,875	2.2
Gastrointestinal preparations	50,914	2.1
Hydrocarbons	49,526	2.1
Chemicals	47,557	2.0
Stimulants and street drugs	46,239	1.9
Anticonvulsants	40,476	1.7
Fumes/gases/vapors	39,586	1.6
Arts/crafts/office supplies	37,990	1.0

Source: 2006 Annual Report of the American Association of Poison Control Centers' National Poison Data System (NPDS), http://www.aapcc.org/DNN/
Note: *Percentages are based on 2,403,539 human exposures.

maintained and that arterial blood gases are stable. Treatment of any developing seizures is important (chapter 15∞), and management of any acid–base disturbances is critical (chapter 31∞). Agents may be used to alter the pH of the urine, thereby facilitating removal of some toxins. *Sodium bicarbonate* produces a more alkaline urine and enhances the excretion of acidic drugs (i.e., aspirin and barbiturates); *ammonium chloride* produces a more acidic urine and enhances the excretion of alkaline drugs (i.e., amphetamines, phencyclidine).

For surface decontamination, it is important to remove the patient's clothing and to cleanse any contaminates from the body. The patient's eyes should be flushed with water, and the hair should be washed with soap and water. If the skin is not injured, alternate soap-and-water and alcohol washes are recommended. If the patient is unable to perform this decontamination alone, the nurse or person providing the decontamination must protect themselves from possible contamination as well.

Syrup of Ipecac has been used primarily to induce vomiting. Ipecac syrup irritates the gastric mucosa and promotes emesis by stimulating the medullary chemoreceptor trigger zone located in the brain. Evidence is sparse indicating that Ipecac actually helps the outcome of poisonings in many cases and may actually cause more harm, such as in cases of caustic poisionings, for example drain cleaners, which may burn tissue again as they are vomited. In fact, the effects of the Ipecac can often be mistaken for the poison itself and delay the effects of other poisoning treatments. Common symptoms experienced by the patient after Ipecac treatment are sedation, lethargy, and diarrhea. Accidental overdose can result when Ipecac is administered at the home. In 2003, this prompted the American Academy of Pediatricians to withdraw their support of Syrup of Ipecac for home use.

Gastric lavage and aspiration may be a course of treatment where the patient has ingested a potentially life-threatening amount of poison. In order to be effective, this procedure must be performed within 60 minutes of ingestion, and if airway protective reflexes are lost, gastric lavage is contraindicated.

Single-dose **activated charcoal** may be administered if the poison is carbon based. Large carbon-based molecules adsorb (adhere) to activated charcoal and minimize or prevent poisons from absorption. Examples of substances that do not adhere very well to charcoal are alcohols, hydrocarbons, cyanides, iron, boron, lithium, heavy metals, corrosives, and organophosphates (nerve agents and pesticides). As with gastric lavage, the effectiveness of activated charcoal decreases with time; the greatest benefit is within 60 minutes of ingestion. Routine use of a cathartic in lieu of or in combination with activated charcoal is not endorsed.

Whole-bowel irrigation may be considered for potentially toxic ingestions of sustained-release or enteric-coated drugs. Patients seem to derive benefit from whole-bowel irrigation after being exposed to potentially toxic ingestions of iron, lead, zinc, or illicit drugs. Whole-bowel irrigation is contraindicated in patients with bowel obstruction, perforation, compromised airway, or hemodynamic instability. The procedure should be used cautiously with debilitated patients or with patients whose medical condition might be further compromised with this treatment. Whole-bowel irrigation decreases the binding capacity of activated charcoal.

Specific antidotes counter the effects of poisons or toxins in a number of cases. General areas of toxicity where antidotes may be effective include heavy metals, radioactive exposure, and overdosing of pharmacologic agents. Throughout the remaining chapters, *Prototype Drug Boxes* highlight a section called *Treatment of Overdose*. This type of drug information is an important topic that nurses should know. In most cases, toxicity treatment includes the more routine elements of nursing care such as health assessment and monitoring vital signs; however, throughout the text, the *Prototype: Treatment of Overdose* boxes will remind the reader of specific antidotes. Table 12.6 summarizes specific antidotes and their use for particular overdosed substances and toxins.

TABLE 12.6	Examples of Specific Antidotes for Overdosed Substances or Toxins	
Generic Name	**Product Name**	**Overdosed Substance or Toxin (Pharmacologic/Toxicity Group)**
acetylcysteine	Mucomyst	Acetaminophen (nonopioid analgesic)
atropine sulfate		Acetylcholine; cholinergic receptor agents; acetylcholinesterase inhibitors (parasympathomimetic)
calcium EDTA	Calcium Disodium Versenate	Lead toxicity (heavy metal poisoning)
deferoxamine	Desferal	Iron toxicity (heavy metal poisoning)
digoxin immune Fab	Digibind	Digoxin; digitoxin (cardiac glycoside)
dimercaprol	BAL in Oil	Arsenic, gold and mercury toxicity (heavy metal poisoning)
flumazenil	Romazicon	Benzodiazepines (sedative–hypnotic)
fomepizole	Antizole	Ethylene glycol toxicity (antifreeze poisoning)
glucagon		Insulin (hypoglycemia)
leucovorin	Wellcovorin	Methotrexate; folic acid blocking agents (antineoplastic/antimetabolite)
naloxone	Narcan	Opioid agents; morphine (opioid analgesic)
neostigmine	Prostigmin	Neuromuscular blocking agents (nondepolarizing blocker)
penetrate calcium trisodium		Radioactive plutonium, americium and curium (radioactive exposure)
penetrate zinc trisodium		Radioactive plutonium, americium and curium (radioactive exposure)
penicillamine	Cuprimine, Depen	Copper, iron, lead, arsenic, gold and mercury toxicity (heavy metal poisoning)
physostigmine	Antilirium	Cholinergic blocking agents; atropine sulfate (anticholinergic)
potassium iodide		Radioactive iodine toxicity (nuclear bomb; radioactive exposure)
pralidoxime	Protopam	Cholinesterase inhibitors; organophosphates; neostigmine; physostigmine (parasympathomimetic)
protamine sulfate		Heparin (parenteral anticoagulant)
prussian blue	Radiogardase	Radioactive cesium-137; nonradioactive thallium (radioactive cesium exposure; thallium poisoning)
succimer	Chemet	Lead, mercury, and arsenic toxicity (heavy metal poisoning)
vitamin K		Coumadin; warfarin (oral anticoagulant)

Chapter REVIEW

KEY CONCEPTS

The numbered key concepts provide a succinct summary of the important points from the corresponding numbered section within the chapter. If any of these points are not clear, refer to the numbered section within the chapter for review.

12.1 Bioterrorism is the deliberate use of a biologic or physical agent to cause panic and mass casualties. The health aspects of biologic and chemical agents have become important public issues.

12.2 Nurses play key roles in emergency preparedness, including providing education, resources, diagnosis and treatment, and planning.

12.3 The Strategic National Stockpile (SNS) is used to rapidly deploy medical necessities to communities experiencing a chemical or biologic attack. The two components are the push package and the vendor-managed inventory.

12.4 Anthrax can enter the body through ingestion or inhalation, or by the cutaneous route. Antibiotic therapy can be successful if given prophylactically or shortly after exposure.

12.5 Viruses such as polio, smallpox, and those causing hemorrhagic fevers are potential biologic weapons. If available, vaccines are the best treatments.

12.6 Chemicals and neurotoxins are potential bioterrorist threats for which there are no specific antidotes.

12.7 Potassium iodide (KI) may be used to block the effects of acute radiation exposure on the thyroid gland, but it is not effective for protecting other organs.

12.8 Among human poison exposures, common pharmacologic agents are at the top of the list. The nurse must be familiar with fundamental elements of toxicity treatment: basic supportive measures, Syrup of Ipecac, gastric lavage and aspiration, activated charcoal, whole-bowel irrigation, and specific antidotes.

NCLEX-RN® REVIEW QUESTIONS

1 The nurse recognizes which of the following to be initial symptoms of inhaled anthrax? (Select all that apply.)
1. Cramping and diarrhea
2. Skin lesions that develop into black scabs
3. Fever
4. Headache
5. Cough and dyspnea

2 Potassium iodine (KI) taken immediately following a nuclear incident can prevent 100% of radioactive iodine from entering which body organ?
1. Brain
2. Thyroid
3. Kidney
4. Liver

3 Soldiers who may have been exposed to nerve gas agents can be expected to display which of these symptoms?
1. Convulsions and loss of consciousness
2. Memory loss and fatigue
3. Malaise and hemorrhaging
4. Fever and headaches

4 Which of these medications is primarily used for the treatment of anthrax?
1. Diphtheria vaccine
2. Amoxicillin (Amoxil)

3. Ciprofloxacin (Cipro)
4. Smallpox vaccine

5 The CDC categorized biologic threats based on their:
1. potential adverse effects.
2. potential impact on public health.
3. potential cost of treatment.
4. potential loss of life.

6 Nurses play a key role in the event of a potential bioterrorist attack including: (Select all that apply.)
1. helping to plan and develop emergency management plans.
2. recognizing and reporting signs and symptoms of chemical or biologic agent exposure, and assisting with treatment.
3. storing antidotes, antibiotics, vaccines, and supplies in their homes.
4. keeping a list of resources such as health and law enforcement agencies and other contacts who would assist in the event of a bioterrorist attack.
5. keeping up-to-date on emergency management protocol and volunteering to become members of a first-response team.

CRITICAL THINKING QUESTIONS

1. Why is the medical community opposed to the mass vaccination of the general public for potential bioterrorist threats such as anthrax and smallpox?

2. Why does the protective effect of KI not extend to body tissues other than the thyroid gland?

3. What is the purpose of the SNS (Strategic National Stockpile)? What is the difference between a "push package" and a VMI (vendor-managed inventory) package?

4. Why do nurses play such a central role in emergency preparedness and treatment of poisonings?

See Appendix D for answers and rationales for all activities.

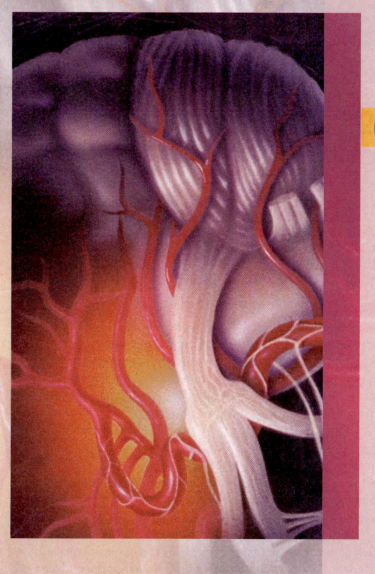

The Nervous System

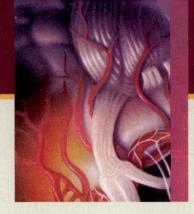

Chapter 13

Drugs Affecting the Autonomic Nervous System

DRUGS AT A GLANCE

LEARNING OUTCOMES

After reading this chapter, the student should be able to:

1. Identify the basic functions of the nervous system.
2. Identify important divisions of the peripheral nervous system.
3. Compare and contrast the actions of the sympathetic and parasympathetic divisions of the autonomic nervous system.
4. Explain the process of synaptic transmission and the neurotransmitters important to the autonomic nervous system.
5. Compare and contrast the types of responses that occur when drugs activate $alpha_1$-, $alpha_2$-, $beta_1$-, or $beta_2$-adrenergic receptors, and nicotinic or muscarinic receptors.
6. Discuss the classification and naming of autonomic drugs based on four possible actions.
7. Describe the nurse's role in the pharmacologic management of patients receiving drugs affecting the autonomic nervous system.
8. For each of the drug classes listed in "Drugs at a Glance," explain the mechanism of drug action, primary actions, and important adverse effects.
9. Use the nursing process to care for patients receiving adrenergic agents, adrenergic-blocking agents, cholinergic agents, and cholinergic-blocking agents.

KEY TERMS

The study of nervous system pharmacology, or *neuropharmacology*, extends over the next eight chapters. Traditionally, neuropharmacology begins with a study of the autonomic nervous system. A firm grasp of autonomic physiology is necessary to understand cardiovascular, renal, respiratory, gastrointestinal, reproductive, and ophthalmic function. Autonomic drugs are important because they mimic involuntary bodily functions. A thorough knowledge of autonomic drugs is essential to the treatment of disorders affecting many body systems, including abnormalities in heart rate and rhythm, hypertension, asthma, glaucoma, and even a runny nose. This chapter serves dual purposes. First, it is a concise review of autonomic nervous system physiology, a subject that is often covered superficially in anatomy and physiology classes. Second, it is an introduction to the four fundamental classes of autonomic drugs: adrenergic agents, cholinergic agents, adrenergic-blocking agents, and cholinergic-blocking agents.

13.1 The Peripheral Nervous System

The nervous system has two major divisions: the **central nervous system (CNS)** and the **peripheral nervous system.** The CNS consists of the brain and spinal cord. The peripheral nervous system consists of all nervous tissue outside the CNS, including sensory and motor neurons. The basic functions of the nervous system are as follows:

- Recognizing changes in the internal and external environments
- Processing and integrating the environmental changes that are perceived
- Reacting to the environmental changes by producing an action or response
- ➤ Figure 13.1 shows the functional divisions of the nervous system. In the peripheral nervous system, neurons either recognize changes to the environment (sensory division) or respond to these changes by moving muscles or secreting chemicals (motor division). The **somatic nervous system** consists of nerves that

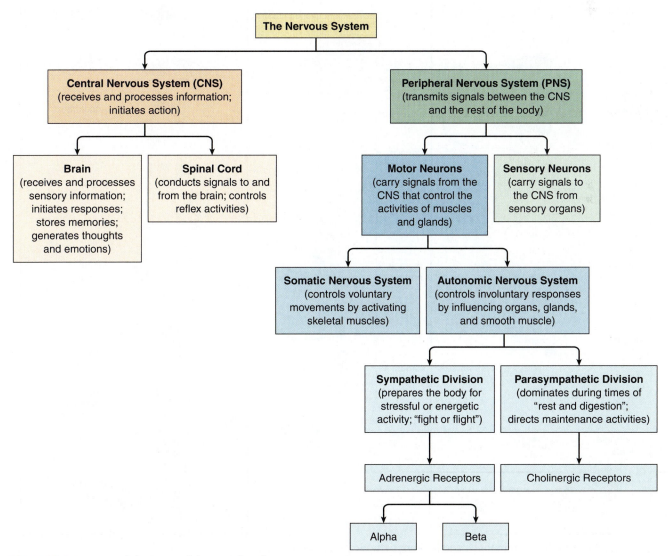

➤ *Figure 13.1* Functional divisions of the peripheral nervous system provide *voluntary* control over skeletal muscle. Nerves of the **autonomic nervous system,** on the other hand, exert *involuntary* control over the contraction of smooth muscle and cardiac muscle, and glandular activity. Organs and tissues regulated by neurons from the autonomic nervous system include the heart, digestive tract, respiratory tract, reproductive tracts, arteries, salivary glands, and portions of the eye.

13.2 The Autonomic Nervous System: Sympathetic and Parasympathetic Divisions

The autonomic nervous system has two divisions: the sympathetic and the parasympathetic nervous systems. With a few exceptions, organs and glands receive nerves from both branches of the autonomic nervous system. The major actions of the two divisions are shown in ➤ Figure 13.2. It is essential that the student learn these general regulatory actions early in the study of pharmacology, because knowledge of autonomic effects is helpful to predict the actions and side effects of many drugs.

The **sympathetic nervous system** is activated under conditions of stress, and produces a set of actions called the **fight-or-flight response.** Activation of this system will ready the body for an immediate response to a potential threat. The heart rate and blood pressure increase, and more blood is shunted to skeletal muscles. The liver immediately produces more glucose for energy. The bronchi dilate to allow more air into the lungs, and the pupils dilate for better vision.

Conversely, the **parasympathetic nervous system** is activated under nonstressful conditions and produces symptoms called the **rest-and-digest response.** Digestive processes are promoted,

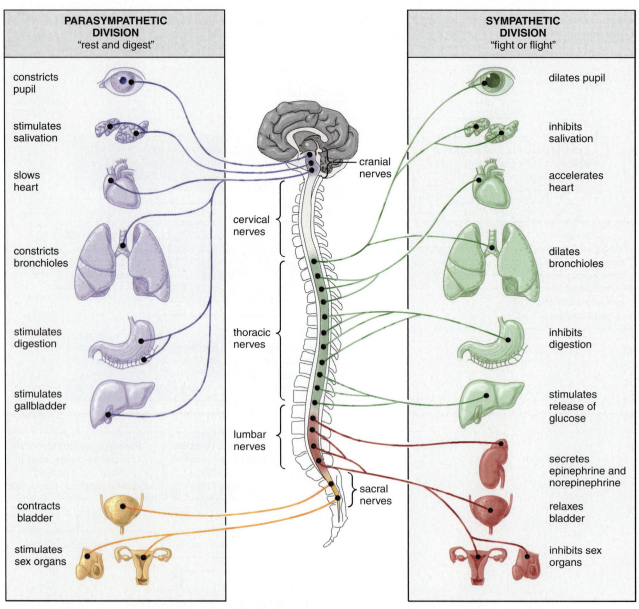

PARASYMPATHETIC DIVISION
"rest and digest"

- constricts pupil
- stimulates salivation
- slows heart
- constricts bronchioles
- stimulates digestion
- stimulates gallbladder
- contracts bladder
- stimulates sex organs

cranial nerves

cervical nerves

thoracic nerves

lumbar nerves

sacral nerves

SYMPATHETIC DIVISION
"fight or flight"

- dilates pupil
- inhibits salivation
- accelerates heart
- dilates bronchioles
- inhibits digestion
- stimulates release of glucose
- secretes epinephrine and norepinephrine
- relaxes bladder
- inhibits sex organs

➤ *Figure 13.2* Effects of the sympathetic and parasympathetic nervous systems
Source: Biology: A Guide to the Natural World, 2nd ed. (p. 558) by David Krogh, 2002, Upper Saddle River, NJ, Prentice Hall. Reprinted by permission.

and heart rate and blood pressure decline. Not as much air is needed, so the bronchi constrict. Generally, most of the actions of the parasympathetic division are the opposite of those of the sympathetic division.

A proper balance of the two autonomic branches is required for body homeostasis. Under most circumstances, the two branches cooperate to achieve a balance of readiness and relaxation. Because the branches produce mostly opposite effects, homeostasis may be achieved by changing one or both branches. For example, heart rate can be increased either by *increasing* the firing of sympathetic nerves or by *decreasing* the firing of parasympathetic nerves. This allows the body a means of fine-tuning its essential organ systems.

The sympathetic and parasympathetic divisions do not always produce opposite effects. For example, the constriction of arterioles is controlled entirely by the sympathetic branch. Sympathetic stimulation causes constriction of arterioles, whereas lack of stimulation causes vasodilation. Sweat glands are also controlled only by sympathetic nerves. In the male reproductive system, the roles are complementary. For example, erection of the penis is a function of the parasympathetic division, and ejaculation is controlled by the sympathetic branch.

13.3 Structure and Function of Autonomic Synapses

For information to be transmitted throughout the nervous system, neurons must communicate with one another, and with muscles and glands. In the autonomic nervous system this communication involves the connection of two neurons, in series. As the action potential travels along the first nerve, it encounters the first **synapse,** or juncture. Because this connection occurs outside the CNS, it is called the **ganglionic synapse.** The basic structure of a ganglionic synapse is shown in ➤ Figure 13.3. The nerve carrying the impulse exiting the spinal cord is called the **preganglionic neuron.** The nerve on the other side of the ganglionic synapse, waiting to receive the impulse, is the **postganglionic neuron.** Beyond the postganglionic neuron is the second synapse. The second synapse occurs at the target tissue.

A large number of drugs affect autonomic function by altering neurotransmitter activity at the second synapse. Some drugs are identical with endogenous neurotransmitters, or have a similar chemical structure, and are able to directly activate the gland or muscle. Others are used to block the activity of natural neurotransmitters. Following are the five general mechanisms by which drugs affect **synaptic transmission.**

- *Drugs may affect the synthesis of the neurotransmitter in the presynaptic nerve:* Drugs that decrease the amount of neurotransmitter synthesis will inhibit autonomic function. Those drugs that increase neurotransmitter synthesis will have the opposite effect.

- *Drugs can prevent the storage of the neurotransmitter in vesicles within the presynaptic nerve:* Prevention of neurotransmitter storage will inhibit autonomic function.

- *Drugs can influence the release of the neurotransmitter from the presynaptic nerve:* Promoting neurotransmitter release will stimulate autonomic function, whereas slowing neurotransmitter release will have the opposite effect.

- *Drugs can prevent the normal destruction or reuptake of the neurotransmitter:* Drugs that cause the neurotransmitter to remain in the synapse for a longer time will stimulate autonomic function.

- *Drugs can bind to the receptor site on the postsynaptic target tissue:* Drugs that bind to postsynaptic receptors and stimulate target tissue will increase autonomic function. Drugs that attach to the postsynaptic targets and prevent the natural neurotransmitter from reaching its receptors will inhibit autonomic function.

The classic study of drugs affecting autonomic function centers around the last two mechanisms. It is important for the student to understand that autonomic drugs are not given to correct physiologic defects in the autonomic nervous system. Compared with other body systems, the autonomic nervous system itself has remarkably little disease. Rather, drugs are used to stimulate or inhibit *target organs* of the autonomic nervous system, such as the heart, lungs, glands, or digestive tract. With few exceptions, the disorder lies in the target organ, not the autonomic nervous system. Thus, when an "autonomic drug" such as norepinephrine (Levarterenol, Levophed) is administered, it does not correct an autonomic disorder; it corrects dysfunction of that target organ naturally stimulated by the autonomic neurotransmitter.

13.4 Norepinephrine and Acetylcholine

The two primary neurotransmitters of the autonomic nervous system are **norepinephrine (NE)** and **acetylcholine (Ach).** A detailed knowledge of the underlying physiology of these neurotransmitters is required for proper understanding of drug action. When reading the following sections, the student should refer to the sites of acetylcholine and norepinephrine action shown in ➤ Figure 13.4.

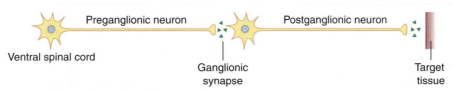

➤ *Figure 13.3* Basic structure of the autonomic pathway

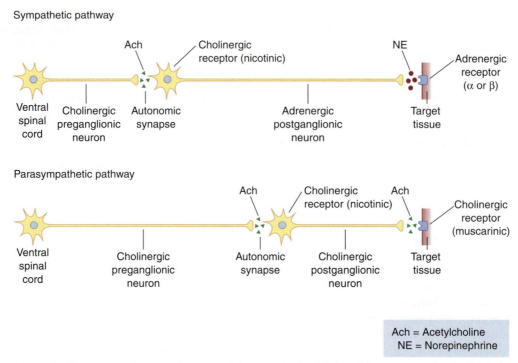

> *Figure 13.4* Receptors in the autonomic nervous system: (a) sympathetic division; (b) parasympathetic division

In the sympathetic nervous system, norepinephrine is the neurotransmitter released at almost all postganglionic nerves. The exception is sweat glands, in which acetylcholine is the neurotransmitter. Norepinephrine belongs to a class of agents called natural **catecholamines**, all of which are involved in neurotransmission. Natural catecholamines also include epinephrine (adrenalin) and dopamine. Examples of synthetic catecholamines are isoproterenol and dobutamine. There are *noncatecholamine* drugs, which have a slightly different chemical structure than the catecholamines, such as ephedrine, phenylephrine, and terbutaline. All of these drugs bind to the same target tissues as adrenalin. The receptors at the ends of postganglionic sympathetic neurons are called **adrenergic**, which comes from the word *adrenalin.*

Adrenergic receptors are of two basic types, **alpha receptors** (α receptors) and **beta receptors** (β receptors). These receptors are further divided into the subtypes alpha$_1$, alpha$_2$, beta$_1$, and beta$_2$. Activation of each receptor subtype results in a characteristic set of physiologic responses, which are generally summarized in Table 13.1.

The significance of these receptor subtypes to pharmacology cannot be overstated. Some drugs are selective and activate only one type of adrenergic receptor, whereas others affect all receptor subtypes. Furthermore, a drug may activate one type of receptor at low doses and begin to affect other receptor subtypes as the dose is increased. Committing the receptor types and their responses to memory is an essential step in learning autonomic pharmacology.

Norepinephrine (NE) is synthesized in the nerve terminal through a series of steps that require the amino acids phenylalanine and tyrosine. The final step of the synthesis involves the conversion of dopamine to norepinephrine. NE is stored in vesicles until an action potential triggers its release into the synaptic cleft. NE then diffuses across the cleft to alpha or beta receptors on the effector organ. The reuptake of NE back into the presynaptic neuron terminates its action. Once reuptake occurs, NE in the nerve terminal may be returned to vesicles for future use, or destroyed enzymatically by **monoamine oxidase (MAO)**. The enzyme catecholamine-O-methyl transferase (COMT) destroys NE at the synaptic cleft. The primary method for termination of NE action is through reuptake. Many drugs affect autonomic function by influencing the synthesis, storage, release, reuptake, or destruction of NE.

The adrenal medulla is a tissue closely associated with the sympathetic nervous system whose anatomic and physiologic arrangement is much different from that of the rest of the sympathetic branch. Early in embryonic life, the adrenal medulla is part of the neural tissue destined to become the sympathetic nervous system. The primitive tissue splits, however, and the adrenal medulla becomes its own functional division. The preganglionic neuron from the spinal cord terminates at the adrenal medulla, and releases the neurotransmitter epinephrine directly into the blood. Once released, epinephrine travels to target organs, where it elicits the classic fight-or-flight symptoms. The action of epinephrine is terminated through hepatic metabolism, rather than reuptake.

Other types of adrenergic receptors exist. Although dopamine was once thought to function only as a chemical precursor to norepinephrine, research has determined that dopamine serves a larger role as a neurotransmitter. Five dopaminergic receptors (D$_1$ through D$_5$) have been discovered in the CNS. Dopaminergic receptors in the CNS are important to the action of certain antipsychotic medicines (chapter 17∞) and in the treatment of Parkinson's disease

TABLE 13.1	Types of Autonomic Receptors		
Neurotransmitter	**Receptor**	**Primary Locations**	**Responses**
norepinephrine (adrenergic)	Alpha$_1$	All sympathetic target organs except the heart	Constriction of blood vessels, dilation of pupils
	Alpha$_2$	Presynaptic adrenergic nerve terminals	Inhibition of release of norepinephrine
	Beta$_1$	Heart and kidneys	Increased heart rate and force of contraction; release of renin
	Beta$_2$	All sympathetic target organs except the heart	Inhibition of smooth muscle
acetylcholine (cholinergic)	Nicotinic	Postganglionic neurons	Stimulation of smooth muscle and gland secretions
	Muscarinic	Heart	Decreased heart rate and force of contraction
		Parasympathetic target: organs other than the heart	Stimulation of smooth muscle and gland secretions

(chapter 20∞). Dopamine receptors in the peripheral nervous system are located in the arterioles of the kidney and other viscera. Although these receptors likely have a role in autonomic function, their therapeutic importance has yet to be fully discovered.

13.5 Acetylcholine and Cholinergic Transmission

Nerves releasing acetylcholine (Ach) are called **cholinergic** nerves. There are two types of cholinergic receptors, which are generally classified after certain chemicals that bind to them (Table 13.1).

- *Nicotinic receptors:* Receptors that were first discovered to bind to nicotine; located at the ganglionic synapse in both the sympathetic and parasympathetic divisions of the autonomic nervous system

- *Muscarinic receptors:* Receptors that were first discovered to bind to muscarine; located on target tissues affected by postganglionic neurons in the parasympathetic nervous system

Early research on laboratory animals found that the actions of Ach at the *ganglia* resemble those of nicotine, the active agent found in tobacco products. Because of this similarity, receptors for Ach in the ganglia are called **nicotinic** receptors. Nicotinic receptors are also present in skeletal muscle, which is controlled by the somatic nervous system. Because these receptors are present in so many locations, drugs affecting nicotinic receptors produce profound effects on both the autonomic and somatic nervous systems. Activation of these cholinergic receptors causes tachycardia, hypertension, and increased tone and motility in the digestive tract. Although nicotinic receptor blockers were some of the first drugs used to treat hypertension, the only current therapeutic application of these agents, known as *ganglionic blockers,* is to produce muscle relaxation during surgical procedures (chapter 19∞). Nicotinic blocking agents have also been used in research to investigate the role of nicotinic receptors in learning and memory.

Activation of acetylcholine receptors affected by *postganglionic* nerve endings in the parasympathetic nervous system results in the classic symptoms of parasympathetic stimulation shown in Figure 13.2. Early research

discovered that these actions closely resemble those produced when a patient ingests the poisonous mushroom *Amanita muscaria.* Because of this similarity, these Ach receptors were named **muscarinic** receptors. Unlike the nicotinic receptors, which have few pharmacologic applications, muscarinic receptors are affected by a number of medications, and these are discussed in subsequent sections of this chapter.

The physiology of acetylcholine affords several mechanisms by which drugs may act. Acetylcholine is synthesized in the presynaptic nerve terminal from choline and acetyl coenzyme A. Once synthesized, Ach is stored in vesicles in the presynaptic neuron. When an action potential reaches the nerve ending, Ach is released into the synaptic cleft, where it diffuses across to find nicotinic or muscarinic receptors. Ach in the synaptic cleft is rapidly destroyed by the enzyme **acetylcholinesterase (AchE),** and choline is reused. The choline is taken up by the presynaptic neuron to make more Ach, and the cycle is repeated. Drugs can affect the formation, release, receptor activation, or destruction of Ach.

AUTONOMIC DRUGS

13.6 Classification and Naming of Autonomic Drugs

Given the opposite actions of the sympathetic and parasympathetic nervous systems, autonomic drugs are classified based on one of four possible actions.

1. *Stimulation of the sympathetic nervous system:* These drugs are called adrenergic agents or **sympathomimetics,** and they produce the classic symptoms of the fight-or-flight response. Natural or synthetic agents that produce a sympathomimetic response include the *catecholamines* and *noncatecholamines.*

2. *Inhibition of the sympathetic nervous system:* These drugs are called adrenergic-blocking agents or **adrenergic antagonists,** and they produce actions *opposite* those of the sympathomimetics. The term **sympatholytics** is another name for adrenergic antagonists.

3. *Stimulation of the parasympathetic nervous system:* These drugs are called cholinergic agents or **parasympathomimetics,** and they produce the characteristic symptoms of the rest-and-digest response.

4. *Inhibition of the parasympathetic nervous system:* These drugs are called cholinergic-blocking agents, **anticholinergics,** parasympatholytics, or muscarinic blockers, and they produce actions *opposite* those of the cholinergic agents.

Students beginning their study of pharmacology often have difficulty understanding the terminology and actions of autonomic drugs. Examination of the four drug classes, however, makes it evident that one group needs to be learned well, because the others are logical extensions of the first. If the fight-or-flight actions of the sympathomimetics are learned, the other three groups can be deduced, because they are either the same or opposite. For example, both the sympathomimetics and the cholinergic-blocking agents increase heart rate and dilate the pupil. The other two groups, the cholinergic agents and the adrenergic-blocking agents, have the opposite effects—slowing heart rate and constricting the pupils. Although this is an oversimplification and exceptions do exist, it is a time-saving means of learning the basic actions and adverse effects of dozens of drugs affecting the autonomic nervous system. It should be emphasized again that mastering the actions and terminology of autonomic drugs early in the study of pharmacology will reap rewards later in the course when these drugs are applied to various systems.

Adrenergic Agents (Sympathomimetics)

The adrenergic agents, also known as sympathomimetics, stimulate the sympathetic nervous system and induce symptoms characteristic of the fight-or-flight response. These drugs have clinical applications in the treatment of shock and hypotension.

13.7 Clinical Applications of Sympathomimetics

Sympathomimetics produce many of the same responses as the anticholinergics. However, because the sympathetic nervous system has alpha and beta subreceptors, the actions of many sympathomimetics are more specific and have wider therapeutic application (Table 13.2).

As mentioned, sympathomimetics may be described chemically as catecholamines or noncatecholamines. The catecholamines share the same biochemical structure as norepinephrine and a short duration of action, and must be administered parenterally. The noncatecholamines can be taken orally and have longer durations of action, because they are not rapidly destroyed by monoamine oxidase or COMT.

Sympathomimetics act either directly or indirectly. Most sympathomimetics act directly by binding to and activating adrenergic receptors. Examples include the three endogenous catecholamines: epinephrine, norepinephrine, and dopamine. Other medications in this class act indirectly, by causing the release of norepinephrine from its vesicles on the presynaptic neuron or by inhibiting the reuptake or de-

TABLE 13.2 Adrenergic Agents (Sympathomimetics)		
Drug	**Primary Receptor Subtype**	**Primary Use**
albuterol (Proventil, Ventolin)	Beta$_2$	Asthma
clonidine (Catapres)	Alpha$_2$ in CNS	Hypertension
dexmedetomidine HCl (Precedex)	Alpha$_2$ in CNS	Sedation
dobutamine (Dobutrex)	Beta$_1$	Cardiac stimulant
dopamine (Intropin)	Alpha$_1$ and beta$_1$	Shock
epinephrine (Adrenalin, others)	Alpha and beta	Cardiac arrest, asthma
formoterol (Foradil)	Beta$_2$	Asthma, COPD
isoproterenol (Isuprel)	Beta$_1$ and beta$_2$	Asthma, dysrhythmias, heart failure
metaproterenol (Alupent)	Beta$_2$	Asthma
metaraminol (Aramine)	Alpha$_1$ and beta$_1$	Shock
methyldopa (Aldomet)	Alpha$_2$ in CNS	Hypertension
midodrine (ProAmatine)	Alpha	Hypertension
norepinephrine (Levarterenol, Levophed)	Alpha and beta$_1$	Shock
oxymetazoline (Afrin and others)	Alpha	Nasal congestion
phenylephrine (Neo-Synephrine)	Alpha	Nasal congestion
pseudoephedrine (Sudafed and others)	Alpha and beta	Nasal congestion
ritodrine (Yutopar)	Beta$_2$	Slowing of uterine contractions
salmeterol (Serevent)	Beta$_2$	Decongestant
terbutaline (Brethine and others)	Beta$_2$	Asthma

struction of NE. Those that act by indirect mechanisms, such as amphetamine or cocaine, are used for their central effects in the brain rather than their autonomic effects. A few agents, such as ephedrine, act by both direct and indirect mechanisms.

Most effects of sympathomimetics are predictable based on their autonomic actions, dependent on which adrenergic receptor subtypes are stimulated. Because the receptor responses are so different, the student will need to memorize the specific subclass(es) of receptors activated by each sympathomimetic. Specific subclasses of receptors and therapeutic applications are as follows:

- Alpha$_1$ receptor: treatment of nasal congestion or hypotension; causes mydriasis during ophthalmic examinations
- Alpha$_2$ receptor: treatment of hypertension through a centrally acting mechanism (Autonomic alpha$_2$ receptors are also located on presynaptic membranes of postganglionic neurons and serve as autoreceptors for naturally occurring NE in the sympathetic nervous system. Activation of alpha$_2$ receptors reduces the release of NE.)
- Beta$_1$ receptor: treatment of cardiac arrest, heart failure, and shock
- Beta$_2$ receptor: treatment of asthma and premature labor contractions

Some sympathomimetics are nonselective, stimulating more than one type of adrenergic receptor. For example, epinephrine stimulates all four types of adrenergic receptors and is used for cardiac arrest and asthma. Pseudoephedrine (Sudafed and others) stimulates both alpha$_1$ and beta$_2$ receptors and is used as a nasal decongestant. Isoproterenol (Isuprel) stimulates both beta$_1$ and beta$_2$ receptors and is used to increase the rate, force, and conduction speed of the heart, and occasionally for asthma. The nonselective drugs generally cause more autonomic-related side effects than the selective agents.

The side effects of the sympathomimetics are mostly extensions of their autonomic actions. Cardiovascular effects such as tachycardia, hypertension, and dysrhythmias are particularly troublesome and may limit therapy. Large doses

---

Pr Prototype Drug | Phenylephrine (Neo-Synephrine)

Therapeutic Class: Nasal decongestant; mydriatic agent; antihypotensive   **Pharmacologic Class:** Adrenergic agent (sympathomimetic)

ACTIONS AND USES

Phenylephrine is a selective alpha-adrenergic agonist that is available in several different formulations, including intranasal, ophthalmic, IM, subcutaneous, and IV. All its actions and indications are extensions of its sympathetic stimulation.

Intranasal Administration: When applied intranasally by spray or drops, phenylephrine reduces nasal congestion by constricting small blood vessels in the nasal mucosa.

Topical Administration: Applied topically to the eye during ophthalmic examinations, phenylephrine can dilate the pupil without causing significant cycloplegia.

Parenteral Administration: The parenteral administration of phenylephrine can reverse acute hypotension caused by spinal anesthesia or vascular shock. Because phenylephrine lacks beta-adrenergic agonist activity, it produces relatively few cardiac side effects at therapeutic doses. Its longer duration of activity and lack of significant cardiac effects gives phenylephrine some advantages over epinephrine or norepinephrine in treating acute hypotension.

ADMINISTRATION ALERTS

- Parenteral administration can cause tissue injury with extravasation.
- Phenylephrine ophthalmic drops may damage soft contact lenses.
- Pregnancy category C

PHARMACOKINETICS

Onset: Immediate IV; 10–15 min IM/subcutaneous

Peak: 5–10 min IV; 15–30 min IV/subcutaneous

Half-life: Less than 15 min IV; 30–60 min IM/subcutaneous

Duration: 15–20 min IV; 30–120 min IM/subcutaneous; 3–6 h topical

ADVERSE EFFECTS

When the drug is used topically or intranasally, side effects are uncommon. Intranasal use can cause burning of the mucosa and rebound congestion if used for prolonged periods (chapter 31 ∞). Ophthalmic preparations can cause narrow-angle glaucoma secondary to their mydriatic effect. High doses can cause reflex bradycardia due to the elevation of blood pressure caused by stimulation of alpha$_1$ receptors.

When used parenterally, the drug should be used with caution in patients with advanced coronary artery disease or hypertension. Anxiety, restlessness, and tremor may occur due to the drug's stimulation effect on the CNS. Patients with hyperthyroidism may experience a severe increase in basal metabolic rate, resulting in increased blood pressure and ventricular tachycardia.

Contraindications: This drug should not be used in patients with acute pancreatitis, heart disease, hepatitis, or narrow-angle glaucoma.

INTERACTIONS

Drug–Drug: Drug interactions may occur with MAO inhibitors, causing a hypertensive crisis. Increased effects may also occur with tricyclic antidepressants, ergot alkaloids, and oxytocin. Inhibitory effects occur with alpha blockers and beta blockers. Phenylephrine is incompatible with iron preparations (ferric salts). Phenylephrine may cause dysrhythmias when taken in combination with digoxin.

Lab Tests: Unknown

Herbal/Food: Unknown

Treatment of Overdose: Overdose may cause tachycardia and hypertension. Treatment with an alpha blocker such as phentolamine (Regitine) may be indicated to decrease blood pressure.

Refer to MyNursingKit for a Nursing Process Focus specific to this drug.

Adrenergic-Blocking Agents

Adrenergic-blocking agents or antagonists inhibit the sympathetic nervous system and produce many of the same rest-and-digest symptoms as the parasympathomimetics. They have wide therapeutic application in the treatment of hypertension.

13.8 Clinical Applications of Adrenergic Antagonists

Adrenergic antagonists act by directly blocking adrenergic receptors. The actions of these agents are specific to either alpha or beta blockade. Medications in this class have great therapeutic application and are the most widely prescribed class of autonomic drugs (Table 13.3).

Alpha-adrenergic antagonists, or simply alpha blockers, are used for their effects on vascular smooth muscle. By relaxing vascular smooth muscle in small arteries, alpha$_1$ blockers such as doxazosin (Cardura) cause vasodilation that results in decreased blood pressure. They may be used either alone or in combination with other agents in the treatment of hypertension (chapter 23∞). A second use is in the treatment of benign prostatic hyperplasia (BPH), due to their ability to increase urine flow by relaxing smooth muscle in the bladder neck, prostate, and urethra (chapter 46∞). The most common adverse effect of alpha blockers is orthostatic hypotension, which occurs when a patient abruptly changes from a recumbent to an upright position. Reflex tachycardia, nasal congestion, and impotence are other important side effects that may occur as a consequence of increased parasympathetic activity.

Beta-adrenergic antagonists may block beta$_1$ receptors, beta$_2$ receptors, or both types of receptors. Regardless of their receptor specificity, all beta blockers are used therapeutically for their effects on the cardiovascular system. Beta blockers decrease the rate and force of contraction of the heart, and slow electrical conduction through the atrioventricular node. Drugs that selectively block beta$_1$ receptors, such as atenolol (Tenormin), are called *cardioselective* agents. Because they have little effect on noncardiac tissue, they exert fewer side effects than nonselective agents such as propranolol (Inderal).

The primary use of beta blockers is in the treatment of hypertension. Although the exact mechanism by which beta blockers reduce blood pressure is not completely understood, it is thought that the reduction may be due to decreased cardiac output or to suppression of renin release by the kidneys. The student should refer to chapter 23∞ for a more comprehensive description of the use of beta blockers in hypertension management.

Beta-adrenergic antagonists have several other important therapeutic applications, discussions of which appear in many chapters in this textbook. By decreasing the cardiac workload, beta blockers can ease the pain associated with migraines (chapter 18∞) and angina pectoris (chapter 25∞). By slowing electrical conduction across the myocardium, beta blockers are useful in treating certain types of dysrhythmias (chapter 26∞). Other therapeutic uses include the treatment of heart failure (chapter 24∞), myocardial infarction (chapter 25∞), and narrow-angle glaucoma (chapter 49∞).

Cholinergic Agents (Parasympathomimetics)

Parasympathomimetics are drugs that mimic action of the parasympathetic nervous system. These cholinergic agents induce the rest-and-digest response.

TABLE 13.3	Adrenergic-Blocking Agents (Antagonists)	
Drug	Primary Receptor Subtype	Primary Use
acebutolol (Sectral)	Beta$_1$	Hypertension, dysrhythmias, angina
atenolol (Tenormin)	Beta$_1$	Hypertension, angina
carteolol (Cartrol)	Beta$_1$ and beta$_2$	Hypertension, glaucoma
carvedilol (Coreg)	Alpha$_1$, beta$_1$, and beta$_2$	Hypertension, heart failure
doxazosin (Cardura)	Alpha$_1$	Hypertension
esmolol (Brevibloc)	Beta$_1$	Hypertension, dysrhythmias
metoprolol (Lopressor, Toprol)	Beta$_1$	Hypertension
nadolol (Corgard)	Beta$_1$ and beta$_2$	Hypertension
phentolamine (Regitine)	Alpha	Severe hypertension
🅟 prazosin (Minipress)	Alpha$_1$	Hypertension
propranolol (Inderal)	Beta$_1$ and beta$_2$	Hypertension, dysrhythmias, heart failure
sotalol (Betapace)	Beta$_1$ and beta$_2$	Dysrhythmias
tamsulosin (Flomax)	Alpha$_1$	Benign prostatic hypertrophy
terazosin (Hytrin)	Alpha$_1$	Hypertension
timolol (Blocadren, Timoptic)	Beta$_1$ and beta$_2$	Hypertension, angina, glaucoma

Note: This is a partial list of adrenergic-blocking drugs. For additional drugs and doses, refer to the chapter containing the primary use.

Pr Prototype Drug | Prazosin *(Minipress)*

Therapeutic Class: Antihypertensive   **Pharmacologic Class:** Adrenergic-blocking agent

ACTIONS AND USES

Prazosin is a selective alpha$_1$-adrenergic antagonist that competes with norepinephrine at its receptors on vascular smooth muscle in arterioles and veins. Its major action is a rapid decrease in peripheral resistance that reduces blood pressure. It has little effect on cardiac output or heart rate, and it causes less reflex tachycardia than some other drugs in this class. Tolerance to prazosin's antihypertensive effect may occur. Its most common use is in combination with other agents, such as beta blockers or diuretics, in the pharmacotherapy of hypertension. Prazosin has a short half-life and is often taken two or three times per day.

ADMINISTRATION ALERTS

- Give a low first dose to avoid severe hypotension.
- Safety during pregnancy (category C) or lactation is not established.

PHARMACOKINETICS

Onset: 2 h

Peak: 2–4 h

Half-life: 2–4 h

Duration: Less than 24 h

ADVERSE EFFECTS

Like other alpha blockers, prazosin tends to cause orthostatic hypotension due to alpha$_1$ inhibition in vascular smooth muscle. In rare cases, this hypotension can cause unconsciousness about 30 minutes after the first dose. To avoid this situation, the first dose should be very low and given at bedtime. Dizziness, drowsiness, or light-headedness may occur. Reflex tachycardia may result from the rapid fall in blood pressure. Alpha blockade may cause nasal congestion or inhibition of ejaculation.

Contraindications: Safety during pregnancy and lactation is not established.

INTERACTIONS

Drug–Drug: Concurrent use of antihypertensives and diuretics results in extremely low blood pressure. Alcohol should be avoided.

Lab Tests: Prazosin increases urinary metabolites of vanillylmandelic acid (VMA) and norepinephrine, which are measured to screen for pheochromocytoma (adrenal tumor). Prazosin will cause false-positive results.

Herbal/Food: Do not use saw palmetto or nettle root products. Saw palmetto blocks alpha$_1$ receptors, resulting in the dilation of blood vessels and a hypotensive response.

Treatment of Overdose: Overdose may cause hypotension. Blood pressure may be elevated by the administration of fluid expanders such as normal saline or vasopressors such as dopamine or dobutamine.

Refer to MyNursingKit for a Nursing Process Focus specific to this drug.

NURSING PROCESS FOCUS   PATIENTS RECEIVING ADRENERGIC-BLOCKER THERAPY

Assessment	Potential Nursing Diagnoses
Baseline assessment prior to administration: - Understand the reason the drug has been prescribed in order to assess for therapeutic effects. - Obtain a complete health history including cardiovascular, cerebrovascular, respiratory disease, or diabetes. Obtain a drug history including allergies, current prescription and OTC drugs, herbal preparations, and alcohol use. Be alert to possible drug interactions. - Evaluate appropriate laboratory findings including electrolytes, glucose, and hepatic and renal function studies. - Obtain baseline weight, vital signs, and cardiac monitoring (e.g., ECG, cardiac output as appropriate.) - For treatment of benign prostatic hypertrophy (BPH), assess urinary output. - Assess the patient's ability to receive and understand instruction. Include the family and caregivers as needed.	- Decreased Cardiac Output (cardiovascular) - Ineffective Tissue Perfusion (cardiopulmonary) - Impaired Gas Exchange (cardiopulmonary) - Ineffective Airway Clearance (asthma) - Impaired Urinary Elimination (BPH) - Activity Intolerance (cardiovascular) - Risk for Falls, Risk for Injury (related to adverse effects of drug therapy) - Risk for Disturbed Sleep Pattern (related to adverse effects of drug therapy) - Sexual Dysfunction (related to adverse effects of drug therapy) - Deficient Knowledge (drug therapy)
Assessment throughout administration: - Assess for desired therapeutic effects dependent on the reason for the drug (e.g., BP within normal range, dysrhythmias/palpitations relieved, greater ease in urination). - Continue frequent and careful monitoring of vital signs, daily weight, and urinary and cardiac output as appropriate, especially if IV administration is used. - Assess for and promptly report adverse effects: bradycardia, hypotension, dysrhythmias, reflex tachycardia (from too-rapid decrease in BP or hypotension), dizziness, headache, and decreased urinary output. Severe hypotension, seizures, and dysrhythmias/palpitations may drug signal toxicity and should be immediately reported.	

(Continued)

NURSING PROCESS FOCUS   **PATIENTS RECEIVING ADRENERGIC-BLOCKER THERAPY** (Continued)

Planning: Patient Goals and Expected Outcomes

The patient will:

- Experience therapeutic effects dependent on the reason the drug is being given (e.g., decreased blood pressure, decreased palpitations, ease of urination).
- Be free from, or experience minimal, adverse effects.
- Verbalize an understanding of the drug's use, adverse effects, and required precautions.
- Demonstrate proper self-administration of the medication (e.g., dose, timing, when to notify provider).

Implementation

Interventions and (Rationales)	Patient and Family Education
Ensuring therapeutic effects: - Continue frequent assessments as described earlier for therapeutic effects dependent on the reason the drug therapy is given. Daily weights should remain at or close to baseline weight. (Pulse, blood pressure, and respiratory rate should be within normal limits or within parameters set by the health care provider. Urinary hesitancy or frequency should be decreased and urine output improved. An increase in weight over 1 kg per day may indicate excessive fluid gain.)	- Teach the patient, family, or caregiver how to monitor the pulse and blood pressure as appropriate. Ensure the proper use and functioning of any home equipment obtained. - Have the patient weigh self daily along with blood pressure and pulse measurements. Report a weight gain or loss of more than 1 kg (approximately 2 lb) in a 24-hour period.
- Follow appropriate administration techniques for ophthalmic doses. (See chapter 3, Principles of Drug Administration for techniques ∞.)	- Instruct the patient, family, or caregiver in proper administration techniques, followed by return-demonstration.
Minimizing adverse effects: - Continue to monitor vital signs. Take blood pressure lying, sitting, and standing to detect orthostatic hypotension. Be particularly cautious with older adults, who are at increased risk for hypotension. Notify the health care provider if the blood pressure or pulse decrease beyond established parameters or if hypotension is accompanied by reflex tachycardia. (Adrenergic drugs decrease heart rate and cause vasodilation, resulting in lowered blood pressure. Orthostatic hypotension may increase the risk of falls or injury. Reflex tachycardia may signal that the blood pressure has dropped too quickly or too substantially.)	- Teach the patient to rise from lying to sitting or standing slowly to avoid dizziness or falls. - Instruct the patient to stop taking medication if blood pressure is 90/60 mmHg or below, or parameters set by the health care provider, and immediately notify the provider.
- Continue cardiac monitoring (e.g., ECG) as ordered for dysrhythmias in the hospitalized patient. (External monitoring devices will detect early signs of adverse effects as well as monitoring for therapeutic effects.)	- Instruct the patient to report palpitations, chest pain, or dyspnea immediately.
- Weigh the patient daily and report a weight gain or loss of 1 kg (approximately 2 lb) or more in a 24-hour period. (Daily weight is an accurate measure of fluid status and takes into account intake, output, and insensible losses. Weight gain or edema may signal that blood pressure has lowered too quickly, stimulating renin release or is an adverse effect.)	- Have the patient weigh self daily, ideally at the same time of day, and record weight along with blood pressure and pulse measurements. Have the patient report a weight gain or loss of more than 1 kg (approximately 2 lb) in a 24-hour period.
- Monitor urine output and symptoms of dysuria such as hesitancy or retention when given for BPH.	- Have the patient promptly report urinary hesitancy, feelings of bladder fullness, or difficulty starting urinary stream.
- Give the first dose of the drug at bedtime. (A first-dose response may result in a greater initial drop in BP than subsequent doses.)	- Instruct the patient to take the first dose of medication at bedtime, immediately before going to bed, and to avoid driving for 12 to 24 hours after the first dose or when the dosage is increased until the effects are known.
- Continue to monitor blood sugar and appropriate lab work. (Adrenergic-blocking drugs affect a wide range of body systems. They may also interfere with some oral diabetic drugs or change the way a hypoglycemic reaction is perceived.)	- Teach the diabetic patient to monitor blood sugar more frequently and to be aware of subtle signs of possible hypoglycemia (e.g., nervousness, irritability). The patient on oral antidiabetic drugs should report any consistent changes in blood sugar levels to the health care provider promptly.
- Assess the patient's mental status and mood. (Adrenergic blockers may cause depression or dysphoria.)	- Teach the patient to report unusual feelings of sadness, despondency, apathy, or depression that may warrant a change in medication.
- Provide for eye comfort such as adequately lighted room. (Adrenergic-blocking drugs can cause miosis and difficulty seeing in low light levels.)	- Caution the patient about driving or other activities in low-light conditions or at night until the effects of drug are known.
- Do not abruptly stop the medication. (Rebound hypertension and tachycardia may occur.)	- Teach the patient, family, or caregiver not to stop the medication abruptly and to call the health care provider if the patient is unable to take the medication for more than 1 day due to illness.

NURSING PROCESS FOCUS PATIENTS RECEIVING ADRENERGIC-BLOCKER THERAPY (Continued)

Implementation

Interventions and (Rationales)	Patient and Family Education
Patient understanding of drug therapy: ■ Use opportunities during administration of medications and during assessments to discuss rationale for drug therapy, desired therapeutic outcomes, most commonly observed adverse effects, parameters for when to call the health care provider, and any necessary monitoring or precautions. (Using time during nursing care helps to optimize and reinforce key teaching areas.)	■ The patient, family, or caregiver should be able to state the reason for the drug; appropriate dose and scheduling; what adverse effects to observe for and when to report; equipment needed as appropriate and how to use that equipment; and the required length of medication therapy needed with any special instructions regarding renewing or continuing prescription as appropriate.
Patient self-administration of drug therapy: ■ When administering medications, instruct the patient, family, or caregiver in the proper self-administration of drugs and ophthalmic drops. (Utilizing time during nurse-administration of these drugs helps to reinforce teaching.)	■ Instruct the patient in proper administration techniques, followed by return-demonstration. ■ The patient, family, or caregiver are able to discuss appropriate dosing and administration needs.

Evaluation of Outcome Criteria

Evaluate the effectiveness of drug therapy by confirming that patient goals and expected outcomes have been met (see "Planning").

See Table 13.3 for a list of drugs to which these nursing actions apply.

13.9 Clinical Applications of Parasympathomimetics

The classic parasympathomimetic is acetylcholine, the endogenous neurotransmitter at cholinergic synapses in the autonomic nervous system. Acetylcholine, however, has almost no therapeutic use because it is rapidly destroyed after administration and produces many side effects. Recall that Ach is the neurotransmitter at the ganglia in both the parasympathetic and sympathetic divisions, and at the neuroeffector junctions in the parasympathetic nervous system, as well as in skeletal muscle. Thus, it is not surprising that administration of Ach or drugs that mimic Ach will have widespread and varied effects on the body.

Parasympathomimetics are divided into two subclasses, direct acting and indirect acting, based on their mechanism of action (Table 13.4). Direct-acting agents, such as bethanechol (Urecholine), bind to cholinergic receptors to produce the rest-and-digest response. Because direct-acting parasympathomimetics are relatively resistant to the destructive effects of the enzyme acetylcholinesterase, they have a longer duration of action than Ach. They are poorly absorbed across the GI tract and generally do not cross the blood–brain barrier. They have little effect on Ach receptors in the ganglia. Because they are moderately selective to muscarinic receptors when used at therapeutic doses, direct-acting parasympathomimetics may also be described as *muscarinic agonists*.

The indirect-acting parasympathomimetics, such as neostigmine (Prostigmin), inhibit the action of AchE. This inhibition allows endogenous Ach to avoid rapid destruction and remain on cholinergic receptors for a longer time, thus prolonging its action. These drugs are called *cholinesterase inhibitors*. Unlike the direct-acting agents, the cholinesterase inhibitors are nonselective and affect all Ach sites: autonomic ganglia, muscarinic receptors, skeletal muscle, and Ach sites in the CNS.

One of the first drugs discovered in this class, physostigmine (Antilirium), was obtained from the dried ripe seeds of *Physostigma venenosum,* a plant found in West Africa. The bean of this plant was used in tribal rituals. As research continued under secrecy during World War II, similar compounds were synthesized that produced potent neurologic effects that could be used during chemical warfare. This class of agents now includes organophosphate insecticides such as malathion and parathion, and toxic nerve gases such as Sarin. Nurses who work in agricultural areas may become quite familiar with the symptoms of acute poisoning with organophosphates. Poisoning results in intense stimulation of the parasympathetic nervous system, which may result in death, if untreated.

Because of their high potential for serious adverse effects, few parasympathomimetics are widely used in pharmacotherapy. Some have clinical applications in ophthalmology, because they reduce intraocular pressure in patients with glaucoma (chapter 49 ∞). Others are used for their stimulatory effects on the smooth muscle of the bowel or urinary tract.

Several drugs in this class are used for their effects on acetylcholine receptors in skeletal muscle or in the CNS, rather than for their parasympathetic action. **Myasthenia gravis** is a disease characterized by destruction of nicotinic receptors in skeletal muscles. Administration of pyridostigmine (Mestinon) or neostigmine (Prostigmin) stimulates skeletal muscle contraction and helps reverse the severe muscle weakness characteristic of this disease. In addition,

TABLE 13.4	Cholinergic Agents (Parasympathomimetics)	
Type	Drug	Primary Use
Direct acting	bethanechol (Duvoid, Urecholine)	To stimulate urination
	cevimeline HCl (Evoxac)	Treatment of dry mouth
	pilocarpine (Isopto Carpine, Salagen)	Glaucoma
Cholinesterase inhibitors (indirect acting)	ambenonium (Mytelase)	Myasthenia gravis
	donepezil (Aricept)	Alzheimer's disease
	edrophonium (Tensilon)	Diagnosis of myasthenia gravis
	galantamine hydrobromide (Razadyne)	Alzheimer's disease
	neostigmine (Prostigmin)	Myasthenia gravis
	physostigmine (Antilirium)	Treatment of severe anticholinergic toxicity
	pyridostigmine (Mestinon)	Myasthenia gravis
	rivastigmine (Exelon)	Alzheimer's disease
	tacrine (Cognex)	Alzheimer's disease

donepezil (Aricept) and tacrine (Cognex) are useful in treating Alzheimer's disease because of their ability to increase the amount of acetylcholine binding to receptors located within the CNS (chapter 20∞).

Cholinergic-Blocking Agents (Anticholinergics)

Cholinergic-blocking agents are drugs that inhibit parasympathetic impulses. Suppressing the parasympathetic division induces symptoms of the fight-or-flight response.

Pr   Prototype Drug | Bethanechol *(Duvoid, Urecholine)*

Therapeutic Class: Nonobstructive urinary retention agent   **Pharmacologic Class:** Muscarinic cholinergic receptor agonist

ACTIONS AND USES
Bethanechol is a direct-acting parasympathomimetic that interacts with muscarinic receptors to cause actions typical of parasympathetic stimulation. Its effects are most noted in the digestive and urinary tracts, where it stimulates smooth-muscle contraction. These actions are useful in increasing smooth-muscle tone and muscular contractions in the GI tract following general anesthesia. In addition, it is used to treat nonobstructive urinary retention in patients with atony of the bladder. Although poorly absorbed from the GI tract, it may be administered orally or by SC injection.

ADMINISTRATION ALERTS
- Never administer IM or IV.
- Oral and subcutaneous doses are *not* interchangeable.
- Monitor blood pressure, pulse, and respirations before administration and for at least 1 hour after subcutaneous administration.
- Pregnancy category C

PHARMACOKINETICS
Onset: 30–90 min PO; 5–15 min subcutaneous
Peak: 60 min PO; 15–30 min subcutaneous
Half-life: 2–4 h PO; less than 60 min subcutaneous
Duration: 6 h PO; 120 min subcutaneous

ADVERSE EFFECTS
The side effects of bethanechol are predicted from its parasympathetic actions. It should be used with extreme caution in patients with disorders that could be aggravated by increased contractions of the digestive tract, such as suspected obstruction, active ulcer, or inflammatory disease. The same caution should be exercised in patients with suspected urinary obstruction or COPD. Side effects include increased salivation, sweating, abdominal cramping, and hypotension that could lead to fainting.

Contraindications: Patients with asthma, epilepsy, or parkinsonism should not use this drug. Safety in pregnancy and lactation and in children younger than 8 years is not established.

INTERACTIONS
Drug–Drug: Drug interactions with bethanechol include increased cholinergic effects from cholinesterase inhibitors and decreased cholinergic effects from procainamide, quinidine, atropine, and epinephrine.

Lab Tests: Bethanechol may cause an increase in serum AST, amylase, and lipase.

Herbal/Food: Cholinergic effects caused by bethanechol may be antagonized by angel's trumpet, jimson weed, or scopalia.

Treatment of Overdose: Atropine sulfate is a specific antidote. Subcutaneous injection of atropine is preferred except in emergencies when the IV route may be used.

Refer to MyNursingKit for a Nursing Process Focus specific to this drug.

NURSING PROCESS FOCUS PATIENTS RECEIVING PARASYMPATHOMIMETIC THERAPY

Assessment	Potential Nursing Diagnoses
Baseline assessment prior to administration: ■ Understand the reason the drug has been prescribed in order to assess for therapeutic effects. ■ Obtain a complete health history including cardiovascular, cerebrovascular, respiratory, musculoskeletal or thyroid diseases, GI or GU obstruction, or diabetes. Obtain a drug history including allergies, current prescription and OTC drugs, and herbal preparations. Be alert to possible drug interactions. ■ Evaluate appropriate laboratory findings such as hepatic or renal function studies. ■ Obtain baseline vital signs, bowel sounds, urinary ouput, muscle strength, and mental status as appropriate. ■ Assess the patient's ability to receive and understand instruction. Include the family and caregivers as needed.	■ Ineffective Airway Clearance (myasthenia gravis) ■ Impaired Physical Mobility (myasthenia gravis) ■ Urinary Retention or Impaired Urinary Elimination (postoperatively, postpartum) ■ Incontinence ■ Risk for Injury (related to adverse effects of drug therapy) ■ Deficient Knowledge (drug therapy)
Assessment throughout administration: ■ Assess for desired therapeutic effects dependent on the reason for the drug (e.g., increased ease of urination, muscle strength and coordination improved, improved mental status). ■ Continue frequent and careful monitoring of vital signs, mental status, bowel sounds, urinary output, and musculoskeletal function as appropriate. ■ Assess for and promptly report adverse effects: bradycardia, hypotension, dysrhythmias, tremors, dizziness, headache, dyspnea, decreased urinary output, abdominal pain, or changes in mental status.	

Planning: Patient Goals and Expected Outcomes

The patient will:
■ Experience therapeutic effects dependent on the reason the drug is being given (e.g., improved physical mobility and coordination, increased ease of urination, improvement in mental status and functioning, and self-care activities).
■ Be free from, or experience minimal, adverse effects.
■ Verbalize an understanding of the drug's use, adverse effects, and required precautions.
■ Demonstrate proper self-administration of the medication (e.g., dose, timing, when to notify provider) and proper ophthalmic drug instillation technique.

Implementation

Interventions and (Rationales)	Patient and Family Education
All Parasympathomimetics	
Ensuring therapeutic effects: ■ Continue frequent assessments as described earlier for therapeutic effects dependent on the reason the drug therapy is given. (Mental status and ability to carry out ADLs has improved; urinary elimination and output is improved; musculoskeletal weakness, ptosis, diplopia, and chewing and swallowing are improved.)	■ Encourage the patient, family, or caregiver to practice supportive measures along with drug therapy to maximize therapeutic effects (e.g., adequate rest periods in myasthenia gravis)
■ Provide supportive nursing measures; e.g., regular toileting schedule, safety measures, etc. (Nursing measures such as assisting patient to normal voiding position will supplement therapeutic drug effects and optimize outcome.)	■ Assess the patient's or family's ability to carry out ADLs at home and explore the need for additional health care referrals. Evaluate home safety needs.
■ Follow appropriate administration techniques for ophthalmic doses. Sustained-release tablets should not be crushed or chewed. Check drug reference material on administration with or without food. (See chapter 3, Principles of Drug Administration for techniques ∞. Sustained-release formulas must dissolve slowly. Food may impair or enhance absorption or prevent adverse effects.)	■ Instruct the patient in proper administration techniques, followed by return-demonstration.

(Continued)

NURSING PROCESS FOCUS   PATIENTS RECEIVING PARASYMPATHOMIMETIC THERAPY *(Continued)*

Implementation

Interventions and (Rationales)	Patient and Family Education
Minimizing adverse effects:	
▪ Monitor for signs of excessive ANS stimulation and notify the health care provider if the pulse is less than 60 beats/min or BP is below established parameters. (Because parasympathomimetic drugs decrease the heart rate and blood pressure, they must be closely monitored to avoid adverse effects. Atropine may be ordered to counteract drug effects.)	▪ Instruct the patient to promptly report tremors, palpitations, changes in blood pressure, dizziness, urinary retention, abdominal pain, or changes in behavior (e.g., confusion, depression, drowsiness). Instruct the patient to report dyspnea, salivation or sweating, or extreme fatigue immediately as these are signs of a potential overdose.
▪ Continue to monitor hepatic function lab work. (Parasympathomimetic drugs may cause liver toxicity and liver enzymes may be monitored weekly for up to 6 weeks.)	▪ Teach the patient, family, or caregiver about the importance of returning for follow-up lab studies.
▪ Carefully calculate and monitor doses. (Careful calculation will avoid overdosage.)	▪ Ensure the patient, family, or caregiver are administering the correct dose by observing return-demonstration.
Patient understanding of drug therapy:	
▪ Use opportunities during administration of medications and during assessments to discuss the rationale for drug therapy, desired therapeutic outcomes, most commonly observed adverse effects, parameters for when to call the health care provider, and any necessary monitoring or precautions. (Using time during nursing care helps to optimize and reinforce key teaching areas.)	▪ The patient, family, or caregiver should be able to state the reason for drug; appropriate dose and scheduling; what adverse effects to observe for and when to report; equipment needed as appropriate and how to use that equipment; and the required length of medication therapy needed with any special instructions regarding renewing or continuing prescription as appropriate.
Patient self-administration of drug therapy:	
▪ When administering the medications, instruct the patient, family, or caregiver in the proper self-administration of drugs and ophthalmic drops. (Utilizing time during nurse-administration of these drugs helps to reinforce teaching.)	▪ Instruct the patient in proper administration techniques, followed by return-demonstration.
	▪ The patient, family, or caregiver are able to discuss appropriate dosing and administration needs.
Direct-Acting Drugs	
▪ Continue frequent monitoring of bowel sounds, and urine output if drugs are given postoperatively or postpartum. (Assessments will detect early signs of adverse effects as well as monitoring for therapeutic effects. Drug onset is in approximately 60 minutes with increased urination and peristalsis following. Drugs are not given if a mechanical obstruction is known or suspected.)	▪ Instruct the patient to have bathroom facilities nearby after taking the drug. The patient may need assistance to the toilet or commode if dizziness occurs.
▪ Provide for eye comfort such as adequately lighted room and appropriate safety measures. (Parasympathomimetic drugs can cause miosis with difficulty seeing in low light levels and blurred vision.)	▪ Caution the patient about driving in low-light conditions, at night, or if vision is blurred. Nightlight use at home and safety measures may be needed to prevent falls.
▪ Help the patient to rise from lying or sitting to standing until drug effects are assessed. (Direct-acting parasympathomimetics may cause significant orthostatic hypotension.)	▪ Instruct the patient to rise from lying or sitting to standing slowly, and to avoid prolonged standing in one place to avoid dizziness or falls.
Cholinesterase Inhibitors	
▪ Continue monitoring musculoskeletal strength, improvement in ptosis or diplopia, and improved chewing and swallowing. (Improvement demonstrates that therapeutic effects have been achieved.)	▪ Teach the patient, family, or caregiver to notify the health care provider if shortness of breath, extreme fatigue, or difficulty with chewing or swallowing occurs or is worsening.
▪ Check drug reference material on administration with or without food. (Some formulations should be taken with food, [e.g., ambenonium], others on an empty stomach [e.g., tacrine]. Food may impair or enhance absorption or prevent adverse effects.)	▪ Teach the patient, family, or caregiver about appropriate scheduling of drug around mealtimes.
▪ Monitor for muscle weakness after the dose is given. (Depending on the time of onset, this symptom indicates cholinergic crisis [overdose], or myasthenic crisis [underdose].)	▪ Instruct the patient to report any severe muscle weakness that occurs 1 hour after taking the drug or if it occurs 3 or more hours after taking the drug.

NURSING PROCESS FOCUS | **PATIENTS RECEIVING PARASYMPATHOMIMETIC THERAPY** *(Continued)*

Implementation

Interventions and (Rationales)	Patient and Family Education
▪ Schedule activities and allow for adequate periods of rest to avoid fatigue. (Excess fatigue can lead to either a cholinergic or myasthenic crisis.)	▪ Instruct the patient to plan activities according to muscle strength and fatigue and to allow for frequent and adequate rest periods. ▪ Instruct the patient to immediately report dyspnea, salivation or sweating, or extreme fatigue.

Evaluation of Outcome Criteria

Evaluate the effectiveness of drug therapy by confirming that the patient goals and expected outcomes have been met (see "Planning").

See Table 13.4 for a list of drugs to which these nursing applications apply.

13.10 Clinical Applications of Anticholinergics

Agents that block the action of acetylcholine are known by a number of names, including anticholinergics, cholinergic blockers, muscarinic antagonists, and parasympatholytics (Table 13.5). Although the term *anticholinergic* is most commonly used, the most accurate term for this class of drugs is muscarinic antagonists, because at therapeutic doses, these drugs are selective for Ach muscarinic receptors, and thus have little effect on Ach nicotinic receptors.

Anticholinergics act by competing with acetylcholine for binding muscarinic receptors. When anticholinergics occupy these receptors, no response is generated at the neuroeffector organs. Suppressing the effects of Ach causes symptoms of sympathetic nervous system activation to predominate. Most therapeutic uses of the anticholinergics are predictable extensions of their parasympathetic-blocking actions: dilation of the pupils, increase in heart rate, drying of secretions, and relaxation of the bronchi.

Note that these are also symptoms of sympathetic activation (fight or flight).

Historically, anticholinergics have been widely used for many different disorders. References to these agents, which are extracted from the deadly nightshade plant, *Atropa belladonna,* date to the ancient Hindus, the Roman Empire, and the Middle Ages. Because of plant's extreme toxicity, extracts of belladonna were sometimes used for intentional poisoning, including suicide, as well as in religious and beautification rituals. The name *belladonna* is Latin for "pretty woman." Roman women applied extracts of belladonna to the face to create the preferred female attributes of the time—pink cheeks and dilated, doelike eyes.

Therapeutic uses of anticholinergics include the following:

- *GI disorders:* These agents decrease the secretion of gastric acid in peptic ulcer disease (chapter 40∞). They also slow intestinal motility and may be useful for reducing the cramping and diarrhea associated with irritable bowel syndrome (chapter 41∞).

TABLE 13.5	Cholinergic-Blocking Agents (Anticholinergics)
Drug	**Primary Use**
atropine (Atro-Pen, Atropair, Atropisol)	Poisoning with anticholinesterase agents, to increase heart rate, dilate pupils
benztropine (Cogentin)	Parkinson's disease, neuroleptic side effects
cyclopentolate (Cyclogyl)	To dilate pupils
dicyclomine (Bentyl, others)	Irritable bowel syndrome
glycopyrrolate (Robinul)	To produce a dry field prior to anesthesia, peptic ulcers
ipratropium (Atrovent)	Asthma
methscopolamine (Pamine)	Motion sickness, ulcers
oxybutynin (Ditropan, Oxytrol)	Incontinence
propantheline (Pro-Banthine)	Irritable bowel syndrome, peptic ulcer
scopolamine (Hyoscine, Transderm-Scop)	Motion sickness, irritable bowel syndrome, adjunct to anesthesia
tiotropium (Spiriva)	Asthma
tolterodine (Detrol)	Overactive bladder with symptoms of urge urinary incontinence, urgency, and frequency
trihexyphenidyl (Artane, others)	Parkinson's disease
tropicamide (Mydiracyl, Tropicacyl)	Mydriasis and cycloplegia for diagnostic procedures

- *Ophthalmic procedures:* Anticholinergics may be used to cause mydriasis or cycloplegia during eye procedures (chapter 49∞).

- *Cardiac rhythm abnormalities:* Anticholinergics can be used to accelerate the heart rate in patients experiencing bradycardia (chapter 26∞).

- *Preanesthesia:* Combined with other agents, anticholinergics can decrease excessive respiratory secretions and reverse the bradycardia caused by anesthetics (chapter 19∞).

- *Asthma:* A few agents, such as ipratropium (Atrovent), are useful in treating asthma, because of their ability to dilate the bronchi (chapter 39∞).

The prototype drug, atropine, is used for several additional medical conditions owing to its effective muscarinic receptor blockade. These applications include reversal of adverse muscarinic effects and treatment of cholinergic agent poisoning, including that caused by overdose of bethanechol (Urecholine), cholinesterase inhibitors, or accidental ingestion of certain types of mushrooms or organophosphate pesticides.

SPECIAL CONSIDERATIONS

Impact of Anticholinergics on Male Sexual Function

A functioning autonomic nervous system is essential for normal male sexual health. The parasympathetic nervous system is necessary for erections, whereas the sympathetic division is responsible for the process of ejaculation. Anticholinergic drugs block transmission of parasympathetic impulses and may interfere with normal erections. Adrenergic antagonists can interfere with the smooth-muscle contractions in the seminal vesicles and penis, resulting in an inability to ejaculate.

For male patients receiving autonomic medications, the nurse should include questions about sexual activity during the assessment process. For patients who are not sexually active, these side effects may be unimportant. For patients who are sexually active, however, drug-induced sexual dysfunction may be a major cause of noncompliance. The patient should be informed to expect such side effects and to report them to the health care provider immediately. In most cases, alternative medications are available that do not affect sexual function. Inform the patient that supportive counseling is available.

Pr Prototype Drug | Atropine *(Atro-Pen, Atropair, Atropisol)*

Therapeutic Class: Antidote for anticholinerase poisoning

Pharmacologic Class: Muscarinic cholinergic receptor antagonist

ACTIONS AND USES

By occupying muscarinic receptors, atropine blocks the parasympathetic actions of Ach and induces symptoms of the fight-or-flight response. Most prominent are increased heart rate, bronchodilation, decreased motility in the GI tract, mydriasis, and decreased secretions from glands. At therapeutic doses, atropine has no effect on nicotinic receptors in ganglia or on skeletal muscle.

Although atropine has been used for centuries for a variety of purposes, its use has declined in recent decades because of the development of safer and more effective medications. Atropine may be used to treat hypermotility diseases of the GI tract such as irritable bowel syndrome, to suppress secretions during surgical procedures, to increase the heart rate in patients with bradycardia, and to dilate the pupil during eye examinations. Once widely used to cause bronchodilation in patients with asthma, atropine is now rarely prescribed for this disorder. Atropine therapy is useful for the treatment of reflexive bradycardia in infants and infantile hypertrophic pyloric stenosis (IHPS).

ADMINISTRATION ALERTS

- Never administer IM.
- Oral and subcutaneous doses are *not* interchangeable.
- Monitor blood pressure, pulse, and respirations before administration and for at least 1 hour after subcutaneous administration.
- Pregnancy category C

PHARMACOKINETICS

Onset: 30 min PO; 5–15 min subcutaneously

Peak: 60–90 min PO; 15–30 min subcutaneously, 30 min IM, 2–4 min IV

Half-life: 4 h PO; 120 min subcutaneously

Duration: 6 h PO; 4 h subcutaneously

ADVERSE EFFECTS

The side effects of atropine limit its therapeutic usefulness and are predictable extensions of its autonomic actions. Expected side effects include dry mouth, constipation, urinary retention, and an increased heart rate. Initial CNS excitement may progress to delirium and even coma.

Contraindications: Atropine is usually contraindicated in patients with glaucoma, because the drug may increase pressure within the eye. Atropine should not be administered to patients with obstructive disorders of the GI tract, paralytic ileus, bladder neck obstruction, benign prostatic hypertrophy, myasthenia gravis, cardiac insufficiency, or acute hemorrhage.

INTERACTIONS

Drug–Drug: Drug interactions with atropine include an increased effect with antihistamines, tricyclic antidepressants, quinidine, and procainamide. Atropine decreases effects of levodopa.

Lab Tests: Unknown

Herbal/Food: Use with caution with herbal supplements, such as aloe, Serona repens (scientific name for saw palmetto), buckthorn, and cascara sagrada (means *sacred bark* in Spanish), which may increase atropine's effect, particularly with chronic use of these herbs.

Treatment of Overdose: Accidental poisoning has occurred in children who eat the colorful, purple berries of the deadly nightshade, mistaking them for cherries. Symptoms of poisoning are those of intense parasympathetic stimulation. Overdose may cause CNS stimulation or depression. A short-acting barbiturate or diazepam (Valium) may be administered to control convulsions. Physostigmine is an antidote for atropine poisoning that quickly reverses the coma caused by large doses of atropine.

Refer to MyNursingKit for a Nursing Process Focus specific to this drug.

Some of the anticholinergics are used for their effects on the CNS, rather than their autonomic actions. Scopolamine (Hyoscine, Transderm-Scop) is used to produce sedation and prevent motion sickness (chapter 41∞); benztropine (Cogentin) is prescribed to reduce the muscular tremor and rigidity associated with Parkinson's disease; and donepezil (Aricept) has a slight memory enhancement effect in patients with Alzheimer's disease (chapter 20∞).

Anticholinergics exhibit a relatively high incidence of side effects. Important adverse effects that limit their usefulness include tachycardia, CNS stimulation, and the tendency to cause urinary retention in men with prostate disorders. Adverse effects such as dry mouth and dry eyes occur due to blockade of muscarinic receptors on salivary glands and lacrimal glands, respectively. Blockade of muscarinic receptors on sweat glands can inhibit sweating, which may lead to hyperthermia. Photophobia can occur because the pupil is unable to constrict in response to bright light. Symptoms of overdose (cholinergic crisis) include fever, visual changes, difficulty swallowing, psychomotor agitation, and/or hallu-cinations. (Use this simile to remember the signs of cholinergic crisis: "Hot as hades, blind as a bat, dry as a bone, mad as a hatter.") The development of safer and more effective drugs has greatly decreased the current use of anticholinergics. An example is ipratropium (Atrovent), a relatively new anticholinergic used for patients with COPD. Because it is delivered via aerosol spray, this agent produces more localized action with fewer systemic side effects than atropine.

HOME & COMMUNITY CONSIDERATIONS

Promoting Safety with Medications That Affect the ANS

Medications affecting the autonomic nervous system are often administered in the home-care setting. It is important that the patient and family understand not only the reason for the medication but also the importance of immediately reporting adverse effects to the health care provider. Emphasize medication compliance to the patient and family. Stress home safety, because many of these drugs may produce side effects that could put the patient at risk for falls or other injuries in the home environment.

NURSING PROCESS FOCUS   PATIENTS RECEIVING ANTICHOLINERGIC THERAPY

Assessment	Potential Nursing Diagnoses
Baseline assessment prior to administration: ■ Understand the reason the drug has been prescribed in order to assess for therapeutic effects. ■ Obtain a complete health history including cardiovascular, cerebrovascular, or respiratory disease, and for acute (narrow-angle) glaucoma. Obtain a drug history including allergies, current prescription and OTC drugs, and herbal preparations. Be alert to possible drug interactions. ■ Evaluate appropriate laboratory findings such as hepatic or renal function studies. ■ Obtain baseline vital signs, urinary output, bowels sounds, and cardiac rhythm if appropriate. ■ Assess the patient's ability to receive and understand instruction. Include the family and caregivers as needed.	■ Decreased Cardiac Output (dysrhythmias) ■ Urinary Retention ■ Constipation ■ Risk for Impaired Body Temperature ■ Risk for Impaired Oral Mucous Membranes ■ Risk for Injury (related to adverse effects of drug therapy) ■ Deficient Knowledge (drug therapy)
Assessment throughout administration: ■ Assess for desired therapeutic effects dependent on the reason for the drug (e.g., increased ease of breathing, cardiac rhythm stable, BP within normal range). ■ Continue frequent and careful monitoring of vital signs, and urinary output and cardiac monitoring as appropriate. ■ Assess for and promptly report adverse effects: tachycardia, hypertension, dysrhythmias, tremors, dizziness, headache, or decreased urinary output. Seizures or ventricular tachycardia may signal drug toxicity and should be immediately reported.	

Planning: Patient Goals and Expected Outcomes

The patient will:

■ Experience therapeutic effects dependent on the reason the drug is being given (e.g., increased ease of breathing, decreased GI motility and cramping).

■ Be free from, or experience minimal, adverse effects.

■ Verbalize an understanding of the drug's use, adverse effects, and required precautions.

■ Demonstrate proper self-administration of the medication (e.g., dose, timing, when to notify provider) and proper use of the inhaler.

(Continued)

NURSING PROCESS FOCUS   PATIENTS RECEIVING ANTICHOLINERGIC THERAPY *(Continued)*

Implementation

Interventions and (Rationales)	Patient and Family Education
Ensuring therapeutic effects:	
▪ Continue frequent assessments as described earlier for therapeutic effects dependent on the reason the drug therapy is given. (Pulse, blood pressure, and respiratory rate should be within normal limits or within parameters set by the health care provider. Gastric motility and cramping have slowed.)	▪ Teach the patient, family, or caregiver how to monitor the pulse and blood pressure. Ensure the proper use and functioning of any home equipment obtained.
▪ Provide supportive nursing measures; e.g., proper positioning for dyspnea; ice chips, fluids, or hard candy for dry mouth, etc. (Nursing measures such as raising the head of the bed during dyspnea will supplement therapeutic drug effects and optimize outcome.)	▪ Instruct the patient that sips of water, ice chips, oral rinses free of alcohol, and hard candies may ease mouth dryness (alcohol-based rinses will dry the mouth further).
▪ Follow appropriate administration techniques for inhalant or ophthalmic doses. (See chapter 3, Principles of Drug Administration for techniques∞.)	▪ Instruct the patient in proper administration techniques, followed by return-demonstration.
Minimizing adverse effects:	
▪ Monitor for signs of excessive ANS stimulation such as drowsiness, blurred vision, tachycardia, dry mouth, urinary hesitancy, and decreased sweating. (Side effects are due to the blockade of muscarinic receptors. Anticholinergics are contraindicated in patients with acute/narrow-angle glaucoma because mydriasis will increase intraocular pressure.)	▪ Instruct the patient to report palpitations, shortness of breath, dizziness, dysphagia, or syncope immediately to the health care provider.
▪ Notify the health care provider if the blood pressure or pulse exceed established parameters. Continue frequent cardiac monitoring as appropriate (e.g., ECG) and urine output. (Because anticholinergic drugs stimulate heart rate and increase the chance for dysrhythmias, they must be closely monitored to avoid adverse effects. External monitoring devices will detect early signs of adverse effects as well as monitoring for therapeutic.)	▪ To allay possible anxiety, teach the patient about the rationale for all equipment used and the need for frequent monitoring as applicable.
▪ Monitor the patient for abdominal distention and auscultate for bowel sounds. Palpate for bladder distention and monitor output. (Anticholinergics may decrease tone and motility of intestinal and bladder smooth muscle.)	▪ Teach the patient about the importance of drinking extra fluids and increasing fiber intake. Instruct the patient to notify the health care provider if difficulty with urination occurs or if constipation is severe.
▪ Minimize exposure to heat and strenuous exercise. (Anticholinergics can inhibit sweat gland secretions. Sweating is necessary for patients to cool down, so the drug can increase their risk for heat exhaustion and heat stroke.)	▪ Instruct the patient to avoid prolonged or strenuous activity in warm or hot environments especially on humid days. Extra-hot showers and hot tubs should also be avoided. Dizziness, change in mental status, pale skin, muscle cramping, and nausea are signs of an impending heat exhaustion or stroke and should be reported immediately.
▪ Provide for eye comfort such as darkened room, soft cloth over eyes, and sunglasses. (Anticholinergic drugs cause mydriasis and photosensitivity to light.)	▪ Instruct the patient that photosensitivity may occur and sunglasses may be needed in bright light or for outside activities. Caution should be taken with driving until drug effects are known.
Patient understanding of drug therapy:	
▪ Use opportunities during administration of medications and during assessments to discuss rationale for drug therapy, desired therapeutic outcomes, most commonly observed adverse effects, parameters for when to call the health care provider, and any necessary monitoring or precautions. (Using time during nursing care helps to optimize and reinforce key teaching areas.)	▪ The patient, family, or caregiver should be able to state the reason for the drug; appropriate dose and scheduling; what adverse effects to observe for and when to report; equipment needed as appropriate and how to use that equipment; and the required length of medication therapy needed with any special instructions regarding renewing or continuing prescription as appropriate.
Patient self-administration of drug therapy:	
▪ When administering the medications, instruct the patient, family, or caregiver in proper self-administration of an inhaler or ophthalmic drops. (Utilizing time during nurse-administration of these drugs helps to reinforce teaching.)	▪ Instruct the patient in proper administration techniques, followed by return-demonstration. ▪ The patient, family, or caregiver are able to discuss appropriate dosing and administration needs.

Evaluation of Outcome Criteria

Evaluate the effectiveness of drug therapy by confirming that patient goals and expected outcomes have been met (see "Planning").

See Table 13.3 for a list of drugs to which these nursing actions apply.

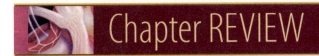

Chapter REVIEW

KEY CONCEPTS

The numbered key concepts provide a succinct summary of the important points from the corresponding numbered section within the chapter. If any of these points are not clear, refer to the numbered section within the chapter for review.

13.1 The peripheral nervous system is divided into a somatic portion, which is under voluntary control, and an autonomic portion, which is involuntary and controls smooth muscle, cardiac muscle, and glandular secretions.

13.2 Stimulation of the sympathetic division of the autonomic nervous system causes symptoms of the fight-or-flight response, whereas stimulation of the parasympathetic branch induces rest-and-digest responses.

13.3 Drugs can affect nervous transmission across a synapse by preventing the synthesis, storage, or release of the neurotransmitter; by preventing the destruction of the neurotransmitter; or by binding neurotransmitters to the receptors.

13.4 Norepinephrine is the primary neurotransmitter released at adrenergic receptors, which are divided into alpha and beta subtypes. Acetylcholine is the other primary neurotransmitter of the autonomic nervous system.

13.5 Acetylcholine is the primary neurotransmitter released at cholinergic receptors (nicotinic and muscarinic) in both the sympathetic and parasympathetic nervous systems. It is also the neurotransmitter at nicotinic receptors in skeletal muscle.

13.6 Autonomic drugs are classified by the receptors they stimulate or block: Sympathomimetics stimulate target tissue innervated by sympathetic nerves, and parasympathomimetics stimulate target tissue innervated by parasympathetic nerves; adrenergic antagonists inhibit functionality of the sympathetic division, whereas anticholinergics inhibit functionality of the parasympathetic branch.

13.7 Sympathomimetics act by directly activating adrenergic receptors, or indirectly by increasing the release of norepinephrine from nerve terminals. They are used primarily for their effects on the heart, bronchial tree, and nasal passages.

13.8 Adrenergic antagonists are used primarily for hypertension and are the most widely prescribed class of autonomic drugs.

13.9 Parasympathomimetics act directly by stimulating cholinergic receptors or indirectly by inhibiting acetylcholinesterase. They have few therapeutic uses because of their numerous side effects.

13.10 Anticholinergics act by blocking the effects of acetylcholine at muscarinic receptors, and are used to dry secretions, treat asthma, and prevent motion sickness.

NCLEX-RN® REVIEW QUESTIONS

1 Following administration of an adrenergic (sympathomimetic) drug, the nurse would assess for which adverse drug effects?
1. Insomnia, nervousness, and hypertension
2. Nausea, vomiting, and hypotension
3. Nervousness, drowsiness, and dyspnea
4. Bronchial dilation, hypotension, and bradycardia

2 Therapeutic uses for anticholinergics include: (Select all that apply.)
1. peptic ulcer disease.
2. bradycardia.
3. decreased sexual function.
4. irritable bowel syndrome.
5. urine retention.

3 Adrenergic-blocking (antagonist) drugs include all of the following adverse reactions except:
1. bronchodilation.
2. tachycardia.
3. edema.
4. heart failure.

4 Elderly patients taking bethanechol (Urecholine) need to be assessed more frequently because of which of the following side effects?
1. Diaphoresis
2. Hypertension
3. Dizziness
4. Urinary retention

5 The patient taking benztropine (Cogentin) should be assessed for:
1. heartburn.
2. constipation.
3. hypothermia.
4. increased gastric motility.

6 The patient taking tacrine (Cognex) should be observant for which of the following adverse effects that may signal a possible overdose has occurred?
1. Excessive sweating, salivation, and drooling
2. Extreme constipation
3. Hypertension and tachycardia
4. Excessively dry eyes and reddened sclera

CRITICAL THINKING QUESTIONS

1. A 24-year-old patient (gravida 3, para 1) is admitted to the labor and delivery unit and states that she is having contractions. She is at 32 weeks gestation. The obstetrician initially begins tocolysis with magnesium sulfate and then switches the patient to terbutaline (Brethine), 5 mg PO every 4 hours around the clock. The nurse recognizes terbutaline as a beta$_2$-adrenergic agent. What nursing assessments should be made with a patient receiving terbutaline therapy? What education does the patient require in relation to terbutaline therapy? How will the nurse evaluate the medication's effectiveness?

2. A 74-year-old female patient underwent a retropubic urethral suspension. She required a Foley catheter for 4 days postoperatively and was still unable to void. She was recatheterized, and a bladder rehabilitation program was begun that included bethanechol (Urecholine). What nursing diagnosis should be considered as a part of this patient's plan of care given this new drug regimen?

3. A 42-year-old male patient was diagnosed with Parkinson's disease 4 years ago. He is being treated with a regimen of amantadine (Symmetrel), an indirect-acting dopaminergic agent, and benztropine mesylate (Cogentin). The nurse recognizes Cogentin as an anticholinergic agent. What should the nurse assess this patient for? Discuss the potential side effects of benztropine that the nurse should assess for in this patient.

See Appendix D for answers and rationales for all activities.

PEARSON

EXPLORE **mynursingkit**

MyNursingKit is your one stop for online chapter review materials and resources. Prepare for success with additional NCLEX®-style practice questions, interactive assignments and activities, web links, animations and videos, and more!

Register your access code from the front of your book at
www.mynursingkit.com.

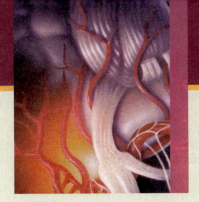

Chapter 14

Drugs for Anxiety and Insomnia

DRUGS AT A GLANCE

LEARNING OUTCOMES

After reading this chapter, the student should be able to:

1. Identify the major types of anxiety disorders.
2. Discuss factors contributing to anxiety and explain some nonpharmacologic therapies used to cope with this disorder.
3. Identify the regions of the brain associated with anxiety, sleep, and wakefulness.
4. Identify the three classes of medications used to treat anxiety and sleep disorders.
5. Explain the pharmacologic management of anxiety and insomnia.
6. Describe the nurse's role in the pharmacologic management of anxiety and insomnia.
7. Identify normal sleep patterns and explain how these might be affected by anxiety and stress.
8. Categorize drugs used for anxiety and insomnia based on their classification and mechanism of action.
9. For each of the classes listed in Drugs at a Glance, know representative drugs and explain their mechanisms of action, primary actions, and important adverse effects.
10. Use the nursing process to care for patients receiving drug therapy for anxiety and insomnia.

KEY TERMS

Patients experience nervousness and tension more often than any other symptoms. Seeking relief from these symptoms, they often turn to a variety of pharmacologic and alternative therapies. Most health care providers agree that even though drugs do not cure the underlying problem, they can provide temporary help to calm patients who are experiencing acute anxiety, or who have simple sleep disorders. This chapter deals with drugs that treat anxiety, cause sedation, or help patients sleep.

ANXIETY DISORDERS

According to the *International Classification of Diseases*, 10th edition (ICD-10), **anxiety** is a state of "apprehension, tension, or uneasiness that stems from the anticipation of danger, the source of which is largely unknown or unrecognized." Anxious individuals can often identify at least some factors that bring on their symptoms. Most people state that their feelings of anxiety are disproportionate to any factual dangers.

14.1 Types of Anxiety Disorders

The anxiety experienced by people faced with a stressful environment is called **situational anxiety.** To a degree, situational anxiety is beneficial because it motivates people to accomplish tasks in a prompt manner—if for no other reason than to eliminate the source of nervousness. Situational stress may be intense, though patients often learn coping mechanisms to deal with the stress without seeking conventional medical intervention.

Generalized anxiety disorder (GAD) is a difficult-to-control, excessive anxiety that lasts 6 months or more. It focuses on a variety of life events or activities, and interferes with normal day-to-day functions. It is by far the most common type of stress disorder, and the one most frequently encountered by the nurse. Symptoms include restlessness, fatigue, muscle tension, nervousness, inability to focus or concentrate, an overwhelming sense of dread, and sleep disturbances. Autonomic signs of sympathetic nervous system activation that accompany anxiety include blood pressure elevation, heart palpitations, varying degrees of respiratory change, and dry mouth. Parasympathetic responses may consist of abdominal cramping, diarrhea, fatigue, and urinary urgency. Women are slightly more likely to experience GAD than men, and its prevalence is highest in the 20–35 age group.

A second category of anxiety, called **panic disorder,** is characterized by intense feelings of immediate apprehension, fearfulness, terror, or impending doom, accompanied by increased autonomic nervous system activity. Although panic attacks usually last less than 10 minutes, patients may describe them as seemingly endless. Up to 5% of the population will experience one or more panic attacks during their lifetime, with women being affected about twice as often as men.

Other categories of anxiety disorders include phobias, obsessive–compulsive disorder, and post-traumatic stress disorder. **Phobias** are fearful feelings attached to situations or objects. Common phobias include fear of snakes, spiders, crowds, or heights. A fear of crowds is termed **social anxiety.** Performers may experience feelings of dread, nervousness, or apprehension termed *performance anxiety*. Some anxiety is normal when a person faces a crowd or performs for a crowd, but extreme fear to the point of phobia is not normal. Phobias compel a patient to avoid the fearful stimulus entirely to the point that his or her behavior is unnatural. Another unnatural behavior is **obsessive–compulsive disorder (OCD).** It involves recurrent, intrusive thoughts or repetitive behaviors that interfere with normal activities or relationships. Common examples include fear of exposure to germs and repetitive hand washing. **Post-traumatic stress disorder (PTSD)** is a type of situational anxiety that develops in response to re-experiencing a previous life event. Traumatic life events such as war, physical or sexual abuse, natural disasters, or murder may lead to a sense of helplessness and re-experiencing of the traumatic event. Hurricane Katrina, as well as the terrorist attack on September 11, 2001, are examples of situations that may trigger PTSD. People who experience these types of traumatic life events are at risk for developing signs and symptoms of PTSD.

14.2 Specific Regions of the Brain Responsible for Anxiety and Wakefulness

Neural systems in the brain associated with anxiety and restlessness include the limbic system and the reticular activating system. These are illustrated in Pharmacotherapy Illustrated 14.1.

The **limbic system** is an area in the middle of the brain responsible for emotional expression, learning, and memory. Signals routed through the limbic system ultimately connect with the hypothalamus. Emotional states associated with this connection include anxiety, fear, anger, aggression, remorse, depression, sexual drive, and euphoria.

The hypothalamus is an important center responsible for unconscious responses to extreme stress such as high blood pressure, elevated respiratory rate, and dilated pupils. These are responses associated with the fight-or-flight response of the autonomic nervous system, as presented in chapter 13∞. The many endocrine functions of the hypothalamus are discussed in chapter 43∞.

The hypothalamus connects with the **reticular formation**, a network of neurons found along the entire length of the brainstem, as shown in Pharmacotherapy Illustrated 14.1. Stimulation of the reticular formation causes heightened alertness and arousal; inhibition causes general drowsiness and the induction of sleep.

The larger area in which the reticular formation is found is called the **reticular activating system (RAS).** This structure projects from the brainstem to the thalamus. The RAS is responsible for sleeping and wakefulness and performs an alerting function for the entire cerebral cortex. It helps a

PHARMACOTHERAPY ILLUSTRATED

14.1   The Reticular Activating System and Related Regions in the Brain Are Important Areas of Focus for Drugs Used to Treat Anxiety and Anxiety-Related Symptoms

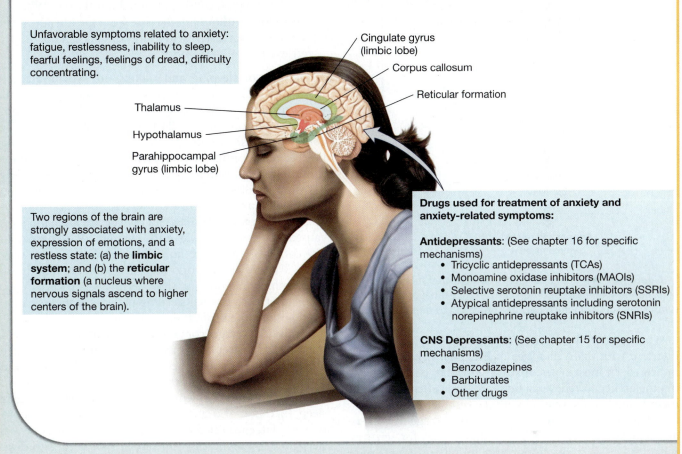

Unfavorable symptoms related to anxiety: fatigue, restlessness, inability to sleep, fearful feelings, feelings of dread, difficulty concentrating.

Cingulate gyrus (limbic lobe)

Corpus callosum

Reticular formation

Thalamus

Hypothalamus

Parahippocampal gyrus (limbic lobe)

Two regions of the brain are strongly associated with anxiety, expression of emotions, and a restless state: (a) the **limbic system**; and (b) the **reticular formation** (a nucleus where nervous signals ascend to higher centers of the brain).

Drugs used for treatment of anxiety and anxiety-related symptoms:

Antidepressants: (See chapter 16 for specific mechanisms)
- Tricyclic antidepressants (TCAs)
- Monoamine oxidase inhibitors (MAOIs)
- Selective serotonin reuptake inhibitors (SSRIs)
- Atypical antidepressants including serotonin norepinephrine reuptake inhibitors (SNRIs)

CNS Depressants: (See chapter 15 for specific mechanisms)
- Benzodiazepines
- Barbiturates
- Other drugs

---

person focus attention on individual tasks by transmitting information to higher brain centers.

If signals are prevented from passing through the RAS, no emotion-related signals are sent to the brain, resulting in a reduction in general brain activity. If signals coming from the hypothalamus are allowed to proceed, then those signals

are further routed through the RAS and on to higher brain centers. This is the neural mechanism thought to be responsible for feelings such as anxiety and fear. It is also the mechanism associated with restlessness and an interrupted sleeping pattern.

14.3 Anxiety Management Through Pharmacologic and Nonpharmacologic Strategies

Although stress itself may be incapacitating, it is often only a symptom of an underlying disorder. It is considered more productive to uncover and address the cause of the anxiety rather than to merely treat the symptoms with medications. Patients should be encouraged to explore and develop nonpharmacologic coping strategies to deal with the underlying causes. Such strategies may include cognitive–behavioral therapy, counseling, biofeedback techniques, meditation, and other complementary therapies. One model for stress management is shown in ➤ Figure 14.1.

PHARMFACTS

Anxiety Disorders
- About 19 million Americans are diagnosed with anxiety every year.
- Other illnesses that commonly coexist with anxiety include depression, eating disorders, and substance abuse.
- The top five causes of anxiety (as listed in order) occur between the ages of 18 and 54:
  1. Phobia
  2. Post-traumatic stress
  3. Generalized anxiety
  4. Obsessive–compulsive feelings
  5. Panic

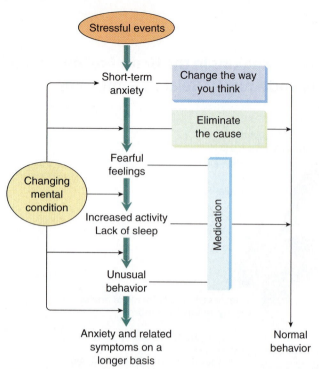

➤ **Figure 14.1** A model of anxiety in which stressful events or a changing mental condition can produce unfavorable symptoms, some of which may be controlled by medication

When anxiety becomes severe enough to significantly interfere with daily activities of life, pharmacotherapy is indicated. In most types of stress, **anxiolytics,** or drugs having the ability to relieve anxiety, are quite effective. These include medications found within a number of therapeutic categories: central nervous system (CNS) agents such as antidepressants and CNS depressants; drugs for seizures (chapter 15∞); emotional and mood disorder drugs (chapter 16∞); antihypertensive agents (chapter 23∞); and antidysrhythmics (chapter 26∞). Anxiolytics provide treatment for all the conditions mentioned in Section 14.1: phobias, post-traumatic stress disorder, generalized anxiety, obsessive–compulsive disorder, and panic attack.

INSOMNIA

Insomnia is a condition characterized by a patient's inability to fall asleep or remain asleep. Pharmacotherapy may be indicated if the sleeplessness interferes with normal daily activities.

14.4 Insomnia and Its Link to Anxiety

Why is it that we need sleep? During an average lifetime, about 33% of the time is spent sleeping, or trying to sleep. Although it is well established that sleep is essential for wellness, scientists are unsure of its function or how much is needed. Following are some theories:

• Inactivity during sleep gives the body time to repair itself.

• Sleep is a function that evolved as a protective mechanism. Throughout history, night-time was the safest time of day.

• Sleep deals with "electrical" charging and discharging of the brain. The brain needs time for processing and filing new information collected throughout the day. When this is done without interference from the outside environment, these vast amounts of data can be retrieved through memory.

The acts of sleeping and waking are synchronized to many different bodily functions. Body temperature, blood pressure, hormone levels, and respiration all fluctuate on a cyclic basis throughout the 24-hour day. When this cycle becomes impaired, pharmacologic or other interventions may be needed to readjust it. Increased levels of the neurotransmitter serotonin help initiate the various processes of sleep.

Insomnia, or sleeplessness, is a disorder sometimes associated with anxiety. There are several major types of insomnia. **Short-term or behavioral insomnia** may be attributed to stress caused by a hectic lifestyle or the inability to resolve day-to-day conflicts within the home environment or the workplace. Worries about work, marriage, children, and health are common reasons for short-term loss of sleep. When stress interrupts normal sleeping patterns, patients cannot sleep because their minds are too active.

Foods or beverages containing stimulants such as caffeine may interrupt sleep. Patients may also find that the use of tobacco products makes them restless and edgy. Alcohol, although often enabling a person to fall asleep, may produce vivid dreams and frequent awakening that prevent restful sleep. Ingestion of a large meal, especially one high in protein and fat, consumed close to bedtime can interfere with sleep, due to the increased metabolic rate needed to digest the food. Certain medications cause CNS stimulation, and these should not be taken immediately before bedtime. Stressful conditions such as too much light, uncomfortable room temperature (especially one that is too warm), snoring, sleep apnea, and recurring nightmares also interfere with sleep. **Long-term insomnia** is often caused by depression, manic disorders, and chronic pain.

COMPLEMENTARY AND ALTERNATIVE THERAPIES

Valerian for Anxiety and Insomnia

Valerian (*Valeriana officinalis*) is a perennial plant grown in Europe, Asia, and North America. Valerian has several substances in its roots that affect the CNS; the exact active chemical has yet to be identified. Valerian has been used to treat nervousness, anxiety, and insomnia for thousands of years and is one of the most widely used herbal CNS depressants. The drug appears to have effects similar to benzodiazepines, such as diazepam (Valium) (Miyasaka, Atallah, & Soares, 2006). The major side effects of valerian are extensions of its therapeutic effects: drowsiness and decreased alertness. Valerian should not be combined with alcohol or other drugs that cause sedation or drowsiness. Note that some people experience a "paradoxical effect" with valerian; that is, they feel nervous or jittery. Although this is not a serious side effect, it should be reported to the health care provider.

PharmFacts

Insomnia

- One third of the world's population has trouble sleeping during part of the year.
- Insomnia is more common in women than in men.
- Patients older than 65 sleep less than any other age group.
- Only about 70% of people with insomnia ever report this problem to their health care providers.
- People buy OTC sleep medications and combination drugs with sleep additives more often than any other drug category. Examples of trade-name products are Anacin PM, Excedrin PM, Nytol, Quiet World, Sleep-Eez, Sominex, Tylenol PM, and Unisom.
- As a natural solution for sleep, some patients consider melatonin or herbal remedies such as valerian or kava (chapter 11 ∞).

Nonpharmacologic means should be attempted prior to initiating drug therapy for sleep disorders. Long-term use of sleep medications is likely to worsen insomnia and may cause physical or psychologic dependence. Some patients experience a phenomenon referred to as **rebound insomnia.** This condition occurs when a sedative drug is discontinued abruptly or after it has been taken for a long time; sleeplessness and symptoms of anxiety then become markedly worse.

Older patients are more likely to experience medication-related sleep problems. Drugs may seem to help the insomnia of an elderly patient for a night or two, only to produce generalized brain dysfunction as the medication accumulates in the system. The agitated patient may then be mistakenly overdosed with further medication. Nurses, especially those who work in geriatric settings, are responsible for making accurate observations and reporting patient responses to drugs so the health care provider can determine the lowest effective maintenance dose. When PRN medication is required for sleep, the nurse needs to conduct an individualized assessment of the individual, as well as follow-up evaluation and documentation of the medication's effect on the patient.

PharmFacts

Insomnia Linked to Insulin Resistance

- Chronic lack of sleep may make people more prone to developing type 2 diabetes, or non–insulin-dependent diabetes mellitus (NIDDM).
- Chronic lack of sleep can provide the impetus for the body to develop a reduced sensitivity to insulin.
- In one study, healthy adults who averaged little more than 5 hours of sleep per night over 8 consecutive nights secreted 50% more insulin than those who averaged 8 hours of sleep per night for the same period. Those who slept less were 40% less sensitive to insulin than those who got more sleep.
- Sleep deprivation (6.5 hours or less per night) may explain why type 2 diabetes is becoming more prevalent.

Complementary and Alternative Therapies

Kava

Kava (*Piper methysticum*) is a shrub native to the South Pacific islands. Kava has active substances in its roots that affect the CNS, and it is frequently used for the treatment of anxiety and insomnia. Recent studies have shown that kava may not be effective for insomnia, but this result may be dose dependent (Kennedy, Little, Haskell, & Scholey, 2006). High-quality research conducted on kava has proven its antianxiety effect (Ernst, 2006). This herb is available as a tincture (alcohol mixture) or tea, or in capsule form. Kava may increase the sedative effects of barbiturates and may interact with a broad range of drugs, including barbiturates, benzodiazepines, and antiparkinsonism agents.

14.5 Use of the Electroencephalogram to Diagnose Sleep and Seizure Disorders

The **electroencephalogram (EEG)** is a tool for diagnosing sleep disorders, seizure activity, depression, and dementia. Four types of brain waves—alpha, beta, delta, and theta—are identified by their shape, frequencies, and height on a graph. Brain waves give the health care provider an idea of how brain activity changes during various stages of sleep and consciousness. For example, alpha waves indicate an awake but drowsy patient. Beta waves indicate an alert patient whose mind is active.

Two distinct types of sleep can be identified with an EEG: nonrapid eye movement (NREM) sleep and rapid eye movement (REM) sleep. There are four progressive stages that advance into REM sleep. The stages of sleep are shown in Table 14.1. After NREM sleep has gone through the four stages, the sequence goes into reverse. Under normal circumstances, after returning from the depths of stage IV back to stage I of NREM, a person will still not awaken. Sleep quality begins to change; it is not as deep, and hormone levels and body temperature begin to rise. At that point, REM sleep occurs. **REM sleep** is often called paradoxical sleep, because the brain wave pattern of this stage is similar to that when persons are drowsy but awake. This is the stage during which dreaming occurs. People with normal sleep patterns move from NREM to REM sleep about every 90 minutes.

Patients who are deprived of stage IV NREM sleep experience depression and a feeling of apathy and fatigue. Stage IV NREM sleep appears to be linked to repair and restoration of the physical body, whereas REM sleep is associated with learning, memory, and the capacity to adjust to changes in the environment. The body requires the dream state associated with REM sleep to keep the psyche functioning normally. When test subjects are deprived of REM sleep, they experience a **sleep debt** and become frightened, irritable, paranoid, and even emotionally disturbed. Judgment is impaired, and reaction time is slowed. It is speculated that to make up for their lack of dreaming, these persons experience far more daydreaming and fantasizing throughout the day.

Pr Prototype Drug | Lorazepam *(Ativan)*

Therapeutic Class: Sedative–hypnotic; anxiolytic; anesthetic adjunct

Pharmacologic Class: Benzodiazepine; GABA$_A$-receptor agonist

ACTIONS AND USES

Lorazepam is a benzodiazepine that acts by potentiating the effects of GABA, an inhibitory neurotransmitter, in the thalamic, hypothalamic, and limbic levels of the CNS. It is one of the most potent benzodiazepines. It has an extended half-life of 10 to 20 hours, which allows for once- or twice-a-day oral dosing. In addition to being used as an anxiolytic, lorazepam is used as a preanesthetic medication to provide sedation, and for the management of status epilepticus.

ADMINISTRATION ALERTS

- When administering IV, monitor respirations every 5 to 15 minutes. Have airway and resuscitative equipment accessible.

- Pregnancy category D

PHARMACOKINETICS
Onset: 1–5 min IV; 15–30 min IM

Peak: 2 h PO; 90 min IM

Half-life: 10–20 h

Duration: Variable

ADVERSE EFFECTS

The most common adverse effects of lorazepam are drowsiness and sedation, which may decrease with time. When given in higher doses or by the IV route, more severe effects may be observed, such as amnesia, weakness, disorientation, ataxia, sleep disturbance, blood pressure changes, blurred vision, double vision, nausea, and vomiting.

Contraindications: This drug should not be used in patients with acute narrow-angle glaucoma, primary depressive disorders, or psychosis, and should be avoided for the management of severe uncontrolled pain.

INTERACTIONS

Drug–Drug: Lorazepam interacts with multiple drugs. For example, concurrent use of CNS depressants, including alcohol, potentiates sedative effects and increases the risk of respiratory depression and death. Lorazepam may contribute to digoxin toxicity by increasing the serum digoxin level. Symptoms include visual changes, nausea, vomiting, dizziness, and confusion.

Lorazepam may decrease the antiparkinsonism effects of levodopa and increase phenytoin levels.

Lab Tests: Unknown

Herbal/Food: Use cautiously with herbal supplements. For example, sedation-producing herbs such as kava, valerian, chamomile, or hops may have an additive effect with medication. Stimulant herbs such as gotu kola and ma huang may reduce the drug's effectiveness.

Treatment of Overdose: If overdose occurs, flumazenil (Romazicon), a specific benzodiazepine receptor antagonist, can be administered to reverse CNS depressant effects.

Refer to MyNursingKit for a Nursing Process Focus specific to this drug.

Other uses include treatment of alcohol withdrawal symptoms (chapter 12∞), central muscle relaxation (chapter 21∞), and as induction agents in general anesthesia (chapter 19∞).

Barbiturates

Barbiturates are drugs derived from barbituric acid. They are powerful CNS depressants prescribed for their sedative, hypnotic, and antiseizure effects that have been used in pharmacotherapy since the early 1900s.

14.9 Use of Barbiturates as Sedatives

Until the discovery of the benzodiazepines, barbiturates were the drugs of choice for treating anxiety and insomnia (see Table 14.5). Although barbiturates are still indicated for several conditions, they are rarely, if ever, prescribed for treating anxiety or insomnia because of significant adverse effects and the availability of more effective medications. The risk of psychologic and physical dependence is high— several are Schedule II drugs. The withdrawal syndrome from barbiturates is extremely severe and can be fatal. Overdose results in profound respiratory depression, hypoten-

LIFESPAN CONSIDERATIONS

Fall Risk in Older Adults and Benzodiazepines

For persons over the age of 65, falls are one of the leading causes of injury-related visits to emergency departments. While multiple risk factors such as visual impairment, urinary incontinence, and physical limitations all contribute to an increase in fall risk, drugs such as the benzodiazepine group have the potential for increasing this risk.

All patients prescribed a benzodiazepine drug should be cautioned about the possibility of oversedation, confusion, or impaired mobility, which may occur even at normal doses. This is especially true for the older patient who is prone to falls. The nurse should also evaluate the safety of the home environment, other risk factors contributing to insomnia (e.g., diuretic use), and explore nondrug options that may be useful in treating the patient's underlying insomnia or anxiety such as short daytime naps to decrease the "sleep debt" or going to bed at the same time each night. Whenever possible, the lowest dose of a benzodiazepine for the shortest amount of time should be used.

---

sion, and shock. Barbiturates have been used to commit suicide, and death due to overdose is not uncommon.

Barbiturates are capable of depressing CNS function at all levels. Like benzodiazepines, barbiturates act by binding to GABA receptor–chloride channel molecules, intensifying the effect of GABA throughout the brain. At low doses they

TABLE 14.5	**Barbiturates for Sedation and Insomnia**	
Drug	Route and Adult Dose (max dose where indicated)	Adverse Effects
SHORT ACTING		
pentobarbital sodium (Nembutal)	Sedative: PO; 20–30 mg bid or qid	Respiratory depression, laryngospasm, apnea
	Hypnotic: PO; 120–200 mg; IM, 150–200 mg	
secobarbital (Seconal)	Sedative: PO; 100–300 mg/day in three divided doses	
	Hypnotic: PO/IM; 100–200 mg	
INTERMEDIATE ACTING		
amobarbital (Amytal)	Sedative: PO; 30–50 mg bid or tid	*Residual sedation*
	Hypnotic: PO/IM; 65–200 mg (max: 500 mg)	Agranulocytosis, angioedema, Stevens–Johnson syndrome, respiratory depression, circulatory collapse, apnea, laryngospasm
aprobarbital (Alurate)	Sedative: PO; 40 mg tid	
	Hypnotic: PO; 40–160 mg	
butabarbital sodium (Butisol)	Sedative: PO; 15–30 mg tid or qid	
	Hypnotic: PO; 50–100 mg at bedtime	
LONG ACTING		
mephobarbital (Mebaral)	Sedative: PO; 32–100 mg tid or qid	*Drowsiness, somnolence*
phenobarbital (Luminal) (see page 172 for the Prototype Drug box ∞)	Sedative: PO; 30–120 mg/day; IV/IM, 100–200 mg/day	Agranulocytosis, respiratory depression, Stevens–Johnson syndrome, exfoliative dermatitis (rare), CNS depression, coma, death
Italics indicate common adverse effects; underlining indicates serious adverse effects.		

reduce anxiety and cause drowsiness. At moderate doses they inhibit seizure activity (chapter 15∞) and promote sleep, presumably by inhibiting brain impulses traveling through the limbic system and the reticular activating system. At higher doses, some barbiturates can induce anesthesia (chapter 19∞).

When taken for prolonged periods, barbiturates stimulate the microsomal enzymes in the liver that metabolize medications. Thus, barbiturates can stimulate their own metabolism, as well as that of hundreds of other drugs that use these enzymes for their breakdown. With repeated use, tolerance develops to the sedative effects of the drug; this includes cross-tolerance to other CNS depressants such as the opioids. Tolerance does not develop, however, to the respiratory depressant effects. (See chapter 15∞, page 177, for Nursing Process Focus: Patients Receiving Antiseizure Drug Therapy.)

Nonbenzodiazepine, Nonbarbiturate CNS Depressants

These drugs reduce anxiety symptoms but are chemically different from the other anxiolytic drug classes.

14.10 Other CNS Depressants for Anxiety and Sleep Disorders

The final group of CNS depressants used for anxiety and sleep disorders consists of miscellaneous agents that are chemically unrelated to either benzodiazepines or barbiturates (see Table 14.6). In addition to nonbenzodiazepine,

nonbarbiturate CNS depressants, other drugs used mainly for treatment of social anxiety symptoms include the antiseizure medication valproate (Depakote), and the beta blockers propranolol (Inderal) and atenolol (Tenormin). Drugs used mainly for insomnia therapy include the newest of all nonbenzodiazepine CNS depressants, zaleplon (Sonata), eszopiclone (Lunesta), and the relatively new drug zolpidem (Ambien). Older CNS depressants such as paraldehyde (Paracetaldehyde), chloral hydrate (Noctec), meprobamate (Equanil), and glutethimide (Doriglute) have only historical interest, because they are so rarely prescribed owing to their potential for serious adverse effects. Buspirone (BuSpar) and zolpidem (Ambien) are commonly prescribed for their anxiolytic effects. Zolpidem (Ambien) and eszopiclone (Lunesta) are used for their hypnotic effects.

The mechanism of action for buspirone (BuSpar) is unclear but appears to be related to D_2 dopamine receptors in the brain. The drug has agonist effects on presynaptic dopamine receptors and a high affinity for serotonin receptors. Buspirone is less likely than benzodiazepines to affect cognitive and motor performance and rarely interacts with other CNS depressants. Common adverse effects include dizziness, headache, and drowsiness. Dependence and withdrawal problems are less of a concern with buspirone. Therapy may take several weeks to achieve optimal results.

Zolpidem (Ambien) is a Schedule IV controlled substance limited to the short-term treatment of insomnia. It is highly specific to the GABA receptor (chapter 15∞) and produces muscle relaxation and anticonvulsant effects only at doses much higher than the hypnotic dose. As with other CNS depressants, it should be used cautiously in patients

Pr Prototype Drug | Zolpidem *(Ambien)*

Therapeutic Class: Sedative–hypnotic   **Pharmacologic Class:** Nonbenzodiazepine GABA$_A$ receptor agonist; nonbenzodiazepine, nonbarbiturate CNS depressant

ACTIONS AND USES
Although it is a nonbenzodiazepine, zolpidem acts in a similar fashion to facilitate GABA-mediated CNS depression in the limbic, thalamic, and hypothalamic regions. It preserves stages III and IV of sleep and has only minor effects on REM sleep. The only indication for zolpidem is for short-term insomnia management (7 to 10 days).

ADMINISTRATION ALERTS
- Because of rapid onset, 7–27 minutes, give immediately before bedtime.
- Pregnancy category B

PHARMACOKINETICS
Onset: 7–27 min
Peak: 0.5–2.3 h
Half-life: 1.7–2.5 h
Duration: 6–8 h

ADVERSE EFFECTS
Adverse effects include daytime sedation, confusion, amnesia, dizziness, depression, nausea, and vomiting.

Contraindications: Lactating women should not take this drug.

INTERACTIONS
Drug–Drug: Drug interactions with zolpidem include an increase in sedation when used concurrently with other CNS depressants, including alcohol. Phenothiazines augment CNS depression.

Lab Tests: Unknown

Herbal/Food: When taken with food, absorption is slowed significantly, and the onset of action may be delayed.

Treatment of Overdose: Generalized symptomatic and supportive measures should be applied with immediate gastric lavage where appropriate. IV fluids should be administered as needed. Use of flumazenil (Romazicon) as a benzodiazepine receptor antagonist may be helpful.

Refer to MyNursingKit for a Nursing Process Focus specific to this drug.

TABLE 14.6	Miscellaneous Drugs for Anxiety and Insomnia	
Drug	Route and Adult Dose (max dose where indicated)	Adverse Effects
NONBENZODIAZEPINE, NONBARBITURATE CNS DEPRESSANTS		
buspirone (BuSpar)	Sedative: PO; 7.5–15 mg in divided doses; may increase by 5 mg/day every 2–3 days if needed (max: 60 mg/day)	*Dizziness, headache, drowsiness, nausea, fatigue, ataxia, vomiting, bitter metallic taste, dry mouth, diarrhea, hypotension*
dexmedetomidine HCl (Precedex)	Sedative: IV; loading dose 1 mcg/kg over 10 min; maintenance dose 0.2–0.7 mcg/kg/hr	Angioedema, cardiac arrest, exfoliative dermatitis (rare); Stevens–Johnson syndrome, anaphylaxis, respiratory failure, coma, sudden death
eszopiclone (Lunesta)	Hypnotic: PO; 2 mg at bedtime; depending on the age, clinical response, and tolerance of the patient, dose may be lowered to 1 mg PO	
ethchlorvynol (Placidyl)	Sedative: PO; 200 mg bid or tid	
	Hypnotic: PO; 500 mg–1 g at bedtime	
remelteon (Rozerem)	Hypnotic: PO; 8 mg at bedtime	
zaleplon (Sonata)	Hypnotic: PO; 10 mg at bedtime (max: 20 mg/day)	
zolpidem (Ambien)	Hypnotic: PO; 5–10 mg at bedtime	
ANTISEIZURE MEDICATION		
valproic acid (Depakene) (see page 176 for the Prototype Drug box ∞)	Social anxiety symptoms: PO; 250 mg tid (max: 60 mg/kg/day)	*Sedation, drowsiness, nausea, vomiting, prolonged bleeding time*
		Deep coma with overdose, liver failure, pancreatitis, prolonged bleeding time, bone marrow suppression
BETA BLOCKERS		
atenolol (Tenormin) (see page 347 for the Prototype Drug box ∞)	Social anxiety symptoms: PO; 25–100 mg/day	*Bradycardia, hypotension, confusion, fatigue, drowsiness*
propranolol (Inderal) (see page 364 for the Prototype Drug box ∞)	Social anxiety symptoms: PO; 40 mg bid (max: 320 mg/day)	Anaphylactic reactions, Stevens–Johnson syndrome, toxic epidermal necrolysis, exfoliative dermatitis, agranulocytosis, laryngospasm, bronchospasm

Italics indicate common adverse effects; underlining indicates serious adverse effects.

with respiratory impairment, in older adults, and when used concurrently with other CNS depressants. Lower dosages may be necessary. Also, because of the rapid onset of this drug (7 to 27 minutes), it should be taken just prior to expected sleep. Because zolpidem is metabolized in the liver and excreted by the kidneys, impaired liver or kidney function can increase serum drug levels. Zolpidem is in pregnancy category B. Zolpidem is used with caution in individuals with a high risk of suicide, because there is a potential for intentional overdose. Adverse reactions are usually minimal (mild nausea, dizziness, diarrhea, daytime drowsiness), but rebound insomnia may occur when the drug is discontinued. Other adverse effects are amnesia and somnambulism (sleepwalking) or other activities that may be performed during sleep (e.g., sleepdriving).

Although structurally unrelated to other drugs used to treat insomnia, eszopiclone (Lunesta) has properties similar to those of zolpidem (Ambien). The effectiveness of eszopiclone has been shown in outpatient and sleep lab studies, but the drug has not directly been compared with zolpidem or other hypnotics. However, eszopiclone's longer elimination half-life, about twice as long as that of zolpidem, may give it an advantage in maintaining sleep and decreasing early-morning awakening. On the other hand, eszopiclone is more likely to cause daytime sedation.

Zaleplon (Sonata) may be useful for people who fall asleep but awake early in the morning, for example, 2:00 a.m. or 3:00 a.m. It is sometimes used for travel purposes and has been advertised by pharmaceutical companies for this purpose.

In 2005, remelteon (Rozerem) was approved by the FDA in a single 8-mg dose. Remelteon is a melatonin receptor agonist, which has been shown to mainly improve sleep induction. It has a relatively short onset of action (30 minutes), and its duration is comparable to the non–extended-release form of zolpidem. The FDA indications for remelteon or zolpidem are not limited to short-term use, because they do not appear to produce dependence or tolerance to the dose.

Drugs not listed in Table 14.6 include diphenhydramine (Benadryl) and hydroxyzine (Vistaril). These are antihistamines that produce drowsiness and may be beneficial in calming patients. They offer the advantage of not causing dependence, although their use is often limited by anticholinergic adverse effects. Diphenhydramine is a common component of OTC sleep aids, such as Nytol and Sominex (chapter 38∞). Doxylamine (Unisom) is another antihistamine medication commonly used as a night-time OTC sleep aid.

NURSING PROCESS FOCUS — PATIENTS RECEIVING DRUGS FOR ANXIETY DISORDERS

Assessment	Potential Nursing Diagnoses
Baseline assessment prior to administration: ■ Understand the reason the drug has been prescribed in order to assess for therapeutic effects. ■ Obtain a complete health history including hepatic, renal, respiratory, cardiovascular or neurologic disease, mental status, narrow-angle glaucoma, and pregnancy or breastfeeding. Obtain a drug history including allergies, current prescription and OTC drugs, herbal preparations, and caffeine and alcohol use. Be alert to possible drug interactions. ■ Assess stress and coping patterns (e.g., existing or perceived stress, duration, coping mechanisms or remedies) ■ Obtain a sleep history (e.g., quality and quantity of sleep, restlessness or frequent wakefulness, snoring or apnea, remedies used for sleep, concerns). ■ Evaluate appropriate laboratory findings (e.g., hepatic or renal function studies). ■ Obtain baseline vital signs and weight. Assess the patient's risk for falls. ■ Assess the patient's ability to receive and understand instruction. Include the family and caregivers as needed.	■ Anxiety ■ Disturbed Sleep Pattern ■ Fatigue ■ Ineffective Coping ■ Activity Intolerance (related to loss of sleep or daytime sleepiness) ■ Deficient Knowledge (drug therapy) ■ Risk for Injury, Risk for Falls (related to adverse effects of drug therapy)
Assessment throughout administration: ■ Assess for desired therapeutic effects (e.g., statements of improvement in anxiety, appetite, ability to carry out ADLs, and sleep patterns normalize). ■ Continue periodic monitoring of liver and renal function studies. ■ Assess vital signs and weight periodically or if symptoms warrant. ■ Assess for and promptly report adverse effects: excessive dizziness, drowsiness, light-headedness, confusion, agitation, palpitations, tachycardia, dizziness or light-headedness, and musculoskeletal weakness.	

(Continued)

NURSING PROCESS FOCUS   PATIENTS RECEIVING DRUGS FOR ANXIETY DISORDERS *(Continued)*

Planning: Patient Goals and Expected Outcomes

The patient will:

- Experience therapeutic effects dependent on the reason the drug is being given (e.g., decreased anxiety, improved sleep patterns).
- Be free from, or experience minimal, adverse effects.
- Verbalize an understanding of the drug's use, adverse effects, and required precautions.
- Demonstrate proper self-administration of the medication (e.g., dose, timing, when to notify provider).

Implementation

Interventions and (Rationales)	Patient and Family Education
Ensuring therapeutic effects:	
▪ Continue assessments as described earlier for therapeutic effects. (If the drug is given for anxiety, the patient reports decreased anxiety, improved sleep and eating habits, improved coping, and ability to carry out ADLs without anxiety. If the drug is given for sleep, the patient reports the ability to fall and remain asleep, and improved daytime wakefulness.)	▪ Assist the patient in developing healthy coping strategies and sleep habits with referral to appropriate health care providers as needed. ▪ Encourage the patient to keep a sleep diary of bedtime, the time involved trying to fall asleep, the quality and quantity of sleep, daytime sleepiness, etc.
Minimizing adverse effects:	
▪ Continue to monitor vital signs, mental status, and coordination and balance periodically. Be particularly cautious with older adults who are at increased risk for falls. (Drugs used for anxiety and sleep may cause excessive drowsiness and dizziness, increasing the risk of falls and injury.)	▪ Teach the patient to rise from lying or sitting to standing slowly to avoid dizziness or falls.
▪ Ensure patient safety, especially in older adults. Observe for light-headedness or dizziness. Monitor ambulation until the effects of drug are known. (Dizziness and drowsiness for a prolonged period of time may occur, dependent on the drug's half-life. Daytime drowsiness may impair walking or the ability to carry out usual ADLs.)	▪ Instruct the patient to call for assistance prior to getting out of bed or attempting to walk alone, and to avoid driving or other activities requiring mental alertness or physical coordination until the effects of the drug are known.
▪ Assess for changes in level of consciousness, disorientation or confusion, or agitation. (Neurologic changes may indicate overmedication or effects of sleep deprivation.)	▪ Instruct the patient or caregiver to immediately report increasing lethargy, disorientation, confusion, changes in behavior or mood, slurred speech, or ataxia.
▪ Assess for changes in visual acuity, blurred vision, loss of peripheral vision, seeing rainbow halos around lights, acute eye pain, or any of these symptoms accompanied by nausea and vomiting and report immediately. (Increased intraoptic pressure in patients with narrow-angle glaucoma may occur in patients taking benzodiazepines.)	▪ Instruct the patient to immediately report any visual changes or eye pain.
▪ Monitor affect and emotional status. (Drug may increase risk of mental depression, especially in patients with suicidal tendencies. Concurrent use of alcohol and other CNS depressants increase the effects and the risk.)	▪ Instruct the patient to report significant mood changes, especially depression, and to avoid alcohol and other CNS depressants while taking the drug.
▪ Encourage appropriate lifestyle changes: lowered caffeine intake including OTC medications that contain caffeine, increased exercise during the day but not immediately before bedtime, limited or no alcohol intake, and smoking cessation. (Healthy lifestyle changes will support and minimize the need for drug therapy. Caffeine and nicotine may decrease the effectiveness of the drug. Alcohol and other CNS depressants may increase the adverse effects of the drugs.)	▪ Encourage the patient to adopt a healthy lifestyle of decreased or abstinence from caffeine, nicotine, and alcohol; and increased exercise. ▪ Advise the patient to discuss all OTC medications with the health care provider to ensure caffeine or alcohol is not included in the formulation.
▪ Avoid abrupt discontinuation of therapy. (Withdrawal symptoms, including rebound anxiety and sleeplessness, are possible with abrupt discontinuation after long-term use.)	▪ Instruct the patient to take the drug exactly as prescribed and to not stop it abruptly.
▪ Assess home storage of medications and identify risks for corrective action. (Overdosage may occur if the patient takes additional doses when drowsy or disoriented from medication effects.)	▪ Instruct the patient that these drugs should not be kept at the bedside to avoid taking additional doses when drowsy.

NURSING PROCESS FOCUS   PATIENTS RECEIVING DRUGS FOR ANXIETY DISORDERS (Continued)

Implementation

Interventions and (Rationales)	Patient and Family Education
■ Assess prior methods of stress reduction or sleep hygiene. Reinforce previously used effective methods and teach new coping skills. (Drug therapy is used for the shortest amount of time possible. Developing other coping skills or improved sleep hygiene may lessen the need for drug therapy.)	■ Teach the patient nonpharmacologic methods for stress relief and for improved sleep hygiene. Refer to appropriate health care providers or support groups as needed.
Patient understanding of drug therapy: ■ Use opportunities during administration of medications and during assessments to discuss the rationale for drug therapy, desired therapeutic outcomes, most commonly observed adverse effects, parameters for when to call the health care provider, and any necessary monitoring or precautions. (Using time during nursing care helps to optimize and reinforce key teaching areas.)	■ The patient should be able to state the reason for the drug; appropriate dose and scheduling; what adverse effects to observe for and when to report; and the anticipated length of medication therapy.
Patient self-administration of drug therapy: ■ When administering the medication, instruct the patient, family, or caregiver in proper self-administration of drug, e.g., taking only amount prescribed. (Utilizing time during nurse-administration of these drugs helps to reinforce teaching.)	■ The patient is able to discuss appropriate dosing and administration needs.

Evaluation of Outcome Criteria

Evaluate the effectiveness of drug therapy by confirming that patient goals and expected outcomes have been met (see "Planning").

See Tables 14.2 and 14.4 for lists of drugs to which these nursing actions apply.

Chapter REVIEW

KEY CONCEPTS

The numbered key concepts provide a succinct summary of the important points from the corresponding numbered section within the chapter. If any of these points are not clear, refer to the numbered section within the chapter for review.

14.1 Generalized anxiety disorder is the most common type of anxiety; phobias, obsessive–compulsive disorder, panic attacks, and post-traumatic stress disorders are other important categories.

14.2 The limbic system and the reticular activating system are specific regions of the brain responsible for anxiety and wakefulness.

14.3 Anxiety can be managed through pharmacologic and nonpharmacologic strategies.

14.4 Insomnia is a sleep disorder that may be caused by anxiety. Nonpharmacologic means should be attempted prior to initiating pharmacotherapy.

14.5 The electroencephalogram records brain waves and is used to diagnose sleep and seizure disorders.

14.6 CNS agents, including anxiolytics, sedatives, and hypnotics, are used to treat anxiety and insomnia.

14.7 When taken properly, antidepressants can reduce symptoms of panic and anxiety. First-line medications include the selective serotonin reuptake inhibitors (SSRIs) and other antidepressants; tricyclic antidepressants (TCAs) and monoamine oxidase inhibitors (MAOIs) are older drug groups.

14.8 Benzodiazepines are drugs of choice for the management of anxiety disorders and insomnia.

14.9 Because of their adverse effects and high potential for dependency, barbiturates are rarely used to treat insomnia.

14.10 Some commonly prescribed agents and CNS depressants not related to the benzodiazepines or barbiturates are used for the treatment of anxiety and sleeplessness.

NCLEX-RN® REVIEW QUESTIONS

1 The nurse should assess a patient who is taking lorazepam (Ativan) for the development of which of these adverse effects?
1. Tachypnea
2. Astigmatism
3. Ataxia
4. Euphoria

2 A patient is receiving temazepam (Restoril). Which of these responses should a nurse expect the patient to have if the medication is achieving the desired affect?
1. The patient sleeps in 3-hour intervals, awakes for a short time, and then falls back to sleep.
2. The patient reports feeling less anxiety during activities of daily living.
3. The patient reports having fewer episodes of panic attacks when stressed.
4. The patient reports sleeping 7 hours without awakening.

3 A 32-year-old female patient has been taking lorazepam (Ativan) for her anxiety and is brought into the emergency department after taking 30 days' worth at one time. The antagonist used in some cases of benzodiazepine overdosage is:
1. epinephrine.
2. atropine.
3. flumazenil.
4. naloxone.

4 A patient has been given instructions about the newly prescribed medication alprazolam (Xanax). Which of these statements, if made by the patient, would indicate that the patient needs further instruction?

1. "I will stop smoking by undergoing hypnosis."
2. "I will not drive immediately after I take this medication."
3. "I will stop the medication when I feel less anxious."
4. "I will take my medication with food if my stomach feels upset."

5 A patient has been taking diazepam (Valium) for 3 months. Which of these statements by the patient would indicate that the outcome of medication therapy has been successful?
1. "I will need to take this medication for the rest of my life."
2. "I feel like I am able to cope with routine stress at my job."
3. "I like this medication. I know that I needed it to treat my anxiety, which is now better, but I think it just makes me feel good, so I am planning to stay on it for quite a while."
4. "I thought this medication would make me think clearly, but I don't feel any change in my feelings."

6 Education given to patients about the use of benzodiazepines should include an emphasis on what important issue?
1. They will be required lifelong to achieve lasting effects.
2. They require frequent blood counts to avoid adverse effects.
3. If the drug is not effective within the first 2 months, it will be stopped immediately.
4. The use of counseling or behavioral techniques in addition to the drug will assist in addressing the underlying disorder.

CRITICAL THINKING QUESTIONS

1. A 58-year-old male patient underwent an emergency coronary artery bypass graft. He suffered complications while in the cardiac intensive care unit and spent 3 days on a ventilator. He is still experiencing a high degree of pain and also states that he cannot fall asleep. The patient has been ordered secobarbital (Seconal) at night for sleep and also has a prescribed opioid analgesic. As the nurse, explain to the student nurse why both medications should be administered.

2. A 42-year-old female patient with ovarian cancer suffered profound nausea and vomiting after her first round of chemotherapy. The oncologist has added lorazepam (Ativan) 2 mg per IV piggyback with ondansetron (Zofran) as part of the prechemotherapy regimen. Consult a drug handbook and discuss the purpose for adding this benzodiazepine.

3. An 82-year-old female patient complains that she "just can't get good rest anymore." She says that she has come to her doctor to get something to help her sleep. What information can the nurse offer this patient regarding the normal changes in sleep patterns associated with aging? What would you recommend for this patient?

See Appendix D for answers and rationales for all activities.

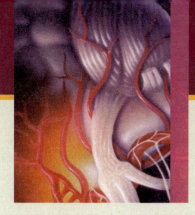

Drugs for Seizures

DRUGS AT A GLANCE

LEARNING OUTCOMES

After reading this chapter, the student should be able to:

1. Compare and contrast the terms *seizures*, *convulsions*, and *epilepsy*.
2. Recognize possible causes of seizures.
3. Relate signs and symptoms to specific types of seizures.
4. Describe the nurse's role in the pharmacologic management of seizures of an acute nature and epilepsy.
5. Explain the importance of patient drug compliance in the pharmacotherapy of epilepsy and seizures.
6. For each of the drug classes listed in Drugs at a Glance, know representative drug examples and explain their mechanism of drug action, primary actions, and important adverse effects.
7. Categorize drugs used in the treatment of seizures based on their classification and mechanism of action.
8. Use the nursing process to care for patients receiving drug therapy for epilepsy and seizures.

KEY TERMS

As the most common neurologic disease, epilepsy affects more than 2 million Americans. By definition, epilepsy is any disorder characterized by recurrent seizures. Symptoms of epilepsy depend on the type of seizure and may include blackout, fainting spells, sensory disturbances, jerking body movements, and temporary loss of memory. This chapter examines the pharmacotherapy used to treat epilepsy and different kinds of seizures.

SEIZURES

A **seizure** or clinically detectable sign of **epilepsy** is a disturbance of electrical activity in the brain that may affect consciousness, motor activity, and sensation. Seizures are caused by abnormal or uncontrolled neuronal discharges. Uncontrolled charges may remain in one focus or propagate to other areas of the brain. As a valuable tool in measuring uncontrolled neuronal activity, the electroencephalogram (EEG) is useful in diagnosing seizure disorders. ➤ Figure 15.1 compares normal and abnormal neuronal tracings.

The terms *seizure* and *convulsion* are not synonymous. **Convulsions** specifically refer to involuntary, violent spasms of the large skeletal muscles of the face, neck, arms, and legs. Although some types of seizures involve convulsions, other seizures do not. Thus, it may be stated that all convulsions are seizures, but not all seizures are convulsions. Because of this difference, drugs described in this chapter will generally be referred to as *antiseizure drugs* rather than *anticonvulsants*. Recognizing also that antiseizure drugs are commonly called *antiepileptic drugs* (AEDs), the term *antiseizure* in this chapter applies to the treatment of all seizure-related symptoms including signs of epilepsy.

15.1 Causes of Seizures

A seizure is really considered symptomatic of an underlying disorder, rather than the disease itself. Triggers include exposure to strobe or flickering lights or the occurrence of small fluid and electrolyte imbalances. Patients appear to have a lower tolerance to environmental triggers, and seizures may occur when patients are sleep deprived.

There are many different etiologies of seizure activity. In some cases, the etiology of seizure may be clear but not in all situations. Seizures represent the most common serious neurologic problem affecting children, with an overall incidence approaching 2% for febrile seizures and 1% for idiopathic epilepsy. Certain medications for mood disorders, psychoses, and local anesthesia when given in high doses may cause seizures, possibly because of increased levels of stimulatory neurotransmitters or toxicity. Seizures may also occur from drug abuse, as with cocaine, or during withdrawal from alcohol or sedative–hypnotic drugs.

Seizures may present as an acute situation, or they may occur on a chronic basis. Seizures that result from an acute complication generally do not recur after the situation has been resolved. On the other hand, if a brain abnormality exists following an acute complication, recurrent seizures are likely. The following are known causes of seizures:

- *Infectious diseases:* Acute infections such as meningitis and encephalitis can cause inflammation in the brain.
- *Trauma:* Physical trauma such as direct blows to the skull may increase intracranial pressure; chemical trauma such as the presence of toxic substances or the ingestion of poisons may cause brain injury.
- *Metabolic disorders:* Changes in fluid and electrolytes such as hypoglycemia, hyponatremia, and water intoxication may cause seizures by altering electrical impulse transmission at the cellular level.
- *Vascular diseases:* Changes in oxygenation such as those caused by respiratory hypoxia and carbon monoxide poisoning, and changes in perfusion such as those caused by hypotension, cerebral vascular accidents, shock, and cardiac dysrhythmias may be causes.
- *Pediatric disorders:* Rapid increase in body temperature may result in a **febrile seizure.**
- *Neoplastic disease:* Tumors, especially rapidly growing ones, may occupy space, increase intracranial pressure, and damage brain tissue by disrupting blood flow.

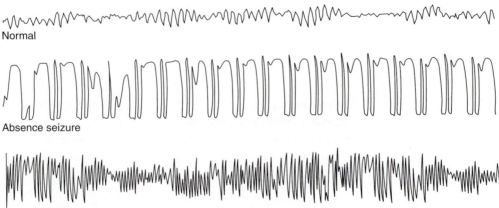

Normal

Absence seizure

Generalized tonic–clonic seizure

➤ **Figure 15.1** EEG recordings showing the differences between normal, absence seizure, and generalized tonic–clonic seizure tracings

An important topic when discussing epilepsy and seizure treatment is pregnancy. Because several antiseizure drugs decrease the effectiveness of oral contraceptives, additional barrier methods of birth control should be practiced to avoid unintended pregnancy. Prior to pregnancy and considering the serious nature of seizures, patients should consult with their health care provider to determine the most appropriate plan of action for seizure control. When patients become pregnant, extreme caution is necessary. Most antiseizure drugs are pregnancy category D. Some antiseizure drugs may cause folate deficiency, a condition correlated with fetal neural tube defects. Vitamin supplements may be necessary. **Eclampsia** is a severe hypertensive disorder of pregnancy, characterized by seizures, coma, and perinatal mortality. Eclampsia is likely to occur from around the 20th week of gestation until at least 1 week after delivery of the baby. Roughly one fourth of patients with eclampsia experience seizures within 72 hours postpartum.

Seizures can have a significant impact on the quality of life. They may cause serious injury if they occur while a person is driving a vehicle or performing a dangerous activity. Almost all states will not grant, or will take away, a driver's license and require a seizure-free period before granting the license. Without successful pharmacotherapy, epilepsy can severely limit participation in school, employment, and social activities and can affect self-esteem. Chronic depression may accompany poorly controlled seizures. Important considerations in nursing care include identifying patients at risk for seizures, documenting the pattern and type of seizure activity, and implementing safety precautions. In collaboration with the patient, the health care provider, pharmacist, and nurse are instrumental in achieving positive therapeutic outcomes. Through a combination of pharmacotherapy, patient–family support, and education, effective seizure control can be achieved in a majority of patients.

15.2 Types of Seizures

The differing presentation of seizures relates to their signs and symptoms. Symptoms may range from sudden, violent shaking and total loss of consciousness to muscle twitching or slight tremor of a limb. Staring into space, altered vision, and difficulty speaking are other behaviors a person may exhibit during a seizure. Determining the cause of recurrent seizures is important for planning appropriate drug selection and treatment options. Proper diagnosis therefore, is essential.

Methods of classifying epilepsy have changed over time. For example, the terms *grand mal* and *petit mal* epilepsy have, for the most part, been replaced by more descriptive and detailed categorization. Epilepsies are typically identified using the International Classification of Epileptic Seizures nomenclature, as partial (focal), generalized, and special epileptic syndromes (see Table 15.1). Types of **partial (focal)** or **generalized seizures** may be recognized based on symptoms observed during a seizure episode. Some symptoms are subtle and reflect the specific nature of neuronal misfiring; others are more complex.

15.3 General Concepts of Antiseizure Pharmacotherapy

The choice of drug for antiseizure pharmacotherapy depends on signs presented by the patient, the patient's previous medical history, and associated pathologies. Once a medication is selected, the patient is placed on a low initial dose. The amount is gradually increased until seizure control is achieved, or until drug side effects prevent additional increases in dose. Serum drug levels may be obtained to assist the health care provider in determining the most effective drug concentration. If seizure activity continues, a different medication is added in small-dose increments while the dose of the first drug is slowly reduced. Because seizures are likely to occur if antiseizure drugs are abruptly withdrawn, the medication is usually discontinued over a period of 6 to 12 weeks.

Traditional and newer antiseizure drugs with indications are shown in Table 15.2. The newer antiseizure drugs offer advantages over the older traditional drugs, mainly because of troublesome side effects. Due to the limited induction of drug-metabolizing enzymes, the pharmacokinetic profiles of the newer antiseizure drugs are less complicated. In addition, the newer antiseizure drugs are generally better tolerated and pose less of a health risk in pregnancy.

One issue of antiseizure drug therapy relates to recent warnings issued by the Food and Drug Administration. In 2008, the FDA analyzed reports from clinical studies involving patients taking a variety of antiseizure medications, mostly newer nontraditional drugs. Patients with epilepsy, bipolar disorder, psychoses, migraines, and neuropathic pain were among the disorders included in the study. Compared to placebo trials, 11 popular antiseizure examples were found to almost double the risk of suicidal behavior and ideation among patients. In a warning issued by the FDA, health care professionals were admonished to carefully *balance clinical need for antiseizure drugs with risk for suicide*. Patients and caregivers were encouraged to pay close attention to changes in mood and *not to make changes in antiseizure regimen* without consulting

LIFESPAN CONSIDERATIONS

Seizure Etiologies Based on Genetics and Age-Related Factors
- The etiologies that trigger the development of childhood epilepsy vary according to age.
- Congenital abnormalities of the CNS, perinatal brain injury, and metabolic imbalances are usually related to seizure activity in neonates, infants, and toddlers.
- Inherited epilepsies, CNS infections, and neurologic degenerative disorders are linked to seizures that have their onset in later childhood.
- Cerebral trauma, cerebrovascular disorders, and neoplastic disease represent the most frequent causes of seizures in the adult population.

TABLE 15.1	Classification of Seizures and Symptoms	
Classification	Type	Symptoms
Partial	Simple partial Complex partial (psychomotor)	■ Olfactory, auditory, and visual hallucinations ■ Intense emotions ■ Twitching of arms, legs, and face ■ Aura (preceding) ■ Brief period of confusion or sleepiness afterward with no memory of seizure (*postictal confusion*) ■ Fumbling with or attempting to remove clothing ■ No response to verbal commands
General	Absence (petit mal) **Atonic** (drop attacks) **Tonic–clonic** (grand mal)	■ Lasting a few seconds ■ Seen most often in children (child stares into space, does not respond to verbal stimulation, may have fluttering eyelids or jerking) ■ Misdiagnosed often (especially in child) as ADD or daydreaming ■ Falling or stumbling for no reason ■ Lasting a few seconds ■ Aura (preceding) ■ Intense muscle contraction (tonic phase) followed by alternating contraction and relaxation of muscles (clonic phase) ■ Crying at beginning as air leaves lungs; loss of bowel/bladder control; shallow breathing with periods of apnea; usually lasting 1–2 minutes ■ Disorientation and deep sleep after seizure (*postictal state*)
Special syndromes	Febrile seizure Myoclonic seizure Status epilepticus	■ Tonic–clonic activity lasting 1–2 minutes ■ Rapid return to consciousness ■ Occurs in children usually between 3 months and 5 years of age ■ Large jerking movements of a major muscle group, such as an arm ■ Falling from a sitting position or dropping what is held ■ Considered a medical emergency ■ Continuous seizure activity, which can lead to coma and death

with their health care provider. The sum of this review indicated that although the older antiseizure drugs have serious clinical drawbacks, so do the newer antiseizure drugs.

Many of the newer antiseizure medications are used in adjunctive therapy. Some drugs are being evaluated for their potential use in monotherapy. In most cases, effective seizure management can be obtained using only a single drug. For some patients, two antiseizure medications may be needed, although unwanted side effects may appear. Some antiseizure drug combinations may actually increase the incidence of seizures. The nurse should consult with current drug guides regarding drug use in monotherapy and compatibility before a second antiseizure drug is added to the regimen.

How Antiseizure Pharmacotherapy Works

The goal of antiseizure pharmacotherapy is to suppress neuronal activity just enough to prevent abnormal or repetitive

PharmFacts

Epilepsy
- The word *epilepsy* is derived from the Greek word *epilepsia*, meaning "to take hold of or to seize."
- About 2 million Americans have epilepsy.
- One of every 100 teenagers has epilepsy.
- Of the U.S. population, 10% will have seizures within their lifetime.
- Most people with seizures are younger than 45 years of age.
- Contrary to popular belief, it is impossible to swallow the tongue during a seizure, and one should never force an object into the mouth of someone who is having a seizure.
- Epilepsy is not a mental illness; children with epilepsy have IQ scores equivalent to those of children without the disorder.
- Famous people who had epilepsy include Julius Caesar, Alexander the Great, Napoleon, Vincent van Gogh, Charles Dickens, Joan of Arc, Socrates, Agatha Christie, Truman Capote, and Richard Burton.
- Among adult alcoholics receiving treatment for withdrawal, over half will experience seizures within 6 hours upon arriving for treatment.

TABLE 15.2	Traditional and Newer Antiseizure Drugs with Indications*				
	PARTIAL SEIZURES	GENERALIZED SEIZURES		SPECIAL	
		Absence	Tonic–Clonic	Myoclonic	
DRUGS THAT POTENTIATE GABA					
diazepam (Valium)		✓	✓	✓	
gabapentin (Neurontin)	✓				
lorazepam (Ativan)			✓		
phenobarbital (Luminal)	✓		✓		
pregabalin (Lyrica)	✓				
primidone (Mysoline)	✓		✓		
tiagabine (Gabitril)	✓				
topiramate (Topamax)	✓		✓	✓	
HYDANTOIN AND NEWER DRUGS					
carbamazepine (Tegretol)	✓		✓		
lamotrigine (Lamictal)	✓	✓	✓	✓	
levetiracetam (Keppra)	✓				
oxcarbazepine (Trileptal)	✓		✓		
phenytoin (Dilantin)	✓		✓		
valproic acid (Depakene)	✓	✓	✓	✓	
zonisamide (Zonegran)	✓	✓	✓	✓	
SUCCINIMIDES					
ethosuximide (Zarontin)		✓			

*Antiseizure drugs approved for use in adjunctive therapy or monotherapy. Check marks include potential uses as well as approved indications.

firing. To this end, there are three general mechanisms by which antiseizure drugs act:

- Stimulating an influx of chloride ions, an effect associated with the neurotransmitter gamma-aminobutyric acid (GABA)
- Delaying an influx of sodium
- Delaying an influx of calcium

Antiseizure pharmacotherapy is directed at controlling the movement of electrolytes across neuronal membranes or affecting neurotransmitter balance. In a resting state, neurons are normally surrounded by a higher concentration of sodium, calcium, and chloride ions. Potassium levels are higher inside the cell. An influx of sodium or calcium into the neuron *enhances* neuronal activity, whereas an influx of chloride ions or an efflux of potassium ions *suppresses* neuronal activity.

Some drugs act by more than one mechanism. This has prompted drug researchers to try to understand more clearly various drug mechanisms and to develop newer better controlled drugs. Recently, a fourth mechanism has been proposed and studied, antagonism of the primary excitatory neurotransmitter glutamate. Glutamate works in concert with the cell's Na^+-K^+ ATPase pump, which helps to restore ion balances across neuronal membranes after fir-

COMPLEMENTARY AND ALTERNATIVE THERAPIES

The Ketogenic Diet for Epilepsy
The ketogenic diet is used when seizures cannot be controlled through pharmacotherapy or when there are unacceptable adverse effects to the medications. Before antiepileptic drugs were developed, this diet was a primary treatment for epilepsy.

The ketogenic diet is a stringently calculated diet that is high in fat and low in carbohydrates and protein. It limits water intake to avoid ketone dilution and carefully controls caloric intake. Each meal has the same ketogenic ratio of 4 g of fat to 1 g of protein and carbohydrate. Extra fat is usually given in the form of cream.

Research suggests that the diet produces a high success rate for certain patients (Cross, 2009). About one third of the children using it become substantially seizure free while one third have their seizures reduced by 50% (Levy & Cooper, 2003). The diet appears to be equally effective for every seizure type. The most frequently reported adverse effects include vomiting, fatigue, constipation, diarrhea, and hunger. Kidney stones, acidosis, and slower growth rates are possible risks. Those interested in trying the diet must consult with their health care provider; this is not a do-it-yourself diet and may be harmful if not carefully monitored by skilled professionals.

ing. Any drug that blocks glutamate activity prevents an influx of positive ions into the cell, so this is consistent with the last two mechanisms.

PHARMACOTHERAPY ILLUSTRATED

15.1 Model of the GABA Receptor–Chloride Channel Molecules in Relationship to Antiseizure Pharmacotherapy

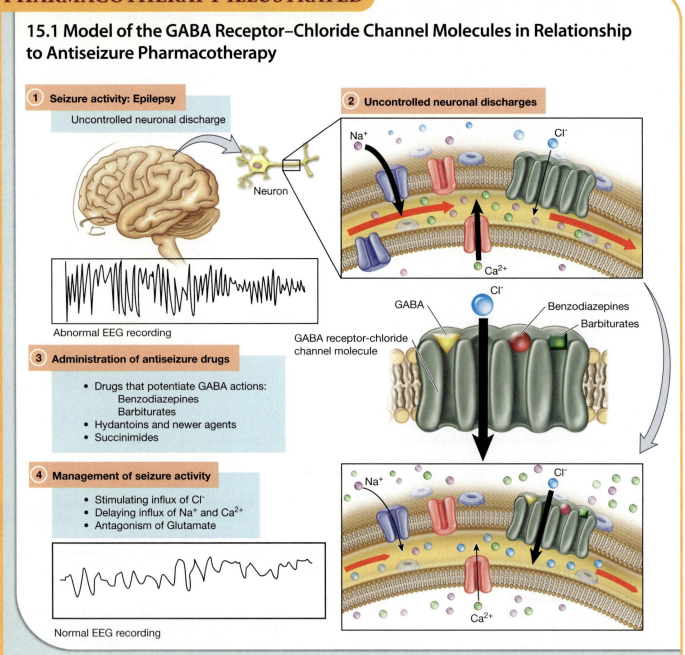

1 Seizure activity: Epilepsy

Uncontrolled neuronal discharge

Neuron

Abnormal EEG recording

2 Uncontrolled neuronal discharges

Na⁺   Cl⁻

Ca²⁺

GABA   Cl⁻   Benzodiazepines   Barbiturates

GABA receptor-chloride channel molecule

3 Administration of antiseizure drugs

- Drugs that potentiate GABA actions:
    Benzodiazepines
    Barbiturates
- Hydantoins and newer agents
- Succinimides

4 Management of seizure activity

- Stimulating influx of Cl⁻
- Delaying influx of Na⁺ and Ca²⁺
- Antagonism of Glutamate

Na⁺   Cl⁻

Ca²⁺

Normal EEG recording

DRUGS THAT POTENTIATE GABA ACTION

Several important antiseizure drugs act by changing the action of **gamma-aminobutyric acid (GABA)**, the primary inhibitory neurotransmitter in the brain. These drugs mimic the effects of GABA by stimulating an influx of chloride ions that interact with the GABA receptor–chloride channel molecule. A model of this receptor is shown in Pharmacotherapy Illustrated 15.1. When the receptor is stimulated, chloride ions move into the cell, and suppress the firing of neurons.

A number of drugs have GABA-related potentiation. Drugs may bind directly to the GABA receptor through specific binding sites. Well-characterized sites have been designated as GABA_A and GABA_B. Drugs may enhance GABA release, or drugs may block the reuptake of GABA into nerve cells and glia. Newer drugs are agents that inhibit GABA degrading enzymes. Barbiturates, benzodiazepines, and several newer drugs reduce seizure activity by intensifying GABA action. The predominate effect of GABA potentiation is CNS depression. These drugs are listed in Table 15.3.

TABLE 15.3	**Antiseizure Drugs That Potentiate GABA Action**	
Drug	Route and Adult Dose (max dose where indicated)	Adverse Effects
BARBITURATES		
amobarbital (Amytal)	IV; 65–500 mg (max: 1 g)	*Somnolence*
mephobarbital (Mebaral)	PO; 400–600 mg/day	Agranulocytosis, Stevens–Johnson syndrome, angioedema, laryngospasm, respiratory depression, CNS depression, coma, death
⊕ phenobarbital (Luminal)	For partial and generalized seizures: PO, 100–300 mg/day; IV/IM, 200–600 mg up to 20 mg/kg	
	For status epilepticus: IV; 15–18 mg/kg in single or divided doses (max: 20 mg/kg)	
primidone (Mysoline)	PO; 250 mg/day, increased by 250 mg/wk up to max of 2 g in two to four divided doses	
BENZODIAZEPINES		
clonazepam (Klonopin)	PO; 1.5 mg/day in three divided doses, increased by 0.5–1.0 mg every 3 days until seizures are controlled	*Drowsiness, sedation, ataxia*
clorazepate (Tranxene)	PO; 7.5 mg tid	Laryngospasm, respiratory depression, cardiovascular collapse, coma
⊕ diazepam (Valium)	IM/IV; 5–10 mg (repeat as needed at 10–15 min intervals up to 30 mg; repeat again as needed every 2–4 h)	
	IV push; administer emulsion at 5 mg/min	
lorazepam (Ativan) (see page 158 for the Prototype Drug box∞)	IV; 4 mg injected slowly at 2 mg/min; if inadequate response after 10 min, may repeat once	
NEWER GABA-RELATED DRUGS		
gabapentin (Neurontin)	For additional therapy: PO, start with 300 mg on day 1; 300 mg bid on day 2; 300 mg tid on day 3; continue to increase over 1 wk to a dose of 1,200 mg/day (400 mg tid); may increase to 1,800–2,400 mg/day	*Drowsiness, dizziness, fatigue, sedation, somnolence, vertigo, ataxia, confusion, asthenia, headache, tremor, nervousness, memory difficulty, difficulty concentrating, psychomotor slowing, nystagmus, paresthesia, nausea, vomiting, anorexia*
pregabalin (Lyrica)	PO; start with 150 mg/day; may be increased up to 300 mg/day within one week (max: 600 mg/day)	Serious disfiguring and debilitating rashes; sudden unexplained death in epilepsy (SUDEP); withdrawal seizures on discontinuation of drug
tiagabine (Gabitril)	PO; start with 4 mg/day; may increase by 4–8 mg/day every week up to 56 mg/day in two to four divided doses	
topiramate (Topamax)	PO; start with 50 mg/day, increased by 50 mg/wk to effectiveness (max: 1,600 mg/day)	
Italics indicate common adverse effects; underlining indicates serious adverse effects.		

Barbiturates

Barbiturates are organic compounds derived from barbituric acid. All derivatives intensify the effect of GABA in the brain and generally depress the firing of CNS neurons.

15.4 Treating Seizures with Barbiturates

The antiseizure properties of phenobarbital were discovered in 1912, and this drug is still commonly prescribed for seizures. As a class, barbiturates generally have a low margin for safety, a high potential for dependence, and they cause profound CNS depression. Phenobarbital, however, is able to suppress abnormal neuronal discharges without causing sedation. It is inexpensive, long acting, and produces a low

incidence of adverse effects. When the drug is given orally, several weeks may be necessary to achieve optimum effects. Phenobarbital is a drug of choice in the pharmacotherapy of neonatal seizures.

Overall barbiturates are effective against all major seizure types except absence seizures. Other than phenobarbital, mephobarbital is occasionally used for epilepsy treatment. Mephobarbital (Mebaral) is converted to phenobarbital in the liver, and offers no significant advantages over phenobarbital. Primidone (Mysoline) has a pharmacologic profile similar to phenobarbital and is among the drugs used effectively to potentiate GABA action.

Amobarbital (Amytal) is an intermediate-acting barbiturate given IM or IV to terminate **status epilepticus.** Unlike phenobarbital, which is a Schedule IV drug, amobarbital is a Schedule II drug and has a higher risk for dependence. As an antiseizure medication, amobarbital is not given orally.

Pr Prototype Drug | Phenobarbital *(Luminal)*

Therapeutic Class: Antiseizure drug; sedative   **Pharmacologic Class:** Barbiturate; GABA$_A$ receptor agonist

ACTIONS AND USES

Phenobarbital is a long-acting barbiturate used for the management of a variety of seizures. It is also used to promote sleep. Phenobarbital should not be used for pain relief, as it may increase a patient's sensitivity to pain.

Phenobarbital acts biochemically by enhancing the action of the GABA neurotransmitter, which is responsible for suppressing abnormal neuronal discharges that can cause epilepsy.

ADMINISTRATION ALERTS

- Parenteral phenobarbital is a soft-tissue irritant. IM injections may produce a local inflammatory reaction. IV administration is rarely used, because extravasation may produce tissue necrosis.
- Controlled substance: Schedule IV
- Pregnancy category D

PHARMACOKINETICS

Onset: 20–60 min PO; 5 min IV

Peak: 8–12 h PO; 30 min IV

Half-life: 2–6 days

Duration: 6–10 h PO; 4–10 h IV

ADVERSE EFFECTS

Phenobarbital is a Schedule IV drug that may cause dependence. Common side effects include drowsiness, vitamin deficiencies (vitamin D; folate, or B$_9$; and B$_{12}$), and laryngospasms. With overdose, phenobarbital may cause severe respiratory depression, CNS depression, coma, and death.

Contraindications: Administration of phenobarbital is inadvisable in cases of hypersensitivity to barbiturates, severe uncontrolled pain, pre-exisiting CNS depression, porphyrias, severe respiratory disease with dyspnea or obstruction, and glaucoma or prostatic hypertrophy.

INTERACTIONS

Drug–Drug: Phenobarbital interacts with many other drugs. For example, it should not be taken with alcohol or other CNS depressants. These substances potentiate barbiturate action, increasing the risk of life-threatening respiratory depression or cardiac arrest. Phenobarbital increases the metabolism of many other drugs, reducing their effectiveness.

Lab Tests: Barbiturates may affect bromsulphalein tests and increase serum phosphatase.

Herbal/Food: Kava and valerian may potentiate sedation.

Treatment of Overdose: There is no specific treatment for overdose. Drug removal may be accomplished by gastric lavage or use of activated charcoal. Hemodialysis may be effective in facilitating removal of phenobarbital from the body. Treatment is supportive and consists mainly of endotracheal intubation and mechanical ventilation. Treatment of bradycardia and hypotension may be necessary.

Refer to MyNursingKit for a Nursing Process Focus specific to this drug.

Benzodiazepines

Like barbiturates, benzodiazepines intensify the effect of GABA in the brain. The benzodiazepines bind directly to the GABA receptor, suppressing abnormal neuronal foci.

15.5 Treating Seizures with Benzodiazepines

Benzodiazepines used in treating epilepsy include clonazepam (Klonopin), clorazepate (Tranxene), lorazepam (Ativan), and diazepam (Valium). Indications include **absence seizures** and **myoclonic seizures**. Parenteral diazepam is used to terminate status epilepticus. Because tolerance may begin to develop after only a few months of therapy with benzodiazepines, seizures may recur unless the dose is periodically adjusted. These drugs are generally not used alone in seizure pharmacotherapy, but instead serve as adjuncts to other antiseizure drugs for short-term seizure control.

The benzodiazepines are one of the most widely prescribed classes of drugs, used not only to control seizures but also for anxiety, skeletal muscle spasms, and alcohol withdrawal symptoms.

DRUGS THAT SUPPRESS SODIUM INFLUX

Several drugs dampen CNS activity by delaying an influx of sodium ions across neuronal membranes. Hydantoins and related antiseizure drugs act by this mechanism.

Hydantoin and Newer Drugs

Sodium channels guide the movement of sodium ions across neuronal membranes into the intracellular space. Sodium ion movement is the major factor that determines whether a neuron will undergo an action potential. If these channels are temporarily inactivated, neuronal activity will be suppressed. With hydantoin and phenytoin-like drugs, sodium channels are not blocked; they are just desensitized. If channels are blocked, neuronal activity completely stops, as occurs with local anesthetic drugs. Several drugs in this group may not desensitize sodium channels directly, but they may affect the threshold of neuronal firing, or they may interfere with transduction of the excitatory neurotransmitter glutamate. These actions are slightly removed from the actual suppression of sodium influx; however, the result (delayed depolarization of the neuron) is the same. These drugs are listed in Table 15.4.

TABLE 15.4	Hydantoins and Related Drugs	
Drug	**Route and Adult Dose (max dose where indicated)**	**Adverse Effects**
HYDANTOINS		
fosphenytoin (Cerebyx)	IV; initial dose 15–20 mg PE*/kg at 100–150 mg PE/min followed by 4–6 mg PE/kg/day	*Somnolence, drowsiness, dizziness, nystagmus, gingival hyperplasia*
ⓟ enytoin (Dilantin)	PO; 15–18 mg/kg or 1-g initial dose; then 300 mg/day in 1–3 divided doses; may be gradually increased 100 mg/week	<u>Agranulocytosis, aplastic anemias; bullous, exfoliative, or purpuric dermatitis; Stevens–Johnson syndrome; toxic epidermal necrolysis; cardiovascular collapse; cardiac arrest</u>
PHENYTOIN-LIKE DRUGS		
carbamazepine (Tegretol)	PO; 200 mg bid, gradually increased to 800–1,200 mg/day in three to four divided doses	*Dizziness, ataxia, somnolence, headache, diplopia, blurred vision, transient indigestion, rhinitis, leukopenia, prolonged bleeding time, nausea, vomiting, anorexia*
felbamate (Felbatol)	Lennox–Gastaut syndrome: PO; start at 15 mg/kg/day in three to four divided doses; may increase 15 mg/kg at weekly intervals to max of 45 mg/kg/day	<u>Agranulocytosis; aplastic anemias; bullous, exfoliative dermatitis; Stevens–Johnson syndrome; toxic epidermal necrolysis; bone marrow depression; acute liver failure; pancreatitis; heart block; respiratory depression</u>
	Partial seizures: PO; start with 1,200 mg/day in three to four divided doses; may increase by 600 mg/day every 2 wk (max: 3,600 mg/day)	
lamotrigine (Lamictal)	PO; 50 mg/day for 2 wk, then 50 mg bid for 2 wk; may increase gradually up to 300–500 mg/day in 2 divided doses (max: 700 mg/day)	
levetiracetam (Keppra)	PO; 500 mg twice daily (max: 3,000 mg total per day)	
oxcarbazepine (Trileptal)	PO; initiation of monotherapy, 300 mg twice daily, increase 300 mg/day every third day up to 1,200 mg/day	
ⓟ valproic acid (Depakene, Depakote)**	PO/IV; 15 mg/kg/day in divided doses when the total daily dose is greater than 250 mg; increase 5–10 mg/kg/day every wk until seizures are controlled (max: 60 mg/kg/day)	
zonisamide (Zonegran)	PO; 100–400 mg/day	

*PE = phenytoin equivalents
**Other formulations of valproic acid include its salts, valproate, and divalproex sodium.
Italics indicate common adverse effects; <u>underlining</u> indicates serious adverse effects.

15.6 Treating Seizures with Hydantoins and Related Drugs

The oldest and most commonly prescribed antiseizure medication is phenytoin (Dilantin). Approved in the 1930s, phenytoin is a broad-spectrum hydantoin drug, useful in treating all types of epilepsy except absence seizures. It provides effective seizure suppression, without the abuse potential or CNS depression associated with barbiturates. Patients vary significantly in their ability to metabolize phenytoin; therefore, dosages are highly individualized. Because of the very narrow range between a therapeutic dose and a toxic dose, patients must be carefully monitored. Phenytoin and fosphenytoin are first-line drugs in the treatment of status epilepticus.

Phenytoin-related drugs are used less frequently. Several widely used drugs share a mechanism of action similar to that of the hydantoins, including carbamazepine (Tegretol), oxcarbazepine (Trileptal), and valproic acid (Depakene, Depakote), which is also available as valproate and divalproex sodium. Because carbamazepine produces fewer adverse effects than phenytoin or phenobarbital, it is a drug of choice for tonic–clonic and partial seizures. Oxcarbazepine is a derivative of carbamazepine, so its treatment profile is similar. Oxcarbazepine is slightly better tolerated than carbamazepine although serious skin and organ hypersensitivity reactions have been noted. Valproic acid is a drug of choice for absence seizures and is used in combination with other drugs for partial seizures. Both carbamazepine and valproic acid are also used for bipolar disorder (chapter 16 ∞).

Newer antiseizure drugs show promise in treatment for a range of disorders including absence seizures, partial seizures, myoclonic seizures, generalized tonic–clonic seizures, and mood disorders. The most common adverse effects of the newer antiseizure drugs are somnolence, drowsiness, dizziness, and blurred vision. Lamotrigine (Lamictal) has a broad spectrum of antiseizure activity, and is FDA-approved for longer-term maintenance of bipolar disorder. This drug's duration of action is greatly affected by other drugs that inhibit or enhance hepatic metabolizing enzymes. Levetiracetam (Keppra) and zonisamide

Pr Prototype Drug | Diazepam *(Valium)*

Therapeutic Class: Antiseizure drug   **Pharmacologic Class:** Benzodiazepine; GABA$_A$ receptor agonist

ACTIONS AND USES

Diazepam binds to the GABA receptor–chloride channels throughout the CNS. It produces its effects by suppressing neuronal activity in the limbic system and subsequent impulses that might be transmitted to the reticular activating system. Effects of this drug are suppression of abnormal neuronal foci that may cause seizures, calming without strong sedation, and skeletal muscle relaxation. When used orally, maximum therapeutic effects may take from 1 to 2 weeks. Tolerance may develop after about 4 weeks. When given IV, effects occur in minutes, and its anticonvulsant effects last about 20 minutes.

ADMINISTRATION ALERTS

- When administering IV, monitor respirations every 5 to 15 minutes. Have airway and resuscitative equipment accessible.
- Pregnancy category D

PHARMACOKINETICS

Onset: 30–60 min PO; 15–30 min IV

Peak: 1–2 h PO; 15 min IM; 1–5 min IV

Half-life: 20–50 h

Duration: 2–3 h PO; 15–60 min IV

ADVERSE EFFECTS

Because of tolerance and dependency, use of diazepam is reserved for short-term seizure control, or for status epilepticus. When given IV, hypotension, muscular weakness, tachycardia, and respiratory depression are common.

Contraindications: When administered in injectable form, this medication should be avoided under the following conditions: shock, coma, depressed vital signs, obstetrical patients, and infants less than 30 days of age. In tablet form, the medication should not be administered to infants less than 6 months of age, to patients with acute narrow-angle glaucoma or untreated open-angle glaucoma, or within 14 days of MAOI therapy.

INTERACTIONS

Drug–Drug: Diazepam should not be taken with alcohol or other CNS depressants because of combined sedation effects. Other drug interactions include cimetidine, oral contraceptives, valproic acid, and metoprolol, which potentiate diazepam's action; and levodopa and barbiturates, which decrease diazepam's action. Diazepam increases the levels of phenytoin in the bloodstream, and may cause phenytoin toxicity.

Lab Tests: Unknown

Herbal/Food: Kava and chamomile may cause an increased effect.

Treatment of Overdose: If an overdose occurs, administer flumazenil (Romazicon), a specific benzodiazepine receptor antagonist to reverse CNS depression.

See chapter 14, page 161∞, Nursing Process Focus: Patients Receiving Drugs for Anxiety Disorders. Refer to MyNursingKit for a Nursing Process Focus specific to this drug.

(Zonegram) are approved for adjunctive therapy of partial seizures in adults. Among the newer antiseizure drugs, levetiracetam is generally less reactive and has less adverse effects than the other antiseizure medications. Conversely, zonisamide is a sulfonamide and can trigger hypersensitivity reactions in some patients. Felbamate (Felbatol) can also cause potentially fatal reactions in patients including aplastic anemia and liver failure.

DRUGS THAT SUPPRESS CALCIUM INFLUX

Neurotransmitters, hormones, and some medications bind to neuronal membranes, stimulating the entry of calcium.

Without calcium influx, neuronal transmission would not be possible. Succinimides delay entry of calcium into neurons by blocking low-threshold calcium channels, increasing the electrical threshold of the neuron and reducing the likelihood that an action potential will be generated. By raising the seizure threshold, succinimides keep neurons from firing too quickly, thus suppressing abnormal foci.

Succinimides

Succinimides are medications that suppress seizures by delaying calcium influx into neurons. They are generally only effective against absence seizures. The succinimides are listed in Table 15.5.

TABLE 15.5	Succinimides	
Drug	Route and Adult Dose (max dose where indicated)	Adverse Effects
ethosuximide (Zarontin)	PO; 250 mg bid, increased every 4–7 days (max: 1.5 g/day)	*Drowsiness, dizziness, ataxia, epigastric distress, weight loss, anorexia, nausea, vomiting*
methsuximide (Celontin)	PO; 300 mg/day; may increase every 4–7 days (max: 1.2 g/day)	
phensuximide (Milontin)	PO; 0.5–1.0 g bid or tid	<u>Agranulocytosis, pancytopenia, aplastic anemia, granulocytopenia</u>

Italics indicate common adverse effects; <u>underlining</u> indicates serious adverse effects.

Pr Prototype Drug | Phenytoin (Dilantin)

Therapeutic Class: Antiseizure drug; antidysrhythmic   **Pharmacologic Class:** Hydantoin; sodium influx–suppressing drug

ACTIONS AND USES

Phenytoin acts by desensitizing sodium channels in the CNS responsible for neuronal responsivity. Desensitization prevents the spread of disruptive electrical charges in the brain that produce seizures. It is effective against most types of seizures except absence seizures. Phenytoin has antidysrhythmic activity similar to that of lidocaine (class IB). An unlabeled use is for digitalis-induced dysrhythmias.

ADMINISTRATION ALERTS

- When administering IV, mix with saline only, and infuse at the maximum rate of 50 mg/min. Mixing with other medications or dextrose solutions produces precipitate.

- Always prime or flush IV lines with saline before hanging phenytoin as a piggyback, since traces of dextrose solution in an existing main IV or piggyback line can cause microscopic precipitate formation, which become emboli if infused. Use an IV line with filter when infusing this drug.

- Phenytoin injectable is a soft-tissue irritant that causes local tissue damage following extravasation. To reduce the risk of soft-tissue damage, do not give IM; inject into a large vein or via a central venous catheter.

- Avoid using hand veins to prevent serious local vasoconstrictive response (purple glove syndrome).

- Pregnancy category D

PHARMACOKINETICS

Onset: Slowly and variably absorbed PO

Peak: 1.5–3 h prompt release; 4–12 h sustained release

Half-life: 22 h

Duration: 15 days

ADVERSE EFFECTS

Phenytoin may cause dysrhythmias, such as bradycardia or ventricular fibrillation, severe hypotension, and hyperglycemia. Severe CNS reactions include headache, nystagmus, ataxia, confusion and slurred speech, paradoxical nervousness, twitching, and insomnia. Peripheral neuropathy may occur with long-term use. Phenytoin can cause multiple blood dyscrasias, including agranulocytosis and aplastic anemia.

This medication may cause severe skin reactions, such as rashes, including exfoliative dermatitis, and Stevens–Johnson syndrome. Connective tissue reactions include lupus erythematosus, hypertrichosis, hirsutism, and gingival hypertrophy.

Contraindications: Patients with hypersensitivity to hydantoin products should be cautious. Rash, seizures due to hypoglycemia, sinus bradycardia, and heart block are contraindications.

INTERACTIONS

Drug–Drug: Phenytoin interacts with many other drugs, including oral anticoagulants, glucocorticoids, H_2 antagonists, antituberculin drugs, and food supplements such as folic acid, calcium, and vitamin D. It impairs the efficacy of drugs such as digitoxin, doxycycline, furosemide, estrogens and oral contraceptives, and theophylline. When combined with tricyclic antidepressants, phenytoin can trigger seizures.

Lab Tests: Hydantoins may produce lower-than-normal values for dexamethasone or metyrapone tests. Phenytoin may increase serum levels of glucose, bromsulphalein, and alkaline phosphatase, and may decrease protein-bound iodine and urinary steroid levels.

Herbal/Food: Herbal laxatives (buckthorn, cascara sagrada, and senna) may increase potassium loss. Ginkgo may reduce the therapeutic effectiveness of phenytoin.

Treatment of Overdose: There is no specific treatment for overdose. Drug removal may be accomplished by gastric lavage, use of activated charcoal, or laxative. Treatment is supportive and consists mainly of maintaining the airway and breathing, monitoring phenytoin blood levels, and appropriately treating adverse symptoms.

Refer to MyNursingKit for a Nursing Process Focus specific to this drug.

15.7 Treating Seizures with Succinimides

Ethosuximide (Zarontin) is the most commonly prescribed drug in this class. It remains a drug of choice for absence seizures, although valproic acid is also effective for these types of seizures. Some of the newer antiseizure drugs, such as lamotrigine (Lamictal) and zonisamide (Zonegran), are being investigated for their roles in treating absence seizures. Lamotrigine has also been found to be effective in patients with partial seizures, usually in combination with other antiseizure medications.

NURSING PROCESS FOCUS   PATIENTS RECEIVING ANTISEIZURE DRUG THERAPY (Continued)

Implementation

Interventions and (Rationales)	Patient and Family Education
▪ Continue to monitor height, weight, and developmental level in pediatric patients. In the school-age child, assess school performance. (Adverse effects of antiseizure drugs or unresolved seizures may hinder normal growth and development.)	▪ Teach the patient's family or caregiver to keep regularly scheduled appointments with the health care provider and report any developmental lags or concerns.
▪ Continue to monitor drug levels, CBC, renal and hepatic function, and pancreatic enzymes. (Antiseizure drugs require periodic drug levels to correlate the level with symptoms. Antiseizure drugs may cause hepatotoxicity and valproic acid may cause pancreatitis as an adverse effect.)	▪ Instruct the patient on the need to return periodically for lab work. ▪ Instruct the patient to carry a wallet identification card or wear medical identification jewelry indicating a seizure disorder and antiseizure medication. ▪ Teach the patient to promptly report any abdominal pain, particularly in the upper quadrants; changes in stool color; yellowing of sclera or skin; or darkened urine.
▪ Assess for changes in the level of consciousness, disorientation or confusion, or agitation. (Neurologic changes may indicate overmedication or adverse drug effects.)	▪ Instruct the patient, family, or caregiver to immediately report increasing lethargy, disorientation, confusion, changes in behavior or mood, slurred speech, or ataxia.
▪ Assess for changes in visual acuity, blurred vision, loss of peripheral vision, seeing rainbow halos around lights, acute eye pain, or any of these symptoms accompanied by nausea and vomiting and report immediately. (Increased intraoptic pressure in patients with narrow-angle glaucoma may occur in patients taking benzodizepines.)	▪ Instruct the patient to immediately report any visual changes or eye pain.
▪ Assess for bruising, bleeding, or signs of infection. (Antiseizure drugs may cause blood dyscrasias and increased chances of bleeding or infection.)	▪ Teach the patient to promptly report any signs of increased bruising, bleeding, or infections (e.g., sore throat and fever, skin rash).
▪ Monitor affect and emotional status. (Antiseizure drugs may increase the risk of mental depression and suicide. Concurrent use of alcohol or other CNS depressants increase the effects and the risk.)	▪ Instruct the patient, family, or caregiver to report significant mood changes, especially depression, and to avoid alcohol and other CNS depressants while taking the drug.
▪ Assess the condition of gums and oral hygiene measures. (Hydantoins and phenytoin-like drugs may cause gingival hyperplasia, increasing the risk of oral infections.)	▪ Instruct the patient to maintain excellent oral hygiene and keep regularly scheduled dental appointments.
▪ Encourage appropriate lifestyle and dietary changes: increased intake of vitamin K, D, folic acid, and vitamin B–rich foods; lowered caffeine intake including OTC medications that contain caffeine; and limited or no alcohol intake. (Caffeine and nicotine may decrease the effectiveness of the benzodiazepines. Barbiturates, drugs with GABA action, and hydantoins and phenytoin-like drugs affect the absorption of vitamins K, D, folic acid, and B vitamins. Alcohol and other CNS depressants may increase the adverse effects of the antiseizure drugs.)	▪ Encourage the patient to decrease or abstain from caffeine, nicotine, and alcohol; and increase intake of folic acid, and vitamins B, D, and K–rich foods. ▪ Advise the patient to discuss all OTC medications with the health care provider to ensure that caffeine or alcohol is not included in the formulation.
▪ Monitor children for paradoxical response to barbiturates. (Hyperactivity may occur.)	▪ Instruct the patient, family, or caregiver to notify the health care provider if the patient exhibits hyperactive behavior.
▪ Assess women of child-bearing age for the possibility of pregnancy, plans for pregnancy, breast-feeding, and contraceptive use. (Antiseizure medications are category D in pregnancy. Barbiturates decrease the effectiveness of oral contraceptives and additional forms of contraception should be used.)	▪ Discuss pregnancy and family planning with women of child-bearing age. Explain the effect of medications on pregnancy and breast-feeding and the need to discuss any pregnancy plans with the health care provider. Discuss the need for additional forms of contraception, including barrier methods, with patients taking barbiturates for seizure control.
▪ Avoid abrupt discontinuation of therapy. (Status epilepticus may occur with abrupt discontinuation.)	▪ Instruct the patient to take the drug exactly as prescribed and to not stop it abruptly.
▪ Assess home storage of medications and identify risks for corrective action. (Overdosage may occur if the patient takes additional doses when drowsy or disoriented from medication effects. Overdosage with barbiturates may prove fatal.)	▪ Instruct the patient that these drugs should not be kept at the bedside and to avoid taking additional doses when drowsy.
▪ Provide emotional support and appropriate referrals as needed. (Treatment with antiseizure drugs may require using combinations of drugs and seizure activity may diminish but may not be resolved. Social isolation and low self-esteem may occur with continued seizure disorder.)	▪ Teach the patient, family, or caregiver about support groups and make appropriate referrals as needed.

Implementation

Interventions and (Rationales)	Patient and Family Education
■ Closely monitor the IV infusion site when using IV antiseizure drugs. All IV drips should be given via infusion pump. (Benzodiazepines, hydantoins, and barbiturates are irritating to the vein. Blanching and pain at the IV site are indicators of extravasation and the IV infusion should be immediately stopped and the provider contacted for further treatment orders. Infusion pumps will allow precise dosing of the medication.)	■ Teach the patient to immediately report pain or burning at the IV site or in extremity with IV.
Patient understanding of drug therapy: ■ Use opportunities during administration of medications and during assessments to discuss the rationale for drug therapy, desired therapeutic outcomes, most commonly observed adverse effects, parameters for when to call the health care provider, and any necessary monitoring or precautions. (Using time during nursing care helps to optimize and reinforce key teaching areas.)	■ The patient should be able to state the reason for the drug; appropriate dose and scheduling; what adverse effects to observe for and when to report; and the anticipated length of medication therapy.
Patient self-administration of drug therapy: ■ When administering the medication, instruct the patient, family, or caregiver in proper self-administration of drug, e.g., take the drug as prescribed and do not substitute brands. (Utilizing time during nurse-administration of these drugs helps to reinforce teaching.)	■ Teach the patient to take the medication as follows: ■ Exactly as ordered and the same manufacturer's brand each time the prescription is filled. (Switching brands may result in differing pharmacokinetics and alterations in seizure control.) ■ Take a missed dose as soon as it is noticed but do not take double or extra doses to "catch up." ■ Take with food to decrease GI upset. ■ Do not abruptly discontinue the medication.

Evaluation of Outcome Criteria

Evaluate the effectiveness of drug therapy by confirming that patient goals and expected outcomes have been met (see "Planning").

See Tables 15.3, 15.4, and 15.5 for lists of drugs to which these nursing actions apply. (See also the Nursing Process Focus table in chapter 14 information related to Benzodiazepine and Nonbenzodiazepine drugs⧜ .)

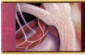

Chapter REVIEW

KEY CONCEPTS

The numbered key concepts provide a succinct summary of the important points from the corresponding numbered section within the chapter. If any of these points are not clear, refer to the numbered section within the chapter for review.

15.1 Seizures are symptomatic of an underlying disorder and are associated with many causes, including head trauma, brain infection, fluid and electrolyte imbalance, hypoxia, stroke, brain tumors, and high fever in children. Pregnancy and quality of life are important issues to consider when discussing epilepsy and seizure management.

15.2 The three broad categories of seizures are partial seizures, generalized seizures, and special epileptic syndromes. Each seizure type has a characteristic set of signs. Control of seizures requires proper diagnosis and drug selection.

15.3 Both traditional and newer antiseizure drugs are indicated for seizures. Both drug classes have serious draw-

backs. Antiseizure drug therapy works by suppressing repetitive and abnormal neuronal firing. Distinct mechanisms include GABA potentiation, delaying an influx of sodium or calcium ions into neurons, and antagonism of the neurotransmitter glutamate. Pharmacotherapy may continue for many years, and antiseizure drugs must be withdrawn gradually to prevent seizure recurrence.

15.4 GABA-potentiating barbiturates, mainly phenobarbital and primidone, are effective against all kinds of seizures except for absence seizures. Phenobarbital is the drug of choice for neonatal seizures.

15.5 Benzodiazepines reduce seizure activity by potentiating GABA action. Their use is limited to short-term therapy for absence seizures, myoclonic seizures, and to terminate status epilepticus.

15.6 Hydantoin and related drugs act by delaying sodium influx into neurons. Phenytoin, carbamazepine, and oxcarbazepine are broad-spectrum drugs used for all types of epilepsy except absence seizures. Valproic acid and lam-

otrigine treat all major types of seizures. Several drugs in this class act by more than one mechanism.

15.7 Succinimides act by delaying calcium influx into neurons. Ethosuximide (Zarontin) is a drug of choice for absence seizures.

NCLEX-RN® REVIEW QUESTIONS

1 The nurse evaluates patient teaching related to causes of seizures. Further teaching is needed if the patient makes which of the following statements?
1. "Seizures can be caused by inflammation of the brain."
2. "Seizures can be caused by low blood sugar."
3. "My relative had seizures because of a large tumor growing in his muscles."
4. "Seizures may occur after a head injury."

2 The nursing student asks the nurse to explain the action of the antiseizure medication, phenytoin. The nurse explains the mechanism of action as:
1. suppression of the influx of chloride into the neuron.
2. stimulation of the influx of calcium into the neuron.
3. suppression of the influx of sodium into the neuron.
4. stimulation of calcium and sodium needed to suppress seizure activity.

3 The nurse recognizes that several chemicals inhibit neurotransmitter function in the brain. The primary inhibitory transmitter in the brain is:
1. sodium.
2. GABA.
3. chloride.
4. calcium.

4 The patient, age 8, is prescribed valproic acid (Depakene) for treatment of a seizure disorder. The nurse should monitor the patient closely for:
1. hyperthermia.
2. vitamin B deficiency.
3. restlessness and agitation.
4. respiratory distress.

5 Discharge teaching for a patient receiving carbamazepine (Tegretol) should include:
1. monitoring blood glucose and reporting decreased levels.
2. expecting a discoloration of contact lenses.
3. immediately reporting unusual bleeding or bruises to the health care provider.
4. expecting a green discoloration of urine.

6 Which of the following medications may be used to treat partial seizures? (Select all that apply.)
1. Phenytoin (Dilantin)
2. Valproic acid (Depakene)
3. Diazepam (Valium)
4. Carbamazepine (Tegretol)
5. Ethosuximide (Zarontin)

CRITICAL THINKING QUESTIONS

1. The nurse practitioner reviews the laboratory results of a 16-year-old patient who presents to the clinic with fatigue and pallor. The patient's hematocrit is 26%, and the nurse notes multiple small petechiae and bruises over the arms and legs. This patient has a generalized tonic–clonic seizure disorder that has been managed well on carbamazepine (Tegretol). Relate the drug regimen to this patient's presentation.

2. A 24-year-old woman is brought to the emergency department by her husband. He tells the triage nurse that his wife has been treated for seizure disorder secondary to a head injury she received in an automobile accident. She takes phenytoin (Dilantin) 100 mg every 8 hours. He relates a history of increasing drowsiness and lethargy in his wife over the past 24 hours. A phenytoin level is performed, and the nurse notes that the results are 24 mcg/dL. Relate the drug regimen to this patient's presentation.

3. The nurse is admitting a 17-year-old female patient with a history of seizure disorder. The patient has broken her leg

in a car accident, in which she was the driver. The patient states that she hates having to take phenytoin (Dilantin), and that she stopped the drug because she could not drive and it was making her angry. Instead of reassuring the patient, the nurse first considers the possible side effects of long-term phenytoin therapy. Explain possible long-term effects of phenytoin therapy and their impact on patient compliance.

See Appendix D for answers and rationales for all activities.

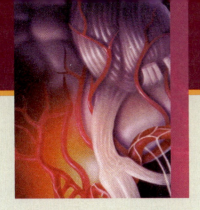

Chapter 16

Drugs for Emotional and Mood Disorders

LEARNING OUTCOMES

After reading this chapter, the student should be able to:

1. Identify the two major categories of mood disorders and their symptoms.
2. Identify the symptoms of attention deficit–hyperactivity disorder.
3. Explain the etiology of major depressive disorder.
4. Discuss the nurse's role in the pharmacologic management of patients with depression, bipolar disorder, or attention deficit–hyperactivity disorder.
5. For each of the drug classes listed in Drugs at a Glance, recognize representative drug examples, explain their mechanism of action, primary actions, and important adverse effects.
6. Categorize drugs used for mood and emotional disorders based on their classification and drug action.
7. Use the nursing process to care for patients receiving drug therapy for mood and emotional disorders.

KEY TERMS

Inappropriate or unusually intense emotions are among the leading causes of mental health disorders. Although mood changes are a normal part of life, when those changes become severe and result in impaired functioning within the family, work environment, or interpersonal relationships, an individual may be diagnosed as having a **mood disorder**. The two major categories of mood disorders are depression and bipolar disorder. A third emotional disorder, attention deficit–hyperactivity disorder, is also included in this chapter.

DEPRESSION

Depression is a disorder characterized by a sad or despondent mood. Many symptoms are associated with depression, including lack of energy, sleep disturbances, abnormal eating patterns, and feelings of despair, guilt, or hopelessness. Depression is the most common mental health disorder of elderly adults, encompassing a variety of physical, emotional, cognitive, and social considerations.

16.1 Characteristics and Forms of Depression

Among the most common forms of mental illness, **major depressive disorder** is estimated to affect 5% to 10% of adults in the United States. The American Psychiatric Association's *Diagnostic and Statistical Manual of Mental Disorders,* 4th edition (DSM-IV), describes the following criteria for diagnosis of a major depressive disorder: a depressed affect plus at least five of the following symptoms lasting for a minimum of 2 weeks:

- Difficulty sleeping or sleeping too much
- Extremely tired; without energy
- Abnormal eating patterns (eating too much or not enough)
- Vague physical symptoms (GI pain, joint/muscle pain, or headaches)
- Inability to concentrate or make decisions
- Feelings of despair, guilt, and misery; lack of self-worth
- Obsessed with death (expressing a wish to die or to commit suicide)
- Avoiding psychosocial and interpersonal interactions
- Lack of interest in personal appearance or sex
- Delusions or hallucinations

The majority of depressed patients are not found in psychiatric hospitals but in mainstream society. For proper diagnosis and treatment to occur, recognition of depression is often a collaborative effort among health care providers. For example, it might be the pharmacist who recognizes that a customer is depressed when he or she buys natural or over-the-counter (OTC) remedies to control anxiety symptoms or to induce sleep. **Dysthymic disorder** is characterized by less se-

vere depressive symptoms that may prevent a person from feeling well or functioning normally. Because depressed patients may be found in multiple settings, every nurse should be proficient in the assessment of patients afflicted with this condition.

Some women experience intense mood shifts associated with hormonal changes during the menstrual cycle, pregnancy, childbirth, and menopause. Up to 80% of women experience **postpartum depression** during the first several weeks after birth of their baby. About 10% of new mothers experience a major depressive episode within 6 months related to the dramatic hormonal shifts that occur during postdelivery. Along with the hormonal changes, additional situational stresses such as responsibilities at home or work, single parenthood, and caring for children or for aging parents, may contribute to the onset of symptoms. If mood is severely depressed and persists long enough, many women will likely benefit from medical treatment, including those with premenstrual dysphoric disorder, depression during pregnancy, postpartum mood disorders, or menopausal distress.

Because of the possible consequences of perinatal mood disorders, some state agencies mandate that all new mothers after giving birth receive information about mood shifts prior to their discharge. Health care providers in obstetrician's offices, pediatric outpatient settings, and family medicine centers are encouraged to conduct routine screening for symptoms of perinatal mood disorders.

During the dark winter months, some patients experience **seasonal affective disorder (SAD)**. This type of depression is associated with enhanced release of the brain neurohormone melatonin due to lower light levels. Exposing patients on a regular basis to specific light therapy may relieve SAD depression and prevent future episodes.

TREATING THE DIVERSE PATIENT

Cultural Influences and the Treatment of Depression

To fully understand any patient who is suffering from depression, sociocultural factors must be fully considered.

- Depression (and other mental illness) is often ignored in many Asian communities because of the tremendous amount of stigma attached to it. Emotions are largely suppressed. Asian patients tend to come to the attention of mental health workers late in the course of their illness, and often have a feeling of hopelessness. It should be noted that Asians and African Americans generally metabolize antidepressants more slowly than other subgroups; therefore, initial doses should be reduced to avoid drug toxicity.

- Alternative therapies such as teas are often used to treat emotional illnesses within some Hispanic American groups; thus, medical help may not be sought for treatment of depression. There is often a stigma attached to mental health problems along with the belief that religious practices will solve mental health problems. Hispanics metabolize antidepressants about the same as other subgroups, although there are reports of greater susceptibility to anticholinergic effects.

- Some people of European origin deny that mental illness exists and therefore believe that depression will subside on its own. Higher doses of antidepressants are often tolerated in this subgroup.

Psychotic depression is characterized by the expression of intense mood shifts and unusual behaviors. Depressive signs and loss of contact with reality, hallucinations, delusions, and disorganized speech patterns are the behaviors observed. For psychotic patients and for patients with extreme mood swings, severe behaviors are often treatable with antipsychotic therapy. See section 16.8 of this chapter and chapter 17∞.

16.2 Assessment and Treatment of Depression

The first step in implementing appropriate treatment for depression is a complete health examination. Certain drugs, such as glucocorticoids, levodopa, and oral contraceptives, can cause the same symptoms as depression, and the health care provider should rule out this possibility. Depression may be mimicked by a variety of medical and neurologic disorders, ranging from B-vitamin deficiencies to thyroid gland problems to early Alzheimer's disease. If physical causes for the depression are ruled out, a psychologic evaluation is often performed to confirm the diagnosis.

During initial health examinations, inquiries should be made about alcohol and drug use, and any thoughts about death or suicide. This exam should include questions about any family history of depressive illness. If other family members have been treated, the nurse should document what therapies they may have received and which were effective or helpful.

To determine a course of treatment, health care providers and nurses assess for well-accepted symptoms of depression. In general, severe depressive illness, particularly that which is recurrent, will require both medication and psychotherapy to achieve the best response. Counseling therapies help patients gain insight into and resolve their problems through verbal interaction with the therapist. Behavioral therapies help patients learn how to obtain more satisfaction and rewards through their own actions and how to unlearn the behavioral patterns that contribute to or result from mood shifts.

Helpful short-term psychotherapies for some forms of depression are *interpersonal* and *cognitive–behavioral therapies*. Interpersonal therapies focus on the patient's disturbed personal relationships that both cause and exacerbate the depression. Cognitive–behavioral therapies help patients change the negative styles of thought and behavior often associated with their depression.

Psychodynamic therapies focus on resolving the patient's internal conflicts. These therapies are often postponed until the depressive symptoms are significantly improved.

In patients unresponsive to pharmacotherapy and with serious and life-threatening mood disorders, **electroconvulsive therapy (ECT)** continues to be a useful treatment. Although ECT is found to be safe, there are still deaths (1 in 10,000 patients). Other serious complications related to seizure activity and anesthesia may be caused by ECT (Janicak, 2002). Recent studies suggest that repetitive transcranial magnetic stimulation (rTMS) is an effective somatic treatment for

major depressive disorder (O'Reardon, 2007). This treatment requires surgical implant of the device. In contrast to ECT, rTMS produces minimal effects on memory, does not require general anesthesia, and is helpful without the overt risk of generalized seizures.

Even with the best professional care, the patient with depression may take a long time to recover. Many individuals with major depression have multiple bouts of the illness over the course of a lifetime. This can take its toll on the patient's family, friends, and other caregivers who may sometimes feel burned out, frustrated, or even depressed themselves. They may experience episodes of anger toward the depressed loved one, only to subsequently suffer reactions of guilt over being angry. Although such feelings are common, they can be distressing, and the caregiver may not know where to turn for help. It is often the nurse who is best able to assist the family members of a person suffering from depression. Family members may need counseling themselves.

ANTIDEPRESSANTS

Drugs used to treat depression are categorized as antidepressants. Antidepressants treat depression by enhancing mood. Over the years, *mood* has come to represent a broader term, encompassing feelings of phobia, obsessive–compulsive behavior, panic, and anxiety. Thus, antidepressants are often prescribed for these disorders as well. Recent studies link depression and anxiety to similar neurotransmitter dysfunction, and both seem to respond to treatment with antidepressant medications (chapter 14∞) Antidepressants are also beneficial in treating psychologic and physical signs of pain (chapter 18∞), especially in patients without major depressive disorder, for example, when mood problems are associated with debilitating conditions such as fibromylagia or muscle spasticity (chapter 21∞).

There is one important warning about antidepressants: In 2004, the U.S. Food and Drug Administration issued an advisory "black box warning" to be included at the beginning of drug package inserts and drug information sheets. The advisory was issued to patients, families, and health professionals to closely monitor adults and children taking antidepressants for warning signs of suicide, especially at the beginning of treatment and when doses are changed. The

PHARMFACTS

Patients with Depressive Symptoms

- Major depression, manic depression, and situational depression are some of the most common mental health challenges worldwide.
- Clinical depression affects more than 19 million Americans each year.
- Fewer than half of those suffering from depression seek medical treatment.
- Most patients consider depression a weakness rather than an illness.
- There is no common age, sex, or ethnic factor related to depression—it can happen to anyone.

FDA further advised that certain signs might be expected among certain patients including anxiety, panic attacks, agitation, irritability, insomnia, impulsivity, hostility, and mania. These warnings apply especially to children, who are at a greater risk for suicidal ideation.

16.3 Mechanism of Action of Antidepressants

Depression is associated with dysfunction of neurotransmitters in regions of the brain connected with focused cognition and emotion. Although medication does not completely restore chemical imbalances, it may help reduce depressive symptoms while the patient develops effective means of coping.

As shown in Pharmacology Illustrated 16.1, antidepressants are theorized to exert effects through actions on specific neurotransmitters in the brain, including norepinephrine, serotonin, and dopamine. The two basic mechanisms of drug action are slowing the reuptake of serotonin and norepinephrine and blocking the enzymatic breakdown of norepinephrine. Within centrally located synaptic terminals, monoamine oxidase (MAO) enzymes normally break down catecholamines and recycle them for further use (chapter 13∞). Making catecholamines more available by either inhibiting MAO enzymes or inhibiting neurotransmitter uptake, enhances activation of adrenergic receptors. The primary classes of antidepressant drugs, listed in Table 16.1, are as follows:

- Tricyclic antidepressants (TCAs)
- Selective serotonin reuptake inhibitors (SSRIs)
- Atypical antidepressants including the serotonin–norepinephrine reuptake inhibitors (SNRIs)
- Monoamine oxidase inhibitors (MAOIs)

Tricyclic Antidepressants

Named for their three-ring chemical structure, **tricyclic antidepressants (TCAs)** were the mainstay of depression pharmacotherapy from the early 1960s until the 1980s, and are still used today.

16.4 Treating Depression with Tricyclic Antidepressants

Tricyclic antidepressants act by inhibiting the presynaptic reuptake of both norepinephrine and serotonin. TCAs are used predominately for major depression and occasionally for milder situational depression. Clomipramine (Anafranil) is approved for treatment of obsessive–compulsive disorder, and other TCAs are sometimes used as unlabeled treatments for panic attacks. One atypical use for TCAs, not related to psychopharmacology, is for the treatment of childhood enuresis (bed-wetting).

Shortly after their approval as antidepressants in the 1950s, it was found that the tricyclic antidepressants produced fewer side effects and were less dangerous than MAO inhibitors.

However, TCAs continued to have some unpleasant and serious side effects. The most common side effect is orthostatic hypotension, due to alpha$_1$ blockade on blood vessels. The most serious adverse effect occurs when TCAs accumulate in cardiac tissue. Although rare, cardiac dysrhythmias can occur.

Sedation is a frequently reported complaint at the initiation of therapy, though patients may become tolerant to this effect after several weeks of treatment. Most drugs have a long half-life, which increases the risk of side effects, especially for patients with delayed excretion. Anticholinergic effects, such as dry mouth, constipation, urinary retention, excessive perspiration, blurred vision, and tachycardia, are common. These effects are less severe if the drug is gradually increased to the therapeutic dose over 2 to 3 weeks. Significant drug interactions can occur with CNS depressants, sympathomimetics, anticholinergics, and MAO inhibitors. Since the advent of newer antidepressants with fewer side effects, TCAs are less frequently used as first-line drugs in the treatment of depression and/or anxiety.

Selective Serotonin Reuptake Inhibitors

Drugs that slow the reuptake of serotonin into presynaptic nerve terminals are called **selective serotonin reuptake inhibitors (SSRIs)**. They have become drugs of choice in the treatment of depression because of their more favorable side-effect profile.

16.5 Treating Depression with SSRIs

Serotonin is a natural indolamine neurotransmitter in the CNS, found in high concentrations within neurons of the hypothalamus, limbic system, medulla, and spinal cord. It is important to several body functions, including cycling between NREM and REM sleep, pain perception, and emotional states. Lack of adequate serotonin in the CNS can lead to depression. Serotonin is metabolized to a less active substance by the enzyme monoamine oxidase (MAO). Serotonin is also known by its chemical name, 5-hydroxytryptamine (5-HT).

In the 1970s, it became increasingly clear that serotonin had a more substantial role in depression than once thought. Clinicians knew that the tricyclic antidepressants altered the sensitivity of serotonin to populations of receptors in the brain, but they did not know how this change was connected with depression. Ongoing efforts to find antidepressants with fewer side effects led to the development of

---

AVOIDING MEDICATION ERRORS

A 23-year-old man was admitted this morning following a suicide attempt when his girlfriend broke up with him. When the nurse enters his room with his medications, he is talking on the telephone with his girlfriend. He makes eye contact with and motions for the nurse to leave his medications on the table so he can take them later. The nurse, not wanting to interrupt his conversation, puts the medications on the table, leaves the room, and charts the medications. What error did the nurse commit and what is the appropriate nursing intervention?

See Appendix D for the suggested answer.

16.1 Antidepressant Therapy Is Directed Toward the Amelioration of Depressive Symptoms

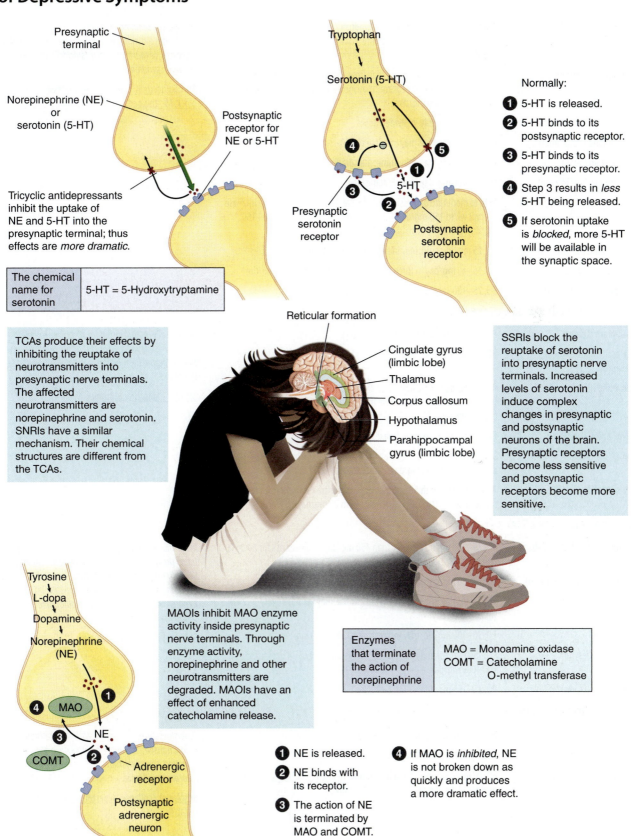

Presynaptic terminal

Norepinephrine (NE) or serotonin (5-HT)

Postsynaptic receptor for NE or 5-HT

Tricyclic antidepressants inhibit the uptake of NE and 5-HT into the presynaptic terminal; thus effects are *more dramatic*.

The chemical name for serotonin	5-HT = 5-Hydroxytryptamine

Tryptophan

Serotonin (5-HT)

5-HT

Presynaptic serotonin receptor

Postsynaptic serotonin receptor

Normally:

1 5-HT is released.

2 5-HT binds to its postsynaptic receptor.

3 5-HT binds to its presynaptic receptor.

4 Step 3 results in *less* 5-HT being released.

5 If serotonin uptake is *blocked*, more 5-HT will be available in the synaptic space.

TCAs produce their effects by inhibiting the reuptake of neurotransmitters into presynaptic nerve terminals. The affected neurotransmitters are norepinephrine and serotonin. SNRIs have a similar mechanism. Their chemical structures are different from the TCAs.

Reticular formation

Cingulate gyrus (limbic lobe)

Thalamus

Corpus callosum

Hypothalamus

Parahippocampal gyrus (limbic lobe)

SSRIs block the reuptake of serotonin into presynaptic nerve terminals. Increased levels of serotonin induce complex changes in presynaptic and postsynaptic neurons of the brain. Presynaptic receptors become less sensitive and postsynaptic receptors become more sensitive.

Tyrosine
↓
L-dopa
↓
Dopamine
↓
Norepinephrine (NE)

MAO

COMT

NE

Adrenergic receptor

Postsynaptic adrenergic neuron

MAOIs inhibit MAO enzyme activity inside presynaptic nerve terminals. Through enzyme activity, norepinephrine and other neurotransmitters are degraded. MAOIs have an effect of enhanced catecholamine release.

Enzymes that terminate the action of norepinephrine	MAO = Monoamine oxidase COMT = Catecholamine O-methyl transferase

1 NE is released.

2 NE binds with its receptor.

3 The action of NE is terminated by MAO and COMT.

4 If MAO is *inhibited*, NE is not broken down as quickly and produces a more dramatic effect.

TABLE 16.1   Antidepressants

Drug	Route and Adult Dose (max dose where indicated)	Adverse Effects
TRICYCLIC ANTIDEPRESSANTS (TCAs)		
amitriptyline (Elavil)	Adult: PO; 75–100 mg/day (may gradually increase to 150–300 mg/day); Geriatric: PO; 10–25 mg at bedtime (may gradually increase to 25–150 mg/day)	*Drowsiness, sedation, dizziness, orthostatic hypotension, dry mouth, constipation, urinary retention, blurred vision, mydriasis, sexual dysfunction, suicidal ideation and serotonin syndrome*
amoxapine (Asendin)	Adult: PO; begin with 100 mg/day (may increase on day 3 to 300 mg/day); Geriatric: PO; 25 mg at bedtime; may increase every 3–7 days to 50–150 mg/day (max: 300 mg/day)	<u>Agranulocytosis, bone marrow depression, seizures, heart block, MI, angioedema of face, tongue, or generalized</u>
clomipramine (Anafranil)	PO; 75–300 mg/day in divided doses	
desipramine (Norpramin)	PO; 75–100 mg/day; may increase to 150–300 mg/day	
doxepin (Sinequan)	PO; 30–150 mg/day at bedtime; may gradually increase to 300 mg/day	
imipramine (Tofranil)	PO; 75–100 mg/day (max: 300 mg/day)	
maprotiline (Ludiomil)	Mild to moderate depression: PO; start at 75 mg/day; gradually increase every 2 wk to 150 mg/day; Severe depression: PO; start at 100–150 mg/day; gradually increase to 300 mg/day	
nortriptyline (Aventyl, Pamelor)	PO; 25 mg tid or qid; may increase to 100–150 mg/day	
protriptyline (Vivactil)	PO; 15–40 mg/day in three to four divided doses (max: 60 mg/day)	
trimipramine (Surmontil)	PO; 75–100 mg/day (max: 300 mg/day)	
SELECTIVE SEROTONIN REUPTAKE INHIBITORS (SSRIs)		
citalopram (Celexa)	PO; start at 20 mg/day (max: 40 mg/day)	*Nausea, dry mouth, insomnia, somnolence, headache, nervousness, anxiety, GI disturbances, dizziness, anorexia, fatigue, sexual dysfunction, suicidal ideation and serotonin syndrome*
escitalopram oxalate (Lexapro)	PO; 10 mg/day; may increase to 20 mg after 1 wk	<u>Stevens–Johnson syndrome</u>
fluoxetine (Prozac)	PO; 20 mg/day in the a.m., may increase by 20 mg/day at weekly intervals (max: 80 mg/day); when stable may switch to a 90-mg sustained-release capsule once weekly (max: 90 mg/wk)	
fluvoxamine (Luvox)	PO; start with 50 mg/day (max: 300 mg/day)	
paroxetine (Paxil)	Depression: PO; 10–50 mg/day (max: 80 mg/day); Obsessive–compulsive disorder: PO; 20–60 mg/day; Panic attacks: PO; 40 mg/day	
sertraline (Zoloft)	Adult: PO; start with 50 mg/day; gradually increase every few weeks to a range of 50–200 mg; Geriatric: start with 25 mg/day	
ATYPICAL ANTIDEPRESSANTS		
bupropion (Wellbutrin; Zyban)	PO; 75–100 mg tid (greater than 450 mg/day increases risk for adverse reactions)	*Insomnia, nausea, dry mouth, constipation, increased blood pressure and heart rate, dizziness, somnolence, sweating, agitation, blurred vision, headache, tremor, vomiting, drowsiness, increased appetite, orthostatic hypotension, sexual dysfunction, suicidal ideation and serotonin syndrome*
duloxetine (Cymbalta) (SNRI)	PO; 40–60 mg/day in one or two divided doses	<u>Stevens–Johnson syndrome</u>
mirtazapine (Remeron)	PO; 15 mg/day in a single dose at bedtime; may increase every 1–2 wk (max: 45 mg/day)	
nefazodone	PO; 50–100 mg bid; may increase up to 300–600 mg/day	
trazodone (Desyrel)	PO; 150 mg/day; may increase by 50 mg/day every 3–4 days up to 400–600 mg/day	
venlafaxine (Effexor) (SNRI)	PO; 25–125 mg tid	
MAO INHIBITORS (MAOIs)		
isocarboxazid (Marplan)	PO; 10–30 mg/day (max: 30 mg/day)	*Drowsiness, insomnia, orthostatic hypotension, blurred vision, nausea, constipation, anorexia, dry mouth, urinary retention, sexual dysfunction, suicidal ideation and serotonin syndrome*
phenelzine (Nardil)	PO; 15 mg tid (max: 90 mg/day)	<u>Respiratory collapse, hypertensive crisis, circulatory collapse</u>
tranylcypromine (Parnate)	PO; 30 mg/day (give 20 mg in a.m. and 10 mg in p.m.); may increase by 10 mg/day at 3-wk intervals up to 60 mg/day	

Italics indicate common adverse effects; <u>underlining</u> indicates serious adverse effects.

MyNursingKit Mechanism in Action: Fluoxetine

MyNursingKit Mechanism in Action: Venlafaxine

Pr Prototype Drug | Imipramine (Tofranil)

Therapeutic Class: Antidepressant; treatment of nocturnal enuresis (bed-wetting) in children   **Pharmacologic Class:** Tricyclic antidepressant

ACTIONS AND USES

Imipramine blocks the reuptake of serotonin and norepinephrine into nerve terminals. It is used mainly for major depression, although it is occasionally used for the treatment of nocturnal enuresis in children. The nurse may find imipramine prescribed for a number of unlabeled uses including intractable pain, anxiety disorders, and withdrawal syndromes from alcohol and cocaine. Therapeutic effectiveness may not occur for 2 or more weeks.

ADMINISTRATION ALERTS

- Paradoxical diaphoresis can be a side effect of TCAs; therefore, diaphoresis may not be a reliable indicator of other disease states such as hypoglycemia.

- Imipramine causes anticholinergic effects and may potentiate effects of anticholinergic drugs administered during surgery.

- Do not discontinue abruptly, because rebound dysphoria, irritability, or sleeplessness may occur.

- Pregnancy category C

PHARMACOKINETICS

Onset: Less than 1 h

Peak: 1–2 h PO; 30 min IM

Half-life: 8–16 h

Duration: Variable

ADVERSE EFFECTS

Side effects include sedation, drowsiness, blurred vision, dry mouth, and cardiovascular symptoms such as dysrhythmias, heart block, and extreme hypertension. Agents that mimic the action of norepinephrine or serotonin should be avoided because imipramine inhibits their metabolism and may produce toxicity. Some patients may experience photosensitivity and hypersensitivity to tricyclic drugs.

Contraindications: This drug should not be used in cases of acute recovery after MI, defects in bundle-branch conduction, narrow-angle glaucoma, and severe renal or hepatic impairment. Patients should not use this drug within 14 days of discontinuing MAOIs.

INTERACTIONS

Drug–Drug: Concurrent use of other CNS depressants, including alcohol, may cause sedation. Cimetidine (Tagamet) may inhibit the metabolism of imipramine, leading to increased serum levels and possible toxicity. Imipramine may reverse the antihypertensive effects of clonidine and potentiate CNS depression. Use of oral contraceptives may increase or decrease imipramine levels. Disulfiram may lead to delirium and tachycardia. Antithyroid agents may produce agranulocytosis. Phenothiazines cause increased anticholinergic and sedative effects. Sympathomimetics may result in cardiac toxicity. Methylphenidate or cimetidine may increase the effects of imipramine and cause toxicity. Phenytoin is less effective when taken with imipramine. MAOIs may result in neuroleptic malignant syndrome.

Lab Tests: Imipramine produces altered blood glucose tests. Elevation of serum bilirubin and alkaline phosphatase is likely.

Herbal/Food: Herbal supplements such as evening primrose oil or ginkgo, may lower the seizure threshold. St. John's wort used concurrently may cause serotonin syndrome.

Treatment of Overdose: There is no specific treatment for overdose. General supportive measures are recommended. Ensure an adequate airway, oxygenation, and ventilation. Monitor cardiac rhythm and vital signs. Gastric lavage may be indicated. Activated charcoal should be administered.

Refer to MyNursingKit for a Nursing Process Focus specific to this drug.

---

an additional category of medications, the selective serotonin reuptake inhibitors (SSRIs).

Whereas the tricyclic class inhibits the reuptake of both norepinephrine and serotonin into presynaptic nerve terminals, the SSRIs selectively target serotonin. Increased levels of serotonin in the synaptic gap induce complex neurotransmitter changes in presynaptic and postsynaptic neurons. Presynaptic receptors become less sensitive, and postsynaptic receptors become more sensitive. This mechanism is illustrated in Pharmacology Illustrated 16.1.

Today, SSRIs have approximately the same efficacy at relieving depression as the MAO inhibitors and the tricyclics. The major advantage of the SSRIs, and the one that makes them drugs of choice, is their greater safety. Sympathomimetic effects (increased heart rate and hypertension) and anticholinergic effects (dry mouth, blurred vision, urinary retention, and constipation) are less common with this drug class. Sedation is also experienced less frequently, and cardiotoxicity is not observed. All drugs in the SSRI class have equal efficacy and similar side effects.

In general, SSRIs elicit a therapeutic response more quickly than TCAs.

One of the most common side effects of SSRIs relates to sexual dysfunction. Up to 70% of both men and women experience decreased libido and lack of ability to reach orgasm. In men, delayed ejaculation and impotence may occur. For patients who are sexually active, these side effects may result in noncompliance with pharmacotherapy. Other common side effects of SSRIs include nausea, headache, weight gain, anxiety, and insomnia. Weight gain may also lead to noncompliance.

Serotonin syndrome (SES) may occur when the patient is taking another medication that affects the metabolism, synthesis, or reuptake of serotonin, causing serotonin to accumulate in the body. Symptoms can begin as early as 2 hours after taking the first dose or as late as several weeks after the initiating pharmacotherapy. SES can be produced by the concurrent administration of an SSRI with a MAOI, a tricyclic antidepressant, lithium, or a number of other medications. Symptoms of SES include mental status changes (confusion, anxiety, restlessness), hypertension, tremors, sweating, hyperpyrexia, or ataxia. Conservative treatment is to discontinue the SSRI and provide supportive care. In severe cases, mechanical ventilation and muscle relaxants may be necessary. If left untreated, death may occur.

Atypical Antidepressants

In terms of classification, the atypical antidepressants do not fit conveniently into the other antidepressant drug classes. Thus, "atypical" in this case really refers to the unique chemical structures represented in the group. These drugs are briefly dealt with here.

Duloxetine (Cymbalta) and venlafaxine (Effexor), sometimes considered to be in their own subgroup, are the **serotonin–norepinephrine reuptake inhibitors (SNRIs).** They specifically inhibit the reabsorption of serotonin and norepinephrine and elevate mood by increasing the levels of these agents in the central nervous system. In many cases, levels of dopamine are also affected with the SNRIs. In addition to being approved in 2004 by the Food and Drug Administration for the treatment of major depression, duloxetine (Cymbalta) was approved for the treatment of neuropathic pain. Venlafaxine (Effexor), more recently used to relieve depressive symptoms, is available in an intermediate-release form that requires two or three doses a day and an extended-release form that allows the patient to take the medication just once a day.

Bupropion (Wellbutrin) not only inhibits the reuptake of serotonin but may also affect the activity of norepinephrine

COMPLEMENTARY AND ALTERNATIVE THERAPIES

St. John's Wort for Depression

One of the most popular herbs in the United States, St. John's wort (*Hypericum perforatum*) is found growing throughout Asia, Europe, and North America. Its modern use is as an antidepressant. It gets its name from a legend that red spots once appeared on its leaves on the anniversary of the beheading of St. John the Baptist. The word *wort* is a British term for "plant."

The primary active ingredients found in St. John's wort are hypericin and hyperforin. Evidence suggests that these substances selectively inhibit serotonin reuptake in certain brain neurons. A number of clinical studies suggest that St. John's wort is an effective treatment for mild to moderate depression, and that it may be just as effective as tricyclic antidepressants and SSRIs (Gastpar, Singer, & Zeller, 2006). Recent analyses also suggest that the herb may be effective for major depression and that it causes fewer adverse effects than traditional drugs (Linde, Berner, & Kriston, 2008). St. John's wort may interact with many medications, including oral contraceptives, warfarin, digoxin, and cyclosporine. It should not be taken concurrently with antidepressant medications.

St. John's wort is well tolerated, producing mild adverse effects such as GI distress, fatigue, and allergic skin reactions. The herb contains compounds that photosensitize the skin; thus, patients should be advised to apply sunscreen or to wear protective clothing when outdoors.

and dopamine. It should be used with caution in patients with seizure disorders because it lowers the seizure threshold. Wellbutrin is marketed as Zyban for use in cessation of smoking. Mirtazapine (Remeron) is used for depression and blocks presynaptic serotonin and norepinephrine re-

---

Pr Prototype Drug | Sertraline *(Zoloft)*

Therapeutic Class: Antidepressant   **Pharmacologic Class:** Selective serotonin reuptake inhibitor (SSRI)

ACTIONS AND USES
Sertraline is used for the treatment of depression, anxiety, obsessive–compulsive disorder, and panic. The antidepressant and anxiolytic properties of this drug can be attributed to its ability to inhibit the reuptake of serotonin in the brain. Other uses include premenstrual dysphoric disorder, post-traumatic stress disorder, and social anxiety disorder. Therapeutic actions include enhancement of mood and improvement of affect with maximum effects observed after several weeks.

ADMINISTRATION ALERTS
- It is recommended that sertraline be given in the morning or evening.
- When administering sertraline as an oral liquid, mix with water, ginger ale, lemon/lime soda, lemonade, or orange juice. Follow manufacturer's instructions.
- Do not give concurrently with a MAO inhibitor or within 14 days of discontinuing MAOI medication.
- Pregnancy category C

> **PHARMACOKINETICS**
> **Onset:** 2–4 wk
> **Peak:** Unknown
> **Half-life:** 24 h
> **Duration:** Variable (extensive binding with serum proteins)

ADVERSE EFFECTS
Adverse effects include agitation, insomnia, headache, dizziness, somnolence, and fatigue. Take extreme precautions in patients with cardiac disease, hepatic impairment, seizure disorders, suicidal ideation, mania, or hypomania.

Contraindications: Concomitant use of sertraline and MAOIs or primozide is not advised. Antabuse should be avoided because of the alcohol content of the drug concentrate.

INTERACTIONS
Drug–Drug: Highly protein bound medications such as digoxin and warfarin should be avoided owing to risk of toxicity and increased blood concentrations leading to increased bleeding. MAOIs may cause neuroleptic malignant syndrome, extreme hypertension, and serotonin syndrome, characterized by headache, agitation, dizziness, fever, diarrhea, sweating, and shivering. Use cautiously with other centrally acting drugs to avoid adverse CNS effects.

Lab Tests: Sertraline results in asymptomatic elevated liver function tests and a slight decrease in uric acid levels.

Herbal/Food: Patients should use precaution if taking St. John's wort or L-tryptophan to avoid serotonin syndrome.

Treatment of Overdose: There is no specific treatment for overdose. Emergency medical attention and general supportive measures may be necessary. Symptoms of overdose include nausea, vomiting, tremor, seizures, agitation, dizziness, hyperactivity, mydriasis, tachycardia, and coma.

Refer to MyNursingKit for a Nursing Process Focus specific to this drug.

ceptors, thereby enhancing release of these neurotransmitters. Nefazodone (available in generic form only) is similar to Remeron. It was originally designed to treat depression, and causes minimal cardiovascular effects, fewer anticholinergic effects, less sedation, and less sexual dysfunction than the other antidepressants. Trazodone (Desyrel) is most frequently used as a sleep aid, rather than as an antidepressant. The high levels of trazodone needed for the amelioration of depression cause excessive sedation in many patients.

Monoamine Oxidase Inhibitors (MAOIs)

The group of drugs called **monoamine oxidase inhibitors (MAOIs)** inhibits monoamine oxidase, the enzyme that terminates the actions of neurotransmitters such as dopamine, norepinephrine, epinephrine, and serotonin. Because of their low safety margin, these drugs are reserved for patients who have not responded to TCAs or SSRIs.

16.6 Treating Depression with MAO Inhibitors

As discussed, the action of norepinephrine at adrenergic synapses is terminated through two means: (1) reuptake into the presynaptic nerve and (2) enzymatic destruction by the enzyme monoamine oxidase (MAO). By decreasing the effectiveness of the enzyme monoamine oxidase, the MAOIs limit the breakdown of norepinephrine, dopamine, and serotonin in the CNS. This creates higher levels of these neurotransmitters in the brain to facilitate neurotransmission and alleviate the symptoms of depression. As shown in Pharmacotherapy Illustrated 16.1, MAO is located within presynaptic nerve terminals.

In the 1950s, the monoamine oxidase inhibitors were the first drugs approved to treat depression. They are just as effective as TCAs and SSRIs in treating depression. However, because of drug–drug and food–drug interactions, hepatotoxicity, and the development of safer antidepressants, MAOIs are now reserved for patients who are not responsive to other antidepressant classes.

Common side effects of the MAOIs include orthostatic hypotension, headache, insomnia, and diarrhea. A primary concern is that these agents interact with a large number of foods and other medications, sometimes with serious effects. A hypertensive crisis can occur when a MAOI is used concurrently with other antidepressants or sympathomimetic drugs. Combining an MAOI with an SSRI can produce serotonin syndrome. If MAOIs are given with antihypertensives, the patient can experience severe hypotension. MAOIs also potentiate the hypoglycemic effects of insulin and oral antidiabetic drugs. Hyperpyrexia (elevation of body temperature) is known to occur in patients taking MAOIs with meperidine (Demerol), dextromethorphan (Pedia Care and others), and TCAs.

A hypertensive crisis can also result from an interaction between MAOIs and foods containing **tyramine,** a form of the amino acid tyrosine. Tyramine is usually degraded by MAO in the intestines. If a patient takes MAOIs however, tyramine enters the bloodstream in high concentrations and displaces norepinephrine within presynaptic nerve terminals. The result is a sudden release of norepinephrine, causing acute hypertension. Symptoms usually occur within minutes of ingesting the food and include occipital headache, stiff neck, flushing, palpitations, diaphoresis, and nausea. Myocardial infarctions and cerebral vascular accidents, though rare, are possible consequences. Calcium channel blockers may be given as an antidote. Because of their serious side effects when taken with food and drugs, MAOIs are rarely used and are limited to patients with symptoms that are resistant to more traditional therapies and to patients who are more likely to comply with food restrictions. Examples of foods containing tyramine are listed in Table 16.2.

BIPOLAR DISORDER

Once known as *manic depression,* **bipolar disorder** is characterized by extreme and opposite moods, episodes of depression that alternate with episodes of mania. Although patients usually experience extreme episodes, periods may shift between

TABLE 16.2	Foods Containing Tyramine		
Fruits	**Dairy Products**	**Alcohol**	**Meats**
Avocados	Cheese (cottage cheese is okay)	Beer	Beef or chicken liver
Bananas	Sour cream	Wines (especially red wines)	Paté
Raisins	Yogurt		Meat extracts
Papaya products, including meat tenderizers			Pickled or kippered herring
Canned figs			Pepperoni
			Salami
			Sausage
			Bologna/hot dogs
Vegetables	**Sauces**	**Yeast**	**Other Foods to Avoid**
Pods of broad beans (fava beans)	Soy sauce	All yeast or yeast extracts	Chocolate

Pr Prototype Drug | Phenelzine *(Nardil)*

Therapeutic Class: Antidepressant   **Pharmacologic Class:** Monoamine oxidase inhibitor (MAOI)

ACTIONS AND USES

Phenelzine produces its effects by irreversible inhibition of monoamine oxidase; therefore, it intensifies the effects of norepinephrine in adrenergic synapses. It is used to manage symptoms of depression not responsive to other types of pharmacotherapy, and is occasionally used for panic disorder. Drug effects may persist for 2 to 3 weeks after therapy is discontinued.

ADMINISTRATION ALERTS

- Washout periods of 2 to 3 weeks are required before introducing other drugs.
- Abrupt discontinuation of this drug may cause rebound hypertension.
- Pregnancy category C

PHARMACOKINETICS
Onset: 2 weeks
Peak: Variable
Half-life: Variable
Duration: 48–96 h

ADVERSE EFFECTS

Common side effects are constipation, dry mouth, orthostatic hypotension, insomnia, nausea, and loss of appetite. It may increase heart rate and neural activity, leading to delirium, mania, anxiety, and convulsions. Severe hypertension may occur when ingesting foods containing tyramine. Seizures, respiratory depression, circulatory collapse, and coma may occur in cases of severe overdose.

Contraindications: Patients with cardiovascular or cerebrovascular disease, hepatic or renal impairment, and pheochromocytoma should not use this drug.

INTERACTIONS

Drug–Drug: Many other drugs affect the action of phenelzine. Concurrent use of tricyclic antidepressants and SSRIs should be avoided because the combination can cause temperature elevation and seizures. Opiates, including meperidine, should be avoided due to increased risk of respiratory failure or hypertensive crisis. Sympathomimetics may precipitate a hypertensive crisis. Caffeine may result in cardiac dysrhythmias and hypertension.

Lab Tests: Phenelzine can produce a slightly false increase in serum bilirubin. Since platelet functioning can be affected, careful attention should be devoted to CBC results.

Herbal/Food: Concurrent use of ginseng may cause headaches, tremors, mania, insomnia, irritability, and visual hallucinations. Concurrent use of ma huang, ephedra, or St. John's wort may result in a hypertensive crisis.

Treatment of Overdose: Intensive symptomatic and supportive treatment may be required. Induction of emesis or gastric lavage with instillation of charcoal slurry may be helpful. Signs and symptoms of CNS stimulation, including seizures, should be treated with IV diazepam, given very slowly. Hypertension should be treated appropriately with calcium channel blockers. Hypotension and vascular collapse should be treated with IV fluids and, if necessary, blood pressure titration with an IV infusion of a dilute pressor agent. Body temperature should be monitored closely, and respiration should be supported with appropriate measures.

Refer to MyNursingKit for a Nursing Process Focus specific to this drug.

---

extremes, or there may be prolonged times when mood is normal. Depressed symptoms and slightly depressed or dysphoric symptoms are the same collection of signs as are referred to earlier in this chapter. Mania is characterized by excessive CNS stimulation that results in symptoms listed in Section 16.7. To be diagnosed with bipolar disorder, manic symptoms must be present for at least 1 week. Hypomania is characterized by the same symptoms, but they are less severe. Mania and hypomania may result from abnormal functioning of neurotransmitters or receptors in the brain. Hypomania may involve an excess of excitatory neurotransmitters (such as norepinephrine or glutamate) or a deficiency of inhibitory neurotransmitters such as gamma-aminobutyric acid (GABA) (chapter 15∞). It is important to distinguish mania from the effects of drug use or abuse and also from schizophrenia (chapter 17∞).

16.7 Characteristics of Bipolar Disorder

During the depressive stages of bipolar disorder, patients exhibit the symptoms of major depression described ear-

lier in this chapter (section 16.1). Patients with bipolar disorder also display signs of **mania**, an emotional state characterized by high psychomotor activity and irritability. Symptoms of mania, as described in the following list, are generally the opposite of depressive symptoms:

- Inflated self-esteem or grandiosity
- Decreased need for sleep (e.g., feels rested after only 3 hours of sleep)
- Increased talkativeness or pressure to keep talking
- Flight of ideas or subjective feeling that thoughts are racing
- Distractibility (i.e., attention too easily drawn to unimportant or irrelevant external stimuli)
- Increased goal-directed activity (either socially, at work or school, or sexually) or psychomotor agitation
- Excessive involvement in pleasurable activities that have a high potential for painful consequences (e.g., unrestrained buying sprees, sexual indiscretions, or foolish business investments)

NURSING PROCESS FOCUS   PATIENTS RECEIVING ANTIDEPRESSANT THERAPY

Assessment	Potential Nursing Diagnoses
Baseline assessment prior to administration: ▪ Understand the reason the drug has been prescribed in order to assess for therapeutic effects. ▪ Obtain a complete health history including hepatic, renal, urologic, cardiovascular, or neurologic disease, current mental status, narrow-angle glaucoma, pregnancy, or breast-feeding. Obtain a drug history including allergies, current prescription and OTC drugs, and herbal preparations. Be alert to possible drug interactions. ▪ Obtain a history of depression or mood disorder, including a family history of same and severity. Use objective screening tools when possible (e.g., Beck Depression Inventory or Geriatric Depression Scale). If symptoms warrant, also consider use of the Mini Mental State Exam for dementia screening. ▪ Obtain baseline vital signs and weight. ▪ Evaluate appropriate laboratory findings (e.g., CBC, electrolytes, glucose, hepatic and renal function studies). ▪ Assess the patient's ability to receive and understand instruction. Include the family and caregivers as needed.	▪ Ineffective Coping ▪ Powerlessness ▪ Anxiety ▪ Disturbed Thought Processes ▪ Sleep Pattern Disturbance ▪ Deficient Self-Care ▪ Imbalanced Nutrition, More or Less Than Body Requirements ▪ Dysfunctional Grieving ▪ Social Isolation, Impaired Social Interaction ▪ Altered Family Processes ▪ Urinary Retention (related to anticholinergic side effects of drug therapy) ▪ Noncompliance (related to adverse drug effects of decreased sexual libido and/or weight gain) ▪ Deficient Knowledge (drug therapy) ▪ Risk for Self-Directed Violence, Risk for Self-Mutilation, Risk for Suicide, Risk for Injury
Assessment throughout administration: ▪ Assess for desired therapeutic effects (e.g., increased mood, lessening depression, increased activity level, return to normal ADLs, appetite and sleep patterns; if used for other uses, e.g., neuropathic pain, assess for appropriate therapeutic effects). ▪ Continue periodic monitoring of CBC, electrolytes, glucose, and hepatic and renal function studies. ▪ Assess vital signs and weight periodically or as symptoms warrant. ▪ Assess for and promptly report adverse effects: dizziness or light-headedness, drowsiness, confusion, agitation, suicidal ideations, palpitations, tachycardia, blurred or double vision, skin rashes, bruising or bleeding, abdominal pain, jaundice, change in color of stool, flank pain, and hematuria.	

Planning: Patient Goals and Expected Outcomes

The patient will:

▪ Experience therapeutic effects dependent on the reason the drug is being given (e.g., increased mood, lessened depression).
▪ Be free from, or experience minimal, adverse effects.
▪ Verbalize an understanding of the drug's use, adverse effects, and required precautions.
▪ Demonstrate proper self-administration of the medication (e.g., dose, timing, when to notify provider).

Implementation

Interventions and (Rationales)	Patient and Family Education
Ensuring therapeutic effects: ▪ Continue assessments as described earlier for therapeutic effects. (Drugs used for depression may take 2 to 8 weeks before full effects are realized. Use objective measures, e.g., Beck Depression Inventory, when possible to help quantify therapeutic results. For outpatient therapy, prescriptions may be limited to 7 days' worth of medication. Have the patient sign a "No Harm/No Suicide" contract as appropriate. When used for anxiety or insomnia, nonpharmacologic measures may be needed until the drug reaches full effects.)	▪ Teach the patient that full effects may not occur for a prolonged period of time but that some improvement should be noticeable after beginning therapy. ▪ Encourage the patient to keep all appointments with the therapist and to discuss ongoing symptoms of depression, reporting any suicidal ideations immediately.

(Continued)

NURSING PROCESS FOCUS   PATIENTS RECEIVING ANTIDEPRESSANT THERAPY *(Continued)*

Implementation

Interventions and (Rationales)	Patient and Family Education
Minimizing adverse effects: ■ Continue to monitor vital signs, mental status, and coordination and balance periodically. Ensure patient safety; monitor ambulation until the effects of the drug are known. Be particularly cautious with older adults who are at increased risk for falls. (Antidepressant drugs may cause drowsiness and dizziness, hypotension, or impaired mental and physical abilities, increasing the risk of falls and injury.)	■ Teach the patient to rise from lying or sitting to standing slowly to avoid dizziness or falls. ■ Instruct the patient to call for assistance prior to getting out of bed or attempting to walk alone, and to avoid driving or other activities requiring mental alertness or physical coordination until effects of the drug are known.
■ Continue to monitor CBC, electrolytes, and renal and hepatic function. (Antidepressant drugs may cause hepatotoxicity as an adverse effect.)	■ Instruct the patient on the need to return periodically for lab work. ■ Teach the patient to promptly report any abdominal pain, particularly in the upper quadrants, changes in stool color, yellowing of sclera or skin, or darkened urine.
■ Assess for changes in level of consciousness, disorientation or confusion, or agitation. (Neurologic changes may indicate under or overmedication, exacerbation of other psychiatric illness, or adverse drug effects.)	■ Instruct the patient, family, or caregiver to immediately report increasing lethargy, disorientation, confusion, changes in behavior or mood, agitation or aggression, slurred speech, or ataxia.
■ Assess for changes in visual acuity, blurred vision, loss of peripheral vision, seeing rainbow halos around lights, acute eye pain, or these symptoms accompanied by nausea and vomiting, and report immediately. (Increased intraoptic pressure in patients with narrow-angle glaucoma may occur in patients taking TCAs.)	■ Instruct the patient to immediately report any visual changes or eye pain.
■ Monitor cardiovascular status. (Early signs of SES and hypertensive crisis with MAOI therapy include rapid increases in blood pressure and pulse.	■ Instruct the patient to immediately report severe headache, dizziness, paresthesias, palpitations, tachycardia, chest pain, nausea or vomiting, diaphoresis, or fever.
■ Assess for bruising, bleeding, or signs of infection. (TCAs may cause blood dyscrasias and increased chances of bleeding or infection.)	■ Teach the patient to promptly report any signs of increased bruising, bleeding, or infections (e.g., sore throat and fever, skin rash).
■ Assess for dry mouth, blurred vision, urinary retention, and sexual dysfunction. (Anticholinergic-like effects and sexual dysfunction, including loss of libido and impotence, are common antidepressant adverse effects. Tolerance to anticholinergic effects usually develops in 2 to 4 weeks.)	■ Teach the patient to use ice chips, frequent sips of water, or chewing gum or hard candy to alleviate dry mouth and to avoid alcohol-based mouthwashes, which may increase dryness. ■ Use of "dry eye" drops and resting eyes periodically may help to decrease dry eye feeling. Teach the patient to report any feelings of scratchiness or eye pain immediately. ■ Instruct the patient to promptly report difficulty with urination, hesitancy, or dysuria. ■ Encourage the patient to discuss concerns about sexual functioning and refer to the health care provider if concerns affect medication compliance. ■ Encourage appropriate lifestyle and dietary changes to reduce the likelihood of weight gain: increased intake of fruits and vegetables, increased activity and exercise levels as depression lifts, abstinence from alcohol, and avoiding large meals before bedtime.
■ For patients taking MAOIs, assess usual dietary intake and provide instruction on foods, beverages, and medications to exclude. (Foods and beverages containing tyramine, alcohol, CNS stimulants and adrenergic-like drugs, narcotics, and other CNS depressants may cause significant adverse effects including hypertensive crisis or profound hypotension.)	■ Instruct the patient, family, or caregiver in dietary and medication restrictions. Provide written and verbal instruction. ■ Instruct the patient to immediately report severe headache, dizziness, paresthesias, palpitations, tachycardia, chest pain, nausea or vomiting, diaphoresis, or fever.
■ Avoid abrupt discontinuation of therapy. (Profound depression, seizures, or withdrawal symptoms may occur with abrupt discontinuation.)	■ Instruct the patient to take the drug exactly as prescribed and to not stop it abruptly.

NURSING PROCESS FOCUS   **PATIENTS RECEIVING ANTIDEPRESSANT THERAPY** *(Continued)*

Implementation

Interventions and (Rationales)	Patient and Family Education
Patient understanding of drug therapy: ■ Use opportunities during administration of medications and during assessments to discuss rationale for drug therapy, desired therapeutic outcomes, most commonly observed adverse effects, parameters for when to call the health care provider, and any necessary monitoring or precautions. (Using time during nursing care helps to optimize and reinforce key teaching areas.)	■ The patient should be able to state the reason for the drug; appropriate dose and scheduling; and what adverse effects to observe for and when to report them.

Patient self-administration of drug therapy:
■ When administering the medication, instruct the patient, family, or caregiver in proper self-administration of drug, e.g., take the drug as prescribed and do not substitute brands. (Utilizing time during nurse-administration of these drugs helps to reinforce teaching.)
	■ Teach the patient to take the medication as follows:
	  ■ Take exactly as ordered and use the same manufacturer's brand each time the prescription is filled. (Switching brands may result in differing pharmacokinetics and alterations in therapeutic effect.)
	  ■ Take a missed dose as soon as it is noticed but do not take double or extra doses to "catch up."
	  ■ Take with food to decrease GI upset.
	  ■ If medication causes drowsiness, take at bedtime.
	  ■ Do not abruptly discontinue medication.

Evaluation of Outcome Criteria

Evaluate effectiveness of drug therapy by confirming that patient goals and expected outcomes have been met (see "Planning").

See Table 16.1 for a list of drugs to which these nursing actions apply.

DRUGS FOR BIPOLAR DISORDER

Drugs for bipolar disorder are called **mood stabilizers**, because they have the ability to moderate extreme shifts in emotions between mania and depression. Antiseizure drugs and atypical antipsychotic drugs are also used for mood stabilization in bipolar patients.

16.8 Pharmacotherapy of Bipolar Disorder

For years, the traditional treatment of bipolar disorder has been lithium (Eskalith), as monotherapy or in combination with other drugs. Lithium was approved in the United States in 1970. Today, in addition to lithium, antiseizure drugs, have emerged as very effective agents employed for mood stabilization (chapter 15∞). For example, valproic acid (Depakene) and carbamazepine (Tegretol) are the antiseizure drugs most often used in the treatment of mania or for rapidly cycling and mixed states of bipolar disease. Lithium remains effective for states of purely manic or purely depressive episodes. For purely depressive episodes however, the newer antiseizure drugs, for example, lamotrigine (Lamictal), may be even more effective than lithium. Lamotrigine is particularly helpful for patients who have experienced chronic depression and have not received effective treatment with the other mood stabilizers. Table 16.3 lists selected drugs used to treat bipolar disorder. In addition to the listed antiseizure agents, gabapentin (Neurontin), oxcarbazepine (Trileptal), topiramate (Topamax), and zon-isamide (Zonegran) all have beneficial effects for mood stabilization (chapter 15∞).

Atypical antipsychotics have been effective mood stabilizers especially for the treatment of acute mania. Clozapine (Clozaril) was the first atypical antipsychotic but carries an increased risk of agranulocytosis. Newer agents with less of risk for agranulocytosis including aripiprazole (Abilify), olanzapine (Zyprexa), quetiapine (Seroquel), risperidone (Risperdal), and ziprasidone (Zeldox), have replaced Clorazil in bipolar treatment. Longer-term stabilization of mood and behavior with atypical antipsychotics is discussed in more detail in chapter 17∞.

Given that lithium is still in use, it is necessary to profile this drug. Lithium has a narrow therapeutic index and is monitored via serum levels every 1 to 3 days when beginning therapy, and every 2 to 3 months thereafter. To ensure therapeutic action, concentrations of lithium in the blood must remain within the range of 0.6 to 1.5 mEq/L. Close monitoring encourages compliance and helps prevent toxicity. Lithium acts like sodium in the body, so conditions in which sodium is lost (e.g., excessive sweating or dehydration) can cause lithium toxicity and serum sodium levels will be monitored along with lithium levels. Lithium overdose may be treated with hemodialysis and supportive care. Baseline studies of renal, cardiac, and thyroid status are indicated, as well as baseline electrolyte studies.

It is not unusual for other drugs to be used in combination with lithium for the control of bipolar disorder. During a patient's depressed stage, tricyclic antidepressants or bupropion (Wellbutrin) may be necessary. During the

TABLE 16.3	Drugs for Bipolar Disorder	
Drug	Route and Adult Dose (max dose where indicated)	Adverse Effects
lithium (Eskalith)	PO; initial: 600 mg tid; maintenance: 300 mg tid (max: 2.4 g/day)	*Headache, lethargy, fatigue, recent memory loss, nausea, vomiting, anorexia, abdominal pain, diarrhea, dry mouth, muscle weakness, hand tremors, reversible leukocytosis, nephrogenic diabetes insipidus* Peripheral circulatory collapse
ANTISEIZURE DRUGS		
carbamazepine (Tegretol)	PO; 200 mg bid, gradually increased to 800–1,200 mg/day in three to four divided doses	*Dizziness, ataxia, somnolence, headache, nausea, diplopia, blurred vision, sedation, drowsiness, nausea, vomiting, prolonged bleeding time* Heart block, aplastic anemia, respiratory depression, exfoliative dermatitis, Stevens–Johnson syndrome, toxic epidermal necrolysis, deep coma, death (with overdose), liver failure, pancreatitis
lamotrigine (Lamictal)	PO; 50 mg/day for 2 weeks, then 50 mg bid for 2 weeks; may increase gradually up to 300–500 mg/day in two divided doses (max: 700 mg/day)	
valproic acid (Depakene) (see page 176 for the Prototype Drug box ∞)	PO; 250 mg tid (max: 60 mg/kg/day)	
ATYPICAL ANTIPSYCHOTIC DRUGS		
aripiprazole (Abilify)	PO; 10–15 mg/day (max: 30 mg/day)	*Tachycardia, transient fever, sedation, dizziness, headache, light-headedness, somnolence, anxiety, nervousness, hostility, insomnia, nausea, vomiting, constipation, parkinsonism, akathisia* Agranulocytosis, neuroleptic malignant syndrome (rare)
olanzapine (Zyprexa)	Adult: PO; start with 5–10 mg/day; may increase by 2.5–5 mg every week (range 10–15 mg/day; max: 20 mg/day). Geriatric: PO; start with 5 mg/day	
quetiapine fumarate (Seroquel)	PO; start with 25 mg bid; may increase to a target dose of 300–400 mg/day in divided doses	
risperidone (Risperdal)	PO; 1–6 mg bid; increase by 2 mg daily to an initial target dose of 6 mg/day	
ziprasidone (Geodon)	PO; 20 mg bid (max: 80 mg bid)	

Italics indicate common adverse effects; underlining indicates serious adverse effects.

Pr Prototype Drug | Lithium *(Eskalith)*

Therapeutic Class: Mood stabilizing drug; bipolar affective disorder drug

Pharmacologic Class: Glutamate inhibitor; serotonin receptor antagonist

ACTIONS AND USES

Although the exact mechanism of action is not clear, lithium has been thought to alter ionic activity and the activities of neurons containing dopamine, norepinephrine, and serotonin by influencing their release, synthesis, and reuptake. More recent studies suggest that lithium may inhibit the action of glutamate, an excitatory neurotransmitter in the synapse. Other promising information indicates that serotonin at the receptor may be blocked and that glycogen synthase kinase-3 beta may be inhibited within the neuron. These actions tend to stabilize a wider range of cellular transduction pathways. Therapeutic actions are stabilization of mood during periods of mania, and antidepressant effects during periods of depression. Lithium has neither antimanic nor antidepressant properties in individuals who do not have bipolar disorder. After taking lithium for 2 to 3 weeks, patients should be able to better concentrate and function in self-care.

ADMINISTRATION ALERTS

- Lithium has a narrow therapeutic/toxic ratio; the risk of toxicity is high.
- Acute overdosage may be treated by hemodialysis.
- Pregnancy category D

PHARMACOKINETICS
Onset: 5–7 days   **Peak:** 10–21 days
Half-life: 20–27 h   **Duration:** Variable

ADVERSE EFFECTS

Lithium may cause dizziness, fatigue, short-term memory loss, increased urination, nausea, vomiting, loss of appetite, abdominal pain, diarrhea, dry mouth, muscular weakness, and slight tremors. Patients should not have a salt-free diet when taking this drug, because it reduces lithium excretion.

Contraindications: This drug is contraindicated in debilitated patients and patients with severe cardiovascular disease, dehydration, or renal disease, and in cases of severe sodium depletion.

INTERACTIONS

Drug–Drug: Some drugs increase the rate at which the kidneys remove lithium from the bloodstream, including diuretics, sodium bicarbonate, and potassium citrate. Other drugs, such as methyldopa and probenecid, inhibit the rate of lithium excretion. Diuretics enhance excretion of sodium and increase the risk of lithium toxicity. Concurrent administration of anticholinergic drugs can cause urinary retention that, coupled with the polyuria effect of lithium, may cause a medical emergency. Alcohol can potentiate drug action.

Lab Tests: Unknown

Herbal/Food: Unknown

Treatment of Overdose: There is no specific treatment for overdose. Treatment is supportive, including gastric lavage, correction of fluid and electrolyte imbalance, and regulation of renal functioning. Hemodialysis is an effective and rapid means of removing the ion from the severely toxic patient; however, recovery time may be prolonged.

NURSING PROCESS FOCUS   PATIENTS RECEIVING THERAPY FOR BIPOLAR DISORDER (ESKALITH)

Assessment	Potential Nursing Diagnoses
Baseline assessment prior to administration: ■ Understand the reason the drug has been prescribed in order to assess for therapeutic effects. ■ Obtain a complete health history including hepatic, renal, cardiovascular, or neurologic disease. Obtain a drug history including allergies, current prescription and OTC drugs, and herbal preparations. Be alert to possible drug interactions. ■ Obtain a history of depression or mood disorder, including a family history of same and severity. Use objective screening tools when possible (e.g., Beck Depression Inventory). ■ Obtain baseline vital signs and weight. ■ Evaluate appropriate laboratory findings (e.g., electrolytes [especially sodium], CBC, hepatic and renal function studies). ■ Assess the patient's ability to receive and understand instruction. Include the family and caregivers as needed.	■ Anxiety ■ Disturbed Thought Processes ■ Sleep Pattern Disturbance ■ Deficient Self-Care ■ Imbalanced Nutrition, More or Less Than Body Requirements (especially sodium) ■ Social Isolation, Impaired Social Interaction ■ Altered Family Processes ■ Deficient Knowledge (drug therapy) ■ Risk for Self-Directed Violence, Risk for Self-Mutilation, Risk for Suicide, Risk for Injury
Assessment throughout administration: ■ Assess for desired therapeutic effects (e.g., stabilized mood, lessening depression, normalized activity levels, appetite, and sleep patterns). ■ Continue periodic monitoring of electrolytes, CBC, and hepatic and renal function studies. Drug levels will be monitored frequently or as symptoms warrant. ■ Continue to monitor vital signs and weight. ■ Assess for and promptly report adverse effects: dizziness, drowsiness, light-headedness, fatigue, muscle weakness, slight tremors, thirst, nausea, vomiting, diarrhea, dry mouth, increased urinary output, short-term memory loss, and tachycardia.	

Planning: Patient Goals and Expected Outcomes

The patient will:
■ Experience therapeutic effects dependent on the reason the drug is being given (e.g., improved and stabilized mood, lessened depression).
■ Be free from, or experience minimal, adverse effects.
■ Verbalize an understanding of the drug's use, adverse effects, and required precautions.
■ Demonstrate proper self-administration of the medication (e.g., dose, timing, when to notify provider).

Implementation

Interventions and (Rationales)	Patient and Family Education
Ensuring therapeutic effects: ■ Continue assessments as described earlier for therapeutic effects. (Lithium may take 2 to 3 weeks before full effects are realized. Use objective measures, e.g., Beck Depression Inventory, when possible to help quantify therapeutic results. Have the patient sign a "No Harm/No Suicide" contract as appropriate.)	■ Teach the patient that full effects may not occur for several weeks but that some improvement should be noticeable after beginning therapy. ■ Encourage the patient to keep all appointments with the therapist and to discuss ongoing symptoms of depression and mania, and immediately report any suicidal ideations.
Minimizing adverse effects: ■ Continue to monitor drug levels, electrolytes (especially sodium), CBC, and renal and hepatic function. Maintain a normal fluid balance. (Lithium is an elemental salt and the body will conserve or lose lithium related to the sodium level. Serum sodium should be drawn with each drug level. Dehydration or overhydration will also result in loss or gain of lithium.)	■ Instruct the patient on the need to return periodically for lab work. ■ Instruct the patient to maintain a normal salt and fluid intake, without unusual or dramatic increases or decreases in normal diet. ■ Teach the patient that conditions such as dehydration may result in abnormal drug levels and to immediately report any symptoms such as thirst, dizziness, confusion, or muscle weakness and to be cautious with exercising or on hot days, as excessive sweating may lead to fluid and sodium loss. Report excessive thirst or urination promptly.

(Continued)

NURSING PROCESS FOCUS   PATIENTS RECEIVING THERAPY FOR BIPOLAR DISORDER (ESKALITH) *(Continued)*

Implementation

Interventions and (Rationales)	Patient and Family Education
■ Weigh the patient daily and report a weight gain or loss of 1 kg (approximately 2 lb) or more in a 24-hour period. Measure intake and output in the hospitalized patient. (Daily weight is an accurate measure of fluid status and takes into account intake, output, and insensible losses. Diuresis is indicated by output significantly greater than intake.)	■ Have the patient weigh self daily, ideally at the same time of day, and record weight. Have the patient report a weight loss or gain of more than 1 kg (approximately 2 lb) in a 24-hour period. ■ Advise the patient to continue to consume enough liquids to remain adequately, but not overly, hydrated. Drinking when thirsty, avoiding alcoholic beverages and caffeine, and ensuring adequate but not excessive salt intake will assist in maintaining a normal fluid and drug balance.
■ Assess for changes in level of consciousness, disorientation or confusion, or agitation. (Neurologic changes may indicate under- or overmedication, exacerbation of other psychiatric illness, or adverse drug effects.)	■ Instruct the patient, family, or caregiver to immediately report increasing lethargy, disorientation, confusion, changes in behavior or mood, agitation or aggression, slurred speech, or ataxia.
■ Monitor renal status, CBC, BUN, creatinine, uric acid, and urinalysis. (Lithium may cause degenerative changes in the kidney, which increases drug toxicity.)	■ Instruct the patient to promptly report decreased urine output, hematuria, or urine sediment; lower abdominal tenderness or flank pain; nausea; or diarrhea to the health care provider.
■ Continue to monitor cardiovascular status including vital signs and apical pulse. (Lithium toxicity may result in cardiac dysrhythmias or angina. Use with caution in patients with a history of coronary artery disease or heart disease.)	■ Instruct the patient to immediately report palpitations, chest pressure, or pain, especially if accompanied by dyspnea; or diaphoresis.
Patient understanding of drug therapy: ■ Use opportunities during administration of medications and during assessments to discuss rationale for drug therapy, desired therapeutic outcomes, most commonly observed adverse effects, parameters for when to call the health care provider, and any necessary monitoring or precautions. (Using time during nursing care helps to optimize and reinforce key teaching areas.)	■ The patient should be able to state the reason for the drug; appropriate dose and scheduling; and what adverse effects to observe for and when to report them.
Patient self-administration of drug therapy: ■ When administering the medication, instruct the patient, family, or caregiver in the proper self-administration of drug, e.g., take the drug as prescribed and do not substitute brands. (Utilizing time during nurse-administration of these drugs helps to reinforce teaching.)	■ Teach the patient to take the medication as follows: 　■ Take exactly as ordered and use the same manufacturer's brand each time the prescription is filled. (Switching brands may result in differing pharmacokinetics and alterations in therapeutic effect). 　■ Take a missed dose as soon as it is noticed but do not take double or extra doses to "catch up." 　■ Take with food to decrease GI upset. 　■ Do not abruptly discontinue medication. ■ Immediately report any increase in dilute urine, diarrhea, fever, or changes in mobility. ■ Drink plenty of fluids to avoid dehydration. ■ Practice reliable contraception and notify your health care provider if pregnancy is planned or suspected.

Evaluation of Outcome Criteria

Evaluate effectiveness of drug therapy by confirming that patient goals and expected outcomes have been met (see "Planning").

manic phases, a benzodiazepine will moderate manic symptoms. In cases of extreme agitation, delusions, or hallucinations, an antipsychotic agent may be indicated. Continued patient compliance is essential to achieving successful pharmacotherapy, because some patients do not perceive their condition as abnormal. To prevent relapse, psychologic therapies and sleep management are considered extremely critical components of bipolar disorder therapy.

PharmFacts

Attention Deficit–Hyperactivity Disorder
■ ADHD is the major reason children are referred for mental health treatment.
■ About half are also diagnosed with oppositional defiant or conduct disorder.
■ About one fourth are also diagnosed with anxiety disorder.
■ About one third are also diagnosed with depression.
■ About one fifth also have a learning disability.

ATTENTION DEFICIT–HYPERACTIVITY DISORDER

A condition characterized by poor attention span, behavior control issues, and/or hyperactivity is called **attention deficit–hyperactivity disorder (ADHD)**. Although the condition is normally diagnosed in childhood, symptoms of ADHD may extend into adulthood.

16.9 Characteristics of ADHD

In reality, ADHD is neither an emotional disorder nor a mood disorder. It is rather a behavioral disorder that affects as many as 5% of all children. Most children diagnosed with this condition are between the ages of 3 and 7 years, and boys are 4 to 8 times more likely to be diagnosed than girls.

ADHD is characterized by developmentally inappropriate behaviors involving difficulty in paying attention or focusing on tasks. ADHD may be diagnosed when the child's hyperactive behaviors significantly interfere with normal play, sleep, or learning activities. Hyperactive children usually have increased motor activity that is manifested by a tendency to be fidgety and impulsive, and to interrupt and talk excessively during their developmental years; therefore, they may not be able to interact with others appropriately at home, school, or on the playground. In boys, the activity levels are usually more overt. Girls show less aggression and impulsiveness but more anxiety, mood swings, social withdrawal, and cognitive and language delays. Girls also tend to be older at the time of diagnosis, so problems and setbacks related to the disorder exist for a longer time before treatment interventions are undertaken. Symptoms of ADHD are described in the following list:

- Easy distractibility
- Failure to receive or follow instructions properly
- Inability to focus on one task at a time and jumping from one activity to another
- Difficulty remembering
- Frequent loss or misplacement of personal items
- Excessive talking and interrupting other children in a group
- Inability to sit still when asked to do so repeatedly
- Impulsiveness
- Sleep disturbance

Most children with ADHD have associated challenges. Many find it difficult to concentrate on tasks assigned in school. Even if children are gifted, their grades may suffer because they have difficulty following a conventional routine; discipline may also be a problem. Teachers are often the first to suggest that a child be examined for ADHD and receive medication when behaviors in the classroom escalate to the point of interfering with learning. A diagnosis is based on psychologic and medical evaluations.

The etiology of ADHD is not clear. For many years, scientists described this disorder as mental brain dysfunction and hyperkinetic syndrome, focusing on abnormal brain function and overactivity. A variety of physical and neurologic disorders have been implicated; only a small percentage of those affected have a known cause. Causes include contact with high levels of lead in childhood and prenatal exposure to alcohol and drugs. Genetic factors may also play a role, although a single gene has not been isolated and a specific mechanism of genetic transmission is not known. The interplay of genetics and environment may be a contributing dynamic. Recent evidence suggests that hyperactivity may be related to a deficit or dysfunction of dopamine, norepinephrine, or serotonin in the reticular activating system of the brain. Although once thought to be the culprits, sugars, chocolate, high-carbohydrate foods and beverages, and certain food additives have been refuted as causative or aggravating factors for ADHD.

The nurse is often involved in the screening and the mental health assessment of children with suspected ADHD. When a child is referred for testing, it is important to remember that both the child and family must be assessed. The family is screened with, or prior to, the child's evaluation. It is the nurse's responsibility to collect comprehensive data about the character and extent of the child's physical, psychologic, and developmental health situation, to formulate the nursing diagnoses, and to create an individualized plan of care. A relevant nursing care plan can be created only if it is based on appropriate communication that fosters rapport and trust.

Once ADHD is diagnosed, the nurse is instrumental in educating the family regarding behavioral strategies that might be used to manage the demands of a child who is hyperactive. For the school-age child, the nurse often serves as the liaison to parents, teachers, and school administrators. The parents and child need to understand the importance of appropriate expectations and behavioral consequences. The child, from an early age and based on his or her developmental level, must be educated about the disorder and understand that there are consequences to inappropriate behavior. Self-esteem must be fostered in the child so that strengths in self-worth can develop. It is important for the child to develop a trusting relationship with health care providers and learn the importance of medication management and compliance.

One third to one half of children diagnosed with ADHD also experience symptoms of attention dysfunction in their adult years. Symptoms of attention deficit disorder (ADD) in adults appear similar to mood disorders. Symptoms include anxiety, mania, restlessness, and depression, which can cause difficulties in interpersonal relationships. Some patients have difficulty holding jobs and may have an increased risk for alcohol and drug abuse. Untreated ADD or ADHD has been linked to low self-esteem, diminished social success, and criminal or violent behaviors.

DRUGS FOR ATTENTION DEFICIT–HYPERACTIVITY DISORDER

The traditional drugs used to treat ADHD in children have been the CNS stimulants. These drugs stimulate specific areas of the central nervous system that heighten alertness and increase focus. Recently, a non-CNS stimulant was approved to treat ADHD. Agents for treating ADHD are listed in Table 16.4.

TABLE 16.4	Drugs for Attention Deficit–Hyperactivity Disorder	
Drug	Route and Adult Dose (max dose where indicated)	Adverse Effects
CNS STIMULANTS		
D- and L-amphetamine racemic mixture (Adderall) (also available as Adderall-XR)	6 years old: PO; 5 mg one or two times/day; may increase by 5 mg at weekly intervals (max: 40 mg/day). 3–5 years old: PO; 2.5 mg one to two times/day; may increase by 2.5 mg at weekly intervals	*Irritability, nervousness, restlessness, insomnia, euphoria, palpitations*
benzphetamine (Didrex)	PO: 25–50 mg 1–3 times per day (max: 150 mg/day)	Sudden death (reported in children with structural cardiac abnormalities), circulatory collapse, exfoliative dermatitis, anorexia, liver failure
dexmethylphenidate (Focalin)	Child older than 6 years: PO: 2.5 mg bid may increase by 2.5–5 mg/week (max: 20 mg/day); 5 mg/day extended release may increase by 5 mg/week	
	Adult: PO: 2.5 mg bid; may increase by 2.5–5 mg/day at weekly intervals (max: 20 mg/day)	
dextroamphetamine (Dexedrine) (also available as DextroStat and Dexedrine Spansules)	3–5 years old: PO; 2.5 mg one or two times/day; may increase by 2.5 mg at weekly intervals	
	6 years old: PO; 5 mg one or two times/day; increase by 5 mg at weekly intervals (max: 40 mg/day)	
lisdexamfetamine (Vyvanse)	PO: 30 mg once daily in the a.m. (max: 70 mg/day)	
methamphetamine (Desoxyn)	6 years old: PO; 2.5–5 mg one or two times/day; may increase by 5 mg at weekly intervals (max: 20–25 mg/day)	
(Pr) methylphenidate (Ritalin)	PO; 5–10 mg before breakfast and lunch, with gradual increase of 5–10 mg/week as needed (max: 60 mg/day)	
NONSTIMULANT FOR ADD/ADHD		
atomoxetine (Strattera)	Adolescents and children less than 70 kg: PO; 0.5 mg/kg/day initially, may be increased every 3 days to a target dose of 1.2 mg/kg given either once in the morning or divided doses in the morning and late afternoon/early evening; may increase to max of 1.4 mg/kg or 100 mg/day, whichever is less	*Headache, insomnia, upper abdominal pain, vomiting, decreased appetite* Severe liver injury (rare)

Italics indicate common adverse effects, underlining indicates serious adverse effects.

(Pr) Prototype Drug | Methylphenidate *(Ritalin)*

Therapeutic Class: Attention deficit–hyperactivity disorder drug

Pharmacologic Class: Central nervous system (CNS) stimulant

ACTIONS AND USES
Methylphenidate activates the reticular activating system, causing heightened alertness in various regions of the brain, particularly those centers associated with focus and attention. Activation is partially achieved by the release of neurotransmitters such as norepinephrine and dopamine. Impulsiveness, hyperactivity, and disruptive behavior are usually reduced within a few weeks. These changes promote improved psychosocial interactions and academic performance. A transdermal, extended release form of methyphenidate was approved in 2006 (Daytrana).

ADMINISTRATION ALERTS
- Sustained-release tablets must be swallowed whole. Breaking or crushing SR tablets causes immediate release of the entire dose.
- Controlled substance: Schedule II drug
- Pregnancy category C

PHARMACOKINETICS
Onset: Less than 60 min

Peak: 2 h; 3–8 sustained release

Half-life: 2–4 h

Duration: 3–6 h; 8 h sustained release; 8–12 h extended release

ADVERSE EFFECTS
In a non-ADHD patient, methylphenidate causes nervousness and insomnia. All patients are at risk for irregular heart beat, high blood pressure, and liver toxicity. Because methylphenidate is a Schedule II drug, it has the potential for causing dependence when used for extended periods. Periodic drug-free "holidays" are recommended to reduce drug dependence and to assess the patient's condition.

Contraindications: Patients with a history of marked anxiety, agitation, psychosis, suicidal ideation, glaucoma, motor tics, or Tourette's disease should not use this drug.

INTERACTIONS
Drug–Drug: Methylphenidate interacts with many drugs. For example, it may decrease the effectiveness of anticonvulsants, anticoagulants, and guanethidine. Concurrent therapy with clonidine may increase adverse effects. Antihypertensives or other CNS stimulants could potentiate the vasoconstrictive action of methylphenidate. MAOIs may produce hypertensive crisis.

Lab Tests: Unknown

Herbal/Food: Administration times relative to meals and meal composition may need individual titration.

Treatment of Overdose: There is no specific treatment for overdose. Signs and symptoms of acute overdose result principally from overstimulation of the CNS and from excessive sympathomimetic effects. Emergency medical attention and general supportive measures may be necessary.

NURSING PROCESS FOCUS   PATIENTS RECEIVING TREATMENT FOR ADHD, ADD

Assessment	Potential Nursing Diagnoses
Baseline assessment prior to administration: ▪ Understand the reason the drug has been prescribed in order to assess for therapeutic effects. ▪ Obtain a complete health history including hepatic, renal, cardiovascular, or neurologic disease, including epilepsy. Obtain a drug history including allergies, current prescription and OTC drugs, and herbal preparations. Be alert to possible drug interactions. ▪ Obtain a social and behavioral history. Use objective screening tools when possible. ▪ Obtain a nutritional history and assess normal sleep patterns. ▪ Obtain baseline vital signs, and height and weight. ▪ Evaluate appropriate laboratory findings (e.g., electrolytes, CBC, hepatic and renal function studies). ▪ Assess the patient's ability to receive and understand instruction. Include the family and caregivers as needed.	▪ Imbalanced Nutrition, Less Than Body Requirements ▪ Disturbed Sleep Pattern ▪ Altered Family Processes ▪ Deficient Knowledge ▪ Risk for Delayed Growth and Development (related to condition or to adverse drug effects) ▪ Risk for Social Isolation, Risk for Impaired Social Interaction
Assessment throughout administration: ▪ Assess for desired therapeutic effects (e.g., increased ability to focus, normalized activity levels with lessened impulsivity, maintenance of normal appetite and sleep patterns). ▪ Continue periodic monitoring of electrolytes, CBC, and hepatic and renal function studies. ▪ Continue to monitor vital signs, and height and weight weekly. ▪ Assess for and promptly report adverse effects: dizziness, light-headedness, anxiety, agitation, excessive physical activity, tachycardia, increased blood pressure, hypertension, and palpitations.	

Planning: Patient Goals and Expected Outcomes

The patient will:
▪ Experience therapeutic effects dependent on the reason the drug is being given (e.g., improved ability to focus, lessened pyschomotor symptoms).
▪ Be free from, or experience minimal, adverse effects.
▪ Verbalize an understanding of the drug's use, adverse effects, and required precautions.
▪ Demonstrate proper self-administration of the medication (e.g., dose, timing, when to notify provider).

Implementation

Interventions and (Rationales)	Patient and Family Education
Ensuring therapeutic effects: ▪ Continue assessments as described earlier for therapeutic effects. (Therapeutic effects include the ability to focus and stay-on-task, lessened impulsivity, and improved social interactions.)	▪ Teach the patient, family, or caregiver to keep a social/behavioral diary. Involve school faculty and other caregivers (e.g., after-school care).
▪ Continue to monitor the pulse and blood pressure on health care visits. (Tachycardia, increased blood pressure, or hypertension may occur if the dose is excessive.)	▪ Teach the patient, family, or caregiver to take the pulse along with weekly height and weight or any time symptoms warrant (e.g., child complains of chest discomfort or palpitations). Assist the patient, family, or caregiver to find pulse location most easily felt and have the patient, family, or caregiver return-demonstrate pulse taking before going home.
▪ Weigh the patient weekly and obtain the patient's height. Report any weight loss or failure to gain weight during the expected growth periods. Assess nutrition and use of other stimulating products (e.g., "energy drinks," caffeinated beverages). (Diminished appetite or anorexia from stimulating effects of the drug, or use of other stimulants, may impair the normal nutrition needed for growth and development.)	▪ Teach the patient, family, or caregiver to obtain height and weight weekly and to report any loss of weight or lack of expected growth. Ensure the proper use and functioning of any home equipment used (e.g., electronic scale). ▪ Discuss the need to avoid or eliminate all foods, beverages, or OTC drugs that contain caffeine or other stimulants.

(Continued)

Implementation

Interventions and (Rationales)	Patient and Family Education
■ Continue to monitor sleep patterns. (Stimulatory effects of drug may affect normal sleeping patterns and may indicate excessive dosage.)	■ Instruct the patient, family, or caregiver to inform the provider of disruption to sleep, increased agitation during the day (possible effect from lack of sleep), or excessive sleepiness during the day. ■ Have the patient take the dose early in the day and before 4:00 p.m. to help alleviate insomnia unless extended-release formulation is used. Take extended-release formulations in the morning.
■ Assess for excessive stimulatory effects: agitation, aggression, tremors, or seizures and report immediately. (Excessive CNS stimulation may cause seizures as an adverse effect.)	■ Instruct the patient, family, or caregiver to immediately report tremors or seizures to the health care provider.
■ Assess the need for continuous medication or need for drug holidays with the patient, family, caregiver, and health care provider based on the social/behavioral diary findings. (Dependent on the degree of behavior, drug holidays over non–school days or vacation periods may be recommended.)	■ Teach the patient, family, or caregiver about the use of drug holidays and explore options. If the drug dose is at the upper range of dose, consider tapering the dose prior to beginning the drug holiday to avoid rebound hyperactivity or agitation.
■ Assess the home environment for medication safety and the need for appropriate interventions. Advise the family on restrictions about prescription renewal. (Methylphenidate is a Schedule II drug and may not be used by any other person than the patient. Safeguard medication in the home to prevent overdosage.)	■ Instruct the patient, family, or caregiver in proper medication storage and the need for the drug to be used by the patient only. ■ Teach the family or caregiver about prescription renewal restrictions (i.e., new prescription each time, no refills, prescription may not be called in) and explore school policies regarding in-school use (e.g., single-dose sent each day, secured blister-pack used if multidoses sent).
Patient understanding of drug therapy: ■ Use opportunities during administration of medications and during assessments to discuss the rationale for drug therapy, desired therapeutic outcomes, most commonly observed adverse effects, parameters for when to call the health care provider, and any necessary monitoring or precautions. (Using time during nursing care helps to optimize and reinforce key teaching areas.)	■ The patient, family, or caregiver should be able to state the reason for the drug; appropriate dose and scheduling; and what adverse effects to observe for and when to report and when to report them.

Patient self-administration of drug therapy:
■ When administering the medication, instruct the patient, family, or caregiver in the proper self-administration of drug, e.g., take the drug as prescribed and do not substitute brands. (Utilizing time during nurse-administration of these drugs helps to reinforce teaching.)
	■ Teach the patient to take the medication as follows:
	  ■ Take exactly as ordered and in the morning to prevent insomnia.
	  ■ Do not take double or extra doses to increase mental focus or to prevent sleepiness. The drug will not achieve these effects but will increase the adverse effects of the drug.
	  ■ Do not abruptly discontinue the medication without consulting the health care provider.

Evaluation of Outcome Criteria

Evaluate effectiveness of drug therapy by confirming that patient goals and expected outcomes have been met (see "Planning").

16.10 Pharmacotherapy of ADHD

The main treatment for ADHD are CNS stimulants. Stimulants reverse many of the symptoms, helping patients focus on tasks. Drugs prescribed for ADHD include D- and L-amphetamine racemic mixture (Adderall), benzphetamine (Didrex), dexmethylphenidate (Focalin), dextroamphetamine (Dexedrine), lisdexamfetamine (Vyvanse), methamphetamine (Desoxyn) and methylphenidate (Ritalin). Intermediate- and longer-release forms of methylphenidate, marketed as Concerta, Metadate, and Methylin, are available. For greater flexibility in dosing, a methylphenidate patch marketed as Daytrana was approved by the FDA in 2006.

Patients taking CNS stimulants must be carefully monitored. CNS stimulants used to treat ADHD may create paradoxical hyperactivity. Adverse reactions include insomnia, nervousness, anorexia, and weight loss. Occasionally, a patient may suffer from dizziness, depression, irritability, nausea, or abdominal pain. CNS stimulants are Schedule II controlled substances and labeled as pregnancy category C. Methylphenidate abuse has been increasing, especially among teens who take the drug to stay awake or as an appetite suppressant to lose weight.

Non-CNS stimulants have been tried for ADHD; however, they exhibit less efficacy. Clonidine (Catapres) is sometimes prescribed when patients are extremely aggressive, active, or have difficulty falling asleep. Atypical antidepressants such as bupropion (Wellbutrin) and tricyclics such as desipramine (Norpramine) and imipramine (Tofranil) are considered second-choice drugs, when CNS stimulants fail to work or are contraindicated.

A recent addition to the treatment of ADHD in children and adults has been atomoxetine (Strattera). Although its exact mechanism is not known, it is classified as a norepinephrine reuptake inhibitor. Patients taking atomoxetine show improved ability to focus on tasks and reduced hyperactivity. Efficacy appears to be equivalent to methylphenidate (Ritalin), although the drug is too new for long-term comparisons. Common side effects include headache, insomnia, upper abdominal pain, decreased appetite, and cough. Unlike methylphenidate, it is not a scheduled drug; thus, parents who are hesitant to place their child on stimulants now have a reasonable alternative. All children treated with atomexetine should be monitored closely for increased risk of suicide ideation.

Chapter REVIEW

KEY CONCEPTS

The numbered key concepts provide a succinct summary of the important points from the corresponding numbered section within the chapter. If any of these points are not clear, refer to the numbered section within the chapter for review.

16.1 Every nurse should be proficient in the assessment of patients with signs of depression. Depression has many forms and characteristics, and its identification and etiology are essential for proper treatment.

16.2 Approaches to treatment of major depression involve a proper health examination, medications, psychotherapeutic techniques, and electroconvulsive or rTMS therapy. There is an important warning from the FDA about antidepressants.

16.3 Antidepressants act by correcting neurotransmitter imbalances in the brain. The two basic mechanisms of action are blocking the enzymatic breakdown of norepinephrine and slowing the reuptake of serotonin. The primary classes of antidepressants are the TCAs, SSRIs, atypical antidepressants, and MAOIs. The serotonin–norepinephrine reuptake inhibitors (SNRIs) are a subgroup of atypical antidepressants recently approved for the relief of depressive symptoms.

16.4 Tricyclic antidepressants are older medications used mainly for the treatment of major depression, obsessive–compulsive disorders, and panic attacks. They have unpleasant and serious side effects.

16.5 SSRIs act by selectively blocking the reuptake of serotonin in nerve terminals. Because of fewer side effects, SSRIs are drugs of choice in the pharmacotherapy of depression. Serotonin syndrome is a serious concern for SSRIs and for other antidepressant drug classes.

16.6 MAOIs are usually prescribed in cases when other antidepressants have not been successful. They have more serious side effects than other antidepressants.

16.7 Patients with bipolar disorder display not only signs of depression but also mania, a state characterized by expressive psychomotor activity and irritability.

16.8 Lithium (Eskalith), antiseizure drugs, and atypical antipsychotic drugs are used to treat bipolar disorder. Lithium is effective for purely manic or purely depressive stages. Antiseizure drugs are more effective in the treatment of mania or for cycling and mixed states of bipolar disorder. Atypical antipsychotics are more effective for the treatment of acute mania and for the longer-term treatment of pyschotic depression.

16.9 Attention deficit–hyperactivity disorder (ADHD) is a common behavioral condition occurring primarily in children and is characterized by difficulty paying attention, hyperactivity, and impulsiveness.

16.10 The most efficacious drugs for symptoms of ADHD are the CNS stimulants such as methylphenidate (Ritalin). A newer, nonstimulant drug, atomoxetine (Strattera), has shown promise in patients with ADHD.

NCLEX-RN® REVIEW QUESTIONS

1 Anticholinergic effects are common adverse effects of antidepressants such as imipramine (Tofranil). These effects may include:
1. psychomotor symptoms.
2. tachycardia, hypertension, and increase in respiratory rate.
3. tardive dyskinesias.
4. blurred vision, dry mouth, and constipation.

2 The parents of a patient receiving methylphenidate (Ritalin) express concern that the health care provider has suggested the child have a "holiday" from the drug. The nurse explains that the drug-free holiday is designed to:
1. reduce the risk of drug toxicity.
2. allow the child's "normal" behavior to return.
3. decrease drug dependence and assess status.
4. prevent hypertensive crisis.

3 Which of the following symptoms would indicate to the nurse that a patient is experiencing lithium toxicity? (Select all that apply.)
1. Diarrhea and ataxia
2. Hypotension and edema
3. Hypertension and dehydration
4. Increased appetite, increased energy, and memory loss
5. Slurred speech and muscle weakness

4 A 17-year-old male has started valproic acid (Depakene) for treatment of bipolar disorder. While he is taking this drug, he should be carefully monitored for:
1. Unusual abdominal pain, especially in the upper quadrant areas
2. An increased susceptibility to infections
3. Lethargy or confusion
4. Unusual bleeding or bruising

5 Which of the following would be a priority component of the teaching plan for a patient prescribed phenelzine (Nardil) for treatment of depression?
1. Headache may occur.
2. Hyperglycemia may occur.
3. Read labels of food and over-the-counter drugs.
4. Monitor blood pressure for hypotension.

6 A patient experiencing moderate depression is placed on sertraline (Zoloft). The nurse should counsel the patient to expect full effects from the drug in:
1. 2–3 days.
2. 1 week.
3. a month or longer.
4. within 24 hours after starting the drug.

CRITICAL THINKING QUESTIONS

1. A 12-year-old girl has been diagnosed with ADHD. Her parents have been reluctant to agree with the pediatrician's recommendation for pharmacologic management; however, the child's performance in school has deteriorated. A school nurse notes that the child has been placed on amphetamine (Adderall), not methylphenidate (Ritalin). Discuss the developmental considerations that might support the use of amphetamine.

2. A 56-year-old female patient has been diagnosed with clinical depression following the death of her husband. She says that she has not been able to sleep for weeks and that she is drinking a lot of coffee. She is also smoking quite a bit. The health care provider prescribes fluoxetine (Prozac). The patient seeks reassurance from the nurse regarding when she should begin feeling "more like myself." How should the nurse respond?

3. A 26-year-old mother of three children comes to the prenatal clinic suspecting a fourth pregnancy. She tells the nurse that she got "real low" after her third baby and that she was prescribed sertraline (Zoloft). She tells the nurse that she is really afraid of "going crazy" if she has to stop taking the drug because of this pregnancy. What concerns should the nurse have?

See Appendix D for answers and rationales for all activities.

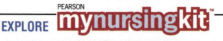

EXPLORE **mynursingkit** PEARSON

MyNursingKit is your one stop for online chapter review materials and resources. Prepare for success with additional NCLEX®-style practice questions, interactive assignments and activities, web links, animations and videos, and more!

Register your access code from the front of your book at
www.mynursingkit.com.

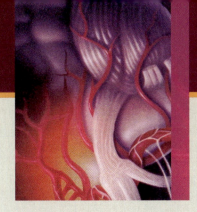

Drugs for Psychoses

LEARNING OUTCOMES

After reading this chapter, the student should be able to:

1. Explain theories for the etiology of schizophrenia.
2. Compare and contrast the positive and negative symptoms of schizophrenia.
3. Discuss the rationale for selecting a specific antipsychotic drug for the treatment of schizophrenia.
4. Explain the importance of patient drug compliance in the pharmacotherapy of schizophrenia.
5. Describe the nurse's role in the pharmacologic management of schizophrenia.
6. Explain the symptoms associated with extrapyramidal side effects of antipsychotic drugs.
7. For each of the drug classes listed in Drugs at a Glance, know representative drug examples, explain their mechanism of action, primary actions, and important adverse effects.
8. Categorize drugs used for psychoses based on their classification and drug action.
9. Use the nursing process to care for patients receiving drug therapy for psychoses.

KEY TERMS

akathisia *page 206*

delusions *page 204*

dopamine type 2 (D₂) receptor *page 204*

dystonia *page 206*

extrapyramidal side effects (EPS) *page 206*

hallucinations *page 204*

illusions *page 204*

negative symptoms *page 204*

neuroleptic *page 206*

neuroleptic malignant syndrome (NMS) *page 206*

paranoia *page 204*

parkinsonism *page 206*

positive symptoms *page 204*

schizoaffective disorder *page 205*

schizophrenia *page 204*

tardive dyskinesia *page 206*

Severe mental illness can be incapacitating for the patient and intensely frustrating for family members and those dealing with the patient on a regular basis. Before the 1950s, patients with acute mental dysfunction were institutionalized, often for their entire lives. With the introduction of chlorpromazine (Thorazine) in the 1950s, and the development of newer drugs, antipsychotic drugs have revolutionized the treatment of mental illness.

17.1 The Nature of Psychoses

A psychosis is a mental health condition characterized by **delusions** (firm ideas and beliefs not founded in reality), **hallucinations** (seeing, hearing, or feeling something that is not there), **illusions** (distorted perceptions of actual sensory stimuli), disorganized behavior, and a difficulty relating to others. Behavior may range from total inactivity to extreme agitation and combativeness. In addition, some patients with psychoses exhibit **paranoia**, an extreme suspicion and delusion that they are being followed, or that others are trying to harm them. Because these patients are unable to distinguish what is real from what is illusion, they are often viewed as medically and legally incompetent.

Psychoses may be classified as *acute* or *chronic*. Acute psychotic episodes occur over hours or days, whereas chronic psychoses develop over months or years. Sometimes a cause may be attributed to the psychosis, such as brain damage, overdoses of certain medications, extreme depression, chronic alcoholism, and drug addiction. Genetic factors are known to play a role in some psychoses. Unfortunately, the vast majority of psychoses have no identifiable cause.

People with psychosis are usually unable to function normally in society without long-term drug therapy. Patients must see their health care provider periodically, and medication must be taken for life. Family members and social support groups are important sources of help for patients who cannot function without continuous drug therapy.

SCHIZOPHRENIA

Schizophrenia is a type of psychosis characterized by abnormal thoughts and thought processes, disordered communication, withdrawal from other people and the outside environment, and a high risk for suicide. Several subtypes of schizophrenic disorders are based on clinical presentation.

17.2 Signs and Symptoms of Schizophrenia

Schizophrenia is the most common psychotic disorder, affecting 1% to 2% of the population. Symptoms generally begin to appear in early adulthood, with a peak incidence in men 15 to 24 years of age, and women 25 to 34 years of age. Patients potentially experience a variety of symptoms that may change over time. The following symptoms may appear quickly or take several months or years to develop.

- Hallucinations, delusions, or paranoia
- Strange behavior, such as communicating in rambling statements or made-up words
- Rapid alternation between extreme hyperactivity and stupor
- Attitude of indifference or detachment toward life activities
- Strange or irrational actions
- Deterioration of personal hygiene, and job or academic performance
- Marked withdrawal from social interactions and interpersonal relationships

When observing patients with schizophrenia, nurses should look for both positive and negative symptoms. **Positive symptoms** are those that *add* on to normal behavior. These include hallucinations, delusions, and a disorganized thought or speech pattern. **Negative symptoms** are those that *subtract* from normal behavior. These symptoms include a lack of interest, motivation, responsiveness, or pleasure in daily activities. Negative symptoms are characteristic of the indifferent personality exhibited by many people with schizophrenia. Proper diagnosis of positive and negative symptoms is important for selection of the appropriate antipsychotic drug.

The cause of schizophrenia has not been determined, although several theories have been proposed. There appears to be a genetic component to schizophrenia, since many patients suffering from schizophrenia have family members who have been afflicted with the same disorder. Another theory suggests the disorder is caused by imbalances in neurotransmitters in specific brain areas. This theory suggests the possibility of overactive dopaminergic pathways in the basal nuclei, an area of the brain that controls motor activity. The basal ganglia with associated nuclei, as shown in ➤ Figure 17.1, are responsible for starting and stopping synchronized motor activity, such as leg and arm motions during walking.

Symptoms of schizophrenia seem to be associated with the **dopamine type 2 (D_2) receptor**. The basal nuclei are particularly rich in D_2 receptors, whereas the cerebrum contains very few. All antipsychotic drugs act by entering dopaminergic

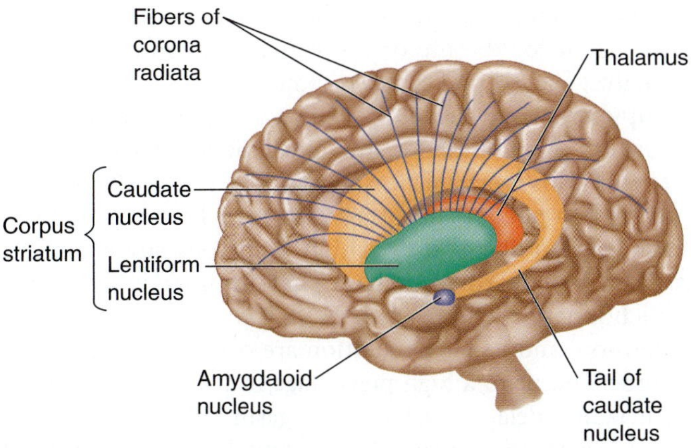

Fibers of
corona
radiata

Thalamus

Caudate
nucleus

Corpus
striatum

Lentiform
nucleus

Amygdaloid
nucleus

Tail of
caudate
nucleus

> *Figure 17.1* Basal ganglia: overstimulation of dopamine receptors may be responsible for schizophrenia

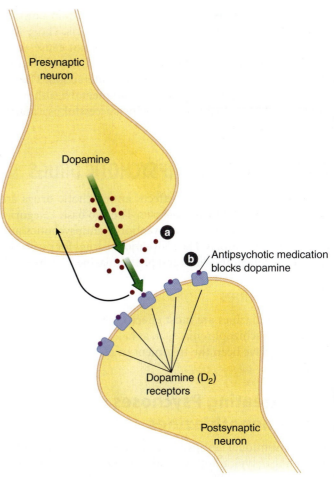

Presynaptic
neuron

Dopamine

Antipsychotic medication
blocks dopamine

Dopamine (D₂)
receptors

Postsynaptic
neuron

> *Figure 17.2* Mechanism of action of antipsychotic drugs: (a) overproduction of dopamine; (b) antipsychotic medication occupies D₂ receptors, preventing dopamine from stimulating the postsynaptic neuron

synapses and competing with dopamine. By blocking a majority of the D_2 receptors, antipsychotic drugs reduce the symptoms of schizophrenia. ➤ Figure 17.2 illustrates antipsychotic drug action at the dopaminergic receptor.

Schizoaffective disorder is a condition in which the patient exhibits symptoms of both schizophrenia and mood disorder. For example, an acute schizoaffective reaction may include distorted perceptions, hallucinations, and delusions, followed by extreme depression. Over time, both positive and negative psychotic symptoms will appear.

Many conditions can cause bizarre behavior, and these should be distinguished from schizophrenia. Chronic use of amphetamines or cocaine can create a paranoid syndrome. Certain complex partial seizures (chapter 15∞) can cause unusual symptoms that are sometimes mistaken for psychoses. Brain neoplasms, infections, or hemorrhage can also cause bizarre, psychotic-like symptoms.

17.3 Pharmacologic Management of Psychoses

Management of severe mental illness is difficult. Many patients do not see their behavior as abnormal, and have diffi-

culty understanding the need for medication. When that medication produces undesirable side effects, such as severe twitching or loss of sexual function, compliance diminishes and patients exhibit symptoms of their pretreatment illness. Agitation, distrust, and extreme frustration are common, as patients cannot comprehend why others are unable to think and see the same as them.

The primary goal for patients with schizophrenia is to reduce psychotic symptoms to a level that allows the patient to maintain normal social relationships, including self-care and interacting with other people. From a pharmacologic perspective, therapy has both a positive and a negative side. Although many symptoms of psychosis can be controlled with current drugs, adverse effects are common and often severe. The antipsychotic drugs do not cure mental illness, and symptoms remain in remission only as long as the patient chooses to take the drug. The relapse rate for patients who discontinue their medication is 60% to 80%.

In terms of efficacy, there is little difference among the various antipsychotic drugs; there is no single drug of choice for schizophrenia. Selection of a specific drug is based on clinician experience, the occurrence of adverse effects, and needs of the patient. For example, patients with

TREATING THE DIVERSE PATIENT

Cultural Views and Treatments of Mental Illness

Some cultures have very different perspectives on the cause of and treatment for mental illness. The foundation of many of these mental health treatments involves herbs and spiritual healing methods. American Indians may be treated by the community traditional "medicine man," who may treat mental symptoms with a sweat lodge and herbs. African Americans may go to a traditional voodoo priest or other healers for treatment, and they frequently use herbs to treat mental symptoms. Hispanics seek treatment from a folk healer, called a *curandero*; and they may use herbs such as chamomile, spearmint, and sweet basil for mental conditions. Members of some cultures may use amulets, or charms that are worn on a string or chain, to protect the wearer from evil spirits that are believed to cause mental illness. Because beliefs can vary widely within cultures themselves, a thorough cultural assessment of feelings and beliefs about health and wellness will assist the health care provider in providing the most appropriate care possible.

psychoses as well as Parkinson's disease need an antipsychotic with minimal extrapyramidal side effects. Those who operate machinery need a drug that does not cause sedation. Men and women who are sexually active may want a drug without negative effects on sexual interaction. The experience and skills of the physician and mental health nurse are particularly valuable in achieving successful psychiatric pharmacotherapy.

CONVENTIONAL ANTIPSYCHOTIC DRUGS

Because of neurologic side effects, antipsychotic drugs are sometimes referred to as **neuroleptics**. The two basic categories of antipsychotic drugs are conventional antipsychotics and atypical antipsychotics. The conventional drugs for psychoses include the phenothiazines and phenothiazine-like drugs.

Phenothiazines

The phenothiazines are most effective at treating the positive signs of schizophrenia, such as hallucinations and delusions, and have been the treatment of choice for psychoses for 50 years.

17.4 Treating Psychoses with Phenothiazines

The conventional antipsychotics, sometimes called first-generation or typical antipsychotics, include the phenothiazine and phenothiazine-like drugs listed in Table 17.1. Within each category, drugs are named by their chemical structure.

The first effective drug used to treat schizophrenia was the low-potency phenothiazine chlorpromazine (Thorazine), approved by the FDA for this use in 1954. A number of phenothiazines are now available to treat mental illness. All block the excitement associated with the positive symptoms of schizophrenia, although they differ in potency and side-effect profiles. Hallucinations and delusions often begin to diminish within days. Other symptoms, however, may require as long as 7 to 8 weeks of pharmacotherapy to improve. Because of the high rate of recurrence of psychotic episodes, pharmacotherapy should be considered long term, often for the life of the patient. Phenothiazines are thought to act by preventing dopamine and serotonin from occupying critical neurologic receptor sites. For the conventional antipsychotics, dopamine has higher affinity for the receptor. This mechanism is illustrated in Figure 17.2.

Although phenothiazines revolutionized the treatment of severe mental illness, they exhibit numerous adverse effects that can limit pharmacotherapy. These are listed in Table 17.2. Anticholinergic effects such as dry mouth, postural hypotension, and urinary retention are common. Ejaculation disorders occur in a high percentage of patients taking phenothiazines; delay in achieving orgasm (in both men and women) is a common cause for noncompliance and menstrual disorders are common. High fence confusion and other signs of **neuroleptic malignant syndrome (NMS)** may occur. Each phenothiazine has a slightly different side-effect spectrum. For example, perphenazine (Phenazine, Trilafon) has a low incidence of anticholinergic effects, whereas chlorpromazine (Thorazine) has a high incidence of anticholinergic effects. Thioridazine (Mellaril) frequently causes sedation, whereas this side effect is less common with trifluoperazine hydrochloride (Stelazine).

Unlike many other drugs whose primary action is on the CNS (e.g., amphetamines, barbiturates, anxiolytics, alcohol), antipsychotic drugs do not cause physical or psychologic dependence. They also have a wide safety margin between a therapeutic and a lethal dose; deaths due to overdoses of antipsychotic drugs are uncommon.

Extrapyramidal effects are a particularly serious set of adverse reactions to antipsychotic drugs. **Extrapyramidal side effects (EPS)** include acute dystonia, akathisia, parkinsonism, and tardive dyskinesia. Acute **dystonias** occur early in the course of pharmacotherapy, and involve severe muscle spasms, particularly of the back, neck, tongue, and face. **Akathisia**, the most common EPS, is an inability to rest or relax. The patient paces, has trouble sitting or remaining still, and has difficulty sleeping. Symptoms of phenothiazine-induced **parkinsonism** include tremor, muscle rigidity, stooped posture, and a shuffling gait. Long-term use of phenothiazines may lead to **tardive dyskinesia**, which is characterized by unusual tongue and face movements such as lip smacking and wormlike motions of

TABLE 17.1	Conventional Antipsychotic Drugs: Phenothiazines	
Drug	Route and Adult Dose (max dose where indicated)	Adverse Effects
🔊 chlorpromazine HCl (Thorazine)	PO; 25–100 mg tid or qid (max: 1,000 mg/day) IM/IV; 25–50 mg (max: 600 mg every 4–6 h)	*Sedation, drowsiness, dizziness, extrapyramidal symptoms, constipation, photosensitivity, orthostatic hypotension, urinary retention*
fluphenazine HCl (Permitil, Prolixin)	PO; 0.5–10 mg/day (max: 20 mg/day)	<u>Agranulocytosis, pancytopenia, anaphylactoid reaction, tardive dyskinesia, neuroleptic malignant syndrome, hypothermia, adynamic ileus, sudden unexplained death</u>
perphenazine (Phenazine, Trilafon)	PO; 4–16 mg bid to qid (max: 64 mg/day)	
prochlorperazine (Compazine)	PO; 0.5–10 mg/day (max: 20 mg/day)	
thioridazine HCl (Mellaril)	PO; 50–100 mg tid (max: 800 mg/day)	
trifluoperazine HCl (originally marketed as Stelazine)	PO; 1–2 mg bid; (max: 20 mg/day) IM; 1–2 mg every 4–6 h (max 10 mg/day)	

Italics indicate common adverse effects; <u>underlining</u> indicates serious adverse effects.

TABLE 17.2 Adverse Effects of Conventional Antipsychotic Drugs

Effect	Description
Acute dystonia	Severe spasms, particularly the back muscles, tongue, and facial muscles; twitching movements
Akathisia	Constant pacing with repetitive, compulsive movements
Anticholinergic effects	Dry mouth, tachycardia, blurred vision
Hypotension	Particularly severe when the patient moves quickly from a recumbent to an upright position
Neuroleptic malignant syndrome	High fever, confusion, muscle rigidity, and high serum creatine kinase; can be fatal
Parkinsonism	Tremor, muscle rigidity, stooped posture, and shuffling gait
Sedation	Usually diminishes with continued therapy
Sexual dysfunction	Impotence and diminished libido
Tardive dyskinesia	Bizarre tongue and face movements such as lip smacking and wormlike motions of the tongue; puffing of cheeks, uncontrolled chewing movements

---

Pr Prototype Drug | Chlorpromazine Hydrochloride *(Thorazine)*

Therapeutic Class: Conventional antipsychotic; schizophrenia drug

Pharmacologic Class: D_2 dopamine receptor antagonist; phenothiazine

ACTIONS AND USES

Chlorpromazine provides symptomatic relief of positive symptoms of schizophrenia and controls manic symptoms in patients with schizoaffective disorder. Many patients must take chlorpromazine for 7 or 8 weeks before they experience improvement. Extreme agitation may be treated with IM or IV injections, which begin to act within minutes. Chlorpromazine can also control severe nausea and vomiting.

ADMINISTRATION ALERTS

- Do not crush or open sustained-release forms.
- When administered IM, give deep IM, only in the upper outer quadrant of the buttocks; the patient should remain supine for 30 to 60 minutes after injection, and then rise slowly.
- The drug must be gradually withdrawn over 2 to 3 weeks, and nausea/vomiting, dizziness, tremors, or dyskinesia may occur.
- IV forms should be used only during surgery or for severe hiccups.
- Pregnancy category C

PHARMACOKINETICS
Onset: 30–60 min
Peak: 2–4 h PO; 15–20 min IM/IV
Half-life: 6 h
Duration: 30 h

ADVERSE EFFECTS

Strong blockade of alpha-adrenergic receptors and weak blockade of cholinergic receptors explain some of chlorpromazine's adverse effects. Common adverse effects are dizziness, drowsiness, and orthostatic hypotension.

Extrapyramidal side effects (EPS) occur more commonly in elderly, female, and pediatric patients who are dehydrated. Neuroleptic malignant syndrome (NMS) may also occur. Patients taking chlorpromazine who are exposed to warmer temperatures should be monitored more closely for symptoms of NMS.

Contraindications: Use is not advised during alcohol withdrawal or when the patient is in a comatose state. Caution should be used with other conditions, including subcortical brain damage, bone marrow depression, and Reye's syndrome. Chlorpromazine is contraindicated in lactation.

INTERACTIONS

Drug–Drug: Chlorpromazine interacts with several drugs. For example, concurrent use with sedative medications such as phenobarbital should be avoided. Taking chlorpromazine with tricyclic antidepressants can elevate blood pressure. Concurrent use of chlorpromazine with antiseizure medication can lower the seizure threshold.

Lab Tests: Chlorpromazine may increase cephalin flocculation and possibly other liver function tests. False-positive results may occur for amylase, 5-hydroxyindole acetic acid, porphobilinogens, urobilinogen, and urine bilirubin. False-positive or false-negative pregnancy tests may result.

Herbal/Food: Kava and St. John's wort may increase the risk and severity of dystonia.

Treatment of Overdose: There is no specific treatment for overdose; patients are treated symptomatically. EPS may be treated with antiparkinsonism drugs, barbiturates, or diphenhydramine (Benadryl). Avoid producing respiratory depression with these treatments.

Refer to MyNursingKit for a Nursing Process Focus specific to this drug.

---

the tongue. If extrapyramidal effects are reported early and the drug is withdrawn or the dosage is reduced, the side effects can be reversible. With higher doses given for prolonged periods, the extrapyramidal symptoms may become permanent. The nurse must be vigilant in observing and reporting EPS, as prevention is the best treatment.

With the conventional antipsychotics, it is not always possible to control the disabling symptoms of schizophrenia without producing some degree of extrapyramidal effects. In these patients, drug therapy may be warranted to treat EPS symptoms. Concurrent pharmacotherapy with an anticholinergic drug may prevent some of the extrapyramidal signs (chapter 13∞). For acute dystonia, benztropine (Cogentin) may be given parenterally. Levodopa (Dopar, Larodopa) is usually avoided, since its ability to increase dopamine function antagonizes the action of the phenothiazines. Beta-adrenergic blockers and benzodiazepines are sometimes given to reduce signs of akathisia.

Nonphenothiazines

The nonphenothiazine antipsychotic medications have equal efficacy as the phenothiazines. Although the incidence of sedation and anticholinergic adverse effects is less, extrapyramidal effects may be common, particularly in older adults.

17.5 Treating Psychoses with Conventional Nonphenothiazine Antipsychotics

The conventional nonphenothiazine antipsychotic class consists of drugs whose chemical structures are dissimilar to the phenothiazines (Table 17.3). Introduced shortly after the phenothiazines, the nonphenothiazines were initially expected to produce fewer side effects. Unfortunately, this appears to not be the case. The spectrum of adverse effects for the nonphenothiazines is identical with that for the phenothiazines, although the degree to which a particular effect occurs depends on the specific drug. In general, the nonphenothiazine drugs cause less sedation and fewer anticholinergic adverse effects than chlorpromazine (Thorazine) but exhibit an equal or even greater incidence of extrapyramidal signs. Concurrent therapy with other CNS depressants must be carefully monitored, because of the potential additive effects.

Drugs in the nonphenothiazine class have the same therapeutic effects and efficacy as the phenothiazines. They are also believed to act by the same mechanism as the phenothiazines, that is, by blocking postsynaptic D_2 dopamine receptors. As a class, they offer no significant advantages over the phenothiazines in the treatment of schizophrenia.

ATYPICAL ANTIPSYCHOTIC DRUGS

Atypical antipsychotics treat both positive and negative symptoms of schizophrenia. They have become drugs of choice for treating psychoses.

Pr Prototype Drug | Haloperidol (Haldol)

Therapeutic Class: Conventional antipsychotic; schizophrenia drug   **Pharmacologic Class:** D_2 dopamine receptor antagonist; nonphenothiazine

ACTIONS AND USES
Haloperidol is classified chemically as a butyrophenone. Its primary use is for the management of acute and chronic psychotic disorders. It may be used to treat patients with Tourette's syndrome and children with severe behavior problems such as unprovoked aggressiveness and explosive hyperexcitability. It is approximately 50 times more potent than chlorpromazine but has equal efficacy in relieving symptoms of schizophrenia. Haldol LA is a long-acting preparation that lasts for approximately 3 weeks following IM or subcutaneous administration. This is particularly beneficial for patients who are uncooperative or unable to take oral medications.

ADMINISTRATION ALERTS
- Do not abruptly discontinue, or severe adverse reactions may occur.
- The patient must take the medication as ordered for therapeutic results to occur.
- If the patient does not comply with oral therapy, injectable extended-release haloperidol should be considered.
- Pregnancy category C

PHARMACOKINETICS
Onset: 30–35 min
Peak: 2–6 h PO; 10–20 min IM
Half-life: 12–37 h PO; 10–19 h IV; 17–25 h IM
Duration: Variable

ADVERSE EFFECTS
Haloperidol produces less sedation and hypotension than chlorpromazine, but the incidence of EPS is high. Older adults are more likely to experience adverse effects and often are prescribed half the adult dose until the adverse effects of therapy can be determined. Although the incidence of NMS is rare, it can occur.

Contraindications: Pharmacotherapy with nonphenothiazines is not advised if the patient is receiving medication for any of the following conditions: Parkinson's disease, seizure disorders, alcoholism, and severe mental depression.

INTERACTIONS
Drug–Drug: Haloperidol interacts with many drugs. For example, the following drugs decrease the effects/absorption of haloperidol: aluminum- and magnesium-containing antacids, levodopa (also increases chances of levodopa toxicity), lithium (increases chance of a severe neurologic toxicity), phenobarbital, phenytoin (also increases chances of phenytoin toxicity), rifampin, and beta blockers (may increase blood levels of haloperidol, thus leading to possible toxicity). Haloperidol inhibits the action of centrally acting antihypertensives.

Lab Tests: Unknown

Herbal/Food: Kava may increase the effect of haloperidol.

Treatment of Overdose: In general, the symptoms of overdose are an exaggeration of known pharmacologic effects and adverse reactions, the most prominent of which would be severe extrapyramidal reactions, hypotension, or sedation. With EPS, antiparkinsonism medication should be administered. Hypotension should be counteracted with IV fluids, plasma, or concentrated albumin, or vasopressor drugs.

Refer to MyNursingKit for a Nursing Process Focus specific to this drug.

TABLE 17.3	Conventional Antipsychotic Drugs: Nonphenothiazines	
Drug	**Route and Adult Dose (max dose where indicated)**	**Adverse Effects**
chlorprothixene (Taractan)	PO; 75–150 mg/day (max: 600 mg/day)	*Sedation, transient drowsiness, extrapyramidal symptoms, tremor, orthostatic hypotension*
haloperidol (Haldol)	PO; 0.2–5 mg bid or tid	
	IM; 2–5 mg every 4 h	Tardive dyskinesia, neuroleptic malignant syndrome, laryngospasm, respiratory depression, hepatotoxicity, acute renal failure, sudden death, agranulocytosis
loxapine succinate (Loxitane)	PO; start with 20 mg/day and rapidly increase to 60–100 mg/day in divided doses (max: 250 mg/day)	
molindone HCl (Moban)	PO; 50–75 mg/day in three to four divided doses; may increase to 100 mg/day in 3–4 days (max: 225 mg/day)	
pimozide (Orap)	PO; 1–2 mg/day in divided doses; gradually increase every other day to 7–16 mg/day (max: 10 mg/day)	
thiothixene HCl (Navane)	PO; 2 mg tid; may increase up to 15 mg/day (max: 60 mg/day)	

Italics indicate common adverse effects; underlining indicates serious adverse effects.

NURSING PROCESS FOCUS   PATIENTS RECEIVING CONVENTIONAL ANTIPSYCHOTIC THERAPY

Assessment	Potential Nursing Diagnoses
Baseline assessment prior to administration:	

Baseline assessment prior to administration:

- Understand the reason the drug has been prescribed in order to assess for therapeutic effects.
- Obtain a complete health history including hepatic, renal, urologic, cardiovascular, respiratory, or neurologic disease (especially Parkinson's disease or seizures), current mental status, pregnancy or breastfeeding. Obtain a drug history including allergies, current prescription and OTC drugs, alcohol use, smoking, and herbal preparations. Be alert to possible drug interactions.
- Obtain a history of depression or mental disorders, including a family history of same and severity.
- Assess for disturbances in thought processes, perception, verbal communication, affect, behavior, interpersonal relationships, and self-care. Use objective screening tools per the health care agency.
- Obtain baseline vital signs and weight.
- Evaluate appropriate laboratory findings (e.g., CBC, electrolytes, glucose, hepatic and renal function studies, drug screening).
- Assess the patient's ability to receive and understand instruction. Include the family and caregivers as needed.

Potential Nursing Diagnoses

- Disturbed Thought Processes
- Disturbed Sensory Perception (auditory, visual)
- Disturbed Personal Identity
- Anxiety (severe, panic)
- Impaired Verbal Communication
- Impaired Social Interaction
- Ineffective Health Maintenance
- Impaired Home Maintenance
- Noncompliance
- Deficient Knowledge (drug therapy)
- Risk for Violence (self-directed, directed at others)
- Risk for Self-Mutilation
- Risk for Disturbed Family Processes, Caregiver Role Strain

Assessment throughout administration:

- Assess for desired therapeutic effects (e.g., normalizing thought processes, lessening delusions, hallucinations, improvement in positive or negative symptoms, ability to return to normal ADLs, improvement in appetite and sleep patterns; if used for other uses, e.g., severe hiccups, assess for appropriate therapeutic effects).
- Continue periodic monitoring of CBC, electrolytes, glucose, hepatic and renal function studies, and therapeutic drug levels.
- Assess vital signs, especially orthostatic blood pressure, and weigh periodically.
- Assess for and promptly report adverse effects: dizziness or light-headedness, confusion, agitation, suicidal ideations, hypotension, tachycardia, increase in temperature, blurred or double vision, skin rashes, bruising or bleeding, abdominal pain, jaundice, change in color of stool, flank pain, and hematuria.
- Assess for and promptly report extrapyramidal (EPS) symptoms including pseudoparkinsonism, acute dystonias, akathisia, and tardive dyskinesias (see "Minimizing adverse effects" in the following section).
- Immediately report signs and symptoms of neuroleptic malignant syndrome (NMS): unstable blood pressure, elevated temperature, diaphoresis, dyspnea, muscle rigidity, and incontinence.

(Continued)

NURSING PROCESS FOCUS | **PATIENTS RECEIVING CONVENTIONAL ANTIPSYCHOTIC THERAPY** *(Continued)*

Planning: Patient Goals and Expected Outcomes

The patient will:

- Experience therapeutic effects dependent on the reason the drug is being given (e.g., lessened positive and negative symptoms, delusions, paranoia, hallucinations).
- Be free from, or experience minimal, adverse effects.
- Verbalize an understanding of the drug's use, adverse effects, and required precautions.
- Demonstrate proper self-administration of the medication (e.g., dose, timing, when to notify provider) when possible.

Implementation

Interventions and (Rationales)	Patient and Family Education
Ensuring therapeutic effects:	
• Continue assessments as described earlier for therapeutic effects. (Drugs used for psychoses and schizophrenia do not cure the underlying disorder but improve positive and negative symptoms of the disorder. Gradual improvement over several weeks to months may be noted.)	• Teach the patient, family, or caregiver that full effects may not occur immediately but that some improvement should be noticeable after beginning therapy. • Supportive, inpatient care may be required during acute, early period of therapy.
• Monitor patient compliance with the drug regimen. (The presence of severe mental disorders may result in noncompliance with medications. Regular, consistent dosing is essential to correcting the underlying disorder. Because the drugs do not cure the underlying disorder, if regular administration is disrupted, symptoms may return abruptly. Intramuscular depot injections may need to be considered if chronic noncompliance continues.)	• Involve the family and caregiver to the extent possible in ensuring the patient remains on regular medication routines. • Ensure that the patient takes the medication as prescribed. *Never* leave medications at the bedside. • Question the possibility of noncompliance if original symptoms or adverse effects suddenly increase in frequency or severity.
Minimizing adverse effects:	
• Continue to monitor vital signs periodically, especially orthostatic blood pressure. Keep patient supine for 30 minutes to 1 hour after giving parenteral medications and recheck blood pressure measurements every 15 to 30 minutes. Ensure patient safety; monitor ambulation until the effects of the drug are known. Be particularly cautious with older adults who are at an increased risk for falls. (Antipsychotic drugs may cause hypotension, increasing the risk of falls and injury.)	• Have the patient rise from lying or sitting to standing slowly to avoid dizziness or falls. • Instruct the patient to call for assistance prior to getting out of bed or attempting to walk alone. For patients on at-home/outpatient medication, avoid driving or other activities requiring mental alertness or physical coordination until effects of the drug are known.

• Continue to monitor motor activity, coordination and balance, and for EPS symptoms, including:
  • Pseudoparkinsonism: tremor, muscle rigidity, stooped posture, bradykinesia (slow to start and shuffling, slow gait)
  • Akathisia: inability to rest and relax, often with pacing
  • Acute dystonias: severe muscle spasms of face, tongue, neck, or back
  • Tardive dyskinesias: "choreoathetoid" movements such as lip smacking, wormlike movements of the tongue, uncontrolled chewing, and grimacing (EPS may be an unavoidable adverse effect of drug therapy but the drug dose will be reduced or stopped, or the medication changed when possible.)
 • Ensure adequate nutrition and fluid intake if tardive dyskinesias are present. (Severe choreoathetoid tongue movement may significantly hinder or prevent adequate nutrition.)
 • Ensure patient safety if pseudoparkinsonism affects gait or if akathisia is present. Acute dystonias may require treatment with other medications to halt spasms. (Bradykinesias, slow-to-start ambulation and slow, shuffling gait, may predispose the patient to falls. Akathisia with pacing may significantly impair the patient's ability to rest and sleep. Additional medications may be required to treat. Anticholinergics or other drugs may be required to stop spasms.)
	• Instruct the patient, family, or caregiver to immediately report EPS symptoms for additional treatment.

NURSING PROCESS FOCUS   PATIENTS RECEIVING CONVENTIONAL ANTIPSYCHOTIC THERAPY *(Continued)*

Implementation

Interventions and (Rationales)	Patient and Family Education
■ Monitor for and immediately report signs and symptoms of NMS: unstable blood pressure, elevated temperature, diaphoresis, dyspnea, muscle rigidity, and incontinence. (NMS is a rare but potentially fatal syndrome that must be recognized and treated immediately.)	■ Instruct the patient, family, or caregiver to immediately report any changes in level of consciousness, elevated temperature, excessive sweating, severe muscle rigidity, increased respirations or shortness of breath, or incontinence.
■ Continue to monitor CBC, electrolytes, renal and hepatic function, and therapeutic drug levels. (Antipsychotic drugs may cause bone marrow depression and hepatotoxicity as adverse effects.)	■ Instruct the patient on the need to return periodically for lab work. ■ Teach the patient to promptly report any abdominal pain, particularly in the upper quadrants, changes in stool color, yellowing of sclera or skin, darkened urine, skin rashes, low-grade fevers, general malaise or changes in behavior or activity level, or redness or swelling around sites of injury.
■ Monitor for anticholinergic effects, including dry mouth, drowsiness, blurred vision, constipation, and urinary retention. Provide symptomatic treatment to ease effects. (Anticholinergic symptoms are common adverse effects of antipsychotic drugs. Tolerance to anticholinergic effects usually develops over time.)	■ Encourage sips of water, ice chips, hard candy, or chewing gum to ease mouth dryness. Avoid alcohol-based mouthwashes, which are drying to the mucosa and which the patient may drink. ■ Increase dietary fiber intake and adequate fluid intake. ■ Report urinary retention to the health care provider promptly.
■ Monitor for sunburning or rashes. (Antipsychotic drugs cause photosensitivity.)	■ Teach the patient, family, or caregiver to apply sunscreen (SPF 15 or above) prior to sun exposure or ensure protective clothing is worn. Promptly report a sunburn to the health care provider.
■ Monitor for alcohol and illegal drug use. (Used concurrently, these cause an increased CNS depressant effect or an exacerbation in psychotic symptoms.)	■ Instruct the patient to avoid alcohol and illegal drug use. Refer the patient to community support groups such as AA or NA as appropriate.
■ Monitor caffeine use. (Use of caffeine-containing substances may negate the effects of antipsychotics.)	■ Teach the patient, family, or caregiver to avoid caffeine-containing beverages, foods, and OTC medications, and to read food labels when in doubt of whether the product contains caffeine.
■ Monitor for smoking. (Heavy smoking may decrease the metabolism of some antipsychotics such as haloperidol, leading to decreased efficacy.)	■ Instruct the patient to stop or decrease smoking. Refer the patient to smoking cessation programs, if indicated.
Patient understanding of drug therapy: ■ Use opportunities during administration of medications and during assessments to discuss rationale for drug therapy, desired therapeutic outcomes, most commonly observed adverse effects, parameters for when to call the health care provider, and any necessary monitoring or precautions. Use brief explanations during times of delusions or hallucinations. (Using time during nursing care helps to optimize and reinforce key teaching areas. Brief, consistent explanations assist to interrupt delusional periods.)	■ The patient, family, or caregiver should be able to state the reason for the drug; appropriate dose and scheduling; and what adverse effects to observe for and when to report them.
Patient self-administration of drug therapy: ■ When administering the medication, instruct the patient, family, or caregiver in proper self-administration of drug, e.g., take the drug as prescribed and do not substitute brands. (Utilizing time during nurse-administration of these drugs helps to reinforce teaching.)	■ Teach the patient, or family, or caregiver to take the medication as follows: ■ Take exactly as ordered and use the same manufacturer's brand each time the prescription is filled. (Switching brands may result in differing pharmacokinetics and alterations in therapeutic effect). ■ Ensure that all medication is taken exactly when and as ordered. Use of a calendar to track doses may be helpful. ■ If the medication causes drowsiness, take at bedtime. Tolerance to anticholinergic effects such as drowsiness usually develops over time. ■ Do not abruptly discontinue the medication.

Evaluation of Outcome Criteria

Evaluate the effectiveness of drug therapy by confirming that patient goals and expected goals have been met (see "Planning").

See Tables 17.1 and 17.3 for lists of drugs to which these nursing actions apply.

17.6 Treating Psychoses with Atypical Antipsychotics

The approval of clozapine (Clozaril), the first atypical antipsychotic, marked the first major advance in the pharmacotherapy of psychoses since the discovery of chlorpromazine decades earlier. Clozapine, and the other drugs in this class, are called second generation, or atypical, because they have a broader spectrum of action than the conventional antipsychotics, controlling both the positive and negative symptoms of schizophrenia (Table 17.4). Furthermore, at therapeutic doses they exhibit their antipsychotic actions without producing the EPS effects of the conventional drugs. Some drugs, such as clozapine, are especially useful for patients in whom other drugs have proved unsuccessful.

The mechanism of action of the atypical drugs is largely unknown, but they are thought to act by blocking several different receptor types in the brain. Like the phenothiazines, the atypical drugs block dopamine D_2 receptors. However, the atypicals also block serotonin (5-HT) and alpha-adrenergic receptors, which is thought to account for some of their properties. Because the atypical drugs are only loosely bound to D_2 receptors, they produce fewer extrapyramidal side effects than the conventional antipsychotics.

Although there are fewer side effects with atypical antipsychotics, adverse effects are still significant, and patients must be carefully monitored. The use of atypical antipsychotics have recently been differentially associated with an increased risk of weight gain, diabetes, and hypertriglyceridemia. In addition, they have been associated with a possible increased risk of cerebrovascular events and higher mortality rates. Although most antipsychotics cause weight gain, the atypical drugs are specifically associated with obesity and its risk factors. Risperidone (risperdal) and some of the other antipsychotic drugs increase prolactin levels, which can lead to menstrual disorders, decreased libido, and osteoporosis in women. In men, high prolactin levels can cause lack of libido and impotence. There is also concern that some atypical drugs alter glucose metabolism, attributing to the onset of type 2 diabetes.

Pr Prototype Drug | Risperidone (Risperdal)

Therapeutic Class: Atypical antipsychotic; schizophrenia drug

Pharmacologic Class: D_2 dopamine receptor antagonist (weaker affinity for D_1 receptors); serotonin (5-HT) receptor antagonist

ACTIONS AND USES

Therapeutic effects of risperidone include treatment and prevention of schizophrenia relapse and expression of bipolar mania symptoms. Risperidone also treats symptoms of irritability in autistic children. Expected results are a reduction of excitment, paranoia, or negative behaviors associated with pyschosis. Effects occur primarily from blockade of dopamine type 2, serotonin type 2, and alpha₂ adrenergic receptors located within the CNS. For a full range of effectiveness, the drug is sometimes combined with lithium (Eskalith, Lithobid) or valproate (Depakene, Depacon). Risperidone is a long-acting preparation, which following IM administration, releases only a small amount. After a 3-week lag, the rest of the drug releases and lasts for approximately 4–6 weeks. PO preparations release sooner and have a 1–2 week onset of action.

ADMINISTRATION ALERTS

- Several weeks are required for therapeutic effectiveness.
- When switching from other antipsychotics, discontinue medications to avoid overlap.
- Pregnancy category C

PHARMACOKINETICS
Onset: 1–2 wk PO; 3 wk IM
Peak: 4–6 wk
Half-life: 20 h
Duration: 6 wk

ADVERSE EFFECTS

Common adverse effects are extrapyrimidal reactions (involuntary shaking of the head, neck, and arms), hyperactivity, fatigue, nausea, dizziness, visual disturbances, fever, and orthostatic hypotension. Risperidone may cause weight gain and hyperglycemia, thus worsening glucose control in diabetic patients.

Contraindications: If older adults with dementia-related psychoses are given risperidone, they are at an increased risk for heart failure, pneumonia, or sudden death. Patients with underlying cardiovascular disease may be especially prone to dysrhythmias and hypotension. Risperidone should be avoided in patients with a history of seizures, suicidal ideations, or kidney/liver disease.

INTERACTIONS

Drug–Drug: Patients taking risperidone should avoid CNS depressants such as alcohol, antihistamines, sedative–hypnotics, or opioid analgesics. These can increase some of the adverse effects of risperidone. Due to inhibition of liver enzymes, other drugs that increase adverse effects of risperidone include SSRIs such as paroxetine (Paxil), sertraline (Zoloft), and fluoxetine (Prozac) and antifungal drugs such as fluconazole (Diflucan), itraconazole (Sporanox), and ketoconazole (Nizoral). Risperidone may interfere with elimination by the kidneys of clozapine (Clozaril), which also increases the risk of adverse reactions.

Lab Tests: Risperidone may cause increased serum prolactin levels and increased ALT (alanine aminotranferease) and AST (aspartate aminotransferase) liver enzyme levels. Other potential lab changes are anemia, thrombocytopenia, leukocytosis, and leukopenia.

Herbal/Food: Use with caution with herbal supplements, such as kava, valerian, or chamomile, which may increase risperidone's CNS depressive effects.

Treatment of Overdose: Activated charcoal, which may be used with sorbitol, may be as or more effective than emesis or gastric lavage, and should be considered in treating overdosage. Establish and maintain an airway; ensure adequate oxygenation and ventilation. Maintain cardiovascular function.

TABLE 17.4	Atypical Antipsychotic Drugs	
Drug	**Route and Adult Dose (max dose where indicated)**	**Adverse Effects**
aripiprazole (Abilify)	PO; 10–15 mg/day (max: 30 mg/day)	*Tachycardia, transient fever, sedation, dizziness, headache, light-headedness, somnolence, anxiety, nervousness, hostility, insomnia, nausea, vomiting, constipation, parkinsonism, akathisia, extrapyramidal symptoms*
clozapine (Clozaril)	PO; start at 25–50 mg/day and titrate to a target dose of 350–450 mg/day in 3 days; may increase further (max: 900 mg/day)	
olanzapine (Zyprexa)	Adult: PO; start with 5–10 mg/day; may increase by 2.5–5 mg every week (range 10–15 mg/day; max: 20 mg/day). Geriatric: PO; start with 5 mg/day	Agranulocytosis, neuroleptic malignant syndrome (rare)
paliperidone (Invega)	PO; 6 mg/day (max: 12 mg/day)	
quetiapine fumarate (Seroquel)	PO; start with 25 mg bid; may increase to a target dose of 300–400 mg/day in divided doses (max: 800 mg/day)	
℗ᵣ risperidone (Risperdal)	PO; 1–6 mg bid; increase by 2 mg daily to an initial target dose of 6 mg/day	
ziprasidone (Geodon)	PO; 20 mg bid (max: 80 mg bid)	
	IM; 10 mg every 2 h (max: 40 mg/day)	

Italics indicate common adverse effects; <u>underlining</u> indicates serious adverse effects.

NURSING PROCESS FOCUS   PATIENTS RECEIVING ATYPICAL ANTIPSYCHOTIC THERAPY

Assessment	Potential Nursing Diagnoses
Baseline assessment prior to administration: ■ Understand the reason the drug has been prescribed in order to assess for therapeutic effects. ■ Obtain a complete health history including hepatic, renal, urologic, cardiovascular, respiratory, or neurologic disease (especially Parkinson's disease or seizures), current mental status, pregnancy, or breast-feeding. Obtain a drug history including allergies, current prescription and OTC drugs, alcohol use, smoking, and herbal preparations. Be alert to possible drug interactions. ■ Obtain a history of depression or mental disorders, including a family history of same and severity. ■ Assess for disturbances in thought processes, perception, verbal communication, affect, behavior, interpersonal relationships, and self-care. Use objective screening tools per the health care agency. ■ Obtain baseline vital signs and weight. ■ Evaluate appropriate laboratory findings (e.g., CBC, electrolytes, glucose, hepatic and renal function studies, lipid levels, drug screening). ■ Assess the patient's ability to receive and understand instruction. Include the family and caregivers as needed.	■ Disturbed Thought Processes ■ Disturbed Sensory Perception (auditory, visual) ■ Disturbed Personal Identity ■ Anxiety (severe, panic) ■ Impaired Verbal Communication ■ Impaired Social Interaction ■ Ineffective Health Maintenance ■ Impaired Home Maintenance ■ Noncompliance ■ Deficient Knowledge (drug therapy) ■ Risk for Violence (self-directed, directed at others) ■ Risk for Self-Mutilation ■ Risk for Disturbed Family Processes, Caregiver Role Strain
Assessment throughout administration: ■ Assess for desired therapeutic effects (e.g., normalizing thought processes, lessening delusions, hallucinations, improvement in positive or negative symptoms, ability to return to normal ADLs, improvement in appetite and sleep patterns). ■ Continue periodic monitoring of CBC, electrolytes, glucose, hepatic and renal function studies, lipid levels, and therapeutic drug levels. ■ Assess vital signs, especially orthostatic blood pressure, and weigh periodically. ■ Assess for and promptly report adverse effects: dizziness or light-headedness, confusion, agitation, suicidal ideations, hypotension, tachycardia, increase in temperature, blurred or double vision, skin rashes, bruising or bleeding, abdominal pain, jaundice, change in color of stool, flank pain, and hematuria. ■ Assess for and promptly report extrapyramidal (EPS) symptoms including pseudoparkinsonism, acute dystonias, akathisia, and tardive dyskinesias (see "Minimizing adverse effects" in the following section). ■ Immediately report signs and symptoms of NMS: unstable blood pressure, elevated temperature, diaphoresis, dyspnea, muscle rigidity, and incontinence.	

(Continued)

NURSING PROCESS FOCUS   PATIENTS RECEIVING ATYPICAL ANTIPSYCHOTIC THERAPY *(Continued)*

Planning: Patient Goals and Expected Outcomes

The patient will:

- Experience therapeutic effects dependent on the reason the drug is being given (e.g., lessened positive and negative symptoms, delusions, paranoia, hallucinations).
- Be free from, or experience minimal, adverse effects.
- Verbalize an understanding of the drug's use, adverse effects, and required precautions.
- Demonstrate proper self-administration of the medication (e.g., dose, timing, when to notify provider) when possible.

Implementation

Interventions and (Rationales)	Patient and Family Education
Ensuring therapeutic effects:	
■ Continue assessments as described earlier for therapeutic effects. (Drugs used for psychoses and schizophrenia do not cure the underlying disorder but improve positive and negative symptoms of the disorder. Gradual improvement over several weeks to months may be noted.)	■ Teach the patient, family, or caregiver that full effects may not occur immediately but that some improvement should be noticeable after beginning therapy. ■ Supportive, inpatient care may be required during the acute, early period of therapy.
■ Monitor patient compliance with the drug regimen. (The presence of severe mental disorders may result in noncompliance with medications. Regular, consistent dosing is essential to correcting the underlying disorder. Because the drugs do not cure the underlying disorder, if regular administration is disrupted, symptoms may return abruptly.)	■ Involve the family and caregiver to the extent possible in ensuring the patient remains on regular medication routines. ■ Ensure that the patient takes the medication as prescribed. *Never* leave medications at the bedside. ■ Question the possibility of noncompliance if original symptoms or adverse effects suddenly increase in frequency or severity.
Minimizing adverse effects:	
■ Continue to monitor vital signs periodically, especially orthostatic blood pressure and for tachycardia. Ensure patient safety; monitor ambulation until the effects of the drug are known. Be particularly cautious with older adults who are at an increased risk for falls. (Antipsychotic drugs may cause hypotension, increasing the risk of falls and injury.)	■ Have the patient rise from lying or sitting to standing slowly to avoid dizziness or falls. ■ Instruct the patient to call for assistance prior to getting out of bed or attempting to walk alone. For patients on at-home/outpatient medication, avoid driving or other activities requiring mental alertness or physical coordination until the effects of the drug are known.
■ Monitor for and immediately report signs and symptoms of NMS: unstable blood pressure, elevated temperature, diaphoresis, dyspnea, muscle rigidity, and incontinence. (NMS is a rare but potentially fatal syndrome that must be recognized and treated immediately.)	■ Instruct the patient, family, or caregiver to immediately report any changes in level of consciousness, elevated temperature, excessive sweating, severe muscle rigidity, increased respirations or shortness of breath, or incontinence.
■ Continue to monitor motor activity, coordination and balance, and for EPS symptoms, including: ■ Pseudoparkinsonism: tremor, muscle rigidity, stooped posture, bradykinesia (slow to start and shuffling, slow gait) ■ Akathisia: inability to rest and relax, often with pacing ■ Acute dystonias: severe muscle spasms of face, tongue, neck, or back ■ Tardive dyskinesias: "choreoathetoid" movements such as lip smacking, wormlike movements of the tongue, uncontrolled chewing, and grimacing (EPS is less common with atypical antipsychotic medications but may occur.) ■ Ensure adequate nutrition and fluid intake if tardive dyskinesias are present. (Severe choreoathetoid tongue movement may significantly hinder or prevent adequate nutrition.) ■ Ensure patient safety if pseudoparkinsonism affects gait or if akathisia is present. Acute dystonias may require treatment with other medications to halt spasms. (Bradykinesias, slow-to-start ambulation and slow, shuffling gait may predispose the patient to falls. Akathisia with pacing may significantly impair the patient's ability to rest and sleep. Additional medications may be required to treat. Anticholinergics or other drugs may be required to stop spasms.)	■ Instruct the patient, family, or caregiver to immediately report EPS symptoms for additional treatment.

NURSING PROCESS FOCUS   PATIENTS RECEIVING ATYPICAL ANTIPSYCHOTIC THERAPY *(Continued)*

Implementation

Interventions and (Rationales)	Patient and Family Education
■ Continue to monitor CBC, electrolytes, glucose, renal and hepatic function, lipid levels, and therapeutic drug levels. (Atypical antipsychotic drugs such as risperidone may cause an increase in glucose levels and clozapine may cause bone marrow depression. Some of the atypical antipsychotics may cause an increase in lipid levels or hyperlipidemia. Hepatic toxicity is an adverse effect possible with all of the antipsychotic drugs.)	■ Instruct the patient on the need to return periodically for lab work. ■ Teach the patient to promptly report any abdominal pain, particularly in the upper quadrants; changes in stool color; yellowing of sclera or skin; darkened urine; skin rashes; low-grade fevers; general malaise or changes in behavior or activity level; or redness or swelling around sites of injury. ■ Teach the diabetic patient, family, or caregiver to monitor the blood sugar more frequently and report consistent elevations to the health care provider.
■ Monitor for anticholinergic effects including dry mouth, drowsiness, blurred vision, constipation, and urinary retention. Provide symptomatic treatment to ease effects. (Anticholinergic symptoms are common adverse effects of antipsychotic drugs. Tolerance to anticholinergic effects usually develops over time.)	■ Encourage sips of water, ice chips, hard candy, or chewing gum to ease mouth dryness. Avoid alcohol-based mouthwashes, which are drying to the mucosa and which the patient may drink. ■ Increase dietary fiber intake and adequate fluid intake. ■ Report urinary retention to the health care provider promptly.
■ Monitor for weight gain, gynecomastia (breast enlargement, tenderness in either gender), and changes in secondary sexual characteristics (e.g., amenorrhea, impotence). (Atypical antipsychotic drugs may cause weight gain and have pituitary effects. Impotence and weight gain may be significant reasons for noncompliance.)	■ Teach the patient, family, or caregiver to weigh the patient daily and report a significant weight gain (over 2 kg, 4 to 5 pounds per week) to the health care provider. ■ Encourage a healthy diet of increased fruits and vegetables, adequate protein intake, and increased exercise. ■ Address sexual concerns in a matter-of-fact manner and refer as appropriate to the health care provider.
■ Monitor for alcohol and illegal drug use. (Used concurrently, these cause an increased CNS depressant effect or an exacerbation in psychotic symptoms.)	■ Instruct the patient to avoid alcohol and illegal drug use. Refer the patient to community support groups such as AA or NA as appropriate.
■ Monitor caffeine use. (Use of caffeine-containing substances may negate the effects of antipsychotics.)	■ Teach the patient, family, or caregiver to avoid caffeine-containing beverages, foods, and OTC medications, and to read food labels when in doubt of whether the product contains caffeine.
■ Monitor for smoking. (Heavy smoking may decrease metabolism of some antipsychotics leading to decreased efficacy.)	■ Instruct the patient to stop or decrease smoking. Refer the patient to smoking cessation programs, if indicated.
Patient understanding of drug therapy: ■ Use opportunities during administration of medications and during assessments to discuss rationale for drug therapy, desired therapeutic outcomes, most commonly observed adverse effects, parameters for when to call the health care provider, and any necessary monitoring or precautions. Use brief explanations during times of delusions or hallucinations. (Using time during nursing care helps to optimize and reinforce key teaching areas. Brief, consistent explanations assist to interrupt delusional periods.)	■ The patient, family, or caregiver should be able to state the reason for the drug; appropriate dose and scheduling; and what adverse effects to observe for and when to report them.

Patient self-administration of drug therapy:
■ When administering the medication, instruct the patient, family, or caregiver in proper self-administration of drug, e.g., take the drug as prescribed and do not substitute brands. (Utilizing time during nurse-administration of these drugs helps to reinforce teaching.).
	■ Teach the patient, family, or caregiver to take the medication as follows:
	  ■ Take exactly as ordered and use the same manufacturer's brand each time the prescription is filled. (Switching brands may result in differing pharmacokinetics and alterations in therapeutic effect).
	  ■ Ensure that all the medication is taken exactly when and as ordered. Use of a calendar to track doses may be helpful.
	  ■ If the medication causes drowsiness, take at bedtime. Tolerance to anticholinergic effects such as drowsiness usually develops over time.
	  ■ Do not abruptly discontinue the medication.

Evaluation of Outcome Criteria

Evaluate the effectiveness of drug therapy by confirming that patient goals and expected outcomes have been met (see "Planning").

See Table 17.4 for a list of drugs to which these nursing actions apply.

17.7 Treating Psychoses with Dopamine System Stabilizers

Due to side effects caused by conventional and atypical antipsychotic medications, a more recent drug class was developed to better meet the needs of patients with psychoses (Bailey, 2003). The newer class is called *dopamine system stabilizers (DSSs)* or dopamine partial agonists. Aripiprazole (Abilify) received FDA approval in 2002 for the treatment of schizophrenia and schizoaffective disorder. Because ari-

piprazole controls both the positive and negative symptoms of schizophrenia, it is grouped in Table 17.4 with the atypical antipsychotic drugs.

Aripiprazole-treated patients appear to exhibit fewer EPS than patients treated with haloperidol (Haldol). Anticholinergic adverse effects are virtually nonexistent. In fact, the incidence of adverse effects generally compared to the other atypical antipsychotic drugs is very low. Notable side effects, however, include headache, nausea/vomiting, fever, constipation, and anxiety.

Chapter REVIEW

KEY CONCEPTS

The numbered key concepts provide a succinct summary of the important points from the corresponding numbered section within the chapter. If any of these points are not clear, refer to the numbered section within the chapter for review.

17.1 Psychoses are severe mental and behavioral disorders characterized by disorganized mental capacity and an inability to recognize reality.

17.2 Schizophrenia is a type of psychosis characterized by abnormal thoughts and thought processes, disordered communication, withdrawal from other people and the environment, and a high risk for suicide.

17.3 Pharmacologic management of psychoses is difficult because the adverse effects of the drugs may be severe, and patients often do not understand the need for medication.

17.4 The phenothiazines have been effectively used for the treatment of psychoses for more than 50 years; however, they have a high incidence of adverse effects. Extrapyra-

midal side effects (EPS) and neuroleptic malignant syndrome (NMS) are two particularly serious conditions.

17.5 The nonphenothiazine conventional antipsychotics have the same therapeutic applications and adverse effects as the phenothiazines.

17.6 Atypical antipsychotics are often preferred because they address both positive and negative symptoms of schizophrenia, and produce less dramatic side effects.

17.7 Dopamine system stabilizers are the newest antipsychotic class. It is hoped that this new class will have the same efficacy as other antipsychotic classes, with fewer serious side effects.

NCLEX-RN® REVIEW QUESTIONS

1 The patient states that he has not taken his antipsychotic drug for the past 2 weeks because it was causing sexual dysfunction. The name *antipsychotic* explains that continuing the medication as prescribed is important because:
1. hypertensive crisis may occur with abrupt withdrawal.
2. muscle twitching may occur.
3. parkinson-like symptoms will occur.
4. symptoms of psychosis are likely to return.

2 Prior to discharge, the nurse provides teaching related to side effects of phenothiazines to the patient, family, or caregiver. Which of the following should be included?
1. The patient may experience withdrawal and slowed activity.
2. Severe muscle spasms may occur early in therapy.
3. Tardive dyskinesia is likely early in therapy.
4. Medications should be taken as prescribed to prevent side effects.

3 A 20-year-old man is admitted to the in-patient psychiatric unit for treatment of acute schizophrenia and is started on risperidone (Risperdal). Therapeutic outcomes of this drug will include:
1. restful sleep, elevated mood, and coping abilities.
2. decreased delusional thinking and lessened auditory/visual hallucinations.
3. orthostatic hypotension, reflex tachycardia, and sedation.
4. relief of anxiety and improved sleep and dietary habits.

4 Nursing implications of the administration of haloperidol (Haldol) to a patient exhibiting psychotic behavior include which of the following? (Select all that apply.)
1. Take 1 hour before or 2 hours after antacids.
2. The incidence of EPS is high.
3. It is therapeutic if ordered on a prn basis.
4. Haldol is contraindicated in Parkinson's disease, seizure disorders, alcoholism, and severe mental depression.
5. Crush the sustained-release form for easier swallowing.

5 Which of the following data collected by the nurse during the history and physical is a contraindication for a patient to receive fluphenazine (Permitil, Prolixin)?
1. Diabetes mellitus
2. Age older than 70
3. Bone marrow depression
4. Hypertension

6 A female, age 39, has been on haloperidol (Haldol) for 3 months for severe psychosis. The nurse is monitoring the patient for the development of acute dystonias with haloperidol, and will monitor for:
1. dry mouth, constipation, and blurred vision.
2. pacing, squirming, or difficulty with gait such as bradykinesia.
3. severe spasms of the muscles of the tongue, face, neck, or back.
4. tremors, wormlike tongue movements, and involuntary lip puckering.

CRITICAL THINKING QUESTIONS

1. A 22-year-old male patient has been on haloperidol (Haldol LA) for 2 weeks for the treatment of schizophrenia. During a follow-up assessment, the nurse notices that the patient keeps rubbing his neck and is complaining of neck spasms. What is the nurse's initial action? What is the potential cause of the sore neck and what would be the potential treatment? What teaching is appropriate for this patient?

2. A 68-year-old patient has been put on olanzapine (Zyprexa) for treatment of acute psychoses. What is a priority of care for this patient? What teaching is important for this patient?

3. A 20-year-old, newly diagnosed patient with schizophrenia has been on chlorpromazine (Thorazine) and is doing well. Today the nurse notices that the patient appears more anxious and is demonstrating increased paranoia. What is the nurse's initial action? What is the potential problem? What patient teaching is important?

See Appendix D for answers and rationales for all activities.

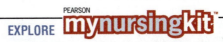

EXPLORE

MyNursingKit is your one stop for online chapter review materials and resources. Prepare for success with additional NCLEX®-style practice questions, interactive assignments and activities, web links, animations and videos, and more!

Register your access code from the front of your book at
www.mynursingkit.com.

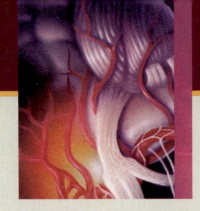

Chapter 18

Drugs for the Control of Pain

LEARNING OUTCOMES

After reading this chapter, the student should be able to:

1. Relate the importance of pain assessment to effective pharmacotherapy.
2. Explain the neural mechanisms at the level of the spinal cord responsible for pain.
3. Explain how pain can be controlled by inhibiting the release of spinal neurotransmitters.
4. Describe the role of nonpharmacologic therapies in pain management.
5. Compare and contrast the types of opioid receptors and their importance in effective management of pain.
6. Explain the role of opioid antagonists in the diagnosis and treatment of acute opioid toxicity.
7. Describe the long-term treatment of opioid dependence.
8. Compare the pharmacotherapeutic approaches of preventing migraines with those of aborting migraines.
9. Describe the nurse's role in the pharmacologic management of patients receiving analgesics and antimigraine drugs.
10. For each of the drug classes listed in Drugs at a Glance, know representative drug examples, and explain the mechanisms of drug action, primary actions, and important adverse effects.
11. Categorize drugs used in the treatment of pain based on their classification and mechanism of action.
12. Use the nursing process to care for patients receiving drug therapy for pain.

Pain is an experience characterized by unpleasant feelings, usually associated with trauma or disease. Since we all experience tissue trauma, pain is a universal experience. At a simplistic level, pain may be viewed as a defense mechanism that helps us to avoid potentially damaging situations and encourages us to seek medical help. Although the neural and chemical mechanisms for pain are fairly straightforward, many psychologic and emotional processes are a part of this experience. Anxiety, fatigue, and depression can increase the perception of pain; positive attitudes and support from caregivers may reduce the perception of pain. For example, some patients tolerate their pain better if they know the source of trauma and the medical courses available to treat their discomfort. There are many options for pain assessment and the treatment of pain-associated disorders.

18.1 Assessment and Classification of Pain

The psychologic reaction to pain is subjective. During physical assessment, the same degree and type of pain that would be described as excruciating or unbearable by one patient, may not even be mentioned by another patient. Several numeric scales and survey instruments are available to help health care providers standardize the patient's conveyance of pain and subsequently measure the progress of drug therapies. Successful pain management depends not only on an accurate assessment of how the patient feels but an understanding of the underlying disorder causing the suffering. Selection of appropriate therapy is dependent on both the nature and characteristic of pain.

Pain may be classified as either acute or chronic. *Acute pain* is an intense pain occurring over a brief period of time, usually from injury to recovery. *Chronic pain* persists over a longer time. Six months is considered the standard. Chronic pain interferes continuously with daily activities, and usually results in feelings of helplessness and hopelessness for the patient.

Pain may also be classified according to its source. Injury to *tissues* produces **nociceptive pain**. This type of pain may be described as *somatic pain* (*sharp*, *localized* sensations) or *visceral pain* (generalized *dull*, *throbbing*, or *aching* sensations). In contrast, **neuropathic pain** results from *injury to the nerves* and is typically described by patients as *burning*, *shooting*, or *numb pain*. Whereas nociceptive pain responds quite well to conventional pain-relief medications, neuropathic pain is more difficult to manage.

18.2 Nonpharmacologic Techniques for Pain Management

Although for most patients, drugs are quite effective at relieving pain, many have significant side effects. For example, at high doses, aspirin causes gastrointestinal (GI) bleeding. Opioids have the potential for dependence and can cause significant drowsiness. To assist patients in obtaining adequate pain relief, nonpharmacologic techniques may be used alone or as an adjunct to pharmacotherapy. When used concurrently with medications, nonpharmacologic techniques may allow for lower doses and possibly fewer drug-related adverse effects. Some techniques used for reducing pain are as follows:

- Acupuncture
- Biofeedback therapy
- Massage
- Heat or cold packs
- Meditation or prayer
- Relaxation therapy
- Art or music therapy
- Imagery
- Chiropractic manipulation
- Hypnosis
- Therapeutic or physical touch
- Transcutaneous electrical nerve stimulation (TENS)
- Energy therapies such as Reiki and Qi gong

Patients with intractable cancer pain sometimes require more invasive techniques as rapidly growing tumors press on vital tissues and nerves. Chemotherapy and surgical treatments for cancer can cause severe pain. Radiation therapy may provide pain relief by shrinking solid tumors that may be pressing on nerves. Surgery may be used to reduce pain by removing the tumor. Then, there is the issue of pain subsequent to the surgery. The treatment of cancer pain usually involves opioids and other adjuvant drugs. Opioid drugs used to relieve cancer pain may require higher than expected doses but given the goal of relieving suffering and improving quality of life, there is no set maximum dose for the amount of drug used in these circumstances.

Injection of alcohol or other neurotoxic substances directly into neuronal tissue is occasionally performed to produce nerve blocks. In many instances, nerve blocks irreversibly stop impulse transmission and have the potential to provide total pain relief.

PharmFacts

Pain

Pain is a common symptom, reflected by the following statistics:

- Every year in America, approximately 16 million people experience chronic arthritic pain.
- More than 31 million adults have reported low back pain, while 19 million people have experienced this pain on a more chronic basis.
- At least 50 million people are fully or partially disabled due to pain.
- More than 50% of adults experience muscle pain each year.
- Up to 40% of people with cancer report moderate to severe pain with treatment.

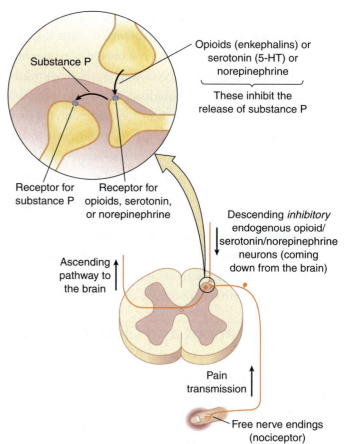

▶ **Figure 18.1** Neural pathways for pain

18.3 The Neural Mechanisms of Pain

The process of pain transmission begins when pain receptors are stimulated. These receptors, called **nociceptors,** are free nerve endings located throughout the body. The nerve impulse signaling pain is sent to the spinal cord by way of two types of sensory neurons, called Aδ and C fibers. **Aδ fibers** are thinly wrapped in myelin, a lipid substance that speeds nerve transmission. **C fibers** are unmyelinated; thus, they carry information more slowly to the brain. Scientists and clinicians believe that Aδ fibers signal sharp, well-defined pain, whereas the C fibers conduct dull, poorly localized pain.

Once pain impulses reach the spinal cord, neurotransmitters are responsible for transmitting the message along to the next set of neurons. A neurotransmitter called **substance P** is thought to be responsible for continuing the pain message, although other neurotransmitter candidates have been proposed. Spinal neurotransmitters are critical because they control whether pain signals continue to the brain. The activity of substance P may be affected by other neurotransmitters released from neurons located within the CNS. One group of neurotransmitters called **endogenous opioids** involves endorphins, dynorphins, and enkephalins. ▶ Figure 18.1 shows one point of contact where endogenous opioids modify spinal sensory information. If pain impulses reach the brain, a person may respond to the sensation with many possible actions, ranging from signaling the skeletal muscles to jerk away from a sharp object, to mental depression, which involves higher brain functioning, e.g., suffering and debilitating thoughts about the pain experience.

The fact that the pain signals begin at nociceptors located within peripheral tissues and proceed throughout the CNS, allows several targets for the pharmacologic intervention. In general, two main classes of pain medications are employed to manage pain, and they act at different locations: The opioids act within the CNS, whereas the nonsteroidal anti-inflammatory drugs (NSAIDs) act at the peripheral tissue level.

OPIOID ANALGESICS

By definition, **analgesics** are medications used to relieve pain. The two basic categories of analgesics are the opioids and the nonopioids. An opioid analgesic is a natural or synthetic morphine-like substance responsible for reducing moderate to severe pain. Opioids are **narcotic** substances, meaning that they produce numbness or stupor-like symptoms.

18.4 Classification of Opioids

Terminology of the narcotic analgesic medications may be confusing. Several of these drugs are obtained from opium, a milky extract from the unripe seeds of the poppy plant, which contains more than 20 different chemicals having pharmacologic activity. Opium consists of 9% to 14% morphine and 0.8% to 2.5% codeine. These natural substances are called **opiates.** In a search for safer analgesics, chemists have created several dozen synthetic drugs with activity similar to that of the opiates. For example, morphine is a natural narcotic; meperidine is a synthetic narcotic. **Opioid** is a general term referring to any of these substances, natural or synthetic, and is often used interchangeably with the term *opiate.*

Narcotic is a general term often used to describe opioid drugs that produce analgesia and CNS depression. In common usage, a narcotic analgesic is the same as an opioid, and the terms are often used interchangeably. In the context of drug enforcement however, the term *narcotic* describes a much broader range of abused illegal drugs such as hallucinogens, heroin, amphetamines, and marijuana. So this is an important fact to remember when relating use of opioids with members of law enforcement.

Opioids exert their actions by interacting with at least six different types of receptors: mu (types one and two), kappa, sigma, delta, and epsilon. From the perspective of pain management, the **mu** and **kappa receptors** are the most important. Drugs that stimulate a particular opioid receptor are called *opioid agonists;* those that block an opioid receptor are called *opioid antagonists.* Responses produced by activation of mu and kappa receptors are listed in Table 18.1.

Some opioid agonists, such as morphine, activate both mu and kappa receptors. Other opioids, such as pentazocine hydrochloride (Talwin), exert mixed opioid agonist–antagonist effects by activating the kappa receptors but blocking the mu receptors. Opioid blockers such as naloxone (Narcan) inhibit both the mu and kappa receptors. This is the body's way of providing for a diverse set of body responses from one substance. ➤ Figure 18.2 illustrates actions resulting from stimulation of mu and kappa receptors.

Opioid Agonists

Narcotic opioid agonists bind to opioid receptors and produce multiple responses throughout the body. Morphine is the prototype drug used to treat severe pain. It is considered the standard by which the effectiveness of other opioids are compared.

18.5 Pharmacotherapy with Opioids

Opioids are the first line of choice for moderate to severe pain (discomfort that cannot be controlled with other "milder" classes of analgesics). More than 20 different opioids are available as medications, which may be classified by similarities in their chemical structures, by their mechanisms of action, or by their effectiveness (Table 18.2). The

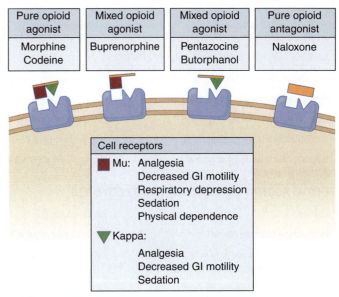

➤ **Figure 18.2** Opioid receptors

most clinically useful classification method is by effectiveness, which places opiates into categories of strong or moderate activity.

Opiates produce many important effects other than analgesia. They are effective at suppressing the cough reflex and at slowing the motility of the GI tract for cases of severe diarrhea. As powerful CNS depressants, opioids can cause sedation, which may either be therapeutic or determined a side effect, depending on the patient's disease state. Some patients experience euphoria and intense relaxation, which are reasons why opiates are sometimes abused. There are many adverse effects, including respiratory depression, sedation, nausea, and vomiting.

All of the narcotic analgesics have the potential to cause physical and psychologic dependence, as discussed in chapter 11∞. Over the years, health care providers and nurses have hesitated to administer the proper amount of opioid analgesics for fear of causing patient dependence or of producing serious adverse effects such as sedation or respiratory depression. Because of this tendency, some patients have not received complete pain relief.

TABLE 18. 1	Responses Produced by Activation of Specific Opioid Receptors	
Response	Mu Receptor	Kappa Receptor
Analgesia	✓	✓
Decreased GI motility	✓	✓
Euphoria	✓	
Miosis		✓
Physical dependence	✓	
Respiratory depression	✓	
Sedation	✓	✓

TABLE 18.2	Opioids for Pain Management	
Drug	Route and Adult Dose (max dose where indicated)	Adverse Effects
OPIOID AGONISTS WITH HIGH EFFECTIVENESS		
hydromorphone hydrochloride (Dilaudid)	PO; 1–4 mg every 4–6 h prn	*Pruritis, constipation, nausea, sedation, drowsiness, dizziness*
levorphanol tartrate (Levo-Dromoran)	PO; 2–3 mg tid—qid prn	
meperidine hydrochloride (Demerol)	PO; 50–150 mg every 3–4 h prn	<u>Anaphylactoid reaction, cardiac arrest, severe respiratory depression or arrest, convulsions</u>
methadone hydrochloride (Dolophine)	PO; 2.5–10 mg every 3–4 h prn	
morphine sulfate (Astramorph PF, Duramorph, others)	PO; 10–30 mg every 4 h prn	
OPIOID AGONISTS WITH MODERATE EFFECTIVENESS		
codeine	PO; 15–60 mg qid	*Sedation, nausea, constipation, dizziness*
hydrocodone bitartrate (Hycodan)	PO; 5–10 mg every 4–6 h prn (max: 15 mg/dose)	<u>Hepatotoxicity, respiratory depression, circulatory collapse, coma</u>
oxycodone hydrochloride (OxyContin); oxycodone terephthalate (Percocet-5, Roxicet, others)	PO; 5–10 mg qid prn	
propoxyphene hydrochloride (Darvon)	PO; 65 mg (HCl form) or 100 mg (napsylate form) every 4 h	
propoxyphene napsylate (Darvon-N)	PRN (max: 390 mg/day HCl; max: 600 mg/day napsylate)	
OPIOID ANTAGONISTS		
nalmefene hydrochloride (Revex)	Subcutaneous/IM/IV; use 1 mg/mL concentration	*Muscle and joint pains, difficulty sleeping, anxiety, headache, nervousness, vomiting, abdominal pain*
	Nonopioid dependent: 0.5 mg/70 kg	
	Opioid dependent: 0.1 mg/70 kg	<u>Hepatotoxicity</u>
naloxone hydrochloride (Narcan)	IV; 0.4–2 mg; may be repeated every 2–3 min up to 10 mg if necessary	
naltrexone hydrochloride (Trexan, ReVia)	PO; 25 mg followed by another 25 mg in 1 h if no withdrawal response (max: 800 mg/day)	
OPIOIDS WITH MIXED AGONIST–ANTAGONIST EFFECTS		
buprenorphine hydrochloride (Buprenex)	IM/IV; 0.3 mg every 6 h (max: 0.6 mg every 4 h)	*Drowsiness, dizziness, light-headedness, euphoria, nausea, clammy skin, sweating, insomnia, abdominal pain, constipation*
butorphanol tartrate (Stadol)	IM; 1–4 mg every 3–4 h prn (max: 4 mg/dose)	
dezocine (Dalgan)	IV; 2.5–10 mg (usually 5 mg) every 2–4 h	<u>Respiratory depression, shock</u>
	IM; 5–10 mg (usually 10 mg) every 3–4 h	
nalbuphine hydrochloride (Nubain)	Subcutaneous/IM/IV; 10–20 mg every 3–6 h prn (max: 160 mg/day)	
pentazocine hydrochloride (Talwin)	PO; 50–100 mg every 3–4 h (max: 600 mg/day)	
	Subcutaneous/IM/IV; 30 mg every 3–4 h (max: 360 mg/day)	

Italics indicate common adverse effects; <u>underlining</u> indicates serious adverse effects.

When used according to accepted medical practice, patients can, and indeed should, receive the pain relief they need without fear of addiction or adverse effects. One method available is **patient-controlled analgesia (PCA)**. In this instance, patients are allowed to self-medicate with opiate medication by the pressing of a button. Safe levels of scheduled pain medication are delivered with an infusion pump.

In the pharmacologic management of pain, it is common practice to combine opioids and nonnarcotic analgesics into a single tablet or capsule. The two classes of analgesics work synergistically to relieve pain, and dose of the opioid can be kept small to avoid dependence and narcotic-related side ef-

fects. With growing concern over the risk of hepatic toxicity related to large doses of acetaminophen, it should be noted that additional doses of *combination* products may raise the dose of acetaminophen or adjuvant drug to unacceptable levels. Additional doses of the combination product should not be used unless the dose of the *nonnarcotic* analgesic does not exceed the recommended dose. As examples, combination analgesics are as follows:

- Vicodin (hydrocodone, 5 mg; acetaminophen, 500 mg)
- Percocet (oxycodone hydrochloride, 7.5 mg; acetaminophen, 325 mg)

- Percodan (oxycodone hydrochloride, 4.5 mg; oxycodone terephthalate, 0.38 mg; aspirin, 325 mg)
- Darvocet-N 50 (propoxyphene napsylate, 50 mg; acetaminophen, 325 mg)
- Empirin with Codeine No. 2 (codeine phosphate, 15 mg; aspirin, 325 mg)
- Tylenol with Codeine (single dose may contain from 15 to 60 mg of codeine phosphate and from 300 to 1,000 mg of acetaminophen)

Some opioids are used primarily for conditions other than general complaints of pain. For example, alfentanil (Alfenta), fentanyl (Sublimaze), remifentanil (Ultiva), and sufentanil (Sufenta) are used for general anesthesia; these are discussed further in chapter 19∞. Codeine is most often prescribed as a cough suppressant and is covered in chapter 38∞. Opioids used in treating diarrhea are presented in chapter 41∞.

Opioid Antagonists

Opioid antagonists are substances that prevent the effects of opioid agonists. Many drugs are considered competitive antagonists because they compete with opioids for access to the opioid receptor.

LIFESPAN CONSIDERATIONS

The Influence of Age on Pain Expression and Perception

Pain control in both children and older adults can be challenging. Knowledge of developmental theories, the aging process, behavioral cues, subtle signs of discomfort, and verbal and nonverbal responses to pain are a must when it comes to effective pain management. Older patients may have a decreased perception of pain or may simply ignore pain as a "natural" consequence of aging. Because these patients frequently go undermedicated, a thorough assessment is needed. As with adults, belief in self-report when assessing for pain in children is important. Developmentally appropriate pain-rating tools are available and should be used on a consistent basis. Comfort measures should also be used.

When administering opioids for pain relief, always monitor patients closely. Smaller doses are usually indicated, and side effects may be heightened. Closely monitor decreased respirations, LOC, and dizziness. Take body weight prior to starting opioid administration and calculate doses accordingly. Keep bed and crib rails raised and the bed in low position at all times to prevent injury from falls. Some opioids, such as meperidine (Demerol), should be used cautiously in children. Many older adults take multiple drugs (polypharmacy), so it is important to obtain a complete list of all medications taken and check for interactions.

Pr Prototype Drug | Morphine *(Astramorph PF, Duramorph, others)*

Therapeutic Class: Opioid analgesic   **Pharmacologic Class:** Opioid receptor agonist

ACTIONS AND USES
Morphine binds with both mu and kappa receptor sites to produce profound analgesia. It causes euphoria, constriction of the pupils, and stimulation of cardiac muscle. It is used for symptomatic relief of serious acute and chronic pain after nonnarcotic analgesics have failed, as preanesthetic medication, to relieve shortness of breath associated with heart failure and pulmonary edema, and for acute chest pain connected with MI.

ADMINISTRATION ALERTS
- The oral solution may be given sublingually.
- The oral solution comes in multiple strengths; carefully observe drug orders and labels before administering.
- Morphine causes peripheral vasodilation, which results in orthostatic hypotension.
- Pregnancy category B (D in long-term use or with high doses)

PHARMACOKINETICS
Onset: Less than 60 min
Peak: 60 min PO; 20–60 min rectally; 50–90 min subcutaneously; 30–60 min IM; 20 min IV
Half-life: 2–3 h
Duration: Up to 7 h

ADVERSE EFFECTS
Morphine may cause dysphoria (restlessness, depression, and anxiety), hallucinations, nausea, constipation, dizziness, and an itching sensation. Overdose may result in severe respiratory depression or cardiac arrest. Tolerance develops to the sedative, nausea-producing, and euphoric effects of the drug. Cross-tolerance also develops between morphine and other opioids such as heroin, methadone, and meperidine. Physical and psychologic dependence develops when high doses are taken for prolonged periods.

Contraindications: Morphine may intensify or mask the pain of gallbladder disease, due to biliary tract spasms. Morphine should also be avoided in cases of acute or severe asthma, GI obstruction, and severe hepatic or renal impairment.

INTERACTIONS
Drug–Drug: Morphine interacts with several drugs. For example, concurrent use of CNS depressants, such as alcohol, other opioids, general anesthetics, sedatives, and antidepressants such as MAO inhibitors and tricyclics potentiates the action of opiates, increasing the risk of severe respiratory depression and death.

Lab Tests: Unknown

Herbal/Food: Yohimbe, kava kava, valerian, and St. John's wort may potentiate the effect of morphine.

Treatment of Overdose: IV administration of naloxone is the specific treatment. Other treatments include activated charcoal, a laxative, and a counteracting narcotic antagonist. Multiple doses may be needed.

Refer to MyNursingKit for a Nursing Process Focus specific to this drug.

NURSING PROCESS FOCUS   PATIENTS RECEIVING OPIOID THERAPY

Assessment	Potential Nursing Diagnoses
Baseline assessment prior to administration: • Understand the reason the drug has been prescribed in order to assess for therapeutic effects. • Obtain a complete health history including cardiovascular, neurologic, respiratory, hepatic, renal, cancer, gallbladder or urologic disease; pregnancy; or breast-feeding. Note recent surgeries or injuries. Obtain a drug history including allergies, current prescription and OTC drugs, and herbal preparations. Be alert to possible drug interactions. • Assess the level of pain. Use objective screening tools when possible (e.g., FLACC [face, limbs, arms, cry, consolability] for infants or very young children, Wong-Baker FACES scale for children, numerical rating scale for adults). Assess history of pain and what has worked successfully or not for the patient in the past. • Obtain baseline vital signs and weight. • Evaluate appropriate laboratory findings (e.g., CBC, hepatic and renal function studies). • Assess the patient's ability to receive and understand instruction. Include the family and caregivers as needed.	• Acute or Chronic Pain (related to injury, disease, or surgical procedure) • Ineffective Breathing Pattern (related to pain or drug therapy, especially when given in the presence of other CNS depressants such as anesthetics postoperatively) • Constipation (related to adverse drug effects) • Deficient Knowledge (related to drug therapy) • Risk for Injury, Risk for Falls (related to adverse drug effects)
Assessment throughout administration: • Assess for desired therapeutic effects (e.g., absent or greatly diminished pain, ability to move more easily without pain, carry out postoperative treatment care). Continue to use a pain-rating scale to quantify the level of improvement. • Continue periodic monitoring of CBC, and hepatic and renal function studies. • Assess vital signs, especially blood pressure, pulse, and respiratory rate. • Assess for and report adverse effects: excessive dizziness, drowsiness, confusion, agitation, hypotension, tachycardia, bradypnea, and pinpoint pupils.	

Planning: Patient Goals and Expected Outcomes

The patient will:
• Experience therapeutic effects dependent on the reason the drug is being given (e.g., absent or decreased pain, ease in movement and postoperative care).
• Be free from, or experience minimal, adverse effects.
• Verbalize an understanding of the drug's use, adverse effects, and required precautions.
• Demonstrate proper self-administration of the medication (e.g., dose, timing, when to notify provider).

Implementation

Interventions and (Rationales)	Patient and Family Education
Ensuring therapeutic effects: • Continue assessments as described earlier for therapeutic effects. Give drug *before* the start of acute pain and encourage regularly scheduled doses for the first 24 to 48 hours postoperatively for adequate postoperative pain relief. Provide additional comfort measures to supplement drug therapy. (Consistent use of a pain rating scale by all providers will help quantify the level of pain relief and lead to better pain control. Watch for subtle signs of pain: hesitancy to move, shallow breaths to avoid increasing pain, grimacing on movement. Encouraging the patient to maintain regular doses during the acute postoperative or pain period may provide better relief than giving "prn" doses on request when pain has increased to the point that medication is needed.)	• Teach the paient that pain relief, rather than merely control, is the goal of therapy. • Encourage the patient to take the drug consistently during the acute postoperative or procedure period rather than requesting only when pain is severe. • Explain the rationale behind the pain rating scale (i.e., it allows consistency among all providers). • Encourage the patient, family, or caregiver to use additional, nonpharmacologic pain relief techniques, e.g., distraction with television or music, backrubs, guided imagery.

Implementation

Interventions and (Rationales)	Patient and Family Education
Minimizing adverse effects:	
▪ Continue to monitor vital signs, especially respirations and pulse oximetry as ordered, postoperatively and in patients with acute pain. For terminal cancer pain, obtain instructions from the oncologist or hospice provider on any dose restrictions. (Respiratory depression is the most common with the first dose of an opioid and when given in the presence of other CNS depressants, e.g., postoperatively when the patient may still be experiencing effects of general anesthesia. Count respirations *before* giving the opioid drug and contact the provider before giving if the respirations are below 12 breaths per minute in the adult patient, or as ordered in the child. Continue to assess the respiratory rate every 15 to 30 minutes for the first 4 hours. For terminal cancer pain, the drug may not be withheld regardless of the respiratory rate, dependent on the provider.)	▪ Encourage the patient to take deep breaths in the postoperative period. ▪ Encourage consistent pain medication usage to increase activity tolerance. ▪ Encourage the patient with terminal cancer to take the dose consistently around the clock with prn doses as required. Advise the family or caregiver on the provider's instructions for adequate pain relief and to contact the provider if any pain remains.
▪ Monitor the blood pressure and pulse periodically or if symptoms warrant. Ensure patient safety; monitor ambulation until the effects of drug are known. Be particularly cautious with older adults who are at an increased risk for falls. (Opioids may cause hypotension as an adverse effect and increase the risk of falls or injuries.)	▪ Teach the patient to rise from lying or sitting to standing slowly to avoid dizziness or falls. ▪ Instruct the patient to call for assistance prior to getting out of bed or attempting to walk alone, and to avoid driving or other activities requiring mental alertness or physical coordination until the effects of the drug are known.
▪ Continue to assess bowel sounds. Increase fluid intake and dietary fiber intake. (Decreased peristalsis is an adverse effect of opioid drugs. Significantly diminished or absent bowels sounds are reported to the health care provider immediately. Additional fluids and fiber may ease constipation but additional medications such as Miralax or Colace may be required.)	▪ Teach the patient to increase fluids to 2 L per day and to increase the intake of dietary fiber such as fruits, vegetables, and whole grains. ▪ Instruct the patient to report severe constipation to the health care provider for additional advice on laxatives or stool softeners.
▪ Monitor for itching or complaints of itching. (Opioids may cause histamine release and itching or a sensation of itching. In severe cases, antihistamines may be required. Assess for itching as an expected side effect versus signs and symptoms of true allergy/anaphylaxis: changes in vital signs especially hypotension and tachycardia, dyspnea, or urticaria.)	▪ Teach the patient to report itching to the health care provider, especially if itching is severe or increasing. ▪ Instruct the patient to immediately report any itching associated with dizziness or light-headedness, difficulty breathing, palpitations, or significant hives.
▪ Assess for changes in level of consciousness, disorientation or confusion, agitation, headache, sluggish or pinpoint pupils, or seizures. (Neurologic changes may indicate overmedication, increased intracranial pressure, or adverse drug effects. Older adults may be at risk for confusion and falls.)	▪ Instruct the patient, family, or caregiver to immediately report increasing lethargy, disorientation, confusion, changes in behavior or mood, agitation or aggression, slurred speech, ataxia, or seizures. ▪ Ensure patient safety if disorientation is present.
▪ Assess for urinary retention, especially in the postoperative period. (Opioids may cause urinary retention as an adverse effect.)	▪ Encourage the patient to move about in bed and to start early ambulation as soon as allowed postoperatively. Assist to a normal voiding position if unable to use bathroom or commode. ▪ Instruct the patient to immediately report an inability to void, increasing bladder pressure, or pain.
▪ Monitor pain relief in patients on patient-controlled analgesia (PCA) pumps. If a basal dose is not given continuously, assess that pain relief is adequate and contact the provider if pain remains present. Teach and encourage the patient to use self-medication control button whenever pain is present, increasing, or before activities. (PCA-administered pain control has greatly improved pain relief for patients with regular dosing but is only effective when taken as needed. Review dosage history and patient symptoms to ensure adequate pain relief. Contact the provider if dose, frequency, or basal dose seems inadequate for relief.)	▪ Instruct the patient, family, or caregiver on the use of the PCA pump. Encourage use on an as-often-as-needed basis and emphasize the limitations present to protect the patient (i.e., overdose is not possible).
Patient understanding of drug therapy:	
▪ Use opportunities during administration of medications and during assessments to discuss the rationale for drug therapy, desired therapeutic outcomes, most commonly observed adverse effects, parameters for when to call the health care provider, and any necessary monitoring or precautions. (Using time during nursing care helps to optimize and reinforce key teaching areas.)	▪ The patient should be able to state the reason for the drug, appropriate dose and scheduling, and what adverse effects to observe for and when to report them.

(Continued)

NURSING PROCESS FOCUS   **PATIENTS RECEIVING OPIOID THERAPY** *(Continued)*

Implementation

Interventions and (Rationales)	Patient and Family Education

Patient self-administration of drug therapy:
 	
▪ When administering the medication, instruct the patient, family, or caregiver in proper self-administration of drug, e.g., take the drug as prescribed when needed. (Utilizing time during nurse-administration of these drugs helps to reinforce teaching.)
	▪ Teach the patient to take the medication as follows:
	  ▪ Before the pain becomes severe and for cancer pain, as consistently as possible.
	  ▪ If using a patient-controlled analgesia (PCA) pump: use the self-dosage button whenever pain begins to increase or before activities such as sitting at the bedside.
	  ▪ Take with food to decrease GI upset.
	  ▪ Because opioids are scheduled drugs (most often C-II through IV), federal law restricts the sale and use of the drug to the person receiving the prescription only. Additional prescriptions may be necessary if the drug is continued beyond the first prescription (e.g., phone-in refills are not allowed for C-II drugs). Do not share with any other person and do not discard any unused drug down drains, flush down the toilet, or place in the garbage. Return any unused drug to the pharmacy or health care provider for proper disposal.

Evaluation of Outcome Criteria

Evaluate effectiveness of drug therapy by confirming that patient goals and expected outcomes have been met (see "Planning").

See Table 18.2 for a list of drugs to which these nursing actions apply.

18.6 Pharmacotherapy with Opioid Antagonists

Opioid overdose can occur as a result of overly aggressive pain therapy or as a result of substance abuse. Any opioid may be abused for its psychoactive effects; however, morphine, meperidine, and heroin are preferred because of their potency. Although heroin is currently available as a legal analgesic in many countries, it is deemed too dangerous for therapeutic use by the FDA and is a major drug of abuse.

Pr Prototype Drug | Naloxone *(Narcan)*

Therapeutic Class: Agent for treatment of acute opioid overdose and misuse

Pharmacologic Class: Opioid receptor antagonist

ACTIONS AND USES
Naloxone is a pure opioid antagonist, blocking both mu and kappa receptors. It is used for complete or partial reversal of opioid effects in emergency situations when acute opioid overdose is suspected. Given intravenously, it begins to reverse opioid-initiated CNS and respiratory depression within minutes. It will immediately cause opioid withdrawal symptoms in patients physically dependent on opioids. It is also used to treat postoperative opioid depression. It is occasionally given as adjunctive therapy to reverse hypotension caused by septic shock.

ADMINISTRATION ALERTS
▪ Administer for a respiratory rate of fewer than 10 breaths/minute. Keep resuscitative equipment accessible.

▪ Pregnancy category B

PHARMACOKINETICS
Onset: 1–2 min IV; 2–5 min IM; 2–5 min subcutaneously

Peak: 5–15 min

Half-life: 60–100 min

Duration: 45 min

ADVERSE EFFECTS
Naloxone itself has minimal toxicity. However, reversal of the effects of opioids may result in rapid loss of analgesia, increased blood pressure, tremors, hyperventilation, nausea and vomiting, and drowsiness.

Contraindications: Naloxone should not be used for respiratory depression caused by nonopioid medications.

INTERACTIONS
Drug–Drug: Drug interactions include a reversal of the analgesic effects of opioid agonists and mixed agonist drugs.

Lab Tests: Unknown

Herbal/Food: Echinacea may increase the risk of hepatotoxicity.

Treatment of Overdose: Naloxone overdose requires the use of oxygen, IV fluids, vasopressors, and other supportive measures as indicated. These treatments may be useful in combination drug overdose (for example, pentazocine with naloxone [Talwin NX]).

Refer to MyNursingKit for a Nursing Process Focus specific to this drug.

Once injected or inhaled, heroin rapidly crosses the blood–brain barrier to enter the brain, where it is metabolized to morphine. Thus, the effects and symptoms of heroin administration are actually caused by the activation of mu and kappa receptors by morphine. The initial effect is an intense euphoria, called a *rush,* followed by several hours of deep relaxation.

Opioid antagonists are blockers of opioid activity. They are often used to reverse the symptoms of opioid addiction, toxicity, and overdose. Symptoms include sedation or respiratory distress. Acute opioid intoxication is a medical emergency, with respiratory depression being the most serious problem. Infusion with the opioid antagonist naloxone (Narcan) may be used to reverse respiratory depression and other acute symptoms. In cases in which the patient is unconscious or unclear which drug has been taken, opioid antagonists may be given to diagnose the overdose. If the opioid antagonist fails to quickly reverse the acute symptoms, the overdose may be attributed to a nonopioid substance.

Opioids with Mixed Agonist–Antagonist Activity

Narcotic opioids that have mixed agonist–antagonist activity stimulate the opioid receptor; thus, they cause analgesia. However, the withdrawal symptoms or adverse effects are not as intense due to partial activity of receptor subtypes.

18.7 Treatment for Opioid Dependence

Although effective at relieving pain, the opioids have a greater risk for dependence than almost any other class of medications. Tolerance develops relatively quickly to the euphoric effects of opioids, causing abusers to escalate their doses and take the drugs more frequently. The higher and more frequent doses rapidly cause physical dependence in opioid abusers.

When physically dependent patients attempt to discontinue drug use, they experience extremely uncomfortable symptoms that convince many to continue their drug-taking behavior to avoid the suffering. As long as the drug is continued, they feel "normal," and many can continue work or social activities. In cases when the drug is abruptly discontinued, the patient experiences about 7 days of withdrawal symptoms before overcoming the physical dependence.

The intense craving characteristic of psychologic dependence may occur for many months, and even years, following discontinuation of opioids. This often results in a return to drug-seeking behavior unless significant support groups are established.

One method of treating opioid dependence has been to switch the patient from IV and inhalation forms of illegal drugs to methadone (Dolophine). Although oral methadone is an opioid, it does not cause the euphoria of the injectable opioids. Methadone also does not cure the dependence, and the patient must continue taking the drug to avoid withdrawal symptoms. This therapy, called **methadone maintenance,** may continue for many months or years, until the patient decides to enter a total withdrawal treatment program. Methadone maintenance allows patients to return to productive work and social relationships without the physical, emotional, and criminal risks of illegal drug use.

A newer treatment option is to administer buprenorphine (Subutex), a mixed opioid agonist–antagonist, by the sublingual route. Buprenorphine is used early in opioid abuse therapy to prevent opioid withdrawal symptoms. Another combination agent, Suboxone, contains both buprenorphine and naloxone, and is used later in the maintenance of opioid addiction.

Health care providers should always be aware that when administering opioids with mixed agonist–antagonist activity, their pain-blocking properties are reduced when administered in combination with opioid agonists. Thus, there may be a tendency to overprescribe mixed opioids, promoting drug misuse. This is true even though in most cases, the potential for causing opioid addiction is lower with mixed agonist–antagonists compared with pure opioid agonists.

NONOPIOID ANALGESICS

The nonopioid analgesics include NSAIDs, acetaminophen, and a few centrally acting drugs. The role of the NSAIDs in the treatment of inflammation and fever is discussed more thoroughly in chapter 33∞. Therefore, there is only brief mention here. Table 18.3 highlights the more common nonopioid analgesics.

Nonsteroidal Anti-Inflammatory Drugs (NSAIDs)

The NSAIDs act by inhibiting pain mediators at the nociceptor level. When tissue is damaged, chemical mediators are released locally, including histamine, potassium ion, hydrogen ion, bradykinin, and prostaglandins. Bradykinin is associated with the sensory impulse of pain. Prostaglandins can induce pain through the formation of free radicals.

18.8 Pharmacotherapy with NSAIDs

Nonsteroidal anti-inflammatory drugs (NSAIDs) inhibit **cyclooxygenase,** an enzyme responsible for the formation of prostaglandins. When cyclooxygenase is inhibited, inflammation and pain are reduced. NSAIDs are drugs of choice for mild to moderate pain, especially for pain associated with inflammation. These drugs have many advantages over the opioids, in that the NSAIDs have antipyretic and anti-inflammatory activity, as well as analgesic properties.

TABLE 18.3	Nonopioid Analgesics	
Drug	**Route and Adult Dose (max dose where indicated)**	**Adverse Effects**
NSAIDs: ASPIRIN AND OTHER SALICYLATES		
Ⓟ aspirin (acetylsalicylic acid, ASA)	PO; 350–650 mg every 4 h (max: 4 g/day)	*Heartburn, stomach pains, ulceration*
choline salicylate (Arthropan)	PO; 435–870 mg (2.5–5 mL) every 4 h	<u>Bronchospasm, anaphylactic shock, hemolytic anemia</u>
salsalate (Disalcid)	PO; 325–3,000 mg/day in divided doses (max: 4 g/day)	
NSAIDs: IBUPROFEN AND RELATED DRUGS		
diclofenac (Cataflam, Voltaren)	PO; 50 mg bid–qid (max: 200 mg/day)	*Indigestion, nausea, occult blood loss, anorexia, headache, drowsiness, dizziness*
diflunisal (Dolobid)	PO; 1,000 mg followed by 500 mg bid–tid	<u>Aplastic anemia, drug-induced peptic ulcer, GI bleeding, agranulocytosis, laryngospasm, laryngeal edema; peripheral edema, anaphylaxis, acute renal failure; vomiting, constipation, diarrhea</u>
etodolac (Lodine)	PO; 200–400 mg tid–qid	
fenoprofen calcium (Nalfon)	PO; 200 mg tid–qid	
flurbiprofen (Ansaid)	PO; 50–100 mg tid–qid (max: 300 mg/day)	
ibuprofen (Advil, Motrin)	PO; 400 mg tid–qid (max: 1,200 mg/day)	
indomethacin (Indocin)	PO; 25–50 mg bid–tid (max: 200 mg/day), or 75 mg sustained release one to two times/day	
ketoprofen (Actron, Orudis)	PO; 12.5–50 mg tid–qid	
ketorolac tromethamine (Toradol)	PO; 10 mg qid prn (max: 40 mg/day)	
mefenamic acid (Ponstel)	PO; Loading dose: 500 mg; Maintenance dose: 250 mg every 6 h prn	
meloxicam (Mobic)	PO; 7.5 mg/day (max: 15 mg/day) 7.5–15 mg daily	
nabumetone (Relafen)	PO; 1,000 mg/day (max: 2,000 mg/day)	
naproxen (Naprosyn, Naprelan)	PO; 500 mg followed by 200–250 mg tid–qid (max: 1,250 mg/day)	
naproxen sodium (Aleve, Anaprox, others)	PO; 250–500 mg bid (max: 1,000 mg/day naproxen)	
ozaprozin (Daypro)	PO; 600–1,200 mg/day (max: 1,800 mg/day)	
piroxicam (Feldene)	PO; 10–20 mg one to two times/day (max: 20 mg/day)	
sulindac (Clinoril)	PO; 150–200 mg bid (max: 400 mg/day)	
tolmetin (Tolectin)	PO; 400 mg tid (max: 2 g/day)	
NSAIDs: COX-2 INHIBITORS		
celecoxib (Celebrex)	PO; 100–200 mg every 6–8 h or 200 mg qid	*Abdominal pain, dizziness, headache, sinusitis, hypersensitivity* <u>Cautious use due to FDA review</u>
ACETAMINOPHEN		
Ⓟ acetaminophen (Tylenol) (see page 472 for the Prototype Drug box ∞)	PO; 325–650 mg every 4–6 h	*Hepatotoxicity in alcoholics* <u>Hepatotoxicity, hepatic coma, acute renal failure</u>
CENTRALLY ACTING DRUGS		
clonidine (Catapres)	PO; 0.1 mg bid–tid (max: 0.8 mg/day)	*Hypotension, dry mouth, constipation, drowsiness, sedation, dizziness, vertigo, fatigue, headache*
tramadol (Ultram)	PO; 50–100 mg every 4–6 h prn (max: 400 mg/day); may start with 25 mg/day, and increase by 25 mg every 3 days up to 200 mg/day	<u>Anaphylactic reaction</u>
ziconotide (Prialt)	Intrathecal 0.1 mcg/h via infusion, may increase by 0.1 mcg/h every 2–3 days (max: 0.8 mcg/h)	

Italics indicate common adverse effects; <u>underlining</u> indicates serious adverse effects.

MyNursingKit | Mechanism in Action: Naproxen

Aspirin, Ibuprofen, and COX-2 Inhibitors

Aspirin and ibuprofen are available OTC and are inexpensive. Ibuprofen and related medications are available in many dif-ferent formulations, including those designed for children. They are safe and produce adverse effects only at high doses.

After tissue damage, prostaglandins are formed with the help of two enzymes called cyclooxygenase type 1 (COX-1)

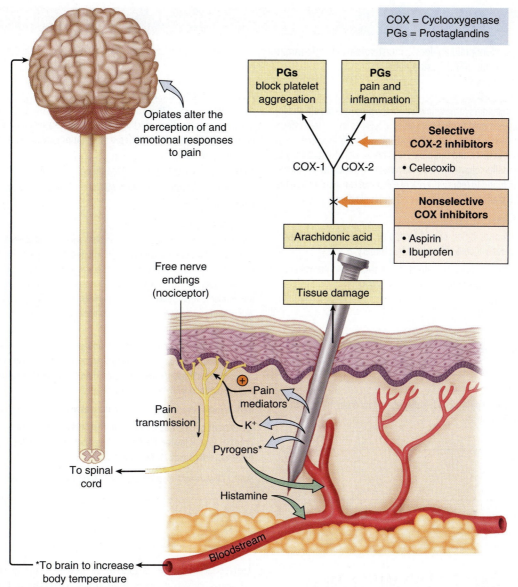

COX = Cyclooxygenase
PGs = Prostaglandins

PGs
block platelet
aggregation

PGs
pain and
inflammation

**Selective
COX-2 inhibitors**

• Celecoxib

COX-1   COX-2

**Nonselective
COX inhibitors**

• Aspirin
• Ibuprofen

Arachidonic acid

Tissue damage

Opiates alter the
perception of and
emotional responses
to pain

Free nerve
endings
(nociceptor)

Pain
transmission

Pain
mediators

K⁺

Pyrogens*

Histamine

To spinal
cord

Bloodstream

*To brain to increase
body temperature

➤ *Figure 18.3* Mechanisms of pain at the nociceptor level

and cyclooxygenase type 2 (COX-2). Aspirin and ibuprofen-related drugs inhibit both COX-1 and COX-2. Thus, COX inhibition is the basis of NSAID therapy. Because the COX-2 enzyme is more specific for the synthesis of inflammatory prostaglandins, the selective COX-2 inhibitors provide more specific and peripheral pain relief. Celecoxib (Celebrex) is the representative COX-2 inhibitor. Other COX-2 inhibitors are available outside of the United States. ➤ Figure 18.3 illustrates the mechanism of pain transmission at the nociceptor level.

Acetaminophen

Acetaminophen is featured as a prototype antipyretic on page 472 in chapter 33∞. Acetaminophen reduces fever by direct action at the level of the hypothalamus and causes dilation of peripheral blood vessels enabling sweating and dissipation of heat. It is the primary alternative to NSAIDs when patients cannot take aspirin or ibuprofen. Acetaminophen does not produce GI bleeding or ulcers, nor does it exhibit cardiotoxicity. Aspirin and acetaminophen have similar efficacies in relieving pain and reducing fever.

Centrally Acting Drugs

Clonidine (Catapres), tramadol (Ultram), and ziconotide (Prialt) are centrally acting analgesics. Of the three drugs, tramadol is the most widely prescribed. Tramadol has weak opioid activity, although it is not thought to relieve pain by this mechanism. Its main action is to inhibit reuptake of norepinephrine and serotonin in spinal neurons. Tramadol is well tolerated, but common adverse effects are vertigo, dizziness, headache, nausea, vomiting, constipation, and lethargy.

Pr Prototype Drug | Aspirin (Acetylsalicylic Acid, ASA)

Therapeutic Class: Nonopioid analgesic; nonsteroidal anti-inflammatory drug (NSAID); antipyretic

Pharmacologic Class: Salicylate; cyclooxygenase (COX) inhibitor

ACTIONS AND USES

Aspirin inhibits prostaglandin synthesis involved in the processes of pain and inflammation and produces mild to moderate relief of fever. It has limited effects on peripheral blood vessels, causing vasodilation and sweating. Aspirin has significant anticoagulant activity, and this property is responsible for its ability to reduce the risk of mortality following MI, and to reduce the incidence of strokes. Aspirin has also been found to reduce the risk of colorectal cancer, although the mechanism by which it affords this protective effect is unknown.

ADMINISTRATION ALERTS

- Platelet aggregation inhibition caused by aspirin is irreversible. Aspirin should be discontinued 1 week prior to elective surgery.
- Aspirin is excreted in the urine and affects urine testing for glucose and other metabolites, such as vanillylmandelic acid (VMA).
- Pregnancy category D

PHARMACOKINETICS
Onset: 1 h
Peak: 2–4 h
Half-life: 15–20 min (aspirin); 2–3 h (salicylate at low dose); more than 20 h (salicylate at high dose)
Duration: 24 h

ADVERSE EFFECTS

At high doses, such as those used to treat severe inflammatory disorders, aspirin may cause gastric discomfort and bleeding because of its antiplatelet effects. Enteric-coated tablets and buffered preparations are available for patients who experience GI side effects.

Contraindications: Because aspirin increases bleeding time, it should not be given to patients receiving anticoagulant therapy such as warfarin, heparin, and plicamycin.

INTERACTIONS

Drug–Drug: Concurrent use of phenobarbital, antacids, and glucocorticoids may decrease aspirin's effects. Aspirin may potentiate the action of oral hypoglycemic drugs. Effects of NSAIDs, uricosuric drugs such as probenecid, beta blockers, spironolactone, and sulfa drugs may be decreased when combined with aspirin. Insulin, methotrexate, phenytoin, sulfonamides, and penicillin may increase effects. When aspirin is taken with alcohol, pyrazolone derivatives, steroids, or other NSAIDs, there is an increased risk for gastric ulcers.

Lab Tests: Aspirin may cause prolonged prothrombin time by decreasing prothrombin production. Aspirin may also interfere with pregnancy tests, and decrease serum levels of cholesterol, potassium, PBI, T_3, and T_4. High salicylate levels may cause abnormalities in liver function tests.

Herbal/Food: Feverfew, garlic, ginger, and ginkgo may increase the risk of bleeding.

Treatment of Overdose: Treatment may include any of the following: activated charcoal, gastric lavage, laxative, or drug therapy for overdose symptoms such as dizziness, drowsiness, abdominal pain, or seizures.

Refer to MyNursingKit for a Nursing Process Focus specific to this drug.

TENSION HEADACHES AND MIGRAINES

Headaches are some of the most common complaints of patients. Living with headaches can interfere with ADLs, thus causing great distress. The pain and inability to focus and concentrate result in work-related absences and difficulties caring for home and family. When the headaches are persistent, or occur as migraines, drug therapy is warranted.

18.9 Classification of Headaches

Of the several varieties of headaches, the most common type is the **tension headache.** This condition occurs when muscles of the head and neck become very tight because of stress, causing a steady and lingering pain. Although quite painful, tension headaches are self-limiting and generally considered an annoyance rather than a medical emergency. Tension headaches can usually be effectively treated with OTC analgesics such as aspirin, ibuprofen, or acetaminophen.

The most painful type of headache is the **migraine,** which is characterized by throbbing or pulsating pain, sometimes preceded by an aura. **Auras** are sensory cues that let the patient know that a migraine attack is coming soon. Examples of sensory cues are jagged lines or flashing lights, or special smells, tastes, or sounds. Most migraines are accompanied by nausea and vomiting. Triggers for migraines include nitrates, monosodium glutamate (MSG)—found in many Asian foods, red wine, perfumes, food additives, caffeine, chocolate, and aspartame. By avoiding foods containing these substances, some patients can prevent the onset of a migraine attack.

PHARMFACTS

Headaches and Migraines
- About 28 million Americans suffer from headaches and migraines.
- Of all migraines, 95% are controlled by drug therapy and other measures.
- Before puberty, more boys have migraines than girls.
- After puberty, women have four to eight times more migraines than men.
- Headaches and migraines appear mostly among people in their 20s and 30s.
- Persons with a family history of headache or migraine have a higher chance of developing these disorders.

NURSING PROCESS FOCUS   PATIENTS RECEIVING NSAID THERAPY

Assessment	Potential Nursing Diagnoses
Baseline assessment prior to administration: • Understand the reason the drug has been prescribed in order to assess for therapeutic effects. • Obtain a complete health history including hepatic, renal, respiratory, cardiovascular, or neurologic disease; pregnancy; or breast-feeding. Obtain a drug history including allergies, current prescription and OTC drugs, herbal preparations, caffeine, nicotine, and alcohol use. Be alert to possible drug interactions. • Obtain baseline vital signs and weight. • Evaluate appropriate laboratory findings (e.g., CBC, coagulation panels, bleeding time, hepatic or renal function studies). • Assess the patient's ability to receive and understand instruction. Include the family and caregiver as needed.	• Pain (Acute or Chronic) • Risk for Injury (related to adverse drug effects)
Assessment throughout administration: • Assess for desired therapeutic effects (e.g., pain is decreased or absent, signs and symptoms of inflammation such as redness or swelling are decreased). • Continue periodic monitoring of CBC, coagulation studies, bleeding time, and hepatic and renal function studies. • Assess vital signs periodically. • Assess for and promptly report adverse effects: symptoms of GI bleeding (dark or "tarry" stools, hematemesis or coffee-ground emesis, blood in the stool), abdominal pain, severe tinnitus, dizziness, drowsiness, light-headedness, confusion, agitation, euphoria or depression, palpitations, tachycardia, hypertension, increased respiratory rate and depth, pulmonary congestion, and edema.	

Planning: Patient Goals and Expected Outcomes

The patient will:
• Experience therapeutic effects (e.g., decreased or absent pain, decreased signs and symptoms of inflammation).
• Be free from, or experience minimal, adverse effects.
• Verbalize an understanding of the drug's use, adverse effects, and required precautions.
• Demonstrate proper self-administration of the medication (e.g., dose, timing, when to notify provider).

Implementation

Interventions and (Rationales)	Patient and Family Education
Ensuring therapeutic effects: • Continue assessments as described earlier for therapeutic effects. (Diminished pain, or signs and symptoms of inflammation contributing to pain should begin after taking first dose and continue to improve. The provider should be notified if the pain increases.)	• Teach the patient to supplement drug therapy with nonpharmacologic measures (e.g., relaxation techniques, diversionary distractions such as television or music) and to report increasing pain unrelieved by drug.
Minimizing adverse effects: • Continue to monitor periodic lab work: hepatic and renal function tests, CBC, and coagulation studies or bleeding time. (Aspirin and salicylates affect platelet aggregation and should be monitored if used long term or if excessive bleeding or bruising is noted. Acetaminophen can be hepatotoxic in large doses or if taken when hepatic dysfunction is present.)	• Instruct the patient on the need to return periodically for lab work if on the drugs long term. • Teach the patient to abstain from alcohol while taking acetaminophen. Men who consume more than two alcoholic beverages per day or women who consume more than one alcoholic beverage per day should consult their health care provider before taking acetaminophen.

(Continued)

NURSING PROCESS FOCUS   PATIENTS RECEIVING NSAID THERAPY (Continued)

Implementation

Interventions and (Rationales)	Patient and Family Education
■ Monitor for abdominal pain, black or tarry stools, blood in the stool, hematemesis or coffee-ground emesis, dizziness, light-headedness, and hypotension, especially if associated with tachycardia. (NSAIDs may cause GI bleeding.)	■ Instruct the patient to immediately report any signs or symptoms of GI bleeding. ■ Teach the patient to take the drug with food or milk to decrease GI irritation and to swallow enteric-coated tablets whole without crushing or breaking. Alcohol use should be avoided or eliminated.
■ Monitor for tinnitus, difficulty hearing, light-headedness, or difficulty with balance and report promptly. (NSAIDs and salicylates may be ototoxic and cause hearing loss.)	■ Instruct the patient to immediately report any signs or symptoms of ringing, humming, buzzing in ears, difficulty with balance, dizziness or vertigo, or nausea.
■ Monitor urine output and renal function studies periodically. (NSAIDs and salicylates may be renal toxic and patients on long-term or high-dose therapy should monitor urine output and have periodic renal function studies.)	■ Instruct the patient on NSAIDs and salicylates to promptly report changes in quantity of urine output, darkening of urine, or edema. ■ Teach the patient on NSAIDs and salicylates to increase fluid intake, especially if fever is present.
■ Avoid the use of aspirin or salicylates in children under 18 unless explicitly ordered by the health care provider. (Aspirin has been associated with an increased risk of Reye's syndrome in children under 18, particularly associated with the flu virus and varicella infections.)	■ Instruct parents to use NSAIDs or acetaminophen in children under 18 for fever or pain control, unless otherwise ordered by the provider. ■ Teach parents to read labels on all OTC medications and to avoid formulations with aspirin or salicylate on the label.
Patient understanding of drug therapy: ■ Use opportunities during administration of medications and during assessments to discuss rationale for drug therapy, desired therapeutic outcomes, most commonly observed adverse effects, parameters for when to call the health care provider, and any necessary monitoring or precautions. (Using time during nursing care helps to optimize and reinforce key teaching areas.)	■ The patient, family, or caregiver should be able to state the reason for the drug; appropriate dose and scheduling; what adverse effects to observe for and when to report; and the anticipated length of medication therapy.
Patient self-administration of drug therapy: ■ When administering the medication, instruct the patient, family, or caregiver in proper self-administration of drug, e.g., with food or milk. (Utilizing time during nurse-administration of these drugs helps to reinforce teaching. Household measuring devices such as teaspoons differ significantly in size and amount and should not be used for pediatric or liquid doses.)	■ The patient, family, or caregiver is able to discuss appropriate dosing and administration needs, including the following: ■ NSAIDs should be taken with food or milk to decrease GI upset. ■ Liquid doses of acetaminophen or NSAIDs should be measured with the enclosed dosage cup, dropper, or spoon. If that measuring device is no longer available, do NOT use a household spoon but obtain another calibrated measuring cup or dropper.

Evaluation of Outcome Criteria

Evaluate the effectiveness of drug therapy by confirming that patient goals and expected outcomes have been met (see "Planning").

See Table 18.3 under "NSAIDS" for a list of drugs to which these nursing actions apply.

18.10 Drug Therapy for Migraine Headaches

There are two primary goals for the pharmacologic therapy of migraines (Table 18.4). The first is to stop migraines in progress, and the second is to prevent migraines from occurring. For the most part, the drugs used to abort migraines are different from those used for prophylaxis. Drug therapy is most effective if begun before a migraine has reached a severe level.

The two major drug classes used as antimigraine drugs, the triptans and the ergot alkaloids, are both serotonin (5-HT) agonists. Serotonergic receptors are found throughout the CNS, and in the cardiovascular and GI systems. At least five receptor subtypes have been identified. In addition to the triptans, other drugs acting at serotonergic receptors include the popular antianxiety drugs fluoxetine (Prozac) and buspirone (BuSpar).

Pharmacotherapy of migraine termination generally begins with acetaminophen or NSAIDs. If OTC analgesics are unable to abort the migraine, the drugs of choice are often the triptans. The first of the triptans, sumatriptan (Imitrex), was marketed in the United States in 1993. These drugs are selective for the 5-HT$_1$-receptor subtype, and they are thought to act by constricting certain intracranial vessels. They are effective in aborting migraines with or without auras. Although oral forms of the triptans are most convenient, patients who experience nausea and vomiting during the migraine may require an alternative dosage form. Intranasal formulations and prefilled syringes of triptans are

TABLE 18.4	**Antimigraine Drugs**	
Drug	Route and Adult Dose (max dose where indicated)	Adverse Effects
ERGOT ALKALOIDS		
dihydroergotamine mesylate (D.H.E. 45, Migranal)	IM; 1 mg; may be repeated at 1-h intervals to a total of 3 mg (max: 6 mg/wk)	*Weakness, nausea, vomiting, abnormal pulse, pruritus*
ergotamine tartrate (Ergostat) ergotamine with caffeine (Cafergot, Ercaf, others)	PO; 1–2 mg followed by 1–2 mg every 30 min until headache stops (max: 6 mg/day or 10 mg/wk)	<u>Delirium, convulsive seizures, intermittent claudication</u>
TRIPTANS		
almotriptan (Axert)	PO; 6.25–12.5 mg; may repeat in 2 h if necessary (max: 2 tabs/day)	*Asthenia, tingling, warming sensation, dizziness, vertigo*
eletriptan (Relpax)	PO; 20–40 mg; may repeat in 2 h if necessary (max: 80 mg/day)	<u>Coronary artery vasospasm, MI, cardiac arrest</u>
frovatriptan (Frova)	PO; 2.5 mg; may repeat in 2 h if necessary (max: 7.5 mg/day)	
naratriptan (Amerge)	PO; 1–2.5 mg; may repeat in 4 h if necessary (max: 5 mg/day)	
rizatriptan (Maxalt)	PO; 5–10 mg; may repeat in 2 h if necessary (max: 30 mg/day); 5 mg with concurrent propranolol (max: 15 mg/day)	
Pr sumatriptan (Imitrex)	PO; 25 mg for 1 dose (max: 100 mg)	
zolmitriptan (Zomig)	PO; 2.5–5 mg; may repeat in 2 h if necessary (max: 10 mg/day)	
ANTISEIZURE DRUGS		
topiramate (Topamax)	PO; start with 50 mg/day, increase by 50 mg/week to effectiveness (max: 1,600 mg/day)	*Nausea, vomiting, sedation, drowsiness, weakness*
valproic acid (Depakene, Depakote)	PO; 250 mg bid (max: 100 mg/day)	<u>Liver failure, bone marrow depression</u>
BETA-ADRENERGIC BLOCKERS		
atenolol (Tenormin) (see page 347 for the Prototype Drug box ∞)	PO; 25–50 mg/day (max: 100 mg/day)	*Bradycardia, hypotension, CHF, confusion, drowsiness, insomnia*
metoprolol (Lopressor)	PO; 50–100 mg one to two times/day (max: 450 mg/day)	<u>Bronchospasm, exfoliative dermatitis, agranulocytosis, membrane irritation, rash, heart block, cardiac arrest, anaphylaxis, Stevens–Johnson Syndrome</u>
propranolol hydrochloride (Inderal) (see page 364 for the Prototype Drug box ∞)	PO; 80–240 mg/day in divided doses; may need 160–240 mg/day	
timolol (Blocadren)	PO; 10 mg bid; may increase to 60 mg/day in two divided doses	
CALCIUM CHANNEL BLOCKERS		
nifedipine (Procardia) (see page 308 for the Prototype Drug box ∞)	PO; 10–20 mg tid (max: 180 mg/day)	*Dizziness, light-headedness, facial flushing, heat sensitivity, diarrhea, peripheral edema, headache, hypotension, constipation*
nimodipine (Nimotop)	PO; 60 mg every 4 h for 21 days; start therapy within 96 hours of subarachnoid hemorrhage	<u>MI, AV block, hepatotoxicity</u>
verapamil hydrochloride (Isoptin) (see page 366 for the Prototype Drug box ∞)	PO; 40–80 mg tid (max: 360 mg/day)	
TRICYCLIC ANTIDEPRESSANTS		
amitriptyline hydrochloride (Elavil)	PO; 75–100 mg/day	*Sedation, drowsiness, orthostatic hypotension, blurred vision, slight mydriasis, dry mouth, urinary retention, constipation*
imipramine (Tofranil) (see page 187 for the Prototype Drug box ∞)	PO; 75–100 mg/day (max: 300 mg/day)	<u>MI, arrythmias, heart block, agranulocytosis, angioedema, bone marrow depression</u>
protriptyline (Vivactil)	PO 15–40 mg/day in three to four divided doses (max: 60 mg/day)	
MISCELLANEOUS DRUGS		
methysergide (Sansert)	PO; 4–8 mg/day in divided doses	*Nausea, vomiting, sedation, drowsiness, weakness, discoloration of urine (for vitamin B$_2$), painful urination*
riboflavin (vitamin B$_2$)	As a supplement: PO; 5–10 mg/day	<u>Shortness of breath</u>
	For deficiency: PO; 5–30 mg/day in divided doses	

Italics indicate common adverse effects; <u>underlining</u> indicates serious adverse effects.

available for patients who are able to self-administer the medication.

For patients who are unresponsive to triptans, the ergot alkaloids may be used to abort migraines. The first purified alkaloid, ergotamine (Ergostat), was isolated from the ergot fungus in 1920, although the actions of the ergot alkaloids had been known for thousands of years. Ergotamine is an inexpensive drug that is available in oral, sublingual, and suppository forms. Modifications of the original molecule have produced a number of other pharmacologically useful drugs, such as dihydroergotamine mesylate (D.H.E. 45, Migranal). Dihydroergotamine is given parenterally and as a nasal spray. Because the ergot alkaloids interact with adrenergic and dopaminergic receptors as well as serotonergic receptors, they produce multiple actions and side effects. Many ergot alkaloids are pregnancy category X drugs.

Drugs for migraine prophylaxis include various classes of drugs that are discussed in other chapters of this textbook. These include antiseizure drugs, beta-adrenergic blockers, calcium channel blockers, and antidepressants. Because all these drugs have the potential to produce side effects, prophylaxis is initiated only if the incidence of migraines is high and the patient is unresponsive to the drugs used to abort migraines. Of the various drugs, the beta blocker propra-

nolol (Inderal) is one of the most commonly prescribed. Amitriptyline (Elavil), an antidepressant, is preferred for patients who may have a mood disorder or suffer from insomnia in addition to their migraines.

COMPLEMENTARY AND ALTERNATIVE THERAPIES

Evening Primrose Oil for Pain

Evening primrose (*Primula biennis*) is a plant native to North America. The oil extracted from the seeds of the plant contains high amounts of gamma linolenic acid, an essential fatty acid that is required by the body for normal growth and development.

Evening primrose oil has been used for a large number of diverse conditions. The strongest scientific evidence is for treating eczema, a condition characterized by inflamed, itchy skin. Some data has suggested that the herb may reduce pain in patients with breast tenderness and rheumatoid arthritis (Little & Parsons, 2000). Although used frequently to treat the symptoms of premenstrual syndrome, research has not shown the herb to be effective for this indication (Dog, 2003). Other claimed uses include diabetic neuropathy, cholesterol reduction, multiple sclerosis, and prevention of stroke; however, scientific evidence is not adequate to support these indications. Evening primrose oil is very safe. There is some concern that it may lower the seizure threshold in patients with epilepsy.

Pr Prototype Drug | Sumatriptan *(Imitrex)*

Therapeutic Class: Antimigraine agent   **Pharmacologic Class:** Triptan; 5-HT (serotonin) receptor agent; vasoconstrictor of intracranial arteries

ACTIONS AND USES

Sumatriptan belongs to a relatively newer group of antimigraine drugs known as the triptans. The triptans act by causing vasoconstriction of cranial arteries; this vasoconstriction is moderately selective and does not usually affect overall blood pressure. This medication is available in oral, intranasal, and subcutaneous forms. Subcutaneous administration terminates migraine attacks in 10 to 20 minutes; the dose may be repeated 60 minutes after the first injection, to a maximum of two doses per day. If taken orally, sumatriptan should be administered as soon as possible after the migraine is suspected or has begun.

ADMINISTRATION ALERTS

- Sumatriptan may produce cardiac ischemia in susceptible persons with no previous cardiac events. Health care providers may opt to administer the initial dose of sumatriptan in the health care setting.

- Sumatriptan's systemic vasoconstrictor activity may cause hypertension and may result in dysrhythmias or myocardial infarction. Keep resuscitative equipment accessible.

- Sumatriptan selectively reduces carotid arterial blood flow. Monitor changes in level of consciousness and observe for seizures.

- Pregnancy category C

PHARMACOKINETICS

Onset: 15 min nasal; 30 min PO; 10 min subcutaneous

Peak: 2 h PO; 12 min subcutaneous, 60–90 min nasal

Half-life: 2 h

Duration: 24–48 h

ADVERSE EFFECTS

Some dizziness, drowsiness, or a warming sensation may be experienced after taking sumatriptan; however, these effects are not normally severe enough to warrant discontinuation of therapy.

Contraindications: Because of its vasoconstricting action, the drug should be used cautiously, if at all, in patients with recent myocardial infarction, or with a history of angina pectoris, hypertension, or diabetes.

INTERACTIONS

Drug–Drug: Sumatriptan interacts with several drugs. For example, an increased effect may occur when taken with monoamine oxidase inhibitors (MAOIs) and selective serotonin reuptake inhibitors (SSRIs). Further vasoconstriction can occur when taken with ergot alkaloids and other triptans.

Lab Tests: Unknown

Herbal/Food: Ginkgo, ginseng, echinacea, and St. John's wort may increase triptan toxicity.

Treatment of Overdose: Treatment may include drug therapy for the following symptoms: weakness, lack of coordination, watery eyes and mouth, tremors, seizures, or breathing problems.

Refer to MyNursingKit for a Nursing Process Focus specific to this drug.

NURSING PROCESS FOCUS PATIENTS RECEIVING TRIPTAN THERAPY

Assessment	Potential Nursing Diagnoses
Baseline assessment prior to administration: ■ Understand the reason the drug has been prescribed in order to assess for therapeutic effects. ■ Obtain a complete health history including cardiovascular, neurologic, hepatic, or renal disease; pregnancy; or breast-feeding. Obtain a drug history including allergies, current prescription and OTC drugs, herbal preparations, caffeine, nicotine, and alcohol use. Be alert to possible drug interactions. ■ Obtain baseline vital signs, apical pulse, level of consciousness, and weight. ■ Assess the level of pain. Use objective screening tools when possible (e.g., Wong-Baker FACES scale for children, numerical rating scale for adults). Assess the history of the pain and what has worked successfully or not for the patient in the past. ■ Evaluate appropriate laboratory findings (e.g., CBC, hepatic or renal function studies). ■ Assess the patient's ability to receive and understand instruction. Include the family and caregivers as needed.	■ Acute Pain ■ Ineffective Health Maintenance (related to inability to manage activities of daily living with chronic pain) ■ Ineffective Coping (related to chronic pain) ■ Deficient Knowledge (drug therapy)
Assessment throughout administration: ■ Assess for desired therapeutic effects (e.g., headache pain is decreased or absent). ■ Continue monitoring level of consciousness and neurologic symptoms (e.g., numbness or tingling). ■ Assess vital signs, especially blood pressure and pulse periodically. ■ Continue periodic monitoring of hepatic and renal function studies. ■ Assess stress and coping patterns for possible symptom correlation (e.g., existing or perceived stress, duration, coping mechanisms or remedies). ■ Assess for and promptly report adverse effects: chest pain or tightness, palpitations, tachycardia, hypertension, dizziness, light-headedness, confusion, and numbness or tingling in extremities.	

Planning: Patient Goals and Expected Outcomes

The patient will:
■ Experience therapeutic effects dependent on the reason the drug is being given (e.g., absent or decreased headache pain, prevention of acute headache pain from migraine attack).
■ Be free from, or experience minimal, adverse effects.
■ Verbalize an understanding of the drug's use, adverse effects, and required precautions.
■ Demonstrate proper self-administration of the medication (e.g., dose, timing, when to notify provider).

Implementation

Interventions and (Rationales)	Patient and Family Education
Ensuring therapeutic effects: ■ Continue assessments as described earlier for therapeutic effects. Give the drug *before* the start of acute pain when possible. (Consistent use of a pain rating scale by all providers will help quantify the level of pain relief and leads to better pain control. Encourage the patient to start the medication before headache becomes severe for better control. Pain relief begins within first several minutes after administration.)	■ Teach the patient that pain relief, rather than merely control, is the goal of therapy. ■ Encourage the patient to take the drug before a headache becomes severe and consistently as ordered. ■ Explain the rationale behind the pain rating scale (i.e., it allows consistency among all providers). ■ Encourage the patient to use additional, nonpharmacologic pain relief techniques, e.g., quiet, darkened, cool room.

(Continued)

NURSING PROCESS FOCUS   PATIENTS RECEIVING TRIPTAN THERAPY *(Continued)*

Implementation

Interventions and (Rationales)	Patient and Family Education
Minimizing adverse effects: ■ Monitor the blood pressure and pulse periodically especially in patients at risk for undiagnosed cardiovascular disease. Cardiovascular status should be monitored frequently following the first dose given. (Triptans cause vasoconstriction. Postmenopausal women, men over 40, smokers, and people with other known CAD risk factors may be at the greatest risk.)	■ Instruct the patient to report any chest pain, tightness, or pulsating activity that is severe or continues following drug dosage.
■ Observe for changes in severity, character, or duration of headache. (Sudden severe headaches of "thunderclap" quality can signal subarachnoid hemorrhage. Headaches that differ in quality and are accompanied by such signs as fever, rash, or stiff neck may herald meningitis.)	■ Instruct the patient to immediately report changes in character or duration of headache or if accompanied by additional symptoms such as fever, rash, or stiff neck.
■ Continue to monitor neurologic status periodically. (Dizziness or light-headedness may be related to headache, an adverse drug effect, or may signal cerebral ischemia.)	■ Instruct the patient to immediately report increasing dizziness, light-headedness, or blurred vision.
■ Monitor dietary intake of foods that contain tyramine, caffeine, alcohol, or other food triggers. (Some foods or beverages may trigger an acute migraine. Correlating symptoms with food or beverages assists in relieving the cause of the headache.)	■ Encourage the patient to keep a food diary and correlate symptoms with specific foods or beverages. Teach the patient to avoid or limit foods containing tyramine, such as pickled foods, beer, wine, and aged cheeses, which are common triggers for migraines.
Patient understanding of drug therapy: ■ Use opportunities during administration of medications and during assessments to discuss the rationale for drug therapy, desired therapeutic outcomes, most commonly observed adverse effects, parameters for when to call the health care provider, and any necessary monitoring or precautions. (Using time during nursing care helps to optimize and reinforce key teaching areas.)	■ The patient should be able to state the reason for the drug; appropriate dose and scheduling; and what adverse effects to observe for and when to report them.
Patient self-administration of drug therapy: ■ When administering the medication, instruct the patient, family, or caregiver in the proper self-administration of drug, e.g., take the drug as prescribed when needed. (Utilizing time during nurse-administration of these drugs helps to reinforce teaching.)	■ Teach the patient to take the medication before the pain becomes severe or at the first symptoms of a migraine if possible. ■ Teach the patient the proper administration of subcutaneous medication, having the patient or caregiver return-demonstrate the technique. (Pain or redness at the injection site is common but usually disappears within an hour after the dose is taken.) ■ Instruct the patient that an appropriate intranasal dose is one spray into ONE nostril unless otherwise ordered by the health care provider.

Evaluation of Outcome Criteria

Evaluate effectiveness of drug therapy by confirming that patient goals and expected outcomes have been met (see "Planning").

See Table 18.4 under "Triptans" for a list of drugs to which these nursing actions apply.

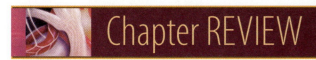

Chapter REVIEW

KEY CONCEPTS

The numbered key concepts provide a succinct summary of the important points from the corresponding numbered section within the chapter. If any of these points are not clear, refer to the numbered section within the chapter for review.

18.1 Pain is assessed and classified as acute or chronic, nociceptor or neuropathic.

18.2 Nonpharmacologic techniques such as massage, biofeedback therapy, and meditation are often important adjuncts to effective pain management.

18.3 Neural mechanisms include pain transmission via Aδ or C fibers and the release of substance P.

18.4 Opioids are natural or synthetic substances extracted from the poppy plant that exert their effects through interaction with mu and kappa receptors.

18.5 Opioids are the drugs of choice for severe pain. They also have other important therapeutic effects including dampening of the cough reflex and slowing of the motility of the GI tract.

18.6 Opioid antagonists may be used to reverse the symptoms of opioid toxicity or overdose, such as sedation and respiratory depression.

18.7 Opioid withdrawal can result in severe symptoms, and dependence is often treated with methadone maintenance and newer drug combination therapies.

18.8 Nonopioid analgesics, such as aspirin, acetaminophen, and the selective COX-2 inhibitors, are effective in treating mild to moderate pain and fever.

18.9 Headaches are classified as tension headaches or migraines. Migraines may be preceded by auras, and symptoms include nausea and vomiting.

18.10 The goals of pharmacotherapy for migraine headaches are to stop migraines in progress and to prevent them from occurring. Triptans, ergot alkaloids, and a number of drugs from other classes are used for migraines.

NCLEX-RN® REVIEW QUESTIONS

1 The nurse teaches the patient relaxation techniques and guided imagery as an adjunct to medication for treatment of pain. The nurse explains that the major benefit of these techniques is that they:
1. are less costly.
2. allow lower doses of drugs with fewer side effects.
3. can be used at home.
4. do not require self-injection.

2 The nurse recognizes that opioid analgesics exert their action by interacting with a variety of opioid receptors. Drugs such as morphine act by:
1. activating kappa and blocking mu receptors.
2. inhibiting mu and kappa receptors.
3. activating mu and kappa receptors.
4. blocking sigma and delta receptors.

3 A patient admitted with hepatitis B is prescribed Vicodin 2 tablets for pain. The appropriate nursing action is to:
1. administer the drug as ordered.
2. administer 1 tablet only.
3. recheck the order with the health care provider.
4. hold the drug until the health care provider arrives.

4 The nurse administers morphine sulfate 4 mg IV to a patient for treatment of severe pain. Which of the following assessments require immediate nursing interventions? (Select all that apply.)
1. The patient's blood pressure is 110/70 mmHg.
2. The patient is drowsy.
3. The patient's pain is unrelieved in 15 minutes.
4. The patient's respiratory rate is 10 breaths per minute.
5. The patient becomes unresponsive.

5 Nursing interventions for a patient receiving opioid analgesics over an extended period should include:
1. referring the patient to a drug treatment center.
2. encouraging increased fluids and fiber in the diet.
3. monitoring for GI bleeding.
4. teaching the patient to self-assess blood pressure.

6 The most appropriate method to ensure adequate pain relief in the immediate postoperative period from an opioid drug would be to:
1. give the drug only when the family members report that the patient is complaining of pain.
2. give the drug every time the patient complains of acute pain.
3. give the drug as consistently as possible for the first 24 to 48 hours.
4. give the drug only when the nurse observes signs and symptoms of pain.

CRITICAL THINKING QUESTIONS

1. A patient is on a patient-controlled analgesia (PCA) pump to manage postoperative pain related to recent orthopedic surgery. The PCA is set to deliver a basal rate of morphine of 6 mg/h. The nurse discovers the patient to be unresponsive with a respiratory rate of 8 breaths per minute and oxygen saturation of 84%. What is the nurse's initial response? What are the nurse's subsequent actions?

2. A 64-year-old patient has had a long-standing history of migraine headaches as well as coronary artery disease, type 2 diabetes, and hypertension. On review of the medical history, the nurse notes that this patient has recently started on sumatriptan (Imitrex), prescribed by the patient's new neurologist. What intervention and teaching should be done for this patient?

3. A 58-year-old patient with a history of a recent MI is on beta-blocker and anticoagulant therapy. The patient also has a history of arthritis, and during a recent flare-up began taking aspirin because it helped control pain in the past. What teaching or recommendation would the nurse have for this patient?

See Appendix D for answers and rationales for all activities.

 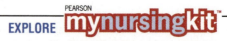

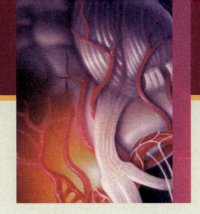

Chapter 19

Drugs for Local and General Anesthesia

LEARNING OUTCOMES

After reading this chapter, the student should be able to:

1. Compare and contrast the five major clinical techniques for administering local anesthetics.
2. Describe differences between the two major chemical classes of local anesthetics.
3. Explain why epinephrine and sodium hydroxide are sometimes included in local anesthetic cartridges.
4. Identify the actions of general anesthetics on the CNS.
5. Compare and contrast the two primary ways that general anesthesia may be induced.
6. Identify the four stages of general anesthesia.
7. For each of the drug classes listed in Drugs at a Glance, know representative drug examples, and explain their mechanisms of action, primary actions, and important adverse effects.
8. Categorize drugs used for anesthesia based on their classification and drug action.
9. Use the nursing process to care for patients who are receiving anesthesia.

KEY TERMS

Anesthesia is a medical procedure performed by administering drugs that cause a loss of sensation. **Local anesthesia** occurs when sensation is lost to a limited part of the body without loss of consciousness. **General anesthesia** requires different classes of drugs that cause loss of sensation to the entire body, usually resulting in a loss of consciousness. This chapter examines drugs used for both local and general anesthesia.

LOCAL ANESTHESIA

Local anesthesia is loss of sensation to a relatively small part of the body without loss of consciousness to the patient. This procedure may be necessary when a relatively brief dental or medical procedure is performed.

19.1 Regional Loss of Sensation Using Local Anesthetics

Although local anesthesia often results in a loss of sensation to a small, limited area, it sometimes affects relatively large portions of the body, such as an entire limb. Thus, some local anesthetic treatments are more accurately called *surface* anesthesia or *regional* anesthesia, depending on how the drugs are administered and their resulting effects.

The five major routes for applying local anesthetics are shown in ▶ Figure 19.1. The method employed is dependent on the location and extent of the desired anesthesia. For example, some local anesthetics are applied topically before a needlestick or for minor skin surgery. Others are used to block sensations to large areas such as a limb or the lower abdomen. The different methods of local and regional anesthesia are summarized in Table 19.1.

Local Anesthetics

Local anesthetics are drugs that produce a rapid loss of sensation to a limited part of the body. They produce their therapeutic effect by blocking the entry of sodium ions into neurons.

19.2 Mechanism of Action of Local Anesthetics

The mechanism of action of local anesthetics is well known. Recall that the concentration of sodium ions is normally higher on the outside of neurons than on the inside. A rapid influx of sodium ions into cells is necessary for neurons to fire.

Local anesthetics act by blocking sodium channels, as illustrated in Pharmacotherapy Illustrated 19.1. Because the blocking of sodium channels is a nonselective process, both sensory and motor impulses are affected. Thus, both sensa-

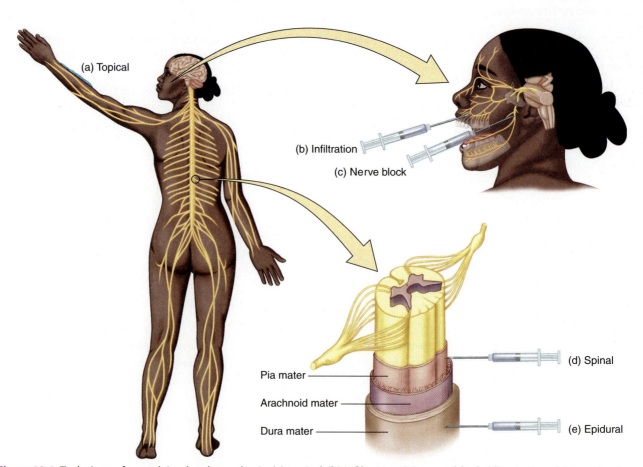

(a) Topical

(b) Infiltration

(c) Nerve block

Pia mater

Arachnoid mater

Dura mater

(d) Spinal

(e) Epidural

▶ *Figure 19.1* Techniques for applying local anesthesia: (a) topical; (b) infiltration; (c) nerve block; (d) spinal; and (e) epidural

TABLE 19.1	Methods of Local Anesthetic Administration	
Route	Formulation/Method	Description
Epidural anesthesia	Injection into the epidural space of the spinal cord	Most commonly used in obstetrics during labor and delivery
Infiltration (field block) anesthesia	Direct injection into tissue immediate to the surgical site	Drug diffuses into tissue to block a specific group of nerves in a small area close to the surgical site
Nerve block anesthesia	Direct injection into tissue that may be distant from the operation site	Drug affects nerve bundles serving the surgical area; used to block sensation in a limb or large area of the face
Spinal anesthesia	Injection into the cerebral spinal fluid (CSF)	Drug affects a large, regional area such as the lower abdomen and legs
Topical (surface) anesthesia	Creams, sprays, suppositories, drops, and lozenges	Applied to mucous membranes including the eyes, lips, gums, nasal membranes, and throat; very safe unless absorbed

tion and muscle activity will temporarily diminish in the area treated with the local anesthetic. Because of their mechanism of action, local anesthetics are called *sodium channel blockers*.

During a medical or surgical procedure, it is essential that the action of the anesthetic last long enough to complete the procedure. Small amounts of epinephrine are sometimes added to the anesthetic solution to constrict blood vessels in the immediate area where the local anesthetic is applied. This keeps the anesthetic in the area longer, thus extending the duration of action of the drug. The addition of epinephrine to lidocaine (Xylocaine), for example, increases the duration of its local anesthetic effect from 20 minutes to as long as 60 minutes. This is important for dental or surgical

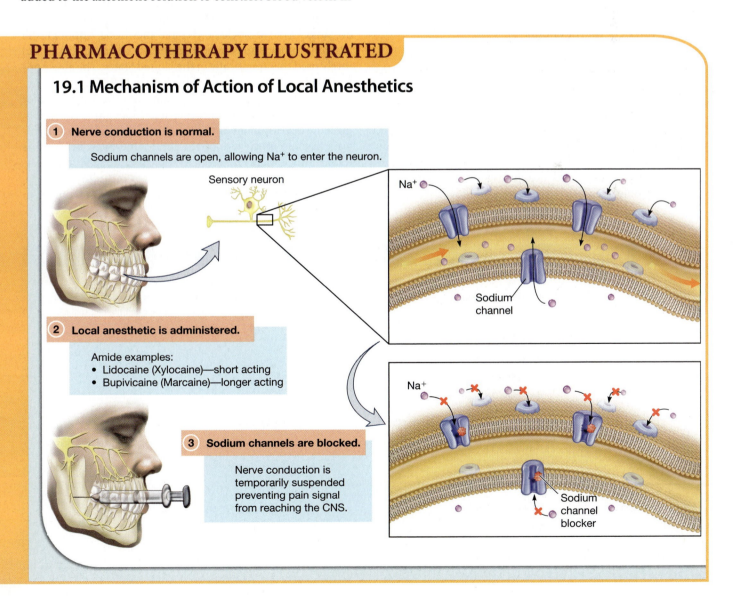

PHARMACOTHERAPY ILLUSTRATED

19.1 Mechanism of Action of Local Anesthetics

1 Nerve conduction is normal.

Sodium channels are open, allowing Na⁺ to enter the neuron.

Sensory neuron

Na⁺

Sodium channel

2 Local anesthetic is administered.

Amide examples:
- Lidocaine (Xylocaine)—short acting
- Bupivicaine (Marcaine)—longer acting

Na⁺

3 Sodium channels are blocked.

Nerve conduction is temporarily suspended preventing pain signal from reaching the CNS.

Sodium channel blocker

procedures that take longer than 20 minutes; otherwise, a second injection of the anesthetic would be necessary.

Sodium hydroxide is sometimes added to anesthetic solutions to increase the effectiveness of the anesthetic in regions that have extensive local infection or abscesses. Bacteria tend to acidify an infected site, and local anesthetics are less effective in this type of environment. Adding alkaline substances such as sodium hydroxide or sodium bicarbonate neutralizes the region and creates a more favorable environment for the anesthetic.

19.3 Classification of Local Anesthetics

Local anesthetics are classified by their chemical structures; the two major classes are **esters** and **amides** (Table 19.2). A small number of miscellaneous agents are neither esters nor amides. As illustrated in ➤ Figure 19.2, the terms *ester* and *amide* refer to types of chemical linkages found within the anesthetic molecules.

Cocaine was the first local anesthetic widely used for medical procedures. Cocaine is a natural ester, found in the leaves of the plant *Erythroxylon coca*, native to the Andes Mountains of Peru. As late as the 1880s, cocaine was routinely used for eye surgery, nerve blocks, and spinal anesthesia. Although still available for local anesthesia, cocaine is a Schedule II drug and rarely used therapeutically in the United States. The abuse potential of cocaine is discussed in chapter 11∞.

Another ester, procaine (Novocain), was the drug of choice for dental procedures from the mid-1900s until the 1960s, until the development of the amide anesthetics led to a significant decline in the use of the drug. One ester, benzocaine (Solarcaine, others) is used as a topical OTC agent for treating a large number of painful conditions, including sunburn, insect bites, hemorrhoids, sore throat, and minor wounds.

TABLE 19.2 Selected Local Anesthetics		
Chemical Classification	Drug	General Adverse Effects
Amides	articaine (Septodont) bupivacaine (Marcaine) dibucaine (Nupercaine, Nupercainal) lidocaine (Xylocaine) prilocaine (Citanest) ropivacaine (Naropin)	<u>Difficulty breathing or swallowing, respiratory depression and arrest, convulsions, anaphylactoid reaction, burning, contact dermatitis</u>
Esters	benzocaine (Americaine, Solarcaine, others) chloroprocaine (Nesacaine) procaine (Novocain) tetracaine (Pontocaine)	*CNS depression* <u>Respiratory arrest, circulatory failure, anaphylactoid reaction</u>
Miscellaneous agents	dyclonine (Dyclone) pramoxine (Tronothane)	*Burning, stinging, sensation at application site* <u>Respiratory or cardiac arrest</u>
Italics indicate common adverse effects; <u>underlining</u> indicates serious adverse effects.		

Type	General formula	Example
Ester	R—C—O—R	Procaine
Amide	R—NH—C—R	Lidocaine

➤ **Figure 19.2** Chemical structures of ester and amide local anesthetics

Amides have largely replaced the esters because they produce fewer side effects and generally have a longer duration of action. Lidocaine (Xylocaine) is the most widely used amide for short surgical procedures requiring local anesthesia.

Adverse effects of local anesthetics are uncommon. Allergy is rare. When it does occur, it is often due to sulfites, which are added as preservatives to prolong the shelf life of the anesthetic, or to methylparaben, which may be added to re-

tard bacterial growth in anesthetic solutions. Early signs of adverse effects of local anesthetics include symptoms of CNS stimulation such as restlessness or anxiety. Later effects, such as drowsiness and unresponsiveness, are due to CNS depression. Cardiovascular effects, including hypotension and dysrhythmias, are possible. Patients with a history of cardiovascular disease are often given forms of local anesthetics that contain no epinephrine to reduce the potential

---

Pr Prototype Drug | Lidocaine (Xylocaine)

Therapeutic Class: Anesthetic (local/topical); antidysrhythmic (class IB)

Pharmacologic Class: Sodium channel blocker; amide

ACTIONS AND USES
Lidocaine, the most frequently used injectable local anesthetic, acts by blocking neuronal pain impulses. It may be injected as a nerve block for spinal and epidural anesthesia. It acts by blocking sodium channels located within the membranes of neurons.

Lidocaine may be given IV, IM, or subcutaneously to treat dysrhythmias, as discussed in chapter 23∞. A topical form is also available.

ADMINISTRATION ALERTS
- Solutions of lidocaine containing preservatives or epinephrine are intended for local anesthesia only, and must never be given parenterally for dysrhythmias.
- Do not apply topical lidocaine to large skin areas or to broken or abraded areas, because significant absorption may occur. Do not allow it to come in contact with the eyes.
- For spinal or epidural block, use only preparations specifically labeled for IV use.
- Pregnancy category B

PHARMACOKINETICS
Onset: 45–90 sec IV; 5–15 min IM; 2–5 min topical

Peak: Less than 30 min

Half-life: 1.5–2 h

Duration: 10–20 min IV; 60–90 min IM; 30–60 min topical; more than 100 min injected for anesthesia

ADVERSE EFFECTS
When lidocaine is used for anesthesia, side effects are uncommon. An early symptom of toxicity is CNS excitement, leading to irritability and confusion. Serious adverse effects include convulsions, respiratory depression, and cardiac arrest. Until the effect of the anesthetic diminishes, patients may injure themselves by biting or chewing areas of the mouth that have no sensation following a dental procedure.

Contraindications: Lidocaine should be avoided in cases of sensitivity to amide-type local anesthetics. Application or injection of lidocaine anesthetic is also contraindicated in the presence of severe trauma or sepsis, blood dyscrasias, dysrhythmias, sinus bradycardia, and severe degrees of heart block.

INTERACTIONS
Drug–Drug: Barbiturates may decrease the activity of lidocaine. Increased effects of lidocaine occur if taken concurrently with cimetidine, quinidine, and beta blockers. If lidocaine is used on a regular basis, its effectiveness may diminish when used with other medications.

Lab Tests: Increased CPK

Herbal/Food: Unknown

Treatment of Overdose: Emergency medical attention is needed because of the many associated substantive symptoms such as breathing difficulty, swelling of the lips, chest pain, irregular heart beat, nausea, vomiting, tremors, and seizure activity.

Refer to MyNursingKit for a Nursing Process Focus specific to this drug.

NURSING PROCESS FOCUS • PATIENTS RECEIVING LOCAL ANESTHESIA

Assessment	Potential Nursing Diagnoses
Baseline assessment prior to administration: ■ Understand the reason the drug has been prescribed in order to assess for therapeutic effects. ■ Obtain a complete health history including cardiovascular, hepatic, renal, respiratory, or neurologic disease; pregnancy; or breast-feeding. Obtain a drug history including allergies, current prescription and OTC drugs, herbal preparations, caffeine, nicotine, and alcohol use. If the patient reports an allergy to "caine" drugs, note the specific reactions the patient experienced. Be alert to possible drug interactions. ■ Obtain baseline vital signs and weight. ■ Assess for areas of broken skin, abrasions, burns, or other wounds in area to be treated with local anesthetic. ■ Evaluate laboratory findings appropriate to the procedure (e.g., CBC, electrolytes, hepatic or renal function studies). ■ Assess the patient's ability to receive and understand instruction. Include the family and caregivers as needed.	■ Pain (related to underlying disease process or condition, secondary to surgery or dental procedure) ■ Deficient Knowledge (drug therapy) ■ Risk for Aspiration ■ Risk for Infection ■ Risk for Injury
Assessment throughout administration: ■ Assess for desired therapeutic effects (e.g., local or regional area numbness). ■ Assess vital signs, especially blood pressure and pulse if regional block is used. Report a BP less than 90/60, pulse above 100, or per parameters as ordered by the health care provider. ■ Assess the local or regional area blocked. Expect blanching in a localized area if the local anesthetic contained epinephrine. If a regional area was blocked, periodically assess the ability to move limbs distal to the block. ■ Assess the level of consciousness if a large regional block was given. Report any increasing drowsiness, dizziness, light-headedness, confusion, or agitation immediately. ■ Assess for and promptly report adverse effects: bradycardia or tachycardia, hypotension or hypertension, and dyspnea.	

Planning: Patient Goals and Expected Outcomes

The patient will:
■ Experience therapeutic effects (e.g., numbness in local or regional area).
■ Be free from, or experience minimal, adverse effects.
■ Verbalize an understanding of the drug's use, adverse effects, and required precautions.
■ Demonstrate proper self-administration of the medication (e.g., dose, timing, when to notify provider).

Implementation

Interventions and (Rationales)	Patient and Family Education
Ensuring therapeutic effects: ■ Continue assessments as described earlier for therapeutic effects. Assess the localized area for numbness and blanching if the local anesthetic included epinephrine. Assess the ability to move limbs distal to the regional anesthetic. (The duration of anesthetic action will depend on the solution used and whether epinephrine is included in the solution. If a large regional area is blocked, e.g., epidural, the patient may regain some motor ability before sensation returns and the return of motor activity signals decreasing levels of anesthesia. An ability to perceive pressure-type sensations may remain during anesthesia and may be alarming to the patient. Epinephrine in the anesthetic solution will constrict localized blood vessels and result in blanching of the area.)	■ Teach the patient that the area may be numb for several hours after the procedure is completed. ■ Teach the patient that it is normal that a slight pressure sensation may remain during anesthesia (e.g., sensation of "tugging" during suturing) but that no pain should be felt. Have the patient alert the health care provider if more than a slight pressure sensation or any pain is noticed during anesthesia. ■ Teach the patient that it is normal to regain some ability to move limbs (e.g., after epidural anesthetic) and movement may return before the ability to feel the movement.

NURSING PROCESS FOCUS   PATIENTS RECEIVING LOCAL ANESTHESIA *(Continued)*

Implementation

Interventions and (Rationales)	Patient and Family Education
Minimizing adverse effects: ■ Continue to monitor vital signs, especially blood pressure and pulse for patients given regional anesthesia. Immediately report a BP below 90/60 or per parameters as ordered by the health care provider, tachycardia or bradycardia, changes in level of consciousness, or dyspnea or decrease in respiratory rate. (Adverse effects of local anesthesia are rare. Regional blocks may cause hypotension with the possibility of reflex tachycardia. Bradycardia, hypotension, decreased level of consciousness, decreased respiratory rate, and dyspnea may signal that the anesthesia has entered the systemic circulation and is acting as a general anesthetic.)	■ Instruct the patient to report any increasing nausea, drowsiness, dizziness, light-headedness, confusion, or anxiety immediately.
■ Caution the patient not to eat, chew gum, or drink until the mouth sensation has returned if local (dental) or oral/throat anesthesia has been used. If throat anesthesia was used, assess the gag reflex before eating. (Local anesthetics are effective for up to 3 hours or more. Biting injuries to oral mucous membranes may occur while tissue is numb. Aspiration of food or liquids is possible until swallowing sensation and gag reflex returns.)	■ Instruct the patient to refrain from eating or drinking for 1 hour or more postanesthesia or until sensation has completely returned to the oral cavity or throat.
■ Ensure patient safety; monitor motor coordination and/or ambulation post–regional block until certain motor movement is unaffected. Be particularly cautious with older adults who are at an increased risk for falls. (Numbness or effects on motor ability post–regional anesthetic may impair movement and increase the risk of falls or injuries.)	■ Instruct the patient to call for assistance prior to getting out of bed or attempting to walk alone post–epidural block, and to avoid driving or other activities requiring physical coordination (e.g., regional upper limb block) until the residual effects of the drug are known.
■ Assess areas of abrasion, burns, or open wounds if a local anesthetic was applied to the area. (Large open or denuded areas may increase the amount of drug absorption into the general circulation. Use sterile technique to apply drug to open areas.)	■ Instruct the patient to report increased redness, swelling, or drainage from open areas under treatment.
■ Read all labels carefully before using parenteral solutions. (Solutions containing epinephrine must *never* be used IV or for local anesthesia in areas of decreased circulation [e.g., fingertips, toes, earlobes] due to vasoconstrictive effects.)	■ Provide an explanation of desired effects of the local anesthetic and the need for postprocedure monitoring.
■ Monitor pain relief in patients post–regional block (e.g., epidural). (Pain sensation will increase as the regional block wears off. Additional pain relief may be required.)	■ Teach the patient to report any discomfort or pain as the anesthesia wears off.
Patient understanding of drug therapy: ■ Use opportunities during administration of medications and during assessments to discuss the rationale for drug therapy, desired therapeutic outcomes, most commonly observed adverse effects, parameters for when to call the health care provider, and any necessary monitoring or precautions. (Using time during nursing care helps to optimize and reinforce key teaching areas.)	■ The patient should be able to state the reason for the drug, anticipated sensations, and adverse effects to observe for and when to report them.
Patient self-administration of drug therapy: ■ When administering the medication, instruct the patient, family, or caregiver in proper self-administration of the drug, e.g., take the drug as prescribed when needed. (Utilizing time during nurse-administration of these drugs helps to reinforce teaching.)	■ Teach the patient to take oral medication (e.g., lidocaine viscous) by swishing and spitting if used for oral cavity or by gargling, and do not swallow unless directed by the health care provider. Apply topical medication in a thin layer to the skin area as directed.

Evaluation of Outcome Criteria

Evaluate the effectiveness of drug therapy by confirming that patient goals and expected outcomes have been met (see "Planning").

See Table 19.2 for a list of drugs to which these nursing actions apply.

effects of this sympathomimetic on the heart and blood pressure. CNS and cardiovascular side effects are not expected unless the local anesthetic is absorbed rapidly or is accidentally injected directly into a blood vessel.

GENERAL ANESTHESIA

General anesthesia is a loss of sensation throughout the entire body, accompanied by a loss of consciousness. General anesthetics are applied when it is necessary for patients to remain still and without pain for a longer time than could be achieved with local anesthetics.

19.4 Characteristics of General Anesthesia

The goal of general anesthesia is to provide a rapid and complete loss of sensation. Signs of general anesthesia include total analgesia and loss of consciousness, memory, and body movement. Although these signs are similar to those of sleeping, general anesthesia and sleep are not exactly the same. General anesthetics depress most nervous activity in the brain, whereas sleeping depresses only very specific areas. In fact, some brain activity actually increases during sleep, as described in chapter 14∞.

General anesthesia is rarely achieved with a single drug. Instead, multiple medications are used to rapidly induce unconsciousness, cause muscle relaxation, and maintain deep anesthesia. This approach, called **balanced anesthesia,** allows a lower dose of inhalation anesthetic, thus making the procedure safer for the patient.

General anesthesia is a progressive process that occurs in distinct phases. The most efficacious medications can quickly induce all four stages, whereas others are able to induce only stage 1. Stage 3 is where most major surgery occurs; thus it is called **surgical anesthesia.** When seeking surgical anesthesia, it is desirable to progress through stage 2 as rapidly as possible, as this stage produces distressing symptoms. These stages are listed in Table 19.3.

TABLE 19.3	Stages of General Anesthesia
Stage	**Characteristics**
1	Loss of pain: The patient loses general sensation but may be awake. This stage proceeds until the patient loses consciousness.
2	Excitement and hyperactivity: The patient may be delirious and try to resist treatment. Heart rate and breathing may become irregular and blood pressure can increase. IV agents are administered here to calm the patient.
3	Surgical anesthesia: Skeletal muscles become relaxed and delirium stabilizes. Cardiovascular and breathing activities stabilize. Eye movements slow and the patient becomes still. Surgery begins here and remains until the procedure ends.
4	Paralysis of the medulla region in the brain (responsible for controlling respiratory and cardiovascular activity): If breathing or the heart stops, death could result. This stage is usually avoided during general anesthesia.

General Anesthetics

General anesthetics are drugs that rapidly produce unconsciousness and total analgesia. These drugs are usually administered by the IV or inhalation routes. To supplement the effects of a general anesthetic, adjunct drugs are given before, during, and after surgery.

19.5 Pharmacotherapy with Inhaled General Anesthetics

There are two primary methods of inducing general anesthesia. *Intravenous* agents are usually administered first because they act within a few seconds. After the patient loses consciousness, *inhaled agents* are used to maintain the anesthesia. During short surgical procedures or those requiring lower stages of anesthesia, the IV agents may be used alone.

Inhaled general anesthetics, listed in Table 19.4, may be gases or volatile liquids. These agents produce their effects by preventing the flow of sodium into neurons in the CNS, thus delaying nerve impulses and producing a dra-

TABLE 19.4	Inhaled General Anesthetics	
Type	**Drug**	**General Adverse Effects**
Gas	🅿 nitrous oxide	*Dizziness, drowsiness, nausea, euphoria, vomiting* <u>Malignant hyperthermia, apnea, cyanosis</u>
Volatile liquid	desflurane (Suprane) enflurane (Ethrane) 🅿 halothane (Fluothane) isoflurane (Forane) methoxyflurane (Penthrane) sevoflurane (Ultane)	*Drowsiness, nausea, vomiting* <u>Myocardial depression, marked hypotension, pulmonary vasoconstriction, hepatotoxicity</u>
Italics indicate common adverse effects; <u>underlining</u> indicates serious adverse effects.		

Pr Prototype Drug | Nitrous Oxide

Therapeutic Class: General anesthetic   **Pharmacologic Class:** Inhalation gaseous agent

ACTIONS AND USES

The main action of nitrous oxide is analgesia caused by suppression of pain mechanisms in the CNS. This agent has a low potency and does not produce a complete loss of consciousness or profound relaxation of skeletal muscle. Because nitrous oxide does not induce surgical anesthesia (stage 3), it is commonly combined with other surgical anesthetic agents. Nitrous oxide is ideal for dental procedures because the patient remains conscious and can follow instructions while experiencing full analgesia.

ADMINISTRATION ALERT

- Establish an IV if one is not already in place in case emergency medications are needed.

PHARMACOKINETICS

Onset: 2–5 min

Peak: Less than 10 min

Half-life: Variable

Duration: Patients recover from anesthesia rapidly after nitrous oxide is discontinued.

ADVERSE EFFECTS

When used in low to moderate doses, nitrous oxide produces few adverse effects. At higher doses, patients exhibit some adverse signs of stage 2 anesthesia such as anxiety, excitement, and combativeness. Lowering the inhaled dose will quickly reverse these adverse effects. As nitrous oxide is exhaled, the patient may temporarily have some difficulty breathing at the end of a procedure. Nausea and vomiting following the procedure are more common with nitrous oxide than with other inhalation anesthetics.

Some general anesthetics infrequently produce liver damage. Nitrous oxide has the potential to be abused by users (sometimes medical personnel) who enjoy the relaxed, sedated state that the drug produces.

Contraindications: This drug is contraindicated in patients with an impaired level of consciousness, head injury, inability to comply with instructions, decompression sickness (nitrogen narcosis, air embolism, air transport), undiagnosed abdominal pain or marked distention, bowel obstruction, hypotension, shock, chronic obstructive pulmonary disease, cyanosis, or chest trauma with pneumothorax.

INTERACTIONS

Drug–Drug: Sympathomimetics and phosphodiesterase inhibitors may exacerbate dysrhythmias.

Lab Tests: Unknown

Herbal/Food: Milk thistle taken before and after anesthesia may lower the potential risk of liver damage. Herbal products such as ginger may also provide therapeutic benefit.

Treatment of Overdose: Metoclopramide may help reduce the symptoms of nausea and vomiting associated with inhalation of nitrous oxide.

Refer to MyNursingKit for a Nursing Process Focus specific to this drug.

---

matic reduction in neural activity. The exact mechanism is not exactly known, although it is likely that gamma-aminobutyric acid (GABA) receptors in the brain are activated. It is not the same mechanism as is known for local anesthetics. There is some inconclusive evidence suggesting that the mechanism may be related to that of some antiseizure drugs. There is no specific receptor that binds to general anesthetics, and they do not seem to affect neurotransmitter release.

Gaseous General Anesthetics

The only gas used routinely for anesthesia is nitrous oxide, commonly called *laughing gas*. Nitrous oxide is used for dental procedures and for brief obstetric and surgical procedures. It may also be used in conjunction with other general anesthetics, making it possible to decrease their dosages with greater effectiveness.

Nitrous oxide should be used cautiously in myasthenia gravis, as it may cause respiratory depression and prolonged hypnotic effects. Patients with cardiovascular disease, especially those with increased intracranial pressure, should be monitored carefully, because the hypnotic effects of the drug may be prolonged or potentiated.

Volatile Liquid General Anesthetics

The volatile anesthetics are liquid at room temperature but are converted into a vapor and inhaled to produce their anesthetic effects. Commonly administered volatile agents are halothane (Fluothane), enflurane (Ethrane), and isoflurane (Forane). The most potent of these is halothane (Fluothane). Some general anesthetics enhance the sensitivity of the heart to drugs such as epinephrine, norepinephrine, dopamine, and serotonin. Most volatile liquids depress cardiovascular and respiratory function. Because it has less effect on the heart and does not damage the liver, isoflurane (Forane) has become the most widely used inhalation anesthetic. The volatile liquids are excreted almost entirely by the lungs, through exhalation.

IV Anesthetics

IV anesthetics are used either alone, for short procedures, or in combination with inhalation anesthetics.

Pr Prototype Drug | Halothane *(Fluothane)*

Therapeutic Class: General anesthetic   **Pharmacologic Class:** Inhalation volatile liquid

ACTIONS AND USES
Halothane produces a potent level of surgical anesthesia that is rapid in onset. Although potent, halothane does not produce as much muscle relaxation or analgesia as other volatile anesthetics. Therefore, halothane is primarily used with other anesthetic agents including muscle relaxants and analgesics. Nitrous oxide is sometimes combined with halothane.

PHARMACOKINETICS
Onset: 2–5 min

Peak: Less than 10 min; the minimum alveolar concentration (MAC) is 0.75%. MAC is reduced in older adults.

Half-life: Variable

Duration: Halothane's duration of action is variable due to its lipid solubility. Patients recover from anesthesia rather rapidly after halothane is discontinued (variable among different age groups; older adults take longer to recover).

ADVERSE EFFECTS
Halothane moderately sensitizes the heart muscle to epinephrine; therefore, dysrhythmias are a concern. This agent lowers blood pressure and the respiration rate. It also overcomes reflex mechanisms that normally keep the contents of the stomach from entering the lungs. Because of potential hepatotoxicity, the use of halothane has declined.

Malignant hyperthermia is a rare but potentially fatal adverse effect triggered by all inhalation anesthetics. It causes muscle rigidity and severe temperature elevation (up to 43°C). This risk is greatest when halothane is used with succinylcholine.

Halothane dilates the cerebral vasculature and may, in certain conditions, increase intracranial pressure.

Contraindications: Halothane is contraindicated in patients with a history of significant or malignant hyperthermia after previous halothane exposure. It should be used with caution in patients with hepatic function impairment, dysrhythmias, head injury, myasthenia gravis, or pheochromocytoma.

INTERACTIONS
Drug–Drug: Excessive hypotension may occur when halothane is combined with antihypertensive drugs. Halothane potentiates the action of nondepolarizing neuromuscular blocking agents.

Levodopa taken concurrently increases the level of dopamine in the CNS, and should be discontinued 6 to 8 hours before halothane administration.

Skeletal muscle weakness, respiratory depression, or apnea may occur if halothane is administered concurrently with polymyxins, lincomycin, or aminoglycosides.

Lab Tests: Unknown

Herbal/Food: Unknown

Treatment of Overdose: No specific therapy is available; patients are treated symptomatically.

Refer to MyNursingKit for a Nursing Process Focus specific to this drug.

HOME & COMMUNITY CONSIDERATIONS

Postanesthesia Follow-Up Care
Patients are kept in the inpatient or outpatient hospital or clinic setting until the effects of an anesthesia are resolved. Patients may return to the home environment following certain outpatient surgeries, dental, and diagnostic procedures using conscious sedation before the effects of the sedation have worn off. Patients are required to have someone with them for 24 hours to monitor and assist their needs. Usually, a follow-up assessment by phone is completed by the nurse or other health care provider within 24 hours. Providing written instructions of all home care required is essential before discharge because vital information may be forgotten if the patient remains groggy.

19.6 Pharmacotherapy with IV Anesthetics

Intravenous anesthetics, listed in Table 19.5, are important supplements to general anesthesia. Although occasionally used alone, they are often administered with inhaled general anesthetics. Concurrent administration of IV and inhaled anesthetics allows the dose of the inhaled agent to be reduced, thus lowering the potential for serious side effects. Furthermore, when IV and inhaled anesthetics are combined, they provide greater analgesia and muscle relaxation than could be provided by the inhaled anesthetic alone. When IV anesthetics are administered alone, they are generally reserved for medical procedures that take less than 15 minutes.

Drugs employed as IV anesthetics include barbiturates, opioids, and benzodiazepines. Opioids offer the advantage of superior analgesia. Combining the opioid fentanyl (Sublimaze) with the antipsychotic agent droperidol (Inapsine) produces a state known as **neuroleptanalgesia**. In this state, patients are conscious, though insensitive to pain and unconnected with surroundings. The premixed combination of these two agents is marketed as Innovar. A similar conscious, dissociated state is produced with ketamine (Ketalar).

NURSING PROCESS FOCUS   PATIENTS RECEIVING GENERAL ANESTHESIA

Assessment	Potential Nursing Diagnoses

Baseline assessment prior to administration:

- Understand the reason the drug has been prescribed in order to assess for therapeutic effects.
- Obtain a complete health history including cardiovascular, respiratory, hepatic, renal, or neurologic disease; pregnancy; or breast-feeding. Obtain a drug history including allergies, current prescription and OTC drugs, herbal preparations, caffeine, nicotine, and alcohol use. Be alert to possible drug interactions.
- Assess for a previous history of anesthesia and note any significant reactions. Obtain a family history of anesthesia problems, particularly related to the use of neuromuscular blockers (e.g., succinylcholine), or any unusual temperature effects related to surgery.
- Obtain baseline vital signs, height, and weight. Note the day/hour the patient last ate or drank.
- Evaluate laboratory findings appropriate to procedure (e.g., CBC, electrolytes, hepatic or renal function studies, MRI or CT scan results).
- Obtain required preoperative paperwork (e.g., informed consent, completed history and physical).
- Administer any preoperative adjunctive drugs (e.g., sedative, analgesic) as ordered.
- Assess the level of anxiety, and any concerns or questions the patient, family, or caregiver may have. Reinforce preoperative teaching, including deep breathing exercises. Provide the family or caregiver with information on the anticipated length of procedure, waiting room area, and telephone and eating availability.
- When working with pediatric patients, allow parents or the caregiver to stay with the child as long as agency policy permits to decrease patient anxiety. Provide simple explanations of the procedure appropriate for the age of the child.
- When working with older adults, note assistive devices (e.g., glasses, hearing aids) and remove only when necessary. Give to the family, caregiver, or provide for safekeeping. Ensure that devices are available in the postoperative period.
- Initiate an intravenous access site if required for the procedure.
- Assess the patient's ability to receive and understand instruction. Include the family and caregivers as needed.

Potential Nursing Diagnoses:
- Anxiety (related to surgical procedure)
- Impaired Gas Exchange
- Ineffective Breathing Pattern
- Decreased Cardiac Output
- Disturbed Sensory Perception
- Nausea (related to adverse drug effects)
- Deficient Knowledge (drug therapy)
- Risk for Injury, Risk for Infection

Assessment throughout administration:

- Assess for desired therapeutic effects (e.g., diminished or loss of consciousness).
- Assess vital signs, especially blood pressure and pulse, frequently. Report a BP less than 90/60, pulse above 100, or per parameters as ordered by the health care provider.
- Maintain operative sterility throughout procedure.
- Assess the level of consciousness in the postoperative period. Continue frequent monitoring of vital signs and pulse oximetry.
- Assess for and promptly report adverse effects: bradycardia or tachycardia, hypotension or hypertension, dyspnea, and rapidly increasing temperature.

Planning: Patient Goals and Expected Outcomes

The patient will:
- Experience therapeutic effects (e.g., adequate anesthesia during procedure).
- Be free from, or experience minimal, adverse effects.
- Verbalize an understanding of the drug's intended use, adverse effects, and required precautions.

(Continued)

NURSING PROCESS FOCUS PATIENTS RECEIVING GENERAL ANESTHESIA (Continued)

Implementation

Interventions and (Rationales)	Patient and Family Education
Ensuring therapeutic effects:	
▪ Continue assessments as described earlier for therapeutic effects. Provide for patient safety during the preoperative and operative period and assess the level of consciousness, vital signs, and return of motor and sensory sensation postoperatively. (The duration of anesthetic action will depend on the drugs used and adjunctive or reversal agents used.)	▪ Provide a quiet environment postoperatively and frequently orient the patient to the postoperative recovery unit.
▪ Assess for shivering in the postoperative period and provide additional blankets or warmth as needed. (General anesthetics depress the CNS and some autonomic activity. As autonomic activity returns, shivering is common. Warm blankets provide comfort during this period.)	▪ Continue to orient the patient in the postoperative period and allay anxiety about shivering.
Minimizing adverse effects:	
▪ Continue to monitor vital signs frequently, including temperature. Report a BP below 90/60 or per parameters as ordered by the health care provider, tachycardia or significant bradycardia, or dyspnea. Report any increase in temperature immediately. (CNS depression will cause decreases in all vital signs but significant bradycardia, hypotension, decreased respiratory rate, or dyspnea should be reported promptly. Malignant hyperthermia associated with succinylcholine is a rare but potentially fatal adverse effect and any increase in temperature above the preoperative baseline should be reported immediately.)	▪ Provide an explanation for all procedures and monitoring to the patient. Continue to reorient the patient to the surroundings frequently in postoperative period.
▪ Provide adequate pain relief in the immediate postoperative period. (General anesthetics do not necessarily provide analgesia, depending on the agent. Adequate pain relief begins ideally in the preoperative period. Assess for nonverbal signs of pain such as restlessness or grimacing as the patient regains consciousness.)	▪ Provide a rationale for pain relief preoperatively and encourage the patient to request pain medication as able. Assure the patient, family, or caregiver that pain needs will be frequently monitored.
▪ Encourage the patient to take deep breaths and move the lower extremities frequently in the postoperative period. (General anesthetics given by inhalation are excreted via the lungs. Deep breathing assists in removing the remaining anesthetic. Early range-of-motion exercises may help prevent venous thrombosis and complications.)	▪ Teach the patient deep breathing exercises in the preoperative period and that early movement of legs will be encouraged in the early postoperative period, unless otherwise ordered by the provider.
▪ Ensure patient safety in the postoperative period. Frequently orient the patient to the surroundings, day and time, and maintain a safe environment. (During the period of anesthesia, consciousness is lost along with the ability to orient to day, time, and person. Confusion related to these effects in the postoperative period is common. Use of safety measures such as side rails and soft restraints may be necessary until the patient regains consciousness.)	
▪ For patients receiving ketamine and other drugs causing neuroleptanalgesia, provide a quiet, calm environment postprocedure. Avoid overstimulating the patient during vital signs, using a soft touch and explanations of all procedures done. (During recovery from neuroleptanalgesia drugs, confusion and misinterpretation of sensory stimulation may cause extreme anxiety, fear, or paranoia. Keep all stimuli to a minimum until patient regains full consciousness.)	▪ Explain the full procedure and required postprocedural care to the patient, family, or caregiver. Alert the family or caregiver that visiting may be restricted during the immediate recovery period in order to minimize sensory stimulation.
Patient understanding of drug therapy:	
▪ Use opportunities during the preoperative period to discuss the rationale for drug therapy, desired therapeutic outcomes, most commonly observed adverse effects, and any necessary monitoring or precautions. (Using time during nursing care helps to optimize and reinforce key teaching areas.)	▪ The patient should be able to state the reason for drug(s), anticipated sensations, and adverse effects to observe for and when to report them.

Evaluation of Outcome Criteria

Evaluate the effectiveness of drug therapy by confirming that patient goals and expected outcomes have been met (see "Planning").

See Tables 19.4 and 19.5 for lists of drugs to which these nursing actions apply.

TABLE 19.5	Intravenous Anesthetics	
Chemical Classification	Drug	General Adverse Effects
Barbiturates and barbiturate-like agents	etomidate (Amidate) methohexital sodium (Brevital) propofol (Diprivan)	*Dizziness, confusion, unsteadiness* <u>Circulatory or respiratory depression with apnea, laryngospasm, anaphylaxis</u>
Benzodiazepines	diazepam (Valium) lorazepam (Ativan) midazolam hydrochloride (Versed)	*Dizziness, decreased alertness, diminished concentration* <u>Cardiovascular collapse, laryngospasm</u>
Opioids	alfentanil hydrochloride (Alfenta) fentanyl citrate (Sublimaze, others) remifentanil hydrochloride (Ultiva) sufentanil citrate (Sufenta)	*Nausea, GI disturbances* <u>Marked CNS depression</u>
Miscellaneous	ketamine (Ketalar)	*Dissociation, increased blood pressure and pulse rate, confusion, excitement*

Italics indicate common adverse effects; <u>underlining</u> indicates serious adverse effects.

Pr Prototype Drug | Thiopental *(Pentothal)*

Therapeutic Class: General anesthetic   **Pharmacologic Class:** Intravenous induction agent; short-acting barbiturate

ACTIONS AND USES

Thiopental is the oldest IV anesthetic. It is used for brief medical procedures and to rapidly induce unconsciousness prior to administering inhaled anesthetics. It is classified as an ultrashort-acting barbiturate, having an onset time of less than 30 seconds and a duration of only 10 to 30 minutes. Unlike some anesthetic agents, it has very low analgesic properties.

ADMINISTRATION ALERT

- Pregnancy category C

PHARMACOKINETICS

Onset: 30–60 sec

Peak: 10–30 min

Half-life: 12 min

Duration: 20–30 min

ADVERSE EFFECTS

Like other barbiturates, thiopental can produce severe respiratory depression when used in high doses. It is used with caution in patients with cardiovascular disease because of its ability to depress the myocardium and cause dysrhythmias. Patients may experience emergence delirium postoperatively. This causes hallucinations, confusion, and excitability.

Contraindications: Thiopental should not be administered to patients with hypersensitivity to barbiturates or with veins unsuitable for IV administration. Variegate porphyria or acute intermittent porphyria are contraindications. In these cases, thiopental or other barbiturates can cause nerve demyelination and CNS lesions, which may lead to pain, weakness, and life-threatening paralysis.

INTERACTIONS

Drug–Drug: Thiopental interacts with many other drugs. For example, use with CNS depressants potentiates respiratory and CNS depression. Phenothiazines increase the risk of hypotension.

Lab Tests: Unknown

Herbal/Food: Kava and valerian may potentiate sedation.

Treatment of Overdose: Because the half-life of thiopental is very brief, overdose is easily managed in the surgical suite by discontinuing the drug and assisting ventilation until respirations return to normal.

Refer to MyNursingKit for a Nursing Process Focus specific to this drug.

19.7 Nonanesthetic Drugs as Adjuncts to Surgery

A number of drugs are used either to complement the effects of general anesthetics or to treat anticipated side effects of the anesthesia. These agents, listed in Table 19.6, are called *adjuncts* to anesthesia. They may be given prior to, during, or after surgery.

The preoperative drugs given to relieve anxiety and to provide mild sedation include barbiturates or benzodiazepines. Opioids such as morphine may be given to counteract pain that the patient will experience after surgery.

TABLE 19.6	Selected Adjuncts to Anesthesia	
Chemical Classification	**Drug**	**General Adverse Effects**
Anticholinergic	atropine	*Dry mouth, urinary retention* Tachycardia, dysrhythmias, paralytic ileus, pharyngitis
Benzodiazepine	midazolam (Versed)	*Drowsiness, slurred speech, tremor* Respiratory depression, laryngospasm
Cholinergic	bethanechol chloride (Duvoid, Urecholine)	*Salivation, abdominal cramping, sweating* Transient complete heart block
Dopamine blocker	droperidol (Inapsine)	*Postoperative drowsiness, extrapyramidal symptoms, hypotension, tachycardia* Laryngospasm, bronchospasm
Neuromuscular blockers	mivacurium (Mivacron) ⓟ succinylcholine (Anectine) tubocurarine	*Muscle fasciculations, bradycardia, hypotension* Respiratory depression, malignant hyperthermia, apnea, circulatory collapse
Opioids	alfentanil hydrochloride (Alfenta) fentanyl citrate (Actiq, Duragesic, Sublimaze, others) fentanyl/droperidol (Innovar) remifentanil hydrochloride (Ultiva) sufentanil citrate (Sufenta)	*Sedation, nausea, GI disturbances* Circulatory depression, cardiac arrest, respiratory depression or arrest, marked CNS depression
Phenothiazine	promethazine (Phenazine, Phenergan, others)	*Blurred vision, dry mouth* Respiratory depression, agranulocytosis
Italics indicate common adverse effects; <u>underlining</u> indicates serious adverse effects.		

Anticholinergics such as atropine may be administered to dry secretions and to suppress the bradycardia caused by some anesthetics.

During surgery, the primary adjuncts are the **neuromuscular blockers** (chapter 20∞). It is necessary to administer drugs that cause skeletal muscles to totally relax in order to carry out surgical procedures safely. Administration of these drugs also allows the amount of anesthetic to be reduced. Neuromuscular blocking agents are classified as *depolarizing* blockers or *nondepolarizing* blockers. The only depolarizing blocker is succinylcholine (Anectine), which works by binding to acetylcholine receptors at neuromuscular junctions to cause total skeletal muscle relaxation. Succinylcholine is used in surgery for ease of tracheal intubation. Mivacurium (Mivacron) is the shortest acting of the nondepolarizing blockers, whereas tubocurarine is a longer-acting neuromuscular blocking agent. The nondepolarizing blockers cause muscle paralysis by competing with acetylcholine for cholinergic receptors at neuromuscular junctions. Once attached to the receptor, the nonpolarizing blockers prevent muscle contraction.

Postoperative drugs include analgesics for pain and antiemetics such as promethazine (Phenergan, others) for the nausea and vomiting that sometimes occur during recovery from the anesthetic. Occasionally a parasympathomimetic such as bethanechol (Urecholine) is administered to stimulate the urinary tract and smooth muscle of the bowel to begin peristalsis following surgery. Bethanechol is featured as a prototype drug in chapter 13∞.

Pr Prototype Drug | Succinylcholine *(Anectine)*

Therapeutic Class: Skeletal muscle paralytic agent; neuromuscular blocker

Pharmacologic Class: Depolarizing blocker; acetylcholine receptor blocking agent

ACTIONS AND USES

Like the natural neurotransmitter acetylcholine, succinylcholine acts on cholinergic receptor sites at neuromuscular junctions. At first, depolarization occurs, and skeletal muscles contract. After repeated contractions, however, the membrane is unable to repolarize as long as the drug stays attached to the receptor. Effects are first noted as muscle weakness and muscle spasms. Eventually, paralysis occurs. Succinylcholine is rapidly broken down by the enzyme cholinesterase; when the IV infusion is stopped, the duration of action is only a few minutes. Use of succinylcholine reduces the amount of general anesthetic needed for procedures. Dantrolene sodium (Dantrium) is a drug used preoperatively or postoperatively to reduce the signs of malignant hyperthermia in susceptible patients.

ADMINISTRATION ALERT

- Pregnancy category C

PHARMACOKINETICS

Onset: 0.5–1 min IV; 2–3 min IM

Peak: Unknown

Half-life: Unknown

Duration: 2–3 min IV; 10–30 min IM

ADVERSE EFFECTS

Succinylcholine can cause complete paralysis of the diaphragm and intercostal muscles; thus, mechanical ventilation is necessary during surgery. Bradycardia and respiratory depression are expected adverse effects. If doses are high, the ganglia are affected, causing tachycardia, hypotension, and urinary retention.

Patients with certain genetic defects may experience a rapid onset of extremely high fever with muscle rigidity—a serious condition known as malignant hyperthermia.

Succinylcholine should be employed with caution in patients with fractures or muscle spasms, because the initial muscle fasciculations may cause additional trauma. Neuromuscular blockade may be prolonged in patients with hypokalemia, hypocalcemia, or low plasma pseudocholinesterase levels.

Contraindications: Succinylcholine should be used with extreme caution in patients with severe burns or trauma, neuromuscular diseases, or glaucoma. Succinylcholine is contraindicated in patients with a family history of malignant hyperthermia or conditions of pulmonary, renal, cardiovascular, metabolic, or hepatic dysfunction.

INTERACTIONS

Drug–Drug: Additive skeletal muscle blockade will occur if succinylcholine is given concurrently with clindamycin, aminoglycosides, furosemide, lithium, quinidine, or lidocaine. The effect of succinylcholine may be increased if given concurrently with phenothiazines, oxytocin, promazine, tacrine, or thiazide diuretics. The effect of succinylcholine is decreased if given with diazepam.

If this drug is given concurrently with halothane or nitrous oxide, an increased risk of bradycardia, dysrhythmias, sinus arrest, apnea, and malignant hyperthermia exists. If succinylcholine is given concurrently with cardiac glycosides, there is increased risk of cardiac dysrhythmias. If narcotics are given concurrently with succinylcholine, there is increased risk of bradycardia and sinus arrest.

Lab Tests: Unknown

Herbal/Food: Unknown

Treatment of Overdose: Treatment may involve drug therapy for the following symptoms: weakness, lack of coordination, watery eyes and mouth, tremors, and seizures. Problems with breathing require emergency medical measures.

Refer to MyNursingKit for a Nursing Process Focus specific to this drug.

 # Chapter REVIEW

KEY CONCEPTS

The numbered key concepts provide a succinct summary of the important points from the corresponding numbered section within the chapter. If any of these points are not clear, refer to the numbered section within the chapter for review.

19.1 Regional loss of sensation is achieved by administering local anesthetics topically or through the infiltration, nerve block, spinal, or epidural routes.

19.2 Local anesthetics act by blocking sodium channels in neurons. Epinephrine is sometimes added to prolong the duration of anesthetic action.

19.3 Local anesthetics are classified as amides or esters. The amides, such as lidocaine (Xylocaine), have generally replaced the esters due to their greater safety.

19.4 General anesthesia produces a complete loss of sensation accompanied by loss of consciousness. This state is usually achieved through the use of multiple medications.

19.5 Inhaled general anesthetics are used to maintain surgical anesthesia. Some, such as nitrous oxide, have low efficacy; whereas others, such as halothane (Fluothane), can induce deep anesthesia.

19.6 IV anesthetics are used either alone, for short procedures, or in combination with inhalation anesthetics.

19.7 Numerous nonanesthetic medications, including opioids, antianxiety agents, barbiturates, and neuromuscular blockers, are administered as adjuncts to surgery.

NCLEX-RN® REVIEW QUESTIONS

1 The patient received lidocaine viscous before a gastroscopy was performed. Priority nursing assessment includes:
1. return of gag reflex.
2. ability to urinate.
3. abdominal pain.
4. ability to stand.

2 The nurse observes a coworker preparing to administer a solution of intravenous lidocaine and epinephrine to a patient with multiple premature ventricular contractions. The appropriate action by the nurse is to:
1. document administration of the drug.
2. notify the nursing supervisor of the error.
3. do nothing; the drug choice is correct.
4. prevent the administration and discuss the need for a solution of lidocaine without epinephrine in this situation.

3 The nurse recognizes that the main action of nitrous oxide is to:
1. provide total relaxation of skeletal muscles.
2. induce loss of consciousness.
3. cause analgesia by suppressing the pain mechanism in the CNS.
4. induce stage 3 anesthesia.

4 The nurse should assess the patient for which of the following side effects if succinylcholine (Anectine) is used as an adjunct to anesthesia? (Select all that apply.)
1. Bradycardia
2. Severe headache
3. Hypertension
4. Respiratory depression
5. Urinary frequency

5 A patient is admitted to the postanesthesia recovery unit (PACU) after receiving ketamine (Ketalar) after his minor orthopedic surgery. In the recovery period, the patient should be:
1. frequently oriented to time, place, and person.
2. kept in a bright environment so there is less drowsiness.
3. assessed for sensory deprivation.
4. placed in a quiet place with low lights and away from noisy patients or equipment.

CRITICAL THINKING QUESTIONS

1. An elderly patient requires local anesthesia for a 3-cm laceration to the distal fourth metacarpal of the left hand. The health care provider requests lidocaine (Xylocaine) 1% with epinephrine. What is the nurse's response?

2. A patient who has a history of heart failure is on digoxin (Lanoxin) and has a history of mild renal failure. The health care provider asks the nurse to prepare succinylcholine (Anectine) IV as an anesthetic for this patient who is having an outpatient procedure. What is the nurse's response?

3. The nurse is reviewing the chart of a patient who has recently had abdominal surgery. The patient is 67 years old, has been on digoxin (Lanoxin), ibuprofen, St. John's wort, and Maalox daily. Which of the information would indi-

cate that this patient may require closer monitoring (and why)? Which is a priority?

See Appendix D for answers and rationales for all activities.

 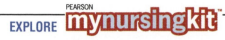

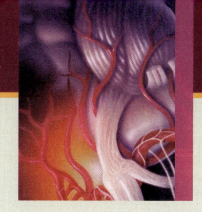

Chapter 20

Drugs for Degenerative Diseases of the Nervous System

LEARNING OUTCOMES

After reading this chapter, the student should be able to:

1. Identify the most common degenerative diseases of the central nervous system (CNS).
2. Describe symptoms of Parkinson's disease.
3. Explain the neurochemical basis for Parkinson's disease, focusing on the roles of dopamine and acetylcholine in the brain.
4. Describe the nurse's role in the pharmacologic management of Parkinson's disease and Alzheimer's disease.
5. Describe symptoms of Alzheimer's disease and explain theories about why these symptoms develop.
6. Explain the goals of pharmacotherapy for Alzheimer's disease and the efficacy of existing medications.
7. Describe the signs and basis for development of multiple sclerosis symptoms.
8. Categorize drugs used in the treatment of Alzheimer's disease, Parkinson's disease, and multiple sclerosis based on their classification and mechanism of action.
9. For each of the drug classes listed in Drugs at a Glance, know representative drug examples, and explain their mechanisms of action, primary action, and important adverse effects.
10. Use the nursing process to care for patients receiving drug therapy for degenerative diseases of the CNS.

KEY TERMS

Degenerative diseases of the CNS are often difficult to deal with pharmacologically. Medications are unable to stop or reverse the progressive nature of these diseases; they can offer only symptomatic relief. Three common debilitating and progressive conditions—Parkinson's disease, Alzheimer's disease, and multiple sclerosis—are the focus of this chapter.

20.1 Degenerative Diseases of the Central Nervous System

Degenerative diseases of the CNS include a diverse set of disorders that differ in their causes and outcomes. Some, such as Huntington's disease, are quite rare, affect younger patients, and are caused by chromosomal defects. Others, such as Alzheimer's disease, affect millions of people (mostly older adults) and have a devastating economic and social impact. Table 20.1 lists the major degenerative disorders of the CNS.

The etiology of most neurologic degenerative diseases is unknown. Most progress from very subtle signs and symptoms early in the course of the disease, to profound neurologic, cognitive, or sensory and motor deficits. In their early stages, these disorders may be quite difficult to diagnose. With the exception of Parkinson's disease, pharmacotherapy provides only minimal benefit. Currently, medication is unable to cure any of the degenerative diseases of the CNS.

PARKINSON'S DISEASE

Parkinson's disease is a degenerative disorder of the CNS caused by death of neurons that produce the brain neurotransmitter dopamine. It is the second most common degenerative disease of the nervous system, affecting more than 1.5 million Americans. Pharmacotherapy is often successful at reducing some of the distressing symptoms of this disease.

20.2 Characteristics of Parkinson's Disease

Parkinson's disease affects primarily patients older than 50 years of age; however, even teenagers can develop the disor-der. Men are affected slightly more than women. The disease is progressive, with the expression of full symptoms often taking many years. The symptoms of Parkinson's disease, or **parkinsonism**, are summarized as follows:

- *Tremors:* The hands and head develop a palsy-like motion or shakiness when at rest; "pill rolling" is a common behavior in progressive states, in which patients rub the thumb and forefinger together as if a pill were between them.

- *Muscle rigidity:* Stiffness may resemble symptoms of arthritis; patients often have difficulty bending over or moving limbs. These symptoms may be less noticeable at first, but progress to become more obvious in later years.

- *Bradykinesia:* The most noticeable of all symptoms, **bradykinesia** is marked by difficulty chewing, swallowing, or speaking. Patients with Parkinson's disease have difficulties initiating movement and controlling fine muscle movements. Walking often becomes difficult. Patients shuffle their feet without taking normal strides.

- *Postural instability:* Patients may be humped over slightly and easily lose their balance. Stumbling results in frequent falls with associated injuries.

PHARMFACTS

Degenerative Diseases of the Central Nervous System

- More than 1.5 million Americans have Parkinson's disease.
- Most patients with Parkinson's disease are older than age 50.
- More than 50% of Parkinson's patients who have difficulty with voluntary movement are younger than 60.
- More men than women develop Parkinson's disease.
- More than 4 million Americans have Alzheimer's disease.
- Alzheimer's disease mainly affects patients older than age 65.
- Of all patients with dementia, 60% to 70% have Alzheimer's disease.
- More than 49,000 Americans die annually of Alzheimer's disease.
- Over 2.5 million people worldwide have multiple sclerosis.
- More than 400,000 Americans have multiple sclerosis.
- More women than men develop multiple sclerosis.
- Multiple sclerosis is five times more prevalent in temperate climates than in tropical climates.

TABLE 20.1	Degenerative Diseases of the Central Nervous System
Disease	Description
Alzheimer's disease	Progressive loss of brain function characterized by memory loss, confusion, and dementia
Amyotrophic lateral sclerosis	Progressive weakness and wasting of muscles caused by destruction of motor neurons
Huntington's chorea	Autosomal-dominant genetic disorder resulting in progressive dementia and involuntary, spasmodic movements of limb and facial muscles
Multiple sclerosis	Demyelination of neurons in the central nervous system (CNS), resulting in progressive weakness, visual disturbances, mood alterations, and cognitive deficits
Parkinson's disease	Progressive loss of dopamine in the CNS causing tremor, muscle rigidity, and abnormal movements and posture

- *Affective flattening:* Patients often have a "masked face" where there is little facial expression or blinking of the eyes.

Although Parkinson's disease is a progressive neurologic disorder primarily affecting muscle movement, other health problems often develop in these patients, including anxiety, depression, sleep disturbances, dementia, and disturbances of the autonomic nervous system such as difficulty urinating and performing sexually. Several theories have been proposed to explain the development of parkinsonism. Because some patients with Parkinson's symptoms have a family history of this disorder, a genetic link is highly probable. Numerous environmental toxins also have been suggested as a cause, but results have been inconclusive. Potentially harmful agents include carbon monoxide, cyanide, manganese, chlorine, and pesticides. Viral infections, head trauma, and stroke have also been proposed as causes of parkinsonism.

Symptoms of parkinsonism develop because of degeneration and destruction of dopamine-producing neurons found within an area of the brain known as the **substantia nigra**. Under normal circumstances, neurons in the substantia nigra supply dopamine to the **corpus striatum**, a region of the brain that controls unconscious muscle movement.

Balance, posture, muscle tone, and involuntary muscle movement depend on the proper balance of the neurotransmitters dopamine (inhibitory) and acetylcholine (stimulatory) in the corpus striatum. If dopamine is absent, acetylcholine has a more dramatic stimulatory effect in this area. For this reason, drug therapy for parkinsonism focuses not only on restoring dopamine function but also on blocking the effect of acetylcholine within the corpus striatum. Thus, when the brain experiences a loss of dopamine within the substantia nigra or an overactive cholinergic influence in the corpus striatum, parkinsonism results.

Extrapyramidal side effects (EPS) develop for the same neurochemical reasons as Parkinson's disease. Recall from chapter 17 ∞ that antipsychotic drugs act through a blockade of dopamine receptors. Treatment with certain antipsychotic drugs may induce parkinsonism-like symptoms, or EPS, by interfering with the same neural pathway and functions affected by the lack of dopamine.

EPS may occur suddenly and become a medical emergency. With acute EPS, patients' muscles may spasm or become "locked up." Fever and confusion are other signs and symptoms of this reaction. If acute EPS occurs in a health care facility, short-term medical treatment can be provided by administering parenteral diphenhydramine (Benadryl). If EPS is recognized outside the health care setting, the patient should immediately be taken to the emergency room, because untreated acute episodes of EPS can be fatal.

Parkinsonism Drugs

Antiparkinsonism agents are given to restore the balance of dopamine and acetylcholine in specific regions of the brain. These drugs include dopaminergic drugs and anticholinergics (cholinergic blockers). Dopaminergic drugs are listed in Table 20.2.

Dopaminergics

These drugs either restore dopamine function or stimulate dopamine receptors located within the brain. Recent efforts have focused on the use of dopamine agonists for the initial treatment of Parkinson's disease.

20.3 Treating Parkinsonism with Dopaminergic Drugs

The goal of pharmacotherapy for Parkinson's disease is to increase the ability of the patient to perform normal daily activities of living (ADLs) such as eating, walking, dressing, and bathing. Although pharmacotherapy does not cure this disorder, symptoms may be dramatically reduced in some patients.

Drug therapy attempts to restore the functional balance of dopamine and acetylcholine in the corpus striatum of the brain. Dopaminergic drugs are used to increase dopamine levels in this region. The drug of choice for parkinsonism is levodopa (Larodopa), a dopaminergic drug that has been used more extensively than any other medication for this disorder. As shown in Pharmacotherapy Illustrated 20.1 (see page 259), levodopa is a precursor of dopamine synthesis. Supplying it directly leads to increased biosynthesis of dopamine within the nerve terminals. Whereas levodopa can cross the blood–brain barrier, dopamine cannot; thus, dopamine itself is not useful for therapy. The effectiveness of levodopa can be "boosted" by combining it with carbidopa. This combination, marketed as Sinemet, makes more levodopa available to enter the CNS.

Several additional approaches to enhancing dopamine are used in treating parkinsonism. Tolcapone (Tasmar), entacapone (Comtan), and selegiline (Carbex, Eldepryl) inhibit enzymes that normally destroy levodopa and dopamine. Selegiline is a monamine oxidase (MAO) inhibitor. Apomorphine (Apokyn), bromocriptine (Parlodel),

---

LIFESPAN CONSIDERATIONS

Living with Alzheimer's and Parkinson's Diseases

Both Alzheimer's and Parkinson's diseases are progressive degenerative neurologic disorders. Whereas Alzheimer's leads to impairments in memory, thinking, and reasoning, Parkinson's can lead to the inability to hold small items because of tremors and rigidity. It is because of these progressive symptoms that patients need all the help and support that caregivers can give. Although nonpharmacologic management such as providing a safe environment can help, medications are available to slow the progression and minimize symptoms. Caregivers will need to provide assistance with ADLs, including making sure that these patients receive their medications.

The side effect of some drugs used to control dementia in patients with Alzheimer's can disrupt sleep. Additionally, many people with dementia often suffer sleep apnea. New research suggests that in addition to providing a routine and structured environment, as little as a few hours of bright light, especially in the evening, may help people living with Alzheimer's maintain a normal sleeping pattern. Patients who received light therapy in the evening also experienced an improvement in their sleep cycle.

TABLE 20.2	Dopaminergic Drugs Used for Parkinsonism	
Drug	Route and Adult Dose (max dose where indicated)	Adverse Effects
amantadine (Symmetrel)	PO; 100 mg 1–2 times/day	*Dizziness, light-headedness, difficulty concentrating, confusion, anxiety, headache, sleep dysfunction, fatigue, nausea, vomiting, constipation, orthostatic hypotension, choreiform and involuntary movements, dystonia, dyskinesia*
apomorphine	SC; 2 mg for the first dose; every few days, doses may be increased by 1 mg (max: 6 mg); if more than 1 week passes between doses, titration should be restarted at 2 mg	
bromocriptine (Parlodel)	PO; 1.25–2.5 mg/day up to 100 mg/day in divided doses	<u>Acute MI, shock, neuroleptic malignant syndrome, agranulocytosis, depression with suicidal tendencies, EPS, fulminant liver failure, severe hepatocellular injury</u>
carbidopa-levodopa (Sinemet)	PO; 1 tablet containing 10 mg carbidopa/100 mg levodopa or 25 mg carbidopa/100 mg levodopa tid (max: 6 tabs/day)	
entacapone (Comtan)	PO; 200 mg given with levodopa-carbidopa up to eight times/day	
Pr levodopa (L-Dopa, Larodopa)	PO; 500 mg–1 g/day; may be increased by 100–750 mg every 3–7 days	
pramipexole dihydrochloride (Mirapex)	PO; Start with 0.125 mg tid for 1 wk; double this dose for the next week; continue to increase by 0.25 mg/dose tid every week to a target dose of 1.5 mg tid	
ropinirole hydrochloride (Requip)	PO; Start with 0.25 mg tid; may increase by 0.25 mg/dose tid every week to a target dose of 1 mg tid	
selegiline hydrochloride (L-Deprenyl, Eldepryl)	PO; 5 mg/dose bid; doses greater than 10 mg/day are potentially toxic	
tolcapone (Tasmar)	PO; 100 mg tid (max: 600 mg/day)	

Italics indicate common adverse effects; <u>underlining</u> indicates serious adverse effects.

pramipexole (Mirapex), and ropinirole (Requip) directly activate the dopamine receptor and are called *dopamine agonists*. Amantadine (Symmetrel), an antiviral agent, causes the release of dopamine from nerve terminals. All these drugs are considered adjuncts to the pharmacotherapy of parkinsonism because they are not as effective as levodopa.

Recent guidelines have focused on dopamine agonists as the initial line of treatment for Parkinson's disease. For example, some studies have purported ropinirole (Requip) to be more than twice as effective in controlling dyskinesia. Patients taking ropinirole alone may also experience less progressive dyskinesia symptoms. However, in terms of activities of daily living (ADLs), some have reported that L-dopa may still better control motor symptoms. Others have suggested that L-dopa taken alone may produce no greater long-term therapeutic advantage than dopamine agonists. Pramipexole (Mirapex) and ropinirole (Requip) have proven to be safe and effective for the initial sole therapy and when combined with L-dopa. The side effects of pramipexole and ropinirole are intense and may include nausea and constipation, headache, orthostatic hypotension, nasal congestion, sudden sleep attacks, and hallucinations.

Other drugs reducing the requirements for L-dopa include the catechol-O-methyl transferase (COMT) inhibitors. Like L-dopa, these agents increase concentrations of existing dopamine in the brain and improve motor fluctuations relating to the wearing-off effect. Examples of this drug class are entacapone (Comtan) and tolcapone (Tasmar). Side effects of COMT inhibitors include mental confusion and hallucinations, nausea and vomiting, cramps, headache, diarrhea, and possible liver damage.

COMPLEMENTARY AND ALTERNATIVE THERAPIES

Ginkgo Biloba for Dementia

The seeds and leaves of ginkgo biloba have been used in traditional Chinese medicine for thousands of years. The tree is planted throughout the world, including the United States. In Western medicine, the focus has been on treating depression and memory loss. In Germany, an extract of ginkgo biloba is approved for the treatment of dementia.

Ginkgo has been shown to improve mental functioning and stabilize Alzheimer's disease. The mechanism of action seems to be related to increasing the blood supply to the brain by dilating blood vessels, decreasing the viscosity of the blood, and modifying the neurotransmitter system (Birks, 2007). Studies concluded that cognitive performance and behavior stabilized or improved for a time period of 6 to 12 months in patients with uncomplicated Alzheimer's disease. Other studies have shown no improvement in the symptoms or progress of Alzheimer's disease (DeKosky, Williamson, Fitzpatrick, Kronmal, Ives, Saxton et al., 2008). Ginkgo is considered safe; however, it may increase the risk of bleeding in patients taking anticoagulants. Other potential uses for ginkgo that are being investigated include asthma, multiple sclerosis, intermittent claudication, sexual dysfunction due to antidepressants, and insulin resistance.

PHARMACOTHERAPY ILLUSTRATED

20.1 Antiparkinson Drugs Focus on Restoring Dopamine Function and Blocking Cholinergic Activity in the Nigrostriatal Pathway

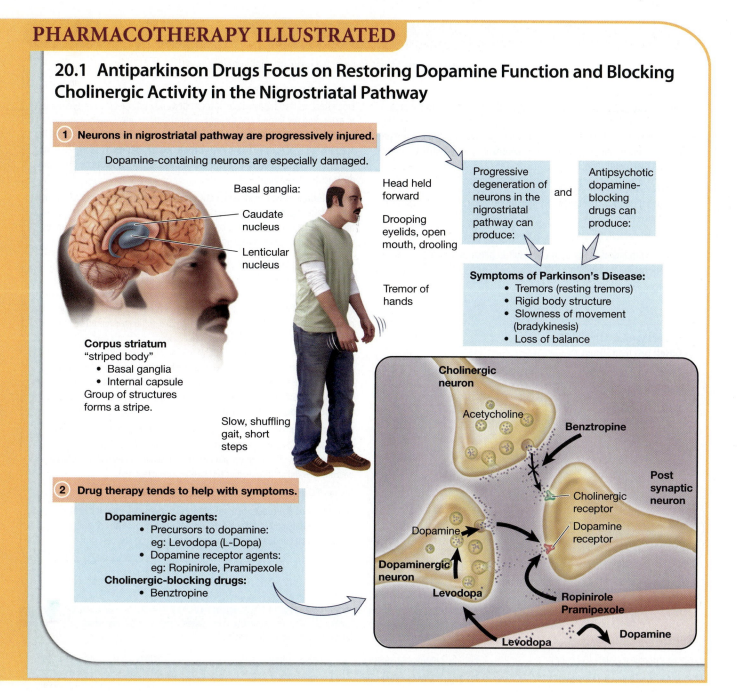

1 Neurons in nigrostriatal pathway are progressively injured.

Dopamine-containing neurons are especially damaged.

Basal ganglia:
Caudate nucleus
Lenticular nucleus

Head held forward

Drooping eyelids, open mouth, drooling

Tremor of hands

Progressive degeneration of neurons in the nigrostriatal pathway can produce:

and

Antipsychotic dopamine-blocking drugs can produce:

Symptoms of Parkinson's Disease:
- Tremors (resting tremors)
- Rigid body structure
- Slowness of movement (bradykinesia)
- Loss of balance

Corpus striatum
"striped body"
- Basal ganglia
- Internal capsule
Group of structures forms a stripe.

Slow, shuffling gait, short steps

2 Drug therapy tends to help with symptoms.

Dopaminergic agents:
- Precursors to dopamine: eg: Levodopa (L-Dopa)
- Dopamine receptor agents: eg: Ropinirole, Pramipexole

Cholinergic-blocking drugs:
- Benztropine

Cholinergic neuron
Acetycholine
Benztropine
Cholinergic receptor
Dopamine receptor
Post synaptic neuron
Dopamine
Dopaminergic neuron
Levodopa
Ropinirole Pramipexole
Levodopa
Dopamine

Anticholinergics

Anticholinergics inhibit the action of acetylcholine in the brain. They are used early in the course of therapy for Parkinsonism disease.

20.4 Treating Parkinsonism with Anticholinergics

A second approach to changing the balance between dopamine and acetylcholine in the brain is to give cholinergic blockers, or anticholinergics. By blocking the effect of acetylcholine, anticholinergics inhibit the overactivity of this neurotransmitter in the corpus striatum of the brain. These agents are listed in Table 20.3.

Anticholinergics such as atropine were the first agents used to treat parkinsonism. The large number of peripheral side effects has limited the uses of this drug class. The anticholinergics now used for parkinsonism are centrally acting and produce fewer side effects. Although anticholinergics act on the CNS, autonomic effects such as dry mouth, blurred vision, tachycardia, urine retention, and constipation are still troublesome. The centrally acting anticholinergics are not as effective as levodopa at relieving the severe symptoms of parkinsonism. They are used early in the course of the disease when symptoms are less severe, in patients who

Pr Prototype Drug | Levodopa *(Larodopa)*

Therapeutic Class: Antiparkinson agent   **Pharmacologic Class:** Dopamine precursor; dopaminergic drug

ACTIONS AND USES

Levodopa restores the neurotransmitter dopamine in extrapyramidal areas of the brain, thus relieving some Parkinson's symptoms. To increase its effect, levodopa is often combined with other medications, such as carbidopa, which prevent its enzymatic breakdown. Up to 6 months may be needed to achieve maximum therapeutic effects.

ADMINISTRATION ALERTS

- The patient may be unable to self-administer medication and may need assistance.
- Administer exactly as ordered.
- Abrupt withdrawal of the drug can result in parkinsonism crisis or neuroleptic malignant syndrome (NMS).
- Pregnancy category C

PHARMACOKINETICS
Onset: Less than 30 min
Peak: 1–3 h
Half-life: 1 h
Duration: Variable

ADVERSE EFFECTS

Side effects of levodopa include uncontrolled and purposeless movements such as extending the fingers and shrugging the shoulders, involuntary movements, loss of appetite, nausea, and vomiting. Muscle twitching and spasmodic winking are early signs of toxicity. Orthostatic hypotension is common in some patients. The drug should be discontinued gradually, because abrupt withdrawal can produce acute parkinsonism.

Contraindications: Levodopa is contraindicated in the treatment of narrow-angle glaucoma, particularly in patients with suspicious pigmented lesions or a history of melanoma. This medication should be avoided in cases of acute psychoses and severe psychoneurosis within 2 weeks of therapy with MAOI.

INTERACTIONS

Drug–Drug: Levodopa interacts with many drugs. For example, tricyclic antidepressants decrease effects of levodopa, increase postural hypotension, and may increase sympathetic activity, with hypertension and sinus tachycardia. Levodopa cannot be used if a MAOI was taken within 14 to 28 days, because concurrent use may precipitate hypertensive crisis. Haloperidol taken concurrently may antagonize the therapeutic effects of levodopa. Methyldopa may increase toxicity. Antihypertensives may cause increased hypotensive effects. Anticonvulsants may decrease the therapeutic effects of levodopa. Antacids containing magnesium, calcium, or sodium bicarbonate may increase levodopa absorption, which could lead to toxicity. Pyridoxine reverses antiparkinsonism effects of levodopa.

Lab Tests: Abnormalities in lab tests may include elevations of liver function tests such as alkaline phosphatase, aspartate aminotransferase (AST), alanine aminotransferase (ALT), lactic dehydrogenase, and bilirubin. Abnormalities in blood urea nitrogen and positive Coombs' test have also been reported.

Herbals/Food: Kava may worsen the symptoms of Parkinson's.

Treatment of Overdose: General supportive measures should be taken along with immediate gastric lavage. Intravenous fluids should be administered judiciously and an adequate airway maintained.

TABLE 20.3	**Anticholinergic Drugs and Drugs with Anticholinergic Activity Used for Parkinsonism**	
Drug	**Route and Adult Dose (max dose where indicated)**	**Adverse Effects**
Pr benztropine mesylate (Cogentin)	PO; 0.5–1 mg/day; gradually increase as needed (max: 6 mg/day)	*Sedation, nausea, constipation, dry mouth, blurred vision, drowsiness, dizziness, tachycardia, hypotension, nervousness*
biperiden hydrochloride (Akineton)	PO; 2 mg one to four times/day	
diphenhydramine hydrochloride (Benadryl) (see page 576 for the Prototype Drug box ∞)	PO; 25–50 mg tid–qid (max: 300 mg/day)	
procyclidine hydrochloride (Kemadrin)	PO; 2.5 mg tid after meals; may be increased to 5 mg tid if tolerated, with an additional 5 mg at bedtime (max: 45–60 mg/day)	Paralytic ileus, cardiovascular collapse
trihexyphenidyl hydrochloride (Artane)	PO; 1 mg on day 1; 2 mg on day 2; then increase by 2 mg every 3–5 days up to 6–10 mg/day (max: 15 mg/day)	

Italics indicate common adverse effects; underlining indicates serious adverse effects.

For the complete nursing process applied to anticholinergic therapy, see Nursing Process Focus: Patients Receiving Anticholinergic Therapy, page 145 in chapter 13∞.

NURSING PROCESS FOCUS   PATIENTS RECEIVING LEVODOPA (LARODOPA) OR LEVODOPA WITH CARBIDOPA (SINEMET)

Assessment	Potential Nursing Diagnoses
Baseline assessment prior to administration: ▪ Understand the reason the drug has been prescribed in order to assess for therapeutic effects. ▪ Obtain a complete health history including cardiovascular, musculoskeletal diseases, or glaucoma. Obtain a drug history including allergies, current prescription and OTC drugs, and herbal preparations. Be alert to possible drug interactions. ▪ Obtain a history of the current disease and symptoms, exacerbating conditions, and ability to carry out ADLs, particularly mobility and eating. ▪ Evaluate appropriate laboratory findings such as hepatic or renal function studies. ▪ Obtain baseline vital signs, bowel sounds, urinary ouput, muscle strength, and mental status as appropriate. ▪ Assess the patient's ability to receive and understand instruction. Include the family or caregivers as needed.	▪ Impaired Physical Mobility ▪ Impaired Swallowing ▪ Impaired Communication (verbal) ▪ Constipation ▪ Self-Care Deficit (feeding, bathing, hygiene, toileting) ▪ Deficient Knowledge (drug therapy) ▪ Risk for Injury, Risk for Falls (related to disease or adverse effects of drug therapy)
Assessment throughout administration: ▪ Assess for desired therapeutic effects dependent on the reason for the drug (e.g., decreased tremors, bradykinesia, rigidity). ▪ Continue periodic monitoring of vital signs, mental status, and motor function. ▪ Assess for and promptly report adverse effects: hypotension, increasing tremors, dizziness, salivation, anorexia, dysphagia, or changes in mental status, including agitation or confusion.	

Planning: Patient Goals and Expected Outcomes

The patient will:

▪ Experience therapeutic effects dependent on the reason the drug is being given (e.g., improved physical mobility and coordination, decreased tremors, rigidity, bradykinesia, and increased ability in self-care activities).

▪ Be free from, or experience minimal, adverse effects.

▪ Verbalize an understanding of the drug's use, adverse effects, and required precautions.

▪ Demonstrate proper self-administration of the medication (e.g., dose, timing, when to notify provider).

Implementation

Interventions and (Rationales)	Patient and Family Education
Ensuring therapeutic effects: ▪ Continue frequent assessments as described earlier for therapeutic effects. Drug therapy may take several weeks or months to have a full effect. Support the patient in self-care activities as necessary until improvement is observed. (The ability to carry out ADLs gradually improves with consistent usage. Continued tremors, rigidity, or other symptoms may require dosage adjustment.)	▪ Teach the patient, family, or caregiver that improvement may be gradual. The patient should report increasing symptoms that are similar to those noted before drug therapy was initiated.
Minimizing adverse effects: ▪ Ensure patient safety; monitor motor coordination and/or ambulation, eating, or other essential motor activities. Be particularly cautious with older adults who are at an increased risk for falls. (Gradual improvement in symptoms may be noticed over time but the drug does not cure the underlying disorder and symptoms may wax and wane over the course of the drug regimen. Particular care with ambulation is required as bradykinesia and rigidity may increase the risk of falls.)	▪ Instruct the patient to call for assistance prior to getting out of bed or attempting to walk alone if bradykinesia, rigidity, or tremors are particularly severe. ▪ Assess the patient's, family's, or caregiver's ability to carry out ADLs at home and explore the need for additional health care referrals. Evaluate home safety needs.

(Continued)

NURSING PROCESS FOCUS   PATIENTS RECEIVING LEVODOPA (LARODOPA) OR LEVODOPA WITH CARBIDOPA (SINEMET) (Continued)

Implementation

Interventions and (Rationales)	Patient and Family Education
▪ Continue to monitor vital signs. Take blood pressure lying, sitting, and standing to detect orthostatic hypotension. Be particularly cautious with older adults, who are at an increased risk for hypotension. Notify the health care provider if blood pressure decreases beyond established parameters or if hypotension is accompanied by reflex tachycardia. (Orthostatic hypotension is a common adverse effect and may increase the risk of falls or injury.)	▪ Teach the patient to rise from lying to sitting or standing slowly to avoid dizziness or falls.
▪ Monitor for behavior changes. (Drug therapy may increase the risk of agitation, confusion, depression, or suicidal thoughts and may cause other mood disturbances such as aggressive behavior.)	▪ Teach the patient, family, or caregiver to watch for and report immediately any signs of changes in behavior or mood such as increased aggression or confusion. Provide additional health care referrals as required for support group, counseling, or respite care.
▪ Carefully evaluate and report dose-related symptoms such as increased tremors and rigidity before the next dose is due or greatly increased symptoms unrelated to the timing of the dose. (The return or gradual increase of symptoms as the next dose comes due may signal a "wearing off" time and the dose may need to be increased, the interval of dosage adjusted, or an adjunctive drug added. A significant and sudden increase in symptoms may signal an overdose or "on–off" phenomenon where symptoms dramatically increase. If symptoms are significant, hospitalization may be required to assess for the rationale behind the exacerbation.)	▪ Instruct the patient, family, or caregiver to be aware of newly occurring muscle twitching, including blepharospasm (in muscles of eyelids), greatly increasing tremors, rigidity, sweating, or other symptoms and to report them immediately. ▪ Encourage the patient, family, or caregiver to maintain a symptom diary if effects seem to diminish as the next dose is due. Review the diary with the patient on each health care visit.
▪ Evaluate nutritional intake. (Absorption of levodopa decreases with high-protein meals or high consumption of foods or vitamins that contain vitamin B_6 [pyridoxine]. Symptoms may dramatically increase if absorption is impaired as dose does not adequately absorb during the time expected.)	▪ Teach the patient to take the medication on an empty stomach or to avoid taking together with a high-protein meal. Avoid excessive consumption of vitamin B_6–rich foods such as such as bananas, wheat germ, fortified cereals, green vegetables, meat, and legumes, and avoid multivitamins that contain vitamin B_6.
▪ Monitor hepatic and renal function labs periodically. (A decrease in these functions may slow the metabolism and excretion of the drug, possibly leading to overdose or toxicity.)	▪ Teach the patient, family, or caregiver about the importance of returning for follow-up lab studies.
▪ Monitor for other drug-related changes. (The drug may cause urine and perspiration to darken in color.)	▪ Advise the patient that urine or sweat may darken and undershirts or dress shields may help to avoid staining of clothing.
Patient understanding of drug therapy: ▪ Use opportunities during administration of medications and during assessments to discuss the rationale for drug therapy, desired therapeutic outcomes, most commonly observed adverse effects, parameters for when to call the health care provider, and any necessary monitoring or precautions. (Using time during nursing care helps to optimize and reinforce key teaching areas.)	▪ The patient, family, or caregiver should be able to state the reason for the drug; appropriate dose and scheduling; and what adverse effects to observe for and when to report.
Patient self-administration of drug therapy: ▪ When administering the medications, instruct the patient, family, or caregiver in the proper self-administration of drugs and the need for regular, consistent dosing. (Utilizing time during nurse-administration of these drugs helps to reinforce teaching.)	▪ Instruct the patient in proper administration guidelines. Encourage the patient, family, or caregiver to maintain a medication log, noting symptoms or adverse effects along with the dose and timing of medications.

Evaluation of Outcome Criteria

Evaluate effectiveness of drug therapy by confirming that patient goals and expected outcomes have been met (see "Planning").

cannot tolerate levodopa, and in combination therapy with other antiparkinsonism drugs.

ALZHEIMER'S DISEASE

Alzheimer's disease is a devastating, progressive, degenerative disease that generally begins after age 60. By age 85, as many as 50% of the population may be affected. Pharmacotherapy has limited success in improving the cognitive function of patients with Alzheimer's disease.

20.5 Characteristics of Alzheimer's Disease

Alzheimer's disease (AD) is responsible for 70% of all dementia. **Dementia** is a degenerative disorder characterized by progressive memory loss, confusion, and an inability to think or communicate effectively. Consciousness and perception are usually unaffected. Known causes of dementia include multiple cerebral infarcts, severe infections, and toxins. Although the cause of most dementia is unknown, it is usually associated with cerebral atrophy or other structural changes within the brain. The patient generally lives 5 to 10 years following diagnosis; AD is the fourth leading cause of death.

Despite extensive, ongoing research, the etiology of Alzheimer's disease remains unknown. The early-onset fa-

milial form of this disorder, accounting for about 10% of cases, is associated with gene defects on chromosome 1, 14, or 21. Chronic inflammation and excess free radicals may cause neuronal damage. Environmental, immunologic, and nutritional factors, as well as viruses, are considered possible sources of brain damage.

Although the cause may be unknown, structural damage in the brain of Alzheimer's patients has been well documented. **Amyloid plaques** and **neurofibrillary tangles,** found within the brain at autopsy, are present in nearly all patients with AD. It is suspected that these structural changes are caused

---

HOME & COMMUNITY CONSIDERATIONS

Caring for Loved Ones with Alzheimer's Disease

The diagnosis of Alzheimer's disease is devastating to the patient and family members alike. Family members must deal with many unexpected changes. The personality of the patient with Alzheimer's disease slowly changes and may include paranoia, anger, and frustration. Many families attempt to care for their loved one at home for as long as possible. A frightening aspect of Alzheimer's disease is the tendency for the patient to wander away. The patient easily becomes lost after leaving the familiarity of the home environment. This tendency to wander is believed to be linked to anxiety on the part of the AD patient who paces or wanders to relieve the tension. Wandering puts the patient at a high risk for severe trauma or death, and it is important for family caregivers to recognize this symptom and ask for assistance promptly.

Pr Prototype Drug | Benztropine *(Cogentin)*

Therapeutic Class: Antiparkinson agent   **Pharmacologic Class:** Centrally acting cholinergic receptor antagonist

ACTIONS AND USES

Benztropine acts by blocking excess cholinergic stimulation of neurons in the corpus striatum. It is used for relief of parkinsonism symptoms and for the treatment of EPS brought on by antipsychotic pharmacotherapy. This medication suppresses tremors but does not affect tardive dyskinesia.

ADMINISTRATION ALERTS

- The patient may be unable to self-administer medication and may need assistance.
- Benztropine may be taken in divided doses, two to four times a day, or the entire day's dose may be taken at bedtime.
- If muscle weakness occurs, the dose should be reduced.
- Pregnancy category C

PHARMACOKINETICS
Onset: 15 min IM/IV; 1 h PO
Peak: 1–2 h
Half-life: 2–3 h
Duration: 6–10 h

ADVERSE EFFECTS

As expected from its autonomic action, benztropine can cause typical anticholinergic side effects such as dry mouth, constipation, and tachycardia. Adverse general effects include sedation, drowsiness, dizziness, restlessness, irritability, nervousness, and insomnia.

Contraindications: Contraindications include narrow-angle glaucoma, myasthenia gravis, and obstructive diseases of the genitourinary and GI tracts.

INTERACTIONS

Drug–Drug: Benztropine interacts with many drugs. For example, benztropine should not be taken with alcohol, tricyclic antidepressants, MAOIs, phenothiazines, procainamide, or quinidine because of combined sedative effects. OTC cold medicines and alcohol should be avoided. Other drugs that enhance dopamine release or activation of the dopamine receptor may produce additive effects. Haloperidol decreases effectiveness.

Antihistamines, phenothiazines, tricyclics, disopyramide phosphate, and quinidine may increase anticholinergic effects, and antidiarrheals may decrease absorption.

Lab Tests: Unknown

Herbal/Food: Unknown

Treatment of Overdose: Physostigmine salicylate, 1 to 2 mg subcutaneously or IV, will reverse symptoms of anticholinergic intoxication. A second injection may be given after 2 hours, if required. Otherwise, treatment is symptomatic and supportive.

Refer to MyNursingKit for a Nursing Process Focus specific to this drug.

Pr Prototype Drug | Donepezil *(Aricept)*

Therapeutic Class: Alzheimer's disease agent   **Pharmacologic Class:** Acetylcholinesterase inhibitor

ACTIONS AND USES

Donepezil is an AchE inhibitor that improves memory in cases of mild to moderate Alzheimer's dementia by enhancing the effects of acetylcholine in neurons in the cerebral cortex that have not yet been damaged. Patients should receive pharmacotherapy for at least 6 months prior to assessing maximum benefits of drug therapy. Improvement in memory may be observed as early as 1 to 4 weeks following medication. The therapeutic effects of donepezil are often short lived, and the degree of improvement is modest, at best. An advantage of donepezil over other drugs in its class is that its long half-life permits it to be given once daily.

ADMINISTRATION ALERTS

- Give medication prior to bedtime.
- Medication is most effective when given on a regular schedule.
- Pregnancy category C

PHARMACOKINETICS
Onset: Less than 20 min
Peak: 3–4 h
Half-life: 70 h
Duration: Variable

ADVERSE EFFECTS

Common side effects of donepezil are vomiting, diarrhea, and darkened urine. CNS side effects include insomnia, syncope, depression, headache, and irritability. Musculoskeletal side effects include muscle cramps, arthritis, and bone fractures. Generalized side effects include headache, fatigue, chest pain, increased libido, hot flashes, urinary incontinence, dehydration, and blurred vision.

Unlike with tacrine, hepatotoxicity has not been observed. Patients with bradycardia, hypotension, asthma, hyperthyroidism, or active peptic ulcer disease should be monitored carefully.

Contraindications: Donepezil is contraindicated in patients with GI bleeding and jaundice.

INTERACTIONS

Drug–Drug: Donepezil will cause anticholinergics to be less effective. Donepezil interacts with several other drugs. For example, bethanechol causes a synergistic effect. Phenobarbital, phenytoin, dexamethasone, and rifampin may speed the elimination of donepezil. Quinidine or ketoconazole may inhibit the metabolism of donepezil. Because donepezil acts by increasing cholinergic activity, two parasympathomimetics should not be administered concurrently.

Lab Tests: Unknown

Herbal/Food: Unknown

Treatment of Overdose: Anticholinergics such as atropine may be used as an antidote for donepezil overdosage. Intravenous atropine sulfate titrated to effect is recommended: an initial dose of 1 to 2 mg IV with subsequent doses based on clinical response.

Refer to MyNursingKit for a Nursing Process Focus specific to this drug.

---

neuronal changes in AD are caused by oxidative cellular damage, antioxidants such as vitamin E are being examined for their effects in AD patients. Other agents currently being examined are anti-inflammatory agents, such as the COX-2 inhibitors, estrogen, and ginkgo biloba.

Agitation occurs in the majority of patients with AD. This may be accompanied by delusions, paranoia, hallucinations, or other psychotic symptoms. Atypical antipsychotic agents such as risperidone (Risperdal) and olanzapine (Zyprexa) may be used to control these episodes. Conventional antipsychotics such as haloperidol (Haldol) are occasionally prescribed, though extrapyramidal side effects often limit their use. The pharmacotherapy of psychosis is presented in chapter 17∞.

Anxiety and depression, although not as common as agitation, may occur in AD patients. Anxiolytics such as buspirone (BuSpar) or some of the benzodiazepines are used to control unease and excessive apprehension (chapter 14∞). Mood stabilizers such as sertraline (Zoloft), citalopram (Celexa), or fluoxetine (Prozac) are given when major depression interferes with daily activities (chapter 16∞).

For the complete nursing process applied to anticholinesterase therapy, see Nursing Process Focus: Patients Receiving Parasympathomimetic Therapy, page 141 in chapter 13∞.

MULTIPLE SCLEROSIS

Multiple sclerosis is a chronic, inflammatory, autoimmune disorder found most prevalent among young adults. Sensory and motor deficits become progressively worse as the patient grows older. If treatments are started early, the frequency of disease symptoms can be slowed and permanent neurologic damage can be delayed.

20.7 Characteristics of Multiple Sclerosis

Multiple sclerosis (MS) is a disorder characterized by damaged myelin located with the CNS. Antibodies slowly target and destroy oligodendrocytes, myelin, and axonal membranes. As axons are destroyed, this impairs the ability of nerves to conduct electrical impulses. Inflammation accompanies damaged tissue, and multiple filamentous plaques called *scleroses* are formed. During the early stages of MS, some axons recover due to partial myelination and the development of alternative circuitry, but as antibodies continue to attack neural tissue, further damage and inflammation lead to neuronal death. Patients often have recurrent episodes of neurologic dysfunction, which progress at a fairly rapid rate.

TABLE 20.5	Disease-Modifying Drugs Used for Multiple Sclerosis	
Drug	Route and Adult Dose (max dose where indicated)	Adverse Effects
IMMUNOMODULATORS		
glatiramer acetate (Copaxone, copolymer-1)	SC; 20 mg/day	*Dizziness, headaches, weakness, confusion, anxiety, mental depression, conjunctivitis, itching, nausea, vomiting, constipation, diarrhea, sexual dysfunction, sweating, menstrual disorders, neutropenia, flulike symptoms, spasticity, pain, reaction at the injection site*
interferon beta-1a (Avonex, Rebif)	IM; 30 mcg once per week	
	SC; 44 mcg three times per week	
interferon beta-1b (Betaseron)	SC; 250 mcg every other day	<u>Seizures, anaphylaxis, hepatotoxicity, spontaneous abortion</u>
natalizumab (Tysabri)	IV; 300 mg infused over 1 h every month	
IMMUNOSUPPRESSANTS		
mitoxantrone (Novantrone)	IV; 12 mg/m^2 every 3 months (lifetime max: 140 mg/m^2)	*Nausea, vomiting, fever, mouth sores, diarrhea, hair loss, anemia; increased susceptibility to infection*
		<u>Cardiotoxicity, dysrhythmia, shortness of breath</u>

Italics indicate common adverse effects; <u>underlining</u> indicates serious adverse effects.

The etiology of multiple sclerosis is unknown. Many clinicians and scientists suspect genetic or microbial factors due to reports that in most cases, MS occurs in regions of colder climate. One theory proposes acquired immunological resistance against pathogenic factors in warmer climates. Microscopic pathogens such as viruses have been suggested, though there is not strong evidence for this theory.

Signs and symptoms associated with axonal injury include fatigue, heat sensitivity, neuropathic pain, spasticity, impaired cognitive ability, disruption of balance and coordination, bowel and bladder symptoms, sexual dysfunction, dizziness, vertigo, visual impairment, and slurred speech. The course of MS is unpredictable, and each patient experiences a variety of symptoms depending on the extent and localization of demyelination.

Drugs for Multiple Sclerosis

There is no cure for MS. Drugs mainly provide relief for patients with recurring symptoms. This is the case for patients diagnosed with **relapse–remitting MS** and **secondary–progressive MS.** Drugs slow progression of the disease and modify associated symptoms. Immunomodulators are the main approach for therapy. These drugs reduce the severity and frequency of symptoms.

If drugs are not successful, as with **progressive–relapsing MS,** the intravenous immunosuppressant mitoxantrone may be considered. Other immunosuppressants (chapter 32∞) may be successful, although these drugs are mainly used for **primary–progressive MS.** With this subtype of MS, symptoms continue to worsen throughout the course of the disease.

Disease-modifying drugs used in the treatment of MS are listed in Table 20.5.

20.8 Treating Multiple Sclerosis with Disease-Modifying Drugs

Currently used for the treatment of *relapse–remitting MS* and *secondary–progressive MS,* immune-modulating drugs are found in two categories: interferon beta (Avonex, Rebif, Betaseron) and glatiramer acetate (Copaxone). Interferon beta is available in two forms, *interferon beta 1a* and *interferon beta 1b.* These products are slightly different and are available as IM medication (Avonex) or SC medication (Rebif and Betaseron). Both formulations reduce the severity of MS symptoms and decrease the number of lesions detected with magnetic resonance imaging (MRI). Although generally well tolerated, the interferons have unfavorable side effects including flulike symptoms (e.g., headaches, fever, chills, muscle aches), anxiety, discomfort experienced at the injection site, and liver toxicity. Due to toxicity concerns and additive effects, caution should be exercised when taking these drugs in combination with chemotherapeutic agents or bone marrow-suppressing drugs.

Glatiramer acetate (Copaxone), formerly known as *copolymer-1,* is a synthetic protein that simulates myelin basic protein, an essential part of the nerve's myelin coating. Since glatiramer acetate resembles myelin, it is thought to curb the body's attack of the myelin covering and reduce the creation of new brain lesions. Copaxone is available in prefilled syringes that can be stored at room temperature for several days. As with the interferons, patients complain of self-injection side effects: redness, pain, swelling, itching, or a lump at the site of injection. Flushing, chest pain, weakness, infection, pain, nausea, joint pain, anxiety, and muscle stiffness are common effects experienced with the immunomodulators.

For *progressive–relapsing MS,* mitoxantrone (Novantrone) is the FDA drug approved for MS patients who have not responded to interferon or glatiramer acetate therapy. Primarily a chemotherapeutic drug, mitoxantrone is substantially more toxic than the immune-modulating drugs. Toxicity is a concern due to irreversible cardiac injury and potential harm to the fetus. Notable adverse side effects are reversible hair loss, GI discomfort (nausea and vomiting), and allergic symptoms (pruritus, rash, hypotension). Some patients experience a harmless blue–green tint to their urine.

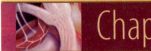

Chapter REVIEW

KEY CONCEPTS

The numbered key concepts provide a succinct summary of the important points from the corresponding numbered section within the chapter. If any of these points are not clear, refer to the numbered section within the chapter for review.

20.1 Degenerative diseases of the nervous system such as Parkinson's disease and Alzheimer's disease cause a progressive loss of neuron function.

20.2 Parkinson's disease is characterized by symptoms of tremors, muscle rigidity, and postural instability and ambulation caused by the destruction of dopamine-producing neurons found within the corpus striatum. The underlying biochemical problem is lack of dopamine activity and a related overactivity of acetylcholine.

20.3 The most commonly used medications for parkinsonism attempt to restore levels of dopamine in the corpus striatum of the brain. Levodopa (Larodopa) is the drug of choice for Parkinson's disease.

20.4 Centrally acting anticholinergic drugs are sometimes used to relieve symptoms of parkinsonism, although they are less effective than levodopa (Larodopa).

20.5 Alzheimer's disease is a progressive, degenerative disease of older adults. Primary symptoms include disorientation, confusion, and memory loss.

20.6 Acetylcholinesterase inhibitors are used to slow the progression of Alzheimer's disease symptoms. These agents have minimal efficacy, and do not cure the dementia.

20.7 MS patients often have recurrent episodes of neurologic dysfunction, which progress at a fairly rapid rate. Symptoms depend on the extent and location of central demyelination.

20.8 Disease-modifying drugs slow the progression of MS and modify associated symptoms. There is no cure for MS.

NCLEX-RN® REVIEW QUESTIONS

1 The family member caring for a patient with Parkinson's disease at home notifies the nurse that the patient is demonstrating a dramatic increase in extrapyramidal symptoms. The nurse should instruct the caregiver to:
1. give diphenhydramine (Benadryl) 25 mg PO.
2. transport the patient to the emergency department.
3. increase the dosage of antiparkinsonism drugs.
4. make an appointment with the health care provider for evaluation.

2 The patient asks what can be expected from drug therapy for treatment of parkinsonism. What is the best response by the nurse?
1. A cure can be expected within 6 months.
2. Symptoms can be reduced and the ability to perform ADLs can be improved.
3. Disease progression will be stopped.
4. EPS will be prevented.

3 Levodopa (Larodopa) is prescribed for a patient with Parkinson's disease. At discharge, which of the following teaching points should the nurse implement?
1. Monitor blood pressure every 2 hours for the first 2 weeks.
2. Expect the urine color to be orange.
3. Report the development of diarrhea.
4. Keep scheduled lab appointments for liver and renal function tests.

4 The nurse discussed the disease process of multiple sclerosis with the patient and caregiver. What does the nurse explain is the cause of MS?
1. The cause is unknown. Amyloid plaques and neurofibrillary tangles have been found in the brain at autopsy.
2. The cause is unknown. Many scars located throughout the brain have been found on MRI scans.
3. Loss of circulation to the brain has been found on MRI scans.
4. Loss of dopamine receptors is thought to occur as a part of the aging process.

5 An overdose of drugs to treat AD may occur if they are taken improperly or if decreased liver or renal function occurs. The nurse assesses the patient for signs of overdose, which include: (Select all that apply.)
1. bradycardia and muscle weakness.
2. tachycardia and hypertension.
3. nausea and vomiting.
4. emotional withdrawal and tachypnea.
5. hypotension and increased muscle strength.

6 An early sign(s) of levodopa toxicity is (are) which of the following?
1. Orthostatic hypotension
2. Drooling
3. Spasmodic eye winking and muscle twitching
4. Nausea, vomiting, and diarrhea

CRITICAL THINKING QUESTIONS

1. A 58-year-old Parkinson's patient is placed on levodopa (Larodopa). In obtaining her health history, the nurse notes that the patient takes Mylanta on a regular basis for mild indigestion, and also takes multivitamins daily (vitamins A, B_6, D, and E). She also has a history of diabetes mellitus type 2. What should the nurse include in teaching for this patient?

2. A patient is on levodopa and benztropine (Cogentin). During a regular office follow-up, the patient tells the nurse that she is going to Arizona in July to visit her grandchildren. What teaching is important for this patient?

3. A 67-year-old Alzheimer's patient is on donepezil (Aricept) and has a history of congestive heart failure, diabetes mellitus type 2, and hypertension. The patient's wife asks the nurse if this new medicine is appropriate for her husband to take. How should the nurse respond? What teaching should be done?

See Appendix D for answers and rationales for all activities.

or brief repeated muscle movements, followed by relaxation of muscle fibers. Relaxation is short lived until charges across the muscle membrane are restored (repolarization). Importantly, patients treated with neuromuscular blockers are able to feel pain. Thus, for surgical procedures, concomitant use of anesthetic agents is essential (chapter 19∞).

An important fact to mention is that neuromuscular blocking agents are different from *ganglionic blocking agents* that target the autonomic nervous system. In this instance, acetylcholine does indeed bind to nicotinic receptors, but the resulting actions are involuntary and do not involve skeletal muscle contraction (chapter 13∞). Ganglionic blockers dampen parasympathetic tone and produce effects like increased heart rate, dry mouth, urinary retention, and reduced gastrointestinal activity. They also dampen sympathetic tone, resulting in reduced sweating and less norepinephrine being released from postsynaptic nerve terminals. As an example, mecamylamine (Inversine) is a ganglionic blocker primarily used to treat patients with essential hypertension (chapter 23∞).

The classic example of a nondepolarizing blocker is tubocurarine. Tubocurarine and related blocking agents are used to relax the muscles of patients being prepared for longer surgical procedures (Table 21.3). Although not preferred for mechanical ventilation or endotracheal intubation, small doses of these agents may be used for intermediate surgical procedures (chapter 19∞). Concerns of tubocurarine-like treatment are over-relaxation of muscles. As examples, normal breathing activity (involving the diaphragm, and glottic and intercostal muscles) and swallowing activity (involving the neck and certain esophageal muscles) require contraction of skeletal muscle.

Depolarizing agents are used primarily to relax the muscles of patients receiving electroconvulsive therapy (ECT) (chapter 15∞) and for shorter surgical procedures, for example, mechanical ventilation and endotracheal intubation (chapter 19∞). Succinylcholine (Anectine, Quelicin) is the prototype example of a depolarizing blocker. Adverse effects include persistent paralysis in some patients, elevated blood levels of potassium, malignant hyperthermia, and postoperative muscle pain. As a specific antidote for persistent paralysis, patients are often given cholinesterase inhibitors. Cholinesterase inhibitors also represent a form of therapy for diagnosis or treatment of myasthenia gravis (chapter 13∞) and for the treatment of Alzheimer's disease (chapter 20∞) and glaucoma (chapter 49∞).

TABLE 21.3	**Neuromuscular Blocking Agents**
Drug	**Duration and Administration Route**
NONDEPOLARIZING BLOCKERS	
atracurium (Tracrium)	Long duration; IV
cisatracurium (Nimbex)	Long duration; IV
mivacurium (Mivacron)	Shorter duration; IV
pancuronium (Pavulon)	Long duration; IV
pipecuronium (Arduan)	Longest duration; IV
rocuronium (Zemuron)	Long duration; IV
tubocurarine	Longest duration; oldest of the nondepolarizing agents; administered IV and IM
vecocuronium (Norcuron)	Long duration; IV
DEPOLARIZING BLOCKERS	
succinylcholine chloride (Anectine, Quelicin) (see page 253 for the Prototype Drug box ∞)	Shortest duration; IV and IM

See chapter 19 ∞, page 253 and MyNursingKit for a Nursing Process Focus specific to neuromuscular blocking agents.

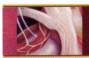
Chapter REVIEW

KEY CONCEPTS

The numbered key concepts provide a succinct summary of the important points from the corresponding numbered section within the chapter. If any of these points are not clear, refer to the numbered section within the chapter for review.

21.1 Muscle spasms, which are involuntary contractions of a muscle or group of muscles, most commonly occur because of localized trauma to the skeletal muscle.

21.2 Muscle spasms can be treated through nonpharmacologic and pharmacologic therapies.

21.3 Many muscle relaxants treat muscle spasms at the level of the CNS by generating their effect within the brain and/or spinal cord, usually by inhibiting upper motor neuron activity, causing sedation, or altering simple reflexes.

21.4 Spasticity, a condition in which selected muscles are continuously contracted, results from damage to the CNS. Ef-

fective treatment for spasticity includes both physical therapy and medications.

21.5 Some antispasmodic drugs used for spasticity act directly on muscle tissue, relieving spasticity by interfering with the release of calcium ions.

21.6 Neuromuscular blocking agents are classified as nondepolarizing blockers and depolarizing blockers. Both agents bind to the acetylcholine nicotinic receptor, relaxing muscles by slightly different mechanisms and duration of action.

NCLEX-RN® REVIEW QUESTIONS

1 Cyclobenzaprine (Cycoflex, Flexeril) is prescribed for a patient with muscle spasms of the lower back. Appropriate nursing intervention would include: (Select all that apply.)
1. assessing the heart rate for tachycardia.
2. providing for patient safety.
3. encouraging frequent ambulation.
4. providing oral suction for excessive oral secretions.
5. assessing for rash.

2 The patient is scheduled to receive botulinum toxin type B (Myobloc) for treatment of muscle spasticity. Patient education needed to prepare the patient for the injections includes that:
1. relief of muscle spasms should occur within several days.
2. drowsiness may occur.
3. a rapid return of energy is to be expected.
4. local anesthesia will be given to decrease the pain of the injections.

3 Prior to administration of cyclobenzaprine (Cycoflex, Flexeril), the nurse notes that the patient's liver enzymes are elevated. The appropriate action would be to:
1. hold the medication and report the elevation to the health care provider.
2. give the medication as ordered.
3. place the lab report on the medical record and await instructions from the health care provider.
4. give the medication as ordered, then collect a blood sample for liver enzymes in 6 hours.

4 A patient who was prescribed cyclobenzaprine (Cycoflex, Flexeril) reports taking propranolol (Inderal) for

blood pressure control. Appropriate nursing interventions include:
1. monitoring neurologic status.
2. giving the drugs concurrently for best results.
3. monitoring closely for hypotension.
4. monitoring renal function.

5 Which of the following statements made by the patient prescribed dantrolene sodium (Dantrium) indicates an understanding of the side effects of the drug?
1. "I will be able to drive myself home from the hospital."
2. "I will not be concerned if I cannot empty my bladder; it's probably my prostate."
3. "I will be able to do my regular work as soon as I get home."
4. "I will report frequent changes in my blood pressure to my doctor."

6 A patient who has been prescribed baclofen (Lioresal) returns to the health care provider after a week of drug therapy, complaining of continued muscle spasms of the lower back. The nurse would assess for:
1. whether the patient has been taking the medication consistently or only when the pain is severe.
2. whether the patient has been consuming alcohol during this time.
3. whether the patient has increased the dosage without consulting the health care provider.
4. whether the patient's log of symptoms indicates the patient is telling the truth.

CRITICAL THINKING QUESTIONS

1. A 46-year-old male quadriplegic patient has been experiencing severe spasticity in the lower extremities, making it difficult for him to maintain position in his electric wheelchair. Prior to the episodes of spasticity, the patient was able to maintain a sitting posture. The risks and benefits of therapy with dantrolene (Dantrium) have been explained to him, and he has decided that the benefits outweigh the risks. What assessments should the nurse make to determine whether the treatment is beneficial?

2. A 52-year-old breast cancer survivor is taking tamoxifen (Nolvadex) and has experienced leg and foot cramps "almost nightly." She states that these cramps have markedly decreased the quality of her sleep and that she is ready to "just stop taking" the tamoxifen to end the leg cramps. The nurse is aware that tamoxifen is considered important in the chemoprevention of breast cancer. What variety of treatment modalities can be offered this patient to promote her comfort and decrease the chance that she will stop therapy?

3. A 32-year-old cotton farmer injured his lower back while unloading a truck at a farm cooperative. His health care provider started him on cyclobenzaprine (Flexeril) 10 mg tid for 7 days and referred him to outpatient physical therapy. After 4 days, the patient reports back to the office nurse that he is constipated and having trouble emptying his bladder. Discuss the cause of these side effects.

See Appendix D for answers and rationales for all activities.

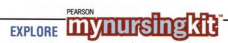

EXPLORE **PEARSON** **mynursingkit™**

MyNursingKit is your one stop for online chapter review materials and resources. Prepare for success with additional NCLEX®-style practice questions, interactive assignments and activities, web links, animations and videos, and more!

Register your access code from the front of your book at
www.mynursingkit.com.

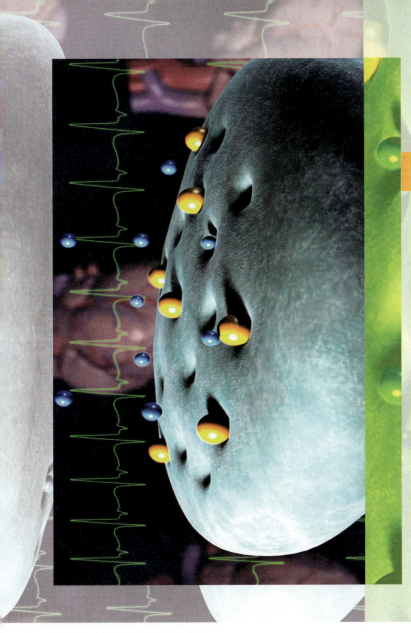

The Cardiovascular and Urinary Systems

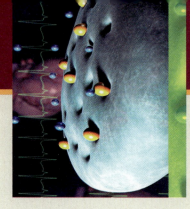

Chapter 22

Drugs for Lipid Disorders

LEARNING OUTCOMES

After reading this chapter, the student should be able to:

1. Summarize the link between high blood cholesterol, LDL levels, and cardiovascular disease.
2. Compare and contrast the different types of lipids.
3. Illustrate how lipids are transported through the blood.
4. Compare and contrast the different types of lipoproteins.
5. Give examples of how cholesterol and LDL levels can be controlled through nonpharmacologic means.
6. For each of the drug classes listed in Drugs at a Glance, know representative drug examples, and explain their mechanisms of action, primary actions, and important adverse effects.
7. Explain the nurse's role in the pharmacologic management of lipid disorders.
8. Use the nursing process to care for patients receiving drug therapy for lipid disorders.

KEY TERMS

esearch during the 1960s and 1970s brought about a nutritional revolution as new knowledge about lipids and their relationship to obesity and cardiovascular disease allowed people to make more intelligent lifestyle choices. Since then, advances in the diagnosis of lipid disorders have helped identify those patients at greatest risk for cardiovascular disease and those most likely to benefit from pharmacologic intervention. Research in pharmacology has led to safe, effective drugs for lowering lipid levels, thus decreasing the risk of cardiovascular-related diseases. As a result of this knowledge and through advancements in pharmacology, the incidence of death due to most cardiovascular diseases has been declining, although cardiovascular disease remains the leading cause of death in the United States.

22.1 Types of Lipids

The three types of lipids important to humans are illustrated in ➤ Figure 22.1. The most common are the **triglycerides,** or neutral fats, which form a large family of different lipids all having three fatty acids attached to a chemical backbone of glycerol. Triglycerides are the major storage form of fat in the body and the only type of lipid that serves as an important energy source. They account for 90% of total lipids in the body.

A second class, the **phospholipids,** is formed when a phosphate group replaces one of the fatty acids in a triglyceride. This class of lipids is essential to building plasma membranes. The best known phospholipids are **lecithins,** which are found in high concentration in egg yolks and soybeans. Once promoted as a natural treatment for high cholesterol levels, controlled studies have not shown lecithin to be of any benefit for this disorder. Likewise, lecithin has been proposed as a remedy for nervous system diseases such as Alzheimer's disease and bipolar disorder, but there is no definite evidence to support these claims.

The third class of lipids is the **steroids,** a diverse group of substances having a common chemical structure called the **sterol nucleus,** or ring structure. Cholesterol is the most widely known of the steroids, and its role in promoting **atherosclerosis** has been clearly demonstrated. Cholesterol is a natural and vital component of plasma membranes. Unlike the triglycerides that provide fuel for the body during times of energy need, cholesterol serves as the building block for a number of essential biochemicals, including vitamin D, bile acids, cortisol, estrogen, and testosterone. Although cholesterol is clearly essential for life, the body needs only minute amounts of it. Moreover, the liver is able to synthesize adequate amounts of cholesterol from other chemicals; it is not necessary to provide additional cholesterol in the diet. Dietary cholesterol is obtained solely from animal products; humans do not metabolize the sterols produced by plants. The American Heart Association recommends intake of less than 300 mg of dietary cholesterol per day.

22.2 Lipoproteins

Because lipid molecules are not soluble in plasma, they must be specially packaged for transport through the blood. To accomplish this transport, the body forms complexes called **lipoproteins,** which consist of various amounts of cholesterol, triglycerides, and phospholipids, along with a protein carrier. The protein component is called an **apoprotein** (*apo-* means "separated from or derived from").

The three most common lipoproteins are classified according to their composition, size, and weight or density, which is due primarily to the amount of apoprotein present in the complex. Each type varies in lipid and apoprotein makeup and serves a different function in transporting lipids from sites of synthesis and absorption to sites of utilization. For example, **high-density lipoprotein (HDL)** contains the most apoprotein, up to 50% by weight. The highest amount of cholesterol is carried by **low-density lipoprotein (LDL).** ➤ Figure 22.2 illustrates the three basic lipoproteins and their compositions.

To understand the pharmacotherapy of lipid disorders, it is important to learn the functions of the major lipoproteins and their roles in transporting cholesterol. LDL transports cholesterol from the liver to the tissues and organs, where it is used to build plasma membranes or to synthesize other steroids. Once in the tissues, cholesterol can also be stored for later use. Storage of cholesterol in the lining of blood vessels, however, is not desirable because it contributes to plaque buildup and atherosclerosis. LDL is often called "bad" cholesterol, because this lipoprotein contributes significantly to plaque deposits and coronary artery disease. **Very low–density lipoprotein (VLDL)** is the primary carrier of triglycerides in the blood. Through a series of steps, VLDL is reduced in size to become LDL. Lowering LDL levels in the blood has been shown to decrease the incidence of coronary artery disease.

HDL is manufactured in the liver and small intestine and assists in the transport of cholesterol away from the body tissues and back to the liver in a process called **reverse cholesterol transport.** The cholesterol component of the HDL is then

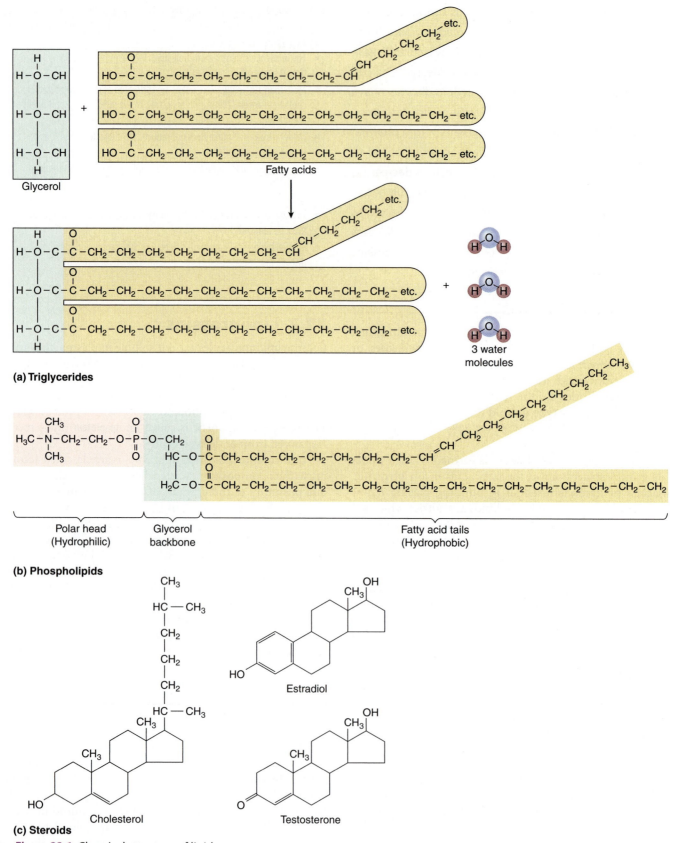

(a) **Triglycerides**

(b) **Phospholipids**

Polar head
(Hydrophilic)

Glycerol
backbone

Fatty acid tails
(Hydrophobic)

Estradiol

Cholesterol

Testosterone

(c) **Steroids**

➤ *Figure 22.1* Chemical structure of lipids

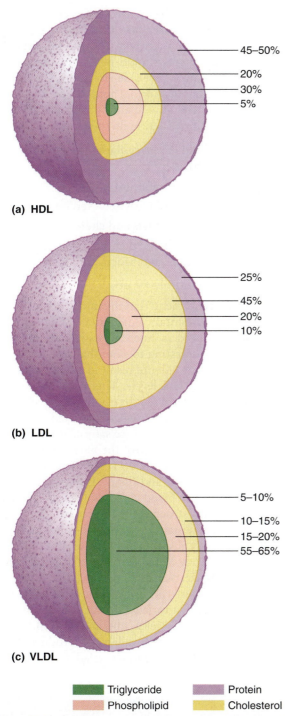

(a) HDL

45–50%
20%
30%
5%

(b) LDL

25%
45%
20%
10%

(c) VLDL

5–10%
10–15%
15–20%
55–65%

Triglyceride   Protein
Phospholipid   Cholesterol

➤ *Figure 22.2* Composition of lipoproteins: (a) HDL; (b) LDL; (c) VLDL

broken down to unite with bile that is subsequently excreted in the feces. Excretion via bile is the only route the body uses to remove cholesterol. Because HDL transports cholesterol for destruction and removes it from the body, it is considered "good" cholesterol.

Several terms are used to describe lipid disorders. **Hyperlipidemia**, the general term meaning "high levels of lipids in the blood," is a major risk factor for cardiovascular disease. Elevated blood cholesterol, or **hypercholesterolemia**, is the type of hyperlipidemia that is most familiar to the general public. **Dyslipidemia** is the term that refers to abnormal (excess or deficient) levels of lipoproteins. Most patients with these disorders are asymptomatic and do not seek medical intervention until cardiovascular disease produces symptoms such as chest pain or signs of hypertension. Statistics suggest that more than half the adult population in the United States have total cholesterol levels above 200 mg/dL and that two thirds of these patients are unaware of their hyperlipidemia.

The etiology of hyperlipidemia may be inherited or acquired. Certainly, diets high in saturated fats and lack of exercise contribute greatly to hyperlipidemia and resulting cardiovascular diseases. However, genetics determines one's ability to metabolize lipids and contributes to high lipid levels in substantial numbers of patients. For most patients, dyslipidemias are the result of a *combination* of genetic and environmental (lifestyle) factors.

22.3 LDL and Cardiovascular Disease

Although high serum cholesterol is associated with cardiovascular disease, it is not adequate to simply measure total cholesterol in the blood. Because some cholesterol is being transported for destruction, a more accurate profile is obtained by measuring LDL and HDL. The goal in maintaining normal cholesterol levels is to maximize the HDL and minimize the LDL. This goal is sometimes stated as a ratio of LDL to HDL. If the ratio is greater than 5.0 (five times more LDL than HDL), the male patient is considered at risk for cardiovascular disease. The normal ratio in women is slightly lower, at 4.5.

Scientists have further divided LDL into subclasses of lipoproteins. For example, one variety found in LDL, called lipoprotein (a), has been strongly associated with plaque formation and heart disease. It is likely that further research will discover other varieties, with the expectation that drugs will be designed to be more selective toward the "bad" lipoproteins. Table 22.1 gives the optimal, borderline, and high laboratory values for each of the major lipids and lipoproteins.

Establishing treatment guidelines for dyslipidemia has been difficult because the condition has no symptoms, and the progression to cardiovascular disease may take decades. Based on ongoing research, the National Cholesterol Education Program (NCEP), an expert panel of the National Heart, Lung, and Blood Institute, periodically revises the recommended treatment guidelines for dyslipidemia. The current guidelines are based on accumulated evidence that reducing "borderline" high cholesterol levels can result in fewer heart attacks and fewer deaths. Optimal levels of LDL cholesterol have been lowered from 130 mg/dL to 100 mg/dL. HDL cholesterol should now be at least 40 mg/dL, compared with the previous 35 mg/dL. In addition, the NCEP guidelines recommend that high cholesterol levels be treated more aggressively in people with diabetes, and that hormone replacement therapy not be considered as an alternative to cholesterol-lowering medications.

TABLE 22.1	Standard Laboratory Lipid Profiles	
Type of Lipid	Laboratory Value (mg/dL)	Standard
Total cholesterol	<200	Desirable
	200–239	Borderline high risk
	>239	High risk
LDL cholesterol	<100	Optimal
	100–129	Near or above optimal
	130–159	Borderline high risk
	160–189	High risk
	>190	Very high risk
HDL cholesterol	<40	Low
	40-59	Borderline high risk
	>60	Desirable
Triglycerides	<150	Normal
	150–199	Borderline high risk
	200–499	High risk
	<500	Very high risk

LIFESPAN CONSIDERATIONS

Pediatric Dyslipidemias

Most people consider dyslipidemia a condition that occurs with advancing age. Dyslipidemias, however, are also a concern for some pediatric patients and multiple research studies have demonstrated that the early stage of atherosclerosis begins in childhood. Children who are most at risk include those with a family history of premature coronary artery disease or dyslipidemia, and those who have hypertension, diabetes, or are obese. Lipid levels fluctuate in children and tend to be higher in girls. Nutritional intervention, regular physical activity, and risk factor management are warranted when the LDL level reaches 110 to 129 mg/dL. More aggressive dietary therapy and pharmacotherapy may be warranted in pediatric patients with LDL levels above 130 mg/dL. The long-term effects of lipid-lowering drugs in children have not been clearly established; therefore, drug therapy is not usually recommended below 10 years of age. The statin class of drugs for lowering lipid levels in adolescents have gained FDA approval, but the concern over rhabdomyolysis has led to a reluctance to prescribe them in all but perhaps extreme cases. Cholestyramine (Questran) and colestipol (Colestid) also have FDA approval for hypercholesterolemia in children, but side effects sometimes result in poor compliance. Until more research into standardized recommendations for pediatric dyslipidemia treatment is completed, dietary changes along with increased exercise levels remain a viable option to help pediatric patients decrease lipid levels.

22.4 Controlling Lipid Levels Through Lifestyle Changes

Lifestyle changes should always be included in any treatment plan for reducing blood lipid levels. Many patients with borderline laboratory values can control their dyslipidemia entirely through nonpharmacologic means. It is important to note that all the lifestyle factors for reducing blood lipid levels also apply to cardiovascular disease in general. Because many patients taking lipid-lowering drugs also have underlying cardiovascular disease, these lifestyle changes are particularly important. To emphasize the importance of lifestyle changes, patients should be taught that *all* drugs used for hyperlipidemia have side effects and, to the extent possible, that maintaining normal lipid values *without* pharmacotherapy should be a therapeutic goal. Following are the most important lipid-reduction lifestyle interventions:

- Monitor blood lipid levels regularly, as recommended by the health care provider.
- Maintain weight at an optimum level.
- Implement a medically supervised exercise plan.
- Reduce dietary saturated fats and cholesterol.
- Increase soluble fiber in the diet, such as that found in oat bran, apples, beans, and broccoli.
- Reduce or eliminate tobacco use.

Nutritionists recommend that the intake of dietary fat be less than 30% of the total caloric intake. Cholesterol intake should be reduced as much as possible and not exceed 300 mg/day. It is interesting to note that restriction of dietary cholesterol alone will not result in a significant reduction in blood cholesterol levels. This is because the liver reacts to a low-cholesterol diet by making more cholesterol and by inhibiting its excretion when saturated fats are present. Thus, the patient must reduce saturated fat in the diet, as well as cholesterol, to control the amount made by the liver and to ultimately lower blood cholesterol levels.

The use of plant sterols and stanols is now recommended by the NCEP to reduce blood cholesterol levels. These plant lipids have a similar structure to cholesterol and therefore compete with that substance for absorption in the digestive tract. When the body absorbs the plant sterols, cholesterol is excreted from the body. When less cholesterol is delivered to the liver, LDL uptake increases, thereby decreasing serum LDL (the "bad" cholesterol) level. Plant sterols and stanols may be obtained from a variety of sources including wheat, corn, rye, oats, and rice, as well as nuts and olive oil. Commercially, stanols and sterols are available in products fortified with Reducol, found in margarines, salad dressings, certain

TREATING THE DIVERSE PATIENT

Cultural Dietary Habits

When different cultural groups prepare food in the way they have been taught by their older family members, it can be difficult to change dietary cholesterol intake. For example, traditional Hispanic cooking may include the use of lard for preparation of frijoles and biscochitos, and for frying tortillas. In addition, foods prepared in traditional ways in the southern and south central United States often include large amounts of butter and oil. Examples include fried okra, fried catfish, and chicken-fried steak. To encourage patients to maintain healthy eating habits while enjoying their cultural cuisine, it is important to offer alternative ideas for preparing traditional foods rather than restricting such foods altogether. Many new ethnic cookbooks are now available with recipes that offer low-fat alternatives to traditional cooking methods and provide tasty alternatives that help reduce overall fat intake.

cereals, and some fruit juices. According to the AHA, the recommended daily intake of plant sterols or stanols is 2 to 3 g.

HMG-CoA REDUCTASE INHIBITORS/STATINS

The statin class of antihyperlipidemics interferes with a critical enzyme in the synthesis of cholesterol. These agents, listed in Table 22.2, are first-line drugs in the treatment of lipid disorders.

22.5 Pharmacotherapy with Statins

In the late 1970s, compounds isolated from various species of fungi were found to inhibit cholesterol production in human cells in the laboratory. This class of drugs, known as the *statins*, has since revolutionized the treatment of lipid disorders. Statins can produce a dramatic 20% to 40% reduction in LDL-cholesterol levels. In addition to dropping the LDL-cholesterol level in the blood, statins can also lower triglyceride and VLDL levels, and raise the level of "good" HDL cholesterol. These effects have been shown to reduce the incidence of serious cardiovascular related events by 25% to 30%.

Cholesterol is manufactured in the liver by a series of more than 25 metabolic steps, beginning with acetyl CoA, a two-carbon unit that is produced in the breakdown of fatty acids. Of the many enzymes involved in this complex pathway, **HMG-CoA reductase** (3-hydroxy-3-methylglutaryl coenzyme A reductase) serves as the primary regulatory site for cholesterol biosynthesis. Under normal conditions, this enzyme is controlled through negative feedback: High levels of LDL cholesterol in the blood will shut down production of HMG-CoA reductase, thus turning off the cholesterol pathway. ➤ Figure 22.3 illustrates selected steps in cholesterol biosynthesis and the importance of HMG-CoA reductase.

The statins act by inhibiting HMG-CoA reductase, which results in less cholesterol biosynthesis. As the liver makes less cholesterol, it responds by making more LDL receptors on the surface of liver cells. The greater number of hepatic LDL receptors increases the removal of LDL from the blood. Blood levels of both LDL and cholesterol are reduced. The drop in lipid levels is not permanent, however, so patients need to remain on these drugs during the remainder of their lives or until their hyperlipidemia can be controlled through dietary or lifestyle changes. Statins have been shown to slow the progression of coronary artery disease

MyNursingKit Natural Methods for Lowering Blood Cholesterol

TABLE 22.2	**Drugs for Dyslipidemias**	
Drug	**Route and Adult Dose (max dose where indicated)**	**Adverse Effects**
HMG-CoA REDUCTASE INHIBITORS		
atorvastatin (Lipitor)	PO; 10–80 mg/day (max: 80 mg/day)	*Headache, dyspepsia, abdominal cramping, myalgia, rash or pruritus*
fluvastatin (Lescol)	PO; 20 mg/day (max: 80 mg/day)	
lovastatin (Mevacor)	PO; 10–20 mg once daily (max: 80 mg/day immediate-release; 60 mg/day extended-release)	Rhabdomyolysis, severe myositis
pitavastatin (Livalo)	PO; 1–4 mg once daily (max: 4 mg/day)	
pravastatin (Pravachol)	PO; 10–40 mg/day (max: 80 mg/day)	
rosuvastatin (Crestor)	PO; 5–40 mg/day (max: 80 mg/day)	
simvastatin (Zocor)	PO; 5–40 mg/day (max: 80 mg/day)	
BILE ACID–BINDING AGENTS		
cholestyramine (Questran)	PO; 4–8 g bid–qid ac and at bedtime	*Constipation, nausea, vomiting, abdominal pain, bloating, dyspepsia*
colesevelam (Welchol)	PO; 1.9 g bid (max: 4.4 g/day)	
colestipol (Colestid)	PO; 5-20 g/day in divided doses	GI tract obstruction, vitamin deficiencies due to poor absorption
FIBRIC ACID AGENTS		
clofibrate (Atromid-S)	PO; 2 g/day in 2 to 4 divided doses	*Abdominal pain, rash, myalgia, fatigue, flulike syndrome, dyspepsia, nausea, vomiting, asthenia*
fenofibrate (Tricor, others)	PO; 54 mg/day (max: 160 mg/day)	
fenofibric acid (Triplix)	PO; 45–135 mg once daily	Cholelithiasis, pancreatitis
gemfibrozil (Lopid)	PO; 600 mg bid (max: 1,500 mg/day)	
OTHER AGENTS		
ezetimibe (Zetia)	Hyperlipidemia: PO; 10 mg/day	*Arthralgia, fatigue, abdominal pain, diarrhea* No serious side effects
niacin (Niac, Nicobid, others)	Hyperlipidemia: PO; 1.5–3.0 g/day in divided doses (max: 6 g/day) Niacin deficiency: PO; 10–20 mg/day	*Flushing, nausea, pruritus, headache, bloating, diarrhea* Dysrhythmias

Italics indicate common adverse effects; underlining indicates serious adverse effects.

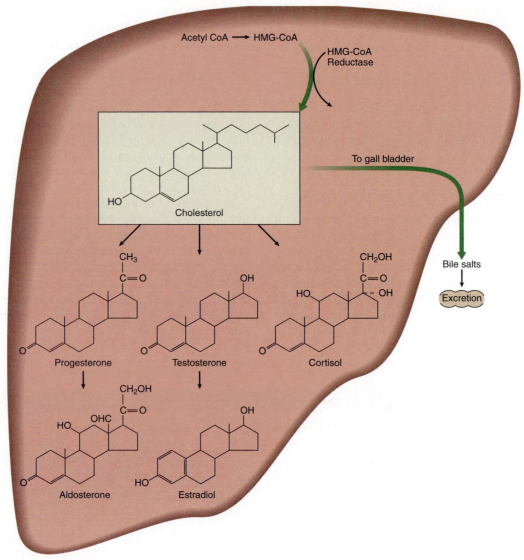

➤ *Figure 22.3* Cholesterol biosynthesis and excretion

and to reduce mortality from cardiovascular disease. The mechanisms of action of the statins and other drugs for dyslipdidemia are illustrated in Pharmacotherapy Illustrated 22.1.

All the statins are given orally and are well tolerated by most patients. Minor side effects include headache, fatigue, muscle or joint pain, and heartburn. Severe myopathy and rhabdomyolysis are rare but serious adverse effects of the statins. **Rhabdomyolysis** is a breakdown of muscle fibers usually due to muscle trauma or ischemia. During rhabdomyolysis, contents of muscle cells spill into the systemic circulation causing potentially fatal acute renal failure. The mechanism by which statins cause this disorder is unknown. Macrolide antibiotics such as erythromycin, azole antifungals, fibric acid agents, and certain immunosuppressants should be avoided during statin therapy, since these interfere with statin metabolism and increase the risk of severe myopathy.

Many statins should be administered in the evening because cholesterol biosynthesis in the body is higher at night. Atorvastatin, pitavastatin, and rosuvastatin have longer half-lives and are effective regardless of the time of day they are taken.

Much research is ongoing to discover additional therapeutic uses of statins. For example, statins block the vasoconstrictive effect of the A-beta protein, a protein associated with Alzheimer's disease. Cholesterol and A-beta protein have similar effects on blood vessels, causing them to constrict. Preliminary research suggests that the statins may protect against dementia by inhibiting the protein and thus slowing dementia caused by blood vessel constriction. Research also suggests that the statins may have the ability to lower the incidence of colorectal cancer. Several attempts have been made to move low doses of certain statins to OTC status; however, the FDA has not approved these applications.

BILE ACID RESINS

Bile acid resins bind bile acids, thus increasing the excretion of cholesterol in the stool. They are sometimes used in combination with the statins. Doses for these agents are listed in Table 22.2.

PHARMACOTHERAPY ILLUSTRATED

22.1 Mechanism of Action of Lipid-Lowering Drugs

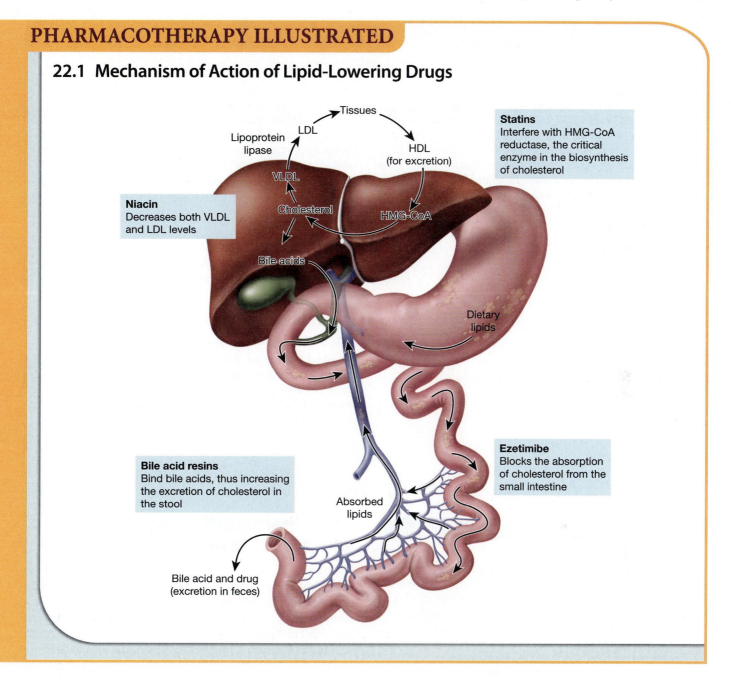

Statins
Interfere with HMG-CoA reductase, the critical enzyme in the biosynthesis of cholesterol

Niacin
Decreases both VLDL and LDL levels

Bile acid resins
Bind bile acids, thus increasing the excretion of cholesterol in the stool

Ezetimibe
Blocks the absorption of cholesterol from the small intestine

Tissues
LDL
Lipoprotein lipase
HDL (for excretion)
VLDL
Cholesterol
HMG-CoA
Bile acids
Dietary lipids
Absorbed lipids
Bile acid and drug (excretion in feces)

22.6 Bile Acid Resins for Reducing Cholesterol and LDL Levels

Prior to the discovery of the statins, the primary means of lowering blood cholesterol was through use of bile acid–binding drugs. These drugs, called **bile acid resins** or sequestrants, bind bile acids, which contain a high concentration of cholesterol. Because of their large size, resins are not absorbed from the small intestine, and the bound bile acids and cholesterol are eliminated in the feces. The liver responds to the loss of cholesterol by making more LDL receptors, which removes even more cholesterol from the blood in a mechanism similar to that of the statin drugs. The bile acid resins are capable of producing a 20% drop in LDL cholesterol. They are no longer considered

first-line drugs for dyslipidemias, although they are sometimes combined with statins for patients who are unable to achieve sufficient response from the statins alone.

The bile acid sequestrants cause more frequent adverse effects than statins. Because they are not absorbed into the systemic circulation, its effects are limited to the GI tract, and include bloating and constipation. In addition to binding bile acids, these agents can bind other drugs, such as digoxin and warfarin, thus increasing the potential for drug–drug interactions.

The newest bile acid–binding agent, colesevelam (Welchol), has more bile acid–binding capacity than the older resins. It is formulated in smaller tablets that are easier to swallow, and fewer tablets are required per day.

Pr Prototype Drug | Atorvastatin *(Lipitor)*

Therapeutic Class: Antihyperlipidemic | **Pharmacologic Class:** HMG-CoA reductase inhibitor, statin

ACTIONS AND USES

The primary indication for atorvastatin is hypercholesterolemia. The statins act by inhibiting HMG-CoA reductase. As the liver makes less cholesterol, it responds by making more LDL receptors on the surface of liver cells. The greater number of LDL receptors in liver cells results in increased removal of LDL from the blood. Blood levels of both LDL and cholesterol are reduced, although at least 2 weeks of therapy is required before these effects are realized. To enhance the drug's therapeutic effects, patients receiving atorvastatin should be placed on a cholesterol-lowering diet. The primary goal in atorvastatin therapy is to reduce the risk of MI and stroke.

ADMINISTRATION ALERTS

- Administer with food to decrease GI discomfort.
- May be taken at any time of the day.
- Pregnancy category X

> **PHARMACOKINETICS**
>
> **Onset:** 2 wk
>
> **Peak:** Plasma concentration, 1–2 h; cholesterol reduction, 2–4 wk
>
> **Half-life:** 14 h (20–30 h for active metabolites)
>
> **Duration:** Unknown

ADVERSE EFFECTS

Adverse effects of atorvastatin rarely cause discontinuation of therapy. Headache and GI complaints such as intestinal cramping, diarrhea, and constipation are common during therapy. A small percentage of patients experience liver damage; thus, hepatic function is monitored during the first few months of therapy. The most serious adverse effect is rhabdomyolysis.

Contraindications: Contraindications include serious liver disease, unexplained persistent elevations of serum transaminases, and prior hypersensitivity to the drug.

INTERACTIONS

Drug–Drug: Atorvastatin interacts with many other drugs. For example, it may increase digoxin levels by 20%, as well as increase levels of norethindrone and ethinyl estradiol (oral contraceptives). Erythromycin may increase atorvastatin levels 40%. Risk of rhabdomyolysis increases with concurrent administration of atorvastatin with macrolide antibiotics, cyclosporine, azole antifungals, and niacin. Ethanol should be avoided during therapy because of its effects on hepatic function.

Lab Tests: May increase serum transaminase and creatine kinase levels.

Herbal/Food: Grapefruit juice inhibits the metabolism of statins, allowing them to reach toxic levels. Red yeast rice contains small amounts of natural statins and may increase the effects of atorvastatin. Because statins also decrease the synthesis of coenzyme Q10 (CoQ10), patients may benefit from CoQ10 supplements. Manifestations of CoQ10 deficiency include high blood pressure, congestive heart failure, and low energy.

Treatment of Overdose: There is no specific treatment for overdose.

Refer to MyNursingKit for a Nursing Process Focus specific to this drug.

COMPLEMENTARY AND ALTERNATIVE THERAPIES

Coenzyme Q10 for Heart Disease

Coenzyme Q10 (CoQ10) is a vitamin-like substance found in most animal cells. It is an essential component in the cell's mitochondria for producing energy or ATP. Because the heart requires high levels of ATP, a sufficient level of CoQ10 is essential to that organ. Foods richest in this substance are pork, sardines, beef heart, salmon, broccoli, spinach, and nuts. Elderly people appear to have an increased need for CoQ10.

Reports of the benefits of CoQ10 for treating heart disease began to emerge in the mid-1960s. Subsequent reports have claimed that CoQ10 may be beneficial in angina pectoris, dysrhythmias, periodontal disease, immune disorders, neurologic disease, obesity, diabetes mellitus, and certain cancers. Considerable research has been conducted on this antioxidant.

Inhibition of the enzyme HMG-CoA reductase by the statins decreases CoQ10 levels. Many of the adverse effects of statins may be due to the decrease in CoQ10 levels, including muscle weakness and rhabdomyolysis. Supplementation with CoQ10 may improve myopathy symptoms (O'Riordan, 2005). Like most dietary supplements, controlled research studies are often lacking and give conflicting results. At this time, evidence to support the use of CoQ10 in treating patients with heart disease, neurologic disorders, or cancer is weak.

NICOTINIC ACID (NIACIN)

Nicotinic acid is a vitamin that is occasionally used to lower lipid levels. It has a number of side effects that limit its use. The dose for nicotinic acid is given in Table 22.2.

22.7 Pharmacotherapy with Nicotinic Acid

Nicotinic acid, or niacin, is a B-complex vitamin. Its ability to lower lipid levels, however, is unrelated to its role as a vitamin because much higher doses are needed to produce its antilipidemic effects. For lowering cholesterol, the usual dose of niacin is 2 to 3 g/day. When taken as a vitamin, the dose is only 25 mg/day. The primary effect of nicotinic acid is to decrease VLDL levels, and because LDL is synthesized from VLDL, the patient experiences a reduction in LDL levels. It also has the desirable effects of reducing triglycerides and increasing HDL levels. As with other lipid-lowering drugs, maximum therapeutic effects may take a month or longer to achieve.

Although effective at reducing LDL levels by as much as 20%, nicotinic acid produces a higher incidence of adverse effects than the statins. Flushing and hot flashes occur in almost every patient. In addition, a variety of uncomfortable intestinal effects such as nausea, excess gas, and diarrhea are commonly reported. More serious adverse effects such as hepatotoxicity and gout are possible. Niacin is not usually prescribed for patients with diabetes mellitus, because the drug can raise fasting blood glucose levels. Because of these adverse effects, nicotinic acid is most often used in lower doses in combination with a statin or bile acid–binding agent. Taking one aspirin tablet 30 minutes prior to niacin administration can reduce uncomfortable flushing in many patients.

Pr Prototype Drug | Cholestyramine *(Questran)*

Therapeutic Class: Antihyperlipidemic **Pharmacologic Class:** Bile acid resin

ACTIONS AND USES

Cholestyramine is a powder that is mixed with fluid before being taken once or twice daily. It is not absorbed or metabolized once it enters the intestine; thus, it does not produce any systemic effects. It may take 30 days or longer to produce its maximum effect. Questran binds with bile acids (containing cholesterol) in an insoluble complex that is excreted in the feces. Cholesterol levels decline due to fecal loss.

ADMINISTRATION ALERTS

- Mix thoroughly with liquid and have the patient drink it immediately to avoid potential irritation or obstruction in the GI tract.
- Give other drugs more than 2 hours before or 4 hours after the patient takes cholestyramine.
- Pregnancy category C

PHARMACOKINETICS
Onset: 24–48 h

Peak: 1–3 wk

Half-life: Unknown

Duration: 2–4 wk

ADVERSE EFFECTS

Although cholestyramine rarely produces serious side effects, patients may experience constipation, bloating, gas, and nausea that sometimes limit its use.

Contraindications: This drug is contraindicated in patients with total biliary obstruction and in those with prior hypersensitivity to the drug.

INTERACTIONS

Drug–Drug: Because cholestyramine can bind to other drugs, such as digoxin, penicillins, thyroid hormone, and thiazide diuretics, and interfere with their absorption, it should not be taken at the same time as these other medications. Cholestyramine may increase the effects of anticoagulants by decreasing the levels of vitamin K in the body.

Lab Tests: Serum aspartate aminotransferase (AST), phosphorus, chloride, and alkaline phosphatase (ALP) levels may increase. Serum calcium, sodium, and potassium levels may decrease.

Herbal/Food: Taking cholestyramine with food may interfere with the absorption of the following essential nutrients: beta-carotene, calcium, folic acid, iron, magnesium, vitamin B_{12}, vitamin D, vitamin E, vitamin K, and zinc. Manifestations of nutrient depletion may include weakened immune system, cardiovascular problems, and osteoporosis.

Treatment of Overdose: There is no specific treatment for overdose.

Refer to MyNursingKit for a Nursing Process Focus specific to this drug.

Because niacin is available without a prescription, patients should be instructed not to attempt self-medication with this drug. One form of niacin available OTC as a vitamin supplement called nicotinamide has no lipid-lowering effects. Patients should be informed that if nicotinic acid is to be used to lower cholesterol, it should be done under medical supervision.

FIBRIC ACID AGENTS

Once widely used to lower lipid levels, the fibric acid agents have been largely replaced by the statins. They are sometimes used in combination with the statins. In addition they remain drugs of choice for treating extremely high triglyceride levels. The fibric acid agents are listed in Table 22.2.

22.8 Pharmacotherapy with Fibric Acid Agents

The first fibric acid agent, clofibrate (Atromid-S), was widely prescribed until a 1978 study determined that it did not reduce mortality from cardiovascular disease. In fact, clofibrate was found to *increase* overall mortality compared with a control group. Although clofibrate is now rarely prescribed, other fibric acid agents, fenofibrate (Tricor), fenofibric acid (Triplix), and gemfibrozil (Lopid), are sometimes indicated for patients with excessive triglyceride and VLDL levels. They are preferred drugs for treating severe hypertriglyceridemia. Combining a fibric acid agent with a statin results in greater decreases in triglyceride levels than

using either drug used alone. The mechanism of action of the fibric acid agents is largely unknown.

CHOLESTEROL ABSORPTION INHIBITORS

In the early 2000s, a new class of drugs was discovered that inhibits the absorption of cholesterol. There is only one drug in this class, ezetimibe (Zetia), which is listed in Table 22.2.

22.9 Pharmacotherapy with Cholesterol Absorption Inhibitors

Cholesterol is absorbed from the intestinal lumen by cells in the jejunum of the small intestine. Ezetimibe blocks this absorption by as much as 50%, causing less cholesterol to enter the blood. Unfortunately, the body responds by synthesizing more cholesterol; thus, a statin may be administered concurrently.

AVOIDING MEDICATION ERRORS

The nurse administers the following oral medications ordered for a 64-year-old man: tetracycline 500 mg bid, digoxin (Lanoxin) 0.25 mg/day, and cholestyramine (Questran) 4 g bid ac and at bed time. At 8:00 a.m., before breakfast, the nurse administers tetracycline 500 mg, digoxin 0.25 mg, and cholestyramine 4 mg. What should the nurse have done differently?

See Appendix D for the suggested answer.

Pr Prototype Drug | Gemfibrozil (Lopid)

Therapeutic Class: Antihyperlipidemic   **Pharmacologic Class:** Fibric acid agent

ACTIONS AND USES

Effects of gemfibrozil include up to a 50% reduction in VLDL with an increase in HDL. The mechanism of achieving this action is unknown. It is less effective than the statins at lowering LDL; thus, it is not a drug of first choice for reducing LDL levels. Gemfibrozil is taken orally at 600 to 1,200 mg/day.

ADMINISTRATION ALERTS

- Administer with meals to decrease GI distress.
- Pregnancy category B

PHARMACOKINETICS

Onset: 1–2 h

Peak: 1–2 h

Half-life: 1.5 h

Duration: 2–4 months

ADVERSE EFFECTS

Gemfibrozil produces few serious adverse effects, but it may increase the likelihood of gallstones and may occasionally affect liver function. The most common adverse effects are GI related: dyspepsia, diarrhea, nausea, and cramping.

Contraindications: Gemfibrozil is contraindicated in patients with hepatic impairment, severe renal dysfunction, or pre-existing gallbladder disease, or those with prior hypersensitivity to the drug.

INTERACTIONS

Drug–Drug: Concurrent use of gemfibrozil with oral anticoagulants may potentiate anticoagulant effects. Concurrent use with statins should be avoided because this increases the risk of myopathy and rhabdomyolysis. Gemfibrozil may increase the effects of certain antidiabetic agents, statins, sulfonylureas, and vitamin K antagonists.

Lab Tests: May increase liver enzyme values, and CPK and serum glucose levels. May decrease hemoglobin (Hgb), hematocrit (Hct), and WBC counts.

Herbal/Food: Fatty foods may decrease the efficacy of gemfibrozil.

Treatment of Overdose: There is no specific treatment for overdose.

Refer to MyNursingKit for a Nursing Process Focus specific to this drug.

When given as monotherapy, ezetimibe produces a modest reduction in LDL of about 20%. Adding a statin to the therapeutic regimen reduces LDL by an *additional* 15% to 20%. Vytorin is a combination tablet containing fixed-dose combinations of ezetimibe and simvastatin. Because bile acid sequestrants inhibit the absorption of ezetimibe, these drugs should not be taken together.

NURSING PROCESS FOCUS   PATIENTS RECEIVING LIPID-LOWERING THERAPY

Assessment	Potential Nursing Diagnoses
Baseline assessment prior to administration: - Understand the reason the drug has been prescribed in order to assess for therapeutic effects. - Obtain a complete health history including cardiovascular, musculoskeletal (pre-existing conditions that might result in muscle or joint pain), gastrointestinal (peptic ulcer disease, hemorrhoids, inflammatory bowel disease, chronic constipation, dysphagia or esophageal strictures), and the possibility of pregnancy. Obtain a drug history including allergies, current prescription and OTC drugs, herbal preparations, and alcohol use. Be alert to possible drug interactions. - Evaluate appropriate laboratory findings, especially liver function studies and lipid profiles. - Assess the patient's ability to receive and understand instruction. Include family and caregivers as needed.	- Imbalanced Nutrition: More than Body Requirements (Fat Intake) - Ineffective Health Maintenance (Individual or Family; dietary and lifestyle changes) - Chronic Pain (related to drug effects) - Deficient Knowledge (drug therapy, dietary and lifestyle changes)
Assessment throughout administration: - Assess for desired therapeutic effects (e.g., lowered total cholesterol, LDL levels, increased HDL levels). - Continue periodic monitoring of lipid profiles, liver function studies, CPK (creatine phosphokinase), and uric acid levels. - Assess for adverse effects: musculoskeletal discomfort, nausea, vomiting, abdominal cramping, diarrhea. Severe musculoskeletal pain, unexplained muscle tenderness accompanied by fever, inability to maintain activities of daily living (ADLs) due to musculoskeletal weakness or pain, unexplained numbness or tingling of extremities, yellowing of sclera or skin, severe constipation, or straining with passing of stools or tarry stools should be reported immediately.	

NURSING PROCESS FOCUS   PATIENTS RECEIVING LIPID-LOWERING THERAPY *(Continued)*

Planning: Patient Goals and Expected Outcomes

The patient will:

- Experience therapeutic effects (e.g., lowered total cholesterol, LDL, increased HDL, normal liver enzymes).
- Be free from, or experience minimal, adverse effects.
- Verbalize an understanding of the drug's use, adverse effects, and required precautions.
- Demonstrate proper self-administration of the medication (e.g., dose, timing, when to notify provider).

Implementation

Interventions and (Rationales)	Patient and Family Education
Ensuring therapeutic effects:	

■ Follow appropriate administration guidelines. (Many of the lipid-lowering drugs have specific administration requirements. For best results, they should be taken at night when cholesterol biosynthesis is at its highest.)	■ Teach the patient to take the drug following appropriate guidelines as follows:
	  ■ *Statins:* Take with evening meal; avoid grapefruit and grapefruit juice, which could inhibit the drug's metabolism, leading to toxic levels.
	  ■ *Bile acid resins:* Take before meals with plenty of fluids, mixing powders or granules thoroughly with liquid. Take other medications 1 hour before, or 4 hours after, the bile acid resin is taken.
	  ■ *Niacin:* Take with cold water to decrease flushing. Take one adult-strength (325 mg) aspirin 30 minutes before the niacin dose.
	  ■ *Fibric acid agents:* Take with a meal.

■ Encourage appropriate lifestyle changes: lowered fat intake, increased exercise, limited alcohol intake, and smoking cessation. Provide for dietitian consultation as needed. (Healthy lifestyle changes will support and minimize the need for drug therapy.)	■ Encourage the patient and family to adopt a healthy lifestyle of low-fat food choices, increased exercise, decreased alcohol consumption, and smoking cessation. ■ Encourage increased intake of omega-3 and coenzyme Q10–rich foods (e.g., fish such as salmon and sardines, nuts, extra-virgin olive and canola oils, beef and chicken). Supplementation may be needed; instruct patient to seek advice of a health care provider before supplements are taken.
Minimizing adverse effects:	
■ Continue to monitor periodic liver function tests and CPK levels. (Abnormal liver function tests or increased CPK levels may indicate drug-induced adverse hepatic effects or myopathy and should be reported.)	■ Instruct the patient on the need to return periodically for lab work.

■ Continue to assess for drug-related symptoms, which may indicate adverse effects are occurring. (Lipid-lowering drugs often adversely affect the liver but may also cause drug-specific adverse effects.)
■ Assess for possibility of increased adverse effects when a combination of lipid-lowering agents are used. (Lipid-lowering agents may be combined for better effects but this increases the risk of adverse effects.)
	■ Teach the patient the importance of reporting signs or symptoms related to adverse drug effects as follows:
	  ■ *Statins:* Report unusual or unexplained muscle tenderness, increasing muscle pain, numbness or tingling of extremities, or effects that hinder normal ADL activities.
	  ■ *Bile acid resins:* Report severe nausea, heartburn, constipation, or straining with passing stools. Any tarry stools or yellowing of sclera or skin should also be reported.
	  ■ *Niacin:* Report flank, joint, or stomach pain, or yellowing of sclera or skin.
	  ■ *Fibric acid agents:* Report unusual bleeding or bruising, right upper quadrant pain, muscle cramping, or changes in the color of the stool.
	■ Instruct the patient taking a combination of lipid-lowering drugs to be alert to symptoms related to adverse effects of <u>both</u> drugs, as above.

■ If long-term therapy is used, ensure adequate intake of fat-soluble vitamins (A, D, E, K) and folic acid in the diet or consider supplementation. (Lipid-lowering drugs may cause depletion or diminished absorption of these nutrients.)	■ Instruct the patient and family about foods high in folic acid and fat-soluble vitamins and about need to consult with the health care provider about possible need for vitamin and folic acid supplementation while on long-term therapy.

(Continued)

NURSING PROCESS FOCUS   PATIENTS RECEIVING LIPID-LOWERING THERAPY *(Continued)*

Implementation

Interventions and (Rationales)	Patient and Family Education
Patient understanding of drug therapy: • Use opportunities during administration of medications and during assessments to discuss rationale for drug therapy, desired therapeutic outcomes, most commonly observed adverse effects, parameters for when to call the health care provider, and any necessary monitoring or precautions. (Using time during nursing care helps to optimize and reinforce key teaching areas.)	• The patient and/or family should be able to state the reason for drug; appropriate dose and scheduling; what adverse effects to observe for and when to report; and the anticipated length of medication therapy.
Patient self-administration of drug therapy: • When administering the medication, instruct the patient and/or family in proper self-administration of drug, e.g., during the evening meal. (Utilizing time during nurse-administration of these drugs helps to reinforce teaching.)	• The patient and family are able to discuss appropriate dosing and administration needs.

Evaluation of Outcome Criteria

Evaluate the effectiveness of drug therapy by confirming that patient goals and expected outcomes have been met (see "Planning").

See Table 22.2 for a list of drugs to which these nursing actions apply.

Chapter REVIEW

KEY CONCEPTS

The numbered key concepts provide a succinct summary of the important points from the corresponding numbered section within the chapter. If any of these points are not clear, refer to the numbered section within the chapter for review.

22.1 Lipids can be classified into three types, based on their chemical structures: triglycerides, phospholipids, and sterols. Triglycerides and cholesterol are blood lipids that can lead to atherosclerotic plaque.

22.2 Lipids are carried through the blood as lipoproteins; VLDL and LDL are associated with an increased incidence of cardiovascular disease, whereas HDL exerts a protective effect.

22.3 Blood lipid profiles are important diagnostic tools in guiding the therapy of dyslipidemias. The optimum levels of the different lipids are reviewed periodically and adjusted based on the results of current research.

22.4 Before starting pharmacotherapy for hyperlipidemia, patients should seek to control the condition through lifestyle changes such as restriction of dietary saturated fats and cholesterol, increased exercise, and smoking cessation.

22.5 Statins inhibit HMG-CoA reductase, a critical enzyme in the biosynthesis of cholesterol. These agents are safe and effective for most patients and are drugs of choice in reducing blood lipid levels.

22.6 The bile acid resins bind bile and cholesterol and accelerate their excretion. These agents can reduce cholesterol and LDL levels but are not drugs of choice due to their frequent adverse effects.

22.7 Nicotinic acid can be effective at lowering LDL cholesterol when given in large amounts. It is not a drug of first choice, but is sometimes combined in smaller doses with other lipid-lowering agents such as the statins.

22.8 Fibric acid agents lower triglyceride levels but have little effect on LDL. They are not drugs of choice because of their potential side effects.

22.9 A newer class of antilipidemic drugs includes ezetimibe, which acts by inhibiting the absorption of cholesterol across the small intestine. Its role in treating hyperlipidemia is in combination with statins to achieve an additive reduction in LDL cholesterol.

NCLEX-RN® REVIEW QUESTIONS

1 The nurse assesses the patient on a statin drug (HMG-CoA reductase inhibitor) for:
1. constipation.
2. muscle or joint pain.
3. hemorrhoids.
4. flushing or "hot flash."

2 When evaluating the effectiveness of lipid-lowering therapy, the nurse would monitor for:
1. increased total cholesterol, LDL, and HDL levels.
2. increased LDL levels and decreased HDL levels.
3. decreased total cholesterol and LDL levels, and increased HDL levels.
4. maintenance of cholesterol, HDL, and LDL levels.

3 The nurse is instructing a patient on home use of nicotinic acid and will include important instructions on how to take the drug. The nurse will teach the patient to:
1. take the drug an hour before meals and with plenty of water.
2. mix the drug thoroughly in water before taking.
3. take other medications 1 hour before or 4 hours after the nicotinic acid.
4. take one aspirin (325 mg) 30 minutes before the nicotinic acid to reduce the incidence of flushing and hot flashes.

4 The nurse teaches the patient with a diagnosis of hyperlipidemia about lipids in the body. The nurse informs the patient that the major storage form of fat in the body is:
1. phospholipids.
2. steroids.
3. triglycerides.
4. lecithins.

5 A patient has been on long-term lipid-lowering therapy. To prevent adverse effects related to the length of therapy and lack of nutrients, the following supplements may be required: (Select all that apply.)
1. Folic acid
2. Vitamins A, D, E, and K
3. Potassium, iodine, and chloride
4. Protein

6 A patient asks the nurse about healthy eating choices to reduce lipid levels in addition to the prescribed use of statin drug therapy. The nurse will instruct the patient that the following are good choices to include in a healthy diet: (Select all that apply.)
1. Broccoli and carrots
2. Almonds and brazil nuts
3. Grapefruit and grapefruit juice
4. Salmon and sardines

CRITICAL THINKING QUESTIONS

1. Identify the plan of care for a patient with hyperlipidemia who has been prescribed atorvastatin (Lipitor).

2. A patient is put on cholestyramine (Questran) for elevated lipids. What teaching is important for this patient?

3. A male diabetic patient presents to the emergency department with complaints of being flushed and having "hot flashes." The patient admits to self-medicating with niacin for elevated lipids. What is the nurse's response?

See Appendix D for answers and rationales for all activities.

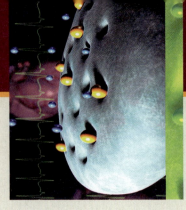

Chapter 23

Drugs for Hypertension

LEARNING OUTCOMES

After reading this chapter, the student should be able to:

1. Explain how hypertension is classified.
2. Summarize the long-term consequences of untreated hypertension.
3. Explain the effects of cardiac output, peripheral resistance, and blood volume on blood pressure.
4. Discuss how the vasomotor center, baroreceptors, chemoreceptors, emotions, and hormones influence blood pressure.
5. Discuss the role of therapeutic lifestyle changes in the management of hypertension.
6. Differentiate between drug classes used for the primary treatment of hypertension and those secondary agents reserved for persistent hypertension.
7. Describe the nurse's role in the pharmacologic management of patients receiving drugs for hypertension.
8. For each of the drug classes listed in Drugs at a Glance, know representative drug examples, and explain their mechanisms of drug action, primary actions, and important adverse effects.
9. Use the nursing process to care for patients receiving antihypertensive drugs.

KEY TERMS

Cardiovascular disease (CVD), which includes all conditions affecting the heart and blood vessels, is the most frequent cause of death in the United States. Hypertension, or high blood pressure, is the most common of the cardiovascular diseases. According to the American Heart Association, high blood pressure is associated with more than 150,000 deaths in the United States each year. Although mild hypertension (HTN) can often be controlled with lifestyle modifications, moderate to severe HTN requires pharmacotherapy.

Because nurses encounter numerous patients with this condition, having an understanding of the underlying principles of antihypertensive therapy is essential. By improving public awareness of hypertension and teaching the importance of early intervention, the nurse can contribute significantly to reducing cardiovascular mortality.

23.1 Definition and Classification of Hypertension

Hypertension (HTN) is defined as the consistent elevation of systemic arterial blood pressure. The diagnosis of chronic HTN is rarely made on a single blood pressure measurement. A patient is said to have HTN if they present with a sustained systolic blood pressure of greater than 140 mmHg or diastolic pressure of greater than 90 to 99 mmHg after multiple measurements are made over several clinic visits.

Many attempts have been made to further define HTN, with the goal of developing guidelines for treatment. In 2003, the National High Blood Pressure Education Program Coordinating Committee of the National Heart, Lung, and Blood Institute of the National Institutes of Health determined the need for updated guidelines that addressed the relationship between blood pressure and the risk of cardiovascular disease. This committee issued The Seventh Report of the Joint National Committee on Prevention, Detection, Evaluation, and Treatment of High Blood Pressure (JNC-7), which has become the standard for treating HTN. The recommendations from Committee Report JNC-7 are summarized in Table 23.1.

In addition to classifying HTN into three categories—prehypertension, Stage 1, and Stage 2—the JNC-7 report issued remarkable data regarding the disease.

- The risk of cardiovascular disease beginning at 115/75 mmHg doubles with each additional increment of 20/10 mmHg.
- Individuals with a systolic blood pressure of 120 to 139 mmHg or a diastolic blood pressure of 80 to 89 mmHg should be considered as prehypertensive. These patients should be strongly encouraged by health care practitioners to adopt health-promoting lifestyle modifications to prevent CVD.
- Patients with prehypertension are at increased risk for progression to HTN; those in the 130 to 139/80 to 89 mmHg blood pressure range are at twice the risk for developing HTN as those with lower values.

Blood pressure changes throughout the life span, gradually and continuously rising from childhood through adulthood. What is considered normal blood pressure at one age may be considered abnormal in someone older or younger. Hypertension has the greatest impact on elderly patients, affecting approximately 30% of those older than 50 years, 64% of men older than age 65, and 75% of women older than age 75.

PharmFacts

Statistics of Hypertension
- Prehypertension (120–139/80–89 mmHg) affects approximately 22% of the adult population, or nearly 45 million people.
- High blood pressure affects more than 73 million U.S. adults, or approximately one in three Americans.
- African American males have the highest rate (51%) of hypertension.
- Among people with HTN, more than 28% do not realize they have the condition.
- Hypertension is the most common complication of pregnancy.
- Approximately 54,000 Americans die of HTN per year; it is a contributing factor in 300,000 additional deaths each year.

TABLE 23.1   Classification and Management of Hypertension in Adults

Blood Pressure Classification	Systolic/Diastolic Blood Pressure (mmHg)	Initial Antihypertensive Therapy	
		Without Compelling Indication*	*With* Compelling Indication*
Normal	119/79 or less	No antihypertensive indicated	No antihypertensive indicated
Prehypertension	120–139/80–89		
Stage 1 Hypertension	140–159/90–99	Thiazide diuretic (for most patients)	Other antihypertensives, as needed
Stage 2 Hypertension	160 or higher/100 or higher	Two-drug combination antihypertensive (for most patients)	

Source: National High Blood Pressure Education Program National Heart, Lung & Blood Institute. (2003). *JNC-7 Express: The Seventh Report of the Joint National Committee on Prevention, Detection, Evaluation, and Treatment of High Blood Pressure.* [on-line] http://www.nhlbi.nih.gov
*Compelling indications include: heart failure, post–myocardial infarction, high risk for coronary artery disease, diabetes, chronic kidney disease, and recurrent stroke prevention

23.2 Factors Responsible for Blood Pressure

Although many factors can influence blood pressure, the three factors responsible for creating the pressure are cardiac output, blood volume, and peripheral resistance. These are shown in ➤ Figure 23.1. An understanding of these factors is essential for relating the pathophysiology of HTN to its pharmacotherapy.

The volume of blood pumped per minute is the **cardiac output.** The higher the cardiac output, the higher the blood pressure. Cardiac output is determined by heart rate and **stroke volume,** the amount of blood pumped by a ventricle in one contraction. This is important to pharmacology, because drugs that change the cardiac output, stroke volume, or heart rate have the potential to influence a patient's blood pressure.

As blood flows at high speeds through the vascular system, it exerts force against the walls of the vessels. Although the inner layer of the blood vessel lining, the endothelium, is extremely smooth, friction reduces the velocity of the blood. This friction in the arteries is called **peripheral resistance.** Arteries have smooth muscle in their walls that, when constricted, will cause the inside diameter or lumen to become smaller, thus creating more resistance and higher pressure. A large number of drugs affect vascular smooth muscle, causing vessels to constrict, thus raising blood pressure. Other drugs cause the smooth muscle to relax, thereby opening the lumen and lowering blood pressure. The role of the autonomic nervous system in controlling peripheral resistance is explained in chapter 13∞.

The third factor responsible for blood pressure is the total amount of blood in the vascular system, or blood volume. Although an average person maintains a relatively constant blood volume of approximately 5 L, this value can change due to many regulatory factors, certain disease states, and pharmacotherapy. More blood in the vascular system will exert additional pressure on the walls of the arteries and raise blood pressure. Drugs are frequently used to adjust blood volume. For example, infusion of intravenous fluids increases blood volume and raises blood pressure. This factor is used to advantage when treating hypotension due to shock (chapter 29∞). In contrast, substances known as **diuretics** can cause fluid loss through urination, thus decreasing blood volume and lowering blood pressure.

23.3 Physiologic Regulation of Blood Pressure

It is critical for the body to maintain a normal range of blood pressure and to have the ability to safely and rapidly change pressure as it proceeds through daily activities such as sleep and exercise. Hypotension can cause dizziness and lack of adequate urine formation, whereas extreme hypertension can cause blood vessels to rupture, or restrict blood flow to critical organs. ➤ Figure 23.2 illustrates how the body maintains homeostasis during periods of blood pressure change.

The central and autonomic nervous systems are intimately involved in regulating blood pressure. On a minute-to-minute basis, a cluster of neurons in the medulla oblongata called the **vasomotor center** regulates blood pressure. Nerves travel from the vasomotor center to the arteries, where the smooth muscle is directed to either constrict (raise blood pressure) or relax (lower blood pressure). Sympathetic outflow from the vasomotor center stimulates alpha$_1$-adrenergic receptors on arterioles, causing vasoconstriction (chapter 13∞).

Receptors in the aorta and the internal carotid artery act as sensors to provide the vasomotor center with vital information on conditions in the vascular system. **Baroreceptors** have the ability to sense pressure within blood vessels, whereas **chemoreceptors** recognize levels of oxygen and carbon dioxide, and the pH in the blood. The vasomotor center reacts to information from baroreceptors and chemoreceptors by raising or lowering blood pressure accordingly. With aging or certain disease states such as diabetes, the baroreceptor response may be diminished.

Emotions can also have a profound effect on blood pressure. Anger and stress can cause blood pressure to rise, whereas mental depression and lethargy may cause it to fall.

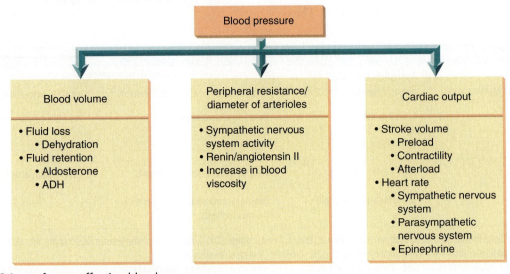

➤ *Figure 23.1* Primary factors affecting blood pressure

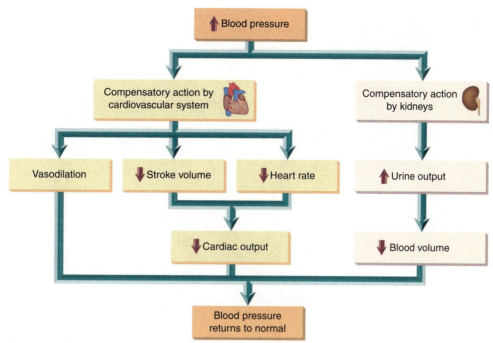

> **Figure 23.2** Blood pressure homeostasis

Strong emotions, if present for a prolonged time period, may become important contributors to chronic hypertension.

A number of hormones and other agents affect blood pressure on a daily basis. When given as medications, some of these agents may have a profound effect on blood pressure. For example, injection of epinephrine or norepinephrine will immediately raise blood pressure. **Antidiuretic hormone (ADH)** is a potent vasoconstrictor that can also increase blood pressure by raising blood volume. ADH is available by parental administration as the drug vasopressin. The **renin–angiotensin–aldosterone system** is particularly important in the pharmacotherapy of hypertension and is discussed in section 23.9. A summary of the various nervous and hormonal factors influencing blood pressure is shown in ➤ Figure 23.3.

23.4 Etiology and Pathogenesis of Hypertension

Hypertension is a complex disease that is caused by a combination of genetic and environmental factors. For the large majority of hypertensive patients, no specific cause can be identified. Hypertension having no identifiable cause is called *primary, idiopathic,* or *essential,* and accounts for 90% of all cases.

In some cases, a specific cause of the HTN *can* be identified. This is called **secondary hypertension**. Certain diseases—such as Cushing's syndrome, hyperthyroidism, and chronic renal disease—cause elevated blood pressure. Certain drugs are also associated with HTN, including corticosteroids, oral contraceptives, and erythropoietin (Epoetin alfa). The therapeutic goal for secondary HTN is to treat or remove the underlying condition that is causing the blood pressure elevation. In many cases, correcting the comorbid condition will cure the associated HTN.

Because chronic HTN may produce no identifiable symptoms, many people are not aware of their condition. Failure to control this condition, however, can result in serious consequences. Four target organs are most often affected by prolonged or improperly controlled HTN: the heart, brain, kidneys, and retina.

One of the most serious consequences of chronic HTN is that the heart must work harder to pump blood to the organs and tissues. The excessive cardiac workload can cause the heart to fail and the lungs to fill with fluid, a condition known as *heart failure* (HF). Drug therapy of HF is covered in chapter 24∞.

High blood pressure over a prolonged period adversely affects the vascular system. Damage to the blood vessels supplying blood and oxygen to the brain can result in transient ischemic attacks and cerebral vascular accidents or strokes. Chronic HTN damages arteries in the kidneys, leading to a progressive loss of renal function. Vessels in the retina can rupture or become occluded, resulting in visual impairment and even blindness.

The importance of treating this disorder in its prehypertensive stage cannot be overstated. If the disease is allowed to progress unchecked, the long-term damage to target organs caused by HTN may be irreversible. This is especially critical in patients with diabetes and those with chronic kidney disease, as these patients are particularly susceptible to the long-term consequences of HTN.

23.5 Nonpharmacologic Management of Hypertension

When a patient is first diagnosed with HTN, a comprehensive medical history is necessary to determine whether the disease can be controlled without the use of drugs. Therapeutic

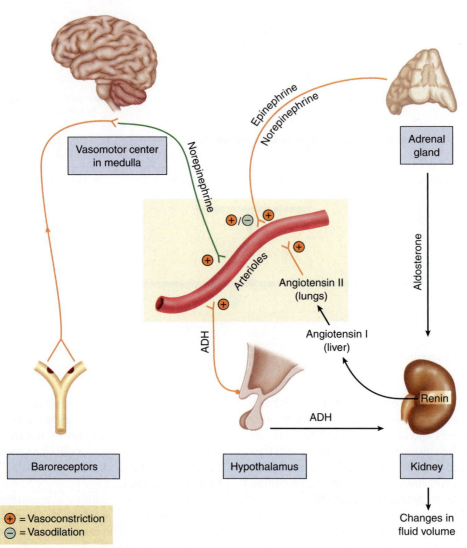

➤ *Figure 23.3* Hormonal and nervous factors influencing blood pressure

lifestyle changes should be recommended for all patients with prehypertension or hypertension. Of greatest importance is maintaining optimum weight, since obesity is closely associated with dyslipidemia and hypertension. Even in obese patients, a 10- to 20-lb weight loss often produces a measurable decrease in blood pressure. Combining a safe weight loss program with proper nutrition can delay the progression from prehypertension to hypertension.

In many cases, implementing positive lifestyle changes may eliminate the need for pharmacotherapy altogether. Even if pharmacotherapy is required, it is important that the patients continue their lifestyle modifications so that dosages can be minimized. The nurse is key to educating patients how to control HTN. Because all blood pressure medications have potential adverse effects, it is important that patients attempt to control their disease through nonpharmacologic means to the greatest extent possible. Important nonpharmacologic methods for controlling hypertension are as follows:

- Limit intake of alcohol.
- Restrict sodium consumption.
- Reduce intake of saturated fat and cholesterol and increase consumption of fresh fruits and vegetables.
- Increase aerobic physical activity.
- Discontinue use of tobacco products.
- Reduce sources of stress and learn to implement coping strategies.
- Maintain optimum weight.

23.6 Factors Affecting the Selection of Antihypertensive Drugs

The goal of antihypertensive therapy is to reduce the morbidity and mortality associated with chronic HTN. Research has confirmed that maintaining blood pressure within normal ranges reduces the risk of hypertension-related diseases such as stroke and heart failure. Several strategies that are used to achieve this goal are summarized in Pharmacotherapy Illustrated 23.1.

The pharmacologic management of hypertension is individualized to the patient's risk factors, comorbid medical conditions, and degree of blood pressure elevation. Patient responses to antihypertensive medications vary widely because of the many complex genetic and environmental factors affecting blood pressure. A large number of antihypertensive drugs are available, and choice of therapy is often based on the experience of the clinician. Although

antihypertensive treatment varies, there are several principles that guide pharmacotherapy.

In most cases, low doses of the initial drug are prescribed and the patient is re-evaluated, after an appropriate time interval. If necessary, dosage is adjusted to maintain optimum blood pressure. The following drug classes are considered primary antihypertensive agents:

- Diuretics
- Angiotensin-converting enzyme (ACE) inhibitors
- Angiotensin II receptor blockers

PHARMACOTHERAPY ILLUSTRATED

23.1 Mechanism of Action of Antihypertensive Drugs

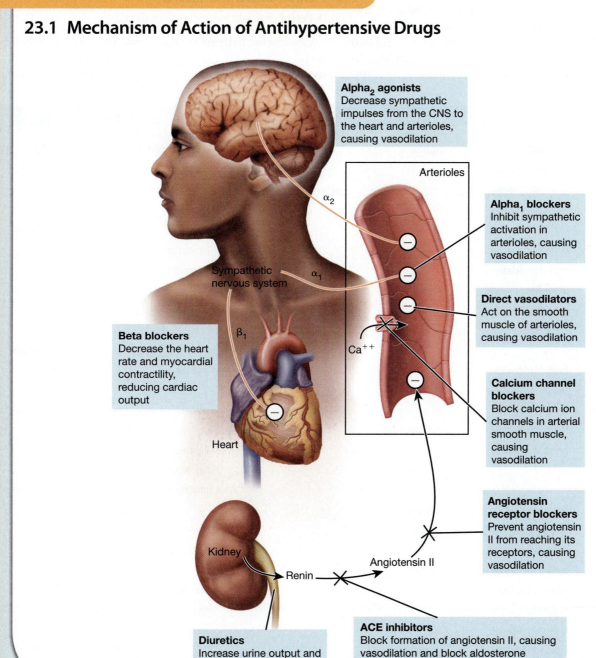

Alpha$_2$ agonists
Decrease sympathetic impulses from the CNS to the heart and arterioles, causing vasodilation

Arterioles

Alpha$_1$ blockers
Inhibit sympathetic activation in arterioles, causing vasodilation

α_2

Sympathetic nervous system

α_1

Direct vasodilators
Act on the smooth muscle of arterioles, causing vasodilation

Ca^{++}

Beta blockers
Decrease the heart rate and myocardial contractility, reducing cardiac output

β_1

Calcium channel blockers
Block calcium ion channels in arterial smooth muscle, causing vasodilation

Heart

Angiotensin receptor blockers
Prevent angiotensin II from reaching its receptors, causing vasodilation

Kidney

Angiotensin II

Renin

Diuretics
Increase urine output and decrease fluid volume

ACE inhibitors
Block formation of angiotensin II, causing vasodilation and block aldosterone secretion, decreasing fluid volume

- Beta-adrenergic antagonists
- Calcium channel blockers

The JNC-7 report recommends thiazide diuretics as the initial drugs for mild to moderate HTN. Patients with a compelling condition, however, may benefit from a second drug, either in combination with the diuretic or in place of the diuretic. The JNC-7 report lists the following as compelling conditions: heart failure, post–myocardial infarction, high risk for coronary artery disease, diabetes, chronic kidney disease, and recurrent stroke prevention.

Prescribing two antihypertensives concurrently results in additive or synergistic blood pressure reduction, and is common practice when managing resistant HTN. This is often necessary when the patient has not responded to the initial medication, has a compelling condition, or has very high, sustained blood pressure. The advantage of using two drugs is that lower doses of each may be used, resulting in fewer side effects and better patient adherence to therapy.

For convenience, drug manufacturers sometimes combine two drugs into a single pill or capsule. The majority of these combinations include a thiazide diuretic, usually hydrochlorothiazide (Microzide). Selected combination antihypertensives are listed in Table 23.2.

Certain antihypertensive classes cause more frequent or serious adverse effects and are generally prescribed only when first-line agents do not produce a satisfactory response. The alternative antihypertensive drug classes include the following:

- Alpha$_1$-adrenergic antagonists
- Alpha$_2$-adrenergic agonists
- Direct-acting vasodilators
- Peripheral adrenergic antagonists

Convincing patients to change established lifestyle habits, spend money on medication, and take drugs on a regular basis when they feel well is often a difficult task for the nurse. Pa-

TABLE 23.2	Combination Drugs for Hypertension				
Trade Name	Thiazide Diuretic	Adrenergic Agent	Potassium-sparing Diuretic	ACE Inhibitor or Angiotensin II Blocker	Other
Accuretic	hydrochlorothiazide			quinapril	
Aldactazide	hydrochlorothiazide		spironolactone		
Avalide	hydrochlorothiazide			irbesartan	
Azor				olmesartan	amlodipine
Benicar HCT	hydrochlorothiazide			olmesartan	
Capozide	hydrochlorothiazide			captopril	
Corzide	bendroflumethiazide	nadolol			
Diovan HCT	hydrochlorothiazide			valsartan	
Dyazide	hydrochlorothiazide		triamterene		
Exforge				valsartan	amlodipine
Hyzaar	hydrochlorothiazide			losartan	
Inderide	hydrochlorothiazide	propranolol			
Lexxel				enalapril	felodipine
Lopressor HCT	hydrochlorothiazide	metoprolol			
Lotensin HCT	hydrochlorothiazide			benazepril	
Lotrel				benazepril	amlodipine
Tarka				trandolapril	verapamil
Tekurna HCT	hydrochlorothiazide	amiloride			
Tenoretic	chlorthalidone	atenolol			
Teveten HCT	hydrochlorothiazide			eprosartan	
Timolide	hydrochlorothiazide	timolol			
Uniretic	hydrochlorothiazide			moexipril	
Vaseretic	hydrochlorothiazide			enalapril	
Zestoretic	hydrochlorothiazide			lisinopril	
Ziac	hydrochlorothiazide	bisoprolol			
*	hydrochlorothiazide				methyldopa

*Available in generic form only

Grape Seed Extract for Hypertension

Grapes and grape seeds have been used for thousands of years. Their primary use has been for cardiovascular conditions such as hypertension (HTN), high blood cholesterol, atherosclerosis, and to generally improve circulation. Some claim that grape seed extract improves wound healing, prevents cancer, and lowers the risk for the long-term consequences of diabetes.

The grape seeds, usually obtained from winemaking, are crushed and placed into tablet, capsule, or liquid forms. Typical doses are 50 to 300 mg/day. Grape seed extract has antioxidant properties. In general, antioxidants improve wound healing and repair cellular injury. Preliminary evidence suggests it may have some benefit in repairing blood vessel damage that could lead to atherosclerosis and HTN. Controlled, long-term studies on the effects of grape seed extracts on HTN have not been conducted. It has few adverse effects but caution should be used if taking anticoagulant drugs because increased bleeding may result. Overall, the benefits of grape seed extract are no different than those of a diet balanced with natural antioxidants (and an occasional glass of red wine).

tients with limited incomes or those who do not have health insurance are especially at risk for adherence. The health care provider should consider generic forms of these drugs to reduce cost and increase adherence to the therapeutic regimen.

Further reducing compliance is the occurrence of undesirable adverse effects. Some of the antihypertensive drugs cause embarrassing side effects such as impotence, which may go unreported. Others cause fatigue and generally make the patient feel sicker than they were before therapy was initiated. The nurse should teach the patient the importance of treating the disease to avoid serious long-term consequences. Furthermore, the nurse should teach patients to report adverse drug effects promptly so that dosage can be adjusted, or the drug changed, and treatment may continue without interruption.

23.7 Treating Hypertension with Diuretics

Diuretics were the first widely prescribed drug class used to treat hypertension in the 1950s. Despite many advances in pharmacotherapy, diuretics are still considered first-line drugs for this disease because they produce few adverse effects and are very effective at controlling mild to moderate hypertension. In addition, clinical research has clearly demonstrated that thiazide diuretics reduce HTN-related morbidity and mortality. Although sometimes used alone, they are frequently prescribed with drugs from other antihypertensive classes to enhance their effectiveness. Diuretics are also used to treat heart failure (chapter 24∞) and kidney disorders (chapter 30∞). Doses for these agents are listed in Table 23.3.

Although many different diuretics are available for HTN, all produce a similar outcome: the reduction of

TABLE 23.3	**Diuretics for Hypertension**	
Drug	Route and Adult Dose (max dose where indicated)	Adverse Effects
POTASSIUM-SPARING DIURETICS		
amiloride (Midamor)	PO; 5–10 mg/day (max: 20 mg/day)	*Minor hyperkalemia, headache, fatigue, gynecomastia (spironolactone)*
eplerenone (Inspra)	PO; 25–50 mg once daily (max: 100 mg/day)	
spironolactone (Aldactone) (see page 242 for the Prototype Drug box ∞)	PO; 25–100 mg 1–2 times/day (max: 400 mg/day)	<u>Dysrhythmias (from hyperkalemia), dehydration, hyponatremia, agranulocytosis, and other blood dyscrasias</u>
triamterene (Dyrenium)	PO; 50–100 mg bid (max: 300 mg/day)	
THIAZIDE AND THIAZIDE-LIKE DIURETICS		
chlorothiazide (Diuril) (see page 423 for the Prototype Drug box ∞)	PO; 250–500 mg/day (max: 2 g/day)	*Minor hypokalemia, fatigue*
chlorthalidone (Hygroton)	PO; 50–100 mg/day (max: 50 mg/day)	<u>Significant hypokalemia, electrolyte depletion, dehydration, hypotension, hyponatremia, hyperglycemia, coma, blood dyscrasias</u>
hydrochlorothiazide (Microzide)	PO; 25–100 mg/day (max: 50 mg/day)	
indapamide (Lozol)	PO; 1.25–5 mg/day (max: 5 mg/day)	
methyclothiazide (Enduron)	PO; 2.5–5 mg once daily (max: 5 mg/day)	
metolazone (Zaroxolyn)	PO; 2.5–10 mg once daily (max: 20 mg/day)	
LOOP/HIGH-CEILING DIURETICS		
bumetanide (Bumex)	PO; 0.5–2.0 mg/day (max: 10 mg/day)	*Minor hypokalemia, postural hypotension, tinnitus, nausea, diarrhea, dizziness, fatigue*
furosemide (Lasix) (see page 330 for the Prototype Drug box ∞)	PO; 20–80 mg/day (max: 600 mg/day)	<u>Significant hypokalemia, blood dyscrasias, dehydration, ototoxicity, electrolyte imbalances, circulatory collapse</u>
torsemide (Demadex)	PO/IV; 10–20 mg/day (max: 200 mg/day)	

Italics indicate common adverse effects; <u>underlining</u> indicates serious adverse effects.

blood volume through the urinary excretion of water and electrolytes. Electrolytes are ions such as sodium (Na^+), calcium (Ca^{2+}), chloride (Cl^-), and potassium (K^+). The mechanisms by which diuretics reduce blood volume differ among the various classes of diuretics and are discussed in chapter 30∞. When a drug changes urine composition or output, electrolyte depletion and dehydration are possible; the specific electrolyte lost is dependent on the mechanism of action of the particular drug. Potassium loss (hypokalemia) is of particular concern for loop and thiazide diuretics.

Thiazide and *thiazide-like* diuretics have been the mainstay for the pharmacotherapy of HTN for decades. The thiazide diuretics are inexpensive, and most are available in generic formulations. They are safe drugs, with urinary potassium loss being the primary adverse effect. The prototype drug in this class, hydrochlorothiazide, is highlighted in this chapter.

Although the *potassium-sparing diuretics* produce only a modest diuresis, their primary advantage is that they do not cause potassium depletion. Thus, they are beneficial when patients are at risk of developing hypokalemia due to their medical condition or the use of thiazide or loop diuretics.

The primary concern when using potassium-sparing diuretics is the possibility of retaining *too much* potassium. Taking potassium supplements with potassium-sparing diuretics may result in dangerously high potassium levels in the blood (hyperkalemia) and lead to cardiac conduction abnormalities. Concurrent use with an ACE inhibitor or angiotensin II receptor blocker significantly increases the potential for the development of hyperkalemia. Spironolactone (Aldactone) is featured as a prototype drug for this class in chapter 30∞.

The *loop diuretics* cause greater diuresis, and thus a greater reduction in blood pressure, than the thiazides or potassium-sparing diuretics. Although this makes them very effective at reducing blood pressure, they are not ideal agents for HTN maintenance therapy. The risk of adverse effects such as hypokalemia and dehydration is greater because of their ability to remove large amounts of fluid from the body in a short time period. Loop diuretics are also ototoxic and may cause deafness. Because they have a higher potential for toxicity, loop diuretics are often reserved for more serious cases of HTN. Furosemide is the only loop diuretic in widespread use, and it is presented as a prototype for heart failure in chapter 24∞.

Pr Prototype Drug | Hydrochlorothiazide *(Microzide)*

Therapeutic Class: Drug for hypertension and edema   **Pharmacologic Class:** Thiazide diuretic

ACTIONS AND USES

Hydrochlorothiazide is the most widely prescribed diuretic for HTN. Like many diuretics, it produces few serious adverse effects and is effective at producing a 10 to 20 mmHg reduction in blood pressure. Patients with severe HTN or a compelling condition may require the addition of a second drug from a different class to control the disease. Hydrochlorothiazide is the most common agent found in fixed-dose combination drugs for HTN. Hydrochlorothiazide is approved to treat ascites, edema, heart failure, HTN, and nephrotic syndrome. Nurses sometimes use HCTZ as an abbreviation for this drug; however, this should be avoided because it causes confusion between hydrochlorothiazide with hydrocortisone.

Hydrochlorothiazide acts on the kidney tubule to decrease the reabsorption of Na^+. Normally, more than 99% of the sodium entering the kidney is reabsorbed by the body. When hydrochlorothiazide blocks this reabsorption, more Na^+ is sent into the urine. When sodium moves across the tubule, water flows with it; thus, blood volume decreases and blood pressure falls. The volume of urine produced is directly proportional to the amount of sodium reabsorption blocked by the diuretic.

ADMINISTRATION ALERT

- Administer the drug early in the day to prevent nocturia.
- Pregnancy category B

PHARMACOKINETICS

Onset: 2 h

Peak: 4 h

Half-life: 45–120 min

Duration: 6–12 h

ADVERSE EFFECTS

Hydrochlorothiazide is well tolerated and exhibits few serious adverse effects. The most common adverse effects are potential electrolyte imbalances due to loss of excessive K^+ and Na^+. Because hypokalemia may cause cardiac conduction abnormalities, patients are usually instructed to increase their potassium intake as a precaution. Hydrochlorothiazide may precipitate gout attacks due to its tendency to cause hyperuricemia.

Contraindications: Contraindications include anuria and prior hypersensitivity to thiazides or sulfonamides. Thiazides are contraindicated in pre-eclampsia or other pregnancy-induced HTN.

INTERACTIONS

Drug–Drug: When given concurrently, other antihypertensives have additive or synergistic effects with hydrochlorothiazide on blood pressure. Thiazides may reduce the effectiveness of anticoagulants, sulfonylureas, and antidiabetic drugs including insulin. Cholestyramine and colestipol decrease the absorption of hydrochlorothiazide and reduce its effectiveness. Hydrochlorothiazide increases the risk of renal toxicity from NSAIDs. Corticosteroids and amphotericin B increase potassium loss when given with hydrochlorothiazide. Hypokalemia caused by hydrochlorothiazide may increase digoxin toxicity. Hydrochlorothiazide decreases the excretion of lithium and can lead to lithium toxicity.

Lab Tests: Hydrochlorothiazide may increase serum glucose, cholesterol, bilirubin, triglyceride, and calcium levels. The drug may decrease serum magnesium, potassium, and sodium levels.

Herbal/Food: Ginkgo biloba may produce a paradoxical increase in blood pressure. Use with hawthorn could result in additive hypotensive effects.

Treatment of Overdose: Overdose is manifested as electrolyte depletion, which is treated with infusions of fluids containing electrolytes. Infusion of fluids will also prevent dehydration and hypotension.

Refer to MyNursingKit for a Nursing Process Focus specific to this drug.

NURSING PROCESS FOCUS   PATIENTS RECEIVING DIURETIC THERAPY

Assessment	Potential Nursing Diagnoses
Baseline assessment prior to administration: ▪ Understand the reason the drug has been prescribed in order to assess for therapeutic effects. ▪ Obtain a complete health history including cardiovascular disease, diabetes, pregnancy, or breast-feeding. Obtain a drug history including allergies, current prescription and OTC drugs, herbal preparations, and alcohol use. Be alert to possible drug interactions. ▪ Evaluate appropriate laboratory findings such as electrolytes, glucose, complete blood count (CBC), hepatic or renal function studies, uric acid levels, and lipid profiles. ▪ Obtain baseline weight, vital signs (especially blood pressure [BP] and pulse), breath sounds, and cardiac monitoring (e.g., ECG, cardiac output) if appropriate. Assess for location and character/amount of edema, if present. Assess baseline hearing and balance.	▪ Deficient Fluid Volume ▪ Fatigue ▪ Decreased Cardiac Output (related to adverse effects of diuretics) ▪ Deficient Knowledge (drug therapy) ▪ Risk for Falls, Risk for Injury (related to hypotension, dizziness associated with adverse effects) ▪ Risk for Functional Incontinence (related to diuretic use) ▪ Risk for Noncompliance (related to adverse effects of drug therapy)
Assessment throughout administration: ▪ Assess for desired therapeutic effects (e.g., lowered systolic and diastolic BP). ▪ Continue periodic monitoring of electrolytes, glucose, CBC, lipid profiles, liver function studies, creatinine, and uric acid levels. ▪ Assess for and promptly report adverse effects: hypotension, palpitations, dizziness, musculoskeletal weakness or cramping, nausea, vomiting, abdominal cramping, diarrhea, headache. Tinnitus or hearing loss, loss of balance or incoordination, severe hypotension accompanied by reflex tachycardiac dysrhythmias, decreased urine output, and weight gain or loss over 1 kg (approximately 2 lb) in a 24-hour period should be reported immediately.	

Planning: Patient Goals and Expected Outcomes

The patient will:
▪ Experience therapeutic effects dependent on the reason the the drug is being given (i.e., decreased blood pressure).
▪ Be free from, or experience minimal, adverse effects.
▪ Verbalize an understanding of the drug's use, adverse effects, and required precautions.
▪ Demonstrate proper self-administration of the medication (e.g., dose, timing, when to notify provider).

Implementation

Interventions and (Rationales)	Patient and Family Education
Ensuring therapeutic effects: ▪ Continue frequent assessments as above for therapeutic effects: blood pressure and pulse are within normal limits or within parameters set by the health care provider. (Systolic and diastolic should return gradually to normal limits without the presence of reflex tachycardia.) ▪ Daily weights should remain at or close to baseline weight. (An increase in weight over 1 kg per day may indicate excessive fluid gain. A decrease of over 1 kg per day may indicate excessive diuresis and dehydration.)	▪ Teach the patient and/or family how to monitor pulse and blood pressure. Ensure proper use and functioning of any home equipment obtained. ▪ Have patient weigh self daily and record weight along with blood pressure and pulse measurements.
▪ Encourage appropriate lifestyle changes. Provide for dietitian consultation as needed. (Healthy lifestyle changes will support and minimize the need for drug therapy.)	▪ Encourage the patient to adopt a healthy lifestyle of low-fat food choices, reduced sodium intake, increased exercise, decreased alcohol consumption, and smoking cessation.
Minimizing adverse effects: ▪ Continue to monitor vital signs. Take blood pressure lying, sitting, and standing to detect orthostatic hypotension. Be cautious with the elderly who are at increased risk for hypotension. (Diuretics reduce circulating blood volume, resulting in lowered blood pressure. Orthostatic hypotension may increase the risk of falls and injury.)	▪ Teach the patient to rise slowly from lying or sitting to standing to avoid dizziness or falls. ▪ Instruct the patient to stop taking the medication if blood pressure is 90/60 mmHg or below, or parameters set by the health care provider, and notify the provider promptly.

(Continued)

Implementation

Interventions and (Rationales)	Patient and Family Education
▪ Continue to monitor electrolytes, glucose, CBC, lipid profiles, liver function studies, creatinine, and uric acid levels. (Most diuretics cause loss of sodium and potassium and may increase lipid, glucose, and uric acid levels.)	▪ Instruct the patient on the need to return periodically for lab work and to inform laboratory personnel of diuretic therapy when providing blood or urine samples. ▪ Advise the patient to carry a wallet identification card or wear medical identification jewelry indicating diuretic therapy.
▪ Continue to monitor hearing and balance, reporting persistent tinnitus or vertigo promptly. (Ototoxicity of cranial nerve VIII may occur, especially with loop diuretics.)	▪ Instruct the patient to report persistent tinnitus, or balance or coordination problems immediately.
▪ Ensure patient safety, especially in the elderly. Observe for light-headedness or dizziness. Monitor ambulation until effects of drug are known. (Dizziness from orthostatic hypotension may occur.)	▪ Instruct the patient to call for assistance prior to getting out of bed or attempting to walk alone, and to avoid driving or other activities requiring mental alertness or physical coordination until effects of the drug are known.
▪ Weigh the patient daily and report a weight gain or loss of 1 kg (approximately 2 lb) or more in a 24-hour period. Measure intake and output in the hospitalized patient. (Daily weight is an accurate measure of fluid status and takes into account intake, output, and insensible losses. Diuresis is indicated by output significantly greater than intake.)	▪ Have the patient weigh self daily, ideally at the same time of day, and record weight along with blood pressure and pulse measurements. Have the patient report a weight loss or gain of more than 1 kg in a 24-hour period. ▪ Advise the patient to continue to consume enough liquids to remain adequately, but not overly hydrated. Drinking when thirsty, avoiding alcoholic beverages, and ensuring adequate but not excessive salt intake will assist in maintaining normal fluid balance. ▪ Teach the patient that excessive heat conditions contribute to excessive sweating, and fluid and electrolyte loss and that extra caution is warranted in these conditions.
▪ Monitor nutritional status and encourage appropriate intake to prevent electrolyte imbalances. (Most diuretics cause sodium and potassium loss. Potassium-sparing diuretics may result in sodium loss but potassium increase.)	▪ Instruct patients taking potassium-*wasting* diuretics (e.g., thiazides, thiazide-like, and loop diuretics) to consume foods high in potassium: fresh fruits such as strawberries and bananas; dried fruits such as apricots and prunes; vegetables and legumes such as tomatoes, beets, and dried beans; juices such as orange, grapefruit or prune; and fresh meats. ▪ Instruct patients taking potassium-*sparing* diuretics to avoid foods high in potassium such as above, not to use salt substitutes (which often contain potassium salts), and to consult with a health care provider before taking vitamin and mineral supplements or specialized sports beverages. (Typical OTC sports beverages, e.g., Gatorade and Powerade, may have lesser amounts of potassium but have high carbohydrate amounts that may lead to increased diuresis, diarrhea, and potential for dehydration from the hyperosmolarity.)
▪ Observe for signs of hyperglycemia. Use with caution in patients with diabetes. (Thiazide, thiazide-like, and loop diuretics can cause hyperglycemia, especially in diabetics.)	▪ Instruct the patient to report signs and symptoms of diabetes mellitus (e.g., polydipsia, polyphagia) or elevated blood sugar to health care provider. Diabetic patients may need to monitor their blood glucose levels more frequently until effects of the diuretic are known.
▪ Observe for sunburning if prolonged sun exposure has occurred. (Some diuretics cause skin photosensitivity.)	▪ Instruct the patient to wear sunscreen and protective clothing if prolonged sun exposure is anticipated.
▪ Observe for signs of infection. (Some diuretics may decrease white blood cell counts and the body's ability to fight infection. Agranulocytosis is a possible adverse effect of diuretic therapy.)	▪ Instruct the patient to report any flulike symptoms: shortness of breath, fever, sore throat, malaise, joint pain, or profound fatigue.
Patient understanding of drug therapy: ▪ Use opportunities during administration of medications and during assessments to discuss the rationale for drug therapy, desired therapeutic outcomes, most common adverse effects, parameters for when to call the health care provider, and any necessary monitoring or precautions. (Using time during nursing care helps to optimize and reinforce key teaching areas.)	▪ The patient and/or caregiver should be able to state the reason for the drug, and appropriate dose and scheduling; what adverse effects to observe for and when to report; and the anticipated length of medication therapy.
Patient self-administration of drug therapy: ▪ When administering the medication, instruct the patient and/or family in the proper self-administration of the drug, e.g., early in the day to prevent disruption of sleep from nocturia. (Proper administration improves the effectiveness of the drug.)	▪ The patient and caregiver are able to discuss appropriate dosing and administration needs.

Evaluation of Outcome Criteria

Evaluate the effectiveness of drug therapy by confirming that patient goals and expected outcomes have been met (see "Planning").

See Table 23.3 for a list of drugs to which these nursing actions apply.

CALCIUM CHANNEL BLOCKERS

Calcium channel blockers (CCBs) exert beneficial effects on the heart and blood vessels by blocking calcium ion channels. They are used in the treatment of HTN and other cardiovascular diseases.

23.8 Treating Hypertension with Calcium Channel Blockers

Calcium channel blockers (CCBs) comprise a group of drugs used to treat angina pectoris, dysrhythmias, and HTN. When CCBs were first approved for the treatment of angina in the early 1980s, it was quickly noted that a "side effect" was the lowering of blood pressure in hypertensive patients. CCBs are usually not used as monotherapy for chronic HTN. They are, however, useful in treating certain populations such as the elderly and African Americans, who are sometimes less responsive to drugs in other antihypertensive classes. Doses for these agents are listed in Table 23.4.

Contraction of muscle is regulated by the amount of calcium ion inside the cell. Muscular contraction occurs when calcium enters the cell through channels in the plasma membrane. CCBs block these channels and inhibit Ca^{2+} from entering the cell, limiting muscular contraction. At low doses, CCBs relax arterial smooth muscle, thus lowering peripheral resistance and decreasing blood pressure. Some

CCBs such as nifedipine (Adalat, Procardia, others) are *selective* for calcium channels in arterioles, whereas others such as verapamil (Calan) affect channels in *both* arterioles and cardiac muscle. CCBs vary in their potency and by the frequency and types of adverse effects produced. Verapamil (Calan, Isoptin, Verelan) is featured as a prototype antidysrhythmic in chapter 26 and diltiazem (Cardizem, Dilacor, Tiamate) as an antianginal in chapter 25.

Two calcium channel blockers, clevidipine (Cleviprex) and nicardipine (Cardene) are important drugs for treating patients who present with serious, life-threatening hypertension. A newer drug approved in 2008, clevidipine is infused until the target blood pressure goal is attained. This drug has an ultrashort half-life of one minute, which allows for rapid adjustments to blood pressure. While clevidipine is indicated only by the IV route for hypertensive emergencies, nicardipine is also available by the oral route for essential hypertension and angina.

23.9 Treating Hypertension with ACE Inhibitors and Angiotensin Receptor Blockers

The renin–angiotensin–aldosterone system (RAAS) is one of the primary homeostatic mechanisms controlling blood pressure and fluid balance in the body. This mechanism is

TABLE 23.4	Calcium Channel Blockers for Hypertension	
Drug	**Route and Adult Dose (max dose where indicated)**	**Adverse Effects**
SELECTIVE: FOR BLOOD VESSELS		
amlodipine (Norvasc)	PO; 5–10 mg once daily (max: 10 mg/day)	*Flushed skin, headache, dizziness, peripheral edema, light-headedness, nausea, constipation, fatigue, weakness, myalgia, arthralgia, impotence, and sexual dysfunction*
felodipine (Plendil)	PO; 5–10 mg/day (max: 20 mg/day)	
isradipine (DynaCirc)	PO; 1.25–10 mg bid (max: 20 mg/day)	
nicardipine (Cardene)	PO; 20–40 mg tid or 30–60 mg; Cardene SR bid (max: 120 mg/day)	<u>Hepatotoxicity, MI, CHF, confusion, mood changes, angioedema (particularly of facial area)</u>
nifedipine (Adalat, Procardia, others)	PO; 10–20 mg tid (max: 180 mg/day)	
nisoldipine (Nisocor)	PO; 10–20 mg bid (max: 60 mg/day)	
NONSELECTIVE: FOR BOTH BLOOD VESSELS AND HEART		
diltiazem (Cardizem, Dilacor, Tiamate) (see page 348 for the Prototype Drug box ∞)	PO; 60–120 mg sustained release bid (max: 540 mg/day)	
verapamil (Calan, Isoptin, Verelan) (see page 366 for the Prototype Drug box ∞)	PO; 80–160 mg tid (max: 480 mg/day)	

Italics indicate common adverse effects; <u>underlining</u> indicates serious adverse effects.

Pr Prototype Drug | Nifedipine *(Adalat, Procardia, others)*

Therapeutic Class: Drug for hypertension and angina   **Pharmacologic Class:** Calcium channel blocker

ACTIONS AND USES

Nifedipine is a CCB generally prescribed for HTN and variant or vasospastic angina. It is occasionally used to treat Raynaud's phenomenon and hypertrophic cardiomyopathy. Nifedipine acts by selectively blocking calcium channels in myocardial and vascular smooth muscle, including those in the coronary arteries. This results in less oxygen utilization by the heart, an increase in cardiac output, and a fall in blood pressure. It is available as capsules and as extended-release tablets (XL).

ADMINISTRATION ALERTS

- Do not administer immediate-release formulations of nifedipine if an impending MI is suspected, or within 2 weeks following a confirmed MI.
- Administer nifedipine capsules or tablets whole. If capsules or extended-release tablets are chewed, divided, or crushed, the entire dose will be delivered at once.
- Pregnancy category C

PHARMACOKINETICS

Onset: 10–30 min PO

Peak: 30 min

Half-life: 2–5 h

Duration: 4–8 h (24 h extended release)

ADVERSE EFFECTS

Adverse effects of nifedipine are generally minor and are related to vasodilation such as headache, dizziness, peripheral edema, and flushing. Immediate-acting forms of nifedipine can cause reflex tachycardia. To avoid rebound hypotension, the drug should be discontinued gradually. In rare cases, nifedipine may cause a paradoxical increase in anginal pain, possibly related to hypotension or heart failure.

Contraindications: The only contraindication is prior hypersensitivity to nifedipine.

INTERACTIONS

Drug–Drug: When given concurrently, other antihypertensives have additive effects with nifedipine on blood pressure. Concurrent use of nifedipine with a beta blocker increases the risk of congestive heart failure. Nifedipine may increase serum levels of digoxin, leading to bradycardia and digoxin toxicity. Alcohol potentiates the vasodilating action of nifedipine, and could lead to syncope caused by a severe drop in blood pressure.

Lab Tests: May increase values for the following lab tests: alkaline phosphatase, LDH, ALT, CPK, and AST.

Herbal/Food: Grapefruit juice may enhance the absorption of nifedipine. Melatonin may increase blood pressure and heart rate.

Treatment of Overdose: The most likely sign of overdosage is hypotension, which is treated with vasopressors. Calcium infusions may be indicated.

Refer to MyNursingKit for a Nursing Process Focus specific to this drug.

NURSING PROCESS FOCUS   PATIENTS RECEIVING CALCIUM CHANNEL BLOCKER THERAPY

Assessment	Potential Nursing Diagnoses
Baseline assessment prior to administration: - Understand the reason the drug has been prescribed in order to assess for therapeutic effects. - Obtain a complete health history including cardiovascular (including MI, heart failure), musculoskeletal (pre-existing conditions that might result in fatigue, weakness, muscle or joint pain), and the possibility of pregnancy. Obtain a drug history including allergies, current prescription and OTC drugs, herbal preparations, and alcohol use. Be alert to possible drug interactions. - Evaluate appropriate laboratory findings, electrolytes, especially potassium level, liver function studies, and lipid profiles. - Obtain baseline weight, vital signs (especially BP and pulse), breath sounds, and cardiac monitoring (e.g., ECG, cardiac output) if appropriate. Assess for location and character/amount of edema, if present.	- Decreased Cardiac Output (disease process) - Fatigue (related to adverse effects of drug therapy) - Altered Tissue Perfusion (related to adverse effects of drug therapy) - Activity Intolerance (related to adverse effects of drug therapy) - Sexual Dysfunction (related to adverse effects of drug therapy) - Deficient Knowledge (drug therapy) - Risk for Falls, Risk for Injury (related to hypotension, dizziness associated with adverse effects)
Assessment throughout administration: - Assess for desired therapeutic effects (e.g., lowered blood pressure within established limits; also lessened or absent angina and dysrhythmias if present). - Continue periodic monitoring of electrolytes, especially potassium. - Assess for adverse effects: nausea, headache, constipation, musculoskeletal fatigue or weakness, flushing, dizziness, or sexual dysfunction. Myalgia, arthralgia, peripheral or facial edema, significant constipation, inability to maintain ADLs due to musculoskeletal weakness or pain, and unexplained numbness or tingling of extremities should be reported immediately to the health care provider.	

NURSING PROCESS FOCUS **PATIENTS RECEIVING CALCIUM CHANNEL BLOCKER THERAPY** *(Continued)*

Planning: Patient Goals and Expected Outcomes

The patient will:

- Experience therapeutic effects (e.g., decreased blood pressure to established parameters).
- Be free from, or experience minimal, adverse effects.
- Verbalize an understanding of the drug's use, adverse effects, and required precautions.
- Demonstrate proper self-administration of the medication (e.g., dose, timing, when to notify provider).

Implementation

Interventions and (Rationales)	Patient and Family Education
Ensuring therapeutic effects:	
Continue frequent assessments as described earlier for therapeutic effects. (Blood pressure and pulse should be within normal limits or within parameters set by health care provider. If drug is given for angina and/or dysrhythmias, significant improvement in reports of pain, palpitations, or ECG demonstrates improvement.)	Teach the patient or family how to monitor pulse and blood pressure. Ensure proper use and functioning of any home equipment obtained.
Encourage appropriate lifestyle changes. Provide for dietitian consultation as needed. (Healthy lifestyle changes will support and minimize the need for drug therapy.)	Encourage the patient to adopt a healthy lifestyle of low-fat food choices, increased exercise, decreased alcohol consumption, and smoking cessation.
Minimizing adverse effects:	
Continue to monitor vital signs. Take blood pressure lying, sitting, and standing to detect orthostatic hypotension. Be cautious with the elderly who are at increased risk for hypotension. (CCBs cause vasodilation, resulting in lowered blood pressure. Orthostatic hypotension may increase the risk of falls and injury.)	Teach the patient to rise slowly from lying or sitting to standing to avoid dizziness or falls. Instruct the patient to stop taking the medication if blood pressure is 90/60 mmHg or below (or according to parameters set by the health care provider) and notify provider promptly.
Continue to monitor periodic electrolyte levels, especially potassium, ECG as appropriate, and hepatic and renal function labs (Hypokalemia may increase the risk of dysrhythmias.)	Instruct the patient on the need to return periodically for lab work or ECGs. Advise the patient to carry a wallet identification card or wear medical identification jewelry indicating CCB therapy.
Ensure patient safety, especially in the elderly. Observe for dizziness. Monitor ambulation until the effects of the drug are known. (Dizziness from orthostatic hypotension may occur.)	Instruct the patient to call for assistance prior to getting out of bed or attempting to walk alone, and to avoid driving or other activities requiring mental alertness or physical coordination until the effects of the drug are known.
Weigh the patient daily and report weight gain or loss of 1 kg or more in a 24-hour period. (Daily weight is an accurate measure of fluid status and takes into account intake, output, and insensible losses.)	Have the patient weigh self daily, ideally at the same time of day, and record weight along with blood pressure and pulse measurements. Have the patient report weight loss or gain of more than 1 kg in a 24-hour period.
Observe for a paradoxical increase in chest pain or angina symptoms. (Severe hypotension may cause this and may indicate blood pressure has decreased too quickly or too substantially.)	Instruct the patient to immediately report chest pain or other angina-like symptoms, especially if symptoms increase.
Monitor for signs of heart failure, such as increasing dyspnea or postural nocturnal dyspnea, rales or "crackles" in lungs, or frothy pink-tinged sputum. (CCBs can decrease myocardial contractility, increasing the risk of heart failure.)	Instruct the patient to immediately report any severe shortness of breath, frothy sputum, profound fatigue, or swelling of extremities as possible signs of heart failure.
Observe for hypersensitivity reaction, and angioedema, especially of facial area.	Instruct the patient to immediately seek medical attention for difficulty breathing, throat tightness, hives or rash, muscle cramps, tremors, or angioedema around the facial area.
Observe for constipation. (CCBs may cause constipation due to decreased peristalsis.)	Instruct the patient to increase fluid and fiber intake to facilitate stool passage. If constipation persists, consider the use of a stool softener or laxative as recommended by the health care provider.

(Continued)

NURSING PROCESS FOCUS	**PATIENTS RECEIVING CALCIUM CHANNEL BLOCKER THERAPY** *(Continued)*

Implementation

Interventions and (Rationales)	Patient and Family Education
Patient understanding of drug therapy: • Use opportunities during the administration of medications and during assessments to discuss rationale for drug therapy, desired therapeutic outcomes, most common adverse effects, parameters for when to call health care provider, and any necessary monitoring or precautions. (Using time during nursing care helps to optimize and reinforce key teaching areas.)	• The patient should be able to state the reason for the drug, appropriate dose, and scheduling; what adverse effects to observe for and when to report; and the anticipated length of medication therapy.
Patient self-administration of drug therapy: • When administering the medication, instruct the patient and/or family in proper self-administration of drug. (Proper administration improves the effectiveness of the drug.)	• The patient should be able to discuss appropriate dosing and administration needs.

Evaluation of Outcome Criteria

Evaluate the effectiveness of drug therapy by confirming that patient goals and expected outcomes have been met (see "Planning").

See Table 23.4 for a list of drugs to which these nursing actions apply.

illustrated in ➤ Figure 23.4. Drugs that affect the RAAS decrease blood pressure and increase urine volume. They are widely used in the pharmacotherapy of HTN, heart failure, and MI. Doses for these drugs are listed in Table 23.5

Renin is an enzyme secreted by specialized cells in the kidney when blood pressure falls, or when there is a decrease in Na^+ flowing through the kidney tubules. Once in the blood, renin converts the inactive liver protein angiotensinogen to angiotensin I. When it passes through the lungs, angiotensin I is converted to **angiotensin II,** one of the most potent natural vasoconstrictors known. The enzyme responsible for the final step in this system is **angiotensin-converting enzyme (ACE).** The intense vasoconstriction of arterioles caused by angiotensin II raises blood pressure by increasing peripheral resistance.

Angiotensin II also stimulates the secretion of **aldosterone,** a hormone from the adrenal cortex. The primary action of aldosterone is to increase sodium ion reabsorption in the kidney. The enhanced sodium reabsorption causes the body to retain water, increasing blood volume and raising blood pressure. Thus, angiotensin II increases blood pressure through two distinct mechanisms: direct vasoconstriction and increased water retention.

First detected in the venom of pit vipers in the 1960s, ACE inhibitors have been approved for HTN since the 1980s. Since then, drugs in this class have become key agents in the treatment of HTN. ACE inhibitors block the effects of angiotensin II, decreasing blood pressure through two mechanisms: lowering peripheral resistance and decreasing blood volume. ACE inhibitors enhance the effects of the thiazide diuretics; thus, drugs from these two classes are often used concurrently in the management of HTN. Some ACE inhibitors have become primary drugs for the treatment of heart failure and myocardial infarction, as discussed in chapters 24 and 27∞, respectively.

Adverse effects of ACE inhibitors are usually minor and include persistent cough and postural hypotension, particularly following the first few doses of the drug. A persistent,

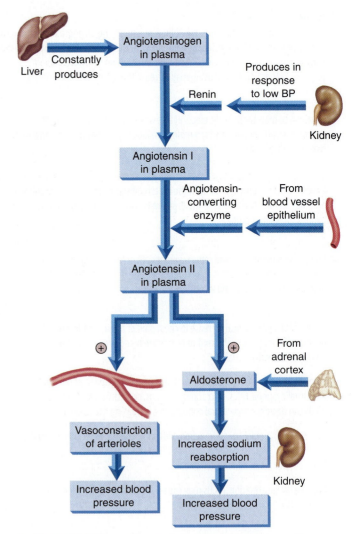

➤ **Figure 23.4** The renin–angiotensin–aldosterone pathway

TABLE 23.5	ACE Inhibitors and Angiotensin II Receptor Blockers for Hypertension	
Drug	Route and Adult Dose (max dose where indicated)	Adverse Effects
ACE INHIBITORS		
benazepril (Lotensin)	PO; 10–40 mg in a single dose or divided doses (max: 40 mg/day)	*Headache, dizziness, orthostatic hypotension, rash*
captopril (Capoten)	PO; 6.25–25 mg tid (max: 450 mg/day)	
enalapril (Vasotec)	PO; 5–40 mg in a single dose or two divided doses (max: 40 mg/day)	<u>Angioedema, acute renal failure, first-dose phenomenon</u>
fosinopril (Monopril)	PO; 5–40 mg/day (max: 80 mg/day)	
lisinopril (Prinivil, Zestoretic, Zestril) (see page 329 for the Prototype Drug box ∞)	PO; 10 mg/day (max: 80 mg/day)	
moexipril (Univasc)	PO; 7.5–30 mg/day (max: 30 mg/day)	
perindopril (Aceon)	PO; 4 mg once daily (max: 16 mg/day)	
quinapril (Accupril)	PO; 10–20 mg/day (max: 80 mg/day)	
ramipril (Altace)	PO; 2.5–5 mg/day (max: 20 mg/day)	
trandolapril (Mavik)	PO; 1–4 mg/day (max: 8 mg/day)	
ANGIOTENSIN II RECEPTOR BLOCKERS		
candesartan (Atacand)	PO; start at 16 mg/day (max: 32 mg/day)	
eprosartan (Teveten)	PO; 600 mg/day or 400 mg qid–bid (max: 800 mg/day)	
irbesartan (Avapro)	PO; 150–300 mg/day (max: 300 mg/day)	
losartan (Cozaar)	PO; 25–50 mg in a single dose or two divided doses (max: 100 mg/day)	
olmesartan (Benicar)	PO; 20–40 mg/day (max: 40 mg/day)	
telmisartan (Micardis)	PO; 40 mg/day (max: 80 mg/day)	
valsartan (Diovan)	PO; 80 mg/day (max: 320 mg/day)	

Italics indicate common adverse effects; <u>underlining</u> indicates serious adverse effects.

dry cough is believed to be caused by accumulation of bradykinin, a proinflammatory substance. Hyperkalemia may occur and can be a major concern for diabetics, those with renal impairment, and patients taking potassium-sparing diuretics. Though rare, the most serious adverse effect of ACE inhibitors is the development of angioedema. Angioedema is swelling around the lips, eyes, throat, and other body regions. In advanced cases, angioedema may lead to airway closure, due to the intense swelling in the neck. When it does occur, angioedema most often develops within hours or days after beginning ACE inhibitor therapy. Late-onset angioedema has been reported after months and even years of treatment with these drugs.

A second method of modifying the RAAS is to block the action of angiotensin II *after* it is formed. The angiotensin II receptor blockers (ARBs) block receptors for angiotensin II in arteriolar smooth muscle and in the adrenal gland, thus causing blood pressure to fall. Their effects of arteriolar dilation and increased sodium excretion by the kidneys are similar to those of the ACE inhibitors. Angiotensin II receptor blockers have relatively few side effects, most of which are related to hypotension. Unlike the ACE inhibitors, they do not cause cough, and angioedema is even more rare with the ARBs. Drugs in this class are usually combined with drugs from other classes in the management of HTN.

A third method of blocking the RAS is to block receptors for aldosterone. The two drugs available that block these re-

ceptors in the kidney are spironolactone (Aldactone) and eplerenone (Inspra). By preventing aldosterone from reaching its receptors in the kidneys, less sodium is reabsorbed and blood pressure falls. These drugs are approved to treat HTN, heart failure, edema, and to reduce morbidity and mortality associated with post-MI in patients with left ventricular dysfunction.

TREATING THE DIVERSE PATIENT

Management of Hypertension in African Americans

The incidence of HTN is significantly higher in African Americans than in other ethnic groups. As expected from this high incidence, African Americans experience greater target-organ damage than other populations. In an effort to reduce the high morbidity and mortality, aggressive antihypertensive therapy may be necessary to overcome resistant HTN in African Americans.

Studies have suggested that certain antihypertensive drug classes are less effective in African Americans. For example monotherapy with ACE inhibitors, angiotensin II receptor blockers or beta-adrenergic antagonists does not reduce blood pressure as much in African Americans, compared to other ethnic groups. Some physicians recommend initiating therapy with two drugs to ensure adequate response. Based on clinical trials in African Americans, the FDA-approved BiDil, a fixed-dose combination of isosorbide dinitrate and hydralazine that appears to be particularly effective at lowering blood pressure in this population.

Pr Prototype Drug | Enalapril *(Vasotec)*

Therapeutic Class: Drug for hypertension and heart failure   **Pharmacologic Class:** ACE inhibitor

ACTIONS AND USES

Enalapril is one of the most frequently prescribed ACE inhibitors for HTN. Unlike captopril (Capoten), the first ACE inhibitor to be marketed, enalapril has a prolonged half-life, which permits administration once or twice daily. It is available as oral tablets and as an IV injection. Enalapril acts by reducing angiotensin II and aldosterone levels to produce a significant reduction in blood pressure with few serious adverse effects. Enalapril may be used as monotherapy or in combination with other antihypertensives. Vaseretic is a fixed-dose combination of enalapril and hydrochlorothiazide.

ADMINISTRATION ALERTS

- May produce a first-dose phenomenon resulting in profound hypotension, which may result in syncope.
- Do not administer if the patient is pregnant. The drug is pregnancy category D.

PHARMACOKINETICS

Onset: 1 h PO; 15 min IV

Peak: 4–8 h PO; 4 h IV

Half-life: 2 h

Duration: 12–24 h PO; 4 h IV

ADVERSE EFFECTS

Unlike diuretics, ACE inhibitors such as enalapril have little effect on electrolyte balance but may cause hyperkalemia. Unlike beta-adrenergic blockers, the ACE inhibitors cause few cardiac adverse effects. Enalapril may cause orthostatic hypotension when the patient moves quickly from a supine to an upright position. A rapid fall in blood pressure may occur following the first dose. Other adverse effects include headache and dizziness. ACE inhibitors can cause life-threatening angioedema, neutropenia, or agranulocytosis.

Contraindications: Enalapril is contraindicated in patients with prior hypersensitivity and should not be administered during pregnancy or lactation.

INTERACTIONS

Drug–Drug: When given concurrently, other antihypertensives have additive effects with enalapril on blood pressure. Thiazide diuretics increase potassium loss. Potassium supplements or potassium-sparing diuretics increase the risk of hyperkalemia. Enalapril may induce lithium toxicity by reducing renal clearance of lithium. NSAIDs may reduce the hypotensive action of ACE inhibitors.

Lab Tests: May increase values of the following: BUN, alkaline phosphatase, serum potassium, serum creatinine, ALT, and AST; may cause a positive ANA titer.

Herbal/Food: Unknown

Treatment of Overdose: The most likely sign of overdosage is hypotension, which may be treated with an IV infusion of normal saline solution.

Refer to MyNursingKit for a Nursing Process Focus specific to this drug.

NURSING PROCESS FOCUS   PATIENTS RECEIVING ANGIOTENSIN-CONVERTING ENZYME (ACE) INHIBITOR AND ANGIOTENSIN RECEPTOR BLOCKER (ARB) THERAPY

Assessment	Potential Nursing Diagnoses
Baseline assessment prior to administration: - Understand the reason the drug has been prescribed in order to assess for therapeutic effects. - Obtain a complete health history including cardiovascular (including MI, heart failure), diabetes, renal disease, and the possibility of pregnancy. Obtain a drug history including allergies, current prescription and OTC drugs, herbal preparations, and alcohol use. Be alert to possible drug interactions. - Evaluate appropriate laboratory findings, electrolytes, especially potassium level, liver function studies, and lipid profiles. - Obtain baseline weight, vital signs (especially BP and pulse), breath sounds, and cardiac monitoring (e.g., ECG, cardiac output) if appropriate. Assess for the location and character/amount of edema, if present.	- Decreased Cardiac Output (disease process) - Altered Tissue Perfusion (related to adverse effects of drug therapy) - Activity Intolerance (related to adverse effects of drug therapy) - Sexual Dysfunction (related to adverse effects of drug therapy) - Deficient Knowledge (drug therapy) - Risk for Falls, Risk for Injury (related to hypotension, dizziness associated with adverse effects) - Risk for Imbalanced Nutrition, More than Body Requirements (potassium intake)
Assessment throughout administration: - Assess for desired therapeutic effects (e.g., lowered blood pressure within established limits). - Continue periodic monitoring of electrolytes, especially potassium. - Assess for adverse effects: headache, cough, orthostatic hypotension, fatigue or weakness, dizziness, symptoms of hyperkalemia, or sexual dysfunction. Angioedema, particularly involving the facial area, should be reported immediately to the health care provider.	

NURSING PROCESS FOCUS	PATIENTS RECEIVING ANGIOTENSIN-CONVERTING ENZYME (ACE) INHIBITOR AND ANGIOTENSIN RECEPTOR BLOCKER (ARB) THERAPY *(Continued)*

Planning: Patient Goals and Expected Outcomes

The patient will:

- Experience therapeutic effects (e.g., decreased blood pressure to established parameters).
- Be free from, or experience minimal, adverse effects.
- Verbalize an understanding of the drug's use, adverse effects, and required precautions.
- Demonstrate proper self-administration of the medication (e.g., dose, timing, when to notify provider).

Implementation

Interventions and (Rationales)	Patient and Family Education
Ensuring therapeutic effects:	
■ Continue frequent assessments as described earlier for therapeutic effects. (Blood pressure and pulse should be within normal limits or within parameters set by health care provider.)	■ Teach the patient, family, or caregiver how to monitor pulse and blood pressure. Ensure proper use and functioning of any home equipment obtained.
■ Encourage appropriate lifestyle changes. Provide for dietitian consultation as needed. (Healthy lifestyle changes will support and minimize the need for drug therapy.)	■ Encourage the patient to adopt a healthy lifestyle of low-fat food choices, increased exercise, decreased alcohol consumption, and smoking cessation.
Minimizing adverse effects:	
■ Continue to monitor vital signs. Take blood pressure lying, sitting, and standing to detect orthostatic hypotension. Be particularly cautious with the first few doses and with the elderly who are at increased risk for hypotension. (ACEIs and ARBs cause vasodilation, resulting in lowered blood pressure. A significant drop in BP may occur with the first few doses. Orthostatic hypotension may increase the risk of falls and injury.)	■ Instruct the patient to take the first dose of the new prescription before bedtime and to use caution during the next few doses until drug effects are known. ■ Teach the patient to rise slowly from lying or sitting to standing to avoid dizziness or falls. ■ Instruct the patient to stop taking the medication if blood pressure is 90/60 mmHg or below, or parameters set by health care provider, and notify the provider promptly.
■ Continue to monitor periodic electrolyte levels, especially potassium, hepatic and renal function labs, and ECG as appropriate. (Hyperkalemia may increase the risk of dysrhythmias.)	■ Instruct the patient on the need to return periodically for lab work. ■ Advise the patient to carry a wallet identification card or wear medical identification jewelry indicating ACEI/ARB therapy.
■ Ensure patient safety, especially in the elderly. Observe for light-headedness or dizziness. Monitor ambulation until effects of drug are known. (Dizziness from orthostatic hypotension may occur.)	■ Instruct the patient to call for assistance prior to getting out of bed or attempting to walk alone, and to avoid driving or other activities requiring mental alertness or physical coordination until the effects of the drug are known.
■ Monitor for persistent dry cough or increasing cough severity. (A change in the severity of the cough may indicate another disease process or may result in the need to consider drugs from other classes.)	■ Teach the patient to anticipate a dry cough that may persist and to use nonpharmacologic measures to treat (e.g., OTC cough lozenges or hard candy, increased fluid intake). ■ Instruct the patient that if the cough becomes troublesome when in supine position, sleep with the head elevated on additional pillows. ■ Advise the patient to consult with the health care provider about the use of antihistamines to relieve a persistent cough unrelieved by nonpharmacologic measures. ■ Instruct the patient to report promptly any change in the severity or frequency of cough. Any cough accompanied by shortness of breath, fever, or chest pain should be reported immediately.
■ Monitor for hyperkalemia. (Reduced aldosterone levels may cause hyperkalemia, especially in patients with diabetes or impaired kidney function.)	■ Instruct the patient on the signs of hyperkalemia (nausea, irregular heartbeat, profound fatigue/muscle weakness, and slow or faint pulse) and to report them immediately. ■ Teach the patient to avoid salt substitutes containing potassium chloride (KCl), consuming snacks advertised as "electrolyte-fortified," specialized sports drinks that contain high-levels of potassium, or excessive intake of foods high in potassium different from their normal diet.

(Continued)

Implementation

Interventions and (Rationales)	Patient and Family Education
Patient understanding of drug therapy: ▪ Use opportunities during administration of medications and during assessments to discuss the rationale for drug therapy, desired therapeutic outcomes, most common adverse effects, parameters for when to call the health care provider, and any necessary monitoring or precautions. (Using time during nursing care helps to optimize and reinforce key teaching areas.)	▪ The patient should be able to state the reason for drug, appropriate dose, and scheduling; what adverse effects to observe for and when to report; and the anticipated length of medication therapy.
Patient self-administration of drug therapy: ▪ When administering the medication, instruct the patient and/or family in proper self-administration of drug, e.g., take the first dose of the new prescription at bedtime. (Proper administration improves the effectiveness of the drug.)	▪ The patient should be able to discuss appropriate dosing and administration needs.

Evaluation of Outcome Criteria

Evaluate the effectiveness of drug therapy by confirming that patient goals and expected outcomes have been met (see "Planning").

See Table 23.5 under "ACE Inhibitors" for a list of drugs to which these nursing actions apply.

23.10 Treating Hypertension with Adrenergic Antagonists

The adrenergic receptor has been a site of pharmacologic action in the treatment of HTN since the first such drugs were developed for this disorder in the 1950s. Blockade of adrenergic receptors results in a number of therapeutic effects on the heart and vessels, and these autonomic drugs are used for a wide variety of cardiovascular disorders. Table 23.6 lists the adrenergic antagonists used for hypertension.

As discussed in chapter 13∞, the autonomic nervous system controls involuntary functions of the body such as heart rate, pupil size, and smooth muscle contraction, including that in the bronchi and arterial walls. Stimulation of the sympathetic division causes fight-or-flight responses such as faster heart rate, an increase in blood pressure, and bronchodilation.

Antihypertensive drugs have been developed that block the sympathetic fight-or-flight response through a number of distinct mechanisms, although all have in common the effect of lowering blood pressure. These mechanisms include the following:

- Blockade of beta$_1$-adrenergic receptors in the heart
- Blockade of alpha$_1$-adrenergic receptors in the arterioles
- Nonselective blockade of both alpha$_1$- and beta-adrenergic receptors
- Stimulation of alpha$_2$-receptors in the brainstem (centrally acting)
- Blockade of peripheral adrenergic neurons

BETA-ADRENERGIC BLOCKERS

Of the subclasses of adrenergic antagonists, only the beta-adrenergic blockers are considered first-line drugs for the pharmacotherapy of HTN. By decreasing the heart rate and contractility, they reduce cardiac output and lower systemic blood pressure. Some of their antihypertensive effect is also caused by blockade of beta$_1$-receptors in the juxtaglomerular apparatus, which inhibits the secretion of renin and the formation of angiotensin II.

Beta blockers have several other important therapeutic applications. By decreasing the cardiac workload, beta blockers can ease the symptoms of angina pectoris. By slowing conduction through the myocardium, beta blockers are able to treat certain types of dysrhythmias. Other therapeutic uses include the treatment of heart failure, myocardial infarction, and migraines. Prototypes of beta-adrenergic antagonists can be found for metoprolol (Lopressor, Toprol) in chapter 24∞, atenolol (Tenormin) in chapter 25∞, propranolol (Inderal) in chapter 26∞, and timolol (Timoptic) in chapter 49∞.

The adverse effects of beta blockers are predictable based on their inhibition of the fight-or-flight response. At low doses, the beta blockers are well tolerated, and serious adverse effects are uncommon. As the dosage is increased, beta blockers will slow the heart rate and cause bronchoconstriction; therefore, they should be used with caution in patients with asthma or heart failure. Many patients report fatigue and activity intolerance at higher doses, because the reduction in heart rate causes the heart to become less responsive to exertion. Less common, though sometimes a major cause of nonadherence, is the effect of beta blockers on male sexual function. These agents can cause decreased libido and erectile dysfunction (impotence). Because abrupt cessation of beta-blocker therapy can result in rebound HTN, angina, and MI, drug doses should be tapered over several weeks.

TABLE 23.6	Adrenergic Antagonists for Hypertension	
Drug	Route and Adult Dose (max dose where indicated)	Adverse Effects
BETA-ADRENERGIC ANTAGONISTS		
acebutolol (Sectral)	PO; 400–800 mg/day (max: 1200 mg/day)	*Fatigue, insomnia, drowsiness, impotence or decreased libido, bradycardia, and confusion*
atenolol (Tenormin): (see page 347 for the Prototype Drug box ∞)	PO; 25–50 mg/day (max: 100 mg/day)	Agranulocytosis, laryngospasm, Stevens–Johnson syndrome, anaphylaxis; if the drug is abruptly withdrawn, palpitations, rebound hypertension, dysrhythmias, MI
betaxolol (Kerlone)	PO; 10–40 mg/day (max: 40 mg/day)	
bisoprolol (Zebeta)	PO; 2.5–5 mg/day (max: 20 mg/day)	
metoprolol (Lopressor, Toprol)	PO; 50–100 mg/day–bid (max: 450 mg/day)	
nadolol (Corgard)	PO; 40 mg/day (max: 320 mg/day)	
pindolol (Visken)	PO; 5 mg bid (max: 60 mg/day)	
propranolol (Inderal) (see page 364 for the Prototype Drug box ∞)	PO; 10–30 mg tid or daily (max: 320 mg/day) IV; 0.5–3.0 mg every 4 hours PRN	
timolol (Timoptic) (see page 771 for the Prototype Drug box ∞)	PO; 10 mg bid (max: 60 mg/day)	
ALPHA₁-ADRENERGIC ANTAGONISTS		
℗ doxazosin (Cardura)	PO; 1 mg at bedtime; may increase to 16 mg/day in a single dose or two divided doses (max: 16 mg/day)	*Orthostatic hypotension, dizziness, headache, fatigue*
prazosin (Minipress) (see page 137 for the Prototype Drug box ∞)	PO; 1 mg at bedtime; may increase to 1 mg bid–tid (max: 20 mg/day)	First-dose phenomenon, tachycardia, dyspnea
terazosin (Hytrin)	PO; 1 mg at bedtime; may increase 1–5 mg/day (max: 20 mg/day)	
ALPHA₂-ADRENERGIC AGONISTS (CENTRALLY ACTING)		
clonidine (Catapres)	PO; 0.1 mg bid–tid (max: 0.8 mg/day)	*Peripheral edema, sedation, depression, headache, dry mouth, decreased libido*
methyldopa (Aldomet)	PO; 250 mg bid or tid (max: 3 g/day)	Hepatotoxicity, hemolytic anemia, granulocytopenia
ALPHA₁- AND BETA BLOCKERS		
carvedilol (Coreg)	PO; 3.125 mg bid (max: 50 mg/day)	*Headache, drowsiness, anxiety, depression, lethargy, impotence*
labetalol (Normodyne, Trandate)	PO; 100 mg bid (max: 1200–2400 mg/day)	Bradycardia, may worsen heart failure and mask symptoms of hypoglycemia
ADRENERGIC NEURON BLOCKERS (PERIPHERALLY ACTING)		
reserpine (Serpasil)	PO; 1.5 mg daily initially; may reduce to 0.1–0.25 mg/day	

Italics indicate common adverse effects; <u>underlining</u> indicates serious adverse effects.

ALPHA₁-ADRENERGIC BLOCKERS

The alpha₁-adrenergic antagonists lower blood pressure directly by blocking sympathetic receptors in arterioles, causing the vessels to dilate. The alpha blockers are not first-line drugs for HTN because long-term clinical trials have shown them to be less effective at reducing the incidence of serious cardiovascular events than diuretics. When used to treat HTN, the alpha blockers are usually used concurrently with other classes of antihypertensives, such as the diuretics. Doxazosin (Cardura) is a prototype antihypertensive included in this chapter. Other prototypes for alpha blockers in this textbook include prazosin (Minipress) in chapter 13∞, and tamsulosin (Flomax) in chapter 46∞.

The alpha₁-adrenergic blockers tend to cause orthostatic hypotension when a person moves quickly from a supine to an upright position. Dizziness, nausea, nervousness, and fatigue are also common.

ALPHA₂-ADRENERGIC AGONISTS

The *alpha₂-adrenergic agonists* decrease the outflow of sympathetic nerve impulses from the CNS to the heart and arterioles. In effect, this produces the same responses as inhibition of the alpha₁ receptor: slowing of the heart rate and conduction velocity, and dilation of the arterioles. The alpha₂ agonists cause sedation, dizziness, and other CNS effects. Abnormalities in sexual function may

Pr　Prototype Drug | Doxazosin *(Cardura)*

Therapeutic Class: Drug for hypertension and BPH　　**Pharmacologic Class:** Alpha$_1$-adrenergic blocker

ACTIONS AND USES

Doxazosin is a selective alpha$_1$-adrenergic blocker available only as tablets. Because it is selective for blocking alpha$_1$ receptors in vascular smooth muscle, it has few adverse effects on other autonomic organs and is preferred over nonselective beta blockers. Doxazosin dilates arteries and veins and is capable of causing a rapid, profound fall in blood pressure. Doxazosin and several other alpha-adrenergic blockers also relax smooth muscle around the prostate gland. Patients who have benign prostatic hyperplasia (BPH) sometimes receive this drug to relieve symptoms of dysuria (chapter 46∞).

ADMINISTRATION ALERTS

- Monitor patients closely for profound hypotension and possible syncope following the first few doses because this drug may produce a first-dose phenomenon.
- The first-dose phenomenon can reoccur when the medication is resumed after a period of withdrawal and with dosage increases.
- Swallow Cardura XL whole: Do not crush, chew, or split the tablet.
- Pregnancy category B

PHARMACOKINETICS
Onset: 2 h
Peak: 2–6 h
Half-life: 9–12 h
Duration: 24 h

ADVERSE EFFECTS

On starting doxazosin therapy, some patients experience serious orthostatic hypotension, although tolerance often develops to this side effect after a few doses. Dizziness and headache are also common adverse effects, although they are rarely severe enough to cause discontinuation of therapy.

Contraindications: Doxazosin is contraindicated in patients with prior hypersensitivity to alpha blockers.

INTERACTIONS

Drug–Drug: When given concurrently, other antihypertensives have additive effects with doxazosin on blood pressure. Oral cimetidine may cause a mild increase (10%) in the half-life of doxazosin.

Lab Tests: Unknown

Herbal/Food: Unknown

Treatment of Overdose: The most likely sign of overdosage is hypotension, which is treated with a vasopressor and/or IV infusion of fluids.

Refer to MyNursingKit for a Nursing Process Focus specific to this drug

NURSING PROCESS FOCUS　　PATIENTS RECEIVING ADRENERGIC-ANTAGONIST THERAPY

Assessment	Potential Nursing Diagnoses
Baseline assessment prior to administration: - Understand the reason the drug has been prescribed in order to assess for therapeutic effects. - Obtain a complete health history including cardiovascular (including MI, heart failure), musculoskeletal (pre-existing conditions that might result in fatigue, weakness, muscle or joint pain), and the possibility of pregnancy. Obtain a drug history including allergies, current prescription and OTC drugs, herbal preparations, and alcohol use. Be alert to possible drug interactions. - Evaluate appropriate laboratory findings, electrolytes, especially potassium level, glucose, hepatic and renal function studies, and lipid profiles. - Obtain baseline weight, vital signs (especially BP and pulse), breath sounds, and cardiac monitoring (e.g., ECG, cardiac output) if appropriate. Assess for the location and character/amount of edema, if present.	- Decreased Cardiac Output (disease process) - Fatigue (related to adverse effects of drug therapy) - Altered Tissue Perfusion (related to adverse effects of drug therapy) - Activity Intolerance (related to adverse effects of drug therapy) - Sexual Dysfunction (related to adverse effects of drug therapy) - Deficient Knowledge (drug therapy) - Risk for Falls, Risk for Injury (related to hypotension, dizziness associated with adverse effects)
Assessment throughout administration: - Assess for desired therapeutic effects (e.g., lowered blood pressure within established limits). - Continue frequent and careful monitoring of vital signs, daily weight, and urinary and cardiac output as appropriate, especially if IV administration is used. - Continue periodic monitoring of electrolytes, especially potassium. - Assess for and promptly report adverse effects: bradycardia, hypotension, dysrhythmias, reflex tachycardia, dizziness, headache, or decreased urinary output. Severe hypotension, seizures, dysrhythmias/palpitations may indicate drug toxicity and should be immediately reported.	

NURSING PROCESS FOCUS   **PATIENTS RECEIVING ADRENERGIC-ANTAGONIST THERAPY** *(Continued)*

Planning: Patient Goals and Expected Outcomes

The patient will:

- Experience therapeutic effects dependent on the reason the drug is being given (e.g., decreased blood pressure).
- Be free from, or experience minimal, adverse effects.
- Verbalize an understanding of the drug's use, adverse effects, and required precautions.
- Demonstrate proper self-administration of the medication (e.g., dose, timing, when to notify provider).

Implementation

Interventions and (Rationales)	Patient and Family Education
Ensuring therapeutic effects:	
• Continue frequent assessments as described earlier for therapeutic effects. Daily weights should remain at or close to baseline weight. (Pulse, blood pressure, and respiratory rate should be within normal limits or within parameters set by the health care provider. An increase in weight over 1 kg (approximately 2 lb) per day may indicate excessive fluid gain.)	• Teach the patient, family, or caregiver how to monitor pulse and blood pressure as appropriate. Ensure proper use and functioning of any home equipment obtained. • Have the patient weigh self daily along with blood pressure and pulse measurements. Report a weight gain or loss of more than 1 kg in a 24-hour period.
• Encourage appropriate lifestyle changes. Provide for dietitian consultation as needed. (Healthy lifestyle changes will support and minimize the need for drug therapy. Adrenergic blockers decrease heart rate and may lead to exercise intolerance. Activity levels should be increased very gradually.)	• Encourage the patient to adopt a healthy lifestyle of low-fat food choices, reduced sodium intake, increased exercise, decreased alcohol consumption, and smoking cessation. • Caution the patient about sudden increases in activity level. Report dizziness, palpitations, or shortness of breath that occurs while exercising.
Minimizing adverse effects:	
• Continue to monitor vital signs. Take blood pressure lying, sitting, and standing to detect orthostatic hypotension. Be cautious with the elderly who are at increased risk for hypotension. Notify the health care provider if blood pressure or pulse decrease beyond established parameters or if hypotension is accompanied by reflex tachycardia. (Adrenergic antagonists decrease heart rate and cause vasodilation, resulting in lowered blood pressure. Orthostatic hypotension may increase the risk of falls or injury. Reflex tachycardia may signal that the blood pressure has dropped too quickly or too substantially.)	• Teach the patient to rise slowly from lying to sitting or standing to avoid dizziness or falls. • Instruct the patient to stop taking medication if blood pressure is 90/60 mmHg or below, or per parameters set by the health care provider, and immediately notify provider.
• Continue cardiac monitoring (e.g., ECG) as ordered for dysrhythmias in the hospitalized patient. (External monitoring devices will detect early signs of adverse effects as well as monitoring for therapeutic effects.)	• Instruct the patient to report palpitations, chest pain, or dyspnea immediately. • To allay possible anxiety, teach the patient the rationale for all equipment used and the need for frequent monitoring.
• Weigh the patient daily and report weight gain or loss of 1 kg or more in a 24-hour period. (Daily weight is an accurate measure of fluid status and takes into account intake, output, and insensible losses.)	• Have the patient weigh self daily, ideally at the same time of day, and record weight along with blood pressure and pulse measurements. Have the patient report a weight gain or loss of more than 1 kg in a 24-hour period.
• Give the first dose of the drug at bedtime. Observe for excessive drowsiness. (A first-dose response may result in a greater initial drop in BP than subsequent doses. Some adrenergic blockers may cause significant drowsiness and are used cautiously in the elderly, who are at risk for falls.)	• Instruct the patient to take the first dose of medication at bedtime and to avoid driving or other hazardous activities for 12 to 24 hours after the first dose, or when the dosage is increased, until effects of the drug are known.
• Continue to monitor blood glucose and appropriate lab work. (Adrenergic-blocking drugs may interfere with some oral diabetic drugs or change the way a hypoglycemic reaction is perceived.)	• Teach diabetic patients to monitor blood sugar more frequently and to be aware of subtle signs of possible hypoglycemia (e.g., nervousness, irritability). Patients on oral antidiabetic drugs should promptly report any consistent changes in their blood sugar levels to the health care provider.
• Assess the patient's mental status and mood. (Adrenergic blockers may cause depression or dysphoria.)	• Teach the patient to report unusual feelings of sadness, despondency, apathy, or depression.

(Continued)

NURSING PROCESS FOCUS   PATIENTS RECEIVING ADRENERGIC-ANTAGONIST THERAPY *(Continued)*

Implementation

Interventions and (Rationales)	Patient and Family Education
■ Provide for eye comfort such as an adequately lighted room. (Adrenergic-blocking drugs can cause miosis and difficulty seeing in low light levels.)	■ Caution the patient about driving or other activities in low-light conditions or at night until the effects of the drug are known.
■ Do not abruptly discontinue the medication. (Rebound hypertension and tachycardia may occur.)	■ Teach the patient, family, or caregiver not to stop medication abruptly and to call the health care provider if patient is unable to take the medication for more than 1 day due to illness.
Patient understanding of drug therapy: ■ Use opportunities during administration of medications and during assessments to discuss rationale for drug therapy, desired therapeutic outcomes, most common adverse effects, parameters for when to call the health care provider, and any necessary monitoring or precautions. (Using time during nursing care helps to optimize and reinforce key teaching areas.)	■ The patient should be able to state the reason for the drug; appropriate dose and scheduling; what adverse effects to observe for and when to report; equipment needed as appropriate and how to use that equipment; and the required length of medication therapy needed with any special instructions regarding renewing or continuing prescription as appropriate.
Patient self-administration of drug therapy: ■ When administering medications, instruct patient and/or family in proper self-administration techniques. (Proper administration improves the effectiveness of the drug.)	■ Instruct the patient in proper administration techniques, followed by return-demonstration. ■ The patient should be able to discuss appropriate dosing and administration needs.

Evaluation of Outcome Criteria

Evaluate the effectiveness of drug therapy by confirming that patient goals and expected outcomes have been met (see "Planning").

See Table 23.6 under "Beta Blockers" for a list of drugs to which these nursing actions apply.

MyNursingKit | Herbal Therapies for Hypertension

occur. Less common, though potentially severe, adverse effects include hemolytic anemia, leukopenia, thrombocytopenia, and lupus. With the exception of methyldopa (Aldomet), which is sometimes a preferred agent for treating HTN occurring during pregnancy, these drugs are rarely prescribed.

ADRENERGIC NEURON BLOCKERS

The earliest drugs for HTN were nonselective agents that blocked nerve transmission at the ganglia or at both alpha- and beta-adrenergic receptors. Although these nonselective agents revolutionized the treatment of HTN, they produced significant adverse effects. The only drug remaining in this class is reserpine, which is rarely used today.

23.11 Treating Hypertension with Direct Vasodilators

Many of the antihypertensive classes discussed thus far lower blood pressure through indirect means by affecting enzymes (ACE inhibitors), autonomic nerves (alpha and beta blockers), or fluid volume (diuretics). It would seem that a more efficient way to reduce blood pressure would be to cause a *direct* relaxation of vascular smooth muscle. Indeed, drugs that directly affect vascular smooth muscle are highly effective at lowering blood pressure but they produce too many adverse effects to be drugs of first choice. These drugs are listed in Table 23.7.

TABLE 23.7	Direct-Acting Vasodilators for Hypertension	
Drug	**Route and Adult Dose (max dose where indicated)**	**Adverse Effects**
ⓟ hydralazine (Apresoline)	PO; 10–50 mg qid (max: 300 mg/day)	*Orthostatic hypotension, fluid retention, headache, palpitations*
minoxidil (Loniten)	PO; 5–40 mg/day (max: 100 mg/day)	<u>Lupuslike reaction (hydralazine), severe hypotension, MI,</u> <u>dysrhythmias, shock</u>
nitroprusside (Nitropress)	IV; 0.3–0.5 mcg/kg/min	
Italics indicate common adverse effects; <u>underlining</u> indicates serious adverse effects.		

Pr Prototype Drug | Hydralazine *(Apresoline)*

Therapeutic Class: Drug for hypertension and heart failure   **Pharmacologic Class:** Direct-acting vasodilator

ACTIONS AND USES

Hydralazine was one of the first oral antihypertensive drugs marketed in the United States. It acts through a direct vasodilation of arterial smooth muscle; it has no effect on veins. Therapy is begun with low doses, which are gradually increased until the desired therapeutic response is obtained. After several months of therapy, tolerance to the drug develops and a dosage increase may be necessary. Although hydralazine produces an effective reduction in blood pressure, drugs in other antihypertensive classes have largely replaced it due to safety concerns. The drug is available as tablets and in parenteral formulations for the treatment of hypertensive emergency.

ADMINISTRATION ALERTS

- Abrupt withdrawal of the drug may cause rebound hypertension and anxiety.
- Pregnancy category C

PHARMACOKINETICS

Onset: 20–30 min PO; 10–30 min IM; 5–20 min IV

Peak: Unknown

Half-life: 3–7 h

Duration: 2–6 h

ADVERSE EFFECTS

Headache, reflex tachycardia, palpitations, flushing, nausea and diarrhea are common, but may resolve as therapy progresses. Patients taking hydralazine often receive a beta-adrenergic blocker to counteract reflex tachycardia. Rarely, the drug may produce a lupuslike syndrome that may persist for 6 months or longer. Sodium and fluid retention is a potentially serious adverse effect. Because of these adverse effects, the use of hydralazine is limited mostly to patients whose HTN cannot be controlled with other, safer medications.

Contraindications: Because of its effects on the heart, hydralazine is contraindicated in patients with angina, rheumatic heart disease, MI, or tachycardia. Patients with lupus should not receive hydralazine, as the drug can worsen symptoms.

INTERACTIONS

Drug–Drug: Administering hydralazine with other antihypertensives may cause severe hypotension. This includes all drug classes used as antihypertensives.

Lab Tests: May produce a false-positive Coombs tests.

Herbal/Food: Unknown

Treatment of Overdose: The most likely sign of overdosage is hypotension, which may be treated with a vasopressor and/or an IV infusion of fluids.

Refer to MyNursingKit for a Nursing Process Focus specific to this drug.

Direct vasodilators produce **reflex tachycardia,** a compensatory response to the sudden decrease in blood pressure caused by the drug. Reflex tachycardia forces the heart to work harder, and blood pressure increases, counteracting the effect of the antihypertensive drug. Patients with coronary artery disease could experience an acute angina attack. Fortunately, reflex tachycardia can be prevented by the concurrent administration of a beta-adrenergic blocker, such as propranolol.

A second potentially serious side effect of direct vasodilator therapy is sodium and water retention. As blood pressure drops, blood flow to the kidneys decreases and renin is released as the body activates the RAAS mechanism. Due to the vasodilation caused by the drug therapy, the angiotensin released does not cause vasoconstriction, but *does* stimulate the release of aldosterone, causing the kidneys to reabsorb sodium and thus water. As the kidney retains more sodium and water, blood volume increases, thus raising blood pressure and canceling the antihypertensive action of the vasodilator. A diuretic may be administered concurrently with a direct vasodilator to prevent fluid retention but warrants extreme caution. Excessive diuresis and lowered blood volume may lead to excessive hypotension and circulatory collapse.

One direct-acting vasodilator, nitroprusside (Nitropress), is a traditional drug of choice for hypertensive emergency, a condition in which diastolic pressure is greater than 120 mmHg, and there is evidence of target-organ damage, usually to the heart, kidney, or brain. This potentially life-threatening condition must be controlled quickly. Nitroprusside, with a half-life of only 2 minutes, has the ability to lower blood pressure almost instantaneously on IV administration. Care must be taken not to decrease blood pressure too quickly because overtreatment can result in hypotension and severe restriction of blood flow to the cerebral, coronary, or renal vascular capillaries. It is essential to continuously monitor patients receiving this drug because the drug is metabolized to cyanide (thiocyanate), which is very toxic to the body. Other drugs for hypertensive emergencies include diazoxide (a direct vasodilator), nicardipine and clevidipine (calcium channel blockers), and enalapril (an ACE inhibitor).

NURSING PROCESS FOCUS   PATIENTS RECEIVING DIRECT VASODILATOR THERAPY

Assessment	Potential Nursing Diagnoses
Baseline assessment prior to administration: ■ Understand the reason the drug has been prescribed in order to assess for therapeutic effects. ■ Obtain a complete health history including cardiovascular (including MI, heart failure), cerebrovascular and neurologic (including level of consciousness, history of CVA, head injury, increased intracranial pressure), respiratory, and the possibility of autoimmune diseases, especially systemic lupus erythematosus. Obtain a drug history including allergies, current prescription and OTC drugs, and herbal preparations. Be alert to possible drug interactions. ■ Evaluate appropriate laboratory findings, electrolytes, especially sodium and potassium levels, hepatic and renal function studies, and lipid profiles. ■ Obtain baseline weight, vital signs, pulse oximetry, breath and heart sounds, and cardiac monitoring (e.g., ECG, cardiac output). Assess the location and character of peripheral edema if present.	■ Decreased Cardiac Output (disease process) ■ Altered Tissue Perfusion (related to adverse effects of drug therapy) ■ Risk for Imbalanced Fluid Volume (related to adverse effects of drug therapy) ■ Risk for Injury (organ systems; related to adverse effects of drug therapy) ■ Risk for Impaired Skin Integrity (related to adverse effects of drug therapy) ■ Deficient Knowledge (drug therapy)
Assessment throughout administration: ■ Assess for desired therapeutic effects (e.g., lowered blood pressure within established limits). ■ Continue frequent and careful monitoring of vital signs, pulse oximetry, urinary and cardiac output, and daily weight, especially if IV administration is used. Blood pressure and pulse must be monitored every 5 minutes or as ordered while on IV infusion of drug. (Invasive monitoring, e.g., arterial lines, are often used for this purpose.) ■ Continue periodic monitoring of electrolytes, especially potassium. ■ Continue frequent physical assessments, particularly neurologic, cardiac, and respiratory systems. ■ Assess for and promptly report adverse effects: excessive hypotension, dysrhythmias, reflex tachycardia, headache, decreased urinary output, peripheral edema, and priapism. Severe hypotension, seizures, and dysrhythmias/palpitations may indicate drug toxicity and should be immediately reported.	

Planning: Patient Goals and Expected Outcomes

The patient will:
■ Experience therapeutic effects dependent on the reason the drug is being given (e.g., decreased blood pressure).
■ Be free from, or experience minimal, adverse effects.
■ Verbalize an understanding of the drug's use, adverse effects, and required precautions.
■ Demonstrate proper self-administration of the medication (e.g., dose, timing, when to notify provider).

Implementation

Interventions and (Rationales)	Patient and Family Education
Ensuring therapeutic effects: ■ Continue frequent assessments as above for therapeutic effects. IV infusion of vasodilators may be titrated frequently to achieve desired effects. Vital signs, cardiac and urinary output, and daily weights should remain within limits set by the health care provider. (Pulse, blood pressure, and respiratory rate should be within normal limits or within acceptable parameters. An increase in weight over 1 kg (approximately 2 lb) per day may indicate excessive fluid gain and may require judicious diuretic therapy.)	■ To allay possible anxiety, teach the patient, family, or caregiver the rationale for all equipment used and the need for frequent monitoring. ■ Teach the patient, family, or caregiver how to monitor pulse and blood pressure as appropriate if patient is on oral therapy at home. Ensure the proper use and functioning of any home equipment obtained. ■ Have the patient weigh self daily along with blood pressure and pulse measurements. Instruct patient to report a weight gain or loss of more than 1 kg in a 24-hour period.

NURSING PROCESS FOCUS | PATIENTS RECEIVING DIRECT VASODILATOR THERAPY *(Continued)*

Implementation

Interventions and (Rationales)	Patient and Family Education
Minimizing adverse effects:	
▪ Continue to monitor vital signs frequently. Be cautious with the elderly, who are at increased risk for hypotension; patients with a pre-existing history of cardiac or cerebrovascular ischemia, which may be worsened by decreased blood pressure; patients with dehydration; and patients with lupus erythematosus. Notify the health care provider immediately if blood pressure or pulse decrease beyond established parameters or if hypotension is accompanied by reflex tachycardia. (Direct-acting vasodilators cause significant vasodilation, resulting in the potential for dramatically and rapidly lowered blood pressure accompanied by reflex tachycardia.)	▪ Instruct the patient to report angina-like symptoms (e.g., chest, arm, back and/or neck pain), palpitations, faintness, dizziness, drowsiness, or headache.
▪ Continue cardiac monitoring (e.g., ECG) and invasive monitoring (e.g., cardiac output, arterial line pressures) as ordered in the hospitalized patient. (Monitoring devices assist in detecting early signs of adverse effects as well as monitoring for therapeutic effects.)	▪ To allay possible anxiety, teach the patient, family, or caregiver the rationale for all equipment used and the need for frequent monitoring.
▪ Continue frequent physical assessments, particularly neurologic, cardiac, and respiratory. Immediately report any changes in level of consciousness, headache, or changes in heart or lung sounds. (Vasodilator therapy may worsen pre-existing neurologic, cardiac, or respiratory conditions as blood pressure drops and perfusion to vital organs diminishes.)	▪ When on oral therapy at home, teach the patient, family, or caregiver to immediately report changes in mental status or level of consciousness, palpitations, dizziness, dyspnea, increasing productive cough (especially if frothy sputum is present).
▪ Weigh the patient daily and report a weight gain or loss of 1 kg or more in a 24-hour period or significant peripheral edema. (Daily weight is an accurate measure of fluid status and takes into account intake, output, and insensible losses.)	▪ When on oral therapy at home, have the patient weigh self daily, ideally at the same time of day, and record weight along with blood pressure and pulse measurements. Have the patient report a weight gain or loss of more than 1 kg in a 24-hour period, or peripheral edema, especially if increasing.
▪ Continue to monitor IV infusion sites frequently. (Direct-acting vasodilators may cause tissue damage if extravasation occurs.)	▪ Instruct the patient to report any burning or stinging pain, swelling, warmth, redness, or tenderness at IV insertion site.
▪ Observe for signs and symptoms of lupus in patients taking vasodilators, particularly hydralazine. (Hydralazine has been linked to drug-induced lupus.)	▪ Instruct the patient to report symptoms such as a "butterfly rash" over the nose and cheeks, muscle aches, and fatigue when taking oral vasodilators, particularly hydralazine.
▪ For oral drug therapy, give the first dose of the drug at bedtime. (A first-dose response may result in a greater initial drop in BP than subsequent doses.)	▪ Instruct the patient to take the first dose of medication at bedtime and to avoid driving or other hazardous activities for 12 to 24 hours after the first dose or when the dosage is increased until effects of the drug are known.
▪ Do not abruptly discontinue the medication. (Rebound hypertension and tachycardia may occur.)	▪ Teach the patient not to stop medication abruptly and to call the health care provider if patient is unable to take medication for more than 1 day due to illness.
▪ Encourage appropriate lifestyle changes. Provide for dietitian consultation as needed. (Healthy lifestyle changes will support and minimize the need for drug therapy. Direct vasodilators decrease blood pressure substantially and concurrent beta blocker use may decrease heart rate. Given alone or together, this may lead to exercise intolerance. Activity levels should be increased very gradually. Alcohol consumption may increase the risk of blood pressure related adverse effects.)	▪ Encourage the patient to adopt a healthy lifestyle of low-fat food choices, reduced sodium intake, increased exercise, decreased alcohol consumption, smoking cessation. ▪ Caution the patient about sudden increases in activity level. Report dizziness, palpitations, or shortness of breath that occurs while exercising.
Patient understanding of drug therapy:	
▪ Use opportunities during administration of medications and during assessments to discuss the rationale for drug therapy, desired therapeutic outcomes, most commonly observed adverse effects, parameters for when to call the health care provider, and any necessary monitoring or precautions. (Using time during nursing care helps to optimize and reinforce key teaching areas.)	▪ The patient should be able to state the reason for the drug; appropriate dose and scheduling; what adverse effects to observe for and when to report; and the anticipated length of medication therapy.

NURSING PROCESS FOCUS   **PATIENTS RECEIVING DIRECT VASODILATOR THERAPY** *(Continued)*

Implementation

Interventions and (Rationales)	Patient and Family Education
Patient self-administration of drug therapy: ■ When administering medications, instruct the patient, family, or caregiver in proper self-administration techniques. (Proper administration improves the effectiveness of the drug.)	■ Instruct the patient in proper administration techniques, followed by return-demonstration. ■ The patient is able to discuss appropriate dosing and administration needs.

Evaluation of Outcome Criteria

Evaluate the effectiveness of drug therapy by confirming that patient goals and expected outcomes have been met (see "Planning").

See Table 23.7 for a list of drugs to which these nursing applications apply.

Chapter REVIEW

KEY CONCEPTS

The numbered key concepts provide a succinct summary of the important points from the corresponding numbered section within the chapter. If any of these points are not clear, refer to the numbered section within the chapter for review.

23.1 High blood pressure is classified as essential (primary) or secondary. Uncontrolled hypertension can lead to chronic and debilitating disorders such as stroke, heart attack, and heart failure.

23.2 The three primary factors controlling blood pressure are cardiac output, peripheral resistance, and blood volume.

23.3 Many factors help regulate blood pressure, including the vasomotor center, baroreceptors and chemoreceptors in the aorta and internal carotid arteries, and the renin–angiotensin system.

23.4 Hypertension has recently been redefined as a sustained blood pressure of 140/90 mmHg after multiple measurements made over several clinic visits. A person with sustained blood pressure of 120–139/80–89 mmHg is said to be prehypertensive, and is at increased risk of developing hypertension.

23.5 Because antihypertensive medications may have uncomfortable side effects, lifestyle changes such as proper diet and exercise should be implemented prior to and during pharmacotherapy to allow lower drug doses.

23.6 Pharmacotherapy of HTN often begins with low doses of a single medication. If this medication proves ineffec-

tive, a second agent from a different class may be added to the regimen.

23.7 Diuretics are often the first-line medications for HTN because they have few side effects and can control minor to moderate hypertension.

23.8 Calcium channel blockers block calcium ions from entering cells and cause smooth muscle in arterioles to relax, thus reducing blood pressure. CCBs have emerged as major drugs in the treatment of hypertension.

23.9 Blocking the renin–angiotensin system prevents the intense vasoconstriction caused by angiotensin II. These drugs also decrease blood volume, which enhances their antihypertensive effect.

23.10 Antihypertensive autonomic agents are available that block alpha$_1$-adrenergic receptors, block beta$_1$- and/or beta$_2$-adrenergic receptors, or stimulate alpha$_2$-adrenergic receptors in the brainstem (centrally acting).

23.11 A few medications lower blood pressure by acting directly to relax arteriolar smooth muscle, but these are not widely used due to their numerous side effects.

NCLEX-RN® REVIEW QUESTIONS

1 The patient has been given a prescription of furosemide (Lasix) as an adjunct to treatment of hypertension and returns for a follow-up check. Which of the following is the most objective data for determining the *effectiveness* of the drug therapy?
1. Absence of edema in lower extremities
2. Weight loss of 6 lb
3. Blood pressure log notes blood pressure 120/70 mmHg to 134/88 mmHg since discharge
4. Frequency of voiding of at least six times per day

2 The nurse prepares to administer hydrochlorothiazide (Microzide) 25 mg to a patient with hypertension. The potassium lab result is 2.5 mEq. The nurse's best action is to:
1. hold the medication and notify the health care provider.
2. administer the drug with orange juice.
3. administer the drug as ordered.
4. give the patient a banana and recheck the potassium level.

3 The patient is on two antihypertensive drugs. The nurse recognizes that the advantage of combination therapy is:
1. the blood pressure will decrease faster.
2. there will be fewer side effects and greater patient compliance.
3. there is less daily medication dosing.
4. combination therapy will treat the patient's other medical conditions.

4 The class of antihypertensives that increases urine production by affecting the renin–angiotensin–aldosterone pathway is the:
1. calcium channel blockers.
2. adrenergic blockers.
3. ACE inhibitors.
4. direct-acting vasodilators.

5 The nurse is preparing to administer the first dose of enalapril (Vasotec). Identify the potential adverse effects of this medication: (Select all that apply.)
1. Reflex hypertension
2. Hyperkalemia
3. Persistent cough
4. Angioedema
5. Hypotension

6 A patient with significant hypertension unresponsive to other medications is given a prescription for hydralazine (Apresoline). An additional prescription of propranolol (Inderal) is also given to the patient. The patient inquires why two drugs are needed. The nurse's best response would be:
1. giving the two drugs together will lower the blood pressure even more than just one alone.
2. the hydralazine may cause tachycardia and the propranolol will help keep the heart rate within normal limits.
3. the propranolol is to prevent lupus erythematosus from developing.
4. direct-acting vasodilators such as hydralazine cause fluid retention and the propranolol will prevent excessive fluid buildup.

CRITICAL THINKING QUESTIONS

1. A 74-year-old patient has a history of hypertension, mild renal failure, and angina. The patient is on a low-sodium, low-protein diet. The most recent BP is 106/84. Should the nurse give the patient benazepril (Lotensin) as scheduled? Provide a rationale for the decision.

2. A patient with diabetes is on atenolol (Tenormin) for hypertension. Identify a teaching plan for this patient.

3. A patient is having a hypertensive crisis (230/130), and the BP needs to be lowered. The patient has an IV drip of nitroprusside (Nitropress) initiated. How much would the nurse want to lower this patient's BP? Identify three nursing interventions that are crucial when administering this medication.

See Appendix D for answers and rationales for all activities.

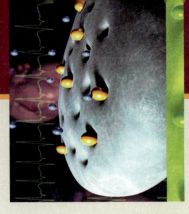

Chapter 24

Drugs for Heart Failure

LEARNING OUTCOMES

After reading this chapter, the student should be able to:

1. Identify the major diseases that accelerate the progression of heart failure.
2. Relate how the symptoms associated with heart failure may be caused by weakened heart muscle and diminished cardiac output.
3. Explain how preload and afterload affect cardiac function.
4. Describe the nurse's role in the pharmacologic management of heart failure.
5. For each of the drug classes listed in Drugs at a Glance, know representative drug examples, and explain their mechanisms of action, primary actions, and important adverse effects.
6. Use the nursing process to care for patients who are receiving drug therapy for heart failure.

KEY TERMS

Heart failure is one of the most common and fatal of the cardiovascular diseases, and its incidence is expected to increase as the population ages. Despite the dramatic decline in mortality for most cardiovascular disease (CVD) that has occurred over the past two decades, the death rate for heart failure has only recently begun to decrease. Although improved treatment of myocardial infarction (MI) and hypertension (HTN) has led to declines in mortality due to heart failure, approximately one in five patients still dies within 1 year of diagnosis of heart failure, and 50% die within 5 years. Historically, this condition was called *congestive* heart failure; however, because not all incidences of this disease are associated with congestion, the more appropriate name is heart failure.

24.1 The Etiology of Heart Failure

Heart failure (HF) is the inability of the ventricles to pump enough blood to meet the body's metabolic demands. Heart failure can be caused by any disorder that affects the heart's ability to receive or eject blood. Whereas weakening of cardiac muscle is a natural consequence of aging, the process can be caused or accelerated by the following:

- Coronary artery disease (CAD)
- Mitral stenosis
- MI
- Chronic HTN
- Diabetes mellitus

Because there is no cure for heart failure, the treatment goals are to prevent, treat, or remove the underlying *causes* when possible. For example, controlling lipid levels and keeping blood pressure within normal limits reduces the incidences of CAD and MI. Maintaining blood glucose within normal values reduces the cardiovascular consequences of uncontrolled diabetes. Thus, for many patients, HF is a preventable condition; controlling associated diseases will greatly reduce the risk of eventual HF. No longer is therapy of HF focused on end stages of the disorder. Pharmacotherapy is now targeted at *prevention* and *slowing the progression* of HF. This change in emphasis has led to significant improvements in survival and the quality of life for patients with HF.

24.2 Cardiovascular Changes in Heart Failure

Although a number of diseases can lead to heart failure, the result is the same: The heart is unable to pump the volume of blood required to meet the metabolic needs of the body. To understand how medications act on the weakened myocardium, it is essential to understand the underlying cardiac physiology.

The right side of the heart receives blood from the venous system and pumps it to the lungs, where the blood receives oxygen and releases carbon dioxide. The blood returns to the left side of the heart, which pumps it to the rest of the body via the aorta. The amount of blood received by the right side should exactly equal that sent out by the left side. If the heart is unable to completely empty the left ventricle, HF may occur. The amount of blood pumped by each ventricle per minute is the **cardiac output**. The relationship between cardiac output and blood pressure is explained in chapter 23∞.

Although many variables affect cardiac output, the two most important factors are preload and afterload. Just before the chambers of the heart contract (systole), they are filled to their maximum capacity with blood. The degree to which the myocardial fibers are stretched just prior to contraction is called **preload**. The more these fibers are stretched, the more forcefully they will contract, a principle called the **Frank–Starling law**. This is somewhat similar to a rubber band; the more it is stretched, the more forcefully it will snap back. The strength of contraction of the heart is called **contractility**. Up to a physiologic limit, *drugs that increase preload and contractility will increase the cardiac output.*

A change in contractility of the heart is called an **inotropic effect**. Drugs that increase contractility are called *positive inotropic agents*. Examples of positive inotropic agents include epinephrine, norepinephrine, thyroid hormone, and dopamine. Drugs that decrease contractility are called *negative inotropic agents*. Examples include quinidine and beta-adrenergic antagonists such as propranolol.

The second important factor affecting cardiac output is **afterload,** the degree of pressure in the aorta that must be overcome for blood to be ejected from the left ventricle. As a simplified example, if the mean arterial pressure in the aorta is 80 mmHg, the left ventricle must generate a minimum of 81 mmHg to open the aortic valve, and even greater pressure to eject the blood from the ventricle and push along the pulse wave through the rest of the systemic circulation. The most common cause of increased afterload is an increase in peripheral resistance due to HTN. As blood pressure increases with HTN, the mean arterial pressure also increases and the force the ventricle has to generate to eject the blood with each heart beat increases. The greater afterload caused by chronic

MyNursingKit | The Beating Heart

PHARMFACTS

Heart Failure

- Heart failure (HF) increases with age. It affects:
  2% of those 40 to 50 years old.
  5% of those 60 to 69 years old.
  10% of those older than age 70.
- More than 57,000 people die of HF each year.
- The incidence of sudden cardiac death is as much as nine times higher in patients with HF than in the general population.
- Heart failure is the most common hospital discharge diagnosis in patients age 65 or older.
- African Americans have one and a half to two times the incidence of HF as whites.
- Heart failure is twice as frequent in hypertensive patients and five times as frequent in persons who have experienced a heart attack.

HTN creates a constant increased workload for the heart. This explains why patients with chronic HTN are more likely to experience HF. *Lowering blood pressure creates less afterload, resulting in less workload for the heart.*

In HF, the myocardium becomes weakened, and the heart cannot eject all the blood it receives. This impairment may occur on the left side, the right side, or on both sides of the heart. If it occurs on the left side, excess blood accumulates in the left ventricle. The wall of the left ventricle thickens and enlarges (hypertrophy) in an attempt to compensate for the increased workload. Over time, changes in the size, shape, and structure of the myocardial cells (myocytes) occur, a process known as **cardiac remodeling.** Because the left ventricle has limits to its ability to compensate for the increased preload, blood "backs up" into the lungs, resulting in the classic symptoms of cough and shortness of breath. Left heart failure is sometimes called *congestive heart failure (CHF).* The pathophysiology of HF is shown in ➤ Figure 24.1.

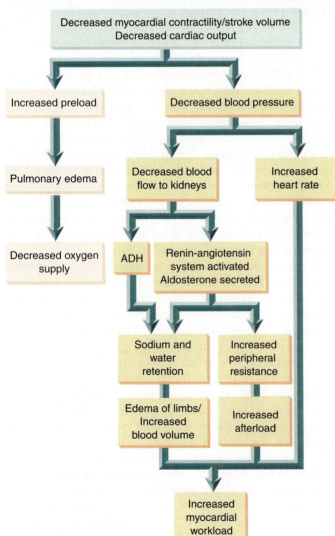

➤ *Figure 24.1* Pathophysiology of heart failure

Although left heart failure is more common, the right side of the heart can also weaken, either simultaneously with the left side or independently of the left side. In right heart failure, the blood backs up into veins, resulting in **peripheral edema** and engorgement of organs such as the liver.

Through proper pharmacotherapy and lifestyle modifications, many patients with HF can be maintained in an asymptomatic state for years. When the heart reaches a stage at which it can no longer handle the workload, *cardiac decompensation* occurs and classic symptoms of HF appear such as dyspnea on exertion, fatigue, pulmonary congestion, and peripheral edema. Lung congestion causes cough and orthopnea (difficulty breathing when recumbent). When pulmonary edema occurs, the patient feels as if he or she is suffocating, and extreme anxiety may result. The condition often worsens at night.

Drugs can relieve the symptoms of heart failure by a number of different mechanisms, including slowing the heart rate, increasing contractility, and reducing the myocardial workload. These mechanisms are shown in Pharmacotherapy Illustrated 24.1.

Over time, the heart may lose its ability to compensate for the increased workload placed upon it. The most common reason why patients experience decompensation is nonadherence with sodium and water restrictions recommended by the health care provider. The second most common reason is nonadherence with drug therapy. The nurse must stress to patients the importance of sodium restriction and drug adherence to maintain a properly functioning heart. Cardiac events such as MI or myocardial ischemia can also precipitate acute HF.

24.3 Treatment of Heart Failure with ACE Inhibitors and Angiotensin Receptor Blockers

ACE inhibitors were approved for the treatment of hypertension in the 1980s. Since then, research studies have clearly demonstrated their ability to slow the progression of heart failure and reduce mortality from this disease. Because of their relative safety, they have replaced digoxin as drugs of choice for the treatment of chronic HF. Indeed, unless specifically contraindicated, all patients with HF and many patients at high risk for HF should receive an ACE inhibitor. The ACE inhibitors used for HF are listed in Table 24.1.

The two primary actions of the ACE inhibitors are to *lower peripheral resistance* (decreased blood pressure) and *inhibit aldosterone secretion* (reduced blood volume). The resultant reduction of arterial blood pressure diminishes the afterload, thus increasing cardiac output. An additional effect of the ACE inhibitors is dilation of veins. This action, which is probably not directly related to their inhibition of angiotensin, decreases pulmonary congestion and reduces peripheral edema. The combined reductions in preload, afterload, and blood volume substantially decrease the work-

PHARMACOTHERAPY ILLUSTRATED

24.1 Mechanisms of Action of Drugs Used for Heart Failure

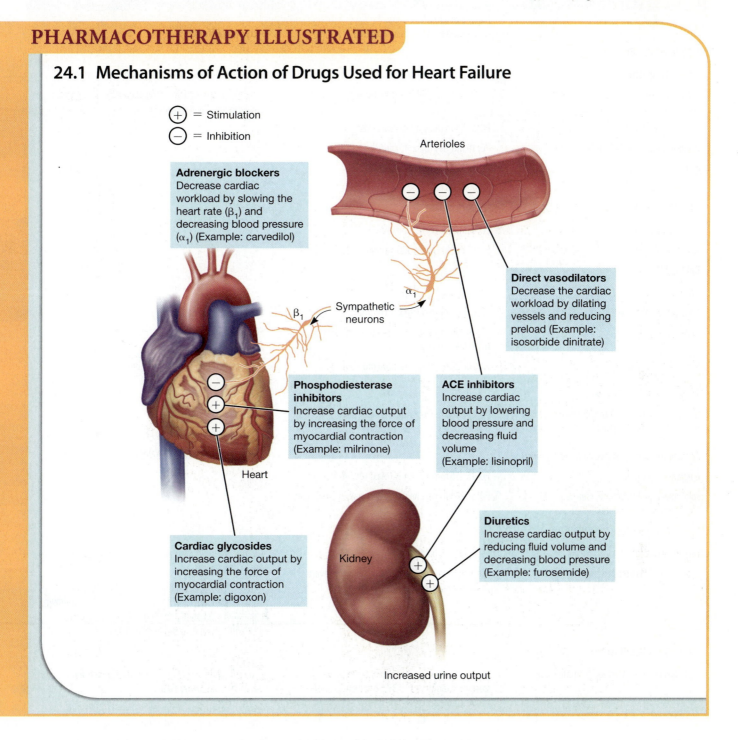

⊕ = Stimulation

⊖ = Inhibition

Arterioles

Adrenergic blockers
Decrease cardiac workload by slowing the heart rate (β_1) and decreasing blood pressure (α_1) (Example: carvedilol)

Direct vasodilators
Decrease the cardiac workload by dilating vessels and reducing preload (Example: isosorbide dinitrate)

α_1

Sympathetic neurons

β_1

Phosphodiesterase inhibitors
Increase cardiac output by increasing the force of myocardial contraction (Example: milrinone)

ACE inhibitors
Increase cardiac output by lowering blood pressure and decreasing fluid volume (Example: lisinopril)

Heart

Cardiac glycosides
Increase cardiac output by increasing the force of myocardial contraction (Example: digoxon)

Diuretics
Increase cardiac output by reducing fluid volume and decreasing blood pressure (Example: furosemide)

Kidney

Increased urine output

load on the heart and allow it to work more efficiently. Patients taking ACE inhibitors experience fewer HF-related symptoms, hospitalizations, and treatment failures. Several ACE inhibitors have been shown to reduce mortality following acute MI when therapy is started soon after the onset of symptoms (chapter 25∞).

Another mechanism for blocking the effects of angiotensin is the use of angiotensin receptor blockers (ARBs). The actions of the ARBs are similar to those of the ACE inhibitors, as would be expected, since both classes inhibit angiotensin. In patients with HF, ARBs show equivalent efficacy to the ACE inhibitors. Valsartan (Diovan) and candesartan (Atacand) were approved to treat HF in 2005. Because research has not yet demonstrated a clear advantage of ARBs over other medications, their use in the treatment of HF is usually reserved for patients unable to tolerate the side effects of ACE inhibitors.

Please refer to Nursing Process Focus: Patients Receiving ACEI (Angiotensin-Covering Enzyme Inhibitor) and ARB (Angiotensin Receptor Blocker) Therapy, page 312 in chapter 23∞, for additional information.

TABLE 24.1 Drugs for Heart Failure

Drug	Route and Adult Dose (max dose where indicated)	Adverse Effects
ACE INHIBITORS		
captopril (Capoten)	PO; 6.25–12.5 mg tid (max: 150 mg/day)	*Headache, dizziness, orthostatic hypotension, cough*
enalapril (Vasotec) (see page 312 for the Prototype Drug box∞)	PO; 2.5 mg qid–bid (max: 40 mg/day)	<u>Severe hypotension (first-dose phenomenon), syncope, angioedema, blood dyscrasias</u>
fosinopril (Monopril)	PO; 5–40 mg/day (max: 40 mg/day)	
ⓟ lisinopril (Prinivil, Zestril)	PO; 10 mg/day (max: 40 mg/day)	
quinapril (Accupril)	PO; 10–20 mg/day (max: 20 mg/day)	
ramipril (Altace)	PO; 2.5–5.0 mg bid (max: 10 mg/day)	
ANGIOTENSIN II RECEPTOR BLOCKERS		
candesartan (Atacand)	PO; 4 mg/day (max: 32 mg/day)	
valsartan (Diovan)	PO; 40 mg bid (max: 320 mg/day)	
DIURETICS		
Loop or High Ceiling		Loop and thiazides:
bumetanide (Bumex)	PO; 0.5–2 mg/day (max: 10 mg/day)	*Electrolyte imbalances, orthostatic hypotension*
furosemide (Lasix)	PO; 20–80 mg in one or more divided doses (max: 600 mg/day)	<u>Severe hypotension, dehydration, hypokalemia, hyponatremia, ototoxicity (loop diuretics)</u>
torsemide (Demadex)	PO; 10–20 mg/day (max: 200 mg/day)	
Thiazide and Thiazide-Like		
hydrochlorothiazide (Microzide) (see page 304 for the Prototype Drug box∞)	PO; 25–200 mg in a single dose or three divided doses (max: 200 mg/day)	Potassium-sparing:
Potassium-Sparing (Aldosterone Antagonist)		*Hyperkalemia, gynecomastia in males, fatigue*
eplerenone (Inspra)	PO; 25–50 mg once daily (max: 100 mg/day)	<u>Dysrhythmias due to hyperkalemia</u>
spironolactone (Aldactone) (see page 424 for the Prototype Drug box∞)	PO; 5–200 mg in divided doses (max: 200 mg/day)	
BETA-ADRENERGIC BLOCKER		
carvedilol (Coreg)	PO; 3.125 mg bid for 2 wk (max: 25–50 mg bid)	*Fatigue, insomnia, drowsiness, impotence or decreased libido, bradycardia, confusion*
ⓟ metoprolol extended release (Toprol-XL)	PO; 25 mg/day for 2 wk; 12.5 mg/day for severe cases (max: 200 mg/day)	<u>Agranulocytosis, laryngospasm, Stevens–Johnson syndrome, anaphylaxis; if the drug is abruptly withdrawn, palpitations, rebound hypertension, life-threatening dysrhythmias, or myocardial ischemia may occur</u>
DIRECT VASODILATOR		
hydralazine with isosorbide dinitrate (BiDil)	PO; 1–2 tablets tid (each tablet contains 20 mg isosorbide dinitrate and 37.5 mg hydralazine) (max: 2 tablets/day)	*Headache, flushing of face, orthostatic hypotension, dizziness, reflex tachycardia* <u>Fainting, severe headache, severe hypotension with overdose, lupuslike reaction (hydralazine)</u>
nesiritide (Natrecor)	IV; 2 mcg/kg bolus followed by continuous infusion at 0.01 mcg/kg/min.	*Hypotension, increased serum creatinine, headache* <u>Dysrhythmias</u>
CARDIAC GLYCOSIDE		
ⓟ digoxin (Digitek, Lanoxin, Lanoxicaps)	PO; 0.125–0.5 mg/day	*Nausea, vomiting, headache, and visual disturbances such as seeing halos, a yellow-green tinge, or blurring* <u>Dysrhythmias, AV block</u>
PHOSPHODIESTERASE INHIBITORS		
inamrinone (Inocor)	IV; 0.75 mg/kg bolus given slowly over 2–3 min; then 5–10 mcg/kg/min (max: 10 mg/kg/day)	*Headache, hypotension* <u>Dysrhythmias</u>
ⓟ milrinone (Primacor)	IV; 50 mcg over 10 min; then 0.375–0.75 mcg/kg/min	

Italics indicate common adverse effects; <u>underlining</u> indicates serious adverse effects.

Pr Prototype Drug | Lisinopril *(Prinivil, Zestril)*

Therapeutic Class: Drug for heart failure and HTN   **Pharmacologic Class:** ACE inhibitor

ACTIONS AND USES
Because of its value in the treatment of both HF and hypertension, lisinopril has become one of the most frequently prescribed drugs. Lisinopril acts by inhibiting angiotensin-converting enzyme and decreasing aldosterone secretion. Blood pressure is decreased and cardiac output is increased. As with other ACE inhibitors, 2 to 3 weeks of therapy may be required to reach maximum effectiveness, and several months of therapy may be needed for cardiac function to return to normal. An additional indication for lisinopril is to improve survival in patients when given within 24 hours of an acute MI. Treatment of migraines is an off-label indication for lisinopril.

ADMINISTRATION ALERTS
- Measure blood pressure just prior to administering lisinopril to be certain that effects are lasting for 24 hours and to determine whether the patient's blood pressure is within acceptable range.
- Safety and efficacy have been established for the use of this medication in children age 6 and older.
- Geriatric patients may have higher blood levels related to renal failure.
- Pregnancy category C (first trimester) or D (second and third trimesters). Use during the second and third trimesters of pregnancy may result in injury or death to the fetus. Discontinue use as soon as pregnancy is suspected.

PHARMACOKINETICS
Onset: 1 h
Peak: 6–8 h
Half-life: 12 h
Duration: 24 h

ADVERSE EFFECTS
Lisinopril is tolerated well by most patients. The most common adverse effects are cough, headache, dizziness, orthostatic hypotension, and rash. Hyperkalemia may occur during therapy; thus, electrolyte levels are usually monitored periodically. Other effects include taste disturbances, chest pain, nausea, vomiting, and diarrhea. Though rare, angioedema is a serious adverse effect.

Contraindications: Lisinopril is contraindicated in patients with hyperkalemia and in those who have previously experienced angioedema caused by ACE inhibitor therapy. It should not be used during pregnancy because it is a category D drug during the second and third trimesters.

INTERACTIONS
Drug–Drug: Indomethacin and other NSAIDs may interact with lisinopril, causing decreased antihypertensive activity. Because of the additive hypotensive action of lisinopril and diuretics, combined therapy with these or other antihypertensive drugs should be carefully monitored. When lisinopril is taken concurrently with potassium-sparing diuretics, hyperkalemia may result. Lisinopril may increase lithium levels and cause lithium toxicity.

Lab Tests: May cause positive ANA titer and increase values of the following: BUN, serum bilirubin, serum alkaline phosphatase, AST, and ALT.

Herbal/Food: Excessive intake of foods rich in potassium and potassium-based salt substitutes should be avoided because of the possibility of hyperkalemia.

Treatment of Overdose: Overdose causes hypotension, which may be treated with the administration of normal saline or a vasopressor.

Refer to MyNursingKit for a Nursing Process Focus specific to this drug.

24.4 Treatment of Heart Failure with Diuretics

Diuretics are common drugs for the treatment of patients with HF because they produce few adverse effects and are effective at increasing urine flow and reducing blood volume, peripheral edema, and pulmonary congestion. When diuretics reduce fluid volume and lower blood pressure, the workload on the heart is reduced, and cardiac output increases. Diuretics are rarely used alone but rather are prescribed in combination with ACE inhibitors or other HF drugs. Because clinical research has not demonstrated their effectiveness in slowing the progression of HF or in decreasing mortality associated with the disease, diuretics are indicated only when there is evidence of fluid retention. In patients presenting with fluid retention, especially with symptoms of severe pulmonary congestion or peripheral edema, diuretics are essential medications. Selected diuretics are listed in Table 24.1. Additional details on diuretics may be found in chapter 30⬥.

Of the diuretic classes, the loop diuretics such as furosemide are most commonly prescribed for HF because of their effectiveness in removing fluid from the body. Loop diuretics are also able to function in patients with renal impairment, an advantage for many patients with decompensated HF. Another major advantage in acute HF is that loop diuretics act quickly, especially IV formulations, which work within minutes.

Thiazide diuretics are also used in the pharmacotherapy of HF. Because they are less effective than the loop diuretics, thiazides are generally reserved for patients with mild to moderate HF. They are sometimes combined with loop diuretics to achieve a more effective diuresis in patients with acute HF.

Potassium-sparing diuretics have limited roles in the treatment of HF because of their low efficacy. Spironolactone, however, is an exception. In addition to being a potassium-sparing diuretic, spironolactone is classified as an *aldosterone antagonist*. Clinical research has demonstrated that spironolactone blocks the deleterious effects of aldosterone on the heart. Spironolactone has been shown to decrease mortality due to sudden death, as well as slow the progression to advanced HF.

Please refer to Nursing Process Focus: Patients Receiving Diuretic Therapy, page 305 in chapter 23⬥, for additional information.

Pr Prototype Drug | Furosemide *(Lasix)*

Therapeutic Class: Drug for heart failure and HTN   **Pharmcologic Class:** Diuretic (loop type)

ACTIONS AND USES

Furosemide is often used in the treatment of acute HF because it has the ability to remove large amounts of excess fluid from the patient in a short period. When given IV, diuresis begins within 5 minutes, giving patients quick relief from their distressing symptoms. Furosemide acts by preventing the reabsorption of sodium and chloride in the loop of Henle region of the nephron. Compared with other diuretics, furosemide is particularly beneficial when cardiac output and renal flow are severely diminished.

ADMINISTRATION ALERTS

- Check the patient's serum potassium levels before administering the drug. If potassium levels are below normal, notify the health care provider before administering.

- Due to the prolonged half-life in premature infants and neonates, the drug must be used with caution.

- Geriatric patients may require lower doses.

- Pregnancy category C

PHARMACOKINETICS

Onset: 30–60 min PO; 5 min IV

Peak: 60–70 min PO; 20–60 min IV

Half-life: 30–60 min

Duration: 6–8 h PO; 2 h IV

ADVERSE EFFECTS

Adverse effects of furosemide, like those of most diuretics, involve potential electrolyte imbalances, the most important of which is hypokalemia. Because furosemide is so effective, fluid loss must be carefully monitored to prevent possible dehydration and hypotension. Hypovolemia may cause orthostatic hypotension and syncope.

Contraindications: Contraindications include hypersensitivity to furosemide or sulfonamides, anuria, hepatic coma, and severe fluid or electrolyte depletion.

INTERACTIONS

Drug–Drug: Because hypokalemia may cause dysrhythmias in patients taking cardiac glycosides, combination therapy with digoxin must be carefully monitored. Concurrent use with corticosteroids, amphotericin B, or other potassium-depleting drugs can result in hypokalemia. When given with lithium, elimination of lithium is decreased, causing a higher risk of toxicity. Furosemide may diminish the hypoglycemic effects of sulfonylureas and insulin.

Lab Tests: Furosemide may increase values for the following: blood glucose, BUN, serum amylase, cholesterol, triglycerides, and serum electrolytes.

Herbal/Food: Unknown

Treatment of Overdose: Overdose will result in hypotension and severe fluid and electrolyte loss. Treatment is supportive, with replacement of fluids and electrolytes, and the possible administration of a vasopressor.

Refer to MyNursingKit for a Nursing Process Focus specific to this drug.

24.5 Treatment of Heart Failure with Cardiac Glycosides

Cardiac glycosides were once used as arrow poisons by African tribes and as medicines by the ancient Egyptians and Romans. Their value in treating heart disorders has been known for over 2,000 years. Extracted from the beautiful flowering plants *Digitalis purpurea* (purple foxglove) and *Digitalis lanata* (white foxglove), drugs from this class are sometimes called *digitalis glycosides*. Until the discovery of ACE inhibitors, cardiac glycosides were the mainstay of HF treatment. Digoxin (Lanoxin) is the only drug in this class available in the United States. The routes and dose for digoxin are listed in Table 24.1.

The primary actions of digoxin are to cause the heart to beat more forcefully (positive inotropic effect) and more slowly, thus improving cardiac output. The reduced heart rate, combined with more forceful contractions, allows for much greater efficiency of the heart.

Although digoxin clearly produces symptomatic improvement in patients, it does not reduce mortality from HF. Because of the development of safer and more effective drugs such as ACE inhibitors, digoxin is now primarily used for more advanced stages of HF, in combination with other agents.

The margin of safety between a therapeutic dose and a toxic dose of digoxin is quite narrow, and severe adverse effects may result from unmonitored treatment. Digitalization refers to a procedure in which the dose of digoxin is gradually increased until tissues become saturated with the drug, and the symptoms of HF diminish. If the patient is critically ill, digitalization can be accomplished rapidly with IV doses in a controlled clinical environment and in which potential adverse effects are carefully monitored. Patients who begin treatment outside the hospital may experience digitalization with digoxin over a period of 7 days, using oral dosing. In either case, the goal is to determine the proper dose of drug that may be administered without undue adverse effects. Frequent serum digoxin levels should be obtained during therapy, and the dosage adjusted based on the laboratory results and the patient's clinical response.

24.6 Treatment of Heart Failure with Beta-Adrenergic Blockers (Antagonists)

Cardiac glycosides and other drugs that produce a positive inotropic effect increase the strength of myocardial contraction and are often used to reverse symptoms of HF. It may seem surprising, then, to find beta-adrenergic blockers—drugs that exhibit a *negative* inotropic effect—prescribed for this disease. Although this class of drugs does indeed

Pr Prototype Drug | Digoxin (Digitek, Lanoxin, Lanoxicaps)

Therapeutic Class: Drug for heart failure   **Pharmacologic Class:** Cardiac glycoside

ACTIONS AND USES

The primary benefit of digoxin is its ability to increase the contractility or strength of myocardial contraction—a positive inotropic action. Digoxin accomplishes this by inhibiting Na^+-K^+ ATPase, the critical enzyme responsible for pumping sodium ions out of the myocardial cell in exchange for potassium ions. As sodium accumulates, calcium ions are released from their storage areas in the cell. The release of calcium ions produces a more forceful contraction of the myocardial fibers.

By increasing myocardial contractility, digoxin directly increases cardiac output, thus alleviating symptoms of HF and improving exercise tolerance. The improved cardiac output results in increased urine production and a desirable reduction in blood volume, relieving distressing symptoms of pulmonary congestion and peripheral edema.

In addition to its positive inotropic effect, digoxin affects impulse conduction in the heart. Digoxin has the ability to suppress the sinoatrial (SA) node and slow electrical conduction through the atrioventricular (AV) node. Because of these actions, digoxin is sometimes used to treat dysrhythmias, as discussed in chapter 26∞.

ADMINISTRATION ALERTS

- Take the apical pulse for 1 full minute, noting rate, rhythm, and quality before administering. If the pulse is below the parameter established by the health care provider (usually 60 beats per minute), withhold the dose and notify the provider.
- Check for recent serum digoxin level results before administering. If the level is higher than the parameter established by the health care provider (usually 1.8 ng/mL), withhold the dose and notify the provider.
- Use with caution in geriatric and pediatric patients because these populations may have inadequate renal and hepatic metabolic enzymes.
- Pregnancy category A

PHARMACOKINETICS

Onset: 30–90 min PO; 5–30 min IV

Peak: 4–6 h PO; 1.5 h IV

Half-life: 3–4 days

Duration: 6–8 days

ADVERSE EFFECTS

The most dangerous adverse effect of digoxin is its ability to create dysrhythmias, particularly in patients who have hypokalemia or impaired renal function. Because diuretics can cause hypokalemia and are often used to treat HF, concurrent use of digoxin and diuretics must be carefully monitored. Other adverse effects of digoxin therapy include nausea, vomiting, fatigue, anorexia, and visual disturbances such as seeing halos, a yellow-green tinge, or blurring. Periodic serum drug levels should be obtained to determine whether the digoxin concentration is within the therapeutic range.

Contraindications: Patients with AV block or ventricular dysrhythmias unrelated to HF should not receive digoxin because the drug may worsen these conditions. Digoxin should be administered with caution to older adults because these patients experience a higher incidence of adverse effects. Patients with renal impairment should receive lower doses of digoxin, because the drug is excreted by this route. The drug should be used with caution in patients with MI, cor pulmonale, or hypothyroidism.

INTERACTIONS

Drug–Drug: Digoxin interacts with many drugs. Concurrent use of digoxin with diuretics can cause hypokalemia and increase the risk of dysrhythmias. Use with ACE inhibitors, spironolactone, or potassium supplements can lead to hyperkalemia and reduce the therapeutic action of digoxin. Administration of digoxin with other positive inotropic agents can cause additive effects on heart contractility. Concurrent use with beta blockers may result in additive bradycardia. Antacids and cholesterol-lowering drugs can decrease the absorption of digoxin. If calcium is administered IV together with digoxin, it can increase the risk of dysrhythmias. Quinidine, verapamil, amiodarone, and alprazolam will decrease the distribution and excretion of digoxin, thus increasing the risk of digoxin toxicity.

Lab Tests: Unknown

Herbal/Food: Ginseng may increase the risk of digoxin toxicity. Ma huang and ephedra may induce dysrhythmias.

Treatment of Overdose: Digoxin overdose can be fatal. Specific therapy involves IV infusion of digoxin immune fab (Digibind), which contains antibodies specific for digoxin.

Refer to MyNursingKit for a Nursing Process Focus specific to this drug.

---

have the potential to worsen HF, they have become standard therapy for many patients with this chronic disorder. Only two beta blockers are approved for the treatment of HF—carvedilol (Coreg) and metoprolol extended release (Toprol-XL). The doses of these agents are listed in Table 24.1.

Patients with HF have excessive activation of the sympathetic nervous system, which damages the heart and leads to progression of the disease. Beta-adrenergic antagonists block the cardiac actions of the sympathetic nervous system, thus slowing the heart rate and reducing blood pressure. Workload on the heart is decreased; after several months of therapy, heart size, shape, and function return to normal in some patients. Extensive clinical research has demonstrated that the

proper use of beta blockers can dramatically reduce the number of HF-associated hospitalizations and deaths.

To benefit patients with HF, however, beta blockers must be administered in a very specific manner. Initial doses must be 1/10 to 1/20 of the target dose. Doses are doubled every 2 weeks until the optimum dose is reached. If therapy is begun with too high a dose, or the dose is increased too rapidly, beta blockers can worsen HF. Beta blockers are rarely used as monotherapy for this disease, but instead are usually combined with other agents, especially ACE inhibitors.

The basic pharmacology of the beta blockers is presented in chapter 13∞. Other uses of the beta-adrenergic blockers are discussed elsewhere in this text: for hypertension in

NURSING PROCESS FOCUS — PATIENTS RECEIVING DIGOXIN THERAPY

Assessment	Potential Nursing Diagnoses
Baseline assessment prior to administration: ■ Understand the reason the drug has been prescribed in order to assess for therapeutic effects. ■ Obtain a complete health history including cardiovascular (including previous MI, heart failure, valvular disease), renal dysfunction, dysrhythmias (especially heart block), and pregnancy or lactation. Obtain a drug history including allergies, current prescription and OTC drugs, herbal preparations, and alcohol use. Be alert to possible drug interactions. ■ Obtain baseline weight, vital signs (especially pulse and BP), breath sounds, and ECG. Assess for location and character of edema if present. ■ Evaluate appropriate laboratory findings, electrolytes, especially potassium level, renal function studies, and lipid profiles.	■ Decreased Cardiac Output (disease process or related to adverse effects of drug therapy) ■ Fatigue (disease process or related to adverse effects of drug therapy) ■ Altered Tissue Perfusion (related to disease process) ■ Activity Intolerance (related to disease process or adverse effects of drug therapy) ■ Deficient Knowledge (drug therapy) ■ Risk for Falls, Risk for Injury (related to adverse effects)
Assessment throughout administration: ■ Assess for desired therapeutic effects (e.g., heart rate and blood pressure return to, or remain within, normal limits; urine output returns to, or is within, normal limits; respiratory congestion (if present) is improved; peripheral edema (if present) is improved; level of consciousness, skin color, capillary refill, and other signs of adequate perfusion are within normal limits; fatigue lessens). ■ Continue periodic monitoring of electrolytes, especially potassium, renal function, and drug levels. ■ Assess for adverse effects: bradycardia, nausea, vomiting, anorexia, visual changes, fatigue, dizziness, or drowsiness. A pulse rate below 60 or above 100, palpitations, significant dizziness or syncope, persistent anorexia or vomiting, and visual changes should be reported to the health care provider immediately. ■ Exercise caution when giving digoxin to the elderly, pediatric patients, or patients with renal insufficiency. Immature or declines in renal function make these populations more susceptible to adverse effects.	

Planning: Patient Goals and Expected Outcomes

The patient will:
■ Experience therapeutic effects (e.g., heart rate and blood pressure remain within established parameters, urine output increases to normal, fatigue lessens, lung sounds clear, peripheral edema decreases).
■ Be free from, or experience minimal, adverse effects.
■ Verbalize an understanding of the drug's use, adverse effects, and required precautions.
■ Demonstrate proper self-administration of the medication (e.g., dose, timing, when to notify provider).

Implementation

Interventions and (Rationales)	Patient and Family Education
Ensuring therapeutic effects: ■ Continue frequent assessments as described earlier for therapeutic effects. (Blood pressure and pulse should return to within normal limits or within parameters set by the provider; urine output returns to within normal limits; peripheral edema decreases; and lung sounds clear.)	■ Teach the patient, family, or caregiver how to monitor pulse and blood pressure. Ensure the proper use and functioning of any home equipment obtained.
■ Encourage appropriate lifestyle changes. Provide for dietitian consultation as needed. (Healthy lifestyle changes will support the benefits of drug therapy.)	■ Encourage the patient to adopt a healthy lifestyle of low-fat food choices, increased exercise, decreased alcohol consumption, and smoking cessation. Provide educational materials on low-fat, low-sodium food choices. ■ Instruct the patient to increase intake of potassium-rich foods such as bananas, apricots, kidney beans, sweet potatoes, and peanut butter.

NURSING PROCESS FOCUS   **PATIENTS RECEIVING DIGOXIN THERAPY** *(Continued)*

Implementation

Interventions and (Rationales)	Patient and Family Education
Minimizing adverse effects: ▪ Continue to monitor vital signs. Take an apical pulse (AP) for 1 full minute before giving the drug. Hold the drug and notify provider if heart rate is below 60 or above 100. Monitor the ECG during digitalization period for dysrhythmias and bradycardia. (Digoxin is a positive inotrope and slows heart rate as it strengthens contractility.)	▪ Teach the patient, family, or caregiver how to take a peripheral pulse before taking the drug. Assist the patient to find the pulse area most convenient and easily felt. Record daily pulse rates and bring record to each health care visit. Instruct the patient to not take the drug if the pulse is below 60 or above 100 and to contact the provider for further direction. If the patient, or family/caregiver buys a stethoscope to take pulse, ensure proper understanding of heart sounds (i.e., "lub-dub" of heartbeat is *ONE* heartbeat), appropriate stethoscope use, and have patient, family, or caregiver return demonstrate.
▪ Continue to monitor periodic electrolyte levels, especially potassium, renal function labs, drug levels, and ECG. (Hypokalemia increases the risk of dysrhythmias. Serum digoxin levels should remain less than 1.8 ng/mL.)	▪ Instruct the patient on the need to return periodically for lab work. ▪ Advise the patient to carry a wallet identification card or wear medical identification jewelry indicating digoxin therapy.
▪ Weigh the patient daily and report a weight gain or loss of 1 kg or more in a 24-hour period. (Daily weight is an accurate measure of fluid status and takes into account intake, output, and insensible losses. Weight gain or edema may signal impending heart failure with reduced organ perfusion, stimulating renin release.)	▪ Have the patient weigh self daily, ideally at the same time of day, and record weight along with pulse measurements. Have the patient report a weight loss or gain of more than 1 kg (approximately 2 lb) in a 24-hour period.
▪ Monitor for signs of worsening heart failure (e.g., increasing dyspnea or postural nocturnal dyspnea, rales or "crackles" in lungs, frothy pink-tinged sputum) and report immediately. (If signs and symptoms worsen, other treatment options may need to be considered.)	▪ Instruct the patient to immediately report any severe shortness of breath, frothy sputum, profound fatigue, or swelling of extremities as possible signs of heart failure.
▪ Report signs of possible digoxin toxicity immediately to the provider and obtain a serum drug level. (Digoxin levels should remain less than 1.8 ng/mL. Signs and symptoms such as bradycardia, nausea and vomiting, anorexia, visual changes, depression or changes in level of consciousness, fatigue, dizziness, or syncope should be reported.)	▪ Instruct the patient or caregiver on signs to report to provider. Encourage the patient to promptly report any significant change in overall health or mental activity.
▪ Use extra caution when measuring the dose of medication ordered and use extreme caution when measuring liquid doses, especially for pediatric patients. (Digoxin has a long half-life and toxic levels may result with only small amounts of additional drug.)	▪ Caution the patient on taking the precise dose of medication ordered, not doubling dose if a dose is missed, and to use extreme caution when measuring liquid doses, especially for pediatric patients.
Patient understanding of drug therapy: ▪ Use opportunities during administration of medications and during assessments to discuss rationale for drug therapy, desired therapeutic outcomes, most common adverse effects, parameters for when to call the provider, and any necessary monitoring or precautions. (Using time during nursing care helps to optimize and reinforce key teaching areas.)	▪ The patient should be able to state the reason for drug; appropriate dose and scheduling; what adverse effects to observe for and when to report; and the anticipated length of medication therapy.
Patient self-administration of drug therapy: ▪ When administering medications, instruct the patient, family, or caregiver in proper self-administration techniques. (Proper administration improves the effectiveness of the drug.)	▪ Instruct the patient in proper administration techniques, followed by return-demonstration. ▪ The patient should be able to discuss appropriate dosing and administration needs.

Evaluation of Outcome Criteria

Evaluate the effectiveness of drug therapy by confirming that patient goals and expected outcomes have been met (see "Planning").

See Table 24.1 under "Cardiac Glycoside" for more information about digoxin.

Pr Prototype Drug | Metoprolol *(Lopressor, Toprol XL)*

Therapeutic Class: Drug for heart failure and HTN   **Pharmacologic Class:** Beta-adrenergic blocker

ACTIONS AND USES

Metoprolol is a selective beta$_1$-adrenergic blocker available in tablet, sustained-release tablet, and IV forms. At higher doses, it may also affect beta$_2$ receptors in bronchial smooth muscle. The drug acts by reducing sympathetic stimulation of the heart, thus decreasing cardiac workload. Metoprolol has been found to slow the progression of HF and to significantly reduce the long-term consequences of the disease. It is usually combined with other HF drugs such as ACE inhibitors. Metoprolol is also approved for angina, HTN, and for reducing cardiac complications following an MI.

ADMINISTRATION ALERTS

- During IV administration, monitor the ECG, blood pressure, and pulse frequently.
- Assess the pulse and blood pressure before oral administration. Hold if the pulse is below 60 beats per minute or if the patient is hypotensive.
- Advise the patient not to crush or chew sustained-release tablets.
- Safety and efficacy in children under age 6 have not been established.
- Doses should be reduced for elderly patients because they are at risk for dizziness and falls.
- Pregnancy category C

> #### PHARMACOKINETICS
> **Onset:** 10–15 min; sustained release, unknown
> **Peak:** 1.5–4 h; 6–12 h sustained release
> **Half-life:** 3–4 h
> **Duration:** 6 h (24 h sustained release)

ADVERSE EFFECTS

Because it is selective for blocking beta$_1$ receptors in the heart, metoprolol has few adverse effects on other autonomic targets and thus is preferred over non-selective beta blockers such as propranolol for patients with respiratory disorders. Adverse effects are generally minor and relate to its autonomic activity, such as slowing of the heart rate and hypotension. Because of its multiple effects on the heart, patients with heart failure should be carefully monitored. Other frequent adverse effects include abnormal sexual function, drowsiness, fatigue, and insomnia.

Contraindications: This drug is contraindicated in patients with asthma, cardiogenic shock, sinus bradycardia, heart block greater than first degree, and overt cardiac failure.

INTERACTIONS

Drug–Drug: Concurrent use with digoxin may result in bradycardia. Oral contraceptives may cause increased metoprolol effects. Use with alcohol or antihypertensives may result in additive hypotension. Metoprolol may enhance the hypoglycemic effects of insulin and oral hypoglycemic agents.

Lab Tests: Metoprolol may increase values for the following: uric acid, lipids, potassium, bilirubin, alkaline phosphatase, creatinine, and antinuclear antibody.

Herbal/Food: Unknown

Treatment of Overdose: Atropine or isoproterenol can be used to reverse bradycardia caused by metoprolol overdose. Hypotension may be reversed by a vasopressor such as parenteral dopamine or dobutamine.

Refer to MyNursingKit for a Nursing Process Focus specific to this drug.

---

chapter 23∞, for dysrhythmias in chapter 26∞, and for angina/myocardial infarction in chapter 25∞.

Please refer to Nursing Process Focus: Patients Receiving Adrenergic-Antagonist Therapy on page 316 in chapter 23∞ for additional information.

24.7 Treatment of Heart Failure with Vasodilators

The two primary drugs in this class, hydralazine (Apresoline) and isosorbide dinitrate (Isordil), act directly to relax blood vessels and lower blood pressure. Hydralazine acts on arterioles. It is an effective antihypertensive drug, although it is not a drug of first choice for this indication. Isosorbide dinitrate (Isordil) is an organic nitrate that acts on veins. The drug is not very effective as monotherapy, and tolerance develops to its actions with continued use.

Because the two drugs act synergistically, isosorbide dinitrate is combined with hydralazine in the treatment of HF. BiDil is a fixed dose combination of 20 mg of isosorbide dinitrate with 37.5 mg of hydralazine. The high incidence of

adverse effects, including reflex tachycardia and orthostatic hypotension, however, limits their use to patients who cannot tolerate ACE inhibitors. Hydralazine is featured as a prototype drug in chapter 23∞. A Nursing Process Focus: Patients Receiving Direct Vasodilator Therapy can be found on page 320 in chapter 13∞.

A third vasodilator used for HF is very different than hydralazine or isosorbide dinitrate. Nesiritide (Natrecor) is a small-peptide hormone, produced through recombinant DNA technology, that is structurally identical to human beta-type natriuretic peptide (hBNP). When heart failure occurs, the ventricles begin to secrete hBNP in response to the increased stretch on the ventricular walls. hBNP enhances diuresis and renal excretion of sodium.

In therapeutic doses, nesiritide causes vasodilation, which contributes to reduced preload. By reducing preload and afterload, the drug compensates for diminished cardiac function. The use of nesiritide is very limited because it can rapidly cause severe hypotension. The drug is given by IV infusion, and patients require continuous monitoring. It is approved only for patients with acutely decompensated heart failure.

24.8 Treatment of Heart Failure with Phosphodiesterase Inhibitors and Other Inotropic Drugs

Advanced HF can be a medical emergency, and prompt, effective treatment is necessary to avoid organ failure or death. In addition to high doses of diuretics, use of positive inotropic drugs is often necessary. The two primary classes of inotropic agents used for decompensated HF are phosphodiesterase inhibitors and beta-adrenergic agonists.

In the 1980s, two drugs became available that block the enzyme **phosphodiesterase** in cardiac and smooth muscle. Blocking phosphodiesterase has the effect of increasing the amount of calcium available for myocardial contraction. The inhibition results in two main actions that benefit patients with HF: a positive inotropic action and vasodilation. Cardiac output is improved because of the increase in contractility and the decrease in left ventricular afterload. The phosphodiesterase inhibitors have a very brief half-life and are occasionally used for the short-term control of acute heart failure. The doses of these agents are listed in Table 24.1.

Because of their toxicity phosphodiesterase inhibitors are reserved for patients who have not responded to ACE inhibitors or cardiac glycosides, and they are generally used for only 2 to 3 days. Prior to 2000, inamrinone was called amrinone. The name was changed to prevent medication errors: The name *amrinone* looked and sounded too similar to amiodarone, an antidysrhythmic drug.

Beta-adrenergic agonists occasionally used for HF include isoproterenol (Isuprel), epinephrine, norepinephrine, dopamine, and dobutamine. Dobutamine has been a traditional drug of choice in this class because it has the ability to increase myocardial contractility rapidly and effectively, with minimal changes to heart rate or blood pressure. This is important because increases in heart rate or blood pressure increase the oxygen demands on the heart and possibly worsen HF. Therapy with dobutamine is usually limited to 72 hours. The two most common adverse effects of beta agonists are tachycardia and dysrhythmias. The basic pharmacology of the beta-adrenergic agonists was presented in chapter 13∞. Epinephrine is featured as a prototype drug for anaphylaxis on page 414 in chapter 29, and dopamine is featured as a prototype drug for shock on page 412 in chapter 29∞.

HOME & COMMUNITY CONSIDERATIONS

Psychosocial Issues and Adherence in Patients with Heart Failure

Patients with depression and lack of social support who have HF have been shown to be less adherent with their drug therapy regimen. Patients are also less likely to implement positive lifestyle modifications when depressed. The nurse should assess these issues in patients with HF and intervene appropriately when warranted. Patients may be referred to cardiac rehabilitation programs, which have been shown to increase adherence. It has been established that lifestyle changes are frequently related to the drug therapy (e.g., reduced sexual desire and performance problems). Many patients weigh the lifestyle changes against the drug's benefits and determine that the adverse effects outweigh the benefits. When patients can no longer maintain what they consider a normal lifestyle, they may become depressed.

COMPLEMENTARY AND ALTERNATIVE THERAPIES

Carnitine for Heart Disease

Carnitine is a natural substance structurally similar to amino acids. Its primary function in metabolism is to move fatty acids from the bloodstream into cells, where carnitine assists in the breakdown of lipids and the production of energy. The best food sources of carnitine are organ meat, fish, muscle meats, and milk products. Carnitine is available as a supplement in several forms, including L-carnitine, D-carnitine, and acetyl-L-carnitine. D-carnitine is associated with potential adverse effects, and should be avoided.

Carnitine has been claimed to enhance energy and sports performance, heart health, memory, immune function, and male fertility. It is sometimes marketed as a "fat burner" for weight reduction.

Carnitine has been extensively studied. There is solid evidence to support supplementation in patients who are deficient in carnitine. Although a normal diet supplies 300 mg per day, certain patients, such as vegetarians or those with heart disease, may need additional amounts. Carnitine supplementation has been shown to improve exercise tolerance in patients with angina. The use of carnitine may prevent the occurrence of dysrhythmias in the early stages of heart disease. Carnitine has also been shown to decrease triglyceride levels while increasing HDL serum levels, thus helping to minimize one of the major risk factors associated with heart disease. Research has not shown carnitine supplementation to be of significant benefit in enhancing sports performance or weight loss.

Pr Prototype Drug | Milrinone *(Primacor)*

Therapeutic Class: Drug for heart failure   **Pharmacologic Class:** Phosphodiesterase inhibitor

ACTIONS AND USES
Of the two phosphodiesterase inhibitors available, milrinone is generally preferred because it has a shorter half-life and fewer side effects. It is given only intravenously and is primarily used for the short-term therapy of advanced HF. The drug has a rapid onset of action. Immediate effects of milrinone include an increased force of myocardial contraction and an increase in cardiac output.

ADMINISTRATION ALERTS
- When this medication is administered IV, a microdrip set and an infusion pump should be used.
- Safety and efficacy have not been established in geriatric and pediatric patients.
- Pregnancy category C

PHARMACOKINETICS
Onset: 2–10 min
Peak: 10 min
Half-life: 3–6 h
Duration: Variable

ADVERSE EFFECTS
The most serious adverse effect of milrinone is ventricular dysrhythmia, which may occur in 1 of every 10 patients taking the drug. The patient's ECG should be monitored continuously during the infusion of the drug. Blood pressure is also continuously monitored during the infusion to prevent hypotension. Less serious side effects include headache, nausea, and vomiting.

Contraindications: The only contraindication to milrinone is previous hypersensitivity to the drug. Milrinone should be used with caution in patients with preexisting dysrhythmias.

INTERACTIONS
Drug–Drug: Milrinone interacts with disopyramide, causing excessive hypotension. Caution should be used when administering milrinone with digoxin, dobutamine, or other inotropic drugs, since their positive inotropic effects on the heart may be additive.

Lab Tests: Unknown

Herbal/Food: Unknown

Treatment of Overdose: Overdose causes hypotension, which is treated with the administration of normal saline or a vasopressor.

Refer to MyNursingKit for a Nursing Process Focus specific to this drug.

 Chapter REVIEW

KEY CONCEPTS

The numbered key concepts provide a succinct summary of the important points from the corresponding numbered section within the chapter. If any of these points are not clear, refer to the numbered section within the chapter for review.

24.1 Heart failure is closely associated with chronic hypertension, coronary artery disease, and diabetes.

24.2 The body attempts to compensate for HF by increasing cardiac output. Preload and afterload are two primary factors determining cardiac output.

24.3 ACE inhibitors reduce symptoms of HF by lowering blood pressure, reducing peripheral edema, and increasing cardiac output. They are drugs of choice for the treatment of HF.

24.4 Diuretics relieve symptoms of HF by reducing fluid overload and decreasing blood pressure.

24.5 Cardiac glycosides increase the force of myocardial contraction and were once drugs of choice for HF. Because of

their low safety margin, and the development of more effective drugs, their use has declined.

24.6 Beta-adrenergic blockers slow the heart rate and decrease blood pressure. They can dramatically reduce hospitalizations and increase the survival of patients with HF.

24.7 Vasodilators can relieve symptoms of HF by reducing preload and decreasing the cardiac workload. Nesiritide (Natrecor) is a newer vasodilator approved for the treatment of acute HF.

24.8 Phosphodiesterase inhibitors and other inotropic agents increase the force of myocardial contraction and improve cardiac output. They are used for the short-term therapy of acute HF.

NCLEX-RN® REVIEW QUESTIONS

1 The patient is prescribed digoxin (Lanoxin) for treatment of HF. Which of the following statements by the patient indicates the need for further teaching?
1. "I may notice my heart rate decrease."
2. "I may feel tired during early treatment."
3. "This drug will help my heart muscle pump less blood."
4. "My heart rate will speed up."

2 The nurse reviews lab studies of a patient receiving digoxin (Lanoxin). Intervention by the nurse is required if the results include a:
1. serum digoxin level of 1.2 ng/dL.
2. serum potassium level of 3.0 mEq/L.
3. hemoglobin of 14.4 g/dL.
4. serum sodium level of 140 mEq/L.

3 Nursing interventions during initial therapy with ACE inhibitors must include:
1. monitoring ECG.
2. monitoring intake and output.
3. monitoring blood pressure.
4. monitoring serum levels.

4 The teaching plan for a patient receiving thiazide diuretics should include:
1. taking the apical pulse.
2. including citrus fruits, melons, and vegetables in the diet.
3. decreasing potassium-rich food in the diet.
4. checking blood pressure three times a day.

5 Lisinopril (Prinivil) is part of the treatment regimen for a patient with HF. The nurse monitors the patient for the side effects of this drug which may include: (Select all that apply.)
1. hyperkalemia.
2. hypokalemia.
3. cough.
4. dizziness.
5. headache.

6 Therapeutic effects of positive inotropic agents given for heart failure include:
1. the heart rate increases to normal, allowing the BP to rise.
2. edema is decreased because of diuretic effects.
3. the BP returns to normal and urine output rises as the heart contracts more forcefully.
4. the heart's conduction system returns to a more regular pattern.

CRITICAL THINKING QUESTIONS

1. A patient is newly diagnosed with mild heart failure. The patient has been started on digoxin (Lanoxin). What objective evidence would indicate that this drug has been effective?

2. A 69-year-old patient has a sudden onset of acute pulmonary edema. The patient has no past cardiac history, is allergic to sulfa antibiotics, and routinely takes no medications. The health care provider orders furosemide (Lasix) to relieve the pulmonary congestion. What interventions are essential in the care of this patient?

3. A patient who is diabetic and hypertensive is started on ACE inhibitors for mild heart failure. What teaching is important for this patient?

See Appendix D for answers and rationales for all activities.

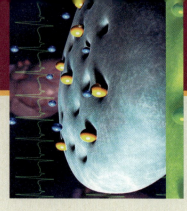

Chapter 25

Drugs for Angina Pectoris and Myocardial Infarction

LEARNING OUTCOMES

After reading this chapter, the student should be able to:

1. Explain the relationship between atherosclerosis and coronary artery disease.
2. Describe factors that affect myocardial oxygen supply and demand.
3. Explain the pathophysiology of angina pectoris and myocardial infarction.
4. Describe the nurse's role in the pharmacologic management of patients with angina and myocardial infarction.
5. Explain mechanisms by which drugs can be used to decrease cardiac oxygen demand and relieve angina pain.
6. Identify classes of drugs that are given to treat the symptoms and complications of myocardial infarction.
7. For each of the drug classes listed in Drugs at a Glance, know representative drug examples, and explain their mechanism of action, primary actions, and important adverse effects.
8. Use the nursing process to care for patients who are receiving drug therapy for angina and myocardial infarction.

KEY TERMS

All tissues and organs of the body are dependent on a continuous arterial supply of oxygen and other vital nutrients to support life and health. With its high metabolic requirements, the heart in particular demands a steady source of oxygen. Should the arterial blood supply become compromised, cardiovascular function may become impaired, resulting in angina pectoris, myocardial infarction (MI), and possibly death. This chapter focuses on the pharmacologic interventions related to angina pectoris and MI.

25.1 Etiology of Coronary Artery Disease and Myocardial Ischemia

The heart, from the moment it begins to function in utero until death, works to distribute oxygen and nutrients via its nonstop pumping action. It is the hardest working organ in the body, functioning continually during both activity and rest. Because the heart is a muscle, it needs a steady supply of nourishment to sustain itself and to maintain the systemic circulation in a balanced state of equilibrium. Any disturbance in blood flow to the vital organs or the myocardium itself—even for brief episodes—can result in life-threatening consequences.

The myocardium receives its blood supply via the right and left coronary arteries, which arise within the aortic sinuses at the base of the aorta. These arteries further diverge into smaller branches that encircle the heart, bringing cardiac muscle a continuous supply of oxygen and nutrients.

Coronary artery disease (CAD) is one of the leading causes of mortality in the United States. The primary defining characteristic of CAD is narrowing or occlusion of a coronary artery. The narrowing deprives cells of needed oxygen and nutrients, a condition known as **myocardial ischemia.** If the ischemia develops over a long period of time, the heart may compensate for its inadequate blood supply, and the patient may experience no symptoms. Indeed, coronary arteries may be occluded as much as 50% or more and cause no symptoms. As CAD progresses, however, the myocardium does not receive enough oxygen to meet the metabolic demands of the heart, and symptoms of angina begin to appear. Persistent myocardial ischemia may lead to heart attack.

The most common etiology of CAD in adults is **atherosclerosis,** the presence of **plaque**—a fatty, fibrous material within the walls of the coronary arteries. Plaque develops progressively over time, producing varying degrees of intravascular narrowing, and a situation that results in partial or total blockage of the vessel. In addition, the plaque impairs normal vessel elasticity, and the coronary vessel is unable to dilate properly when the myocardium needs additional blood or oxygen, such as during periods of exercise. Plaque accumulation occurs gradually, over periods of 40 to 50 years in some individuals, but actually begins to accrue early in life. The development of atherosclerosis is illustrated in ➤ Figure 25.1.

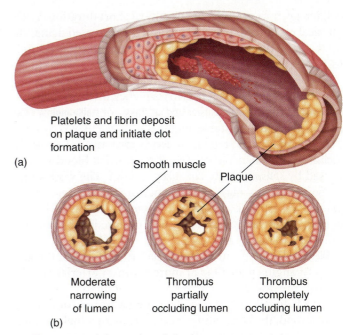

Platelets and fibrin deposit on plaque and initiate clot formation

(a)

Smooth muscle

Plaque

Moderate narrowing of lumen

Thrombus partially occluding lumen

Thrombus completely occluding lumen

(b)

➤ **Figure 25.1** Atherosclerosis in the coronary arteries
Source: Mulvihill et al., Human Diseases: A Systematic Approach, 6th ed., © 2006, p. 115. Reprinted by permission of Pearson Education, Inc., Upper Saddle River, NJ.

ANGINA PECTORIS

Angina pectoris is acute chest pain caused by insufficient oxygen to a portion of the myocardium. More than 6 million Americans have angina pectoris, with over 350,000 new cases occurring each year. It is more prevalent in those over 55 years of age.

25.2 Pathogenesis of Angina Pectoris

The classic presentation of angina pectoris is steady, intense pain in the anterior chest, sometimes accompanied by a crushing or constricting sensation. The discomfort may radiate to the left shoulder and proceed down the left arm and it may extend posterior to the thoracic spine or move upward to the jaw. In some patients, the pain is experienced in the midepigastrium or abdominal area. Recent studies indicate that women do not always present with the classic symptoms of angina. In women, gastric distress, nausea and vomiting, a burning sensation in the chest or chest wall, overwhelming fatigue, and sweating may be more common symptoms. For most patients, the discomfort is accompanied by severe emotional distress—a feeling of panic with fear of impending death. There is usually pallor, dyspnea with cyanosis, diaphoresis, tachycardia, and elevated blood pressure.

Angina pain is usually precipitated by physical exertion or emotional excitement—events associated with *increased myocardial oxygen demand.* Narrowed coronary arteries containing atherosclerotic deposits prevent the proper flow of oxygen and nutrients to the stressed cardiac muscle.

Angina pectoris episodes are usually of short duration. With physical rest and/or stress reduction, the increased demands on the heart diminish, and the discomfort subsides within 5 to 10 minutes.

There are several types of angina. When angina occurrences are fairly predictable as to frequency, intensity, and duration, the condition is described as classic or **stable angina.** The pain associated with stable angina is usually relieved by rest.

A second type of angina, known as **vasospastic** or **Prinzmetal's angina** occurs when the decreased myocardial blood flow is caused by *spasms* of the coronary arteries. The vessels undergoing spasms may or may not contain atherosclerotic plaque. Vasospastic angina pain occurs most often during periods of rest, although it may occur unpredictably, and be unrelated to rest or activity.

Silent angina is a form of the disease that occurs in the absence of angina pain. One or more coronary arteries are occluded, but the patient remains asymptomatic. Although the mechanisms underlying silent angina are not completely understood, the condition is associated with a high risk for acute MI and sudden death.

When episodes of angina arise more frequently, become more intense, and occur during periods of rest, the condition is called **unstable angina.** Unstable angina is a type of acute coronary syndrome in which a portion of plaque within a coronary artery ruptures. A thrombus quickly builds on the displaced plaque, and the artery becomes in serious danger of occlusion. This condition is a medical emergency requiring aggressive medical intervention because it is associated with an increased risk for MI.

Angina pain often parallels the signs and symptomatology of a heart attack. It is extremely important that the health care provider be able to accurately identify the characteristics that differentiate the two conditions, because the pharmacologic interventions related to angina differ considerably from those of MI. Angina, although painful and distressing, rarely leads to a fatal outcome, and the chest pain is usually immediately relieved by nitroglycerin. Myocardial infarction, however, carries a high mortality rate if appropriate treatment is delayed. Pharmacologic intervention must be initiated immediately and systematically maintained in the event of MI.

The nurse should understand that a number of conditions—many unrelated to cardiac pathology—may cause chest pain. These include gallstones, peptic ulcer disease, esophageal reflux, biliary disease, pneumonia, musculoskeletal injuries, and certain cancers. When a person presents with chest pain, the foremost objective for the health care provider is to quickly determine the cause of the pain so that proper, effective interventions can be delivered.

25.3 Nonpharmacologic Management of Angina

A combination of variables influence the development and progression of CAD, including dietary patterns and lifestyle choices. The nurse is instrumental in teaching patients how to prevent CAD as well as how to lower the rate of recur-

---

PHARMFACTS

Angina Pectoris

- Over 9 million Americans have angina pectoris; 500,000 new cases occur each year.
- 20% of the deaths due to cardiovascular disease are attributed to smoking.

Myocardial Infarction

- More than 1.1 million Americans experience a new or recurrent MI each year.
- About one third of the patients experiencing MIs will die from them.
- About 60% of the patients who died suddenly of MI had no previous symptoms of the disease.
- More than 20% of men and 40% of women will die from MI within 1 year after being diagnosed.

---

rence of angina episodes. Such support includes the formulation of a comprehensive plan of care that incorporates psychosocial support and an individualized teaching plan. The patient needs to understand the causes of angina, identify the conditions and situations that trigger it, and develop motivation to modify behaviors associated with the disease.

Listing therapeutic lifestyle behaviors that modify the development and progression of cardiovascular disease (CVD) may seem repetitious, as the student has encountered these same factors in chapters on hypertension, hyperlipidemia, and heart disease. However, the importance of prevention and management of CVD through nonpharmacologic means cannot be overemphasized. Practicing healthy lifestyle habits can *prevent* CAD in many individuals and *slow the progression* of the disease in those who have plaque buildup. The following factors have been shown to reduce the incidence of CAD:

- Limit alcohol consumption to small amounts.
- Eliminate foods high in cholesterol or saturated fats.
- Keep blood cholesterol and other lipid indicators within the normal ranges.
- Do not use tobacco.
- Keep blood pressure within the normal range.
- Exercise regularly and maintain optimum weight.
- Keep blood glucose levels within normal range.
- Limit salt (sodium) intake.

When the coronary arteries are significantly obstructed, the two most common interventions are **percutaneous transluminal coronary angioplasty (PTCA)**, with stent insertion, and **coronary artery bypass graft (CABG) surgery.** PTCA is a procedure whereby the area of narrowing is dilated using either a balloon catheter or a laser. Because the artery may return to its original narrowed state after the procedure, a stent is sometimes used in conjunction with a balloon angioplasty. Angioplasty with stenting typically relieves 90% of the original blockage in the artery. The patient usually receives aspirin therapy 2 hours prior to the procedure and heparin for 24 hours after

The Influence of Gender and Ethnicity on Angina

Angina occurs more frequently in females than males, but the prevalence of MI is higher among men than women. Among ethnic groups, the incidence of angina is highest amongst African Americans, followed by Hispanic Americans and Caucasians, and lowest in Asian populations. African American females have twice the risk of angina compared with African American males.

Because women may not experience angina pain the same way as men do, any epigastric or chest area pain, especially occurring with exertion, should be investigated as possible angina. Some women may also minimize their discomfort, delaying treatment. Several recent studies have suggested that women and people from South Asia with angina may have worse clinical outcomes. Until more definitive studies are conducted, patients of any gender or ethnicity should be encouraged to seek immediate attention for chest discomfort occurring with exertion or emotional stress and not delay possible treatment.

Cardiopulmonary Resuscitation (CPR) and Other Education for Heart Disease

Coronary heart disease is the number-one killer in the United States. For this reason it is imperative that individuals learn CPR and encourage others to become certified. In addition, nurses are in a valuable position to educate those in their communities on methods to lower their risks for coronary heart disease. Education pertaining to positive lifestyle changes, controlling hypertension, and smoking cessation are all important issues to decrease an individual's risk. Lifestyle changes such as decreasing dietary fat intake, increasing intake of fruit and vegetables, and participating in regular exercise are essential to limiting one's risk for coronary heart disease.

the completion of angioplasty to minimize the risk of thrombus formation.

Coronary bypass surgery is reserved for severe cases of coronary blockage that cannot be dealt with by less invasive treatment modalities. A portion of a vein from the leg or chest is used to create a "bypass artery." One end of the graft is sewn to the aorta and the other end to the coronary artery beyond the narrowed area. Blood from the aorta then flows through the new grafted vessel to the heart muscle, "bypassing" the blockage in the coronary artery. The result is increased blood flow to the heart muscle, which reduces angina and the risk of MI.

25.4 Pharmacologic Management of Angina

There are several desired therapeutic outcomes for a patient receiving pharmacotherapy for angina. A primary goal is to reduce the intensity and frequency of angina episodes. Additionally, successful pharmacotherapy should improve exercise tolerance and allow the patient to participate more actively in activities of daily living. Long-term goals include extending the patient's life span by preventing serious consequences of ischemic heart disease such as dysrhythmias, heart failure, and MI. To be most effective, pharmacotherapy must be accompanied by therapeutic lifestyle changes that promote a healthy heart.

Although various drug classes are used to treat the disease, antianginal medications may be placed into two basic categories: those that *terminate* an acute angina episode in progress, and those that decrease the *frequency* of angina episodes. The primary means by which antianginal drugs accomplish these goals is to reduce the myocardial demand for oxygen. This may be accomplished by the following mechanisms:

- Slowing the heart rate
- Dilating veins so the heart receives less blood (reduced preload)
- Causing the heart to contract with less force (reduced contractility)
- Lowering blood pressure, thus offering the heart less resistance when ejecting blood from its chambers (reduced afterload)

The pharmacotherapy of angina uses three classes of drugs: organic nitrates, beta-adrenergic antagonists, and calcium channel blockers. Rapid-acting organic nitrates are drugs of choice for *terminating* acute angina pain. Beta-adrenergic blockers are drugs of choice for preventing angina pain, although calcium channel blockers are used when beta blockers are not tolerated well by a patient. Long-acting nitrates, given by the oral or transdermal routes, are effective alternatives. Persistent angina requires drugs from two or more classes, such as a beta-adrenergic blocker combined with a long-acting nitrate or calcium channel blocker. Pharmacotherapy Illustrated 25.1 illustrates the mechanisms of action of drugs used to prevent and treat coronary artery disease.

Approved in 2006, ranolazine (Ranexa) is a newer drug for angina. Ranolazine is believed to act by shifting the metabolism of cardiac muscle cells so that they utilize glucose as the primary energy source rather than fatty acids. This decreases the metabolic rate and oxygen demands of myocardial cells. Thus, this is the only antianginal that acts through its *metabolic* effects, rather than *hemodynamic* effects: Ranolazine does not change heart rate or blood pressure. The drug is well tolerated, with dizziness, nausea, constipation, and headache being the most frequently reported adverse effects. It is used to prevent anginal episodes: It will not terminate an acute attack. The drug is only approved for chronic angina that has not responded to other drugs.

ORGANIC NITRATES

After their medicinal properties were discovered in 1857, the organic nitrates became the mainstay for the treatment of angina. Their mechanism of action is the result of the formation of nitric acid, a potent vasodilator, in vascular smooth muscle.

PHARMACOTHERAPY ILLUSTRATED

25.1 Mechanisms of Action of Drugs Used to Treat Angina

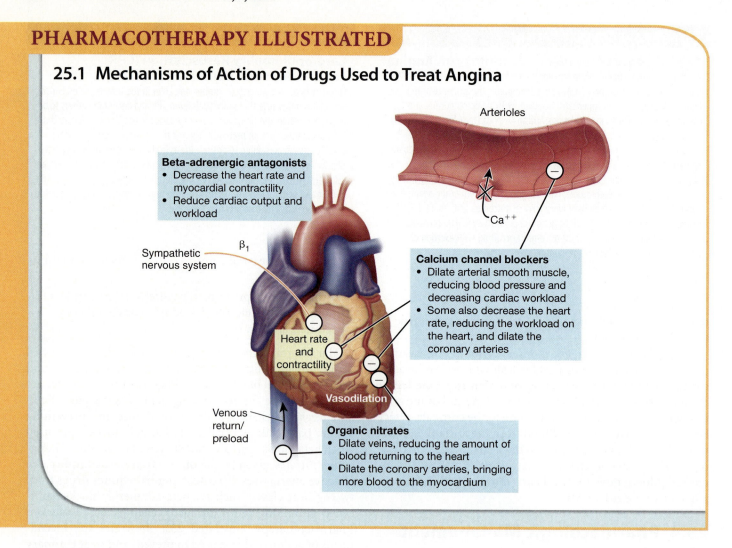

Beta-adrenergic antagonists
- Decrease the heart rate and myocardial contractility
- Reduce cardiac output and workload

Sympathetic nervous system

β_1

Heart rate and contractility

Venous return/ preload

Arterioles

Ca^{++}

Calcium channel blockers
- Dilate arterial smooth muscle, reducing blood pressure and decreasing cardiac workload
- Some also decrease the heart rate, reducing the workload on the heart, and dilate the coronary arteries

Vasodilation

Organic nitrates
- Dilate veins, reducing the amount of blood returning to the heart
- Dilate the coronary arteries, bringing more blood to the myocardium

25.5 Treating Angina with Organic Nitrates

The primary therapeutic action of the organic nitrates is their ability to relax both arterial and venous smooth muscle. Dilation of veins reduces the amount of blood returning to the heart (preload), so the chambers contain a smaller volume. With less blood for the ventricles to pump, cardiac output is reduced and the workload on the heart is decreased, thereby lowering myocardial oxygen demand. The therapeutic outcome is that chest pain is alleviated and episodes of angina become less frequent. The organic nitrates are shown in Table 25.1.

Organic nitrates also have the ability to dilate coronary arteries, which was once thought to be their primary mechanism of action. It seems logical that dilating a partially occluded coronary artery would allow more oxygen to reach the ischemic tissue. Although this effect does indeed occur, it is no longer considered the primary mechanism of nitrate action in *stable* angina. This action, however, is crucial in treating *vasospastic* angina, in which the chest pain is caused by coronary artery spasm. The organic nitrates can relax these spasms, allowing more oxygen to reach the myocardium, thereby terminating the pain.

Organic nitrates are of two types, short acting and long acting. The short-acting nitrates, such as nitroglycerin, are taken sublingually to quickly terminate an acute angina episode. Long-acting nitrates, such as isosorbide dinitrate (Dilatate, Isordil), are taken orally or delivered through a transdermal patch to decrease the frequency and severity of angina episodes. Long-acting organic nitrates are also occasionally used to treat symptoms of heart failure, and their role in the treatment of this disease is discussed in chapter 24 ∞.

Tolerance is a common and potentially serious problem with the long-acting organic nitrates. The magnitude of the tolerance depends on the dosage and the frequency of drug administration. Although tolerance develops rapidly, after only 24 hours of therapy in some patients, it also disappears rapidly when the drug is withheld. Patients are often instructed to remove the transdermal patch for 6 to 12 hours each day or withhold the night-time dose of the oral medications to delay the development of tolerance. Because the oxygen demands of the heart during sleep are diminished, the patient with stable angina experiences few angina episodes during this drug-free interval.

TABLE 25.1	Selected Drugs for Angina and Myocardial Infarction	
Drug	Route and Adult Dose (max dose where indicated)	Adverse Effects
ORGANIC NITRATES		
amyl nitrite	Inhalation; 1 ampule (0.18–0.3 ml) PRN	*Headache, postural hypotension, flushing of face, dizziness, rash (transdermal patch), tolerance*
isosorbide dinitrate (Dilatate, Isordil)	PO; 2.5–30 mg qid (max: 480 mg/day)	
isosorbide mononitrate (Imdur, Ismo, Monoket)	PO; 20 mg qid (max: 240 mg/day with sustained release)	<u>Anaphylaxis, circulatory collapse due to hypotension, syncope due to orthostatic hypotension</u>
ⓟ nitroglycerin (Nitrostat, Nitro-Dur, Nitro-Bid, others)	SL; 1 tablet (0.3–0.6 mg) or 1 spray (0.4–0.8 mg) every 3–5 min (max: three doses in 15 min)	
BETA-ADRENERGIC BLOCKERS		
acebutolol (Sectral)	PO; 400–800 mg daily (max: 1,200 mg/day)	*Fatigue, insomnia, drowsiness, impotence or decreased libido, bradycardia, and confusion*
ⓟ atenolol (Tenormin)	PO; 25–50 mg/day (max: 100 mg/day)	
metoprolol (Lopressor, Toprol XL)	PO; 100 mg bid (max: 400 mg/day)	<u>Agranulocytosis, laryngospasm, Stevens–Johnson syndrome, anaphylaxis; if the drug is abruptly withdrawn, palpitations, rebound hypertension, life-threatening dysrhythmias, or MI may occur</u>
nadolol (Corgard)	PO; 40 mg daily (max: 240 mg/day)	
propranolol (Inderal, Inderal LA) (see page 364 for the Prototype Drug box ∞)	PO; 10–20 mg bid–tid (max: 320 mg/day)	
timolol maleate (Betimol) (see page 771 for the Prototype Drug box ∞)	PO; 15–45 mg tid (max: 60 mg/day)	
CALCIUM CHANNEL BLOCKERS		
amlodipine (Norvasc)	PO; 5–10 mg/day (max: 10 mg/day)	*Flushed skin, headache, dizziness, peripheral edema, light-headedness, nausea, diarrhea*
bepridil (Vascor)	PO; 200 mg/day (max: 360 mg/day)	
diltiazem (Cardizem, Cartia XT, Dilacor XR, Taztia XT, Tiazac)	PO; regular release; 30 mg tid–qid (max: 480 mg/day) Extended release; 20–240 mg bid (max: 540 mg/day)	<u>Hepatotoxicity, MI, CHF, confusion, mood changes</u>
nicardipine (Cardene)	PO; 20–40 mg tid or 30–60 mg SR bid (max: 120 mg/day)	
nifedipine (Adalat, Procardia, others) (see page 308 for the Prototype Drug box ∞)	PO; 10–20 mg tid (max: 180 mg/day)	
verapamil (Calan, Covera-HS, Isoptin SR, Verelan) (see page 366 for the Prototype Drug box ∞)	Extended release: 30–90 mg once daily PO; 80 mg tid–qid (max: 480 mg/day)	

Italics indicate common adverse effects; <u>underlining</u> indicates serious adverse effects.

BETA-ADRENERGIC BLOCKERS (ANTAGONISTS)

25.6 Treating Angina with Beta-Adrenergic Blockers

Beta-adrenergic antagonists or blockers reduce the cardiac workload by slowing the heart rate and reducing contractility. These drugs are as effective as the organic nitrates in decreasing the frequency and severity of angina episodes caused by exertion. Unlike the organic nitrates, tolerance does not develop to the antianginal effects of the beta blockers. They are ideal for patients who have both hypertension *and* coronary artery disease because of their antihypertensive action. They are considered drugs of choice for the prophylaxis of stable angina. Beta-adrenergic antagonists are not effective for treating vasospastic angina and may in fact worsen this condition. The beta-blockers used for angina are listed in Table 25.1. Beta blockers are widely used in medicine, and additional details may be found in chapters 13, 23, 24, and 26 ∞.

Please refer to Nursing Process Focus: Patients Receiving Adrenergic-Antagonist Therapy on page 316 in chapter 23 ∞ for additional information.

CALCIUM CHANNEL BLOCKERS

25.7 Treating Angina with Calcium Channel Blockers

Blockade of calcium channels has a number of effects on the heart, most of which are similar to those of beta blockers. Like beta blockers, calcium channel blockers (CCBs) are used for a number of cardiovascular conditions, including hypertension (chapter 23 ∞) and dysrhythmias (chapter 26 ∞). The calcium channel blockers used for angina are shown in Table 25.1.

Pr Prototype Drug | Nitroglycerin *(Nitrostat, Nitro-Bid, Nitro-Dur, others)*

Therapeutic Class: Antianginal drug   **Pharmacologic Class:** Organic nitrate, vasodilator

ACTIONS AND USES

Nitroglycerin, the oldest and most widely used organic nitrate, can be delivered by a number of different routes: sublingual, oral, translingual, IV, transmucosal, transdermal, topical, and extended-release forms. It may be taken while an acute angina episode is in progress or just prior to physical activity. When given sublingually, it reaches peak plasma levels in 2 to 4 minutes, thus terminating angina pain rapidly. Chest pain that does not respond within 10 to 15 minutes after two or three doses of sublingual nitroglycerin may indicate MI, and emergency medical services should be contacted. The transdermal and oral sustained release forms are for prophylaxis only, since they have a relatively slow onset of action.

ADMINISTRATION ALERTS

- For IV administration, use a glass IV bottle and special IV tubing, because plastic absorbs nitrates significantly, thus reducing the patient dose.
- Cover the IV bottle to reduce the degradation of nitrates due to light exposure.
- Use gloves when applying nitroglycerin paste or ointment to prevent self-administration.
- Pregnancy category C

PHARMACOKINETICS

Onset: 1–3 min sublingual; 2–5 min buccal; 40–60 min transdermal patch

Peak: 4–8 min sublingual; 4–10 min buccal; 1–2 h transdermal patch

Half-life: 1–4 min

Duration: 30–60 min sublingual; 2 h buccal; 18–24 h transdermal patch

ADVERSE EFFECTS

The adverse effects of nitroglycerin are usually cardiovascular in nature and rarely life threatening. Because nitroglycerin can dilate cerebral vessels, headache is a common side effect and may be severe. Occasionally, the venous dilation caused by nitroglycerin produces reflex tachycardia. Some health care providers prescribe a beta-adrenergic blocker to diminish this undesirable increase in heart rate. Many of the side effects of nitroglycerin diminish after a few doses.

Contraindications: Nitroglycerin should not be given to patients with preexisting hypotension or with high intracranial pressure or head trauma. Drugs in this class are contraindicated in pericardial tamponade and constrictive pericarditis because the heart cannot increase cardiac output to maintain blood pressure when vasodilation occurs. Sustained-release forms should not be given to patients with glaucoma because they may increase intraocular pressure. Dehydration or hypovolemia should be corrected before nitroglycerin is administered; otherwise, serious hypotension may result.

INTERACTIONS

Drug–Drug: Concurrent use with phosphodiesterase-5 inhibitors (sildenafil [Viagra], vardenafil [Levitra], or tadalafil [Cialis]) may cause life-threatening hypotension and cardiovascular collapse. Use with alcohol and antihypertensive drugs may cause additive hypotension.

Lab Tests: Nitroglycerin may increase values of urinary catecholamines and VMA concentrations.

Herbal/Food: Unknown

Treatment of Overdose: Hypotension may be reversed with administration of IV normal saline. If methemoglobinemia is suspected, methylene blue may be administered.

NURSING PROCESS FOCUS   PATIENTS RECEIVING NITROGLYCERIN

Assessment	Potential Nursing Diagnoses
Baseline assessment prior to administration: - Understand the reason the drug has been prescribed in order to assess for therapeutic effects. - Obtain a complete health history including cardiovascular (including previous MI, heart failure, valvular disease), cerebrovascular and neurologic (including level of consciousness, history of cardiovascular accident [CVA], head injury, increased intracranial pressure), renal or hepatic dysfunction, dysrhythmias, and pregnancy or lactation. Obtain a drug history including allergies, current prescription and OTC drugs, herbal preparations, and alcohol use. Be aware that use of erectile dysfunction drugs within the past 24 to 48 hours may cause profound and prolonged hypotension when nitrates are administered. Be alert to possible drug interactions. - Obtain baseline weight, vital signs (especially blood pressure [BP] and pulse), and ECG. Assess for location and character of angina if currently present. - Evaluate appropriate laboratory findings, electrolytes, renal function studies, and lipid profiles. Troponin and/or creatine kinase lab tests may be ordered to rule out MI.	- Decreased Cardiac Output (disease process or related to adverse effects of drug therapy) - Altered Tissue Perfusion (related to disease process) - Pain (headache, related to adverse effects of drug therapy) - Fatigue (disease process or related to adverse effects of drug therapy) - Activity Intolerance (related to disease process or adverse effects of drug therapy) - Deficient Knowledge (drug therapy) - Risk for Falls, Risk for Injury (related to adverse effects)

NURSING PROCESS FOCUS   PATIENTS RECEIVING NITROGLYCERIN (Continued)

Assessment	Potential Nursing Diagnoses
Assessment throughout administration: ▪ Assess for desired therapeutic effects (e.g., chest pain has subsided or has significantly lessened), heart rate and blood pressure remain within normal limits, and ECG remains within normal limits without signs of ischemia or infarct. ▪ Continue periodic monitoring of ECG for ischemia or infarct. ▪ Continue frequent monitoring of blood pressure and pulse whenever IV nitrates are used or when giving rapid-acting (e.g., sublingual) nitrates. With sublingual nitrates, take BP before *and* 5 minutes after giving the dose and hold drug if BP is less than 90/60, pulse is over 100 (or parameters as ordered). ▪ Assess for and promptly report adverse effects: excessive hypotension, dysrhythmias, reflex tachycardia (from too-rapid decrease in BP or significant hypotension), headache that does not subside within 15–20 minutes or when accompanied by neurologic changes, or decreased urinary output. Severe hypotension, seizures, dysrhythmias should be reported immediately. Chest pain remaining present after three sublingual nitroglycerin tablets given 5 minutes apart should be reported immediately, even if pain has lessened, as this may be a sign of impending ischemia or infarction.	

Planning: Patient Goals and Expected Outcomes

The patient will:
- Experience therapeutic effects (e.g., angina subsides or substantially diminishes, heart rate and blood pressure remain within established parameters, ECG is within normal limits).
- Be free from, or experience minimal, adverse effects.
- Verbalize an understanding of the drug's use, adverse effects, and required precautions.
- Demonstrate proper self-administration of the medication (e.g., dose, timing, when to notify provider).

Implementation

Interventions and (Rationales)	Patient and Family Education
Ensuring therapeutic effects: ▪ Continue frequent assessments as above for therapeutic effects. (As vasodilation occurs from nitrates, preload and afterload diminish, decreasing the workload of the heart and decreasing myocardial oxygenation needs; chest pain diminishes.)	▪ Ask the patient to briefly describe the location and character of pain (use pain rating scale for rapid assessment) prior to and after giving nitrates to assess for the extent of relief.
▪ Continue to monitor ECG, blood pressure, and pulse. (Nitrates cause vasodilation and possible hypotension. BP assessment aids in determining drug frequency and dose. ECG monitoring helps detect adverse effects such as reflex tachycardia, ischemia, or infarction.)	▪ Teach the patient, family, or caregiver how to monitor pulse and blood pressure. Ensure the proper use and functioning of any home equipment obtained.
▪ Evaluate the need for adjunctive treatment with health care provider for angina prevention and treatment (e.g., beta blockers, aspirin therapy) or further cardiac studies. (Patients with unstable angina may require adjunctive drug therapy or definitive cardiac studies to determine the need for other treatment options.)	▪ Encourage the patient to discuss any changes in character, severity, or frequency of angina episodes with provider. Instruct the patient not to take daily aspirin without discussing with the health care provider first.
▪ For patients on transdermal nitroglycerin patches, remove the patch for 6–12 hours at night, or as directed by health care provider. (This helps prevent or delay the development of tolerance to nitrates. Removing the patch at night, when cardiac workload is lessened, helps avoid possible anginal attacks during the daytime when workload is greater.)	▪ Instruct the patient on the proper use of nitroglycerin and rationale for removing transdermal patches. Also instruct the patient on transdermal patches to always remove the old patch, cleanse the skin underneath gently, and to rotate sites before applying a new patch.
▪ Encourage appropriate lifestyle changes. Provide for dietitian consultation as needed. (Healthy lifestyle changes will support the benefits of drug therapy.)	▪ Encourage the patient to adopt a healthy lifestyle of low-fat food choices, increased exercise, decreased alcohol consumption, and smoking cessation. Provide educational materials on low-fat, low-sodium food choices.

(Continued)

NURSING PROCESS FOCUS **PATIENTS RECEIVING NITROGLYCERIN** *(Continued)*

Implementation

Interventions and (Rationales)	Patient and Family Education
Minimizing adverse effects: ▪ Continue to monitor vital signs frequently. Be cautious with the elderly who are at increased risk for hypotension; and patients with a pre-existing history of cardiac or cerebrovascular disease, or recent head injury, which may be worsened by vasodilation. Notify the health care provider immediately if angina remains unrelieved or if blood pressure or pulse decrease beyond established parameters or if hypotension is accompanied by reflex tachycardia. (Nitrates may cause vasodilation, resulting in the potential for hypotension accompanied by reflex tachycardia. Reflex tachycardia increases myocardial oxygen demand, worsening angina.)	▪ Instruct the patient to report dizziness, faintness, palpitations, or headache unrelieved after taking nonnarcotic analgesics (e.g., acetaminophen). ▪ Instruct the patient on nitrates to rise from lying to sitting or standing slowly to avoid dizziness or falls, especially if taking sublingual nitrates, or until drug effects are known.
▪ Continue cardiac monitoring (e.g., ECG) if IV nitrates are administered. (Monitoring devices assist in detecting early signs of adverse effects of drug therapy, myocardial ischemia or infarction, as well as monitoring for therapeutic effects.)	▪ To allay possible anxiety, teach the patient the rationale for all equipment used and the need for frequent monitoring.
▪ Continue frequent physical assessments, particularly neurologic, cardiac, and respiratory. Immediately report any changes in level of consciousness, headache, or changes in heart or lung sounds. (Nitrate therapy may worsen pre-existing neurologic, cardiac, or respiratory conditions as blood pressure drops and perfusion to vital organs diminishes. Lung congestion may signal impending heart failure.)	▪ When on oral therapy at home, instruct the patient to immediately report changes in mental status or level of consciousness, palpitations, dizziness, dyspnea, or increasing productive cough, especially if frothy sputum is present, and seek medical attention.
▪ Review the medications taken by the patient before discharge, and review all prescription as well as OTC medications with the patient. Current use of erectile dysfunction drugs is contraindicated with nitrates. (Erectile dysfunction drugs lower BP and when combined with nitrates, can result in severe and prolonged hypotension.)	▪ Instruct the patient to not take sildenafil (Viagra), vardenafil (Levitra), or tadalafil (Cialis) while taking nitrates and to discuss treatment options for erectile dysfunction with the health care provider.
Patient understanding of drug therapy: ▪ Use opportunities during administration of medications and during assessments to discuss the rationale for drug therapy, desired therapeutic outcomes, most common adverse effects, parameters for when to call the health care provider, and any necessary monitoring or precautions. (Using time during nursing care helps to optimize and reinforce key teaching areas.)	▪ The patient should be able to state the reason for drug; appropriate dose and scheduling; what adverse effects to observe for and when to report; equipment needed as appropriate and how to use that equipment; and the required length of medication therapy needed with any special instructions regarding renewing or continuing prescription as appropriate.
Patient self-administration of drug therapy: ▪ When administering medications, instruct the patient, family, or caregiver in proper self-administration of drugs and when to contact provider. (Proper administration increases the effectiveness of the drug.)	▪ The patient should be able to state how to use sublingual nitroglycerin at home: 　▪ Take one nitroglycerin (NTG) tablet under the tongue for angina/chest pain. Remain seated or lay down to avoid dizziness or falls. 　▪ If chest pain continues, repeat one NTG tablet, under the tongue, in 5 minutes. 　▪ If chest pain continues, repeat NTG, under the tongue, in 5 minutes. 　▪ If chest pain continues, even if reduced, do not take further NTG unless specifically directed by health care provider. Call EMS system (e.g., 911) for assistance. Do *not* drive self to emergency room. ▪ If blood pressure monitoring equipment is available at home, have the patient, family, or caregiver take blood pressure prior to second and third nitroglycerin doses. Hold the drug and contact EMS if BP is less than 90/60 mmHg.

Evaluation of Outcome Criteria

Evaluate the effectiveness of drug therapy by confirming that patient goals and expected outcomes have been met (see "Planning").

Pr Prototype Drug | Atenolol (Tenormin)

Therapeutic Class: Antianginal drug   **Pharmacologic Class:** Beta-adrenergic blocker

ACTIONS AND USES

Atenolol is one of the most frequently prescribed drugs in the United States due to its relative safety and effectiveness in treating a number of chronic disorders, including heart failure, hypertension, angina, and MI. The drug selectively blocks beta$_1$-adrenergic receptors in the heart. Its effectiveness in treating angina is attributed to its ability to slow heart rate and reduce contractility, both of which lower myocardial oxygen demand. As with other beta blockers, therapy generally begins with low doses, which are gradually increased until the therapeutic effect is achieved. Because of its 7- to 9-hour half-life, it may be taken once daily.

ADMINISTRATION ALERTS

- During IV administration, monitor ECG continuously; blood pressure and pulse should be assessed before, during, and after the dose is administered.
- Assess pulse and blood pressure before oral administration. Hold if the pulse is below 60 beats per minute or if the patient is hypotensive.
- Atenolol may precipitate bronchospasm in susceptible patients with initial doses.
- Pregnancy category D

PHARMACOKINETICS

Onset: 1 h
Peak: 2–4 h
Half-life: 1–4 min
Duration: 24 h

ADVERSE EFFECTS

Being a cardioselective beta$_1$-adrenergic blocker, atenolol has few adverse effects on the lung. The most frequently reported adverse effects of atenolol include fatigue, weakness, bradycardia, and hypotension.

Contraindications: Because atenolol slows heart rate, it should not be used in patients with severe bradycardia, AV heart block, cardiogenic shock, or decompensated heart failure. Due to its vasodilation effects, it is contraindicated in patients with severe hypotension.

INTERACTIONS

Drug–Drug: Concurrent use with calcium channel blockers may result in excessive cardiac suppression. Use with digoxin may slow AV conduction, leading to heart block. Concurrent use of atenolol with other antihypertensives may result in additive hypotension. Anticholinergics may cause decreased absorption from the GI tract.

Lab Tests: Atenolol may increase values of the following blood tests: uric acid, lipids, potassium, creatinine, and antinuclear antibody.

Herbal/Food: Unknown

Treatment of Overdose: The most serious symptoms of atenolol overdose are hypotension and bradycardia. Atropine or isoproterenol may be used to reverse bradycardia. Atenolol can be removed from the systemic circulation by hemodialysis.

Refer to MyNursingKit for a Nursing Process Focus specific to this drug.

CCBs have several cardiovascular actions that benefit the patient with angina. Most important, CCBs relax arteriolar smooth muscle, thus lowering blood pressure. This reduction in afterload decreases myocardial oxygen demand. Some of the CCBs also slow conduction velocity through the heart, decreasing heart rate and contributing to the reduced cardiac workload. An additional effect of the CCBs is their ability to dilate the coronary arteries and bring more oxygen to the myocardium. This is especially important in patients with vasospastic angina. Because they are able to relieve the acute vasospasms of variant angina, CCBs are considered drugs of choice for this condition. For stable angina, they may be used as monotherapy in patients unable to tolerate beta blockers. In patients with persistent symptoms, CCBs may be combined with organic nitrates or beta blockers.

Please refer to Nursing Process Focus: Patients Receiving Calcium Channel Blocker Therapy, page 308 in chapter 23∞, for the complete Nursing Process applied to patients receiving calcium channel blockers.

MYOCARDIAL INFARCTION

Heart attacks or **myocardial infarctions (MIs)** are responsible for a substantial number of deaths each year. Some patients die before reaching a medical facility for treatment, and many others die within 48 hours following the initial MI. Clearly, MI is a serious and frightening disease and one responsible for a large percentage of sudden deaths.

25.8 Diagnosis of Myocardial Infarction

The primary cause of MI is advanced coronary artery disease. Plaque buildup can severely narrow one or more branches of the coronary arteries. Pieces of unstable plaque can break off and lodge in a small vessel serving a portion of the myocardium. Exposed plaque activates the coagulation cascade, resulting in platelet aggregation and adherence (chapter 27∞). A new clot quickly builds on the existing plaque, making obstruction of the vessel imminent.

Deprived of its oxygen supply, the affected area of myocardium becomes ischemic, and myocytes begin to die in about 20 minutes unless the blood supply is quickly restored. Necrosis of myocardial tissue, which may be irreversible, releases certain "marker" enzymes, which can be measured in the blood to confirm the patient has experienced an MI.

Extreme chest pain is usually the first symptom of MI, and the one that drives most patients to seek medical attention. An electrocardiogram can give important clues as to the extent and location of the MI. The infarcted region of the myocardium is nonconducting and may produce abnormalities of Q waves, T waves, and S-T segments (chapter 26∞). Laboratory test results are used to aid in diagnosis and monitor

Pr Prototype Drug | Diltiazem (*Cardizem, Cartia XT, Dilacor XR, Taztia XT, Tiazac*)

Therapeutic Class: Antianginal drug   **Pharmacologic Class:** Calcium channel blocker

ACTIONS AND USES

Like other calcium channel blockers, diltiazem inhibits the transport of calcium into myocardial cells. It has the ability to relax both coronary and peripheral blood vessels, bringing more oxygen to the myocardium and reducing cardiac workload. It is useful in the treatment of atrial dysrhythmias and hypertension, as well as stable and vasospastic angina. When given as sustained-release capsules, it is administered once daily.

ADMINISTRATION ALERTS

- During IV administration, the patient must be continuously monitored, and cardioversion equipment must be available.
- Extended-release tablets and capsules should not be crushed or split.
- Pregnancy category C

PHARMACOKINETICS

Onset: 30–60 min (2–3 h sustained release)

Peak: 2–3 h (6–11 h sustained release)

Half-life: 3.5–9 h

Duration: 6–8 h (12 h sustained release)

ADVERSE EFFECTS

Adverse effects of diltiazem are generally not serious and are related to vasodilation: headache, dizziness, and edema of the ankles and feet. Abrupt withdrawal may precipitate an acute anginal episode.

Contraindications: Diltiazem is contraindicated in patients with AV heart block, sick sinus syndrome, severe hypotension, or bleeding aneurysm, or those undergoing intracranial surgery. This drug should be used with caution in patients with renal or hepatic impairment.

INTERACTIONS

Drug–Drug: Concurrent use of diltiazem with other cardiovascular drugs, particularly digoxin or beta-adrenergic blockers, may cause partial or complete heart block, heart failure, or dysrhythmias. Diltiazem may increase digoxin or quinidine levels when taken concurrently. Additive hypotension may occur if used with ethanol, beta blockers, or antihypertensives.

Lab Tests: Unknown

Herbal/Food: St. John's wort and ginseng may decrease the effectiveness of diltiazem. Garlic, hawthorn, and goldenseal may increase the antihypertensive effect of diltiazem.

Treatment of Overdose: Atropine or isoproterenol may be used to reverse bradycardia cause by diltiazem overdose. Hypotension may be reversed by a vasopressor such as dopamine or dobutamine. Calcium chloride can be administered by slow IV push to reverse hypotension or heart block induced by CCBs.

Refer to MyNursingKit for a Nursing Process Focus specific to this drug.

---

progress after an MI. Table 25.2 describes some of these important laboratory values.

Early diagnosis of MI, and prompt initiation of pharmacotherapy, can significantly reduce mortality and the long-term disability associated with MI. The pharmacologic goals for treating a patient with an acute MI are as follows:

- Restore blood supply (reperfusion) to the damaged myocardium as quickly as possible through the use of thrombolytics.
- Reduce myocardial oxygen demand with organic nitrates, beta blockers, or CCBs to prevent additional infarctions.
- Control or prevent MI-associated dysrhythmias with beta blockers or other antidysrhythmics.
- Reduce post-MI mortality with aspirin, beta blockers, and ACE inhibitors.
- Manage severe MI pain and associated anxiety with narcotic analgesics.

THROMBOLYTICS

In treating MI, thrombolytic therapy is administered to dissolve clots obstructing the coronary arteries, thus restoring circulation to the myocardium. Dosages and descriptions of the various thrombolytics are given in chapter 27 on page 383 .

25.9 Treating Myocardial Infarction with Thrombolytics

Quick restoration of cardiac circulation with thrombolytic medications reduces mortality caused by acute MI. After the clot is successfully dissolved, anticoagulant therapy is initiated to prevent the formation of additional clots. ➤ Figure 25.2 illustrates the pathogenesis and treatment of MI.

Thrombolytics are most effective when administered from 20 minutes to 12 hours after the onset of MI symptoms. If administered after 24 hours, the drugs are mostly ineffective. In addition, research has suggested that patients older than age 75 do not experience reduced mortality from these drugs. Because thrombolytic therapy is expensive and has the potential to produce serious adverse effects, it is important to identify circumstances that contribute to successful therapy. The development of clinical practice guidelines to identify those patients who benefit most from thrombolytic therapy is an ongoing process.

Thrombolytics have a narrow margin of safety between dissolving clots and producing serious adverse effects. Although therapy is usually targeted to a single thrombus in a specific artery, once infused in the blood, the drugs travel to all vessels and may cause adverse effects anywhere in the body. The primary risk of thrombolytics is excessive bleeding due to interference with the normal clotting process. Vital signs must be monitored continuously; signs of bleeding

TABLE 25.2	Changes in Blood Test Values Following Acute MI			
Blood Test	Initial Elevation After MI	Peak Elevation After MI	Duration of Elevation	Normal Range
CK (creatine kinase)	3–8 h	12–24 h	2–4 days	22–198 units/L (values vary widely between labs and among testing protocols)
ESR (erythrocyte sedimentation rate)	first week		several weeks	males: 1–13 mm/hr females: 1–20 mm/hr
glucose			duration of stress response	fasting: 80–120 mg/dL
LDH (lactate dehydrogenase)	8–72 h	3–6 days	8–14 days	50–150 units/L
myoglobin	1–3 h	4–6 h	1–2 days	0–85 ng/mL
troponin I	2–4 h	24–36 h	7–10 days	3.1 mcg/L
troponin T	2–4 h	24–36 h	10–14 days	0.01–0.1 ng/L
WBC (white blood cell count)	few hours		3–7 days	$4.8–10.8 \times 10^3$ mcg/L

call for discontinuation of therapy. Because these drugs are rapidly destroyed in the blood, stopping the infusion normally results in the rapid termination of adverse effects.

Please refer to Nursing Process Focus: Patients Receiving Thrombolytic Therapy, page 384 in chapter 27∞ for the complete Nursing Process applied to patients receiving thrombolytic therapy.

25.10 Drugs for Symptoms and Complications of Acute Myocardial Infarction

The most immediate needs of the patient with MI are to ensure that the heart continues functioning and that permanent damage from the infarction is minimized. In addition to thrombolytic therapy to restore perfusion to the myocardium, drugs from several other classes are administered soon after the onset of symptoms, to prevent reinfarction and ultimately to reduce mortality from the episode.

ANTIPLATELET AND ANTICOAGULANT DRUGS

Unless contraindicated, 160 to 325 mg of aspirin is given as soon as an MI is suspected. Aspirin use in the weeks following an acute MI dramatically reduces mortality, probably due to its antiplatelet action. The low doses used in maintenance therapy (75–150 mg/day) rarely cause GI bleeding.

The adenosine diphosphate (ADP)–receptor blockers clopidogrel (Plavix) and ticlopidine (Ticlid) are effective antiplatelet agents that are approved for the prevention of thrombotic stroke and MI. Because these drugs are considerably more expensive than aspirin, they are usually considered for patients allergic to aspirin or who are at risk for GI bleeding from aspirin.

Glycoprotein IIb/IIIa inhibitors are antiplatelet agents with a mechanism of action distinct from that of aspirin. These

agents are sometimes indicated for unstable angina or MI, or for patients undergoing PTCA. The most common drug in this class, abciximab (ReoPro), is infused at the time of PTCA, and continued for 12 hours after the procedure is completed.

On diagnosis of MI in the emergency room, patients are immediately placed on the anticoagulant heparin to prevent additional thrombi from forming. Heparin therapy is generally continued for 48 hours, or until PTCA is completed, at which time patients are switched to warfarin (Coumadin). An alternative is to administer a low molecular weight heparin, such as enoxaparin (Lovenox). The student should refer to chapter 27∞ for a comparison of the different coagulation modifiers and the dosages for these medications.

COMPLEMENTARY AND ALTERNATIVE THERAPIES

Ginseng and Cardiovascular Disease

Ginseng is one of the oldest known herbal remedies. *Panax ginseng* is distributed throughout China, Korea, and Siberia, whereas *Panax quinquefolius* is native to Canada and the United States. There are differences in chemical composition between the two species of ginseng; American ginseng is not considered equivalent to Siberian ginseng. The plant's popularity has led to its extinction from certain regions, and much of the commercial ginseng is now grown commercially.

Ginseng has been used for centuries to promote general wellness, boost immune function, and reduce fatigue. There are some claims that the herb lowers blood glucose and can help in the management of hypertension.

Ginseng is thought to have calcium channel antagonist actions. The herb appears to improve blood flow to the heart in times of low oxygen supply, such as with myocardial ischemia. Some research has shown that ginseng lowers blood sugar levels in patients with type 2 diabetes. In addition, some studies have found ginseng to boost the immune system. The nurse should caution clients who take ginseng, because herb–drug interactions are possible with calcium channel blockers, oral hypoglycemics, warfarin, and loop diuretics.

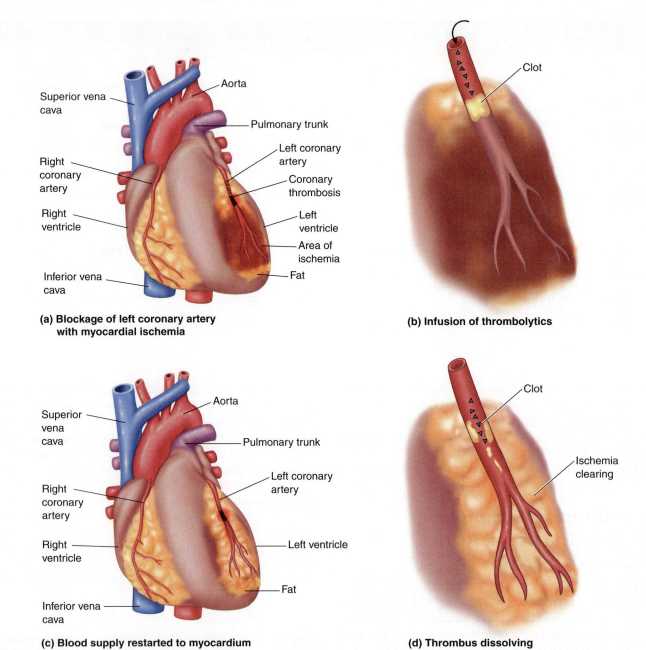

(a) Blockage of left coronary artery with myocardial ischemia

(b) Infusion of thrombolytics

(c) Blood supply restarted to myocardium

(d) Thrombus dissolving

➤ *Figure 25.2* Blockage and reperfusion following myocardial infarction: (a) blockage of left coronary artery with myocardial ischemia; (b) infusion of thrombolytics; (c) blood supply returning to myocardium; (d) thrombus dissolving and ischemia clearing
Source: Figures (a) and (c): Mulvihill et al., Human Diseases: A Systematic Approach, *6th ed., © 2006, p. 105. Reprinted by permission of Pearson Education, Inc., Upper Saddle River, NJ.*

NITRATES

The value of organic nitrates in treating angina was discussed in Section 25.6. Nitrates have additional uses in the patient with a suspected MI. At the initial onset of chest pain, sublingual nitroglycerin is administered to assist in the diagnosis, and three doses may be taken 5 minutes apart. Pain that persists 5 to 10 minutes after the initial dose may indicate an MI, and the patient should seek immediate medical assistance.

Patients with persistent pain, heart failure, or severe hypertension may receive IV nitroglycerin for 24 hours following the onset of pain. The arterial and venous dilation produced by the drug reduces myocardial oxygen demand. Organic nitrates also relieve coronary artery vasospasm, which may be present during the acute stage of MI. On the patient's discharge from the hospital, organic nitrates are discontinued, unless they are needed for relief of stable angina pain.

BETA-ADRENERGIC BLOCKERS

Beta blockers reduce myocardial oxygen demand, which is critical for patients experiencing a recent MI. In addition, they slow impulse conduction through the heart, thereby

Pr Prototype Drug | Reteplase *(Retavase)*

Therapeutic Class: Drug for dissolving blood clots   **Pharmacologic Class:** Thrombolytic

ACTIONS AND USES

Prepared through recombinant DNA technology, reteplase acts by cleaving plasminogen to form plasmin. Plasmin then degrades the fibrin matrix of thrombi. Like other drugs in this class, reteplase should be given as soon as possible after the onset of MI symptoms. Administered by IV bolus, it usually acts within 20 minutes. A second bolus may be injected 30 minutes after the first, if needed to clear the thrombus. After the clot has been dissolved, therapy with heparin or an alternative anticoagulant is started to prevent additional clots from forming. Reteplase may be used off-label to treat acute and chronic deep vein thrombosis and occluded catheters.

ADMINISTRATION ALERTS

- Reconstitute the drug immediately prior to use with diluent provided by manufacturer; swirl to mix—do not shake.
- Do not give any other drug simultaneously through the same IV line.
- Reteplase and heparin are incompatible and must never be combined in the same solution.
- Pregnancy category C

PHARMACOKINETICS

Onset: Immediate
Peak: Unknown
Half-life: 13–16 min
Duration: Unknown

ADVERSE EFFECTS

The most serious adverse effect of reteplase is abnormal bleeding. Bleeding may be prolonged at injection sites and catheter insertion sites. Dysrhythmias may occur during myocardial reperfusion.

Contraindications: Reteplase is contraindicated in patients with active bleeding or history of CVA, or who have had recent surgical procedures.

INTERACTIONS

Drug–Drug: Concurrent therapy with aspirin, anticoagulants, and platelet aggregation inhibitors will produce an additive anticoagulant effect and increase the risk of bleeding.

Lab Tests: Reteplase degrades plasminogen in blood samples, thus decreasing serum plasminogen and fibrinogen levels.

Herbal/Food: Ginkgo biloba should be avoided because it may increase the risk of bleeding.

Treatment of Overdose: There is no specific treatment for overdose.

Refer to MyNursingKit for a Nursing Process Focus specific to this drug.

---

suppressing dysrhythmias, which are serious and sometimes fatal complications following an MI. Research has clearly demonstrated that beta blockers can reduce MI-associated mortality if they are administered within 8 hours of MI onset. These drugs may initially be administered IV in the hospital, and later switched to oral dosing for home therapy. Unless contraindicated, beta-blocker therapy continues for the remainder of the patient's life. For patients unable to tolerate beta blockers, calcium channel blockers are an alternative.

ANGIOTENSIN-CONVERTING ENZYME (ACE) INHIBITORS

Clinical research has demonstrated increased survival for patients administered the ACE inhibitors captopril (Capoten) or lisinopril (Prinivil, Zestoretic) following an acute MI. These drugs are most effective when therapy is started within 24 hours after the onset of symptoms. Oral doses are normally begun after thrombolytic therapy is completed and the patient's condition has stabilized. IV therapy may be used during the early stages of MI pharmacotherapy.

PAIN MANAGEMENT

The pain associated with an MI can be debilitating. Pain control is essential to ensure patient comfort and to reduce stress. Opioids such as morphine sulfate or fentanyl are given to ease extreme pain and to sedate the anxious patient. Pharmacology of the opioids was presented in chapter 18∞.

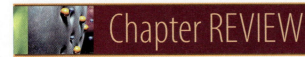

Chapter REVIEW

KEY CONCEPTS

The numbered key concepts provide a succinct summary of the important points from the corresponding numbered section within the chapter. If any of these points are not clear, refer to the numbered section within the chapter for review.

25.1 The myocardium requires a continuous supply of oxygen from the coronary arteries to function properly. Coronary artery disease, which includes both angina and myocardial infarction, is caused by narrowing of the arterial lumen due to atherosclerotic plaque.

25.2 Angina pectoris is the narrowing of a coronary artery, resulting in a lack of sufficient oxygen to the heart muscle. Chest pain on emotional or physical exertion is the most characteristic symptom, although some forms of angina do not cause pain.

25.3 Angina management may include nonpharmacologic therapies such as diet and lifestyle modifications, angioplasty, or surgery.

25.4 Goals for the pharmacotherapy of angina are to terminate acute attacks and prevent future episodes. They are usually achieved by reducing cardiac workload.

25.5 The organic nitrates relieve angina by dilating veins and coronary arteries. They are drugs of choice for terminating acute episodes of stable angina.

25.6 Beta-adrenergic blockers relieve anginal pain by decreasing the oxygen demands on the heart. They are drugs of choice for prophylaxis of stable angina.

25.7 Calcium channel blockers relieve angina by dilating the coronary vessels and reducing the workload on the heart. They are drugs of first choice for treating vasospastic angina.

25.8 The early diagnosis of myocardial infarction increases chances of survival. Early pharmacotherapy with antidysrhythmics targeted reducing the workload on the heart and inhibiting fatal dysrhythmias.

25.9 If given within hours after the onset of MI, thrombolytic agents can dissolve clots and restore perfusion to affected regions of the myocardium.

25.10 A number of additional drugs are used to treat the symptoms and complications of acute MI. These include antiplatelet and anticoagulant agents, beta blockers, glycoprotein IIB/IIIA inhibitors, analgesics, and ACE inhibitors.

NCLEX-RN® REVIEW QUESTIONS

1 The patient is being discharged with nitroglycerin (Nitrostat). Patient education would include the instructions:
1. "Swallow 3 tablets immediately for pain and call 911."
2. "Put one tablet under your tongue for chest pain. If pain does not subside, you may repeat in 5 minutes, taking no more than three tablets."
3. "Call your physician when you have chest pain. He will tell you how many tablets to take."
4. "Place three tablets under your tongue and call 911."

2 A primary mechanism of action that makes nitrates useful for a patient with angina includes:
1. they increase heart rate to increase cardiac output.
2. they increase preload so more blood is available to be pumped to the circulatory system.
3. they increase contractility so the heart works more effectively.
4. they decrease afterload so the workload of the heart is decreased.

3 The nurse recognizes that the mechanism of action of beta-adrenergic blockers in the treatment of angina is:
1. slowed heart rate and decreased contractility.
2. increased contractility and heart rate.
3. relaxation of arterial and venous smooth muscle.
4. decreased peripheral resistance.

4 The patient should remove the transdermal nitroglycerin patch at night to:
1. prevent overdose.
2. prevent adverse reactions.
3. ensure the dosage is appropriate.
4. delay development of tolerance.

5 Put the following nursing interventions in order for a patient who is experiencing chest pain.
1. Administer nitroglycerin sublingually.
2. Assess heart rate and blood pressure.
3. Assess the location, quality, and intensity of pain.
4. Document interventions and outcomes.

6 Erectile dysfunction drugs such as sildenafil (Viagra) are contraindicated in patients taking nitrates for angina because:
1. they contain nitrates, resulting in an overdose.
2. they decrease blood pressure and may result in prolonged and severe hypotension when combined with nitrates.
3. they will adequately treat the patient's angina as well as erectile dysfunction.
4. they will increase the possibility of nitrate tolerance developing and should be avoided unless other drugs can be used.

CRITICAL THINKING QUESTIONS

1. A patient on the medical unit is complaining of chest pain (4 on a scale of 10), has a history of angina, and is requesting his PRN nitroglycerin spray. The patient's blood pressure is 96/60 mmHg at present. Identify what the nurse should do.

2. A patient is recovering from an acute MI and has been put on atenolol (Tenormin). What teaching should the patient receive prior to discharge from the hospital?

3. A patient with chest pain has been given the calcium channel blocker diltiazem (Cardizem) IV for a heart rate of 118 beats per minute. Blood pressure at this time is 100/60 mmHg. What precautions should the nurse take?

See Appendix D for answers and rationales for all activities.

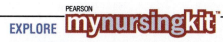

EXPLORE **PEARSON mynursingkit**

MyNursingKit is your one stop for online chapter review materials and resources. Prepare for success with additional NCLEX®-style practice questions, interactive assignments and activities, web links, animations and videos, and more!

Register your access code from the front of your book at **www.mynursingkit.com**.

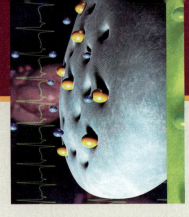

Chapter 26

Drugs for Dysrhythmias

LEARNING OUTCOMES

After reading this chapter, the student should be able to:

1. Explain how rhythm abnormalities can affect cardiac function.
2. Illustrate the flow of electrical impulses through the normal heart.
3. Classify dysrhythmias based on their location and type of rhythm abnormality.
4. Explain how an action potential is controlled by the flow of sodium, potassium, and calcium ions across the myocardial membrane.
5. Identify the importance of nonpharmacologic therapies in the treatment of dysrhythmias.
6. Identify the general mechanisms of action of antidysrhythmic drugs.
7. Describe the nurse's role in the pharmacologic management of patients with dysrhythmias.
8. Know representative drug examples for each of the drug classes listed in Drugs at a Glance, and explain their mechanisms of action, primary actions, and important adverse effects.
9. Use the nursing process to care for patients receiving drug therapy for dysrhythmias.

KEY TERMS

Dysrhythmias are abnormalities of electrical conduction that may result in alterations in heart rate or cardiac rhythm. Sometimes called *arrhythmias,* they encompass a number of different disorders that range from harmless to life threatening. Diagnosis is often difficult because patients often must be connected to an electrocardiograph (ECG) and be experiencing symptoms in order to determine the exact type of rhythm disorder. Proper diagnosis and optimum pharmacotherapy can significantly affect the frequency of dysrhythmias and their consequences.

26.1 Etiology and Classification of Dysrhythmias

Whereas some dysrhythmias produce no symptoms and have negligible effects on cardiac function, others are life threatening and require immediate treatment. Typical symptoms include dizziness, weakness, decreased exercise tolerance, shortness of breath, and fainting. Patients may report palpitations or a sensation that their heart has skipped a beat. Persistent dysrhythmias are associated with increased risk of stroke and heart failure. Severe dysrhythmias may result in sudden death. Because asymptomatic patients may not seek medical attention, it is difficult to estimate the frequency of the disease, although it is likely that dysrhythmias are quite common in the population.

Dysrhythmias are classified by a number of different methods. The simplest method is to name dysrhythmias according to the *type* of rhythm abnormality produced and their *locations.* Dysrhythmias that originate in the atria are sometimes referred to as *supraventricular.* Atrial **fibrillation**, a complete disorganization of rhythm, is the most common type of dysrhythmia. Those that originate in the ventricles are generally more serious, as they are more likely to interfere with the normal function of the heart. A summary of common dysrhythmias and a brief description of each abnormality are given in Table 26.1. Although a correct diagnosis of the type of dysrhythmia is sometimes difficult, it is essential for effective treatment.

Dysrhythmias can occur in both healthy and diseased hearts. Although the actual cause of most dysrhythmias is elusive, they are closely associated with certain conditions, primarily heart disease and myocardial infarction. The following are diseases and conditions associated with dysrhythmias:

- Hypertension (HTN)
- Cardiac valve disease such as mitral stenosis
- Coronary artery disease
- Medications such as digoxin
- Low potassium levels in the blood
- Myocardial infarction
- Stroke
- Diabetes mellitus
- Congestive heart failure

26.2 Conduction Pathways in the Myocardium

Although there are many types of dysrhythmias, all have in common a defect in the *generation* or *conduction* of electrical impulses across the myocardium. These electrical impulses, or **action potentials,** carry the signal for cardiac muscle cells to contract and are precisely coordinated for the chambers to

---

PHARMFACTS

Dysrhythmias

- Dysrhythmias are responsible for more than 44,000 deaths each year.
- Atrial dysrhythmias occur more commonly in men than in women.
- The incidence of atrial dysrhythmias increases with age. They affect:
  <0.5% of those aged 25 to 35.
  1.5% of those up to age 60.
  9% of those over age 75.
- About 15% of strokes occur in patients with atrial dysrhythmias.
- A large majority of sudden cardiac deaths are believed to be caused by ventricular dysrhythmias.
- Atrial fibrillation affects 1.5 to 2.2 million people in the United States.

MyNursingKit | Childhood Dysrhythmias

TABLE 26.1 Types of Dysrhythmias

Name of Dysrhythmia	Description
Atrial or ventricular tachycardia	Rapid heart beat greater than 100 beats per minute in adults; ventricular tachycardia is more serious than atrial tachycardia
Atrial or ventricular flutter	Rapid, regular heartbeats; may range between 200–300 beats/min; atrial may require treatment but is not usually fatal; ventricular flutter requires immediate treatment
Atrial or ventricular fibrillation	Very rapid, uncoordinated beats; complete disorganization of rhythm resulting in lack of adequate cardiac contraction; requires immediate treatment
Heart block	Area of nonconduction in the myocardium; may be partial or complete; classified as first, second, or third degree
Premature atrial or premature ventricular contractions (PVCs)	An extra beat often originating from a source other than the SA node; not normally serious unless it occurs in high frequency
Sinus bradycardia	Slow heartbeat, less than 60 beats per minute; may require a pacemaker

beat in a synchronized manner. For the heart to function properly, the atria must contract simultaneously, sending their blood into the ventricles. Following atrial contraction, the right and left ventricles then must contract simultaneously. Lack of synchronization of the atria and ventricles or of the right and left sides of the heart may have profound consequences. The total time for the electrical impulse to travel across the heart is about 0.22 second. The normal conduction pathway in the heart is illustrated in ➤ Figure 26.1.

Control of synchronization begins in a small area of tissue in the wall of the right atrium known as the **sinoatrial (SA) node.** The SA node or *pacemaker* of the heart has a property called **automaticity,** the ability of certain cells to spontaneously generate an action potential. The SA node generates a new action potential approximately 75 times per minute under resting conditions, with a normal range of 60 to 100 beats per minute. This is referred to as the normal **sinus rhythm.** The SA node is greatly influenced by the activity of the sympathetic and parasympathetic divisions of the autonomic nervous system.

On leaving the SA node, the action potential travels quickly across both atria to the **atrioventricular (AV) node.** The AV node also has the property of automaticity, although less so than the SA node. Should the SA node malfunction, the AV node has the ability to spontaneously generate action potentials and continue the heart's contraction at a rate of 40 to 60 beats per minute. Impulse conduction through the AV node, compared with other areas in the heart, is slow. This allows the atrial contraction enough time to completely empty blood into the ventricles, thereby optimizing cardiac output.

As the action potential leaves the AV node, it travels rapidly to the **atrioventricular bundle,** or *bundle of His.* The impulse is then conducted down the right and left **bundle branches** to the **Purkinje fibers,** which carry the action potential to all regions of the ventricles almost simultaneously. Should the SA and AV nodes become nonfunctional, cells in the AV bundle and Purkinje fibers can continue to generate myocardial contractions at a rate of about 30 beats per minute.

Although action potentials normally begin at the SA node and spread across the myocardium in a coordinated manner, other regions of the heart may begin to initiate beats. These areas, known as **ectopic foci** or **ectopic pacemakers,** may send impulses across the myocardium that compete with those from the normal conduction pathway. Although healthy hearts often experience an extra beat without incident, ectopic foci in diseased hearts have the potential to cause the types of dysrhythmias noted in Table 26.1.

It is important to understand that the underlying purpose of this conduction system is to keep the heart beating in a regular, synchronized manner so that cardiac output can be maintained. Some dysrhythmias occur sporadically, elicit no symptoms, and do not affect cardiac output. These types of abnormalities may go unnoticed by the patient, and rarely require treatment. Others, however, profoundly affect cardiac output, result in patient symptoms, and have the potential to produce serious if not mortal consequences. It is these types of dysrhythmias that require pharmacotherapy.

26.3 The Electrocardiograph

The wave of electrical activity across the myocardium can be measured using the electrocardiograph. The graphic recording from this device, or **electrocardiogram (ECG),** is useful in diagnosing many types of heart conditions, including dysrhythmias.

Three distinct waves are produced by a normal ECG: the P wave, the QRS complex, and the T wave. Changes to the wave patterns or in their timing can reveal certain pathologies. For example, a long PR interval suggests a heart block, and a flat T wave indicates ischemia to the myocardium. Elevated ST segments are used to guide the pharmacotherapy of MI. A normal ECG and its relationship to impulse conduction in the heart is shown in ➤ Figure 26.2.

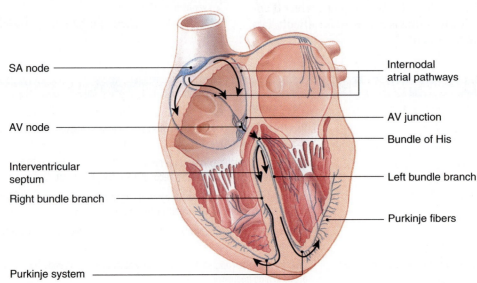

➤ *Figure 26.1* Normal conduction pathway in the heart
Source: Pearson Education/PH College.

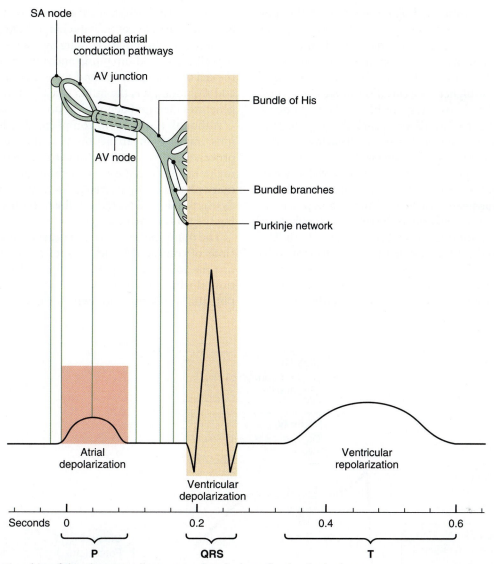

> ➤ *Figure 26.2* Relationship of the electrocardiogram to electrical conduction in the heart
> *Source: Pearson Education/PH College.*

26.4 Nonpharmacologic Therapy of Dysrhythmias

The therapeutic goals of antidysrhythmic pharmacotherapy are to prevent or terminate dysrhythmias in order to reduce the risks of sudden death, stroke, or other complications resulting from the disease. Because these drugs can cause serious adverse effects, antidysrhythmics are normally reserved for patients experiencing symptoms of dysrhythmia or for those whose condition cannot be controlled by other means. Treating asymptomatic dysrhythmias with medications provides little or no benefit to the patient. Health care providers use several nonpharmacologic strategies to eliminate dysrhythmias.

The more serious types of dysrhythmias are corrected through electrical shock of the heart, with treatments such as elective **cardioversion** and **defibrillation**. The electrical shock momentarily stops all electrical impulses in the heart, both normal and abnormal. The temporary cessation of electri-

cal activity often allows the SA node to automatically return conduction to a normal sinus rhythm.

Other types of nonpharmacologic treatment include identification and destruction of the myocardial cells responsible for the abnormal conduction through a surgical procedure called *catheter ablation*. Cardiac pacemakers are sometimes implanted to correct the types of dysrhythmias that cause the heart to beat too slowly. **Implantable cardioverter defibrillators (ICD)** are placed in patients to restore normal rhythm by either pacing the heart or giving it an electric shock when dysrhythmias occur. In addition, the ICD is capable of storing information regarding the heart rhythm for the health care provider to evaluate.

26.5 Phases of the Myocardial Action Potential

Because most antidysrhythmic drugs act by interfering with myocardial action potentials, a firm grasp of this phenomenon is necessary for understanding drug mechanisms. Action potentials occur in both neurons and cardiac muscle cells due to differences in the concentration of certain ions found inside and outside the cell. Under resting conditions, Na^+ and Ca^{2+} are found in higher concentrations *outside* myocardial cells, and K^+ is found in higher concentration *inside* these cells. These imbalances are, in part, responsible for the slight negative charge (80 to 90 mV) inside a myocardial cell membrane relative to the outside of the membrane. A cell having this negative membrane potential is called **polarized.**

An action potential begins when **sodium ion channels** located in the plasma membrane open and Na^+ rushes *into* the cell producing a rapid **depolarization,** or loss of membrane potential. During this period, Ca^{2+} also enters the cell through **calcium ion channels,** although the influx is slower than that of sodium. The entry of Ca^{2+} into the cells is a signal for the release of additional intracellular calcium that is held in storage inside the sarcoplasmic reticulum. It is this large increase in intracellular Ca^{2+} that is responsible for the contraction of cardiac muscle.

During depolarization, the inside of the plasma membrane temporarily reverses its charge, becoming positive. The cell returns to its polarized state by the removal of Na^+ from the cell via the sodium pump and movement of K^+ back into the cell through **potassium ion channels.** In cells located in the SA and AV nodes, it is the influx of Ca^{2+}, rather than Na^+, that generates the rapid depolarization of the membrane.

Although it may seem complicated to learn the different ions involved in an action potential, understanding the process is very important to cardiac pharmacology. Blocking potassium, sodium, or calcium ion channels is the primary pharmacologic strategy used to prevent or terminate dysrhythmias. ➤ Figure 26.3 illustrates the flow of ions during the action potential.

The pumping action of the heart requires alternating periods of contraction and relaxation. There is a brief period of time following depolarization, and most of repolarization, during which the cell cannot initiate another action potential. This time, known as the **refractory period,** ensures

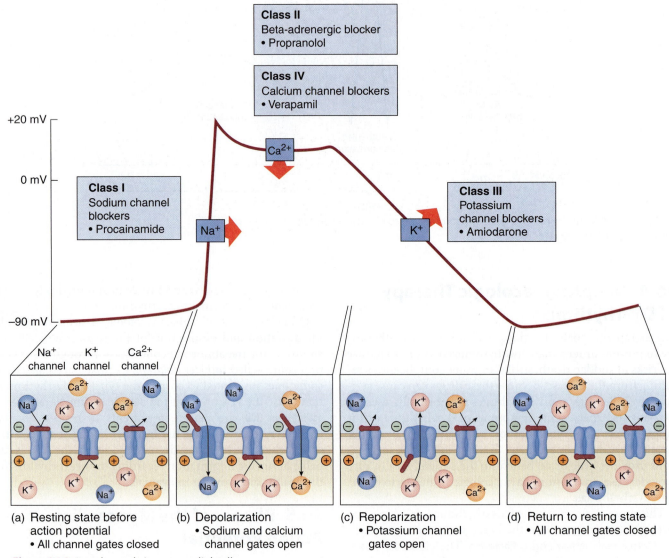

➤ *Figure 26.3* Ion channels in myocardial cells

that the myocardial cell finishes contracting before a second action potential begins. Some antidysrhythmic agents produce their effects by prolonging the refractory period.

26.6 Mechanisms and Classification of Antidysrhythmic Drugs

Antidysrhythmic drugs act by altering specific electrophysiologic properties of the heart. They do this through two basic mechanisms: blocking flow through ion channels (conduction) or altering autonomic activity (automaticity).

Antidysrhythmic drugs are grouped according to the stage in which they affect the action potential. These drugs fall into four primary classes, referred to as classes I, II, III, and IV, and a fifth group that includes miscellaneous drugs not acting by one of the first four mechanisms. The five categories of antidysrhythmics and their mechanisms are listed in Table 26.2.

The use of antidysrhythmic drugs has significantly declined in recent years. Research studies have found that the use of antidysrhythmic medications for prophylaxis can actually *increase* patient mortality. This is because there is a narrow margin between a therapeutic effect and a toxic effect with drugs that affect cardiac rhythm. They have the ability not only to *correct* dysrhythmias but also to worsen or even *create* new dysrhythmias. These prodysrhythmic effects have resulted in less use of drugs in class I and increased use of drugs in class II and class III (specifically, amiodarone).

Another reason for the decline in antidysrhythmic drug use is the success of nonpharmacologic techniques. Research has demonstrated that catheter ablation and implantable defibrillators are more successful in managing certain types of dysrhythmias than is the prophylactic use of medications.

SODIUM CHANNEL BLOCKERS (CLASS I)

The first medical use of quinidine, a sodium channel blocker, was recorded in the 18th century. Doses for the sodium channel blockers, the largest class of antidysrhythmics, are listed in Table 26.3.

26.7 Treating Dysrhythmias with Sodium Channel Blockers

Sodium channel blockers, the class I drugs, are divided into three subgroups, IA, IB, and IC, based on subtle differences in their mechanism of action. Because the action potential is dependent on the opening of sodium ion channels, a blockade of these channels will prevent depolarization. The spread of the action potential across the myocardium will slow, and areas of ectopic pacemaker activity will be suppressed.

The sodium channel blockers are similar in structure and action to local anesthetics. In fact, lidocaine is a class I antidysrhythmic that is a prototype local anesthetic in chapter 19∞. This anesthetic-like action slows impulse conduction across the heart. Some class I antidysrhythmics, such as quinidine and procainamide, are effective against many different types of dysrhythmias. The remaining class I drugs are more specific, and indicated only for life-threatening ventricular dysrhythmias. Although a prototype for many decades, quinidine is rarely used today due to the availability of safer antidysrhythmics.

All the sodium channel blockers have the potential to create new dysrhythmias or worsen existing ones. The reduced heart rate caused by the drug can cause hypotension, dizziness, and syncope. During pharmacotherapy, the ECG should be monitored for signs of cardiotoxicity, such as increases in the PR and QT intervals and widening of QRS complex. Some class I drugs have significant anticholinergic effects such as dry mouth, constipation, and urinary retention. Special precautions should be taken with older adults, because anticholinergic side effects may worsen urinary hesitancy in patients with prostate enlargement. Lidocaine can cause CNS toxicity such as drowsiness, confusion, and convulsions.

TABLE 26.2	Classification of Antidysrhythmics		
Class	**Actions**		**Indications**
I: Sodium channel blockers			
IA example: procainamide	Delays repolarization; slows conduction velocity; increases duration of the action potential		Atrial fibrillation, premature atrial contractions, PVCs, ventricular tachycardia
IB example: lidocaine	Accelerates repolarization; slows conduction velocity; decreases duration of action potential		Severe ventricular dysrhythmias
IC example: flecainide	No significant effect on repolarization; slows conduction velocity		Severe ventricular dysrhythmias
II: Beta-adrenergic antagonists example: propranolol	Slows conduction velocity; decreases automaticity; prolongs refractory period		Atrial flutter and fibrillation, tachydysrhythmia, ventricular dysrhythmias
III: Potassium channel blockers example: amiodarone	Slows repolarization; increases duration of action potential; prolongs refractory period		Severe atrial and ventricular dysrhythmias
IV: Calcium channel blockers example: verapamil	Slows conduction velocity; decreases contractility; prolongs refractory period		Paroxysmal supraventricular tachycardia, supraventricular tachydysrhythmia

TABLE 26.3 Antidysrhythmic Drugs

Drug	Route and Adult Dose (max dose where indicated)	Adverse Effects
CLASS IA: SODIUM CHANNEL BLOCKERS		
disopyramide (Norpace)	PO; 100–200 mg qid (max: 1,200–1,600 mg/day); therapeutic serum drug level is 2–5 mcg/mL	*Nausea, vomiting, diarrhea, dry mouth, urinary retention*
ⓟ procainamide (Procanbid)	PO; 1 g loading dose followed by 250–500 mg bid	May produce new dysrhythmias or worsen existing ones; hypotension, blood dyscrasias (quinidine) and lupus (procainamide)
	IV; 15–18 mg/kg as loading dose by slow infusion over 30 min followed by 1–4 mg/min as maintenance dose by continuous infusion	
quinidine gluconate	PO; 200–600 mg tid–qid (max: 3–4 g/day)	
quinidine sulfate	PO; 200–400 mg tid–qid (max: 3–4 g/day); therapeutic serum drug level is 2–5 mcg/mL	
CLASS IB: SODIUM CHANNEL BLOCKERS		
lidocaine (Xylocaine) (see page 243 for the Prototype Drug box ∞)	IV; 1–4 mg/min infusion rate (max: 3 mg/kg per 5–10 min)	*Nausea, vomiting, drowsiness, dizziness, lethargy*
mexiletine (Mexitil)	PO; 200–300 mg tid (max: 1,200 mg/day)	May produce new dysrhythmias or worsen existing ones; hypotension, bradycardia, CNS toxicity (lidocaine), malignant hyperthermia (lidocaine), status epilepticus if abruptly withdrawn (phenytoin)
phenytoin (Dilantin, Phenytek) (see page 175 for the Prototype Drug box ∞)	PO; 100–200 mg tid (max: 625 mg/day)	
	IV; 50–100 mg every 10–15 min until dysrhythmia is terminated (max: 1 g/day)	
CLASS IC: SODIUM CHANNEL BLOCKERS		
flecainide (Tambocor)	PO; 100 mg bid (max: 400 mg/day)	*Nausea, vomiting, dizziness, headache*
propafenone (Rythmol)	PO; 150–300 mg tid (max: 900 mg/day)	May produce new dysrhythmias or worsen existing ones; hypotension, bradycardia
CLASS II: BETA-ADRENERGIC BLOCKERS		
acebutolol (Sectral)	PO; 200–600 mg bid (max: 1,200 mg/day)	*Fatigue, insomnia, drowsiness, impotence or decreased libido, bradycardia, and confusion*
esmolol (Brevibloc)	IV; 50 mcg/kg/min maintenance dose (max: 200 mcg/kg/min)	Agranulocytosis, laryngospasm, Stevens–Johnson syndrome, anaphylaxis; if the drug is abruptly withdrawn, palpitations, rebound hypertension, life-threatening dysrhythmias, or myocardial ischemia may occur
ⓟ propranolol (Inderal, InnoPran XL)	PO; 10–30 mg tid–qid (max: 480 mg/day) IV; 0.5–3.1 mg every 4 hours	
CLASS III: POTASSIUM CHANNEL BLOCKERS		
ⓟ amiodarone (Cordarone, Pacerone)	PO; 400–600 mg/day (max: 1,600 mg/day as loading dose)	*Blurred vision (amiodarone), photosensitivity, nausea, vomiting, anorexia*
dofetilide (Tikosyn)	PO; 125–500 mcg bid based on creatinine clearance	May produce new dysrhythmias or worsen existing ones; hypotension, bradycardia, pneumonia-like syndrome (amiodarone), angioedema (dofetilide), CNS toxicity (ibutilide)
dronedarone (Multaq)	PO; 400 mg bid	
ibutilide (Corvert)	IV; 1 mg infused over 10 min	
sotalol* (Betapace, Betapace AF, Sorine)	PO; 80 mg bid (max: 320 mg/day)	
CLASS IV: CALCIUM CHANNEL BLOCKERS		
diltiazem (Cardizem, Cartia XT, Dilacor XR, Taztia XT, Tiazac) (see page 348 for the Prototype Drug box ∞)	IV; 5–10 mg/h continuous infusion for a maximum of 24 h (max: 15 mg/h)	*Flushed skin, headache, dizziness, peripheral edema, light-headedness, nausea, diarrhea*
ⓟ verapamil (Calan, Covera-HS, Isoptin SR, Verelan) (see page 366 for the Prototype Drug box ∞)	PO; 240–480 mg/day IV; 5–10 mg direct: may repeat in 15–30 min if needed	Hepatotoxicity, MI, CHF, confusion, mood changes
MISCELLANEOUS ANTIDYSRHYTHMICS		
adenosine (Adenocard, Adenoscan)	IV; 6–12 mg given as a bolus injection every 1–2 min as needed (max: 12 mg/dose)	*Facial flushing, dyspnea, chest warmth* May produce new dysrhythmias or worsen existing ones
digoxin (Digitek, Lanoxin, Lanoxicaps) (see page 331 for the Prototype Drug box ∞)	PO; 0.125–0.5 mg qid; therapeutic serum drug level is 0.8–2 ng/mL	*Nausea, vomiting, headache, and visual disturbances* May produce new dysrhythmias or worsen existing ones

Italics indicate common adverse effects; underlining indicates serious adverse effects.

*Sotalol is a beta blocker, but because its cardiac effects are similar to those of amiodarone, it is considered a class III drug.

Pr Prototype Drug | Procainamide *(Procanbid)*

Therapeutic Class: Antidysrhythmic   **Pharmacologic Class:** Sodium channel blocker/class IA

ACTIONS AND USES

Procainamide is an older drug, approved in 1950, that is chemically related to the local anesthetic procaine. Procainamide blocks sodium ion channels in myocardial cells, thus reducing automaticity and slowing conduction of the action potential across the myocardium. This slight delay in conduction velocity prolongs the refractory period and can suppress dysrhythmias. Procainamide is referred to as a broad-spectrum drug because it has the ability to correct many different types of atrial and ventricular dysrhythmias. The most common dosage form is the extended release tablet; however, procainamide is also available in capsule, IV, and IM formulations. The therapeutic serum drug level is 4 to 8 mcg/mL. The use of procainamide has declined significantly due to the development of more specific and safer drugs.

ADMINISTRATION ALERTS

- Use the supine position during IV administration because severe hypotension may occur.
- Do not break or crush extended-release tablets.
- Pregnancy category C

PHARMACOKINETICS (PO)
Onset: 30 min
Peak: 1–1.5 h
Half-life: 3 h
Duration: 3 h (8 h sustained release)

ADVERSE EFFECTS

Nausea, vomiting, abdominal pain, hypotension, and headache are common during procainamide therapy. High doses may produce CNS effects such as confusion or psychosis. Like all antidysrhythmic drugs, procainamide has the ability to produce new dysrhythmias or worsen existing ones. A lupus-like syndrome may occur in 30% to 50% of patients taking the drug over a year.

Contraindications: Procainamide is contraindicated in patients with complete AV block, severe CHF, blood dyscrasias, and myasthenia gravis.

INTERACTIONS

Drug–Drug: Additive cardiac depressant effects may occur if procainamide is administered with other antidysrhythmics. Additive anticholinergic side effects will occur if procainamide is used concurrently with anticholinergic drugs.

Lab Tests: Procainamide may increase values for the following: AST, ALT, serum alkaline phosphatase, LDH, and serum bilirubin. False-positive Coombs test and ANA titers may occur.

Herbal/Food: Unknown

Treatment of Overdose: Supportive treatment is targeted to reversing hypotension with vasopressors and preventing or treating procainamide-induced dysrhythmias.

Refer to MyNursingKit for a Nursing Process Focus specific to this drug.

NURSING PROCESS FOCUS   PATIENTS RECEIVING ANTIDYSRHYTHMIC DRUGS

Assessment	Potential Nursing Diagnoses
Baseline assessment prior to administration: - Understand the reason the drug has been prescribed in order to assess for therapeutic effects (e.g., atrial, ventricular dysrhythmias). - Obtain a complete health history including cardiovascular (including previous dysrhythmias, HTN, MI, heart failure), and the possibility of pregnancy. Obtain a drug history including allergies, current prescription and OTC drugs, herbal preparations, and alcohol use. Be alert to possible drug interactions. - Obtain baseline weight, vital signs (especially BP and pulse), ECG (rate and rhythm), cardiac monitoring (such as cardiac output if appropriate), and breath sounds. Assess for location and character/amount of edema, if present. - Evaluate appropriate laboratory findings, electrolytes, especially potassium level, renal and liver function studies, and lipid profiles.	- Decreased Cardiac Output (related to dysrhythmias, disease processes, or to adverse effects of drug therapy) - Altered Tissue Perfusion (related to dysrhythmias, disease processes, or to adverse effects of drug therapy) - Anxiety (related to dysrhythmias) - Fatigue (related to dysrhythmias or to adverse effects of drug therapy) - Activity Intolerance (related to adverse effects of drug therapy) - Sexual Dysfunction (related to adverse effects of drug therapy) - Deficient Knowledge (drug therapy) - Risk for Falls, Risk for Injury (related to hypotension, dizziness associated with dysrhythmias, or to adverse effects of drug therapy)
Assessment throughout administration: - Assess for desired therapeutic effects (e.g., control or elimination of dysrhythmia, blood pressure and pulse within established limits). - Continue frequent monitoring of ECG (continuous if hospitalized). Check pulse quality, volume, and regularity along with ECG. Assess for complaints of palpitations and correlate symptoms with ECG findings. - Continue periodic monitoring of electrolytes, especially potassium. - Assess for adverse effects: dizziness, hypotension, nausea, vomiting, headache, fatigue or weakness, flushing, or sexual dysfunction. Bradycardia, tachycardia, or new or different dysrhythmias should be reported to the health care provider immediately.	

(Continued)

NURSING PROCESS FOCUS   PATIENTS RECEIVING ANTIDYSRHYTHMIC DRUGS *(Continued)*

Planning: Patient Goals and Expected Outcomes

The patient will:

- Experience therapeutic effects dependent on the reason the drug is being given (e.g., decreased dysrhythmias, and blood pressure and pulse within normal limits).
- Be free from, or experience minimal, adverse effects.
- Verbalize an understanding of the drug's use, adverse effects, and required precautions.
- Demonstrate proper self-administration of the medication (e.g., dose, timing, when to notify health care provider).

Implementation

Interventions and (Rationales)	Patient and Family Education
Ensuring therapeutic effects: - Continue frequent assessments as above for therapeutic effects. (Dysrhythmias have diminished or are eliminated. Blood pressure and pulse should be within normal limits or within parameters set by health care provider.)	- To allay possible anxiety, teach the patient, family, or caregiver the rationale for all equipment used and the need for frequent monitoring.
- Encourage appropriate lifestyle changes. Provide for dietitian consultation as needed. (Healthy lifestyle changes will support and minimize the need for drug therapy.)	- Encourage the patient to adopt a healthy lifestyle of low-fat food choices, increased exercise, decreased caffeine and alcohol consumption, and smoking cessation.
Minimizing adverse effects: - Continue to monitor ECG and pulse for quality and volume. Take pulse for 1 full minute to assess for regularity. Continue to assess for complaints of palpitations, correlating palpitations or pulse irregularities with ECG. (Not all dysrhythmias are symptomatic. Correlating symptoms with the ECG may help determine the need for further symptom management.)	- Teach the patient, family, or caregiver how to take a peripheral pulse for 1 full minute before taking the drug. Assist the patient to find the pulse area that is most convenient and easily felt. Record daily pulse rates and regularity and bring record to each health care visit. Instruct the patient to notify the health care provider if pulse is below 60 or above 100, there is a noticeable change in regularity from previously felt, or if palpitations develop or worsen.
- Take blood pressure lying, sitting, and standing to detect orthostatic hypotension. Be cautious with the first few doses of the drug and with the elderly who are at increased risk for hypotension. (Antidysrhythmic drugs may cause hypotension. A first-dose effect may occur with a significant drop in BP with the first few doses. Orthostatic hypotension may increase the risk of falls and injury.)	- Teach the patient to rise slowly from lying or sitting to standing to avoid dizziness or falls. - Instruct the patient to take the first dose of the new prescription before bedtime and to be cautious during the next few doses until drug effects are known. - Teach the patient, family, or caregiver how to monitor blood pressure if required. Ensure proper use and functioning of any home equipment obtained. - Instruct the patient to notify the health care provider if blood pressure is 90/60 mmHg or below, or per parameters set by health care provider.
- Continue to monitor periodic electrolyte levels, especially potassium, renal function labs, and drug levels as needed. (Hypokalemia increases the risk of dysrhythmias. Inadequate, or high levels of antidysrhythmic drug may lead to increased or more lethal dysrhythmias.)	- Instruct the patient on the need to return periodically for lab work. - Advise the patient to carry a wallet identification card or wear medical identification jewelry indicating antidysrhythmic therapy.
- Weigh the patient daily and report a weight gain or loss of 1 kg or more in a 24-hour period. Continue to assess for edema, noting location and character. (Daily weight is an accurate measure of fluid status and takes into account intake, output, and insensible losses. Weight gain or edema may indicate adverse drug effects or worsening cardiovascular disease processes.)	- Have the patient weigh self daily, ideally at the same time of day, and record weight along with pulse measurements. Have the patient report a weight loss or gain of more than 1 kg (approximately 2 lb) in a 24-hour period.
- Monitor for breath sounds and heart sounds (e.g., increasing dyspnea or postural nocturnal dyspnea, rales or "crackles" in lungs, frothy pink-tinged sputum, murmurs or extra heart sounds) and report immediately. (Increasing lung congestion or new or worsening heart murmurs may indicate impending heart failure. Potassium-channel blockers are associated with pulmonary toxicity.)	- Instruct the patient to immediately report any severe shortness of breath, frothy sputum, profound fatigue, or swelling of extremities as possible signs of heart failure or pulmonary toxicity.
- Report any visual changes, skin rashes, sunburning to the health care provider. (Potassium-channel blockers may cause photosensitivity, skin rashes, and blurred vision.)	- Teach the patient to report any vision changes promptly and to maintain regular eye examinations. - Teach the patient of importance to wear protective clothing and apply sunscreen regularly during periods of sun exposure.

NURSING PROCESS FOCUS **PATIENTS RECEIVING ANTIDYSRHYTHMIC DRUGS** (Continued)

Implementation

Interventions and (Rationales)	Patient and Family Education
Patient understanding of drug therapy: ■ Use opportunities during administration of medications and during assessments to discuss rationale for drug therapy, desired therapeutic outcomes, most common adverse effects, parameters for when to call health care provider, and any necessary monitoring or precautions. (Using time during nursing care helps to optimize and reinforce key teaching areas.)	■ The patient and/or family should be able to state the reason for drug; appropriate dose and scheduling; what adverse effects to observe for and when to report; equipment needed as appropriate and how to use that equipment; and the required length of medication therapy needed with any special instructions regarding renewing or continuing prescription as appropriate.
Patient self-administration of drug therapy: ■ When administering medications, instruct the patient, family, or caregiver in proper self-administration techniques. (Proper administration increases the effectiveness of the drug.)	■ Teach the patient to take drugs as evenly spaced apart as possible and not to double dose if a dose is missed. ■ Teach the patient not to discontinue the medication abruptly and to call the health care provider if the patient is unable to take medication for more than 1 day due to illness. ■ The patient is able to discuss appropriate dosing and administration needs.

Evaluation of Outcome Criteria

Evaluate the effectiveness of drug therapy by confirming that patient goals and expected outcomes have been met (see "Planning").

See Table 26.3 for a list of drugs (classes I–IV) to which these nursing actions apply. See also Nursing Process Focus tables, chapter 23 ∞ *, for information related to specific categories of antidysrhythmic drugs (e.g., calcium channel blockers).*

BETA-ADRENERGIC ANTAGONISTS/BLOCKERS (CLASS II)

Beta-adrenergic antagonists are widely used for cardiovascular disorders, including hypertension, MI, heart failure, and dysrhythmias. Their ability to slow the heart rate and conduction velocity can suppress several types of dysrhythmias. The beta blockers are listed in Table 26.3.

26.8 Treating Dysrhythmias with Beta-Adrenergic Antagonists

As expected from their effects on the autonomic nervous system, beta-adrenergic blockers slow the heart rate and decrease conduction velocity through the AV node. Myocardial automaticity is reduced, and many types of dysrhythmias are stabilized. These effects are primarily caused by blockade of calcium ion channels in the SA and AV nodes, although these drugs also block sodium ion channels in the atria and ventricles.

The main value of beta blockers as antidysrhythmic agents is to treat atrial dysrhythmias associated with heart failure. In post-MI patients, beta blockers decrease the likelihood of sudden death due to their antidysrhythmic effects. The basic pharmacology of beta-adrenergic antagonists is explained in chapter 13 ∞.

Only a few beta blockers are approved for dysrhythmias, because of the potential for serious adverse effects. Blockade of beta receptors in the heart may result in bradycardia, and hypotension may cause dizziness and possible syncope. Those beta blockers that affect beta$_2$-adrenergic receptors

will also affect the lung, possibly causing bronchospasm. This is of particular concern in patients with asthma, or in elderly patients with chronic obstructive pulmonary disease (COPD). Abrupt discontinuation of beta blockers can lead to dysrhythmias and hypertension.

POTASSIUM CHANNEL BLOCKERS (CLASS III)

Although a small class of drugs, the potassium channel blockers have important applications in the treatment of dysrhythmias. These drugs prolong the duration of the action potential and reduce automaticity. The potassium channel blockers are listed in Table 26.3.

26.9 Treating Dysrhythmias with Potassium Channel Blockers

After the action potential has passed and the myocardial cell is in a depolarized state, repolarization depends on replacement of potassium inside the cell. By blocking potassium

TREATING THE DIVERSE PATIENT

Asian Patients' Sensitivity to Propranolol

Studies have shown that Asians may metabolize propranolol more quickly than Caucasians, probably due to a lack of specific drug metabolizing enzyme (mephenytoin hydroxylase). Because of this genetic difference, the drug has a significantly greater effect on heart rate in many patients of Asian descent. The nurse should assess this population for possible overdosage, and monitor for possible adverse reactions due to high drug levels.

Pr Prototype Drug | Propranolol *(Inderal, InnoPran XL)*

Therapeutic Class: Class II antidysrhythmic   **Pharmacologic Class:** Beta-adrenergic antagonist

ACTIONS AND USES

Propranolol is a nonselective beta-adrenergic blocker, affecting beta$_1$ receptors in the heart, and beta$_2$ receptors in pulmonary and vascular smooth muscle. Propranolol reduces heart rate, slows myocardial conduction velocity, and lowers blood pressure. Propranolol is most effective in treating tachycardia that is caused by excessive sympathetic stimulation. It is approved to treat a wide variety of diseases, including hypertension, angina, and migraine headaches, and for prevention of MI. The drug is available in tablet, extended-release capsules, and IV formulations.

ADMINISTRATION ALERTS

- Abrupt discontinuation may cause MI, severe hypertension, and ventricular dysrhythmias.
- Swallow extended-release tablets whole: Do not crush or chew contents.
- If pulse is less than 60 beats per minute, notify the health care provider.
- Pregnancy category C

PHARMACOKINETICS (PO)
Onset: 0.5–1 h
Peak: 1–2 h (6 h extended release)
Half-life: 3–5 h
Duration: 6–12 h (24 h extended release)

ADVERSE EFFECTS

Common adverse effects of propranolol include fatigue, hypotension, and bradycardia. Because of the ability of propranolol to slow the heart rate, patients with serious cardiac disorders such as heart failure must be carefully monitored. Adverse effects such as diminished libido and impotence may result in nonadherence in male patients. Propranolol should be used cautiously in diabetics due to its hypoglycemic effects and because it may "mask" the symptoms of hypoglycemia as the adrenergic "fight-or-flight" to hypoglycemia is blocked. This drug should be used with caution in patients with reduced renal output, because the drug may accumulate to toxic levels in the blood and cause dysrhythmias.

Contraindications: Because of its depressive effects on the heart, propranolol is contraindicated in patients with cardiogenic shock, sinus bradycardia, greater than first-degree heart block, and heart failure. Because it constricts smooth muscle in the airways, the drug is contraindicated in patients with COPD or asthma.

INTERACTIONS

Drug–Drug: Concurrent administration with other beta blockers may produce additive effects on the heart, and bradycardia or hypotension may result. Because both propranolol and calcium channel blockers suppress myocardial contractility, concurrent use may lead to additive bradycardia. Phenothiazines can add to the hypotensive effects of propranolol. Propranolol should not be given within 2 weeks of an MAO inhibitor, as severe bradycardia and hypotension could result. Use of ethanol or antacids containing aluminum hydroxide gel will slow the absorption of propranolol and reduce its therapeutic effects. Administration of beta-adrenergic agonists such as albuterol (Proventil) will antagonize the actions of propranolol.

Lab Tests: Propranolol may give a false increase for urinary catecholamines.

Herbal/Food: Unknown

Treatment of Overdose: Treatment is targeted to reversing hypotension with vasopressors, and bradycardia with atropine or isoproterenol. Intravenous glucagon reverses the cardiac depression caused by beta blocker overdose by enhancing myocardial contractility, increasing heart rate, and improving AV node conduction.

Refer to MyNursingKit for a Nursing Process Focus specific to this drug.

---

channels, the class III antidysrhythmics delay repolarization of the myocardial cells and lengthen the refractory period, which tends to stabilize dysrhythmias. Most drugs in this class have multiple actions and also affect adrenergic receptors or sodium channels. For example, in addition to blocking potassium channels, sotalol (Betapace, Betapace AF, Sorine) is considered a beta-adrenergic blocker.

The potassium channel blockers are reserved for serious dysrhythmias. Amiodarone (Cordarone, Pacerone) is one of the more frequently used drugs in this class, and is featured as the class III antidysrhythmic. It may be used to treat many different types of atrial and ventricular dysrhythmias. Dofetilide (Tikosyn) and ibutilide (Corvert) are given to terminate atrial flutter or fibrillation. Sotalol (Betapace, Betapace AF, Sorine) is approved for specific types of atrial and ventricular dysrhythmias, when safer drugs have failed to terminate the dysrhythmia.

Drugs in this class have limited uses because of potentially serious adverse effects. Like other antidysrhythmics, potas-

sium channel blockers slow the heart rate, resulting in serious bradycardia and possible hypotension. These adverse effects occur in a significant number of patients. These agents can worsen dysrhythmias, especially following the first few doses. Older adults with preexisting heart failure must be carefully monitored because they are particularly at risk for adverse cardiac effects of potassium channel blockers.

Amiodarone can produce pulmonary toxicity in a significant number of patients. Sotalol and ibutilide can produce torsades de pointes, a type of ventricular tachycardia that can become rapidly fatal if not recognized and treated. Treatment of torsades de pointes includes IV magnesium sulfate or potassium chloride.

In 2009, a new potassium channel blocker was approved. Dronedarone (Multaq) is chemically similar to amiodarone but is claimed to have a reduced incidence of adverse effects. Like sotalol, dronedarone has multiple actions on the heart. Dronedarone is approved for the treatment of paroxysmal or persistent atrial fibrillation or flutter. The labeling in-

Pr Prototype Drug | Amiodarone *(Cordarone, Pacerone)*

Therapeutic Class: Class III antidysrhythmic **Pharmacologic Class:** Potassium channel blocker

ACTIONS AND USES

Amiodarone is structurally similar to thyroid hormone. It is approved for the treatment of resistant ventricular tachycardia that may prove life threatening, and it has become a drug of choice for the treatment of atrial dysrhythmias in patients with heart failure. In addition to blocking potassium ion channels, some of this drug's actions on the heart relate to its blockade of sodium ion channels. Amiodarone is available as oral tablets and as an IV infusion. IV infusions are limited to short-term therapy, normally only 2 to 4 days. When given orally, its onset of action may take several weeks. Its effects, however, can last 4 to 8 weeks after the drug is discontinued, since it has an extended half-life that may exceed 100 days. The therapeutic serum level of amiodarone is 0.5 to 2.5 mcg/mL.

ADMINISTRATION ALERTS

- Hypokalemia and hypomagnesemia should be corrected prior to initiating therapy.
- Pregnancy category D

PHARMACOKINETICS (PO)
Onset: 2–3 d to 1–3 wk
Peak: 3–7 h
Half-life: 15–100 days
Duration: 10–150 days

ADVERSE EFFECTS

The most serious adverse effect from amiodarone occurs in the lung, with the drug causing a pneumonia-like syndrome. Amiodarone may also cause blurred vision, rashes, photosensitivity, nausea, vomiting, anorexia, fatigue, dizziness, and hypotension. Because this medication is concentrated by certain tissues and has a prolonged half-life, adverse effects may be slow to resolve.

Contraindications: Amiodarone is contraindicated in patients with severe bradycardia, cardiogenic shock, sick sinus syndrome, severe sinus node dysfunction, or third-degree AV block.

INTERACTIONS

Drug–Drug: Amiodarone can increase serum digoxin levels by as much as 70%. Amiodarone greatly enhances the actions of anticoagulants: Thus, the dose of warfarin must be cut by as much as half. Use with beta-adrenergic blockers or calcium channel blockers may cause or worsen sinus bradycardia, sinus arrest, or AV block. Amiodarone may increase phenytoin levels two- to threefold.

Lab Tests: May increase values for the following tests: nuclear antibody, ALT, AST, and serum alkaline phosphatase, T_4.

Herbal/Food: Use with echinacea may cause an increased risk of hepatotoxicity. Aloe may cause an increased effect of amiodarone.

Treatment of Overdose: Treatment of amiodarone overdose is targeted to reversing hypotension with vasopressors, and bradycardia with atropine or isoproterenol.

Refer to MyNursingKit for a Nursing Process Focus specific to this drug.

---

cludes a boxed warning stating that dronedarone increases the risk of death and is contraindicated in patients with serious heart failure.

CALCIUM CHANNEL BLOCKERS (CLASS IV)

Like beta blockers, the calcium channel blockers are widely prescribed for various cardiovascular disorders. By slowing conduction velocity, they are able to stabilize certain dysrhythmias. Doses for the antidysrhythmic calcium channel blockers are listed in Table 26.3.

26.10 Treating Dysrhythmias with Calcium Channel Blockers

Although about 10 calcium channel blockers (CCBs) are available to treat cardiovascular diseases, only a limited number have been approved for dysrhythmias. A few CCBs such as diltiazem (Cardizem) and verapamil (Calan) block calcium ion channels in both the heart and arterioles; the remainder are specific to calcium channels in vascular smooth muscle. Diltiazem is a prototype drug for the treatment of angina, as discussed in chapter 25∞. The basic pharmacology of this drug class is presented in chapter 23∞.

Blockade of calcium ion channels has a number of effects on the heart, most of which are similar to those of beta-adrenergic blockers. Effects include reduced automaticity in the SA node and slowed impulse conduction through the AV node. This slows the heart rate and prolongs the refractory period. Calcium channel blockers are only effective against supraventricular dysrhythmias.

Calcium channel blockers are safe medications that are well tolerated by most patients. As with other antidysrhythmics, bradycardia and hypotension are frequent adverse effects. Because the cardiac effects of CCBs are almost identical with those of beta-adrenergic blockers, patients concurrently taking drugs from both classes are especially at risk for bradycardia and possible heart failure. Because older patients often have multiple cardiovascular disorders, such as hypertension, heart failure, and dysrhythmias, it is not unusual to find elderly patients taking drugs from multiple classes.

AVOIDING MEDICATION ERRORS

During a morning assessment, the nurse observes that a surgical patient has developed an irregular heart rate of 120 beats per minute. The nurse notifies the resident physician, who orders a stat electrocardiogram. A ventricular dysrhythmia is detected and the physician tells the nurse to administer lidocaine 150 mg as a single bolus to be followed by a continuous infusion of 1 g of lidocaine in 500 mL of 5% dextrose in water. The nurse is not sure what the usual loading dose is. What should the nurse do?

See Appendix D for the suggested answer.

Pr Prototype Drug | Verapamil *(Calan, Covera-HS, Isoptin SR, Verelan)*

Therapeutic Class: Class IV antidysrhythmic   **Pharmacologic Class:** Calcium channel blocker

ACTIONS AND USES

Verapamil was the first CCB approved by the FDA. The drug acts by inhibiting the flow of calcium ions both into myocardial cells and in vascular smooth muscle. In the heart, this action slows conduction velocity and stabilizes dysrhythmias. In the vessels, calcium channel blockade lowers blood pressure, reducing cardiac workload. Verapamil also dilates the coronary arteries, an action that is important when the drug is used to treat angina (chapter 25∞). The drug is available in oral, oral extended-release, and IV formulations. The therapeutic serum level is 0.08 to 0.3 mcg/mL.

ADMINISTRATION ALERTS

- Swallow the capsule whole: Do not open or allow patients to chew the contents.
- For IV administration, inspect the drug preparation to make sure the solution is clear and colorless.
- Pregnancy category C

> **PHARMACOKINETICS (PO)**
> **Onset:** 1–2 h
> **Peak:** 30–90 min (4–8 h extended release)
> **Half-life:** 2–8 h
> **Duration:** 3–7 h PO (24 h extended release)

ADVERSE EFFECTS

Adverse effects are generally minor and include headache, constipation, and hypotension. Because verapamil can cause bradycardia, patients with heart failure should be carefully monitored.

Contraindications: Verapamil is contraindicated in patients with AV heart block, sick sinus syndrome, severe hypotension, or bleeding aneurysm, or those undergoing intracranial surgery. Use with caution in patients with renal or hepatic impairment.

INTERACTIONS

Drug–Drug: Verapamil has the ability to elevate blood levels of digoxin (Digitek, Lanoxin, Lanoxicaps). Since digoxin and verapamil both slow conduction through the AV node, their concurrent use must be carefully monitored to avoid bradycardia. Use with antihypertensive drugs, including beta blockers, may cause additive hypotension.

Lab Tests: Unknown

Herbal/Food: Grapefruit juice may increase verapamil levels. Hawthorn may have additive hypotensive effects.

Treatment of Overdose: Treatment of verapamil overdose is targeted to reversing hypotension with vasopressors. Calcium salts such as calcium chloride may be administered to increase the amount of calcium available to the myocardium and arterioles.

Refer to MyNursingKit for a Nursing Process Focus specific to this drug.

26.11 Miscellaneous Drugs for Dysrhythmias

Two other drugs, adenosine (Adenocard, Adenoscan) and digoxin (Digitek, Lanoxin, Lanoxicaps), are occasionally used to treat specific dysrhythmias, but do not act by the mechanisms previously described. These miscellaneous agents are listed in Table 26.3.

Adenosine (Adenocard, Adenoscan) is a naturally occurring nucleoside. When given as a 1- to 2-second bolus IV injection, adenosine terminates serious atrial tachycardia by slowing conduction through the AV node and decreasing automaticity of the SA node. Its primary indication is a specific dysrhythmia known as paroxysmal supraventricular tachycardia (PSVT), for which it is a drug of choice. It is also used to assist in the diagnosis of coronary artery disease or dysrhythmias in patients who are unable to undergo an exercise stress test. Although dyspnea is common, adverse effects are generally self-limiting because of its 10-second half-life.

Although digoxin is primarily used to treat heart failure, it is also prescribed for certain types of atrial dysrhythmias due to its ability to decrease automaticity of the SA node and slow conduction through the AV node. Because excessive levels of digoxin can produce serious dysrhythmias, and interactions with other medications are common, patients must be carefully monitored during therapy. Additional information on the mechanism of action and the adverse effects of digoxin may be found in chapter 24∞, where this drug is featured as a prototype cardiac glycoside for heart failure.

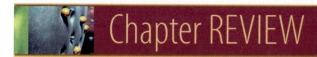

Chapter REVIEW

KEY CONCEPTS

The numbered key concepts provide a succinct summary of the important points from the corresponding numbered section within the chapter. If any of these points are not clear, refer to the numbered section within the chapter for review.

26.1 The frequency of dysrhythmias in the population is difficult to predict because many patients experience no symptoms. Persistent or severe dysrhythmias may be lethal. Dysrhythmias are classified by the location (atrial or ventricular) or type (flutter, fibrillation, or block) of rhythm abnormality produced.

26.2 The electrical conduction pathway from the SA node, to the AV node, to the bundle branches and Purkinje fibers keeps the heart beating in a synchronized manner. Some myocardial cells in these regions have the property of automaticity.

26.3 The electrocardiograph may be used to record electrophysiologic events in the heart and to diagnose dysrhythmias.

26.4 Nonpharmacologic therapy of dysrhythmias, including cardioversion, ablation, and implantable cardioverter defibrillators, are often the treatments of choice.

26.5 Changes in sodium and potassium levels generate the action potential in myocardial cells. Depolarization occurs when sodium (and calcium) rushes in; repolarization occurs when sodium ions are removed and potassium ions are restored inside the cell.

26.6 Antidysrhythmic drugs are classified by their mechanism of action, namely, classes I through IV. The use of antidysrhythmic drugs has been declining.

26.7 Sodium channel blockers, the largest group of antidysrhythmics, act by slowing the rate of impulse conduction across the heart.

26.8 Beta-adrenergic blockers act by reducing automaticity as well as by slowing conduction velocity across the myocardium.

26.9 Potassium channel blockers act by prolonging the refractory period of the heart.

26.10 Calcium channel blockers act by reducing automaticity and by slowing myocardial conduction velocity. Their actions and effects are similar to those of the beta blockers.

26.11 Digoxin and adenosine are used for specific dysrhythmias but do not act by blocking ion channels.

NCLEX-RN® REVIEW QUESTIONS

1 A type I diabetic on insulin reports that he takes propranolol (Inderal) for his hypertension. This raises a concern and the nurse will teach the patient to check glucose levels more frequently because:
1. the beta blocker can produce insulin resistance.
2. the two agents used together will increase the risk of ketoacidosis.
3. propranolol will increase insulin requirements by antagonizing the effects at the receptors.
4. the beta blocker can mask symptoms of hypoglycemia.

2 When monitoring for therapeutic effect of any antidysrhythmic agent, the nurse would be sure to assess:
1. pulse.
2. blood pressure.
3. drug level.
4. hourly urine output.

3 Because of its effect on the heart, verapamil (Calan, Covera-HS, Isoptin SR, Verelan) should be used with extra caution or is contraindicated in patients with:
1. hypertension.
2. tachycardia.

3. heart failure.
4. angina.

4 Common adverse effects of antidysrhythmic medications include: (Select all that apply.)
1. hypotension.
2. hypertension.
3. dizziness.
4. weakness.
5. panic attacks.

5 A patient is given a prescription for propranolol (Inderal) 40 mg bid. The <u>most</u> important instruction for the nurse to give this patient is:
1. take this medication on an empty stomach, as food interferes with its absorption.
2. do not stop taking this medication abruptly; the dosage must be decreased gradually if it is discontinued.
3. if the patient experiences any disturbances in hearing, the patient should notify the health care provider immediately.
4. the patient may become very sleepy while taking this medication; do not drive.

6 A patient was admitted from the emergency department after receiving treatment for dysrhythmias and will be started on amiodarone (Cordarone, Pacerone) because of lack of therapeutic effects from his other antidysrhythmic therapy. When the nurse checks with him in the afternoon, he complains of feeling lightheaded and dizzy. The nurse will first assess:

1. whether there is the possibility of sleep deprivation from the stress of admission to the hospital.

2. whether an allergic reaction is occurring with anticholinergic-like symptoms.

3. whether the amiodarone level is not yet therapeutic enough to treat the dysrhythmias.

4. whether the patient's pulse and blood pressure are within normal limits.

CRITICAL THINKING QUESTIONS

1. A patient with a history of COPD and tachycardia has recently been placed on propranolol (Inderal) to control the tachydysrhythmia. What is a priority for the nurse in monitoring this patient?

2. A patient is started on amiodarone (Cordarone, Pacerone) for cardiac dysrhythmias. This patient is also on digoxin (Digitek, Lanoxin, Lanoxicaps), warfarin (Coumadin), and insulin. What is a priority teaching for this patient?

3. A patient is on verapamil (Calan, Covera-HS, Isoptin SR, Verelan) and digoxin (Digitek, Lanoxin, Lanoxicaps). What is a priority that this patient needs to be monitored for?

See Appendix D for answers and rationales for all activities.

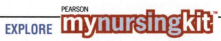

EXPLORE

MyNursingKit is your one stop for online chapter review materials and resources. Prepare for success with additional NCLEX®-style practice questions, interactive assignments and activities, web links, animations and videos, and more!

Register your access code from the front of your book at
www.mynursingkit.com.

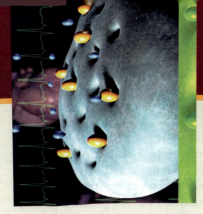

Chapter 27

Drugs for Coagulation Disorders

LEARNING OUTCOMES

After reading this chapter, the student should be able to:

1. Illustrate the major steps of hemostasis and fibrinolysis.
2. Describe thromboembolic disorders that are indications for coagulation modifiers.
3. Identify the primary mechanisms by which coagulation modifier drugs act.
4. Explain how laboratory testing of coagulation parameters is used to monitor anticoagulant pharmacotherapy.
5. Describe the nurse's role in the pharmacologic management of coagulation disorders.
6. For each of the classes listed in Drugs at a Glance, know representative drug examples, and explain the mechanism of drug action, primary actions, and important adverse effects.
7. Use the nursing process to care for patients receiving drug therapy for coagulation disorders.

KEY TERMS

Pr Prototype Drug | Warfarin *(Coumadin)*

Therapeutic Class: Anticoagulant (oral)   **Pharmacologic Class:** Vitamin K antagonist

ACTIONS AND USES

Indications for warfarin therapy include the prevention of CVA, MI, DVT, and pulmonary embolism in patients undergoing hip or knee surgery, or in those with long-term indwelling central venous catheters or prosthetic heart valves. The drug may be given to prevent thromboembolic events in high-risk patients following an MI or an atrial fibrillation episode.

Unlike with heparin, the anticoagulant activity of warfarin can take several days to reach its maximum effect. This explains why heparin and warfarin therapy are overlapped. Warfarin inhibits the action of vitamin K. Without adequate vitamin K, the synthesis of clotting factors II, VII, IX, and X is diminished. Because these clotting factors are normally circulating in the blood, it takes several days for their plasma levels to fall, and for the anticoagulant effect of warfarin to appear. Another reason for the slow onset is that 99% of the warfarin is bound to plasma proteins and is thus unavailable to produce its effect. The therapeutic range of serum warfarin levels varies from 1 to 10 mcg/mL, to achieve an INR value of 2.0 to 3.0.

ADMINISTRATION ALERTS

- If life-threatening bleeding occurs during therapy, the anticoagulant effects of warfarin can be reduced by IM or subcutaneous administration of its antagonist, vitamin K_1.
- Pregnancy category X

PHARMACOKINETICS (PO)

Onset: 2–7 days

Peak: 0.5–3 days

Half-life: 0.5–3 days

Duration: 3–5 days

ADVERSE EFFECTS

The most serious adverse effect of warfarin is abnormal bleeding. On discontinuation of therapy, the anticoagulant activity of warfarin may persist for up to 10 days.

Contraindications: Patients with recent trauma, active internal bleeding, bleeding disorders, intracranial hemorrhage, severe hypertension, bacterial endocarditis, or severe hepatic or renal impairment should not take warfarin.

INTERACTIONS

Drug–Drug: Extensive protein binding is responsible for numerous drug–drug interactions, including an increased effect of warfarin with alcohol, NSAIDs, diuretics, SSRIs and other antidepressants, steroids, antibiotics and vaccines, and vitamins (e.g., vitamin K). During warfarin therapy, the patient should not take any other prescription or OTC drugs unless approved by the health care provider.

Lab Tests: Unknown

Herbal/Food: Use of warfarin with herbal supplements such as green tea, ginkgo, feverfew, garlic, cranberry, chamomile, and ginger may increase the risk of bleeding.

Treatment of Overdose: The specific treatment for overdose is oral or parenteral administration of vitamin K_1. When administered IV, vitamin K_1 can reverse the anticoagulant effects of warfarin within 6 hours.

Refer to MyNursingKit for a Nursing Process Focus specific to this drug.

NURSING PROCESS FOCUS   PATIENTS RECEIVING ANTICOAGULANT THERAPY

Assessment	Potential Nursing Diagnoses
Baseline assessment prior to administration: - Understand the reason the drug has been prescribed in order to assess for therapeutic effects (e.g., prevention of thrombosis from developing when phlebitis is present). - Obtain a complete health history including cardiovascular (including HTN, MI, heart failure) and peripheral vascular disease (including thrombophlebitis), respiratory (including previous pulmonary embolism), neurologic (including recent head injury, CVA), hepatic or renal disease, diabetes, peptic ulcer disease, hypercholesterolemia, and the possibility of alcoholism or pregnancy. Ask women of menstrual age about length and heaviness of usual menstrual flow. Obtain a drug history including allergies, current prescription and OTC drugs, herbal preparations, and alcohol use. Be alert to possible drug interactions. - Obtain baseline weight, vital signs, ECG (if appropriate), and breath sounds. Assess for presence, quality, location of angina, and for presence of dyspnea or chest pain. Assess extremities for symptoms of thrombophlebitis (e.g., warmth, swelling, tenderness in calf, positive Homan's sign) and for location and character/amount of edema, if present. - Evaluate appropriate laboratory findings (e.g., aPTT, aPT, and/or INR), complete blood count (CBC), renal and liver function studies, arterial blood gases (ABGs) as appropriate, and lipid profiles.	- Pain (related to thrombosis and lessened perfusion) - Ineffective Tissue Perfusion (related to decreased circulation in affected area) - Impaired Skin Integrity (in lower extremities related to ineffective tissue perfusion) - Anxiety (related to possible hospitalization, uncertainty over seriousness of illness) - Deficient Knowledge (drug therapy) - Risk for Injury (bleeding, related to adverse effects of anticoagulant therapy)

NURSING PROCESS FOCUS PATIENTS RECEIVING ANTICOAGULANT THERAPY *(Continued)*

Assessment	Potential Nursing Diagnoses
Assessment throughout administration: ■ Assess for desired therapeutic effects (e.g., area of phlebitis exhibits signs of improvement with no symptoms of thrombosis formation; signs and symptoms of existing thrombosis show gradual improvement: e.g., previous anginal or peripheral extremity pain has diminished or is eliminated; peripheral pulses are improving in quality and volume). ■ Continue periodic monitoring of appropriate lab values (e.g., aPTT, PT, and/or INR). ■ Assess for adverse effects: bleeding at IV sites, wounds, excessive ecchymosis, petechiae, hematuria, black/tarry stools, rectal bleeding, "coffee-ground" emesis, epistaxis, bleeding from gums, hemoptysis, prolonged and/or heavy menstrual flow, and for occult bleeding, such as pallor, dizziness, hypotension, tachycardia, abdominal pain, areas of abdominal wall swelling or firmness, lumbar pain, or decreased level of consciousness.	

Planning: Patient Goals and Expected Outcomes

The patient will:
- Experience therapeutic effects dependent on the reason the drug is being given (e.g., prevention of thrombosis or limited extension of existing thrombosis).
- Be free from, or experience minimal, adverse effects.
- Verbalize an understanding of the drug's use, adverse effects, and required precautions.
- Demonstrate proper self-administration of the medication (e.g., dose, timing, when to notify provider).

Implementation

Interventions and (Rationales)	Patient and Family Education
Ensuring therapeutic effects: ■ Continue frequent assessments as described earlier for therapeutic effects, e.g., existing area of phlebitis exhibits signs of improvement; signs and symptoms of existing thrombosis show gradual improvement; and peripheral pulses are improving in quality and volume. (Anticoagulants help prevent the formation of thrombi or prevent existing thrombi from increasing in size.)	■ To allay possible anxiety, teach the patient, family, or caregiver the rationale for all equipment used (e.g., antiembolic stockings, intermittent pneumatic sequential compression devices) and the need for frequent monitoring.
■ Encourage early ambulation postoperatively in the hospitalized patient and active range of motion (ROM) if the patient is on bedrest or has limited mobility. Perform passive ROM in patients who are unable to perform active ROM. (Early ambulation and ROM prevents venous stasis and thrombosis formation, lessening the need for anticoagulant therapy.)	■ Assist the patient with ambulation postoperatively and teach active ROM. Teach the patient, family, or caregiver how to perform passive ROM exercises for patients who are unable to perform active ROM.
■ Assess the patient's lifestyle and occasions of travel over extended lengths of time. (Prolonged sitting during air or car travel may limit blood flow to lower extremities and venous return, promoting the formation of thrombi. Frequent stretching and ambulating, and increasing fluids to maintain normal osmolarity/viscosity may decrease thrombosis formation and lessen the need for anticoagulant therapy.)	■ Educate patients and consumers about thrombosis prevention during travel: periodic stretching, short periods of ambulation, avoid sitting for prolonged periods, and increasing fluid intake.
■ Encourage appropriate lifestyle changes. Provide for dietitian consultation as needed. (Smoking increases platelet aggregation and promotes the formation of thrombi. Healthy lifestyle changes will support and minimize the need for drug therapy.)	■ Encourage the patient to adopt a healthy lifestyle of low-fat food choices, increased exercise, decreased caffeine and alcohol consumption, and smoking cessation. Provide for appropriate consultation (e.g., dietitian) as needed.
Minimizing adverse effects: ■ Monitor for signs and symptoms of excessive visible bleeding: bleeding at IV sites, wounds, excessive ecchymosis, petechiae, hematuria, black/tarry stools, rectal bleeding, "coffee-ground" emesis, epistaxis, bleeding from gums, hemoptysis, prolonged and/or heavy menstrual flow, and for occult bleeding. (Frequent assessment for both visible and occult bleeding is necessary to prevent hemorrhage and to start early corrective treatment as appropriate.)	■ Teach the patient, family, or caregiver signs and symptoms of excessive bleeding, including occult bleeding. If external bleeding occurs, pressure over the site should be held up to 15 minutes. If bleeding continues, is severe, or is accompanied by dizziness or syncope, immediate medical attention (e.g., 911) should be obtained. ■ Women of menstrual age should report excessively heavy or prolonged menstrual bleeding and should keep a "pad count" and report to the health care provider.

(Continued)

NURSING PROCESS FOCUS   PATIENTS RECEIVING ANTICOAGULANT THERAPY *(Continued)*

Implementation

Interventions and (Rationales)	Patient and Family Education
• Continue to monitor frequent labs (aPTT, aPT, and/or INR), CBC, and platelets. (Therapeutic aPTT and aPT levels are usually 1.5–2.5 times the normal control value. INR is usually 2–3.5 or 4. Values below the norm indicate below-therapeutic levels of the drug; values above the norm indicate a high potential for bleeding and hemorrhage. CBC, especially RBC, Hgb and Hct, and platelet levels should remain within normal limits. Decreasing values on the CBC may indicate excessive bleeding and the need to assess for location.)	• Instruct patient on need to return periodically for lab work and to alert lab personnel that anticoagulant therapy is being used. • Instruct the patient to carry a wallet identification card or wear medical identification jewelry indicating anticoagulant therapy.
• Continue to monitor peripheral pulses for quality and volume, and complaints of angina or chest pain, especially if new or of sudden onset or accompanied by dyspnea. (Monitoring for new or sudden onset of pain is necessary to ensure prompt treatment of possible emboli.)	• Teach the patient to report any sudden pain in chest, legs or calves, dyspnea, or new-onset anginal pain immediately.
• Minimize opportunities for injury or bleeding where possible: avoid IM injections, provide soft toothbrush, and be cautious when providing care, especially with elderly who have more fragile skin. (Anticoagulants raise the risk of bleeding and causes of even minor bleeding should be avoided when possible.)	• Instruct the patient on ways to minimize opportunities for injury or bleeding where possible: • Switch to a soft toothbrush and inspect gums after brushing. • Use an electric razor if possible or be cautious with a safety razor, holding prolonged pressure over small nicks. • Be cautious with food preparation, especially when cutting food. • Avoid contact sports, amusement park rides, or other physical activities that may cause intense or violent bumping, jostling, or injury. • Frequently assess elderly family members on anticoagulant therapy who have more fragile skin and may experience skin tears or ecchymosis more frequently.
• Closely evaluate all new prescriptions or use of OTC medications for drug interactions. (Many drugs interact with anticoagulants, increasing the chance for bleeding. All OTC medications containing salicylates, e.g., aspirin, are contraindicated.)	• Instruct the patient to consult the health care provider before taking any new prescription or OTC medication, including herbal preparations.
• Maintain normal diet, avoiding increases or decreases in vitamin K–rich foods (e.g., asparagus, broccoli, cabbage, cauliflower, kale) and limit or eliminate alcohol intake. (Vitamin K is necessary for the synthesis of clotting agents. Sudden increases or decreases in dietary intake of vitamin K–rich foods may increase or decrease the effectiveness of anticoagulants, particularly oral anticoagulant therapy. Excessive intake of alcohol, over two drinks per day in men or one in women, may alter the effectiveness of oral anticoagulants.)	• Teach the patient to maintain a normal diet, avoiding increases or decreases in vitamin K–rich foods and limit or eliminate alcohol intake. Vitamin K supplements, and protein supplement drinks (e.g., Ensure, or Boost) that often have vitamin K added should also be avoided. • Advise patients to avoid excessive intake of alcohol while on oral anticoagulants.
• Assess for any symptoms of hepatitis (e.g., darkening urine, light or clay-colored stools, itchy skin, jaundice of sclera or skin, abdominal pain especially in right upper quadrant [RUQ]) in patients receiving oral anticoagulant therapy. (Drug-induced hepatitis is a possible adverse effect of oral anticoagulant therapy.)	• Instruct the patient to report any signs of possible hepatitis immediately, especially abdominal discomfort that localizes to the RUQ.
Patient understanding of drug therapy: • Use opportunities during administration of medications and during assessments to discuss rationale for drug therapy, desired therapeutic outcomes, most common adverse effects, parameters for when to call health care provider, and any necessary monitoring or precautions. (Using time during nursing care helps to optimize and reinforce key teaching areas.)	• The patient should be able to state the reason for drug; appropriate dose and scheduling; what adverse effects to observe for and when to report; equipment needed as appropriate and how to use that equipment; and the required length of medication therapy needed with any special instructions regarding renewing or continuing prescription as appropriate.

NURSING PROCESS FOCUS   PATIENTS RECEIVING ANTICOAGULANT THERAPY (Continued)

Implementation

Interventions and (Rationales)	Patient and Family Education

Patient self-administration of drug therapy:
■ When administering medications, instruct the patient, family, or caregiver in proper self-administration techniques followed by return demonstration. (Proper drug administration increases the effectiveness of the drug.)
	■ Teach the patient, family, or caregiver in proper self-administration techniques:
	  ■ Injections of heparin or LMWH should be administered in the fatty layers of the abdomen or just above the iliac crest avoiding the periumbilical area by 5 cm (2 in.).
	  ■ Skin is drawn up ("pinched") and needle is inserted at a 90-degree angle.
	  ■ Injection is given without aspirating for blood return.
	  ■ Release skin and hold slight pressure to site but do not massage area.
	■ Have patient, family, or caregiver return-demonstrate technique until proper technique is used and they are comfortable giving injection.
	■ Teach the patient on oral anticoagulants to take the medication at the same time each day.

Evaluation of Outcome Criteria

Evaluate the effectiveness of drug therapy by confirming that patient goals and expected outcomes have been met (see "Planning").

See Table 27.3 for a list of drugs to which these nursing actions apply.

antiplatelet agents are used to prevent clot formation in arteries. The antiplatelet agents are listed in Table 27.4.

27.6 Pharmacotherapy with Antiplatelet Drugs

Platelets are a key component of hemostasis: too few platelets or diminished platelet function can profoundly in-

crease bleeding time. The following four types of drugs are classified as antiplatelet agents:

1. Aspirin
2. ADP receptor blockers
3. Glycoprotein IIb/IIIa receptor antagonists
4. Agents for intermittent claudication

TABLE 27.4	**Antiplatelet Agents**	
Drug	**Route and Adult Dose (max dose where indicated)**	**Adverse Effects**
aspirin (ASA, acetylsalicylic acid) (see page 230 for the Prototype Drug box ∞)	PO; 80 mg/day to 650 mg bid	*Nausea, vomiting, diarrhea, abdominal pain* <u>Increased clotting time, GI bleeding (aspirin), CNS effects (dipyridamole), anaphylaxis (aspirin)</u>
dipyridamole (Persantine)	PO; 75–100 mg qid	
ADP RECEPTOR BLOCKERS		
clopidogrel (Plavix)	PO; 75 mg/day	*Dyspepsia, abdominal pain, rash, and diarrhea* <u>Increased clotting time, GI bleeding, blood dyscrasias</u>
prasugrel (Effient)	PO; 60 mg loading dose followed by 10 mg/day	
ticlopidine (Ticlid)	PO; 250 mg bid (max: 500 mg/day)	
GLYCOPROTEIN IIB/IIIA RECEPTOR ANTAGONISTS		
abciximab (ReoPro)	IV; 0.25 mg/kg initial bolus over 5 min; then 10 mcg/kg/min for 12 h (max: 10 mcg/min)	*Dyspepsia, dizziness, pain at injection site, hypotension, bradycardia, minor bleeding* <u>Hemorrhage, thrombocytopenia</u>
eptifibatide (Integrilin)	IV; 180 mcg/kg initial bolus over 1–2 min; then 2 mcg/kg/min for 24–72 h	
tirofiban (Aggrastat)	IV; 0.4 mcg/kg/min for 30 min; then 0.1 mcg/kg/min for 12–24 h	
AGENTS FOR INTERMITTENT CLAUDICATION		
cilostazol (Pletal)	PO; 100 mg bid	*Dyspepsia, nausea, vomiting, dizziness, myalgia, headache* <u>Tachycardia and palpitations (cilostazol), CNS effects (pentoxifylline), heart failure, MI</u>
pentoxifylline (Trental)	PO; 400 mg tid	

Italics indicate common adverse effects; <u>underlining</u> indicates serious adverse effects.

Aspirin deserves special mention as an antiplatelet agent. Because it is available over the counter, patients may not consider aspirin a potent medication; however, its anticoagulant activity is well documented. Aspirin acts by binding irreversibly to the enzyme cyclooxygenase in platelets. This binding inhibits the formation of thromboxane A$_2$, a powerful inducer of platelet aggregation. The anticoagulant effect of a single dose of aspirin may persist for as long as a week. Concurrent use of aspirin with other coagulation modifiers should be avoided, unless approved by the prescriber. Aspirin is featured as a drug prototype for pain relief in chapter 18∞, and is also indicated for prevention of strokes and MI in chapter 25∞, and reduction of inflammation in chapter 33∞.

The ADP receptor blockers are a small group of drugs that irreversibly alter the plasma membrane of platelets. This alteration changes the binding of ADP to its receptor on platelets so they are unable to receive the chemical signals required for them to aggregate. Both ticlopidine (Ticlid) and clopidogrel (Plavix) are given orally to prevent thrombi formation in patients who have experienced a recent thromboembolic event such as a stroke or MI. Ticlopidine can cause life-threatening neutropenia and agranulocytosis. Clopidogrel is considerably safer, having adverse effects comparable to those of aspirin. Prasugrel (Effient) is a newer ADP receptor blocker, approved in 2009. It is indicated to reduce thrombotic events in patients with acute coronary syndromes who undergo PCI.

Glycoprotein IIb/IIIa receptor antagonists are relatively new additions to the treatment of thromboembolic disease.

Glycoprotein IIb/IIIa is an enzyme necessary for platelet aggregation. These drugs are used to prevent thrombi in patients experiencing a recent MI, stroke, or percutaneous transluminal coronary angioplasty (PTCA). Although these drugs are the most effective antiplatelet agents, they are very expensive. Another major disadvantage is that they can be given only by the IV route.

Intermittent claudication (IC) is a condition caused by lack of sufficient blood flow to skeletal muscles in the lower limbs. Ischemia of skeletal muscles causes severe pain on walking, particularly in the calf muscles. Although some of the therapies for myocardial ischemia are beneficial in treating IC, two drugs are approved *only* for this disorder. Pentoxifylline (Trental) acts on RBCs to reduce their viscosity and increase their flexibility, thus allowing them to enter vessels that are partially occluded and reduce hypoxia and pain in the muscle. Pentoxifylline also has antiplatelet action. Cilostazol (Pletal) inhibits platelet aggregation and promotes vasodilation, which brings additional blood to ischemic muscles. Both drugs are given orally and show only modest improvement in IC symptoms. Exercise and therapeutic lifestyle changes are necessary for maximum benefit.

AVOIDING MEDICATION ERRORS

A breast-feeding mother develops thrombophlebitis. Warfarin (Coumadin) 2 mg once a day is ordered. What should the nurse question about this order?

See Appendix D for the suggested answer.

Pr Prototype Drug | Clopidogrel *(Plavix)*

Therapeutic Class: Antiplatelet drug   **Pharmacologic Class:** ADP receptor blocker

ACTIONS AND USES
Clopidogrel is indicated for the prevention of thromboembolic events in patients with a recent history of MI, CVA, or peripheral artery disease. It is also approved for thrombi prophylaxis in patients with unstable angina, including those who are receiving vascular bypass procedures or angioplasty. It may be given off-label to prevent thrombi formation in patients with coronary artery stents, and to prevent postoperative deep vein thromboses. Because the drug is expensive, it is usually prescribed for patients unable to tolerate aspirin, which has similar anticoagulant activity. It is given orally.

Clopidogrel prolongs bleeding time by inhibiting platelet aggregation directly inhibiting ADP binding to its receptor. This binding is irreversible and the platelet will be affected for the remainder of its life span.

ADMINISTRATION ALERTS
- Tablets should not be crushed or split.
- Discontinue drug at least 5 days prior to surgery.
- Pregnancy category B

PHARMACOKINETICS (PO)
Onset: 1–2 h
Peak: 2 h
Half-life: 8 h
Duration: Unknown

ADVERSE EFFECTS
Clopidogrel is generally well tolerated. Frequent adverse effects include flulike syndrome, headache, dizziness, and rash or pruritus. Like other coagulation modifiers, bleeding is a potential adverse event.

Contraindications: Clopidogrel is contraindicated in patients with active bleeding.

INTERACTIONS
Drug–Drug: Use with anticoagulants, other antiplatelet agents, thrombolytic agents, or NSAIDS, including aspirin, will increase the risk of bleeding. Barbiturates, rifampin, or carbamazepine may increase the anticoagulant activity of clopidogrel. The azole antifungals, protease inhibitors, erythromycin, verapamil, or zafirlukast may diminish the antiplatelet actions of clopidogrel.

Lab Tests: Clopidogrel prolongs bleeding time.

Herbal/Food: Herbal supplements that affect coagulation such as feverfew, green tea, ginkgo, fish oil, ginger, or garlic may increase the risk of bleeding.

Treatment of Overdose: In cases of poisoning, platelet transfusions may be necessary to prevent hemorrhage.

Refer to MyNursingKit for a Nursing Process Focus specific to this drug.

NURSING PROCESS FOCUS — PATIENTS RECEIVING ANTIPLATELET THERAPY

Assessment	Potential Nursing Diagnoses
Baseline assessment prior to administration: ■ Understand the reason the drug has been prescribed in order to assess for therapeutic effects (e.g., decreased risk of development of CVAs and MI). ■ Obtain a complete health history including cardiovascular (including HTN, MI, PTCA with stent placement) and peripheral vascular disease, respiratory (including previous pulmonary embolism), neurologic (including recent head injury and CVA), hepatic or renal disease, diabetes, peptic ulcer disease, hypercholesterolemia, and the possibility of alcoholism or pregnancy. Ask women of menstrual age about the length and heaviness of usual menstrual flow. Obtain a drug history including allergies, current prescription and OTC drugs, herbal preparations, and alcohol use. Be alert to possible drug interactions. ■ Obtain baseline weight, vital signs, ECG (if appropriate), and breath sounds. Assess for presence, quality, location of angina, and for presence of dyspnea or chest pain. Assess extremities for symptoms of thrombophlebitis (e.g., warmth, swelling, tenderness in calf, positive Homan's sign) and for location and character/amount of edema, if present. ■ Evaluate appropriate laboratory findings (e.g., bleeding time), CBC and platelets, renal and liver function studies, and lipid profiles.	■ Ineffective Tissue Perfusion (related to decreased circulation in affected area) ■ Impaired Skin Integrity (in lower extremities related to ineffective tissue perfusion) ■ Deficient Knowledge (drug therapy) ■ Risk for Injury (bleeding, related to adverse effects of antiplatelet therapy)
Assessment throughout administration: ■ Assess for desired therapeutic effects (e.g., no symptoms of thrombosis formation). ■ Continue periodic monitoring of appropriate lab values (e.g., CBC, platelets, bleeding time). ■ Assess for adverse effects: oozing from open wound sites, ecchymosis, petechiae, epistaxis, bleeding from gums, and for occult bleeding, such as pallor, dizziness, hypotension, tachycardia, abdominal pain, areas of abdominal wall swelling or firmness, lumbar pain, or decreased level of consciousness.	

Planning: Patient Goals and Expected Outcomes

The patient will:
■ Experience therapeutic effects dependent on the reason the drug is being given (e.g., prevention of CVA due to thrombosis).
■ Be free from, or experience minimal, adverse effects.
■ Verbalize an understanding of the drug's use, adverse effects, and required precautions.
■ Demonstrate proper self-administration of the medication (e.g., dose, timing, when to notify provider).

Implementation

Interventions and (Rationales)	Patient and Family Education
Ensuring therapeutic effects: ■ Continue assessments as described earlier for therapeutic effects, e.g., no symptoms of thrombotic stroke; signs and symptoms due to existing peripheral arterial insufficiency show gradual improvement, such as previous peripheral extremity pain has diminished or is eliminated; or peripheral pulses are improving in quality and volume. (Antiplatelet drugs help prevent the formation of thrombi, particularly in the arterial system.)	■ Teach patients of disease symptoms to observe for, dependent on the reason the drug has been ordered (e.g., sudden onset of weakness affecting one side or limb [CVA]; cold, pale extremity without peripheral pulses [arterial occlusion]).
■ Encourage appropriate lifestyle changes. Provide for dietitian consultation as needed. (Smoking increases platelet aggregation and promotes the formation of thrombi. Healthy lifestyle changes will support and minimize the need for drug therapy.)	■ Encourage the patient to adopt a healthy lifestyle of low-fat food choices, increased exercise, and decreased caffeine and alcohol consumption. Provide for appropriate consultation (e.g., dietitian) as needed. ■ Provide information on smoking cessation and emphasize the risk that smoking poses in vascular diseases.

(Continued)

Implementation

Interventions and (Rationales)	Patient and Family Education
Minimizing adverse effects: ■ Monitor for signs and symptoms of bleeding: oozing at IV sites or wounds, ecchymosis, petechiae, hematuria, black/tarry stools, rectal bleeding, "coffee-ground" emesis, epistaxis, bleeding from gums, prolonged and/or heavy menstrual flow, and for occult bleeding, such as pallor, dizziness, hypotension, tachycardia, abdominal pain, areas of abdominal wall swelling or firmness, lumbar pain, or decreased level of consciousness. (The risk of bleeding from antiplatelet therapy is not as severe as it is for anticoagulants, but it should be monitored while the patient is on antiplatelet therapy.)	■ Teach the patient or caregiver signs and symptoms of excessive bleeding, including occult bleeding, and to report any concerns to the health care provider promptly. ■ Women of menstrual age should report excessively heavy or prolonged menstrual bleeding and keep a "pad count" and report to the health care provider.
■ Continue to monitor labs, including CBC, platelets, and lipid levels. (CBC and platelet levels should remain within normal limits. Many patients with arterial disease have concurrent lipid disorders and may need additional treatment. Decreasing values on the CBC may indicate excessive bleeding and the need to assess for location.)	■ Instruct the patient on the need to return periodically for lab work and to alert lab personnel that antiplatelet therapy is being used. ■ Instruct the patient to carry a wallet identification card or wear medical identification jewelry indicating antiplatelet therapy.
■ Continue to monitor peripheral pulses for quality and volume, complaints of angina or chest pain, especially if new or of sudden onset or accompanied by dyspnea. (Monitoring for new or sudden onset of pain is necessary to ensure prompt treatment of possible emboli.)	■ Teach the patient, family, or caregiver to report any sudden pain in chest, legs, or calves; dyspnea; or new-onset anginal pain immediately.
■ Minimize opportunities for injury or bleeding where possible: avoid IM injections, provide soft toothbrush, and be cautious when providing care, especially with the elderly who have more fragile skin. (Antiplatelet drugs raise the risk of bleeding and potential causes of bleeding should be avoided when possible.)	■ Instruct the patient on ways to minimize opportunities for injury or bleeding where possible: ■ Switch to a soft toothbrush and inspect gums after brushing. ■ Use an electric razor if possible or be extra cautious with a safety razor, holding prolonged pressure over small nicks. ■ Be cautious with food preparation, especially when cutting food. ■ Avoid contact sports, amusement park rides, or other physical activities that may cause intense or violent bumping, jostling, or injury. ■ Frequently assess elderly family members on antiplatelet therapy who have more fragile skin and may experience skin tears or ecchymoses more frequently.
■ Closely evaluate all new prescriptions or use of OTC medications for drug interactions. (Many drugs interact with antiplatelets, increasing the chance for bleeding. All OTC medications containing salicylates, e.g., aspirin, and NSAIDs, e.g., ibuprofen, should not be taken unless otherwise ordered by a health care provider.)	■ Instruct the patient to consult the health care provider before taking any new prescription or OTC medication, including herbal preparations.
■ Maintain a normal diet and limit alcohol intake. (Excessive intake of alcohol, over two drinks a day in men or one in women, may alter the effectiveness of antiplatelet drugs and increase the risk of bleeding.)	■ Teach the patient to maintain a normal diet, avoiding excessive intake of alcohol. Provide for dietary consultation as needed.
Patient understanding of drug therapy: ■ Use opportunities during administration of medications and during assessments to discuss the rationale for drug therapy, desired therapeutic outcomes, most common adverse effects, parameters for when to call the health care provider, and any necessary monitoring or precautions. (Using time during nursing care helps to optimize and reinforce key teaching areas.)	■ The patient should be able to state reason for drug; appropriate dose and scheduling; what adverse effects to observe for and when to report; equipment needed as appropriate and how to use that equipment; and the required length of medication therapy needed with any special instructions regarding renewing or continuing prescription as appropriate.
Patient self-administration of drug therapy: ■ When administering medications, instruct the patient, family, or caregiver in proper self-administration techniques. (Proper administration will increase the effectiveness of the drug.)	■ Teach the patient, family, or caregiver in proper self-administration techniques.

Evaluation of Outcome Criteria

Evaluate the effectiveness of drug therapy by confirming that patient goals and expected outcomes have been met (see "Planning").

See Table 27.4 for a list of drugs to which these nursing actions apply.

TABLE 27.5	Thrombolytics	
Drug	**Route and Adult Dose (max dose where indicated)**	**Adverse Effects**
⏺ alteplase (Activase, TPA)	IV; 60 mg initially then 20 mg/h infused over next 2 h	*Superficial bleeding at injection sites, allergic reactions*
reteplase (Retavase) (see page 351 for the Prototype Drug box ∞)	IV; 10 units over 2 min; repeat dose in 30 min	<u>Serious internal bleeding, intracranial hemorrhage, hypertension</u>
streptokinase (Kabikinase)	IV; 250,000–1.5 million units over 60 min	
tenecteplase (TNKase)	IV; 30–50 mg infused over 5 seconds	
Italics indicate common adverse effects; <u>underlining</u> indicates serious adverse effects.		

THROMBOLYTICS

It is often mistakenly believed that the purpose of anticoagulants such as heparin or warfarin (Coumadin) is to digest and remove pre-existing clots, but this is not the case. A totally different class of drugs, the thrombolytics, is needed for this purpose. The thrombolytics are listed in Table 27.5.

27.7 Pharmacotherapy with Thrombolytics

Thrombolytics promote fibrinolysis, or clot destruction, by converting plasminogen to plasmin. The enzyme plasmin digests fibrin and breaks down fibrinogen, prothrombin, and other plasma proteins and clotting factors. Unlike the anticoagulants, which can only *prevent* clots, thrombolytics actually *dissolve* the insoluble fibrin within the clot. These agents are administered for disorders in which an intravascular clot has already formed, such as in acute MI, pulmonary embolism, acute ischemic CVA, and DVT.

The goal of thrombolytic therapy is to quickly restore blood flow to the tissue served by the blocked vessel. Delays in re-establishing circulation may result in ischemia and permanent tissue damage. The therapeutic effect of thrombolytics is greater when they are administered as soon as possible after clot formation occurs, preferably within 4 hours.

Because clotting is a natural and desirable process to prevent excessive bleeding, thrombolytics have a narrow margin of safety between dissolving "normal" and "abnormal"

Pr Prototype Drug | Alteplase *(Activase)*

Therapeutic Class: Drug for dissolving clots | **Pharmacologic Class:** Thrombolytic

ACTIONS AND USES

Produced through recombinant DNA technology, alteplase is identical to the enzyme human tissue plasminogen activator (TPA). As with other thrombolytics, the primary action of alteplase is to convert plasminogen to plasmin, which then dissolves fibrin clots. To achieve maximum effect, therapy should begin immediately after the onset of symptoms. Alteplase does not exhibit the allergic reactions seen with streptokinase. Alteplase is a drug of choice for the treatment of CVA due to thrombus and is used off-label to restore the patency of IV catheters.

ADMINISTRATION ALERTS

- Drug must be given within 12 hours of onset of symptoms of MI and within 3 hours of thrombotic CVA for maximum effectiveness.
- Avoid parenteral injections during alteplase infusion to decrease risk of bleeding.
- Pregnancy category C

PHARMACOKINETICS
Onset: Immediate
Peak: 5–10 min after infusion is discontinued
Half-life: 30 min
Duration: 3 h

ADVERSE EFFECTS

The most common adverse effect of alteplase is bleeding, which may occur superficially at needle puncture sites or internally. Intracranial bleeding is a rare, though possible, adverse effect. Signs of bleeding such as spontaneous ecchymoses, hematomas, or epistaxis should immediately be reported to the health care provider.

Contraindications: Alteplase is contraindicated in active internal bleeding, history of CVA within the past 2 months, recent trauma or surgery, severe uncontrolled hypertension, intracranial neoplasm, or arteriovenous malformation.

INTERACTIONS

Drug–Drug: Concurrent use with anticoagulants, antiplatelet agents, or NSAIDs, including aspirin, may increase the risk of bleeding.

Lab Tests: Alteplase will increase PT and aPTT.

Herbal/Food: Use with supplements that affect coagulation such as feverfew, green tea, ginkgo, fish oil, ginger, or garlic should be avoided, since they may increase the risk of bleeding.

Treatment of Overdose: There is no specific treatment for overdose.

Refer to MyNursingKit for a Nursing Process Focus specific to this drug.

NURSING PROCESS FOCUS   PATIENTS RECEIVING THROMBOLYTIC THERAPY

Assessment	Potential Nursing Diagnoses
Baseline assessment prior to administration: ▪ Understand the reason the drug has been prescribed in order to assess for therapeutic effects (e.g., treatment of MI, CVA, pulmonary embolism). ▪ Obtain a complete health history including cardiovascular, peripheral vascular disease, respiratory, neurologic (including recent head injury), recent surgeries or injuries, hepatic or renal disease, diabetes, peptic ulcer disease, recent childbirth (within 10 days), or the possibility of pregnancy. Obtain a drug history including allergies, current prescription and OTC drugs, herbal preparations, and alcohol use. Be alert to possible drug interactions. ▪ Obtain baseline weight, vital signs, ECG, and breath sounds. Assess the presence, quality, and location of angina, and for presence of dyspnea or chest pain. Assess neurologic status. ▪ Evaluate laboratory findings (aPTT, aPT, INR, bleeding time), CBC and platelets, renal and liver function studies, ABGs (arterial blood gas) as appropriate, and lipid profiles. Support the patient during other required tests (e.g., CT or MRI prior to thrombolytic therapy for CVA). ▪ Establish all monitoring equipment and necessary lines or arrange for their insertion (e.g., ECG monitoring, IV, Foley catheter, arterial line).	▪ Pain (related to thrombosis and lessened perfusion) ▪ Ineffective Tissue Perfusion (related to decreased circulation in affected area) ▪ Impaired Gas Exchange (pulmonary emboli) ▪ Impaired Skin Integrity (in lower extremities related to ineffective tissue perfusion) ▪ Anxiety (related to condition, hospitalization) ▪ Deficient Knowledge (drug therapy) ▪ Risk for Injury (bleeding and hemorrhage, related to adverse effects of thrombolytic therapy)
Assessment throughout administration: ▪ Continue frequent assessments for therapeutic effects (e.g., angina has diminished significantly or is eliminated and ECG findings within normal limits, respiratory effort and ABGs significantly improved). ▪ Continue frequent monitoring of appropriate lab values (e.g., Hgb, Hct, platelets, RBC, urinalyis, ABGs). ▪ Monitor vital signs and ECG every 15 minutes during the first hour of infusion, and then every 30 minutes during the remainder of infusion and for the first 8 hours. ▪ Assess for adverse effects: bleeding at IV sites, wounds, excessive ecchymosis, petechiae, hematuria, black/tarry stools, rectal bleeding, "coffee-ground" emesis, epistaxis, bleeding from gums, hemoptysis, dysrhythmias, and for occult bleeding, such as pallor, dizziness, hypotension, tachycardia, abdominal pain, areas of abdominal wall swelling or firmness, lumbar pain, or decreased level of consciousness. ▪ Monitor neurologic status frequently, especially if thrombolytics are used for CVA.	

Planning: Patient Goals and Expected Outcomes

The patient will:

▪ Experience therapeutic effects dependent on the reason the drug is being given (e.g., reperfusion of coronary arteries).

▪ Be free from, or experience minimal, adverse effects.

▪ Verbalize an understanding of the drug's use, adverse effects, and required precautions.

▪ Demonstrate proper self-administration of necessary post-thrombolytic medications (e.g., dose, timing, when to notify provider).

Implementation

Interventions and (Rationales)	Patient and Family Education
Ensuring therapeutic effects: ▪ Continue frequent assessments as described earlier for therapeutic effects, e.g., previous angina has diminished significantly or is eliminated and ECG findings show decrease in ischemia. (Thrombolytics rapidly dissolve existing clots to allow re-perfusion of the affected area.)	▪ Teach the patient about all procedures and their necessity prior to beginning thrombolytic therapy. ▪ To allay anxiety, teach the patient, family, or caregiver the rationale for all equipment used.
▪ Post-therapy, encourage appropriate lifestyle changes. Provide for dietitian consultation as needed. (Smoking increases platelet aggregation and promotes the formation of thrombi. Healthy lifestyle changes will support and minimize the need for future drug therapy.)	▪ Encourage the patient to adopt a healthy lifestyle of low-fat food choices, increased exercise, decreased caffeine and alcohol consumption, and smoking cessation. Provide for appropriate consultation (e.g., dietitian) as needed.

NURSING PROCESS FOCUS   PATIENTS RECEIVING THROMBOLYTIC THERAPY (Continued)

Implementation

Interventions and (Rationales)	Patient and Family Education
Minimizing adverse effects:	
▪ Monitor frequently for signs and symptoms of excessive bleeding, such as pallor, hypotension, tachycardia, dizziness, sudden severe headache, lumbar pain, or decreased level of consciousness. (Frequent assessment for both visible and occult bleeding is necessary to prevent extensive hemorrhage and to start early corrective treatment as possible. Bleeding risk is elevated up to 2 to 4 days post-treatment and if the patient is maintained on anticoagulant or antiplatelet therapy post-thrombolytics.)	▪ Allay anxiety by reassuring the patient and explaining rationale for frequent monitoring. Provide adequate pain relief as appropriate.
▪ Monitor vital signs and ECG every 15 minutes during the first hour of infusion, and then every 30 minutes during remainder of infusion and for the first 8 hours. Report any dysrhythmias immediately. (Obtaining vital signs frequently will assess for adverse effects of the drug including hypotension and tachycardia associated with bleeding and for dysrhythmias. Dysrhythmias may occur postperfusion of the coronary arteries or may be associated with adverse effects.)	▪ To allay possible anxiety, teach the patient, family, or caregiver the rationale for all equipment used and the need for frequent monitoring. ▪ Teach the patient to report any palpitations, dyspnea, or angina postinfusion.
▪ Maintain the patient on bedrest and with limited activity during the infusion. (Limited physical activity and bedrest decrease the chance for bruising, injury, and bleeding.)	▪ Provide an explanation and rationale that activity will be limited during infusion and for up to 8 hours post-treatment.
▪ Monitor neurologic status frequently, especially if thrombolytics are used for CVA. (A sudden change in neurologic status or sudden severe headache is a possible sign of an intracranial bleed with increased intracranial pressure.)	▪ To allay possible anxiety, teach the patient the rationale for the frequent assessments and provide reassurance. ▪ Instruct the family or caregiver to report any change in the patient's mental status or level of consciousness during the postinfusion period immediately.
▪ Avoid invasive procedures during the infusion and up to 8 hours postinfusion. (Any puncture site or site of invasive procedure will create an additional site for bleeding. Whenever an invasive procedure must be used, the site must be maintained under pressure for 30 minutes or longer to prevent hemorrhage.)	▪ Teach the patient that after any required procedures, pressure will be maintained to the site for a prolonged period of time.
▪ Continue to monitor lab work (Hgb, Hct, platelet counts, and bleeding time) frequently post-treatment. Periodic CBC and ABGs may also be monitored. Activity may be limited during this postinfusion time period. (The risk of bleeding remains high for 2 to 4 days postinfusion.)	▪ Provide an explanation for the need for activity restriction and frequent monitoring during this time.
Patient understanding of drug therapy:	
▪ Use opportunities during administration of thrombolytic therapy to explain the rationale for drug therapy, desired therapeutic outcomes, required monitoring for adverse effects, and precautions that will be taken during the infusion and in the immediate postinfusion time period. (Using time during nursing care helps to reassure the patient and allay anxiety.) ▪ Provide support and reassurance to the family and caregivers during the time of treatment. (Providing support, reassurance, and appropriate referrals, e.g., pastoral care or social service support, assists family members in a stressful situation.)	▪ The patient should have an understanding of the rationale behind thrombolytic therapy, equipment, and monitoring that will be used, and the care required in the postinfusion period. ▪ Allow family members time to discuss fears, concerns, and provide referral to appropriate support and ancillary providers as appropriate.
Patient self-administration of drug therapy:	
▪ Provide education during the postinfusion period about required medical care follow-up, postinfusion drug therapy [e.g., anticoagulants or antiplatelet drugs], and lifestyle changes. (Utilizing time during nursing care helps to reinforce teaching and assess for any questions or concerns the patient, family, or caregiver may have.)	▪ Teach the patient, family, or caregiver in proper self-administration techniques of anticoagulants or antiplatelet drugs as appropriate.

Evaluation of Outcome Criteria

Evaluate the effectiveness of drug therapy by confirming that patient goals and expected outcomes have been met (see "Planning").

See Table 27.5 for a list of drugs to which these nursing actions apply.

TABLE 27.6	Hemostatics	
Drug	Route and Adult Dose (max dose where indicated)	Adverse Effects
ⓟ aminocaproic acid (Amicar)	IV; 4–5 g for 1 h, then 1–1.25 g/h until bleeding is controlled	*Allergic skin reactions, headache*
aprotinin (Trasylol)	IV; 2 million KIU (loading dose) followed by 500,000 KIU/h during procedure	<u>Anaphylaxis, thrombosis. bronchospasm, nephrotoxicity</u>
tranexamic acid (Cyklokapron, Lysteda)	IV; 10 mg/kg, three to four times daily for 2 to 8 days	
	PO; Two 650 mg tablets, three times daily for a maximum of 5 days	

Italics indicate common adverse effects; <u>underlining</u> indicates serious adverse effects.

clots. Vital signs must be monitored continuously, and signs of bleeding call for discontinuation of therapy. Because these drugs are rapidly destroyed in the bloodstream, discontinuation of the infusion normally results in the immediate termination of thrombolytic activity. After the clot is successfully dissolved with the thrombolytic, therapy with a coagulation modifier is generally initiated to prevent the reformation of clots.

Since the discovery of streptokinase, the first thrombolytic, there have been a number of subsequent generations of thrombolytics. The newer drugs such as tenecteplase (TNKase) have a more rapid onset and longer duration and are reported to have fewer side effects than older drugs in this class. TPA, marketed as alteplase (Activase), has replaced urokinase as the drug of choice in clearing thrombosed central intravenous lines. Because urokinase was obtained from pooled human donors and had a small risk for being contaminated with viruses, it was removed from the market.

HEMOSTATICS

Hemostatics, also called *antifibrinolytics,* have an action opposite that of anticoagulants: They shorten bleeding time. The class name *hemostatics* comes from the drugs' ability to slow blood flow. They are used to prevent excessive bleeding following surgical procedures.

27.8 Pharmacotherapy with Hemostatics

The final class of coagulation modifiers, the hemostatics, is a small group of drugs used to prevent and treat excessive bleeding from surgical sites. In addition, an oral form of tranexamic acid (Lysteda) was approved in 2009 for the treatment of heavy menstrual bleeding. All the hemostatics have very specific indications for use, and none are commonly prescribed. Although their mechanisms differ, all drugs in this class prevent fibrin from dissolving, thus enhancing the stability of the clot. The hemostatics are listed in Table 27.6.

ⓟ Prototype Drug | Aminocaproic Acid *(Amicar)*

Therapeutic Class: Clot stabilizer   **Pharmacologic Class:** Hemostatic/antifibrinolytic

ACTIONS AND USES

Aminocaproic acid is prescribed in situations in which there is excessive bleeding because clots are being dissolved prematurely. The drug acts by inactivating plasminogen, the precursor of the enzyme plasmin that digests the fibrin clot. During acute hemorrhage, the drug can be given IV to reduce bleeding in 1 to 2 hours. It is also available in tablet form. It is most commonly prescribed following surgery to reduce postoperative bleeding. The therapeutic serum level is 100 to 400 mcg/mL.

ADMINISTRATION ALERTS

- Aminocaproic acid may cause hypotension and bradycardia when given IV. Assess vital signs frequently and place the patient on a cardiac monitor to assess for dysrhythmias.
- Pregnancy category C

> **PHARMACOKINETICS (PO)**
> **Onset:** Unknown
> **Peak:** 2 h
> **Half-life:** Unknown
> **Duration:** Unknown

ADVERSE EFFECTS

Because aminocaproic acid tends to stabilize clots, it should be used cautiously in patients with a history of thromboembolic disease. Rapid IV administration may cause hypotension and/or bradycardia. Side effects are generally mild.

Contraindications: Aminocaproic acid is contraindicated in patients with disseminated intravascular clotting or severe renal impairment.

INTERACTIONS

Drug–Drug: Hypercoagulation may occur with concurrent use of estrogens and oral contraceptives.

Lab Tests: Unknown

Herbal/Food: Unknown

Treatment of Overdose: There is no treatment for overdose.

Refer to MyNursingKit for a Nursing Process Focus specific to this drug.

Chapter REVIEW

KEY CONCEPTS

The numbered key concepts provide a succinct summary of the important points from the corresponding numbered section within the chapter. If any of these points are not clear, refer to the numbered section within the chapter for review.

27.1 Hemostasis is a complex process involving multiple steps and a large number of enzymes and clotting factors. The final product is a fibrin clot that stops blood loss.

27.2 Fibrinolysis, or removal of a blood clot, is an enzymatic process initiated by the release of TPA. Plasmin digests the fibrin strands, thus restoring circulation to the injured area.

27.3 Diseases of hemostasis include thromboembolic disorders caused by thrombi and emboli, thrombocytopenia, and bleeding disorders such as hemophilia and von Willebrand's disease.

27.4 The normal coagulation process can be modified by a number of different mechanisms, including inhibiting specific clotting factors, dissolving fibrin, and inhibiting platelet function.

27.5 Anticoagulants are used to prevent thrombi from forming or enlarging. The primary drugs in this category are heparin (parenteral) and warfarin (oral), although low-molecular-weight heparins and thrombin inhibitors are also available.

27.6 Several drugs prolong bleeding time by interfering with the aggregation of platelets. Antiplatelet drugs include aspirin, ADP blockers, glycoprotein IIb/IIIa receptor antagonists, and miscellaneous agents for treating intermittent claudication.

27.7 Thrombolytics are used to dissolve existing intravascular clots in patients with MI or CVA.

27.8 Hemostatics or antifibrinolytics are used to promote the formation of clots in patients with excessive bleeding from surgical sites.

NCLEX-RN® REVIEW QUESTIONS

1 The nurse's understanding of the clotting mechanism is important in administering anticoagulant drugs. The nurse understands that which of the following clotting factors are formed after injury to the vessels?
1. Fibrin, vitamin K
2. Thromboplastin, fibrinogen
3. Prothrombin, thrombin
4. Thrombin, fibrin

2 The patient receiving heparin therapy asks how the "blood thinner" works. The best response by the nurse would be:
1. "heparin makes the blood less thick."
2. "heparin does not thin the blood but prevents clots from forming as easily in the blood vessels."
3. "heparin decreases the number of platelets so that blood clots more slowly."
4. "heparin dissolves the clot."

3 Nursing interventions for a patient receiving enoxaparin (Lovenox) may include: (Select all that apply.)
1. teaching the patient or family to give subcutaneous injections at home.
2. teaching the patient or family not to take any OTC drugs without first consulting with the health care provider.
3. teaching the patient to observe for unexplained bleeding such as pink, red, or dark brown urine or bloody gums.

4. teaching the patient to monitor for the development of DVT.
5. teaching the importance of drinking grapefruit juice daily.

4 The nurse receives the patient's lab values throughout warfarin drug therapy. The expected therapeutic level is:
1. aPTT of three to four times the normal control value.
2. aPTT one to two times the patient's baseline level.
3. aPT one to two times the patient's last result.
4. aPT one and a half to two and a half times the control value.

5 A patient is receiving a thrombolytic agent, alteplase (Activase), following an acute myocardial infarction. Which condition is most likely attributed to thrombolytic therapy with this agent?
1. Skin rash with urticaria
2. Wheezing with labored respirations
3. Bruising and epistaxis
4. Temperature elevation of 100.8 °F

6 A patient has started clopidogrel (Plavix) after experiencing a TIA (transient ischemic attack). The desired therapeutic effects of this drug will be:
1. anti-inflammatory and antipyretic effects.
2. to reduce the risk of a stroke from a blood clot.
3. analgesic as well as clot-dissolving effects.
4. to stop clots from becoming emboli.

CRITICAL THINKING QUESTIONS

1. The nurse is working on a medical unit in which a patient suddenly develops left-sided weakness and garbled speech. The nurse calls the health care provider, who diagnoses the patient with a CVA and orders heparin 5,000 units IV and a heparin drip to run at 1,000 units per hour. What should the nurse do?

2. A patient has had an acute MI and has received alteplase (Activase) to lyse the clot. What nursing actions should have been taken prior to administering the medication to the patient?

3. A patient is receiving enoxaparin subcutaneously after being diagnosed with thrombophlebitis. What precautions should be taken when giving this medication?

See Appendix D for answers and rationales for all activities.

EXPLORE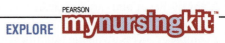

MyNursingKit is your one stop for online chapter review materials and resources. Prepare for success with additional NCLEX®-style practice questions, interactive assignments and activities, web links, animations and videos, and more!

Register your access code from the front of your book at
www.mynursingkit.com.

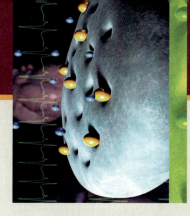

Chapter 28

Drugs for Hematopoietic Disorders

LEARNING OUTCOMES

After reading this chapter, the student should be able to:

1. Describe the process of hematopoiesis.
2. Explain how hematopoiesis is regulated.
3. Explain why hematopoietic agents are often administered to patients following chemotherapy or organ transplant.
4. Explain the functions of colony-stimulating factors.
5. Classify types of anemia based on their causes.
6. Identify the role of intrinsic factor in the absorption of vitamin B$_{12}$.
7. Describe the metabolism, storage, and transfer of iron in the body.
8. Describe the nurse's role in the pharmacologic management of hematopoietic disorders.
9. For each of the drug classes listed in Drugs at a Glance, know representative drugs, and explain their mechanism of drug action, primary actions, and important adverse effects.
10. Use the nursing process to care for patients who are receiving drug therapy for hematopoietic disorders.

KEY TERMS

The blood serves all other cells in the body and is the only fluid tissue. Because of its diverse functions, diseases affecting blood constituents have widespread effects on the body. Correspondingly, drugs for treating blood disorders will affect cells in many different tissues. This chapter will examine medications used to enhance the functions of erythrocytes, leukocytes, and platelets. Pharmacology of the hematopoietic system is a small, though emerging, branch of medicine.

28.1 Hematopoiesis

Blood is a highly dynamic tissue; more than 200 billion new blood cells are formed every day. The process of blood cell formation is called **hematopoiesis,** or hemopoiesis. Hematopoiesis occurs primarily in red bone marrow and requires B vitamins, vitamin C, copper, iron, and other nutrients.

Hematopoiesis is responsive to the demands of the body. For example, the production of white blood cells can increase to 10 times normal in response to infection. The number of red blood cells can increase as much as 5 times normal in response to blood loss or hypoxia. Homeostatic control of hematopoiesis is influenced by a number of hormones and growth factors, which allow for points of pharmacologic intervention. The process of hematopoiesis is illustrated in ➤ Figure 28.1.

Hematopoiesis begins with a **stem cell,** which is capable of maturing into any type of blood cell. The specific path taken by the stem cell, whether it becomes an erythrocyte, leukocyte, or platelet, depends on the internal needs of the body. These needs are transmitted to the stem cells by way of hormones and other regulatory substances. These control substances include erythropoietin and chemicals secreted by leukocytes known as colony-stimulating factors. Through recombinant DNA technology, some of these regulatory agents are now available in sufficient quantities to be used as medications.

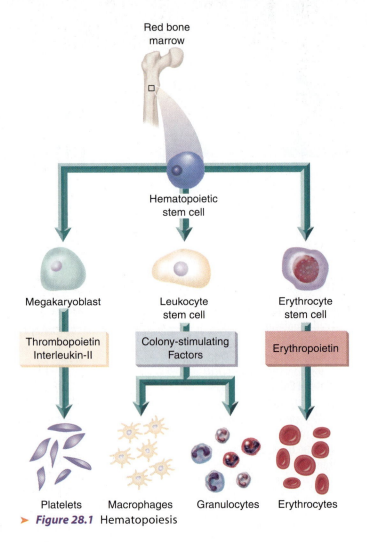

➤ **Figure 28.1** Hematopoiesis

The management of hematopoietic diseases often involves simply replacing a deficient substance that is essential to hematopoiesis. In some cases, the drug is identical to, or very closely resembles, the deficient factor. For example, the drug epoetin alfa (Epogen, Procrit) is identical to the natural hormone erythropoietin and stimulates the production of red blood cells in the same manner. As another example, administration of antianemic agents such as ferrous sulfate or vitamin B_{12} supplies factors that may be deficient in some patients.

Some of the hematopoietic drugs have become important adjunct medications in the treatment of cancer. Antineoplastic drugs often are toxic to bone marrow and cause dramatic reductions in circulating erythrocytes, WBCs, and platelets. Hematopoietic drugs may be used to boost blood cell counts in these patients.

HEMATOPOIETIC GROWTH FACTORS

Natural hormones that promote some aspect of blood formation are called *hematopoietic growth factors.* Several growth factors, shown in Table 28.1, are used pharmacologically to stimulate erythrocyte, leukocyte, or platelet production.

PHARMFACTS

Hematopoietic Disorders

- A pregnant woman's body produces 45% more blood because it contains nutrients and oxygen for the growing fetus. The greatest increase in blood production occurs around week 20 of pregnancy.
- A deficiency of vitamin B_{12}, folate, or vitamin B_6 may increase the blood level of homocysteine, an amino acid normally found in the blood. An elevated blood level of homocysteine is a risk factor for heart disease and stroke.
- Vegetarians who do not eat meats, fish, eggs, milk, or milk products are at high risk for developing vitamin B_{12} deficiency. Vegetarians may find adequate amounts in fortified cereals, nutritional supplements, or yeast.
- Administration of folic acid during pregnancy has been found to reduce neural tube birth defects in the newborn.
- Heavy menstrual periods may result in considerable iron loss.

TABLE 28.1	Hematopoietic Growth Factors	
Drug	Route and Adult Dose (max dose where indicated)	Adverse Effects
darbepoetin alfa (Aranesp)	Subcutaneous/IV; 0.45 mcg/kg once per wk	*Headache, fever, nausea, diarrhea, insomnia, cough, upper respiratory infection, edema*
℗ epoetin alfa (Epogen, Procrit)	Subcutaneous/IV; 3–500 units/kg/dose three times/wk, usually starting with 50–100 units/kg/dose until target Hct range of 30–33% (max: 36%) is reached. Hct should not increase by more than four points in any 2-wk period.	Hypertension, seizures, heart failure, MI
COLONY-STIMULATING FACTORS		
℗ filgrastim (Neupogen): granulocyte-CSF	IV; 5 mcg/kg/day by 30-min infusion, may increase by 5 mcg/kg/day (max: 30 mcg/kg/day); 5 mcg/kg/day subcutaneous as single dose, may increase by 5 mcg/kg/day (max: 20 mcg/kg/day)	*Flulike syndrome, fever, dyspnea, nausea, vomiting, bone pain (sargramostim)*
pegfilgrastim (Neulasta)	Subcutaneous; 6 mg once per chemotherapy cycle at least 24 h after chemotherapy	Bone pain, arthralgia, thrombocytopenia, cutaneous vasculitis, pericardial effusion, (sargramostim), tachycardia (sargramostim)
sargramostim (Leukine): granulocyte-macrophage-CSF	IV; 250 mcg/m²/day infused over 2 h for 21 days, begin 2–4 h after bone marrow transfusion and not less than 24 h after last dose of chemotherapy or 12 h after last radiation therapy	
PLATELET ENHANCERS		
oprelvekin (Neumega)	Subcutaneous; 50 mcg/kg once daily starting 6–24 h after completing chemotherapy for 14–21 days or until platelet count is at least 50,000/mcL	*Edema, fever, headache, dizziness, dyspnea, fatigue, rash, nausea, vomiting*
		Tachycardia, febrile neutropenia, pleural effusion, anaphylaxis, dysrhythmias, candidiasis
eltrombopag (Promacta)	PO; 50 mg once daily (max: 75 mg/day)	*Arthralgia, myalgia, paresthesia, insomnia*
romiplostim (Nplate)	subcutaneous; 1 mcg/kg (max; 10 mcg/kg/wk)	Bone marrow fibrosis, thromboembolism, hematologic malignancy, hepatotoxicity (eltrombopag)

Italics indicate common adverse effects; <u>underlining</u> indicates serious adverse effects.

28.2 Pharmacotherapy with Erythropoietin

The process of red blood cell formation, or *erythropoiesis*, is regulated primarily by the hormone **erythropoietin**. Secreted by the kidney, erythropoietin travels to the bone marrow, where it interacts with receptors on hematopoietic stem cells with the message to increase erythrocyte production. Erythropoietin also stimulates the production of hemoglobin, which is required for a functional erythrocyte.

The primary signal for the increased secretion of erythropoietin is a reduction in oxygen reaching the kidneys. Serum levels of erythropoietin may increase as much as 1,000-fold in response to severe hypoxia. Hemorrhage, chronic obstructive pulmonary disease, anemia, or high altitudes may cause this hypoxia.

Erythropoietin is marketed as epoetin alfa (Epogen, Procrit). Darbepoetin alfa (Aranesp) is a newer agent that is closely related to epoetin alfa. It has the same action, effectiveness, and safety profile; however, it has a two to three times longer duration of action that allows it to be administered once weekly. Darbepoetin alfa is approved for the treatment of anemia associated with chemotherapy or chronic renal failure. It should be noted that when given as an adjunctive agent in cancer treatment, the anemia must be secondary to the *chemotherapy*, not the *cancer* itself. Research has shown that the administration of these drugs

LIFESPAN CONSIDERATIONS

Epoetin Alfa as the New "Blood Doping"

"Blood doping," withdrawing blood from an athlete and then re-transfusing it before a competitive sporting event, has been used by some athletes in an attempt to gain a competitive edge. With increased RBCs and higher hemoglobin, the oxygen-carrying capacity of the blood is thought to increase, boosting endurance. Because the blood used is the athlete's own, pre-event drug screening does not detect foreign drugs or substances. Charges of blood doping are difficult to prove because athletes can naturally boost RBC and hemoglobin levels by training at high altitudes, which stimulates RBC production. Blood doping, however, comes with a price. The increased blood volume and viscosity have led to hypertension, thrombosis, and death.

Blood doping has changed with the availability of epoetin alfa. Because epoetin stimulates RBC production, the athlete may need to withdraw less blood initially and then rely on epoetin to boost RBCs even more post–retransfusion, or epoetin may be used alone. Because it may be used weeks before a sporting event, drug and substance tests may again be negative. The physical consequences of blood doping such as hypertension, thrombosis, or death remain. Adolescents participating in competitive sports activities may attempt to emulate professional sports figures or may have heard about epoetin and question its advantages. The nurse plays a key role in providing accurate information about epoetin and counseling adolescents about the risks and adverse effects of epoetin or any other sports-enhancing drugs.

does not benefit patients when the anemia is caused by the malignancy; in fact, mortality is *increased* in these patients by the administration of the drug.

Pr Prototype Drug | Epoetin Alfa *(Epogen, Procrit)*

Therapeutic Class: Drug for anemia   **Pharmacologic Class:** Hematopoietic growth factor, erythropoietin

ACTIONS AND USES

Epoetin alfa is made through recombinant DNA technology and is functionally identical to human erythropoietin. Because of its ability to stimulate erythropoiesis, epoetin alfa is effective in treating disorders caused by a deficiency in red blood cell formation. Patients with chronic renal failure often cannot secrete enough endogenous erythropoietin, and benefit from epoetin administration. Epoetin is sometimes given to patients undergoing cancer chemotherapy to counteract the anemia caused by antineoplastic agents. It is occasionally prescribed for patients prior to blood transfusions or surgery, and to treat anemia in HIV-infected patients. Epoetin alfa is usually administered by the subcutaneous route three times per week until a therapeutic response is achieved (usually 2 to 6 weeks).

ADMINISTRATION ALERTS

- The subcutaneous route is generally preferred over IV, since lower doses are needed and absorption is slower.
- Do not shake the vial, because this may deactivate the drug. Visibly inspect the solution for particulate matter.
- Pregnancy category C

PHARMACOKINETICS (SUBCUTANEOUS)
Onset: 7–14 days
Peak: Unknown
Half-life: 413 h
Duration: Unknown

ADVERSE EFFECTS

Epoetin alfa has several FDA boxed warnings that include the following:

- The drug may increase the risk of serious cardiovascular events, thromboembolic events, and mortality.
- The drug may shorten survival time and promote tumor progression in patients with certain cancers such as breast, cervical, and lung cancer.
- The drug may increase mortality and serious cardiovascular events in patients with chronic renal failure.
- The drug may increase the risk for deep vein thrombosis (DVT) in perisurgery patients not receiving anticoagulant prophylaxis.

Hypertension may occur in as many as 30% of patients receiving the drug, and a concurrent antihypertensive drug may be indicated. Other frequent adverse effects include headache, fever, nausea, diarrhea, and edema.

Patients taking epoetin alfa who are on dialysis may require increased doses of heparin to maintain adequate anticoagulation. Transient ischemic attacks (TIAs), heart attacks, and strokes have occurred in chronic renal failure patients on dialysis being treated with epoetin alfa.

The effectiveness of epoetin alfa will be greatly reduced in patients with iron deficiency or other vitamin-depleted states. Most patients receive iron supplements during therapy to compensate for the increased red blood cell production.

Contraindications: Contraindications include uncontrolled hypertension, and known hypersensitivity to mammalian cell products. Care must be taken not to administer epoetin alfa to patients with *myeloid* malignancies such as myelogenous leukemia because the drug may increase tumor growth.

INTERACTIONS

Drug–Drug: There are no clinically significant drug interactions with epoetin alfa.

Lab Tests: Unknown

Herbal/Food: Unknown

Treatment of Overdose: Overdose may lead to polycythemia (too many erythrocytes), which can be corrected by phlebotomy.

Refer to MyNursingKit for a Nursing Process Focus specific to this drug.

NURSING PROCESS FOCUS   PATIENTS RECEIVING EPOETIN ALFA

Assessment	Potential Nursing Diagnoses
Baseline assessment prior to administration: - Understand the reason the drug has been prescribed in order to assess for therapeutic effects (e.g., anemia secondary to chronic renal failure, cancer treatment). - Obtain a complete health history including cardiovascular (including HTN, MI) and peripheral vascular disease, respiratory (including previous pulmonary embolism), neurologic (including CVA), or hepatic or renal disease. Obtain a drug history including allergies, current prescription and OTC drugs, herbal preparations, and alcohol use. Be alert to possible drug interactions. - Obtain baseline weight and vital signs, especially blood pressure. - Evaluate appropriate laboratory findings (e.g., CBC, aPTT, INR, transferrin and serum ferritin levels, renal and liver function studies).	- Ineffective Tissue Perfusion (related to underlying disorder) - Activity Intolerance (related to underlying disorder) - Fatigue (related to underlying disorder) - Deficient Knowledge (drug therapy) - Risk for Injury (related to adverse drug effects)

NURSING PROCESS FOCUS   PATIENTS RECEIVING EPOETIN ALFA *(Continued)*

Assessment	Potential Nursing Diagnoses
Assessment throughout administration: ■ Continue assessment for therapeutic effects (e.g., Hct, RBC count significantly improved, patient's activity level and general sense of well-being has improved). ■ Continue frequent monitoring of appropriate lab values (e.g., CBC, aPTT, INR). ■ Monitor vital signs frequently, especially blood pressure, during the first 2 weeks of therapy. ■ Assess for adverse effects: HTN, headache, neurologic changes in level of consciousness or premonitory signs and symptoms of seizure activity, angina, signs of thrombosis development in peripheral extremities.	

Planning: Patient Goals and Expected Outcomes

The patient will:
- Experience therapeutic effects dependent on the reason the drug is being given (e.g., experience increase in activity level, less fatigue and shortness of breath on exertion).
- Be free from, or experience minimal, adverse effects.
- Verbalize an understanding of the drug's use, adverse effects, and required precautions.
- Demonstrate proper self-administration of the medication (e.g., dose, timing, when to notify provider).

Implementation

Interventions and (Rationales)	Patient and Family Education
Ensuring therapeutic effects: ■ Continue frequent assessments as above for therapeutic effects. (RBC count increases rapidly in first 2 weeks of therapy. CBC and platelet count should show continued improvement. Blood pressure and pulse should remain within normal limits or within parameters set by the health care provider.)	■ Instruct the patient on the need to return frequently for follow-up lab work.
■ Encourage adequate rest periods and adequate fluid intake. (The patient may be significantly fatigued due to low Hbg and Hct. Adequate fluid intake helps maintain adequate fluid balance as Hct levels rise.)	■ Encourage the patient to rest when fatigued and to space activities throughout the day to allow for adequate rest periods. ■ Encourage intake of water and non-hyperosmolar beverages.
Minimizing adverse effects: ■ Continue to monitor for adverse effects, especially HTN, peripheral thrombosis, or seizure activity. (As Hct rapidly increases during the first 2 weeks of therapy, HTN or seizures may occur. Peripheral thrombosis, including coronary or cerebral, may also occur.)	■ Teach the patient, family, or caregiver how to monitor pulse and blood pressure as appropriate. Ensure the proper use and functioning of any home equipment obtained. ■ Instruct the patient, family, or caregiver to report headache (especially if sudden onset or severe), changes in level of consciousness, weakness or numbness in extremities, or premonitory signs of seizure activity (e.g., aura), angina, or symptoms of peripheral thrombosis (e.g., leg pain, pale extremity, diminished peripheral pulses).
■ Assess transportation needs of the patient and refer to appropriate resources as needed. (Driving may be restricted up to 90 days after initiation of drug therapy.)	■ Advise the patient to consult with the health care provider about driving or other hazardous activities during the first several months of drug therapy.
■ Continue to monitor aPTT prior to dialysis in patients with chronic renal failure. (The heparin dose during dialysis may need to be increased as the Hct increases.)	■ Explain any changes in medication routine to the patient and provide a rationale.
■ When administering to premature infants, use preservative-free formulations. (Epoetin alfa may contain preservatives such as benzyl alcohol, which may cause "fetal gasping syndrome.")	■ To allay anxiety, offer parents rationales for all treatments provided for the infant.
■ Encourage adequate dietary intake of iron, folic acid, and vitamin B_{12}. Provide dietary consult as needed. Consider nutritional supplements of these nutrients if the diet is inadequate. (The response to epoetin alfa may be decreased if blood levels of iron, folic acid, and vitamin B_{12} are deficient.)	■ Teach the patient to maintain a healthy diet with adequate amounts of iron, folic acid, and vitamin B_{12} (e.g., found in meats, dairy, eggs, fortified cereals and breads, leafy green vegetables, citrus fruits, dried beans and peas).

(Continued)

NURSING PROCESS FOCUS   PATIENTS RECEIVING EPOETIN ALFA (Continued)

Implementation

Interventions and (Rationales)	Patient and Family Education
Patient understanding of drug therapy: ■ Use opportunities during administration of medications and during assessments to discuss rationale for drug therapy, desired therapeutic outcomes, most common adverse effects, parameters for when to notify the health care provider, and any necessary monitoring or precautions. (Using time during nursing care helps to optimize and reinforce key teaching areas.)	■ The patient should be able to state the reason for the drug, appropriate dose and scheduling; what adverse effects to observe for and when to report; and the anticipated length of medication therapy.
Patient self-administration of drug therapy: ■ When administering medications, instruct the patient, family, or caregiver in proper self-administration techniques followed by return demonstration. (Proper administration increases the effectiveness of the drug.) Proper technique includes: ■ The vial should be gently rotated to mix contents and never shaken. Vials are kept under refrigeration and should be gently warmed in the hand. ■ All vials are for one-time use only and any remaining amount should be discarded. ■ If indwelling subcutaneous soft catheter (e.g., Insuflon soft catheter), the patient, family, or caregiver should be taught appropriate site care, insertion technique as appropriate, or schedule for rotating sites.	■ Teach the patient, family, or caregiver in proper self-administration techniques. If indwelling soft catheter (e.g., Insuflon soft catheter) is left in place for injections, teach the patient the proper care of the site, catheter, and any schedule for rotating sites. ■ Have the patient, family, or caregiver return-demonstrate technique until the proper technique is used and they are comfortable giving the injection.

Evaluation of Outcome Criteria

Evaluate the effectiveness of drug therapy by confirming that patient goals and expected outcomes have been met (see "Planning").

28.3 Pharmacotherapy with Colony-Stimulating Factors

Regulation of white blood cell (WBC) production, or *leukopoiesis*, is more complicated than erythropoiesis because there are different types of leukocytes in the blood. Pharmacologically, the most important substances controlling production are **colony-stimulating factors (CSFs)**. Also called leukopoietic growth factors, the CSFs comprise a small group of drugs that stimulate the growth and differentiation of one or more types of leukocytes. Doses for these medications are listed in Table 28.1.

When the body receives a bacterial challenge, the production of CSFs increases rapidly. The CSFs are active at very low concentrations; each stem cell stimulated by these growth factors is capable of producing as many as 1,000 mature leukocytes. The CSFs not only increase the production of *new* leukocytes, they also activate *existing* white blood cells. Examples of enhanced functions include increased migration of leukocytes to the bacteria, increased antibody toxicity, and increased phagocytosis.

CSFs are named according to the types of blood cells that they stimulate. For example, granulocyte colony-stimulating factor (G-CSF) increases the production of neutrophils, the most common type of granulocyte. Granulocyte/macrophage colony-stimulating factor (GM-CSF) stimulates both neutrophil and macrophage production. The process of identifying the many endogenous CSFs, determining their normal functions, and discovering their potential value as therapeutic agents is an emerging area of pharmacology.

The goal of CSF pharmaotherapy is to produce a rapid increase in the number of neutrophils in patients who have suppressed immune systems. CSF therapy shortens the length of time patients are susceptible to life-threatening infections due to low numbers of neutrophils (neutropenia). Indications include patients undergoing chemotherapy or receiving bone marrow or stem cell transplants, or who have certain malignancies. By raising neutrophil counts, CSFs can assist in keeping antineoplastic dosing regimens on schedule (and more effective).

Filgrastim (Neupogen) is similar to natural G-CSF and is primarily used for chronic neutropenia or neutropenia secondary to chemotherapy. Pegfilgrastim (Neulasta) is a form of filgrastim bonded to a molecule of polyethylene glycol (PEG). The PEG decreases the renal excretion of the molecule, allowing it to remain in the body with a sustained duration of action. Sargramostim (Leukine) is similar to natural GM-CSF and is used to treat neutropenia in patients treated for acute myelogenous leukemia, and patients who are having autologous bone marrow transplantation.

28.4 Pharmacotherapy with Platelet Enhancers

The production of platelets, or *thrombocytopoiesis*, begins when megakaryocytes in the bone marrow start shedding membrane-bound packets. These packets enter the bloodstream and become platelets. A single megakaryocyte can produce thousands of platelets.

Pr Prototype Drug | Filgrastim *(Neupogen)*

Therapeutic Class: Drug for increasing neutrophil production   **Pharmacologic Class:** Colony stimulating factor

ACTIONS AND USES

Filgrastim is human G-CSF produced through recombinant DNA technology. Its two primary actions are to increase neutrophil production in the bone marrow and to enhance the phagocytic and cytotoxic functions of existing neutrophils. This is particularly important for patients with neutropenia, which often is associated with severe bacterial and fungal infections. Administration of filgrastim will shorten the length of time of neutropenia in cancer patients whose bone marrow has been suppressed by antineoplastic agents or in patients following bone marrow or stem cell transplants. It may also be used in patients with AIDS-related immunosuppression. It is administered subcutaneously or by slow IV infusion.

ADMINISTRATION ALERTS

- Do not administer within 24 hours before or after chemotherapy with cytotoxic agents because this will greatly decrease the effectiveness of filgrastim.
- Pregnancy category C

PHARMACOKINETICS (SUBCUTANEOUS)
Onset: 4 h
Peak: 2–8 h
Half-life: 3.5 h
Duration: 1 wk

ADVERSE EFFECTS

Although filgrastim is well tolerated, the drug is associated with potentially serious adverse effects and close monitoring is required. Bone pain may occur in up to 33% of patients receiving filgrastim. A small percentage of patients may develop an allergic reaction. Frequent laboratory tests are necessary to ensure that excessive numbers of neutrophils, or leukocytosis, does not occur. Leukocyte counts higher than 100,000 cells/mm^3 increase the risk of serious adverse effects such as respiratory failure, intracranial hemorrhage, retinal hemorrhage, and MI. Fatal rupture of the spleen has occurred in a small number of patients.

Contraindications: The only contraindication is hypersensitivity to *E. coli* proteins because this microbe is used to produce the recombinant drug.

INTERACTIONS

Drug–Drug: Because antineoplastic drugs and colony-stimulating factors produce opposite effects, filgrastim is not administered until at least 24 hours after a chemotherapy session.

Lab Tests: Values for the following may be increased: leukocyte alkaline phosphatase, serum alkaline phosphatase, uric acid, and LDH.

Herbal/Food: Unknown

Treatment of Overdose: There is no treatment for overdose.

Refer to MyNursingKit for a Nursing Process Focus specific to this drug.

NURSING PROCESS FOCUS   PATIENTS RECEIVING COLONY-STIMULATING FACTORS

Assessment	Potential Nursing Diagnoses
Baseline assessment prior to administration: - Understand the reason the drug has been prescribed in order to assess for therapeutic effects (e.g., neutropenia, leukopenia, secondary to cancer treatment, HIV, post–bone marrow transplant). - Obtain a complete health history including recent or current infections, recent surgeries, injuries or wounds, yeast infections (e.g., thrush), vaccination history, cardiac conditions (e.g., dyrhythmias, CHF), or respiratory, renal, and hepatic conditions. Obtain a drug history including allergies, current prescription and OTC drugs, herbal preparations, and alcohol use. Be alert to possible drug interactions. - Obtain baseline weight and vital signs. Assess level of fatigue. - Evaluate appropriate laboratory findings (e.g., CBC, WBC or absolute neutrophil count [ANC]), renal and liver function studies, uric acid levels, and ECG. [ANC = Total WBC count multiplied by the total percentage of neutrophils (segs plus bands); e.g., WBC 5000 × (0.45 segmented neutrophils + 0.05 banded neutrophils) = 5000 × 0.5 = ANC of 2500.]	- Anxiety (related to concerns about seriousness of underlying disorder; insurance/financial concerns) - Fear (related to concerns about seriousness of underlying disorder; insurance/financial concerns) - Activity Intolerance (related to underlying disorder or drug treatment of disorder) - Fatigue (related to underlying disorder or drug treatment of disorder) - Deficient Knowledge (drug therapy) - Risk for Infection (related to underlying disorder or drug treatment of disorder) - Risk for Impaired Oral Mucous Membranes (related to drug treatment or disorder) - Risk for Caregiver Role Strain (family and caregivers)
Assessment throughout administration: - Continue assessment for therapeutic effects (e.g., CBC and WBC or ANC has increased, no signs or symptoms of infection). - Continue frequent monitoring of appropriate lab values (e.g., CBC, WBC or ANC, Hct, platelet count, renal and hepatic labs, uric acid levels). - Monitor vital signs and level of fatigue. - Assess for adverse effects: bone pain (especially lower back, posterior iliac crests, and sternum), fever, nausea, anorexia, hyperuricemia, anemia, ST depression on ECG, angina, respiratory distress, and allergic reaction. Continue to assess for infection and fatigue related to drug treatment (e.g., chemotherapy).	

(Continued)

NURSING PROCESS FOCUS   PATIENTS RECEIVING COLONY-STIMULATING FACTORS *(Continued)*

Planning: Patient Goals and Expected Outcomes

The patient will:

- Experience therapeutic effects dependent on the reason the drug is being given (e.g., experience increase WBC/ANC level, no signs or symptoms of infection).
- Be free from, or experience minimal, adverse effects.
- Verbalize an understanding of the drug's use, adverse effects, and required precautions.
- Demonstrate proper self-administration of the medication (e.g., dose, timing, when to notify provider).

Implementation

Interventions and (Rationales)	Patient and Family Education
Ensuring therapeutic effects: - Continue frequent assessments as described earlier for therapeutic effects. (A rise in WBC and/or ANC counts will depend on condition treated, e.g., depth and length of nadir from cytotoxic chemotherapy.)	- Instruct the patient on the need to return frequently for follow-up lab work.
- Encourage adequate rest periods and adequate fluid intake. (Patient may be significantly fatigued due to the drug therapy for the disease condition. Adequate fluid intake helps maintain adequate urinary output and prevent UTIs.)	- Encourage the patient to rest when fatigued and to space activities throughout the day to allow for adequate rest periods. - Encourage the intake of water and non-hyperosmolar beverages, and drinking whenever thirsty.
Minimizing adverse effects: - Continue to monitor for adverse effects: bone pain (especially lower back, posterior iliac crests, and sternum), fever, nausea, anorexia, hyperuricemia, anemia, ST depression on ECG, angina, respiratory distress, and allergic reaction. Continue to assess for infection and fatigue related to drug treatment, e.g., chemotherapy. (Bone pain tends to occur 2 to 3 days prior to rise in circulating WBC due to the production of WBCs in bone marrow. ST segment depression on ECG may occur with potential for serious dysrhythmias. Respiratory distress may develop after the administration of sargramostim and should be reported immediately. Hyperuricemia may cause goutlike conditions.)	- Instruct the patient to report any severe bone pain not relieved by nonnarcotic analgesics. - Teach the patient to immediately report any palpitations, dizziness, angina, or dyspnea. - Gout-prone patients should report signs and symptoms of gout and increase fluid intake to enhance the renal elimination of uric acid.

- Maintain meticulous infection control measures. Report any signs and symptoms of infections or fever immediately. (The patient will continue to be at risk for infections until WBC/ANC levels rise. Opportunistic infections such as yeast and viruses such as herpes simplex may occur. Parameters will be set by health care provider for reporting fever, e.g., any temperature over 100.5°F, dependent on the underlying disease condition and drug therapy.)	- Instruct the patient in hygiene and infection control measures such as:
	  - Frequent handwashing.
	  - Avoiding crowded indoor places.
	  - Avoiding people with known infections or young children who have a higher risk of having an infection.
	  - Cooking food thoroughly, allowing the family or caregiver to prepare raw foods and to clean up, but the patient should not consume raw fruits or vegetables.
	- Teach the patient to report any fever and symptoms of infection such as: wounds with redness or drainage, increasing cough, increasing fatigue, white patches on oral mucous membranes or white and itchy vaginal discharge, or itchy blister-like vesicles on skin.

- Monitor ECG periodically for ST segment depression or dysrhythmias and report immediately. (Sargramostim may cause significant ST depression with potential for serious dysrhythmias, especially in patients with previous cardiac conditions.)	- Teach the patient to report any palpitations, dizziness, or angina immediately.
- Monitor for signs of dyspnea or respiratory distress, especially when accompanied by tachycardia and hypotension, and report immediately. (Sargramostim may cause respiratory distress as granulocyte counts rise, especially in patients with pre-existing respiratory disorders.)	- Teach the patient to report any dyspnea, respiratory distress, palpitations, or dizziness immediately.
- Monitor for signs and symptoms of allergic-type reactions. (The patient may be hypersensitive to proteins from *E. coli* used to develop the drug.)	- Teach the patient to report symptoms of allergic reaction such as rash, urticaria, wheezing, and dyspnea immediately.
- Monitor hepatic status during drug administration period. (Filgrastim may cause an elevation in liver enzymes.)	- Instruct the patient to report any significant itching, yellowing of sclera or skin, darkened urine, or light or clay-colored stools.

NURSING PROCESS FOCUS   PATIENTS RECEIVING COLONY-STIMULATING FACTORS *(Continued)*

Implementation

Interventions and (Rationales)	Patient and Family Education
■ Stop administration when WBC counts reach the level determined by the health care provider. (Filgrastim may be stopped when neutrophil counts reach 10,000/mm³; sargramostim may be stopped when neutrophil counts reach 20,000/mm³ or as ordered by the health care provider.)	■ Teach the patient about the importance of returning regularly for lab work.
Patient understanding of drug therapy: ■ Use opportunities during administration of medications and during assessments to discuss the rationale for drug therapy, desired therapeutic outcomes, most common adverse effects, parameters for when to call the health care provider, and any necessary monitoring or precautions. (Using time during nursing care helps to optimize and reinforce key teaching areas.)	■ The patient, family, or caregiver should be able to state the reason for the drug, appropriate dose and scheduling; what adverse effects to observe for and when to report; and the anticipated length of medication therapy.

Patient self-administration of drug therapy:
■ When administering medications, instruct the patient, family, or caregiver in proper self-administration techniques followed by return demonstration. (Proper administration increases the effectiveness of the drug.) Proper technique includes:
  ■ Vial should be gently rotated to mix contents and never shaken. Vials are kept under refrigeration and should be gently warmed in the hand.
  ■ All vials are for one-time use only and any remaining amount should be discarded.
  ■ If indwelling subcutaneous soft catheter (e.g., Insuflon soft catheter) is used, the patient should be taught appropriate site care, insertion technique as appropriate, or schedule for rotating sites.
	■ Teach the patient, family, or caregiver in proper self-administration techniques. If indwelling soft catheter (e.g., Insuflon soft catheter) is left in place for injections, teach the patient, family, or caregiver the proper care of site, catheter, and any schedule for rotating sites.
	■ Have the patient, family, or caregiver return-demonstrate the technique until the proper technique is used and they are comfortable giving the injection.

Evaluation of Outcome Criteria

Evaluate the effectiveness of drug therapy by confirming that patient goals and expected outcomes have been met (see "Planning").

Megakaryocyte activity is controlled by the hormone **thrombopoietin**, which is produced by the liver. Thrombopoietin is not available as a medication, although it is currently undergoing clinical trials.

The oldest and most widely available drug to enhance platelet production is oprelvekin (Neumega). (Produced through recombinant DNA technology, oprelvekin stimulates the production of megakaryocytes and thrombopoietin. Oprelvekin is functionally equivalent to interleukin-11 (IL-11), a substance secreted by monocytes and lymphocytes that signals cells in the immune system to respond to an infection.

Oprelvekin is used to enhance the production of platelets in patients who are at risk for thrombocytopenia caused by cancer chemotherapy. The drug shortens the time that the patient is thrombocytopenic and very susceptible to adverse bleeding events. The onset of action is 5 to 9 days, and therapy generally continues until the platelet count returns to greater than 50,000/mm³. Platelet counts will remain elevated for about 7 days after the last dose. Oprelvekin is given only only by the SC route. The primary adverse effect is fluid retention, which occurs in about 60% of patients and can be a concern for patients with pre-existing cardiovascular or renal disease. Visual impairment may occur during therapy. Nursing care for patients receiving treatment with oprelvekin is similar to care for patients receiving the colony-stimulating factors for WBCs.

In 2008 two new platelet enhancers were approved. Romiplostim (Nplate) and eltrombopag (Promacta) are approved to improve platelet function in patients with chronic immune (idiopathic) thrombocytopenia purpura (ITP). Chronic ITP is a disorder characterized by inadequate platelet production and/or increased platelet destruction. Patients with ITP experience a high risk for bruising and bleeding, which may occur anywhere in the body. Both drugs increase the number of platelets by activating the natural receptor for thrombopoietin. Eltrombopag is an oral agent whereas romiplostim is given by the subcutaneous route.

ANEMIAS

Anemia is a condition in which red blood cells have a diminished capacity to deliver oxygen to tissues. Although there are many different causes of anemia, they fall into one of the following categories:

- Erythrocyte loss due to hemorrhage
- Increased erythrocyte destruction
- Impaired erythrocyte production

TABLE 28.2	Classification of Anemia	
Morphology	Description	Examples
Macrocytic–normochromic	Large, abnormally shaped erythrocytes with normal hemoglobin concentration	Pernicious anemia, folate-deficiency anemia
Microcytic–hypochromic	Small, abnormally shaped erythrocytes with decreased hemoglobin concentration	Iron-deficiency anemia, thalassemia
Normocytic–normochromic	Destruction or depletion of normal erythroblasts or mature erythrocytes	Aplastic anemia, hemorrhagic anemia, sickle-cell anemia, hemolytic anemia

Anemia is considered a sign of an underlying disorder, rather than a distinct disease. For therapy to be successful, the underlying pathology must be identified and treated.

28.5 Classification of Anemias

Classification of anemia is generally based on a description of the erythrocyte's size and color. Sizes are described as normal (normocytic), small (microcytic), or large (macrocytic). Color is based on the amount of hemoglobin present and is described as normal red (normochromic) or light red (hypochromic). This classification is shown in Table 28.2.

Although each type of anemia has specific characteristics, all have common signs and symptoms. If the anemia occurs gradually, the patient may remain asymptomatic, except during periods of physical exercise. As the condition progresses, the patient often exhibits pallor, which is a paleness of the skin and mucous membranes due to hemoglobin deficiency. Decreased exercise tolerance, fatigue, and lethargy occur because insufficient oxygen reaches muscles. Dizziness and fainting are common as the brain does not receive enough oxygen to function properly. The respiratory and cardiovascular systems compensate for the oxygen depletion by increasing respiration rate and heart rate. Chronic or severe disease can result in heart failure.

ANTIANEMIC AGENTS

Depending on the type of anemia, several vitamins and minerals may be given to enhance the oxygen-carrying capacity of blood. The most common antianemic agents are cyanocobalamin (CaloMist, Nascobal), folic acid (Folvite, others), and ferrous sulfate (Feosol, others). These agents are listed in Table 28.3.

28.6 Pharmacotherapy with Vitamin B₁₂ and Folic Acid

Vitamin B_{12} is an essential component of two coenzymes that are required for actively growing and dividing cells. Vitamin B_{12} is not synthesized by either plants or animals; only bacteria can make this substance. Because only minuscule amounts of vitamin B_{12} are required (3 mcg/day), deficiency of this vitamin is usually not due to insufficient dietary intake. Instead, the most common cause of vitamin B_{12} deficiency is absence of **intrinsic factor,** a protein secreted by stomach cells. Intrinsic factor is required for vitamin B_{12} to be absorbed from the intestine. ➤ Figure 28.2 illustrates the metabolism of vitamin B_{12}. Inflammatory diseases of the stomach or surgical removal of the stomach may result in deficiency of intrinsic factor. Inflammatory diseases of the small intestine

MyNursingKit   Raw Liver for Breakfast?

TABLE 28.3	Antianemic Agents	
Drug	Route and Adult Dose (max dose where indicated)	Adverse Effects
cyanocobalamin (CaloMist, Nascobal)	IM/deep subcutaneous; 30 mcg/day for 5–10 days; then 100–200 mcg/mo	*Diarrhea, hypokalemia, rash* <u>Anaphylaxis</u>
folic acid (Folvite)	PO/IM/subcutaneous/IV; less than 1 mg/day	No adverse effects
IRON SALTS		
ferrous fumarate (Feostat, others)	PO; 200 mg tid or qid	*Nausea, heartburn, constipation, dark stools*
ferrous gluconate (Fergon)	PO; 325–600 mg qid; may be gradually increased to 650 mg qid as needed and tolerated	<u>Cardiovascular collapse, aggravation of peptic ulcers or ulcerative colitis, hepatic necrosis, anaphylaxis (iron dextran)</u>
ferrous sulfate (Feosol, others)	PO; 750–1500 mg/day in 1–3 divided doses	
ferumoxytol (Feraheme)	IV; single dose of 510 mg followed by a second 510 mg dose 3 to 8 days later	
iron dextran (Dexferrum)	IM/IV; dose is individualized and determined from a table supplied by the drug manufacturer that correlates body weight to hemoglobin values (max: 100 mg within 24 h)	

Italics indicate common adverse effects; <u>underlining</u> indicates serious adverse effects.

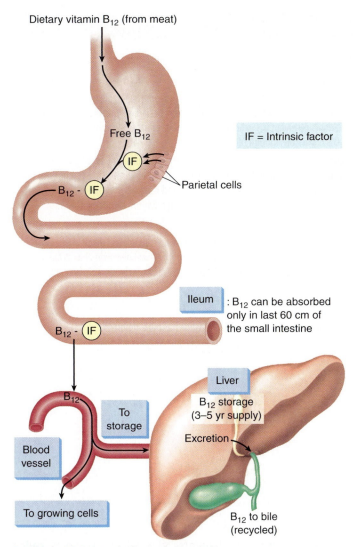

Dietary vitamin B₁₂ (from meat)

Free B₁₂

IF = Intrinsic factor

IF

B₁₂ - IF   Parietal cells

Ileum : B₁₂ can be absorbed only in last 60 cm of the small intestine

B₁₂ - IF

Liver
B₁₂ storage
(3–5 yr supply)

Excretion

B₁₂

To storage

Blood vessel

To growing cells

B₁₂ to bile (recycled)

> *Figure 28.2* Metabolism of vitamin B₁₂

RESEARCH SHOWS

Folic Acid Supplements Prior to Pregnancy

The Question: Does folic acid reduce the incidence of neural tube defects if taken prior to pregnancy? It has been established for several decades that folic acid deficiency during pregnancy increases the risk of neural tube defects in the newborn, and that receiving adequate amounts during pregnancy can reduce the risk. However, does folic acid exert this protective effect if taken prior to pregnancy?

The Study: The authors reviewed studies performed since 1996. Research supported the conclusion that folic acid supplementation during the periconceptional period did indeed reduce the risk of neural tube defects. Furthermore, supplementation with 0.4 mcg was not associated with any adverse effects.

Nursing Implications: Half of all pregnancies are unplanned. Thus, the nurse should recommend folic acid supplementation for all women with a reasonable possibility of pregnancy.

Source: Wolff, T., Takacs-Witkop, K., Miller, M. & Syed, S (2009). Folic Acid Supplementation for the Prevention of Neural Tube Defects: An Update of the Evidence for the U.S. Preventive Services Task Force. Annals of Internal Medicine 150: 632–639.

that affect food and nutrient absorption may also cause vitamin B₁₂ deficiency. Because vitamin B₁₂ is found primarily in foods of animal origin, strict vegetarians may require careful meal planning or a vitamin supplement to prevent deficiency.

The most profound consequence of vitamin B₁₂ deficiency is a condition called **pernicious** or **megaloblastic anemia**, which affects both the hematologic and nervous systems. The hematopoietic stem cells produce abnormally large erythrocytes that do not fully mature. Red blood cells are most affected, though lack of maturation of all blood cell types may occur in severe disease. The symptoms of pernicious anemia are often nonspecific and develop slowly, sometimes over decades. Nervous system symptoms may include memory loss, confusion, unsteadiness, tingling or numbness in the limbs, delusions, mood disturbances, and even hallucinations in severe deficiencies. Permanent nervous system damage may result if the disease remains untreated. Pharmacotherapy includes the administration of cyanocobalamin, a form of vitamin B₁₂ (see the prototype drug feature in this chapter).

Folic acid, or **folate,** is a B-complex vitamin that is essential for normal DNA and RNA synthesis. As with B₁₂ deficiency, insufficient folic acid can manifest itself as anemia.

In fact, the metabolism of vitamin B₁₂ and folic acid are intricately linked; a B₁₂ deficiency will create a lack of activated folic acid.

Folic acid does not require intrinsic factor for intestinal absorption, and the most common cause of folate deficiency is insufficient dietary intake. This is often observed in patients with chronic alcoholism because their diets are often deficient in this nutrient, and alcohol interferes with folate metabolism in the liver. Fad diets and malabsorption disorders of the small intestine can also result in folate anemia. Hematopoietic signs of folate deficiency are the same as those for B₁₂ deficiency; however, no neurologic signs are present. Folate deficiency during pregnancy has been linked to neural birth defects such as spina bifida.

Treatment of mild deficiency or prophylaxis of folate deficiency is accomplished by increasing the dietary intake of folic acid by including fresh green vegetables, dried beans, and wheat products. In cases when adequate dietary intake cannot be achieved, therapy with folate sodium (Folvite) or folic acid is warranted. Folic acid is discussed further in chapter 42∞, where it is a drug prototype for water-soluble vitamins.

28.7 Pharmacotherapy with Iron

Iron is a mineral essential to the function of several mitochondrial enzymes involved in metabolism and energy production in the cell. Most iron in the body, 60% to 80%, is associated with hemoglobin inside erythrocytes. Because free iron is toxic, the body binds the mineral to the protein complexes **ferritin, hemosiderin,** and **transferrin.** Ferritin and hemosiderin maintain iron stores *inside* cells, whereas transferrin *transports* iron to sites in the body where it is needed.

After erythrocytes die, nearly all the iron in their hemoglobin is incorporated into transferrin and recycled for later use. Because of this efficient recycling, only about 1 mg of iron is excreted from the body per day, making daily dietary

Pr Prototype Drug | Cyanocobalamin *(Calomist, Nascobal)*

Therapeutic Class: Drug for anemia   **Pharmacologic Class:** Vitamin supplement

ACTIONS AND USES

Cyanocobalamin is a purified form of vitamin B_{12} that is indicated for patients with vitamin B_{12} deficiency anemia. Treatment is most often by weekly, biweekly, or monthly IM or subcutaneous injections. Oral vitamin B_{12} formulations are available primarily as vitamin supplementation, although they are only effective in patients who have sufficient amounts of intrinsic factor. Intranasal spray formulations are available that provide for daily (Calomist) or once-weekly (Nascobal) dosage. Because these intranasal formulations exhibit variable absorption and bioavailability, they are used for *maintenance therapy* after normal vitamin B_{12} levels have been restored by parenteral preparations.

Parenteral administration rapidly reverses most signs and symptoms of B_{12} deficiency, usually within a few days or weeks. If the disease has been prolonged, symptoms may take longer to resolve, and some neurologic damage may be permanent. In most cases, treatment must often be maintained for the remainder of the patient's life.

ADMINISTRATION ALERTS

- If PO preparations are mixed with fruit juices, administer quickly because ascorbic acid affects the stability of vitamin B_{12}.
- Pregnancy category A (C when used parenterally)

PHARMACOKINETICS

Onset: Days to weeks

Peak: 8–12 h (PO), 1–2 h (intranasal), and 1 h (IV)

Half-life: 6 days

Duration: Unknown

ADVERSE EFFECTS

Adverse effects from cyanocobalamin are uncommon. Hypokalemia is possible; thus, serum potassium levels are monitored periodically. A small percentage of patients receiving B_{12} exhibit rashes, itching, or other signs of allergy. Anaphylaxis is possible, though rare.

Contraindications: Contraindications include sensitivity to cobalt and folic acid–deficiency anemia. Cyanocobalamin is contraindicated in patients with severe pulmonary disease and should be used cautiously in patients with heart disease because of the potential for sodium retention caused by the drug.

INTERACTIONS

Drug–Drug: Drug interactions with cyanocobalamin include a decrease in absorption when given concurrently with alcohol, aminosalicylic acid, neomycin, and colchicine. Chloramphenicol may interfere with therapeutic response to cyanocobalamin.

Lab Tests: Unknown

Herbal/Food: Unknown

Treatment of Overdose: No overdosage has been reported.

Refer to MyNursingKit for a Nursing Process Focus specific to this drug.

---

iron requirements in most individuals quite small. Iron balance is maintained by the increased absorption of the mineral from the proximal small intestine during periods of deficiency. Because iron is found in greater quantities in meat products, vegetarians are at higher risk of iron-deficiency anemia.

Iron deficiency is the most common cause of anemia. More than 50% of patients diagnosed with iron deficiency anemia have GI bleeding, such as may occur from GI malignancies or chronic peptic ulcer disease. In the United States and Canada, iron deficiency most commonly occurs in women of childbearing age due to blood losses during menses and pregnancy. These conditions may require more than the recommended daily allowance (RDA) of iron (chapter 42∞). The most significant effect of iron deficiency is a reduction in erythropoiesis, resulting in symptoms of anemia.

Mild iron-deficiency anemia may be prevented or corrected by increasing the intake of iron-rich foods, such as fish, red meat, fortified cereal, and whole-grain breads. For more severe deficiencies, ferrous sulfate (Feosol, others), ferrous gluconate (Fergon), and ferrous fumarate (Feostat, others)

are used as iron supplements. Slow-release products, called iron carbonyl (Feosol-caps, Ferronyl), are more expensive but are less dangerous following accidental exposure in children because there is a longer period for intervention before toxic effects materialize. Iron dextran (Dexferrum) is a parenteral supplement that may be used when the patient is unable to take oral preparations. Because iron oxidizes vitamin C, many iron supplements contain this vitamin. Vitamin C also is believed to enhance iron absorption. Depending on the degree of iron depletion and the amount of iron supplement that can be tolerated by the patient without significant side effects, 3 to 6 months of therapy may be required.

In 2009, the FDA approved a new iron salt. Ferumoxytol (Feraheme) is approved to treat iron deficiency associated with chronic kidney disease (with or without dialysis). The drug consists of iron oxide protected by a carbohydrate shell. The shell remains intact until the drug enters macrophages, whereby the iron is released to its storage depots. The advantage of ferumoxytol over existing iron salts is that it can be administrated safely by the IV route and can raise iron levels more rapidly.

Pr Prototype Drug | Ferrous Sulfate (Feosol, others)

Therapeutic Class: Agent for anemia   **Pharmacologic Class:** Iron supplement

ACTIONS AND USES

Ferrous sulfate is an iron supplement containing 20% to 30% elemental iron. It is available in a wide variety of dosage forms to prevent or rapidly reverse symptoms of iron-deficiency anemia. Other forms of iron include ferrous fumarate, which contains 33% elemental iron, and ferrous gluconate, which contains 12% elemental iron. The doses of these various preparations are based on their iron content. In general, patients with iron deficiency respond rapidly to the administration of ferrous sulfate. Although a positive therapeutic response may be achieved in 48 hours, therapy may continue for several months to replenish the storage depots for iron.

Laboratory evaluation of hemoglobin (Hgb) or hematocrit (Hct) values is conducted regularly, as excess iron is toxic. Although a positive therapeutic response may be achieved in 48 hours, therapy may continue for several months.

ADMINISTRATION ALERTS

- When administering IV, be careful to prevent infiltration, as iron is highly irritating to tissues.
- Use the Z-track method (deep muscle) when giving IM.
- Do not crush tablet or empty contents of capsule when administering.
- Do not give tablets or capsules within 1 hour of bedtime.
- Pregnancy category A

PHARMACOKINETICS

Because iron is a natural substance, it is difficult to obtain pharmacokinetic values.

ADVERSE EFFECTS

The most frequent adverse effect of ferrous sulfate is GI upset. Taking the drug with food will diminish GI symptoms but can decrease the absorption of iron by 50% to 70%. In addition, antacids should not be taken with ferrous sulfate because they also reduce absorption of the mineral. Ideally, iron preparations should be administered 1 hour before or 2 hours after a meal. Iron preparations may darken stools, but this is a harmless side effect. Constipation is common; therefore, an increase in dietary fiber may be indicated. Excessive doses of iron are very toxic, and patients should be advised to take the medication exactly as directed.

Contraindications: Iron salts drugs should not be used in hemolytic anemia without documentation of iron deficiency because iron will not correct this condition and it may build to toxic levels. The drug should not be administered to patients with hemochromatosis, peptic ulcer, regional enteritis, or ulcerative colitis.

INTERACTIONS

Drug–Drug: Absorption is reduced when oral iron salts are given concurrently with antacids, proton-pump inhibitors, or calcium supplements. Iron decreases the absorption of tetracyclines, fluoroquinolones, and etidronate. To prevent possible interactions, it is advisable to take iron supplements 1 to 2 hours before or after other medications.

Lab Tests: Ferrous sulfate may decrease serum calcium level and increase serum bilirubin.

Herbal/Food: Food, especially dairy products, will inhibit absorption of ferrous sulfate. Foods high in vitamin C such as orange juice and strawberries can increase the absorption of iron.

Treatment of Overdose: The antidote for acute iron intoxication is deferoxamine (Desferal). This parenteral agent binds iron, which is subsequently removed by the kidneys, turning the urine a reddish brown color.

Refer to MyNursingKit for a Nursing Process Focus specific to this drug.

NURSING PROCESS FOCUS | PATIENTS RECEIVING TREATMENT FOR ANEMIA (FOLIC ACID, VITAMIN B₁₂, FERROUS SULFATE)

Assessment	Potential Nursing Diagnoses
Baseline assessment prior to administration: - Understand the reason the drug has been prescribed in order to assess for therapeutic effects (e.g., type of anemia: secondary to inflammatory bowel disease, lack of vitamin B₁₂, etc). - Obtain a complete health history including cardiovascular, GI, hepatic, or renal disease. Obtain a drug history including allergies, current prescription and OTC drugs, and herbal preparations. Be alert to possible drug interactions. Obtain a dietary history, including alcohol use. - Obtain baseline weight and vital signs. Assess fatigue level. - Evaluate appropriate laboratory findings (e.g., CBC, electrolytes, transferrin and serum ferritin levels, renal and liver function studies.)	- Ineffective Tissue Perfusion (related to underlying disorder) - Activity Intolerance (related to underlying disorder) - Fatigue (related to underlying disorder) - Imbalanced Nutrition, Less Than Body Requirements (related to lack of intake or lack of absorption of nutrients) - Deficient Knowledge (drug therapy) - Risk for Injury (related to underlying disorder or adverse drug effects)
Assessment throughout administration: - Continue assessment for therapeutic effects (e.g., Hct, RBC count improved, patient's activity level, and general sense of well-being). - Continue monitoring of appropriate lab values (e.g., CBC, electrolytes, hepatic, and renal function). - Assess for adverse effects: itching, skin rash, hypokalemia, nausea, vomiting, heartburn, constipation, black stools (iron preparations), or allergic reactions.	

(Continued)

Planning: Patient Goals and Expected Outcomes

The patient will:

- Experience therapeutic effects dependent on the reason the drug is being given (e.g., experience increase in activity level, less fatigue and shortness of breath on exertion).
- Be free from, or experience minimal, adverse effects.
- Verbalize an understanding of the drug's use, adverse effects, and required precautions.
- Demonstrate proper self-administration of the medication (e.g., dose, timing, when to notify provider).

Implementation

Interventions and (Rationales)	Patient and Family Education
Ensuring therapeutic effects:	
▪ Continue assessments as described earlier for therapeutic effects. (RBC and Hct counts may rise over 3 to 6 months. Note gradually increasing levels of activity and less complaints of fatigue as counts rise.)	▪ Instruct the patient on the need to return for periodic lab work.

▪ Encourage adequate dietary intake of nutrient whenever possible. Consider long-term supplementation as appropriate. (Maintaining a healthy diet may decrease the need for long-term supplementation or will enhance therapeutic effects.)	▪ Teach the patient to increase intake of folic acid, vitamin B$_{12}$, and iron-rich foods such as:
	  ▪ Folic acid: leafy green vegetables, citrus fruits, and dried beans and peas
	  ▪ Vitamin B$_{12}$: fish, meat, poultry, eggs, milk and milk products, and fortified breakfast cereals
	  ▪ Iron: meats, fish, poultry, lentils, and beans

▪ Follow appropriate administration guidelines. (Following appropriate administration techniques maximizes absorption for enhanced therapeutic effect. Oral formulations may require special administration requirements.)	▪ Teach the patient specific administration guidelines, including:
	  ▪ Folic acid: May be taken on empty stomach or with food.
	  ▪ Vitamin B$_{12}$: Must be given IM in cases of pernicious anemia. Take oral formulations with meals.
	  ▪ Iron: Take on empty stomach. Liquid preparations should be sipped through a straw with the straw held toward the back of the mouth to avoid staining teeth. Increasing intake of Vitamin C–rich foods may also enhance iron absorption.

Minimizing adverse effects:	
▪ Continue to monitor for adverse effects, including skin rash, hypokalemia, nausea, vomiting, constipation, heartburn, staining of teeth, black stools (iron preparations), or allergic reactions. (Hypokalemia and subsequent significant dysrhythmias may occur with Vitamin B$_{12}$ administration. Staining of the teeth from liquid oral preparations and black stools may occur with iron.)	▪ Instruct the patient to monitor for signs and symptoms of hypokalemia (e.g., muscle weakness or cramping, palpitations) and to report promptly. ▪ Teach the patient to increase fluid and fiber intake as part of a healthy diet while on iron preparations and to dilute oral liquid formulations and sip through straw placed in the back of the mouth.
▪ Plan activities to allow for periods of rest to help patient conserve energy. (Fatigue from anemia due to decreased Hgb levels is common.)	▪ Encourage the patient to rest when fatigued and to space activities throughout the day to allow for adequate rest periods.
Patient understanding of drug therapy:	
▪ Use opportunities during administration of medications and during assessments to discuss rationale for drug therapy, desired therapeutic outcomes, most common adverse effects, parameters for when to call the health care provider, and any necessary monitoring or precautions. (Using time during nursing care helps to optimize and reinforce key teaching areas.)	▪ The patient, family, or caregiver should be able to state reason for drug; appropriate dose and scheduling; what adverse effects to observe for and when to report; and the anticipated length of medication therapy.
Patient self-administration of drug therapy:	
▪ When administering medications, instruct the patient, family, or caregiver in proper self-administration techniques as described earlier and of proper intramuscular injection technique for Vitamin B$_{12}$ followed by return demonstration. (Proper administration will increase the effectiveness of the drug.)	▪ The patient should be able to discuss appropriate dosing and any special administration techniques required related to drug taken. ▪ Have the patient, family, or caregiver return-demonstrate the technique until the proper technique is used and they are comfortable giving the injection.
▪ Keep all vitamins and iron preparations out of the reach of young children. (Iron poisoning may be fatal in young children.)	▪ Teach the patient to keep iron preparations and vitamins containing iron, in a secure place if young children are present in the home.

Evaluation of Outcome Criteria

Evaluate the effectiveness of drug therapy by confirming that patient goals and expected outcomes have been met (see "Planning").

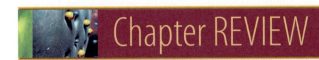

Chapter REVIEW

KEY CONCEPTS

The numbered key concepts provide a succinct summary of the important points from the corresponding numbered section within the chapter. If any of these points are not clear, refer to the numbered section within the chapter for review.

28.1 Hematopoiesis is the process of blood cell production that begins with primitive stem cells that reside in bone marrow. Homeostatic control of hematopoiesis is maintained through hormones and growth factors.

28.2 Erythropoietin is a hormone that stimulates the production of red blood cells when the body experiences hemorrhage or hypoxia. Epoetin alfa is a synthetic form of erythropoietin used to treat specific anemias.

28.3 Colony-stimulating factors (CSFs) are growth factors that stimulate the production of leukocytes. They are used to reduce the duration of neutropenia in patients undergoing chemotherapy or organ transplantation.

28.4 Platelet enhancers stimulate the activity of megakaryocytes and thrombopoietin, and increase the production

of platelets. Oprelvekin, the only drug in this class, is prescribed for patients with thrombocytopenia.

28.5 Anemias are disorders in which the oxygen-carrying capacity of the blood is reduced owing to hemorrhage, excessive erythrocyte destruction, or insufficient erythrocyte synthesis.

28.6 Deficiencies in either vitamin B_{12} or folic acid can lead to pernicious anemia. Treatment with cyanocobalamin can reverse symptoms of pernicious anemia in many patients, although some degree of nervous system damage may be permanent.

28.7 Iron deficiency is the most common cause of nutritional anemia and can be successfully treated with iron supplements.

NCLEX-RN® REVIEW QUESTIONS

1 An elderly patient diagnosed with iron-deficiency anemia will be taking ferrous sulfate (Feosol, others) orally. The nurse will teach required administration guidelines to the patient, including: (Select all that apply.)
1. take the tablets on an empty stomach if possible.
2. increase fluid intake and increase dietary fiber while taking this medication.
3. if liquid preparations are used, dilute with water or juice and sip through a straw placed in the back of the mouth.
4. crush or dissolve sustained-release tablets in water if they are too big to swallow.

2 Erythropoietin regulates the process of red blood cell (RBC) formation. The nurse understands this mechanism is activated by a reduction of oxygen reaching the:
1. brain.
2. heart.
3. kidneys.
4. lungs.

3 The patient with a diagnosis of cancer is receiving epoetin alfa (Epogen, Procrit) as part of the treatment regimen. The nurse evaluates the effectiveness of this drug by:
1. assessing the patient's energy level.
2. monitoring the patient's hematocrit and hemoglobin level.
3. monitoring the patient's blood pressure.
4. assessing the patient's level of consciousness.

4 The nursing plan of care for a patient receiving epoetin alfa (Epogen, Procrit) should include careful monitoring for symptoms of:
1. angina, or a change in level of consciousness.
2. severe hypotension.
3. impaired liver function.
4. severe diarrhea.

5 To best monitor for therapeutic effects from filgrastim (Neupogen), the nurse will monitor:
1. Hgb and Hct.
2. WBC or ANC counts.
3. electrolytes.
4. RBC count.

6 The nursing plan of care for a patient receiving filgrastim (Neupogen) should include:
1. frequent observations for infection.
2. frequent monitoring of vital signs, especially blood pressure.
3. periodic ECG monitoring.
4. intake and output measurements.

CRITICAL THINKING QUESTIONS

1. A patient newly diagnosed with renal failure asks the nurse why he must receive injections of epoetin alfa (Epogen, Procrit). Develop teaching points to describe the indications for this drug.

2. A patient is receiving filgrastim (Neupogen). What nursing interventions are appropriate to safely administer this drug and provide patient safety throughout therapy?

3. A patient is receiving ferrous sulfate (Feosol, others). What teaching should the nurse provide to this patient?

See Appendix D for answers and rationales for all activities.

EXPLORE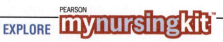

MyNursingKit is your one stop for online chapter review materials and resources. Prepare for success with additional NCLEX®-style practice questions, interactive assignments and activities, web links, animations and videos, and more!

Register your access code from the front of your book at
www.mynursingkit.com.

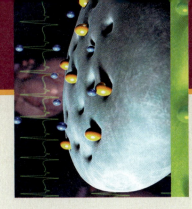

Drugs for Shock

LEARNING OUTCOMES

After reading this chapter, the student should be able to:

1. Compare and contrast the different types of shock.
2. Relate the general symptoms of shock to their physiologic causes.
3. Explain the initial treatment priorities for a patient who is in shock.
4. Compare and contrast the use of colloids and crystalloids in fluid replacement therapy.
5. List the drugs used in the pharmacotherapy of anaphylaxis and discuss their indications.
6. For each of the classes shown in Drugs at a Glance, know representative drug examples, and explain their mechanism of action, primary actions, and important adverse effects.
7. Use the steps of the nursing process to care for patients who are receiving drug therapy for shock.

KEY TERMS

hock is a condition in which vital tissues and organs are not receiving enough blood to function properly. Without adequate oxygen and other nutrients, cells cannot carry out normal metabolic processes. Shock is a medical emergency; failure to reverse the causes and symptoms of shock may lead to irreversible organ damage and death. This chapter examines how drugs are used to aid in the treatment of different types of shock.

29.1 Characteristics of Shock

Shock is a collection of signs and symptoms, many of which are nonspecific. Although symptoms vary among the different kinds of shock, some similarities exist. The patient appears pale and may claim to feel sick or weak without reporting specific complaints. Behavioral changes are often some of the earliest symptoms and may include restlessness, anxiety, confusion, depression, and apathy. Lack of sufficient blood flow to the brain may cause unconsciousness. Thirst is a common complaint. The skin may feel cold or clammy. Without immediate treatment, multiple body systems will be affected and respiratory or renal failure may result. ➤ Figure 29.1 shows common symptoms of a patient in shock.

The central problem in most types of shock is the inability of the cardiovascular system to send sufficient blood to the vital organs, with the heart and brain being affected early in the progression of the disease. Assessing the patient's cardiovascular status will provide important clues for a diagnosis of shock. Blood pressure is usually low and cardiac output diminished. Heart rate may be rapid with a weak, thready pulse. Breathing is usually rapid and shallow. ➤ Figure 29.2 (page 407) illustrates the physiologic changes that occur during circulatory shock.

29.2 Causes of Shock

Shock is often classified by naming the underlying pathologic process or organ system causing the disease. Table 29.1 describes the different types of shock and their primary causes.

The diagnosis of shock is rarely based on nonspecific symptoms. A careful medical history, however, may give the nurse valuable clues as to what type of shock may be present. For example, obvious trauma or bleeding would suggest **hypovolemic shock**, related to volume depletion. If trauma to the brain or spinal cord is evident, **neurogenic shock**, a type of distributive shock caused by a sudden loss of nerve impulse communication, may be suspected. A history of heart disease would suggest **cardiogenic shock**, which is caused by inadequate cardiac output due to pump failure. A recent infection may indicate **septic shock**, a type of distributive shock caused by the presence of bacteria and toxins in the blood. A history of allergy with a sudden onset of symptoms following food or drug intake may suggest **anaphylactic shock**, the most severe type I allergic response. The pharmacotherapy of anaphylaxis is included in Section 29.7 (page 413).

29.3 Treatment Priorities for a Patient with Shock

Shock is treated as a medical emergency, and the first goal is to provide basic life support. Rapid identification of the underlying cause followed by aggressive treatment, is essential, because the patient's condition may deteriorate rapidly without specific, emergency measures. It is critical to use the initial nursing

Neurologic
• Restlessness
• Anxiety
• Lethargy
• Confusion

Skin
• Pale
• Clammy
• Cool

Cardiovascular
• Tachycardia
• Thready pulse
• Low cardiac output
• Low blood pressure

Respiratory
• Rapid breathing
• Shallow respiration

Metabolism
• Low temperature
• Thirst
• Acidosis
• Low urine output

➤ *Figure 29.1* Symptoms of a patient in shock

PHARMFACTS

Shock
- Cardiogenic shock, because it responds poorly to treatment, is the most lethal form of shock and has an 80% to 100% mortality rate.
- Hypovolemic shock carries a 10% to 31% mortality rate.
- With anaphylactic or distributive shock, death can ensue within minutes if treatment is not available to treat the condition: Neurogenic shock is a form of distributive shock.
- It is estimated that 500 to 1,000 cases of fatal anaphylactic shock occur each year in the United States.
- Septic shock, usually caused by gram-negative bacteria, has a mortality rate of 40% to 70% but can be as high as 90%, depending on the causative organism.

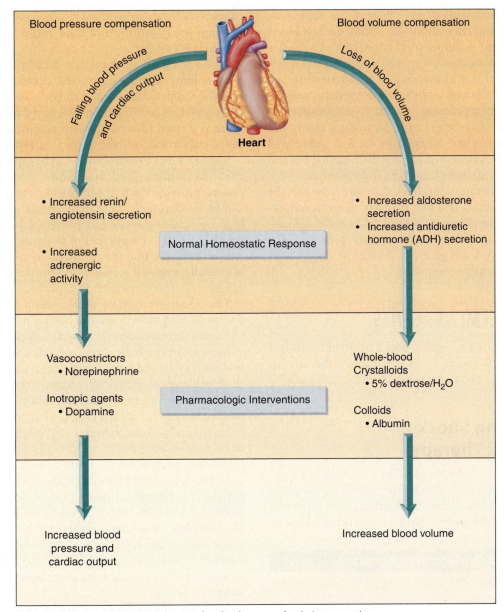

> *Figure 29.2* Physiologic changes during circulatory shock: pharmacologic intervention

TABLE 29.1	**Common Types of Shock**	
Type of Shock	Definition	Underlying Pathology
Anaphylactic	Acute allergic reaction	Severe reaction to an allergen such as penicillin, nuts, shellfish, or animal proteins
Cardiogenic	Failure of the heart to pump sufficient blood to tissues	Left heart failure, myocardial ischemia, MI, dysrhythmias, pulmonary embolism, or myocardial or pericardial infection
Hypovolemic	Loss of blood volume	Hemorrhage, burns, excessive diuresis, or severe vomiting or diarrhea
Neurogenic	Vasodilation due to overstimulation of the parasympathetic nervous system or understimulation of the sympathetic nervous system	Trauma to the spinal cord or medulla, severe emotional stress or pain, or drugs that depress the central nervous system
Septic	Multiple organ dysfunction as a result of pathogenic organisms in the blood; often a precursor to acute respiratory distress syndrome and disseminated intravascular coagulation	Widespread inflammatory response to bacterial, fungal, or parasitic infection

interventions of maintaining the ABCs of life support—airway, breathing, and circulation—to sustain normal blood pressure. The patient is immediately connected to a cardiac monitor, and a pulse oximeter is applied. More invasive monitoring (e.g., arterial line monitoring of blood pressure and pulse rate) is often required and should be started as soon as feasible. Unless contraindicated, oxygen is administered at 15 L/min via a nonrebreather mask. Neurologic status and level of consciousness are carefully monitored. Additional nursing interventions consist of keeping the patient quiet and warm and offering psychologic support and reassurance.

The remaining therapies for shock depend on the specific cause of the condition. The two primary pharmacotherapeutic goals are to restore normal fluid volume and composition and to maintain adequate blood pressure. For anaphylaxis, an additional goal is to prevent or stop the hypersensitive inflammatory response.

FLUID REPLACEMENT AGENTS

Various drugs are used to replace blood or other fluids lost during hypovolemic shock. Fluid replacement therapy includes blood, blood products, colloids, and crystalloids, as listed in Table 29.2.

29.4 Treating Shock with IV Fluid Therapy

Hypovolemic shock can be triggered by a number of conditions, including hemorrhage, extensive burns, severe dehydration, persistent vomiting or diarrhea, and intensive diuretic therapy. If the patient has lost significant blood or other body fluids, immediate maintenance of blood volume through the IV infusion of fluid and electrolytes or blood products is essential.

Blood or blood products may be administered to restore fluid volume, depending on the clinical situation. Whole blood is indicated for the treatment of acute, massive blood loss (depletion of more than 30% of the total volume) when there is a need to replace plasma volume *and* supply red blood cells to increase the oxygen-carrying capacity.

A single unit of whole blood can be separated into its specific constituents (red and white blood cells, platelets, plasma proteins, fresh frozen plasma, and globulins), which can be used to treat more than one patient. The supply of blood products, however, depends on human donors and requires careful crossmatching to ensure compatibility between the donor and the recipient. In addition, although it is carefully screened, whole blood has the potential to transmit serious infections such as hepatitis or HIV.

The administration of whole blood to expand volume and to sustain blood pressure has been largely replaced by the use of fluid infusion therapy. Drugs used to expand fluid volume are of two basic types: colloids and crystalloids. Colloid and crystalloid infusions are often used when up to one third of an adult's blood volume has been lost.

Colloids are proteins or other large molecules that stay suspended in the blood for a long period because they are too large to easily cross membranes. While circulating, they draw water molecules from the cells and tissues into the blood vessels through their ability to increase plasma oncotic pressure. Blood-product colloids include normal human serum albumin, plasma protein fraction, and serum globulins. The non–blood-product colloids are dextran (40, 70, and high molecular weight) and hetastarch (Hespan). These agents are administered to provide life-sustaining support following massive hemorrhage and to treat shock, as well as to treat burns, acute liver failure, and neonatal hemolytic disease.

Crystalloids are IV solutions that contain electrolytes in concentrations resembling those of plasma. Unlike colloids, crystalloid solutions can readily leave the blood and enter cells. They are used to replace fluids that have been lost and to promote urine output. Common crystalloids used in shock include normal saline, lactated Ringer's, Plasmalyte, and hypertonic saline. Additional information on the role of crystalloids and colloids in correcting fluid balance disorders is included in chapter 31∞.

TABLE 29.2	Fluid Replacement Agents
Agent	**Examples**
Blood products	• whole blood • plasma protein fraction • fresh frozen plasma • packed red blood cells
Colloids	• plasma protein fraction (Plasmanate, Plasma-Plex, Plasmatein, PPF, Protenate) • dextran 40 (Gentran 40, Hyskon, Rheomacrodex) or dextran 70 (Macrodex) • hetastarch (Hespan) • normal serum albumin, human (Albuminar, Albutein, Buminate, Plasbumin)
Crystalloids	• normal saline (0.9% sodium chloride) • lactated Ringer's • Plasmalyte • hypertonic saline (3% sodium chloride) • 5% dextrose in water (D5W)*
*Not used for shock	

VASOCONSTRICTORS/VASOPRESSORS

In some types of shock, the most serious medical challenge facing the patient is hypotension, which may become so profound as to cause collapse of the circulatory system. Vasoconstrictors are drugs for maintaining blood pressure when vasodilation has caused hypotension but fluids have not been lost (i.e., anaphylactic shock) and when fluid replacement therapy have proved ineffective. These medications are listed in Table 29.3.

Pr Prototype Drug | Normal Serum Albumin *(Albuminar, Plasbumin, others)*

Therapeutic Class: Fluid replacement agent   **Pharmacologic Class:** Blood product, colloid

ACTIONS AND USES

Normal serum albumin is a protein extracted from whole blood, plasma, or placental human plasma. Albumin naturally comprises about 60% of all blood proteins. Its normal functions are to maintain plasma oncotic pressure and to shuttle certain substances through the blood, including fatty acids, certain hormones and a substantial number of drug molecules. After extraction from blood or plasma, albumin is sterilized to remove possible contamination by the hepatitis viruses or HIV.

Administered IV, albumin increases the oncotic pressure of the blood and causes fluid to move from the tissues to the general circulation. It is used to restore plasma volume in hypovolemic shock, or to restore blood proteins in patients with hypoproteinemia, which frequently occurs in patients with hepatic cirrhosis. It has an immediate onset of action and is available in concentrations of 5% and 25%.

ADMINISTRATION ALERTS

- Infuse higher concentrations more slowly because the risk of a large, rapid fluid shift is greater.
- Use a large-gauge (16- to 20-gauge) IV cannula for administration of the drug.
- Pregnancy category C

PHARMACOKINETICS
Because albumin is a natural substance, it is not possible to obtain pharmacokinetic values for supplements.

ADVERSE EFFECTS

Because albumin is a natural blood product, the patient may have antibodies to the donor albumin and allergic reactions are possible. However, coagulation factors, antibodies, and most other blood proteins have been removed; therefore, the incidence of allergic reactions from albumin is not high. Signs of allergy include fever, chills, rash, dyspnea, and possibly hypotension. Protein overload may occur if excessive amounts of albumin are infused.

Contraindications: Contraindications include severe anemia or cardiac failure in the presence of normal or increased intravascular volume, and allergy to albumin.

INTERACTIONS
Drug–Drug: Unknown

Lab Tests: Normal serum albumin may increase serum alkaline phosphatase.

Herbal/Food: Unknown

Treatment of Overdose: There is no treatment for overdose.

Refer to MyNursingKit for a Nursing Process Focus specific to this drug.

29.5 Treating Shock with Vasoconstrictors/Vasopressors

In the early stages of shock, the body compensates for the initial fall in blood pressure by activating the sympathetic nervous system. This sympathetic activity produces vasoconstriction, which raises blood pressure and increases the rate and force of myocardial contractions. The purpose of these compensatory measures is to maintain blood flow to vital organs such as the heart and brain, and to decrease flow to other organs, including the kidneys and liver.

The body's ability to compensate is limited, however, and profound hypotension may develop as shock progresses. In severe cases, fluid replacement agents alone are not effective at raising blood pressure, and other medications are indicated. Sympathomimetic vasoconstrictors, also known as

TABLE 29.3	Vasoconstrictors and Inotropic Drugs for Shock	
Drug	**Route and Adult Dose (max dose where indicated)**	**Adverse Effects**
digoxin (Lanoxin, Lanoxicaps) (see page 331 for the Prototype Drug box ∞)	IV; digitalizing dose 2.5–5 mcg every 6 hours for 24 h; maintenance dose 0.125–0.5 mg/day	*Nausea, vomiting, headache, and visual disturbances such as halos, a yellow/green tinge, or blurring* Dysrhythmias, AV block
dobutamine (Dobutrex)	IV; infused at a rate of 2.5–40 mcg/kg/min for a max of 72 h	*Palpitations, tingling or coldness of extremities, nervousness, changes in blood pressure (hypotension or hypertension)* Tachycardia or bradycardia (overdose), hypertension, dysrhythmias, necrosis at injection site, severe hypertension
⊕ dopamine (Dopastat, Intropin)	IV; 2–5 mcg/kg/min initial dose; may be increased to 20–50 mcg/kg/min	
⊕ epinephrine (Adrenalin)	Subcutaneousl 0.1–0.5 mL of 1:100 every 10–15 min; IV 0.1–0.25 mL of 1:1000 every 10–15 min	
⊕ norepinephrine (Levophed)	IV; initial 0.5–1 mcg/min, titrate to response; usual range 8–30 mcg/min	
phenylephrine (Neo-Synephrine, others) (see page 133 for the Prototype Drug box ∞)	IV; 0.1–0.18 mg/min until pressure stabilizes, then 0.04–0.06 mg/min for maintenance	
Italics indicate common adverse effects; <u>underlining</u> indicates serious adverse effects.		

NURSING PROCESS FOCUS   PATIENTS RECEIVING IV FLUID REPLACEMENT THERAPY FOR SHOCK

Assessment	Potential Nursing Diagnoses
Baseline assessment prior to administration: • Understand the reason the drug has been prescribed in order to assess for therapeutic effects (e.g., type of shock). • Obtain a complete health history including cardiovascular (including HTN, MI), neurologic (including CVA or head injury), burns, endocrine, and hepatic or renal disease. Obtain a drug history including allergies, current prescription and OTC drugs, and herbal preparations. Be alert to possible drug interactions. • Obtain baseline weight and vital signs, level of consciousness, breath sounds, and urinary and cardiac output. • Evaluate appropriate laboratory findings (e.g., Hgb and Hct, WBC count, electrolytes, arterial blood gases, total protein and albumin levels, aPTT, aPT or INR, blood cultures, renal and liver function studies).	• Decreased Cardiac Output (cardiovascular) • Ineffective Tissue Perfusion (cardiopulmonary, septic shock) • Impaired Gas Exchange (cardiopulmonary) • Ineffective Airway Clearance (anaphylaxis) • Deficient Fluid Volume (volume loss, third-spacing) • Anxiety or Fear (related to concerns about severity of condition) • Deficient Knowledge (drug therapy) • Risk for Injury (related to adverse effects of drug therapy or administration) • Risk for Excessive Fluid Volume (related to drug therapy)
Assessment throughout administration: • Assess for desired therapeutic effects dependent on the reason for the drug (e.g., BP, pulse, cardiac output return to within acceptable range, adequate urine output). • Continue frequent and careful monitoring of vital signs, and urinary and cardiac output as appropriate. • Assess for and promptly report adverse effects: tachycardia, hypertension, dysrhythmias, decreasing level of consciousness, increasing dyspnea, lung congestion, pink-tinged frothy sputum, decreased urinary output, or allergic reactions.	

Planning: Patient Goals and Expected Outcomes

The patient will:
• Experience therapeutic effects dependent on the reason the drug is being given (e.g., improved blood pressure, cardiac and urine output within normal limits).
• Be free from, or experience minimal, adverse effects.
• Verbalize an understanding of the drug's use, adverse effects, and required precautions.

Implementation

Interventions and (Rationales)	Patient and Family Education
Ensuring therapeutic effects: • Continue frequent assessments as above for therapeutic effects dependent on the reason the drug therapy is given. (Pulse, blood pressure, and respiratory rate should be within normal limits or within parameters set by the health care provider, and ABGs and/or pulse oximetry are within acceptable parameters. Cardiac output is within normal limits and urine output has increased.)	• To allay anxiety, teach the patient and family about the rationale for all equipment used and the need for frequent monitoring.
• Provide supportive nursing measures; e.g., moistening lips if patient is intubated, explanations for all procedures, and frequent orientation. (Supportive nursing measures help to decrease patient, family, and caregiver anxiety and supplement therapeutic drug effects to optimize outcome. Patient may be intubated and/or sedated.)	• Explain all procedures to the patient before beginning. Provide frequent assurance and verbal stimuli if the patient is intubated.
Minimizing adverse effects: • Monitor for signs of fluid volume excess, e.g., increasing BP, hypertension, tachycardia, bounding pulse, confusion, decreasing level of consciousness. Continue frequent cardiac monitoring, e.g., ECG, and cardiac output and urine output. (Because of the critical condition of the patient in shock, a delicate balance between fluid volume excess and deficit exists. Frequent assessments must be made to detect and avoid adverse effects. External and invasive monitoring devices will detect early signs of adverse effects as well as monitoring for therapeutic effects.)	• Instruct the patient to report palpitations, shortness of breath, chest pain, dyspnea, or headache immediately. • Continue to explain to the patient the rationale for all equipment used, procedures completed, and the need for frequent monitoring.
• Frequently monitor CBC, electrolyte, aPTT, and aPT or INR levels. (Crystalloid solutions may cause electrolyte imbalances. Colloid solutions may reduce normal blood coagulation.)	• To allay anxiety, teach the patient, family, and caregiver about the rationale for frequent monitoring of lab values.

NURSING PROCESS FOCUS PATIENTS RECEIVING IV FLUID REPLACEMENT THERAPY FOR SHOCK *(Continued)*

Implementation

Interventions and (Rationales)	Patient and Family Education
▪ Weigh patient daily and report weight gain or loss of 1 kg (approximately 2 lb) or more in a 24-hour period. (Daily weight is an accurate measure of fluid status and takes into account intake, output, and insensible losses. Weight gain or edema may signal excessive fluid volume.)	▪ Explain to the patient the rationale for all equipment used for weighing the patient and the need for frequent monitoring.
▪ Closely monitor for signs and symptoms of allergy if colloids are used. (Blood or blood products, and colloids cause allergic and anaphylactic reactions.)	▪ Instruct the patient to report dyspnea, itching, feelings of throat tightness, palpitations, chest pain or tightening, or headache immediately.
Patient understanding of drug therapy: ▪ Use opportunities during administration of medications and during assessments to discuss the rationale for drug therapy, desired therapeutic outcomes, and any necessary monitoring or precautions. (Using time during nursing care helps to optimize and reinforce supportive drug treatment and care.)	▪ The patient and/or family should be able to state an understanding of the reason for the drug, equipment used, the possible length of medication therapy needed, and any supportive treatments that will be given. ▪ Continue to provide supportive care to the family or caregiver due to the stressful nature of the patient's condition. Provide referral to appropriate resources (e.g., pastoral care, social services).

Evaluation of Outcome Criteria

Evaluate the effectiveness of drug therapy by confirming that patient goals and expected outcomes have been met (see "Planning").

See Table 29.2 for a list of the drugs to which these nursing actions apply.

See also Nursing Process Focus tables, chapter 13 for information related to adrenergic drugs (vasoconstrictors/vasopressors), and chapter 24 for positive inotropic agents used in the treatment of shock ∞.

Pr Prototype Drug | Norepinephrine *(Levophed)*

Therapeutic Class: Drug for shock   **Pharmacologic Class:** Nonselective adrenergic agonist: vasopressor

ACTIONS AND USES
Norepinephrine is a sympathomimetic that acts directly on alpha-adrenergic receptors in vascular smooth muscle to immediately raise blood pressure. To a lesser degree, it also stimulates beta$_1$-receptors in the heart, thus producing a positive inotropic response that may increase cardiac output. Its primary indications are acute shock and cardiac arrest. Norepinephrine is the vasopressor of choice for septic shock because research has demonstrated that it significantly decreases mortality. It is given by the IV route and has a duration of only 1 to 2 minutes after the infusion is terminated.

ADMINISTRATION ALERTS
- Start an infusion only after ensuring the patency of the IV. Monitor the flow rate continuously.
- If extravasation occurs, administer phentolamine to the area of infiltration as soon as possible.
- Do not abruptly discontinue infusion.
- Pregnancy category D

> **PHARMACOKINETICS**
> **Onset:** 1–2 min
> **Peak:** 1–2 min
> **Half-life:** Unknown
> **Duration:** Unknown

ADVERSE EFFECTS
Norepinephrine is a powerful vasoconstrictor; thus, continuous monitoring of the patient's blood pressure is required to prevent the development of hypertension. When first administered, reflex bradycardia is sometimes experienced. It also has the ability to produce various types of dysrhythmias, although less so than other vasopressors. If extravasation occurs, the drug may cause serious skin and soft tissue injury. Blurred vision and photophobia are signs of overdose.

Contraindications: Norepinephrine should not be administered to patients who are experiencing hypotension due to blood volume deficits because vasoconstriction already exists in such patients. Norepinephrine may cause additional, severe peripheral and visceral vasoconstriction with decreased urine output. Norepinephrine is not usually given to patients with mesenteric or peripheral vascular thrombosis, because there is an increased risk of increasing ischemia and worsening the infarction.

INTERACTIONS
Drug–Drug: Alpha and beta blockers may antagonize the drug's vasopressor effects. Conversely, ergot alkaloids and tricyclic antidepressants may potentiate vasopressor effects. Digoxin, halothane, and cyclopropane may increase the risk of dysrhythmias.

Lab Tests: Unknown

Herbal/Food: Unknown

Treatment of Overdose: Discontinuing the infusion usually results in a rapid reversal of adverse effects such as hypertension.

Refer to MyNursingKit for a Nursing Process Focus specific to this drug.

vasopressors, are used to stabilize blood pressure in shock patients. When given intravenously, these drugs have rapid onsets with short durations, and will immediately raise blood pressure. Because of adverse effects and potential organ damage due to the rapid and intense vasoconstriction, vasopressors are used only after fluid and electrolyte restoration has failed to raise blood pressure. These drugs are considered critical care agents: The infusions are continuously monitored and adjusted to ensure the desired therapeutic effect has been achieved without significant adverse effects. Therapy is discontinued as soon as the patient's condition stabilizes. Discontinuation of vasopressor therapy is always gradual, due to the possibility of rebound hypotension and undesirable cardiac effects.

Vasopressors used to treat shock include dopamine (Dopastat, Intropin), norepinephrine (Levophed), phenylephrine (Neo-Synephrine, others), and epinephrine. Because dopamine also affects the strength of myocardial contraction, it is considered both a vasopressor and an inotropic agent (see Section 29.6). Epinephrine is usually associated with the treatment of anaphylaxis (Section 29.7). The basic pharmacology of the sympathomimetics is presented in chapter 13∞.

INOTROPIC DRUGS

Inotropic agents, also called *cardiotonic drugs,* increase the force of contraction of the heart. In the treatment of shock, they are used to increase the cardiac output. The inotropic agents are listed in Table 29.3.

29.6 Treating Shock with Inotropic Agents

As shock progresses, the heart may begin to fail; cardiac output decreases, lowering the amount of blood reaching vital tissues and deepening the degree of shock. **Inotropic agents** have the potential to reverse the cardiac symptoms of shock by increasing the strength of myocardial contraction. For example, digoxin (Lanoxin) increases myocardial contractility and cardiac output, thus quickly bringing critical tissues their essential oxygen. Chapter 22∞ should be reviewed, because digoxin and other medications prescribed for heart failure are sometimes used for the treatment of shock.

Dobutamine (Dobutrex) is a selective beta$_1$-adrenergic agent that has value in the short-term treatment of certain

---

Pr Prototype Drug | Dopamine *(Dopastat, Intropin)*

Therapeutic Class: Drug for shock   **Pharmacologic Class:** Nonselective adrenergic agonist; inotropic agent

ACTIONS AND USES
Dopamine is the immediate metabolic precursor to norepinephrine. Although dopamine is classified as a sympathomimetic, its mechanism of action is dependent on the dose. At low doses, the drug selectively stimulates dopaminergic receptors, especially in the kidneys, leading to vasodilation and an increased blood flow through the kidneys. This makes dopamine of particular value in treating hypovolemic and cardiogenic shock. At higher doses, dopamine stimulates beta$_1$-adrenergic receptors, causing the heart to beat more forcefully and increasing cardiac output. Another beneficial effect of dopamine when given in higher doses is its ability to stimulate alpha-adrenergic receptors, thus causing vasoconstriction and raising blood pressure.

ADMINISTRATION ALERTS
- Give this drug as a continuous infusion only.
- Ensure the patency of the IV prior to beginning the infusion.
- Because there are different dosage ranges based on the desired therapeutic effect, always double-check drug calculations before giving the drug.
- If extravasation occurs, administer phentolamine to the area of infiltration as soon as possible.
- Pregnancy category C

PHARMACOKINETICS
Onset: 1–2 min
Peak: Unknown
Half-life: 2 min
Duration: Less than 10 min

ADVERSE EFFECTS
Because of its profound effects on the cardiovascular system, patients receiving dopamine must be continuously monitored for signs of dysrhythmias and hypertension. Adverse effects are normally self-limiting because of the short half-life of the drug. Dopamine is a vesicant drug that can cause severe, irreversible skin and soft tissue damage if the drug infiltrates.

Contraindications: Dopamine is contraindicated in patients with pheochromocytoma or ventricular fibrillation.

INTERACTIONS
Drug–Drug: Concurrent administration with MAO inhibitors or ergot alkaloids increase alpha-adrenergic effects. Phenytoin may decrease dopamine action. Beta blockers may inhibit the inotropic effects of dopamine. Alpha blockers inhibit peripheral vasoconstriction. Digoxin and many anesthetics increase the risk of dysrhythmias.

Lab Tests: Unknown

Herbal/Food: Unknown

Treatment of Overdose: Discontinuing the infusion usually results in rapid reversal of adverse effects such as hypertension. The short-acting alpha-adrenergic blocker phentolamine may be administered to stabilize the patient's condition.

Refer to MyNursingKit for a Nursing Process Focus specific to this drug.

types of shock, due to its ability to cause the heart to beat more forcefully. Dobutamine is especially beneficial when the primary cause of shock is related to heart failure, rather than hypovolemia. The resulting increase in cardiac output assists in maintaining blood flow to vital organs. Dobutamine has a half-life of only 2 minutes and is given only as an IV infusion.

Dopamine (Dopastat, Intropin) activates both beta- and alpha-adrenergic receptors. It is primarily used in shock conditions to increase blood pressure by causing peripheral vasoconstriction (alpha$_1$ activation) and increasing the force of myocardial contraction (beta$_1$ activation). Dopamine has the potential to cause dysrhythmias and is given only as an IV infusion.

ANAPHYLAXIS

Anaphylaxis is a potentially fatal condition in which body defenses produce a hyperresponse to a foreign substance known as an *antigen* or *allergen*. On first exposure, the allergen produces no symptoms; however, the body responds by becoming highly sensitized for a subsequent exposure. During anaphylaxis, the body responds quickly, often just minutes after exposure to the allergen, by releasing massive amounts of histamine and other mediators of the inflammatory response. The patient may experience itching, hives, and a tightness in the throat or chest. Swelling occurs around the larynx, causing a nonproductive cough and the voice to become hoarse. As anaphylaxis progresses, the patient experiences a rapid fall in blood pressure and difficulty breathing due to bronchoconstriction. The hypotension causes reflex tachycardia. Without medical intervention, anaphylaxis leads to a profound state of shock, which is often fatal. ➤ Figure 29.3 illustrates the symptoms of anaphylaxis.

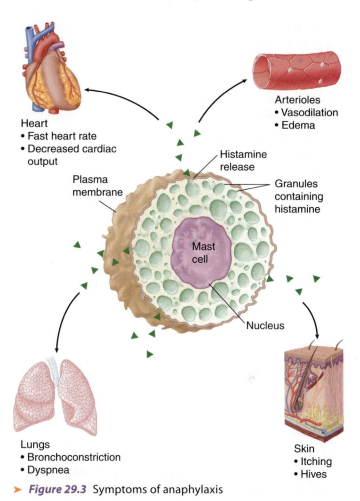

Heart
- Fast heart rate
- Decreased cardiac output

Arterioles
- Vasodilation
- Edema

Histamine release

Plasma membrane

Granules containing histamine

Mast cell

Nucleus

Lungs
- Bronchoconstriction
- Dyspnea

Skin
- Itching
- Hives

➤ *Figure 29.3* Symptoms of anaphylaxis

29.7 Pharmacotherapy of Anaphylaxis

The pharmacotherapy of anaphylaxis is symptomatic and involves supporting the cardiovascular system and preventing further hyperresponse by body defenses. Various medications are used to treat the symptoms of anaphylaxis, depending on the severity of the symptoms.

Epinephrine, 1:1000, given subcutaneously or IM, is an initial drug of choice because it causes vasoconstriction and can rapidly relieve symptoms of bronchoconstriction. If necessary, the dose may be repeated up to three times at 10- to 15-minute intervals. Crystalloids or colloids may be needed to prevent shock if the patient presents with volume depletion. Antihistamines such as diphenhydramine (Benadryl) may be administered IM or IV to prevent further release of histamine. A bronchodilator such as albuterol (Ventolin, Proventil) is often administered by inhalation to relieve the acute shortness of breath caused by histamine release. High-flow oxygen is usually administered. Systemic glucocorticoids such as hydrocortisone are given to dampen the *delayed* inflammatory response that may occur several hours after the initial event.

Nearly all drugs have the capability to *cause* anaphylaxis. Although this is a rare adverse drug effect, the nurse must be

---

prepared to quickly deal with anaphylaxis by understanding the indications and doses of the various drugs on the emergency cart. The most common drugs causing anaphylaxis include the following:

- Antibiotics, especially penicillins, cephalosporins, and sulfonamides
- NSAIDs, such as aspirin, ibuprofen, and naproxen
- ACE inhibitors
- Opioid analgesics
- Iodine-based contrast media used for radiographic exams

Although obtaining a patient history of drug allergy is helpful in predicting some adverse drug reactions, anaphylaxis may occur without a previously reported incident. However, previous severe hypersensitivity to a drug is always a contraindication to the future use of that or closely related drugs in the same class. Unless the drug is the only one available to treat the patient's condition, the drug should not be administered.

If a drug must be given for which the patient has a known allergy, the patient may be *pretreated* with antihistamines or glucocorticoids to suppress the inflammatory response. If time permits, patients may be desensitized. Desensitization

for penicillin and cephalosporin allergy, which takes about 6 hours, has been shown to be effective in preventing severe allergic reactions to these antibiotics. A typical desensitization regimen would involve administering an initial dose of 0.01 mg of the antibiotic and observing the patient for allergy. The dose may then be doubled every 15 to 20 minutes until the full dose has been achieved. Desensitization has also been achieved for patients with aspirin-induced asthma who require aspirin therapy for another condition.

HOME & COMMUNITY CONSIDERATIONS

Recurrent Anaphylaxis

Patients with a history of recurrent anaphylaxis may be prescribed epinephrine to be self-administered intramuscularly via an automatic injectable device (EpiPen). Instruct these patients regarding safe "pen" storage and disposal and the proper injection technique. Encourage patients to use the medication-free "trainer" auto-inject pen to practice the technique. Advise patients to expect some medication to remain in the pen following injection and to report all episodes requiring pen usage to their health care provider. Advise patients to wear a medical alert bracelet or necklace stating "allergy" and to carry a medication allergy list in wallet or purse.

MyNursingKit | Mechanism in Action: Epinephrine

Pr Prototype Drug | Epinephrine *(Adrenalin)*

Therapeutic Class: Drug for anaphylaxis and shock   **Pharmacologic Class:** Nonselective adrenergic agonist; vasopressor

ACTIONS AND USES

Subcutaneous or IV epinephrine is a drug of choice for anaphylaxis because it can reverse many of the distressing symptoms within minutes. Epinephrine is a nonselective adrenergic agonist, stimulating both alpha- and beta-adrenergic receptors. Almost immediately after injection, blood pressure rises due to stimulation of alpha$_1$ receptors. Activation of beta$_2$ receptors in the bronchi opens the airways and relieves the patient's shortness of breath. Cardiac output increases due to stimulation of beta$_1$ receptors in the heart. In addition to the SC and IM routes, topical, inhalation, and ophthalmic preparations are available. The intracardiac route is used for cardiopulmonary resuscitation under extreme conditions, usually during open cardiac massage, or when no other route is possible.

ADMINISTRATION ALERTS

- Parenteral epinephrine is an irritant that may cause tissue damage if extravasation occurs.
- Pregnancy category C

PHARMACOKINETICS

Onset: 3–5 min (subcutaneous); 5–10 min (IM)

Peak: 20 min

Half-life: Unknown

Duration: 1–4 h

ADVERSE EFFECTS

The most common adverse effects of epinephrine are nervousness, tremors, palpitations, tachycardia, dizziness, headache, and stinging/burning at the site of application. When administered parenterally, hypertension, and dysrhythmias may occur rapidly; therefore, the patient should be monitored carefully following injection.

Contraindications: In life-threatening conditions such as anaphylaxis, there are no absolute contraindications for the use of epinephrine. The drug must be used with caution, however, in patients with dysrhythmias, cerebrovascular insufficiency, hyperthyroidism, narrow-angle glaucoma, hypertension, or coronary ischemia, because epinephrine may worsen these conditions.

INTERACTIONS

Drug–Drug: Epinephrine may result in hypotension if used with phenothiazines or oxytocin. There may be additive cardiovascular effects with other sympathomimetics. MAO inhibitors, tricyclic antidepressants, and alpha- and beta-adrenergic agents inhibit the actions of epinephrine. Epinephrine will decrease the effects of beta blockers. Some general anesthetics may sensitize the heart to the effects of epinephrine.

Lab Tests: Epinephrine may decrease serum potassium level.

Herbal/Food: Unknown

Treatment of Overdose: Overdose may be serious, and alpha- and beta-adrenergic blockers are indicated. If blood pressure remains high, a vasodilator may be administered.

Refer to MyNursingKit for a Nursing Process Focus specific to this drug.

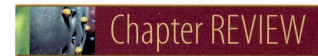

Chapter REVIEW

KEY CONCEPTS

The numbered key concepts provide a succinct summary of the important points from the corresponding numbered section within the chapter. If any of these points are not clear, refer to the numbered section within the chapter for review.

29.1 Shock is a clinical syndrome characterized by the inability of the cardiovascular system to pump enough blood to meet the metabolic needs of the tissues. Key body systems affected by shock are the nervous, renal, and cardiovascular systems.

29.2 Shock is often classified by the underlying pathologic process or by the organ system that is primarily affected, including cardiogenic, hypovolemic, neurogenic, septic, and anaphylactic shock.

29.3 The initial treatment of shock involves administration of basic life support, replacement of lost fluid, and maintenance of blood pressure.

29.4 During hypovolemic shock, crystalloids replace lost fluids and electrolytes; colloids expand plasma volume and maintain blood pressure. Whole blood may be indicated in cases of massive hemorrhage.

29.5 Vasopressors are critical care drugs sometimes needed during severe shock to maintain blood pressure. These drugs are sympathomimetics that strongly constrict the arteries and immediately raise blood pressure.

29.6 Inotropic drugs are useful in reversing the decreased cardiac output resulting from shock by increasing the strength of myocardial contraction.

29.7 Anaphylaxis is a serious hypersensitivity response to an allergen that is treated with a large number of different drugs, including sympathomimetics, antihistamines, and glucocorticoids. Common drugs such as penicillins, cephalosporins, NSAIDs, and ACE inhibitors may cause anaphylaxis.

NCLEX-RN® REVIEW QUESTIONS

1 The patient in hypovolemic shock is prescribed an infusion of lactated Ringer's. The nurse recognizes the function of this fluid in the treatment of shock is to: (Select all that apply.)
1. replace fluid and promote urine output.
2. draw water into cells.
3. draw water from cells to blood vessels.
4. maintain vascular volume.

2 The nurse evaluates the effectiveness of dopamine therapy for a patient in shock. Which of the following may indicate treatment is successful? (Select all that apply.)
1. Improved urine output
2. Increased blood pressure
3. Breath sounds are diminished
4. Slight hypotension occurs
5. Peripheral pulses are intact

3 Dobutamine (Dobutrex) is used to treat a patient experiencing cardiogenic shock. Nursing intervention includes:
1. monitoring for fluid overload.
2. monitoring for cardiac dysrhythmias.
3. monitoring respiratory status.
4. monitoring for hypotension.

4 Teaching for a patient receiving plasma protein fraction (Plasmanate) should include reporting which of the following possible adverse reactions?
1. Unusual bleeding
2. Hyperglycemia
3. Anaphylactic reaction
4. Hypotension

5 Nursing assessment of a patient receiving normal serum albumin for treatment of shock should include:
1. assessing breath sounds.
2. monitoring glucose.
3. monitoring potassium level.
4. monitoring hemoglobin and hematocrit.

6 A patient is receiving a crystalloid infusion (lactated Ringer's) for treatment of hypovolemic shock. Because of concerns for fluid volume overload, the nurse will frequently monitor: (Select all that apply.)
1. breath sounds.
2. potassium, glucose, and sodium levels.
3. daily weight.
4. level of consciousness.
5. aPTT, aPT, INR.

CRITICAL THINKING QUESTIONS

1. A patient is on a norepinephrine (Levophed) drip for cardiogenic shock with a blood pressure of 84/40 mmHg. Why is this patient on this medication? What nursing assessments should occur? When and how should the norepinephrine drip be discontinued?

2. The health care provider orders 3 L of 0.9% normal saline (NS) for a 22-year-old patient with vomiting and diarrhea, and a heart rate of 122 bpm and blood pressure of 102/54 mmHg. Is this an appropriate IV solution for this patient? Why or why not?

3. A patient with a severe head injury has been put on an IV drip of dextrose 5% water running at 150 mL/h. The nurse receives this transfer patient and is reviewing the health care provider's orders. Is the IV solution appropriate for this patient? Why or why not?

See Appendix D for answers and rationales for all activities.

 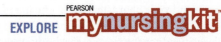

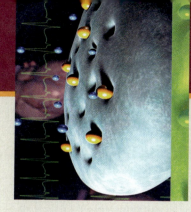

Diuretic Therapy and Drugs for Renal Failure

LEARNING OUTCOMES

After reading this chapter, the student should be able to:

1. Explain the role of the kidneys in maintaining fluid, electrolyte, and acid–base balance.
2. Explain the processes that change the composition of filtrate as it travels through the nephron.
3. Describe the adjustments in pharmacotherapy that must be considered in patients with renal failure.
4. Identify indications for diuretics.
5. Describe the general adverse effects of diuretic pharmacotherapy.
6. Compare and contrast the loop, thiazide, and potassium-sparing diuretics.
7. Describe the nurse's role in the pharmacologic management of renal failure, and in diuretic therapy.
8. For each of the classes shown in Drugs at a Glance, know representative drugs, and explain the mechanism of drug action, primary actions, and important adverse effects.
9. Use the nursing process to care for patients who are receiving drug therapy for renal failure, and diuretic therapy.

KEY TERMS

carbonic anhydrase *page 424*
diuretic *page 420*
filtrate *page 418*

nephron *page 418*
reabsorption *page 418*
renal failure *page 418*

secretion *page 418*
urinalysis *page 418*

The kidneys serve an amazing role in maintaining homeostasis. By filtering a volume equivalent to all the body's extracellular fluid every 100 minutes, the kidneys are able to make immediate adjustments to fluid volume, electrolyte composition, and acid–base balance. This chapter examines diuretics, agents that increase urine output, and other drugs used to treat kidney failure. Chapter 31∞ presents additional agents for treating fluid, electrolyte, and acid–base imbalances.

30.1 Functions of the Kidneys

When most people think of the kidneys, they think of excretion. Although this is certainly true, the kidneys have many other homeostatic functions. The kidneys are the primary organs for regulating fluid balance, electrolyte composition, and acid–base balance of body fluids. They also secrete the enzyme renin, which helps regulate blood pressure (chapter 23∞) and erythropoietin, a hormone that stimulates red blood cell production (chapter 28∞). In addition, the kidneys are responsible for the production of calcitriol, the active form of vitamin D, which helps maintain bone homeostasis (chapter 47∞). It is not surprising that our overall health is strongly dependent on proper functioning of the kidneys.

The urinary system consists of two kidneys, two ureters, one urinary bladder, and a urethra. Each kidney contains more than 1 million **nephrons,** the functional units of the kidney. Blood enters the nephron through the large renal arteries and is filtered through a semipermeable membrane known as the glomerulus. Water and other small molecules readily pass through the glomerulus and enter Bowman's capsule, the first section of the nephron, and then the proximal tubule. Once in the nephron, the fluid is called **filtrate.** After leaving the proximal tubule, the filtrate travels through the loop of Henle and, subsequently, the distal tubule. Nephrons empty their filtrate into common collecting ducts, and then into larger and larger collecting structures inside the kidney. Fluid leaving the collecting ducts and entering subsequent portions of the kidney is called *urine.* Parts of the nephron are illustrated in ➤ Figure 30.1.

MyNursingKit Nephrology Channel

MyNursingKit Basic Function of the Kidney Animation

PharmFacts

Renal Disorders
- Although more than 17,000 kidney transplants are performed annually, more than 70,000 people are on a waiting list for a replacement kidney.
- One of every 750 people is born with a single kidney. A single kidney is larger and more vulnerable to injury from heavy contact sports.
- About 260,000 Americans suffer from chronic kidney failure, and 50,000 die annually from causes related to the disease.
- Type 2 diabetes is the leading cause of chronic kidney failure, accounting for 30% to 40% of all new cases each year.
- Hypertension is the second leading cause of chronic kidney failure, accounting for about 25% of all new cases each year.

Many drugs are small enough to pass through the pores of the glomerulus and enter the filtrate. If the drug is bound to plasma proteins, however, it will be too large, and will continue circulating in the blood.

30.2 Renal Reabsorption and Secretion

When filtrate enters Bowman's capsule, its composition is very similar to that of plasma. Plasma proteins such as albumin, however, are too large to pass through the filter and will not be present in the filtrate or in the urine of healthy patients. If these proteins *do* appear in urine, it means they were able to pass through the filter due to kidney pathology.

As filtrate travels through the nephron, its composition changes dramatically. Some substances in the filtrate cross the walls of the nephron to reenter the blood, a process known as tubular **reabsorption.** Water is the most important molecule reabsorbed in the tubule. For every 180 L of water entering the filtrate each day, approximately 178.5 L is reabsorbed, leaving only 1.5 L to be excreted in the urine. Glucose, amino acids, and essential ions such as sodium, chloride, calcium, and bicarbonate are also reabsorbed.

Certain ions and molecules too large to pass through Bowman's capsule may still enter the urine by crossing from the blood to the filtrate in a process called tubular **secretion.** Potassium, phosphate, hydrogen, and ammonium ions enter the filtrate through active secretion. Acidic drugs secreted in the proximal tubule include penicillin G, ampicillin, sulfisoxazole, nonsteroidal anti-inflammatory drugs (NSAIDs), and furosemide: Basic drugs include procainamide, epinephrine, dopamine, neostigmine, and trimethoprim.

Reabsorption and secretion are critical to the pharmacokinetics of drugs. Some drugs are reabsorbed, whereas others are secreted into the filtrate. For example, approximately 90% of a dose of penicillin G enters the urine through secretion. When the kidney is damaged, reabsorption and secretion mechanisms are impaired and serum drug levels may be dramatically affected. The processes of reabsorption and secretion are illustrated in Figure 30.1.

RENAL FAILURE

Renal failure is a decrease in the kidneys' ability to maintain electrolyte and fluid balance and to excrete waste products. The cause of renal failure may be due to pathology within the kidney itself or the result of disorders in other body systems. The primary treatment goals for a patient with renal failure are to maintain blood flow through the kidneys and adequate urine output.

30.3 Diagnosis and Pharmacotherapy of Renal Failure

Before pharmacotherapy may be considered in a patient with renal failure, an assessment of the degree of kidney impairment is necessary. The basic diagnostic test is a **urinalysis,**

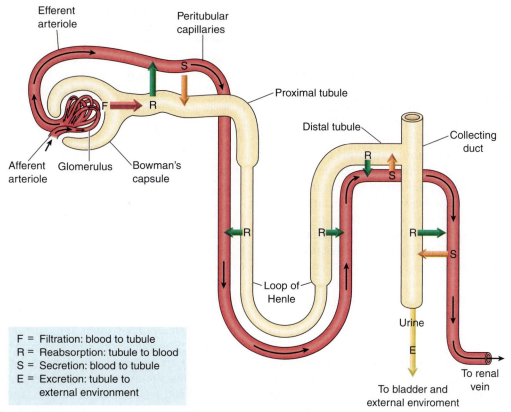

Efferent arteriole
Peritubular capillaries
Proximal tubule
Distal tubule
Collecting duct
Afferent arteriole
Glomerulus
Bowman's capsule
Loop of Henle
Urine
To bladder and external enviroment
To renal vein

F = Filtration: blood to tubule
R = Reabsorption: tubule to blood
S = Secretion: blood to tubule
E = Excretion: tubule to external environment

➤ *Figure 30.1* The nephron

which examines urine for the presence of blood cells, proteins, pH, specific gravity, ketones, glucose, and microorganisms. The urinalysis can detect proteinuria and albuminuria, which are the primary measures of structural kidney damage. Although it is easy to perform, the urinalysis is nonspecific: Many diseases can cause abnormal urinalysis values. Serum creatinine is an additional measure for detecting kidney disease. To provide a more definitive diagnosis, diagnostic imaging such as computed tomography, sonography, or magnetic resonance imaging may be necessary. Renal biopsy may be performed to obtain a more specific diagnosis.

The best marker for estimating kidney function is the *glomerular filtration rate (GFR)*, which is the volume of filtrate passing through Bowman capsules per minute. The GFR can be used to predict the onset and progression of kidney failure, and provides an indication of the ability of the kidneys to excrete drugs from the body. A progressive decline in GFR indicates a decline in the number of functioning nephrons. As nephrons "die," however, the remaining healthy nephrons have the ability to compensate by increasing their filtration capacity. Thus, patients with significant kidney damage may exhibit no symptoms until 50% or more of the nephrons have "died" and the GFR falls to less than half its normal value.

Renal failure is classified as acute or chronic, depending on its onset. Acute renal failure requires immediate treatment because retention of nitrogenous waste products in the body such as urea and creatinine can result in death if untreated. The most frequent cause of acute renal failure is renal hypoperfusion, which is lack of sufficient blood flow

through the kidneys. Hypoperfusion can lead to permanent destruction to kidney cells and nephrons. To correct this type of renal failure, the cause of the hypoperfusion must be quickly identified and corrected. Potential causes include heart failure, dysrhythmias, hemorrhage, toxins, and dehydration. Because pharmacotherapy with nephrotoxic drugs can also lead to either acute or chronic renal failure, it is good practice for the nurse to remember common nephrotoxic drugs, which are listed in Table 30.1. Patients receiving these medications must receive frequent kidney function tests.

TABLE 30.1	Nephrotoxic Drugs
Drug or Class	**Indication**
Aminoglycosides	Infection
Amphotericin B	Systemic antifungal infection
Angiotensin-converting enzyme (ACE) inhibitors	HTN, heart failure
Cisplatin/carboplatin	Cancer
Cyclosporine/tacrolimus	Immunosuppression
Foscarnet	Viral infection
Nonsteroidal anti-inflammatory drugs (NSAIDs)	Inflammation
Pentamidine	Infection (*Pneumocystis*)
Radiographic contrast agents	Diagnosis of kidney and vascular disorders

Chronic renal failure occurs over a period of months or years. Over half of the patients with chronic renal failure have a medical history of longstanding hypertension (HTN) or diabetes mellitus. Because of the long, gradual development period and nonspecific symptoms, chronic renal failure may go undiagnosed for many years. By the time the disease is diagnosed, impairment may be irreversible. In end-stage renal disease (ESRD), dialysis and kidney transplantation become treatment alternatives.

Pharmacotherapy of renal failure attempts to cure the cause of the dysfunction. Diuretics are given to increase urine output, and cardiovascular drugs are administered to treat underlying HTN or heart failure. Dietary management is often necessary to prevent worsening of renal impairment. Depending on the stage of the disease, dietary management may include protein restriction and reduction of sodium, potassium, phosphorus, and magnesium intake. For diabetic patients, control of blood glucose through intensive insulin therapy may reduce the risk of renal damage. Selected pharmacologic agents used to prevent and treat kidney failure are summarized in Table 30.2.

The nurse serves a key role in recognizing and responding to renal failure. Once a diagnosis is established, all nephrotoxic medications should be either discontinued or used with extreme caution. Because the kidneys excrete most drugs or their metabolites, medications will require a significant dosage reduction in patients with moderate to severe renal failure. The importance of this cannot be overemphasized: *Administering the "average" dose to a patient in severe renal failure can have fatal consequences.*

DIURETICS

Diuretics are drugs that alter the volume and/or composition of body fluids. They are indicated for the treatment of HTN, heart failure, and disorders characterized by accumulation of edema fluid.

30.4 Mechanisms of Action of Diuretics

A **diuretic** is a drug that increases urine output. The goal of most diuretic therapy is to reverse abnormal fluid retention by the body. Excretion of excess fluid in the body is particularly desirable in the following conditions:

- Hypertension
- Heart failure
- Kidney failure
- Liver failure or cirrhosis
- Pulmonary edema

The most common mechanism by which diuretics act is by blocking sodium (Na^+) reabsorption in the nephron, thus sending more Na^+ to the urine. Chloride ions (Cl^-) follow sodium. Because water molecules also travel with sodium ions, blocking the reabsorption of Na^+ will increase the volume of urination, or diuresis. Diuretics may affect the renal excretion of other ions, including magnesium, potassium, phosphate, calcium, and bicarbonate ions.

Diuretics are classified into three major groups, and one miscellaneous group, based on differences in their chemical structures and mechanism of action. Some drugs, such as furosemide (Lasix), act by preventing the reabsorption of Na^+ in the loop of Henle; thus, they are called *loop* diuretics. Because of the abundance of Na^+ in the filtrate within the loop of Henle, drugs in this class are capable of producing large increases in urine output. Other drugs, such as the *thiazides,* act by blocking Na^+ in the distal tubule. Because most Na^+ has already been reabsorbed from the filtrate by the time it reaches the distal tubule, the thiazides produce less diuresis than furosemide and other loop diuretics. The third major class is named *potassium sparing,* because these diuretics have minimal effect on potassium (K^+) excretion. Miscellaneous agents include the osmotic diuretics and carbonic anhydrase inhibitors. The sites in the nephron at which the various diuretics act are shown in Pharmacotherapy Illustrated 30.1.

TABLE 30.2	Pharmacologic Management of Renal Failure	
Complication	**Pathogenesis**	**Treatment**
Anemia	Kidneys are unable to synthesize enough erythropoietin for red blood cell production	Epoetin alfa (Procrit, Epogen)
Hyperkalemia	Kidneys are unable to adequately excrete potassium	Dietary restriction of potassium; polystyrene sulfate (Kayexalate) with sorbitol
Hyperphosphatemia	Kidneys are unable to adequately excrete phosphate	Dietary restriction of phosphate; phosphate binders such as calcium carbonate (Os-Cal 500, others), calcium acetate (Calphron, PhosLo), lanthanum carbonate (Fosrenol), or sevelamer (Renagel)
Hypervolemia	Kidneys are unable to excrete sufficient sodium and water, leading to water retention	Dietary restriction of sodium; loop diuretics in acute conditions, thiazide diuretics in mild conditions
Hypocalcemia	Hyperphosphatemia leads to loss of calcium	Usually corrected by reversing the hyperphosphatemia, but additional calcium supplements may be necessary
Metabolic acidosis	Kidneys are unable to adequately excrete metabolic acids	Sodium bicarbonate or sodium citrate

PHARMACOTHERAPY ILLUSTRATED

30.1 Mechanisms of Action of Diuretics

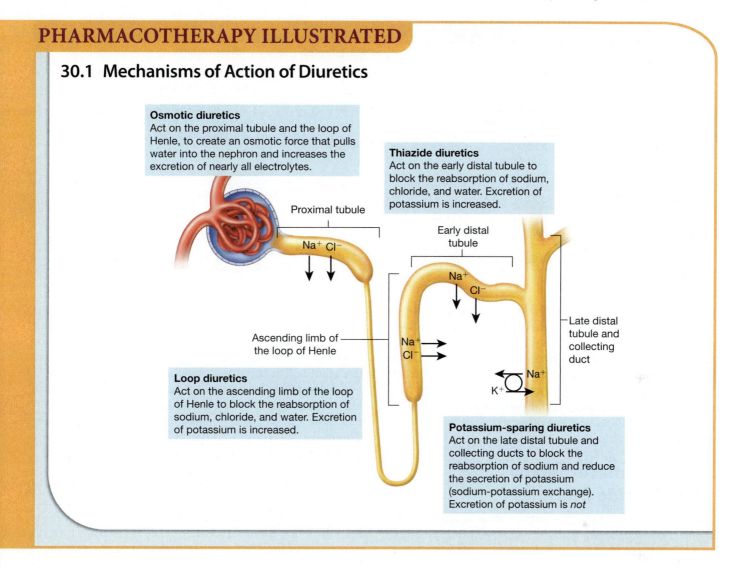

Osmotic diuretics
Act on the proximal tubule and the loop of Henle, to create an osmotic force that pulls water into the nephron and increases the excretion of nearly all electrolytes.

Thiazide diuretics
Act on the early distal tubule to block the reabsorption of sodium, chloride, and water. Excretion of potassium is increased.

Proximal tubule

Early distal tubule

Ascending limb of the loop of Henle

Late distal tubule and collecting duct

Loop diuretics
Act on the ascending limb of the loop of Henle to block the reabsorption of sodium, chloride, and water. Excretion of potassium is increased.

Potassium-sparing diuretics
Act on the late distal tubule and collecting ducts to block the reabsorption of sodium and reduce the secretion of potassium (sodium-potassium exchange). Excretion of potassium is *not*

It is common practice to combine two or more drugs in the pharmacotherapy of HTN and fluid retention disorders. The diuretics are frequently a component of fixed-dose combinations with drugs from other classes. The primary rationales for combination therapy are that the incidence of adverse effects is decreased and the pharmacologic effects (such as diuresis or reduction in blood pressure) may be enhanced. For patient convenience, some of these drugs are combined in single-tablet formulations. Over 25 different fixed-dose combinations are available to treat HTN (Table 23.2∞). Examples of single-tablet diuretic combinations that include diuretics include the following:

- Aldactazide: hydrochlorothiazide and spironolactone
- Dyazide: hydrochlorothiazide and triamterene
- Zestoretic: hydrochlorothiazide and lisinopril

30.5 Pharmacotherapy with Loop Diuretics

The most effective diuretics are the *loop* or *high-ceiling* diuretics. Drugs in this class act by blocking the reabsorption of Na^+ and Cl^- in the loop of Henle. When given IV, they have the ability to cause large amounts of fluid to be excreted by the kidney in a very short time. Loop diuretics are used to reduce the edema associated with heart failure, hepatic cirrhosis, or chronic renal failure. Furosemide and torsemide are also approved for HTN. Doses for the loop diuretics are listed in Table 30.3.

Furosemide is the most frequently prescribed loop diuretic. A prototype feature for furosemide was given in chapter 24∞. Unlike the thiazide diuretics, furosemide is able to increase urine output even when blood flow to the kidneys is diminished, which makes it of particular value in patients with renal failure. Torsemide has a longer half-life than furosemide, which offers the advantage of once-a-day dosing. Bumetanide (Bumex) is 40 times more potent than furosemide but has a shorter duration of action.

The rapid excretion of large amounts of fluid has the potential to produce serious adverse effects, including dehydration and electrolyte imbalances. Signs of dehydration include thirst, dry mouth, weight loss, and headache. Hypotension, dizziness, and fainting can result from the rapid fluid loss. Potassium depletion can be serious and cause dysrhythmias;

TABLE 30.3	**Loop Diuretics**	
Drug	Route and Adult Dose (max dose where indicated)	Adverse Effects
bumetanide (Bumex)	PO; 0.5–2 mg/day, may repeat at 4- to 5-h intervals if needed (max: 10 mg/day) IV/IM; 0.5–1 mg over 1–2 min, repeated every 2–3 hours PRN (max: 10 mg/day)	*Minor hypokalemia, postural hypotension, tinnitus, nausea, diarrhea, dizziness, fatigue* Significant hypokalemia, blood dyscrasias, dehydration, ototoxicity, electrolyte imbalances, circulatory collapse
ethacrynic acid (Edecrin)	PO; 50–100 mg 1–2 times/day, may increase by 25–50 mg PRN (max: 400 mg/day). IV; 0.5–1 mg/kg or 50 mg (max: 100 mg/dose)	
furosemide (Lasix) (see page 330 for the Prototype Drug box ∞)	PO; 20–80 mg in single or divided doses (max: 600 mg/day) IV/IM; 20–40 mg in single or divided doses up to 600 mg/day	
torsemide (Demadex)	PO/IV; 10–20 mg/day (max: 200 mg/day)	

Italics indicate common adverse effects; underlining indicates serious adverse effects.

potassium supplements may be prescribed to prevent hypokalemia. Potassium loss is of particular concern to patients who are also taking digoxin (Lanoxin) because these patients may experience dysrhythmias. Although rare, ototoxicity is possible, and other ototoxic drugs such as the aminoglycoside antibiotics should be avoided during loop diuretic therapy. Because of the potential for serious adverse effects, the loop diuretics are normally reserved for patients with moderate to severe fluid retention, or when other diuretics have failed to achieve therapeutic goals.

30.6 Pharmacotherapy with Thiazide Diuretics

The thiazides constitute the largest, most frequently prescribed class of diuretics. These drugs act on the distal tubule to block Na^+ reabsorption and increase K^+ and water excre-

tion. Their primary use is for the treatment of mild to moderate hypertension; however, they are also indicated for edema due to mild to moderate heart failure, liver failure, and renal failure. They are less effective at producing diuresis than the loop diuretics and they are ineffective in patients with severe renal failure. The thiazide diuretics are listed in Table 30.4.

All the thiazide diuretics are available by the oral route and have equivalent efficacy and safety profiles. They differ, however, in their potency and duration of action. Three drugs—chlorthalidone (Hygroton), indapamide (Lozol), and metolazone (Zaroxolyn)—are not true thiazides, although they are included with this drug class because they have similar mechanisms of action and adverse effects.

The adverse effects of thiazides are similar to those of the loop diuretics, though their frequency is less, and they do not cause ototoxicity. Dehydration and excessive loss of

TABLE 30.4	**Thiazide and Thiazide-Like Diuretics**	
Drug	Route and Adult Dose (max dose where indicated)	Adverse Effects
SHORT ACTING		
℗ chlorothiazide (Diuril)	PO; 250 mg–1 g/day IV; 250 mg–1 g/day in single or two divided doses	*Minor hypokalemia, fatigue* Significant hypokalemia, electrolyte depletion, dehydration, hypotension, hyponatremia, hyperglycemia, coma, blood dyscrasias
hydrochlorothiazide (Microzide) (see page 304 for the Prototype Drug box ∞)	PO; 25–100 mg/day as single or divided dose (max: 50 mg/day for HTN; 100 mg/day for edema)	
INTERMEDIATE ACTING		
bendroflumethiazide and nadolol (Corzide)	PO; 1 tablet/day (40–80 mg nadolol/5 mg bendroflumethiazide)	
metolazone (Zaroxolyn)	PO; 2.5–10 mg once daily (max: 5 mg/day for HTN; 20 mg/day for edema)	
LONG ACTING		
chlorthalidone (Hygroton)	PO; 50–100 mg/day (max: 50 mg/day for HTN; 200 mg/day for edema)	
indapamide (Lozol)	PO; 1.25–2.5 mg once daily (max: 5 mg/day)	
methyclothiazide (Aquatensen, Enduron)	PO; 2.5–10 mg/day (max: 5 mg/day for HTN; 10 mg/day for edema)	

Italics indicate common adverse effects; underlining indicates serious adverse effects.

Na$^+$, K$^+$, or Cl$^-$ may occur with overtreatment. Concurrent therapy with digoxin requires careful monitoring to prevent dysrhythmias due to potassium loss. Potassium supplements may be indicated during thiazide therapy to prevent hypokalemia. Diabetic patients should be aware that thiazide diuretics sometimes raise blood glucose levels.

30.7 Pharmacotherapy with Potassium-Sparing Diuretics

Hypokalemia is one of the most serious adverse effects of the thiazide and loop diuretics. The therapeutic advantage of the potassium-sparing diuretics is that increased diuresis can be obtained without affecting blood K$^+$ levels. Doses for the potassium-sparing diuretics are listed in Table 30.5. There are two distinct mechanisms by which these drugs act.

Normally, sodium and potassium are exchanged in the distal tubule; Na$^+$ is reabsorbed back into the blood, and K$^+$ is secreted into the distal tubule. Triamterene and amiloride block this exchange, causing Na$^+$ to stay in the tubule and ultimately leave through the urine. When Na$^+$ is blocked, the body retains more K$^+$. Because most of the Na$^+$ has already been removed before the filtrate reaches the distal tubule, these potassium-sparing diuretics produce only a mild diuresis. Their primary use is in combination with thiazide or loop diuretics to minimize potassium loss.

The third potassium-sparing diuretic, spironolactone, acts by blocking the actions of the hormone aldosterone. It is sometimes called an *aldosterone antagonist,* and may be used to treat hyperaldosteronism. Blocking aldosterone enhances the *excretion* of Na$^+$ and the *retention* of K$^+$. Like the other two drugs in this diuretic class, spironolactone produces only a weak diuresis. Unlike the other two, spironolactone has been found to significantly reduce mortality in patients with heart failure (chapter 24∞). Eplerenone (Inspra) is a newer aldosterone antagonist that is claimed to exhibit fewer adverse effects than spironolactone.

Patients taking potassium-sparing diuretics should *not* take potassium supplements or be advised to add potassium-rich foods to their diet. Intake of excess potassium when taking these medications may lead to hyperkalemia.

Pr Prototype Drug | Chlorothiazide *(Diuril)*

Therapeutic Class: Antihypertensive, agent for reducing edema   **Pharmacologic Class:** Thiazide diuretic

ACTIONS AND USES

The most common indication for chlorothiazide is mild to moderate HTN. It may be combined with other antihypertensives in the multidrug therapy of severe HTN. It is also prescribed to treat fluid retention due to heart failure, liver disease, and corticosteroid or estrogen therapy. When the drug is given orally, it may take as long as 4 weeks to obtain the *optimum* therapeutic effect.

ADMINISTRATION ALERTS

- Give oral doses in the morning to prevent interrupted sleep due to nocturia.
- Give IV at a rate of 0.5 g over 5 min when administering intermittently.
- When administering IV, take special care to avoid extravasation, because this drug is highly irritating to tissues.
- Pregnancy category C

> #### PHARMACOKINETICS
> **Onset:** 2 h PO; 15 min IV
> **Peak:** 3–6 h PO; 30 min IV
> **Half-life:** 45–120 min
> **Duration:** 6–12 h PO; 2 h IV

ADVERSE EFFECTS

Excess loss of water and electrolytes can occur during chlorothiazide pharmacotherapy. Symptoms include thirst, weakness, lethargy, muscle cramping, hypotension, and tachycardia. Because of the potentially serious consequences of hypokalemia, patients concurrently taking digoxin should be carefully monitored. The intake of potassium-rich foods should be increased, and K$^+$ supplements may be indicated.

Contraindications: This drug is contraindicated in patients with anuria, hypokalemia, severe hepatic or renal impairment, and hypersensitivity to sulfonamides.

INTERACTIONS

Drug–Drug: When given concurrently with other antihypertensives, additive effects on blood pressure will occur. When chlorothiazide is administered with amphotericin B or corticosteroids, the risk for hypokalemic effects increases. Antidiabetic medications such as sulfonylureas and insulin may be less effective when taken with chlorothiazide. Cholestyramine and colestipol decrease the absorption of chlorothiazide. Concurrent administration with digoxin may cause toxicity due to increased potassium and magnesium loss. Alcohol potentiates the hypotensive action of some thiazide diuretics, and caffeine may increase diuresis.

Lab Tests: Chlorothiazide may increase serum amylase values and sulfobromophthalein (SBP) retention. May decrease protein-bound iodine (PBI) values and interfere with urine steroid determination.

Herbal/Food: Absorption of chlorothiazide is increased when taken with food. Licorice and oral aloe, in large amounts, may worsen hypokalemia. When used with chlorothiazide, ginkgo biloba may increase blood pressure. Use with hawthorn may result in additive hypotensive effects.

Treatment of Overdose: Treatment includes fluid and electrolyte infusions and drugs used to raise blood pressure.

Refer to MyNursingKit for a Nursing Process Focus specific to this drug.

TABLE 30.5   Potassium-Sparing Diuretics

Drug	Route and Adult Dose (max dose where indicated)	Adverse Effects
amiloride (Midamor)	PO; 5 mg/day (max: 20 mg/day)	*Minor hyperkalemia, headache, fatigue, gynecomastia*
eplerenone (Inspra)	PO; 25–50 mg once daily (max: 100 mg/day for HTN; 50 mg/day for heart failure)	
(Pr) spironolactone (Aldactone)	PO; 25–100 mg 1–2 times/day (max: 400 mg/day)	<u>Dysrhythmias (from hyperkalemia), dehydration, hyponatremia, agranulocytosis, and other blood dyscrasias</u>
triamterene (Dyrenium)	PO; 50–100 mg bid (max: 300 mg/day)	

Italics indicate common adverse effects; <u>underlining</u> indicates serious adverse effects.

30.8 Miscellaneous Diuretics for Specific Indications

A few miscellaneous diuretics, listed in Table 30.6, have limited and specific indications. Two of these drugs inhibit **carbonic anhydrase,** an enzyme that affects acid–base balance by its ability to form carbonic acid from water and carbon dioxide. Acetazolamide (Diamox) is a carbonic anhydrase inhibitor used to decrease intraocular fluid pressure in patients with open-angle glaucoma (chapter 49∞). In addition to its diuretic effect, acetazolamide has applications as an anticonvulsant and in treating motion sickness and glaucoma. It has also been used to treat acute mountain sickness in patients at very high altitudes. The carbonic anhydrase inhibitors are not commonly used as diuretics, because they produce only a weak diuresis and can contribute to metabolic acidosis.

The osmotic diuretics also have very specific applications. For example, mannitol is used to maintain urine flow in patients with acute renal failure or during prolonged surgery. Since this agent is not reabsorbed in the tubule, it is able to maintain the flow of filtrate even in cases with severe renal hypoperfusion. Mannitol can also be used to lower intraocular pressure in certain types of glaucoma, although it is used for this purpose only when safer agents have failed to produce an effect. It is a highly potent diuretic that is given only by the IV route. Unlike other diuretics that draw excess fluid away from tissue spaces, mannitol can worsen

---

(Pr) Prototype Drug | Spironolactone (Aldactone)

Therapeutic Class: Antihypertensive, drug for reducing edema

Pharmacologic Class: Potassium-sparing diuretic, aldosterone antagonist

ACTIONS AND USES

Spironolactone, the most frequently prescribed potassium-sparing diuretic is primarily used to treat mild HTN, often in combination with other antihypertensives. It may be used to reduce edema associated with kidney or liver disease and it is effective in slowing the progression of heart failure.

Spironolactone acts by inhibiting aldosterone, the hormone secreted by the adrenal cortex that is responsible for increasing the renal reabsorption of Na^+ in exchange for K^+, thus causing water retention. When aldosterone is blocked by spironolactone, Na^+ and water excretion is increased and the body retains more potassium. Spironolactone may also be used to treat primary hyperaldosteronism. It is available in tablet form, and as a fixed-dose combination with hydrochlorothiazide.

ADMINISTRATION ALERTS
- Give with food to increase the absorption of the drug.
- Do not give K^+ supplements.
- Pregnancy category D

PHARMACOKINETICS
Onset: 1–2 days
Peak: 2–3 days
Half-life: 12–24 h
Duration: 2–3 days or more

ADVERSE EFFECTS

Spironolactone does such an efficient job of retaining K^+ that hyperkalemia may develop. The risk of hyperkalemia is increased if the patient takes potassium supplements or is concurrently taking ACE inhibitors. Signs and symptoms of hyperkalemia include muscle weakness, fatigue, and bradycardia. In men, spironolactone can cause gynecomastia, impotence, and diminished libido. Women may experience menstrual irregularities, hirsutism, and breast tenderness. When serum potassium levels are monitored carefully and maintained within normal values, adverse effects from spironolactone are uncommon.

Contraindications: Spironolactone is contraindicated in patients with anuria, significant impairment of renal function, or hyperkalemia. Spironolactone is contraindicated during pregnancy and lactation.

INTERACTIONS

Drug–Drug: When spironolactone is combined with ammonium chloride, acidosis may occur. Aspirin and other salicylates may decrease the diuretic effect of the medication. Concurrent use with digoxin may decrease the effects of digoxin. When taken with potassium supplements, ACE inhibitors, and ARBs, hyperkalemia may result. Concurrent use with antihypertensives will result in an additive hypotensive effect.

Lab Tests: Spironolactone may increase plasma cortisol values, and may interfere with serum glucose determination.

Herbal/Food: Use with hawthorn may result in additive hypotensive effects.

Treatment of Overdose: Treatment is supportive and may include agents to replace fluid and electrolytes lost through diuresis, and drugs to raise blood pressure.

Refer to MyNursingKit for a Nursing Process Focus specific to this drug.

TABLE 30.6	**Miscellaneous Diuretics**	
Drug	Route and Adult Dose (max dose where indicated)	Adverse Effects
CARBONIC ANHYDRASE INHIBITORS		
acetazolamide (Diamox)	PO; 250–375 mg/day	*Electrolyte imbalances, fatigue, nausea, vomiting, dizziness*
methazolamide (Neptazane)	PO; 50–100 mg bid–tid	<u>Dehydration, blood dyscrasias, pancytopenia, flaccid paralysis, hemolytic anemia, aplastic anemia</u>
OSMOTIC DIURETICS		
glycerin (Colace, Osmoglyn)	PO; 1.0–1.8 g/kg, 1–2 h before ocular surgery	*Electrolyte imbalances, fatigue, nausea, vomiting, dizziness*
mannitol (Osmitrol)	IV; 100 g infused over 2–6 h	<u>Hyponatremia, edema, convulsions, tachycardia</u>
urea (Ureaphil)	IV; 1.0–1.5 g/kg over 1–2.5 h	
Italics indicate common adverse effects, <u>underlining</u> indicates serious adverse effects.		

NURSING PROCESS FOCUS   PATIENTS RECEIVING DIURETIC THERAPY

Assessment	Potential Nursing Diagnoses
Baseline assessment prior to administration: ■ Understand the reason the drug has been prescribed in order to assess for therapeutic effects. ■ Obtain a complete health history including cardiovascular disease, diabetes, and pregnancy or breastfeeding. Obtain a drug history including allergies, current prescription and OTC drugs, herbal preparations, use of digoxin, lithium, or antihypertensive drugs, and alcohol use. Be alert to possible drug interactions. ■ Evaluate appropriate laboratory findings such as electrolytes, glucose, CBC, hepatic or renal function studies, uric acid levels, and lipid profiles. ■ Obtain baseline weight, vital signs (especially BP and pulse), breath sounds, and cardiac monitoring (e.g., ECG, cardiac output) if appropriate. Assess for location and character/amount of edema, if present. Assess baseline hearing and balance.	■ Deficient Fluid Volume (related to adverse effects of diuretics) ■ Fatigue ■ Decreased Cardiac Output (related to adverse effects of diuretics) ■ Deficient Knowledge (drug therapy) ■ Risk for Falls, Risk for Injury (related to hypotension, dizziness associated with adverse effects) ■ Risk for Functional Incontinence (related to diuretic use) ■ Risk for Noncompliance (related to adverse effects of drug therapy)
Assessment throughout administration: ■ Assess for desired therapeutic effects (e.g., adequate urine output, lowered BP if given for HTN). ■ Continue periodic monitoring of electrolytes, glucose, CBC, lipid profiles, liver function studies, creatinine, and uric acid levels. ■ Assess for and promptly report adverse effects: hypotension, palpitations, dizziness, musculoskeletal weakness or cramping, nausea, vomiting, abdominal cramping, diarrhea, or headache. Tinnitus or hearing loss, loss of balance or incoordination, severe hypotension accompanied by reflex tachycardiac dysrhythmias, decreased urine output, and weight gain or loss over 1 kg (approximately 2 lb) in a 24-hour period should be reported immediately.	

Planning: Patient Goals and Expected Outcomes

The patient will:

■ Experience therapeutic effects dependent on the reason the drug is being given (e.g., decreased blood pressure).

■ Be free from, or experience minimal, adverse effects.

■ Verbalize an understanding of the drug's use, adverse effects, and required precautions.

■ Demonstrate proper self-administration of the medication (e.g., dose, timing, when to notify provider).

(Continued)

NURSING PROCESS FOCUS   **PATIENTS RECEIVING DIURETIC THERAPY** *(Continued)*

Implementation

Interventions and (Rationales)	Patient and Family Education
Ensuring therapeutic effects:	
▪ Continue frequent assessments as described earlier for therapeutic effects: urine output is increased, blood pressure and pulse are within normal limits or within parameters set by the health care provider. (Diuresis may be moderate to extreme depending on the type of diuretic given. BP should be within normal limits without the presence of reflex tachycardia.) ▪ Daily weights should remain at or close to baseline weight. (An increase in weight over 1 kg per day may indicate excessive fluid gain. A decrease of over 1 kg per day may indicate excessive diuresis and dehydration.)	▪ Teach the patient, family, or caregiver how to monitor pulse and blood pressure. Ensure the proper use and functioning of any home equipment obtained. ▪ Have the patient weigh self daily and record weight along with blood pressure and pulse measurements.
Minimizing adverse effects:	
▪ Continue to monitor vital signs. Take blood pressure lying, sitting, and standing to detect orthostatic hypotension. Be cautious with the elderly who are at increased risk for hypotension. (Diuretics reduce circulating blood volume, resulting in lowered blood pressure. Orthostatic hypotension may increase the risk of falls.)	▪ Teach the patient to rise from lying or sitting to standing slowly to avoid dizziness or falls. ▪ Instruct the patient to stop taking the medication if blood pressure is 90/60 mmHg or below, or parameters set by the health care provider, and promptly notify the provider.
▪ Continue to monitor electrolytes, glucose, CBC, lipid profiles, liver function studies, creatinine, and uric acid levels. (Most diuretics cause loss of Na^+ and K^+ and may increase lipid, glucose, and uric acid levels.)	▪ Instruct the patient on the need to return periodically for lab work and to inform laboratory personnel of diuretic therapy when providing blood or urine samples. ▪ Advise the patient to carry a wallet identification card or wear medical identification jewelry indicating diuretic therapy.
▪ Continue to monitor hearing and balance, reporting persistent tinnitus or vertigo promptly. (Ototoxicity may occur, especially with loop diuretics.)	▪ Have the patient report persistent tinnitus, and balance or coordination problems immediately.
▪ Ensure patient safety, especially in the elderly. Observe for dizziness. Monitor ambulation until effects of drug are known. (Dizziness from orthostatic hypotension may occur.)	▪ Instruct the patient to call for assistance prior to getting out of bed or attempting to walk alone, and to avoid driving or other activities requiring mental alertness or physical coordination until the effects of the drug are known.
▪ Weigh the patient daily and report significant weight gains or losses. Measure intake and output in the hospitalized patient. (Daily weight is an accurate measure of fluid status and takes into account intake, output, and insensible losses. Diuresis is indicated by output significantly greater than intake.)	▪ Have the patient weigh self daily, ideally at the same time of day. Have the patient report a weight loss or gain of more than 1 kg (approximately 2 lb) in a 24-hour period. ▪ Advise the patient to continue to consume enough liquids to remain adequately, but not overly hydrated. Drinking when thirsty, avoiding alcoholic beverages, and ensuring adequate but not excessive salt intake will assist in maintaining normal fluid balance. ▪ Teach the patient that excessive heat conditions contribute to excessive sweating and fluid and electrolyte loss, and extra caution is warranted in these conditions.
▪ Monitor nutritional status and encourage appropriate intake to prevent electrolyte imbalances. (Electrolyte imbalances may occur with diuretics. Most diuretics cause Na^+ and K^+ loss. Potassium-sparing diuretics may result in Na^+ loss but K^+ increase.)	▪ Instruct the patient taking potassium-*wasting* diuretics (e.g., thiazides, thiazide-like, and loop diuretics) to consume foods high in potassium: fresh fruits such as strawberries and bananas; dried fruits such as apricots and prunes; vegetables and legumes such as tomatoes, beets, and dried beans; juices such as orange, grapefruit or prune; and fresh meats. ▪ Instruct the patient taking potassium-*sparing* diuretics to avoid foods high in K^+ such as described earlier, not to use salt substitutes (which often contain K^+ salts), and to consult with a health care provider before taking vitamin and mineral supplements or specialized sports beverages. (Typical OTC sports beverages, e.g., Gatorade and Powerade, may have lesser amounts of potassium but have high carbohydrate amounts, which may lead to increased diuresis, diarrhea, and the potential for dehydration from the hyperosmolarity.)

NURSING PROCESS FOCUS   PATIENTS RECEIVING DIURETIC THERAPY *(Continued)*

Implementation

Interventions and (Rationales)	Patient and Family Education
▪ Observe for signs of hypokalemia or hyperkalemia. Use with caution in patients taking corticosteroids, ACE inhibitors, angiotensin-receptor blockers (ARBs), digoxin, or lithium. Report symptoms to the health care provider promptly. (Thiazide, thiazide-like, and loop diuretics can cause hypokalemia; potassium-sparing diuretics may cause hyperkalemia. Concurrent use with corticosteroids may increase the risk of hypokalemia. Concurrent use with ACE inhibitors or ARBs may increase the risk of hyperkalemia. Concurrent use with digoxin increases the risk of potentially fatal dysrhythmias and concurrent use with lithium may cause toxic levels of the drug.)	▪ Instruct patient to report signs and symptoms of hypokalemia or hyperkalemia immediately to the health care provider. ▪ Teach the patient to follow recommended dietary intake of high- or low-potassium foods as appropriate to the type of diuretic taken to avoid hypokalemia or hyperkalemia.
▪ Observe for signs of hyperglycemia. Use with caution in patients with diabetes. (Thiazide, thiazide-like, and loop diuretics may cause hyperglycemia, especially in diabetics.)	▪ Instruct the patient to report signs and symptoms of diabetes mellitus (e.g., polydipsia, polyphagia) or elevated blood sugar to the health care provider. Diabetic patients may need to monitor their blood glucose levels more frequently until the effects of the diuretic are known.
▪ Observe for symptoms of gout. (Diuretics may cause hyperuricemia, which may result in goutlike conditions including warmth, pain, tenderness, swelling, and redness around joints, arthritis-like symptoms, and limited movement in affected joints.)	▪ Instruct the patient to promptly report signs and symptoms of gout to the health care provider. ▪ Teach the gout-prone patient to increase fluid intake, and avoid shellfish, organ meats (e.g., liver, kidneys), alcohol, and high-fructose beverages.
▪ Observe for sunburning if prolonged sun exposure has occurred. (Many diuretics cause photosensitivity and an increased risk of sunburning.)	▪ Instruct the patient to wear sunscreen and protective clothing if prolonged sun exposure is anticipated.
▪ Observe for signs of infection. (Some diuretics may decrease white blood cell counts. Agranulocytosis is a possible adverse effect of diuretic therapy.)	▪ Instruct the patient to report any flulike symptoms: shortness of breath, fever, sore throat, malaise, joint pain, or profound fatigue.
Patient understanding of drug therapy: ▪ Use opportunities during administration of medications and during assessments to discuss the rationale for drug therapy, desired therapeutic outcomes, most common adverse effects, parameters for when to call the health care provider, and any necessary monitoring or precautions. (Using time during nursing care helps to optimize and reinforce key teaching areas.)	▪ The patient, family, or caregiver should be able to state the reason for the drug; appropriate dose and scheduling; what adverse effects to observe for and when to report; and the anticipated length of medication therapy.
Patient self-administration of drug therapy: ▪ When administering the medication, instruct the patient, family, or caregiver in the proper self-administration of the drug, e.g., early in the day to prevent disruption of sleep from nocturia. (Proper administration increases the effectiveness of the drug.)	▪ The patient, family, or caregiver is able to discuss appropriate dosing and administration needs.

Evaluation of Outcome Criteria

Evaluate the effectiveness of drug therapy by confirming that patient goals and expected outcomes have been met (see "Planning").

See Tables 30.1 through 30.4 for lists of drugs to which these nursing actions apply.

edema and thus must be used with caution in patients with pre-existing heart failure or pulmonary edema. The exception is the brain: Mannitol and urea can reduce intracranial pressure due to cerebral edema. Osmotic diuretics are rarely drugs of first choice due to their potential toxicity.

Chapter REVIEW

KEY CONCEPTS

The numbered key concepts provide a succinct summary of the important points from the corresponding numbered section within the chapter. If any of these points are not clear, refer to the numbered section within the chapter for review.

30.1 The kidneys regulate fluid volume, electrolytes, and acid–base balance.

30.2 The three major processes of urine formation are filtration, reabsorption, and secretion. As filtrate travels through the nephron, its composition changes dramatically as a result of the processes of reabsorption and secretion.

30.3 The dosage levels for most medications must be adjusted in patients with renal failure. Diuretics may be used to maintain urine output while the cause of the renal impairment is treated.

30.4 Diuretics are drugs that increase urine output, usually by blocking sodium reabsorption. The three primary classes are loop, thiazide, and potassium-sparing diuretics.

30.5 The most efficacious diuretics are the loop or high-ceiling agents, which block the reabsorption of sodium in the loop of Henle.

30.6 The thiazides act by blocking sodium reabsorption in the distal tubule of the nephron, and are the most widely prescribed class of diuretics.

30.7 Though less effective than the loop diuretics, potassium-sparing diuretics are used in combination with other agents, and help prevent hypokalemia.

30.8 Several less commonly prescribed classes such as the osmotic diuretics and the carbonic anhydrase inhibitors have specific indications in reducing intraocular fluid pressure (acetazolamide) or reversing severe renal hypoperfusion (mannitol).

NCLEX-RN® REVIEW QUESTIONS

1 Which of the following actions by the nurse is most important when caring for a patient with renal disease?
1. Identify medications that have the potential for nephrotoxicity.
2. Check the specific gravity of the urine daily.
3. Eliminate potassium-rich foods from the diet.
4. Encourage the patient to void every 4 hours.

2 The patient admitted for congestive heart failure (CHF) is receiving digoxin (Lanoxin) and furosemide (Lasix). Which of the following laboratory levels should the nurse carefully monitor?
1. Potassium
2. Creatinine
3. Calcium
4. Sodium

3 Which of the following clinical manifestations may indicate the patient is experiencing hypokalemia?
1. Hypertension
2. Polydipsia
3. Cardiac dysrhythmias
4. Diarrhea

4 Which of the following medications must be used with caution in patients with a history of CHF?
1. Acetazolamide (Diamox)
2. Mannitol (Osmitrol)
3. Bumetanide (Bumex)
4. Ethacrynic acid (Edecrin)

5 The nurse recognizes which of the disorders as a cause of chronic renal failure? (Select all that apply.)
1. Chronic urinary tract infections
2. Diabetes mellitus
3. Congenital malformation
4. Hypertension
5. Hypotension

6 A patient with a history of CHF will be started on the potassium-sparing diuretic, spironolactone (Aldactone). Which of the following drug groups should *not* be used, or used with extreme caution in patients taking potassium-sparing diuretics?
1. NSAIDs
2. Corticosteroids
3. Loop diuretics
4. ACE inhibitors or ARBs

CRITICAL THINKING QUESTIONS

1. A 43-year-old man is diagnosed with hypertension following an annual physical examination. The patient is thin and states that he engages in fairly regular exercise, but he describes his job as highly stressful. He also has a positive family history for hypertension and stroke. The health care provider initiates therapy with losartan (Cozaar). After 2 months, the patient has noted no appreciable difference in blood pressure values. The health care provider switches the patient to combination losartan and hydrochlorothiazide (Hyzaar), which proves to be very effective. Why is the new therapy more effective?

2. A 78-year-old woman is admitted to the intensive care unit with a diagnosis of heart failure. The nurse administers furosemide (Lasix) 40 mg IV push. What assessments should the nurse make to determine the effectiveness of this therapy?

3. A 17-year-old male patient is admitted to the ICU following a car–train collision. The patient sustained a depressed skull fracture and is on a ventilator. Two days after surgery, there are obvious signs of increasing intracranial pressure. The nurse administers 32 g of a 15% solution of mannitol (Osmitrol) per IV over 30 minutes. The patient's mother asks the nurse to explain why her son needs this drug. What explanation should the nurse offer?

See Appendix D for answers and rationales for all activities.

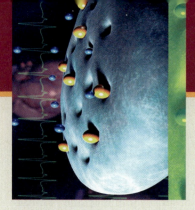

Chapter 31

Drugs for Fluid Balance, Electrolyte, and Acid–Base Disorders

LEARNING OUTCOMES

After reading this chapter, the student should be able to:

1. Describe conditions for which IV fluid therapy may be indicated.
2. Explain how changes in the osmolality or tonicity of a fluid can cause water to move to a different compartment.
3. Compare and contrast the use of colloids and crystalloids in IV therapy.
4. Explain the importance of electrolyte balance in the body.
5. Explain the pharmacotherapy of sodium and potassium imbalances.
6. Discuss common causes of alkalosis and acidosis and the medications used to treat these disorders.
7. Describe the nurse's role in the pharmacologic management of fluid balance, electrolyte, and acid–base disorders.
8. For each of the classes listed in Drugs at a Glance, know representative drugs, and explain the mechanism of drug action, primary actions, and important adverse effects.
9. Use the nursing process to care for patients who are receiving drug therapy for fluid balance, electrolyte, and acid–base disorders.

KEY TERMS

acidosis *page 440*
alkalosis *page 441*
anion *page 436*
buffer *page 440*
cation *page 436*
colloids *page 436*

crystalloids *page 432*
electrolytes *page 436*
extracellular fluid (ECF) compartment *page 431*
hyperkalemia *page 438*
hypernatremia *page 437*
hypokalemia *page 438*

hyponatremia *page 437*
intracellular fluid (ICF) compartment *page 431*
osmolality *page 431*
osmosis *page 431*
pH *page 440*
tonicity *page 431*

The volume and composition of fluids in the body must be maintained within narrow limits. Excess fluid volume can lead to hypertension, congestive heart failure, or peripheral edema, whereas depletion results in dehydration and perhaps shock. Body fluids must also contain specific amounts of essential ions or electrolytes, and be maintained at particular pH values. Accumulation of excess acids or bases can change the pH of body fluids and rapidly result in death if left untreated. This chapter will examine drugs used to reverse fluid balance, electrolyte, or acid–base disorders.

FLUID BALANCE

Body fluids travel between compartments, which are separated by semipermeable membranes. Control of water balance in the various compartments is essential to homeostasis. Fluid imbalances are frequent indications for pharmacotherapy.

31.1 Body Fluid Compartments

The greatest bulk of body fluid consists of water, which serves as the universal solvent in which most nutrients, electrolytes, and minerals are dissolved. Water alone is responsible for about 60% of the total body weight in a middle-age adult. A newborn may contain 80% water, whereas an older adult may contain only 40%.

In a simple model, water in the body can be located in one of two places, or compartments. The **intracellular fluid (ICF) compartment,** which contains water that is *inside* cells, accounts for about two thirds of the total body water. The remaining one third of body fluid resides *outside* cells in the **extracellular fluid (ECF) compartment.** The ECF compartment is further divided into two parts: fluid in the *plasma,* or *intravascular space,* and fluid in the *interstitial spaces* between cells. The re-

lationship between these fluid compartments is illustrated in ➤ Figure 31.1.

A continuous exchange and mixing of fluids occurs between the various compartments, which are separated by membranes. For example, the plasma membranes of cells separate the ICF from the ECF. The capillary membranes separate plasma from the interstitial fluid. Although water travels freely among the compartments, the movement of large molecules and those with electrical charges is governed by processes of diffusion and active transport. Movement of ions and drugs across membranes is a primary concern of pharmacokinetics (chapter 5∞).

31.2 Osmolality, Tonicity, and the Movement of Body Fluids

Osmolality and tonicity are two related terms central to understanding fluid balance in the body. Large changes in the osmolality or tonicity of a body fluid can cause significant shifts in water balance between compartments. The nurse will often administer IV fluids to compensate for these changes.

The **osmolality** of a fluid is determined by the number of dissolved particles, or solutes, in 1 kg (1 L) of water. In most body fluids, three solutes determine the osmolality: sodium, glucose, and urea. Sodium is the greatest contributor to osmolality due to its abundance in most body fluids. The normal osmolality of body fluids ranges from 275 to 295 milliosmols per kilogram (mOsm/kg).

The term **tonicity** is sometimes used interchangeably with osmolality, although they are somewhat different. Tonicity is the ability of a solution to cause a change in water movement across a membrane due to osmotic forces. Whereas osmolality is a laboratory value that can be precisely measured, tonicity is a general term used to describe the *relative* concentration of IV fluids. The tonicity of the plasma is used as the reference point when administering IV solutions: Normal plasma is considered isotonic. Solutions that are isotonic have the same concentration of solutes (same osmolality) as plasma. *Hypertonic* solutions contain a greater concentration of solutes than plasma, whereas *hypotonic* solutions have a lesser concentration of solutes than plasma.

Through **osmosis,** water moves from areas of low solute concentration (low osmolality), to areas of high solute concentration (high osmolality). If a *hypertonic* (hyperosmolar) IV solution is administered, the plasma gains more solutes than the interstitial fluid. Water will move, by osmosis, from the interstitial fluid compartment to the plasma compartment. This type of fluid shift removes water from cells and can result in dehydration. Water will move in the opposite direction, from plasma to interstitial fluid, if a *hypotonic* solution is administered. This type of fluid shift could result in hypotension due to movement of water out of the vascular system. Isotonic solutions will produce no net fluid shift. These movements are illustrated in ➤ Figure 31.2.

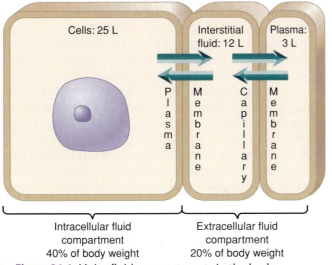

Cells: 25 L | Interstitial fluid: 12 L | Plasma: 3 L

Plasma Membrane Capillary Membrane

Intracellular fluid compartment
40% of body weight

Extracellular fluid compartment
20% of body weight

➤ **Figure 31.1** Major fluid compartments in the body

Type of infusion	Movement of Fluid ▲ = solute	Result

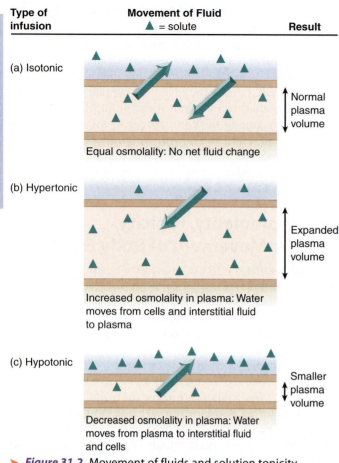

(a) Isotonic — Normal plasma volume

Equal osmolality: No net fluid change

(b) Hypertonic — Expanded plasma volume

Increased osmolality in plasma: Water moves from cells and interstitial fluid to plasma

(c) Hypotonic — Smaller plasma volume

Decreased osmolality in plasma: Water moves from plasma to interstitial fluid and cells

➤ **Figure 31.2** Movement of fluids and solution tonicity

31.3 Regulation of Fluid Intake and Output

The average adult has a water *intake* of approximately 2500 mL/day, most of which comes from food and beverages. Water *output* is achieved through the kidneys, lungs, skin, feces, and sweat. To maintain water balance, water intake must equal water output. Net gains or losses of water can be estimated by changes in total body weight.

The most important physiologic regulator of fluid intake is the thirst mechanism. The sensation of thirst occurs when osmoreceptors in the hypothalamus sense that the ECF has become hypertonic. Saliva secretion diminishes and the mouth dries, driving the individual to drink liquids. As the ingested water is absorbed, the osmolality of the ECF falls and the thirst center in the hypothalamus is no longer stimulated.

The kidneys are the primary regulators of fluid output. Through activation of the renin–angiotensin–aldosterone system (chapter 23∞), the hormone aldosterone is secreted by the adrenal cortex. Aldosterone causes the kidneys to retain additional sodium and water in the body, thus increasing the osmolality of the ECF. A second hormone, antidiuretic hormone (ADH), is released during periods of high plasma osmolality. ADH acts directly on the distal tubules of the kidney to increase water reabsorption. This increased water in the intravascular space dilutes the plasma, thus lowering its osmolality.

Failure to maintain proper balance between intake and output can result in fluid balance disorders that are indications for pharmacologic intervention. Fluid *deficit* disorders can cause dehydration or shock, which are treated by administering oral or intravenous (IV) fluids. Fluid *excess* disorders are treated with diuretics (chapter 30∞). In the treatment of fluid imbalances, the ultimate goal is to diagnose and correct the *cause* of the disorder while administering supporting fluids and medications to stabilize the patient.

FLUID REPLACEMENT AGENTS

Net loss of fluids from the body can result in dehydration and shock. IV fluid therapy is used to maintain blood volume and support blood pressure.

31.4 Intravenous Therapy with Crystalloids and Colloids

When fluid output exceeds fluid intake, volume deficits may result. Shock, dehydration, or electrolyte loss may occur; large deficits are fatal, unless treated. The following are some common reasons for fluid depletion:

- Loss of GI fluids due to vomiting, diarrhea, chronic laxative use, or GI suctioning
- Excessive sweating during hot weather, athletic activity, or prolonged fever
- Severe burns
- Hemorrhage
- Excessive diuresis due to diuretic therapy or uncontrolled diabetic ketoacidosis

The immediate goal in treating a volume deficit disorder is to replace the depleted fluid. In nonacute circumstances, this may be achieved by drinking more liquids or by administering fluids via a feeding tube. In acute situations, IV fluid therapy is indicated. Regardless of the route, careful attention must be paid to restoring normal levels of blood elements and electrolytes, as well as fluid volume.

Intravenous replacement fluids are of two basic types: crystalloids and colloids. **Crystalloids** are IV solutions that contain electrolytes and other agents that closely mimic the body's extracellular fluid. They are used to replace depleted fluids, and to promote urine output. Crystalloid solutions are capable of quickly diffusing across membranes, leaving the plasma and entering the interstitial fluid and ICF. It is estimated that two thirds of infused crystalloids will distribute in the interstitial space. Isotonic, hypotonic, and hypertonic solutions are available. Sodium is the most common crystalloid added to solutions. Some crystalloids contain dextrose, a form of glucose, commonly in concentrations of 2.5%, 5%, or 10%. Dextrose is added to provide nutritional value: 1 L of 5% dextrose supplies 170 calories. In addition, water is formed during the metabolism of dextrose, enhancing the rehydration of the patient. When dextrose is infused, it is metabolized, and the solution becomes hypotonic. Selected crystalloids are listed in Table 31.1.

Infusion of crystalloids will increase total fluid volume in the body, but the *compartment* that is most expanded depends on the solute (sodium) concentration of the fluid administered. *Isotonic* crystalloids can expand the circulating *intravascular* fluid volume without causing major fluid shifts between compartments. Isotonic crystalloids such as normal saline are often used to treat fluid loss due to vomiting, diarrhea, or surgical procedures, especially when the blood pressure is low. Because isotonic crystalloids can rapidly expand circulating blood volume, care must be taken not to create fluid overload in the patient.

Infusion of *hypertonic* crystalloids expands plasma volume by drawing water away from the cells and tissues. These agents may be used to relieve cellular edema, especially cerebral edema. When patients are dehydrated and have hypertonic plasma, a solution that is initially hypertonic, may be infused, such as D5 0.45% NS that matches the tonicity of the plasma. This allows the fluid to enter the vascular compartment without causing a net fluid loss or gain in the cells. As the dextrose is subsequently metabolized, the solution

TABLE 31.1 Selected Crystalloid IV Solutions

Drug	Tonicity
Normal saline (0.9% NaCl)	Isotonic
Hypertonic saline (3% NaCl)	Hypertonic
Hypotonic saline (0.45% NaCl)	Hypotonic
Lactated Ringer's	Isotonic
Plasma-Lyte 148	Isotonic
Plasma-Lyte 56	Hypotonic
DEXTROSE SOLUTIONS	
5% dextrose in water (D5W)	Isotonic*
5% dextrose in normal saline	Hypertonic
5% dextrose in 0.2% saline	Isotonic
5% dextrose in lactated Ringer's	Hypertonic
5% dextrose in plasma-Lyte 56	Hypertonic

*Because dextrose is metabolized quickly, the solution is sometimes considered hypotonic.

Pr Prototype Drug | Dextran 40 *(Gentran 40, others)*

Therapeutic Class: Plasma volume expander   **Pharmacologic Class:** Colloid

ACTIONS AND USES

Dextran 40 is a polysaccharide that is too large to pass through capillary walls. It is similar to dextran 70, except dextran 40 has a lower molecular weight. Dextran 40 acts by raising the osmotic pressure of the blood, thereby causing fluid to move from the interstitial spaces of the tissues to the intravascular space (blood). Given as an IV infusion, it has the capability of expanding plasma volume within minutes after administration. Cardiovascular responses include increased blood pressure, increased cardiac output, and improved venous return to the heart. Dextran 40 is excreted rapidly by the kidneys. Indications include fluid replacement for patients experiencing hypovolemic shock due to hemorrhage, surgery, or severe burns. When given for acute shock, it is infused as rapidly as possible until blood volume is restored.

Dextran 40 also reduces platelet adhesiveness and improves blood flow, through its ability to reduce blood viscosity. These properties have led to its use in preventing deep vein thromboses and pulmonary emboli.

ADMINISTRATION ALERTS

- Emergency administration may be given 1.2 to 2.4 g/min.
- Nonemergency administration should be infused no faster than 240 mg/min.
- Discard unused portions once opened because dextran contains no preservatives.
- Pregnancy category C

PHARMACOKINETICS

Onset: Several minutes

Peak: Unknown

Half-life: Unknown

Duration: 12–24 h

ADVERSE EFFECTS

Vital signs should be monitored continuously during dextran 40 infusions to prevent hypertension caused by plasma volume expansion. Signs of fluid overload include tachycardia, peripheral edema, distended neck veins, dyspnea, or cough. A small percentage of patients are allergic to dextran 40, with urticaria being the most common sign.

Contraindications: Dextran 40 is contraindicated in patients with renal failure or severe dehydration. Other contraindications include severe CHF and hypervolemic disorders.

INTERACTIONS

Drug–Drug: There are no clinically significant interactions.

Lab Tests: Dextran 40 may prolong bleeding time.

Herbal/Food: Unknown

Treatment of Overdose: For patients with normal renal function, discontinuation of the infusion will result in reduction of adverse effects. Patients with renal impairment may benefit from the administration of an osmotic diuretic.

Refer to MyNursingKit for a Nursing Process Focus specific to this drug.

NURSING PROCESS FOCUS   PATIENTS RECEIVING IV FLUID AND ELECTROLYTE REPLACEMENT THERAPY

Assessment	Potential Nursing Diagnoses
Baseline assessment prior to administration: • Understand the reason the drug has been prescribed in order to assess for therapeutic effects (e.g., replacement therapy, treatment of shock). • Obtain a complete health history including cardiovascular (including HTN, MI), neurologic (including CVA or head injury), burns, endocrine, and hepatic or renal disease. Obtain a drug history including allergies, current prescription and OTC drugs, and herbal preparations. Be alert to possible drug interactions. • Obtain baseline weight and vital signs, level of consciousness (LOC), breath sounds, and urinary output as appropriate. • Evaluate appropriate laboratory findings (e.g., electrolytes, CBC, urine specific gravity and urinalysis, BUN and creatinine, total protein and albumin levels, aPTT, aPT or INR, renal and liver function studies).	• Deficient Fluid Volume • Decreased Cardiac Output • Fatigue • Activity Intolerance • Deficient Knowledge (drug therapy) • Risk for Falls, Risk for Injury (related to hypotension, dizziness associated with adverse effects) • Risk for Excessive Fluid Volume (related to drug therapy) • Risk for Ineffective Health Maintenance (regarding drug effects and dietary needs)
Assessment throughout administration: • Assess for desired therapeutic effects (e.g., electrolyte values return to within normal range, adequate urine output). • Continue monitoring of vital signs, urinary output, and LOC as appropriate. • Assess for and promptly report adverse effects: tachycardia, HTN, dysrhythmias, decreasing LOC, increasing dyspnea, lung congestion, pink-tinged frothy sputum, decreased urinary output, muscle weakness or cramping, or allergic reactions.	

Planning: Patient Goals and Expected Outcomes

The patient will:
• Experience therapeutic effects dependent on the reason the drug is being given (e.g., increased urinary output and relief of dehydration, electrolyte values within normal limits).
• Be free from, or experience minimal, adverse effects.
• Verbalize an understanding of the drug's use, adverse effects, and required precautions.
• Demonstrate proper self-administration of the medication (e.g., dose, timing, when to notify provider).

Implementation

Interventions and (Rationales)	Patient and Family Education
Ensuring therapeutic effects: • Continue frequent assessments as described earlier for therapeutic effects. Assist the patient with obtaining fluids and with eating as needed. (Urinary output is within normal limits. Electrolyte balance is restored. The elderly, infants, and patients who cannot access fluids or eat by themselves, e.g., post-CVA, are at increased risk for fluid and electrolyte imbalance.)	• Teach the patient to continue to consume enough liquids to remain adequately, but not overly hydrated. Drinking when thirsty, avoiding alcoholic beverages, maintaining a healthy diet, and ensuring adequate but not excessive salt intake will assist in maintaining normal fluid and electrolyte balance. • Have the patient weigh self daily and record weight along with blood pressure and pulse measurements as appropriate. • Teach the patient, family, or caregiver how to monitor pulse and blood pressure if needed. Ensure proper use and functioning of any home equipment obtained.
Minimizing adverse effects: • Monitor for signs of fluid volume excess or deficit, e.g., increasing BP (excess), decreasing BP (deficit), tachycardia, changes in quality of pulse (bounding or thready). Monitor for signs of potential electrolyte imbalance including nausea, vomiting, GI cramping, diarrhea, muscle weakness, cramping or twitching, paresthesias, and irritability. Confusion, decreasing LOC, increasing hypotension or HTN especially if associated with tachycardia, decreased urine output, and seizures are reported immediately. (Many fluid and electrolyte imbalances have similar symptoms. When assessing the patient for adverse effects, consider past history, drug history, and current condition and medications to correlate symptoms to possible causes.)	• Instruct the patient to report changes in muscle strength or function; numbness and tingling in lips, fingers, arms or legs; palpitations; dizziness; nausea or vomiting; GI cramping; or decreased urination.

Implementation

Interventions and (Rationales)	Patient and Family Education
■ Frequently monitor CBC, electrolytes, aPTT, and aPT or INR levels. (Crystalloid solutions may cause electrolyte imbalances. Colloid solutions may reduce normal blood coagulation. Frequent monitoring of electrolyte levels while on replacement therapy may be needed to ensure therapeutic effects.)	■ Instruct the patient on the need to return periodically for lab work
■ Continue to monitor vital signs. Take blood pressure lying, sitting, and standing to detect orthostatic hypotension. Be cautious with the elderly who are at increased risk for hypotension. (Dehydration and electrolyte imbalances may cause dizziness and hypotension. Orthostatic hypotension may increase the risk of injury.)	■ Teach the patient to rise from lying or sitting to standing slowly to avoid dizziness or falls.
■ Ensure patient safety, especially in the elderly. Observe for dizziness and monitor or assist with ambulation as needed. (Dizziness from electrolyte imbalances or orthostatic hypotension may occur.)	■ Instruct the patient to call for assistance prior to getting out of bed or attempting to walk alone, and to avoid driving or other activities requiring mental alertness or physical coordination if needed.
■ Weigh the patient daily and report a weight gain or loss of 1 kg (approximately 2 lb) or more in a 24-hour period. (Daily weight is an accurate measure of fluid status and takes into account intake, output, and insensible losses. Weight gain or edema may signal excessive fluid volume or electrolyte imbalances.)	■ Have the patient weigh self daily, ideally at the same time of day, and record weight along with blood pressure and pulse measurements. Have the patient report significant weight loss or gain. ■ Teach the patient that excessive heat conditions contribute to excessive sweating and fluid and electrolyte loss, and extra caution is warranted in these conditions.
■ Closely monitor for signs and symptoms of allergy if colloids are used. (Colloids may cause allergic and anaphylactic reactions.)	■ Instruct the patient to immediately report dyspnea, itching, feelings of throat tightness, palpitations, chest pain or tightening, or headache.
■ Closely monitor IV sites closely when infusing potassium or ammonium. Double-check doses with another nurse before giving. (Potassium and ammonium are irritating to the vessel and phlebitis may result. Potassium is a "high-alert" medication and double-checking doses before administering prevents medication errors.)	■ Instruct the patient to report any irritation, pain, redness, or swelling at the IV site or in the arm where the drug is infusing.
■ Monitor nutritional status and encourage appropriate fluid intake to prevent electrolyte imbalances. (Electrolyte imbalances may occur due to inadequate nutrition or fluid intake as well as from drug therapy, e.g., diuretics.)	■ Teach the patient to consume enough liquids to remain adequately, but not overly, hydrated. ■ Instruct the patient with hypokalemia to consume foods high in K^+: fresh fruits such as strawberries and bananas; dried fruits such as apricots and prunes; vegetables and legumes such as tomatoes, beets, and dried beans; juices such as orange, grapefruit or prune; and fresh meats. Instruct the patient with hyperkalemia to avoid the foods mentioned earlier (for hypokalemia) as well as salt substitutes (which often contain potassium salts), and to consult with a health care provider before taking vitamin and mineral supplements or specialized sports beverages. (Typical OTC sports beverages, e.g., Gatorade and Powerade, may have lesser amounts of potassium but have high carbohydrate amounts, which may lead to increased diuresis, diarrhea, and the potential for dehydration from the hyperosmolarity.)
Patient understanding of drug therapy: ■ Use opportunities during administration of medications and during assessments to discuss rationale for drug therapy, desired therapeutic outcomes, and any necessary monitoring or precautions. (Using time during nursing care helps to optimize and reinforce supportive drug treatment and care.)	■ The patient, family, or caregiver should be able to state the reason for the drug; appropriate dose and scheduling; what adverse effects to observe for and when to report; and the anticipated length of medication therapy.
Patient self-administration of drug therapy: ■ When administering the medication, instruct the patient, family, or caregiver in proper self-administration of drug, e.g., early in the day to prevent disruption of sleep from nocturia. (Proper administration will increase the effectiveness of the drug.)	■ The patient and family or caregiver are able to discuss appropriate dosing and administration needs.

Evaluation of Outcome Criteria

Evaluate the effectiveness of drug therapy by confirming that patient goals and expected outcomes have been met (see "Planning").

See Tables 31.1, 31.2, and 31.4 for a list of the drugs to which these nursing actions apply.

becomes hypotonic. This hypotonic solution then causes water to shift into the intracellular space, relieving the dehydration within the cells. A solution of 3% normal saline is hypertonic and usually reserved for treating severe hyponatremia (Na < 115 mEq/L). Excessive use is avoided because it can lead to expansion of the intravascular (plasma) compartment and a risk of hypertension.

Hypotonic crystalloids will cause water to move out of the plasma to the tissues and cells in the *intracellular* compartment; thus, these solutions are not considered efficient plasma volume expanders. Hypotonic crystalloids are indicated for patients with hypernatremia and cellular dehydration. Care must be taken not to cause depletion of the intravascular compartment (hypotension) or too much expansion of the intracellular compartment (peripheral edema). Patients who are dehydrated with *low* blood pressure should be given normal saline; patients who are dehydrated with *normal* blood pressure should be given a hypotonic solution.

Colloids are proteins, starches, or other large molecules that remain in the blood for a long time because they are too large to easily cross the capillary membranes. While circulating, they have the same effect as hypertonic solutions, drawing water molecules from the cells and tissues into the plasma through their ability to increase plasma osmolality and osmotic pressure. Sometimes called *plasma volume expanders,* these solutions are particularly important in treating hypovolemic shock due to burns, hemorrhage, or surgery.

The most commonly used colloid is normal serum albumin, which is featured as a prototype drug for shock in chapter 29∞. Several colloid products contain dextran, a synthetic polysaccharide. Dextran infusions can double the plasma volume within a few minutes, though its effects last only about 12 hours. Plasma protein fraction is a natural volume expander that contains 83% albumin and 17% plasma globulins. Plasma protein fraction and albumin are also indicated in patients with hypoproteinemia. Hetastarch is a synthetic colloid with properties similar to those of 5% albumin, but with an extended duration of action. Selected colloid solutions are listed in Table 31.2.

ELECTROLYTES

Electrolytes are small charged molecules essential to homeostasis. Too little or too much of an electrolyte can result in serious complications and must be quickly corrected. Table 31.3 describes electrolytes that are important to human physiology.

31.5 Physiologic Role of Electrolytes

Minerals are inorganic substances needed in very small amounts to maintain homeostasis (chapter 42∞). Minerals are held together by ionic bonds and dissociate or ionize when placed in water. The resulting ions have positive or negative charges and are able to conduct electricity, hence the name **electrolyte.** Positively charged electrolytes are called **cations**; those with a negative charge are **anions.** Electrolyte levels are measured in units of milliequivalents per liter (mEq/L).

Electrolytes are essential to many body functions, including nerve conduction, membrane permeability, muscle contraction, water balance, and bone growth and remodeling. Levels of electrolytes in body fluids are maintained within very narrow ranges, primarily by the kidneys and GI tract. As electrolytes are lost due to normal excretory functions, they must be replaced by adequate intake; otherwise, electrolyte imbalances will result. Although imbalances can occur with any ion, Na^+, K^+, and Ca^{2+} are of greatest importance. The major body electrolyte imbalance states and their treatments are listed in Table 31.4. Calcium, phosphorous, and magnesium imbalances are discussed in chapter 42∞; the role of calcium in bone homeostasis is presented in chapter 47∞.

An electrolyte imbalance is a sign of an underlying medical condition that needs attention. Imbalances are associated with a large number of disorders, with renal impairment being the most common cause. In some cases, drug therapy itself can cause the electrolyte imbalance. For example, aggressive therapy with loop diuretics such as furosemide (Lasix) can rapidly deplete the body of sodium and potassium. The therapeutic goal is to quickly correct the electrolyte imbalance while the underlying condition is being diagnosed and treated. Treatments for electrolyte imbalances depend upon the severity of the condition and range from simple adjustments in dietary intake to rapid electrolyte infusions. Serum electrolyte levels must be carefully monitored during therapy to prevent imbalances in the *opposite* direction; levels can change rapidly from hypo-concentrations to hyper-concentrations.

TABLE 31.2	Selected Colloid IV Solutions (Plasma Volume Expanders)
Drug	**Tonicity**
5% albumin	Isotonic
Dextran 40 in normal saline	Isotonic
Dextran 40 in D5W	Isotonic
Dextran 70 in normal saline	Isotonic
Hetastarch 6% in normal saline	Isotonic
Plasma protein fraction	Isotonic

TABLE 31.3	Electrolytes Important to Human Physiology		
Compound	**Formula**	**Cation**	**Anion**
Calcium chloride	$CaCl_2$	Ca^{2+}	$2Cl^-$
Disodium phosphate	Na_2HPO_4	$2Na^+$	HPO_4^{2-}
Potassium chloride	KCl	K^+	Cl^-
Sodium bicarbonate	$NaHCO_3$	Na^+	HCO_3^-
Sodium chloride	NaCl	Na^+	Cl^-
Sodium sulfate	Na_2SO_4	$2Na^+$	SO_4^{2-}

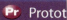

TABLE 31.4	**Electrolyte Imbalances**		
Ion	Condition	Abnormal Serum Value (mEq/L)	Supportive Treatment*
Calcium	Hypercalcemia	>11	Hypotonic fluid or calcitonin
	Hypocalcemia	<4	Calcium supplements or vitamin D
Chloride	Hyperchloremia	>112	Hypotonic fluid
	Hypochloremia	<95	Hypertonic salt solution
Magnesium	Hypermagnesemia	>4	Hypotonic fluid
	Hypomagnesemia	<0.8	Magnesium supplements
Phosphate	Hyperphosphatemia	>6	Dietary phosphate restriction
	Hypophosphatemia	<1	Phosphate supplements
Potassium	Hyperkalemia	>5	Hypotonic fluid, buffers, or dietary potassium restriction
	Hypokalemia	<3.5	Potassium supplements
Sodium	Hypernatremia	>145	Hypotonic fluid or dietary sodium restriction
	Hyponatremia	<135	Hypertonic salt solution or sodium supplement

*For all electrolyte imbalances, the primary therapeutic goal is to identify and correct the *cause* of the imbalance.

31.6 Pharmacotherapy of Sodium Imbalances

Sodium is the major electrolyte in extracellular fluid. Because of sodium's central roles in neuromuscular physiology, acid–base balance, and overall fluid distribution, sodium imbalances can have serious consequences. Although definite sodium monitors or sensors have yet to be discovered in the body, the regulation of sodium balance is well understood.

Sodium balance and water balance are intimately connected. As Na^+ levels increase in a body fluid, solute particles accumulate, and the osmolality increases. Water will move toward this area of relatively high osmolality. In simplest terms, water travels toward or with Na^+. The physiologic consequences of this relationship cannot be overstated: As the Na^+ and water content of plasma increases, so does blood volume and blood pressure. Thus, Na^+ movement provides an important link between water retention, blood volume, and blood pressure.

In healthy individuals, sodium *intake* is equal to sodium *output,* which is regulated by the kidneys. High levels of aldosterone secreted by the adrenal cortex promote Na^+ and water retention by the kidneys, as well as K^+ excretion. Inhibition of aldosterone promotes sodium and water excretion. When a patient ingests high amounts of sodium, aldosterone secretion decreases, thus allowing excess Na^+ enter the urine. This relationship is illustrated in ➤ Figure 31.3.

Sodium excess, or **hypernatremia,** occurs when the serum sodium level rises above 145 mEq/L. The most common cause of hypernatremia is decreased Na^+ excretion, due to kidney pathology. Hypernatremia may also be caused by excessive intake of sodium, either through dietary consumption or by overtreatment with IV fluids containing sodium chloride or sodium bicarbonate. Another cause of hypernatremia is high net water losses, such as occur from inadequate water intake, watery diarrhea, fever, or burns. High doses of glucocorticoids or estrogens also promote Na^+ retention.

A high serum sodium level increases the osmolality of the plasma, drawing fluid from interstitial spaces and cells, thus causing cellular dehydration. Manifestations of hypernatremia include thirst, fatigue, weakness, muscle twitching, convulsions, altered mental status, and a decreased level of consciousness. For minor hypernatremia, a low-salt diet may be effective in returning serum sodium to normal levels. In patients with acute hypernatremia, however, the treatment goal is to rapidly return the osmolality of the plasma to normal. If the patient is hypovolemic, infusing hypotonic fluids such as 5% dextrose or 0.45% NaCl will increase plasma volume while at the same time reducing plasma osmolality. If the patient is hypervolemic, diuretics may be used to remove Na^+ and fluid from the body.

Sodium deficiency, or **hyponatremia,** is a serum sodium level less than 135 mEq/L. Hyponatremia may occur through *excessive dilution* of the plasma, caused by excessive ADH secretion or administration of hypotonic IV solutions. Hyponatremia may also result from *increased sodium loss* due to disorders of the skin, GI tract, or kidneys. Significant loss of sodium by the skin may occur in burn patients, and in those experiencing excessive sweating or prolonged fever. Gastrointestinal sodium losses may occur from vomiting, diarrhea, or GI suctioning, and renal Na^+ loss may occur with diuretic use and in certain advanced kidney disorders. Early symptoms of hyponatremia include nausea, vomiting, anorexia, and abdominal cramping. Later signs include altered neurologicl function such as confusion, lethargy, convulsions, coma, and muscle twitching or tremors. Hyponatremia caused by excessive dilution is treated with loop diuretics (chapter 30). These drugs will cause an isotonic diuresis, thus removing the fluid overload that caused the hyponatremia. Hyponatremia caused by Na^+ loss may be treated with oral or parenteral sodium chloride, or with IV fluids containing salt, such as normal saline or lactated Ringer's.

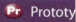

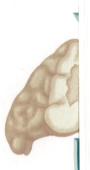

TABLE 32.2	Selected Vaccines and Their Schedules
Vaccine	**Schedule and Age**
diphtheria, tetanus, and pertussis (Daptacel, DPaT, Infanrix, Tripedia)	IM; 0.5 mL at ages 2 mo, 4 mo, 6 mo, and 18 mo
haemophilus influenza type B conjugate (ActHIB, HibTITER, PedvaxHIB) Comvax is a combination of haemophilus and hepatitis B vaccines.	IM; 0.5 mL at ages 2 mo, 4 mo, 6 mo, and 15 mo; children aged 12–14 mo who have not been vaccinated receive a single dose
hepatitis A (Havrix, VAQTA)	Children: IM; 0.5 mL at age 12 mo, followed by a booster 6 mo to 12 mo later Adults: 1 mL followed by a booster 6 mo to 12 mo later
hepatitis B (Engerix-B, Recombivax HB) Twinrix is a combination of hepatitis A and hepatitis B vaccines.	Children: 2.5–5 mcg at birth; then 0.5 mL at 1–4 mo and 6–18 mo Adults: 0.5 mL in three doses, with the second dose 30 days after the first, and the final dose 6 mo after the first
human papillomavirus (Gardasil)	Children (females): IM; 0.5 mL with first dose at age 11 or 12 years Administer second dose 2 months after the first dose and the third dose 6 months after the first dose (at least 24 weeks after the first dose)
influenza vaccine (Afluria, Fluarix, FluLaval, Fluvirin, Fluzone)	Children: IM two doses 1 mo apart; then annual dose Adults: IM single annual dose or intranasal (FluMist)
measles, mumps, and rubella (MMR II) Proquad is a combination of MMR and varicella vaccines.	Subcutaneous; 0.5 mL single dose at age 15 mo to puberty First dose at age 12–15 mo Second dose at age 4–6 yr
pneumococcal, polyvalent (Pneumovax 23), or 7-valent (Prevnar)	Adults (Pneumovax 23 or Pnu-Immune 23): subcutaneous or IM; 0.5 mL as a single dose Children (Prevnar): IM; four doses at ages 2 mo, 4 mo, 6 mo, and 12–15 mo
poliovirus, inactivated (IPOL)	Children: subcutaneous; 0.5 mL at ages 4–8 wk, 2–4 mo, and 6–12 mo
rotavirus (Rotarix, RotaTeq)	Children: Oral; three 2 mL doses at 2 mo, 4 mo, and 6 mo (Rotarix does not require a dose at 6 mo)
varicella (Varivax)	Patients 12 mo and older: subcutaneous; 0.5 mL, two doses given 4–8 wk apart Younger than 12 mo: 0.5 mL as a single dose

➤ *Figure 31.3*

31.7 Pha
of Potass

Potassium, the
important role
maintaining a
carefully balan
nal excretion. I
by the actions
nal excretion
every sodium
secreted into th
be maintained
pokalemia are
ous neuromus

only a few such medications are available. These agents include interferons and interleukins produced by recombinant DNA technology. Immunostimulants are listed in Table 32.3.

32.5 Pharmacotherapy with Biologic Response Modifiers

When challenged by specific antigens, certain cells in the immune system secrete cytokines that help defend against the invading organisms. These natural cytokines have been identified, and through recombinant DNA technology, sufficient quantities have been produced to treat certain disorders. Sometimes called **biologic response modifiers,** some of these agents boost specific functions of the immune system. Biologic response modifiers that enhance hematopoiesis, such as colony-stimulating factors, epoetin alfa, and oprelvekin (Neumega), were presented in chapter 28.

Interferons (IFNs) are cytokines secreted by lymphocytes and macrophages that have been infected with a virus. After secretion, interferons attach to uninfected cells and signal them to secrete antiviral proteins. Part of the nonspecific defense system, IFNs slow the spread of viral infections and enhance the activity of existing leukocytes. These drugs have antiviral, anticancer, and anti-inflammatory properties. The actions of interferons include modulation of immune functions such as increasing phagocytosis and enhancing the cytotoxic activity of T cells.

The class of IFNs having the greatest clinical utility is the alpha interferons, for which six different formulations are available. These include IFN alfa-2b, IFN alfa-n3, IFN alfa-n1, pegIFN alfa-2a, and pegIFN alfa-2b (note that when used as medications, the spelling is changed from alpha to alfa). In the two peg formulations the inert molecule polyethylene glycol is attached to the interferon. This addition extends the half-life of the drug to allow for once-weekly dosing. Indications for IFN alfa therapy include hairy cell leukemia, AIDS-related Kaposi's sarcoma, non-Hodgkin's lymphoma, and chronic hepatitis virus B or C infections. The use of IFN alfa in the pharmacotherapy of hepatitis is presented in chapter 36.

Pr Prototype Drug | Hepatitis B Vaccine *(Engerix-B, Recombivax HB)*

Therapeutic Class: Vaccine   **Pharmacologic Class:** Vaccine

ACTIONS AND USES

Hepatitis B vaccine is used to provide active immunity in individuals who are at risk for exposure to hepatitis B virus (HBV). It is indicated for infants born to HBV-positive mothers, and those at high risk for exposure to HBV-infected blood, including nurses, physicians, dentists, dental hygienists, morticians, and paramedics. Because HBV infection is extremely difficult to treat, it is prudent for all health care workers to receive HBV vaccine before beginning their clinical education, unless contraindicated. The vaccine is also indicated for all persons who engage in high-risk sexual practices, such as heterosexual activity with multiple partners, female prostitutes, or homosexual or bisexual practices or persons who repeatedly contract sexually transmitted infections. HBV vaccine does *not* provide protection against exposure to other (non-B) hepatitis viruses. HBV vaccine is produced through recombinant DNA technology using yeast cells. It is not prepared from human blood.

Hepatitis B vaccination requires three IM injections; the second dose is given 1 month after the first, and the third dose 6 months after the first dose. The drug is nearly 100% effective in providing immunity to HBV. The effectiveness of the vaccine in producing immunity in adults declines with age.

ADMINISTRATION ALERTS

- In adults, use the deltoid muscle for the injection site, unless contraindicated.

- Because none of the formulas of *Recombivax HB* contain a preservative, once the single-dose vial has been penetrated, the withdrawn vaccine should be used promptly, and the vial discarded.

- Epinephrine (1:1,000) should be immediately available to treat a possible anaphylactic reaction.

- Pregnancy category C

PHARMACOKINETICS
Onset: 2 wk

Peak: 6 mo

Half-life: Unknown

Duration: 5 to 7 y

ADVERSE EFFECTS

The most common adverse effects from HBV vaccination are pain at the injection site and mild to moderate fever and chills. Approximately 15% of patients will experience systemic effects, usually fatigue, dizziness, fever, and headache. Hypersensitivity reactions such as urticaria or anaphylaxis are possible.

Contraindications: This vaccine is contraindicated in patients with hypersensitivity to yeast or HBV vaccine. Patients who demonstrated severe hypersensitivity to the first dose of the vaccine should not receive subsequent doses. The drug should be administered with caution in patients with fever or active infections, or those with compromised cardiopulmonary status.

INTERACTIONS

Drug–Drug: Unknown

Lab Tests: Unknown

Herbal/Food: Unknown

Treatment of Overdose: Overdoses have not been recorded.

Refer to MyNursingKit for a Nursing Process Focus specific to this drug.

Interferon beta consists of two different formulations, beta-1a and beta-1b, which are primarily reserved for the treatment of severe multiple sclerosis (chapter 20∞). A third drug in this class, IFN gamma-1b, has limited clinical application in the treatment of chronic granulomatous disease and severe osteopetrosis.

Interleukins (ILs) are another class of cytokines, synthesized primarily by lymphocytes, monocytes, and macrophages that enhance the capabilities of the immune system. The ILs have widespread effects on immune function including stimulation of cytotoxic T-cell activity against tumor cells, increased B-cell and plasma cell production, and promotion of inflammation. At least 30 different ILs have been identified, though only a few are available as medications. Interleukin-2, derived from T helper lymphocytes, promotes the proliferation of both T lymphocytes and activated B lymphocytes. It is available as aldesleukin (Proleukin), which is approved for the treatment of metastatic renal carcinoma. Aldesleukin

COMPLEMENTARY AND ALTERNATIVE THERAPIES

Echinacea for Boosting the Immune System

Echinacea purpurea, or purple coneflower, is a popular botanical native to the midwestern United States and central Canada. The flowers, leaves, and stems of this plant are harvested and dried. Preparations include dried powder, tincture, fluid extracts, and teas. No single ingredient seems to be responsible for the herb's activity; a large number of potentially active chemicals have been identified from the extracts.

Echinacea was used by Native Americans to treat various wounds and injuries. Echinacea is believed to boost the immune system by increasing phagocytosis and inhibiting the bacterial enzyme hyaluronidase. Some substances in echinacea appear to have antiviral activity; thus, the herb is sometimes taken to treat the common cold and influenza—an indication for which it has received official approval in Germany. In general, echinacea is used as a supportive treatment for any disease involving inflammation and to enhance the immune system. Side effects are rare; however, it may interfere with drugs that have immunosuppressant effects.

TABLE 32.3 Immunostimulants

Drug	Route and Adult Dose (max dose where indicated)	Adverse Effects
aldesleukin (Proleukin): interleukin-2	IV; 600,000 units/kg (0.037 mg/kg) every 8 h by a 15-min IV infusion for a total of 14 doses	*Flulike symptoms (fever, chills, malaise), rash, anemia, nausea, vomiting, diarrhea, confusion, agitation, dyspnea* <u>Cardiac arrest, hypotension, tachycardia, thrombocytopenia, oliguria, anuria, pulmonary edema</u>
Bacillus Calmette-Guérin (BCG) vaccine (Tice, TheraCys)	Intradermal (Tice); 0.1 mL as vaccine Intravesical (TheraCys); bladder instillation for bladder carcinoma	*Flulike symptoms (fever, chills, malaise), dysuria, hematuria, anemia* <u>Thrombocytopenia, cystitis, UTI</u>
INTERFERONS		
Pr interferon alfa-2b (Intron-A)	IM/subcutaneous; hairy cell leukemia: 2 million units/m² three times/wk Kaposi's sarcoma: 30 million units/m² 3 times/wk Hepatitis: 3 million units/m² three times/wk for 18–24 mo	*Flulike symptoms, myalgia, fatigue, headache, anorexia, diarrhea* <u>Myelosuppression, thrombocytopenia, suicide ideation, seizures (interferon beta), MI (interferon gamma), anaphylaxis, hepatotoxicity</u>
interferon alfacon-1 (Infergen)	Subcutaneous: 9 mcg three times/wk	
interferon alfa-n3 (Alferon N)	Intralesional: 0.05 mL (250,000 IU) per wart twice/wk for up to 8 wk	
interferon beta-1a (Avonex, Rebif)	IM (Avonex); 30 mcg/wk Subcutaneous (Rebif); 44 mcg three times/wk	
interferon beta-1b (Betaseron)	Subcutaneous; 0.25 mg (8 million units) every other day	
peginterferon alfa-2a (Pegasys)	Subcutaneous; 180 mcg/wk for 48 wk	
peginterferon alfa-2b (Peg-Intron)	Subcutaneous; 1.5 mcg/kg/wk	

Italics indicate common adverse effects; <u>underlining</u> indicates serious adverse effects.

Pr Prototype Drug | Interferon alfa-2b (Intron-A)

Therapeutic Class: Immunostimulant   **Pharmacologic Class:** Interferon, biologic response modifier

ACTIONS AND USES

Interferon alfa-2b is a biologic response modifier prepared by recombinant DNA technology that is approved to treat cancers (hairy cell leukemia, malignant melanoma, non-Hodgkin's lymphoma, AIDS-related Kaposi's sarcoma), as well as viral infections (human papilloma virus, chronic hepatitis virus B and C). Off-label indications may include chronic myelogenous leukemia, bladder cancer, herpes simplex virus, renal cell cancer, varicella-zoster virus, and West Nile virus. It is available for IV, IM, and subcutaneous administration.

Rebetron is a combination drug containing IFN alfa 2b and ribavirin, an antiviral agent. Rebetron is indicated for pharmacotherapy of hepatitis C infection. Peginterferon alfa-2b (Peg-Intron) has a molecule of PEG attached to the interferon molecule, which gives the drug an extended half-life. Peginterferon alfa-2b is only approved to treat chronic hepatitis C virus infections, although it may be used off-label to treat chronic hepatitis B infections and neoplastic disease.

ADMINISTRATION ALERTS

- The drug should be administered under the careful guidance of a health care provider experienced with its use.
- Subcutaneous administration is recommended for patients at risk for bleeding (platelet count less than 50,000/mm³)
- Pregnancy category C

PHARMACOKINETICS
Onset: Unknown
Peak: 3–12 h (IM)
Half-life: 2 h
Duration: Unknown

ADVERSE EFFECTS

A flulike syndrome of fever, chills, dizziness, and fatigue occurs in 50% or patients, although this usually diminishes as therapy progresses. Headache, nausea, vomiting, diarrhea, and anorexia are relatively common. Depression and suicidal ideation have been reported and may be severe enough to require discontinuation of the drug. With prolonged therapy, serious toxicity such as immunosuppression, hepatotoxicity, and neurotoxicity may be observed.

Contraindications: Contraindications include hypersensitivity to interferons, autoimmune hepatitis, and hepatic decompensation. Neonates and infants should not receive this drug because it contains benzyl alcohol, which is associated with an increased incidence of neurologic and other serious complications in these age groups.

INTERACTIONS

Drug–Drug: Use with ethanol may cause excessive drowsiness and dehydration. There is additive myelosuppression with antineoplastics. Zidovudine may increase hematologic toxicity.

Lab Tests: Large declines in hematocrit, leukocyte counts, and platelet counts may occur after 3–5 days of therapy. Hepatic enzymes may become elevated during IFN therapy and may require discontinuation of the drug. Interferon alfa-2b may elevate triglyceride levels.

Herbal/Food: Unknown

Treatment of Overdose: Overdose may cause lethargy and coma. Treatment is by general supportive measures.

Refer to MyNursingKit for a Nursing Process Focus specific to this drug.

NURSING PROCESS FOCUS   PATIENTS RECEIVING IMMUNOSTIMULANT THERAPY

Assessment	Potential Nursing Diagnoses
Baseline assessment prior to administration: ■ Understand the reason the drug has been prescribed in order to assess for therapeutic effects. ■ Obtain a complete health history including previous history of actual disease (e.g., chickenpox), hepatic, renal, cardiovascular, neurologic, or autoimmune disease, HIV infection, fever or active infections, pregnancy or breastfeeding, and previous allergic response to immunizations or to products contained within immunization (e.g., yeast sensitivity, sensitivity to eggs or albumin products). Obtain a drug history, especially the use of immunosuppressants or corticosteroids. ■ Obtain an immunization history and any unusual reactions or responses that occurred. ■ Obtain baseline vital signs, especially temperature. ■ Evaluate appropriate laboratory findings (e.g., CBC, platelets, electrolytes, titers, hepatic and renal labs).	■ Health Seeking Behaviors (expressed desire to obtain vaccinations) ■ Ineffective Health Maintenance (related to failure to complete immunization schedule) ■ Deficient Knowledge (vaccination schedule, recommendations) ■ Risk for Injury (related to drug adverse effects)
Assessment throughout administration: ■ Assess for patient adherence to recommended immunization schedule (e.g., need for repeated immunizations, boosters in adults). ■ Continue periodic monitoring of CBC, and liver and renal function studies as appropriate. ■ Assess vital signs, especially temperature. ■ Assess for and immediately report adverse effects: fever, dizziness, confusion, muscle weakness, tachycardia, hypotension, syncope, dyspnea, pulmonary congestion, skin rashes, bruising or bleeding, or anaphylactic reactions.	

Planning: Patient Goals and Expected Outcomes

The patient will:
■ Experience therapeutic effects dependent on the reason the drug is being given (e.g., active immunity).
■ Be free from, or experience minimal, adverse effects.
■ Verbalize an understanding of the drug's use, adverse effects, and required precautions.
■ Demonstrate proper self-administration of the medication (e.g., dose, timing, when to notify provider).

Implementation

Interventions and (Rationales)	Patient and Family Education
Ensuring therapeutic effects: ■ Continue assessments as described earlier for therapeutic effects. (The patient should adhere to the recommended immunization schedule. Periodic titers may be needed to confirm immunity, especially in individuals who are over 60 or those who are immunosuppressed.)	■ Teach the patient and family or caregiver to keep vaccination records and to remain current with required immunizations. ■ Encourage older adults to have titers drawn to confirm immunity.
■ For patients traveling overseas, obtain immunization recommendations for destination country. (Current recommendations may be found on the CDC Traveler's Health web site.)	■ Teach the patient to consult the CDC Traveler's website before planning overseas travel and to consult with the health care provider about risks and required immunizations.
Minimizing adverse effects: ■ Continue to monitor vital signs, especially temperature, and neurologic status. (Immunizations and immunostimulants may cause dermatologic, cardiovascular, and neurologic adverse effects. An increase in temperature, localized ulcerations or signs of infection at injection site, tachycardia or palpitations, dizziness, or changes in level of consciousness may indicate significant adverse effects.) ■ Report all significant adverse effects to the health care provider for reporting to VAERS—Vaccine Adverse Event Reporting System.	■ Teach the patient to immediately report any fever over 101° or as instructed by the health care provider, changes in consciousness such as drowsiness or disorientation, dyspnea, or tachycardia or palpitations.

(Continued)

NURSING PROCESS FOCUS   PATIENTS RECEIVING IMMUNOSTIMULANT THERAPY *(Continued)*

Implementation

Interventions and (Rationales)	Patient and Family Education
▪ Treat minor side effects symptomatically. (Minor adverse effects may be treated with acetaminophen or as ordered by the health care provider for low-grade fevers less than 101°F, for localized tenderness, or for minor arthralgias and malaise. Cool compresses to injection site may help alleviate malaise, fever, or injection site soreness.)	▪ Teach the patient to treat minor symptoms as needed but to report adverse effects (as described earlier).
▪ Assess for possibility of pregnancy, previous history of organ transplantation, and home environment including significantly immunocompromised patients at home, e.g., from chemotherapy, before giving live virus immunizations. (Some live vaccinations continue to be shed from the patient in the postvaccination period and may be transmitted to immunocompromised patients in the home environment. Pregnancy is a contraindication for vaccination with the live viruses and women who become pregnant within 3 months of immunization with a live vaccine should consult their health care provider.)	▪ Teach the patient to alert their health care providers to any home situation that may require deferral of live vaccinations before vaccination is given. Women who are pregnant or who become pregnant within the first 3 months after vaccination should consult with their health care provider.
▪ Avoid or defer immunizations in any patient with a fever, autoimmune disease, or those taking corticosteroids. (Fever may make it more difficult to discern drug reaction versus an infectious process. Immune response to vaccine may be over- or undertherapeutic and an increased risk of adverse effects may result.)	▪ Explain to the patient the need to defer vaccinations under certain conditions and ensure that follow-up appointments are made as appropriate to maintain currency with immunizations.
▪ Assess the patient for previous use of BCG vaccine and consult with the health care provider before giving PPD ("Mantoux") skin testing for TB. (BCG stimulates immunity to the tuberculosis and recent vaccination may cause an adverse reaction to PPD injection or result in a false positive reaction.)	▪ Teach the patient that previous use of BCG may result in a false-positive TB test, an unusual reaction to the PPD ("Mantoux") test, or that other testing may be required to confirm or refute current infection.
▪ Monitor for signs of opportunistic and superinfections, or an increase in bruising or bleeding in patients receiving interferon therapy. (Myelosuppression may occur, increasing the risk of infections and bleeding.)	▪ Instruct the patient to immediately report fever, increasing malaise and weakness, gingivitis or white patches in mouth, vaginal yeast infections, increase in bruising, or prolonged or excessive bleeding to the provider.
▪ Continue to monitor neurologic and mental status in the patient receiving interferon therapy. (Psychosis, depression, and suicidal ideations are potential adverse effects of interferon use.)	▪ Instruct the patient, family, or caregiver to immediately report increasing lethargy, disorientation, confusion, changes in behavior or mood, agitation or aggression, slurred speech, or ataxia.
Patient understanding of drug therapy: ▪ Use opportunities during administration of medications and during assessments to discuss rationale for drug therapy, desired therapeutic outcomes, most common adverse effects, parameters for when to call the health care provider, and any necessary monitoring or precautions. (Using time during nursing care helps to optimize and reinforce key teaching areas.)	▪ The patient should be able to state the reason for the drug; appropriate dose and scheduling; and what adverse effects to observe for and when to report them.

Patient self-administration of drug therapy:
▪ Specific to interferons, when administering the medication, instruct the patient, family, or caregiver in the proper self-administration of the drug. (Proper administration will increase the effectiveness of the drug.)
	▪ Teach the patient to take the medication as follows:
	  ▪ Reconstitute the powder (if applicable) with supplied diluent and gently rotate the vial between the palms, do not shake. Check solution to be sure it is clear and has no particules.
	  ▪ Discard solution as instructed by the health care provider (some vials remain available for use up to 30 days, others are for single-use only). Single-use syringes should be discarded after use, even if solution remains.
	  ▪ Do not change manufacturer's brands without consulting with the health care provider.
	▪ Have the patient, family, or caregiver return-demonstrate the injection technique until they are comfortable with administering drug.

Evaluation of Outcome Criteria

Evaluate the effectiveness of drug therapy by confirming that patient goals and expected outcomes have been met (see "Planning").

See Table 32.3 for a list of drugs to which these nursing actions apply.

must be administered in multiple, brief IV infusions because of its short half-life. Therapy is sometimes limited by capillary leak syndrome, a serious condition in which plasma proteins and other substances leave the blood and enter the interstitial spaces because of "leaky" capillaries. Interleukin-11, which is derived from bone marrow cells, is a growth factor with multiple hematopoietic effects. It is marketed as oprelvekin (Neumega) for its ability to stimulate platelet production in immunosuppressed patients (chapter 28∞).

In addition to interferons and interleukins, a few additional biologic response modifiers are available to enhance the immune system. Levamisole (Ergamisole) is used to stimulate the production of B cells, T cells, and macrophages in patients with colon cancer. Bacillus Calmette–Guérin (BCG) vaccine (Tice, TheraCys) is an attenuated strain of *Mycobacterium bovis* used for the pharmacotherapy of certain types of bladder cancer.

IMMUNOSUPPRESSANTS

Drugs used to inhibit the immune response are called *immunosuppressants*. They are used for patients receiving transplanted tissues or organs, and to treat severe inflammatory disorders. These agents are listed in Table 32.4.

32.6 Immunosuppressants for Preventing Transplant Rejection and for Treating Inflammation

The immune response is normally viewed as a lifesaver that protects individuals from a host of pathogens in the environment. For those receiving organ or tissue transplants, however, the immune response is the enemy. Transplanted organs from donors always contain antigens that trigger the immune response. This response, called **transplant rejection,** is often acute; antibodies can destroy transplanted tissue within a few days. The cell-mediated branch of the immune system responds more slowly to the transplant, attacking it about 2 weeks following surgery. Even if the organ survives these challenges, chronic rejection of the transplant may occur months or even years after surgery.

Immunosuppressants are drugs given to dampen the immune response. One or more immunosuppressants are administered at the time of transplantation and are continued for several months following surgery. In some cases, they are continued indefinitely at low doses. Transplantation would be impossible without the use of effective immunosuppressant drugs. In addition, these agents may be prescribed for severe cases of rheumatoid arthritis or other inflammatory autoimmune diseases.

Although the mechanisms of action of the immunosuppressant drugs differ, all suppress some aspect of T-cell function. Some act nonselectively by inhibiting all aspects of the immune system. Other, newer drugs suppress only specific aspects of the immune response. Obviously, the nonselective agents will provide more widespread immunosuppression, but carry greater risk of adverse effects.

Because the immunosuppressants are toxic to bone marrow, they are capable of producing serious adverse effects. During immunosuppressant therapy, the patient will be susceptible to infection from all types of pathogens: viral, bacterial, fungal, or protozoan. Infections are common and the patient must be protected from situations for which exposure to pathogens is likely. Prophylactic therapy with anti-infectives may become necessary if immune function becomes excessively suppressed. Long-term survivors of transplants are also at high risk of developing cancers, especially lymphoma, skin cancer, cervical cancer, and Kaposi's sarcoma.

Drug classes that have immunosuppressant activity include glucocorticoids, antimetabolites, antibodies, and calcineurin inhibitors. The glucocorticoids are potent inhibitors of inflammation and are discussed in detail in chapters 33 and 43∞. They are often drugs of choice in the short-term therapy of severe inflammation. Antimetabolites such as sirolimus (Rapamune) and azathioprine (Imuran) inhibit aspects of lymphocyte replication. By binding to the intracellular messenger **calcineurin,** cyclosporine (Sandimmune, Neoral) and tacrolimus (Prograf) disrupt T cell function. The calcineurin inhibitors are of value in treating psoriasis, an inflammatory disorder of the skin (chapter 48∞).

Recall from Section 32.2 that antibodies are proteins produced by the immune system to defend against microbes. In fact, Section 32.3 discussed how infusion of antibodies can provide passive immunity. It may seem puzzling, then, to learn that certain antibodies may be administered to patients to *suppress* the immune response. How is this possible?

When animals such as mice are injected with human T cells or T-cell protein receptors, the animal recognizes these as foreign and produces antibodies against them. When purified and injected into humans, these mouse antibodies will attack T cells (or T-cell receptors). Four of these antibodies are used as immunosuppressants. For example, muromonab-CD3 (Orthoclone OKT3) is administered to prevent rejection of kidney, heart, and liver transplants, and to deplete the bone marrow of T cells prior to marrow transplant. Basiliximab (Simulect) and daclizumab (Zenapax) are given to prevent acute rejection of kidney transplants. Infliximab (Remicade) is used to suppress the severe inflammation that often accompanies autoimmune disorders such as Crohn's disease and rheumatoid arthritis. Note that the suffix "ab" in the generic name refers to antibody. Because some drugs in this monoclonal antibody class are used as antineoplastics, the student should refer to chapter 37∞.

MyNursingKit | Xenotransplants

AVOIDING MEDICATION ERRORS

An order was written to administer methotrexate 10 mg once a day for an elderly patient with rheumatoid arthritis. Explain why the nurse should question this medication order.

See Appendix D for the suggested answer.

TABLE 32.4	Immunosuppressants	
Drug	**Route and Adult Dose (max dose where indicated)**	**Adverse Effects**
ANTIBODIES		
basiliximab (Simulect)	IV; 20 mg times two doses (first dose 2 h before surgery; second dose 4 days after transplant)	*Local reactions at injection site (pain, erythema, myalgia), influenza-like symptoms (malaise, fever, chills), headache, dizziness*
daclizumab (Zenapax)	IV; 1 mg/kg start first dose no more than 24 h prior to transplant, then repeat every 14 days for four more doses	Anaphylaxis, hypertension, infections (may occur in many different body systems), renal impairment (basiliximab), pulmonary edema (muromonab-CD3 and lymphocyte immune globulin), herpes simplex or cytomegalovirus infections (muromonab-CD3)
infliximab (Remicade)	IV; 3–5 mg/kg followed by the same dose at 2 and 6 weeks	
lymphocyte immune globulin or antithymocyte globulin, (Atgam)	IV; 10–30 mg/kg/day	
muromonab-CD3 (Orthoclone OKT3)	IV; 5 mg/day administered for 10–14 days	
ANTIMETABOLITES AND CYTOTOXIC AGENTS		
anakinra (Kineret)	Subcutaneous; 100 mg once daily	*Injection site reactions* Leukopenia, infections, malignancy
azathioprine (Imuran)	PO/IV; 3–5 mg/kg/day initially; may be able to reduce to 1–3 mg/kg/day	*Nausea, vomiting, anorexia* Severe nausea and vomiting, bone marrow suppression, thrombocytopenia, infections, malignancy, hepatotoxicity
cyclophosphamide (Cytoxan) (see page 556 for the Prototype Drug box ∞)	PO; Initial: 1–5 mg/kg/day. Maintenance: 1–5 mg/kg every 7–10 days IV; 40–50 mg/kg in divided doses over 2–5 days up to 100 mg/kg	*Nausea, vomiting, anorexia, neutropenia, alopecia* Anaphylaxis, leukopenia, pulmonary emboli, interstitial pulmonary fibrosis, toxic epidermal necrolysis, Stevens–Johnson syndrome, hemorrhagic cystitis, nephrotoxicity
etanercept (Enbrel)	Subcutaneous; 25 mg twice/wk or 0.08 mg/kg or 50 mg once/wk	*Local reactions at injection site (pain, erythema, myalgia), abdominal pain, vomiting, headache* Infections, pancytopenia, MI, heart failure, heart failure, malignancy
methotrexate (Rheumatrex, Trexall) (see page 558 for the Prototype Drug box ∞)	PO: 15–30 mg/day for 5 days; repeat every 12 wk for three courses	*Headache, glossitis, gingivitis, mild leukopenia, nausea* Ulcerative stomatitis, myelosuppression, aplastic anemia, hepatic cirrhosis, nephrotoxicity, sudden death, pulmonary fibrosis or pneumonia
mycophenolate (CellCept, Myfortic)	PO/IV; 720 mg bid in combination with corticosteroids and cyclosporine, within 24 h of transplant	*Peripheral edema, diarrhea, headache, tremor, dyspepsia, abdominal pain* UTI, leukopenia, anemia, thrombocytopenia, sepsis, hypertension
sirolimus (Rapamune)	PO; 6-mg loading dose immediately after transplant, then 2 mg/day	*Hypercholesterolemia, rash, arthralgia, diarrhea, nausea, vomiting, asthenia, back pain, weight gain, hyperlipidemia* Hypertension, leukopenia, anemia, thrombocytopenia, sepsis, secondary infections, malignancy
temsirolimus (Torisel)	IV; 25 mg once weekly over 30–60 min	*Rash, asthenia, mucositis, nausea, edema, anorexia, hyperglycemia, hyperlipidemia* Anemia, anaphylaxis, infections, interstitial lung disease or pneumonia, birth defects
thalidomide (Thalomid)	PO; 100–300 mg/day (max: 400 mg/day) times at least 2 wk	*Rash, mild leukopenia, fever, dizziness, diarrhea, malaise, drowsiness* Toxic epidermal necrolysis, birth defects (pregnancy category X), orthostatic hypotension, neutropenia, peripheral neuropathy

TABLE 32.4	**Immunosuppressants** (Continued)		
Drug	**Route and Adult Dose (max dose where indicated)**	**Adverse Effects**
CALCINEURIN INHIBITORS		
(Pr) cyclosporine (Neoral, Sandimmune)	PO; initial dose 14–18 mg/kg just prior to surgery; after 2 weeks, then 5–10 mg/kg/day	*Hirsutism, tremor, vomiting* Hypertension, MI, nephrotoxicity, hyperkalemia, seizures, paresthesia, hepatotoxicity
tacrolimus (Prograf)	PO; 0.15–0.3 mg/kg/day in two divided doses every 12 h; give first oral dose 8–12 h after discontinuing IV therapy IV; 0.03–0.05 mg/kg/day as continuous infusion; start no sooner than 6 h after transplant and continue until patient can take oral therapy	*Oliguria, nausea, constipation, diarrhea, headache, abdominal pain, insomnia, peripheral edema, fever* Infections, hypertension, nephrotoxicity, neurotoxicity (tremors, paresthesia, psychosis), hyperkalemia, anemia, hyperglycemia

Italics indicate common adverse effects; underlining indicates serious adverse effects.

(Pr) **Prototype Drug** | **Cyclosporine** (*Neoral, Sandimmune*)

Therapeutic Class: Immunosuppressant   **Pharmacologic Class:** Calcineurin inhibitor

ACTIONS AND USES

Cyclosporine is a complex chemical obtained from a soil fungus that inhibits helper T cells. Compared to some of the other immunosuppressants, cyclosporine is less toxic to bone marrow cells. When prescribed for transplant recipients, it is often used in combination with high doses of a glucocorticoid such as prednisone. Cyclosporine is approved for the prophylaxis of kidney, heart, and liver transplant rejection; psoriasis; and xerophthalmia, an eye condition of diminished tear production caused by ocular inflammation. An IV form is available for transplant rejection and for severe cases of ulcerative colitis or Crohn's disease.

ADMINISTRATION ALERTS

- Neoral (microemulsion) and Sandimmune are not bioequivalent and cannot be used interchangeably without close supervision by the health care provider.
- Pregnancy category C

PHARMACOKINETICS
Onset: 7–14 days
Peak: 3–4 h
Half-life: 16–27 h
Duration: Unknown

ADVERSE EFFECTS

The primary adverse effect of cyclosporine occurs in the kidneys, with up to 75% of patients experiencing reduction in urine output. Over half the patients taking the drug will experience hypertension and tremor. Other common side effects are headache, gingival hyperplasia, and elevated hepatic enzymes. Although opportunistic infections occur during cyclosporine therapy, they are fewer than with some of the other immunosuppressants. Periodic blood counts are necessary to ensure that WBCs do not fall below 4,000, or platelets below 75,000. Long-term therapy increases the risk of malignancy, especially lymphomas and skin cancers.

Contraindications: The only contraindication is prior hypersensitivity to the drug.

INTERACTIONS

Drug–Drug: Drugs that decrease cyclosporine levels include phenytoin, phenobarbital, carbamazepine, and rifampin. Azole antifungal drugs, ACE inhibitors, NSAIDs, and macrolide antibiotics may increase cyclosporine levels.

Lab Tests: Cyclosporine may increase serum triglycerides and uric acid. It may decrease hepatic enzymes and urinary function test values.

Herbal/Food: Grapefruit juice can raise cyclosporine levels by 50–200%. This drug should be used with caution with herbal immune-stimulating supplements such as astragalus and echinacea, which may interfere with immunosuppressants.

Treatment of Overdose: There is no specific treatment for overdose.

Refer to MyNursingKit for a Nursing Process Focus specific to this drug.

NURSING PROCESS FOCUS   PATIENTS RECEIVING IMMUNOSUPPRESSANT THERAPY

Assessment	Potential Nursing Diagnoses
Baseline assessment prior to administration: - Understand the reason the drug has been prescribed in order to assess for therapeutic effects. - Obtain a complete health history including previous history or current case of cancer; fever or active infections (especially herpes, varicella, and CMV); hepatic, renal, cardiovascular, neurologic, or autoimmune disease; dermatologic conditions; HIV infection; and pregnancy or breastfeeding. Obtain a drug history, especially the use of corticosteroids. - Obtain a dietary history, especially the intake of grapefruit juice. - Obtain baseline vital signs, especially blood pressure and temperature, and height and weight. - Assess oral and dental health. - Evaluate appropriate laboratory findings (e.g., CBC, platelets, electrolytes, glucose, hepatic and renal labs, lipid levels).	- Anxiety or Fear (related to concerns about condition, treatment) - Ineffective Therapeutic Regimen Management (related to complexity of disease, treatment) - Social Isolation - Deficient Knowledge (drug therapy) - Risk for Infection - Risk for Injury - Risk for Impaired Oral Mucous Membranes (related to drug treatment)
Assessment throughout administration: - Assess for desired therapeutic effects (e.g., no signs or symptoms of transplant rejection, severe inflammatory response or autoimmune responses are suppressed). - Continue monitoring of CBC, platelets, electrolytes, glucose, liver and renal function studies, and lipid levels. - Assess vital signs, especially blood pressure and temperature. - Assess for and immediately report adverse effects: fever, chills, visible signs of infection, nausea, vomiting, dizziness, confusion, muscle weakness, tremors, tachycardia, hypertension, angina, syncope, dyspnea, pulmonary congestion, skin rashes, bruising or bleeding, or decreased urine output.	

Planning: Patient Goals and Expected Outcomes

The patient will:

- Experience therapeutic effects dependent on the reason the drug is being given (e.g., free from signs of transplant rejection, excessive/autoimmune response limited and decreasing).
- Be free from, or experience minimal, adverse effects.
- Verbalize an understanding of the drug's use, adverse effects, and required precautions.
- Demonstrate proper self-administration of the medication (e.g., dose, timing, when to notify provider).

Implementation

Interventions and (Rationales)	Patient and Family Education
Ensuring therapeutic effects: - Continue assessments as described earlier for therapeutic effects. (Monitoring will be specific to transplant, e.g., maintenance of urine output. Severe inflammatory conditions and autoimmune disorders should show gradually lessening inflammation and pain.)	- Advise the patient on the treatment/condition-specific monitoring requirements (e.g., urine output, improvement of movement in joints with lessened swelling).
Minimizing adverse effects: - Continue to monitor vital signs, especially blood pressure and temperature. (Immunosuppressant drugs may cause hypertension and increase the risk of infections.)	- Teach the patient how to monitor blood pressure. Ensure the proper use and functioning of any home equipment obtained. The patient should report blood pressure over 140/90 mmHg or per parameters set by the health care provider. Chest pain or pressure should be reported immediately. - Teach the patient to report any fever over 101°F or as instructed by the health care provider.

Interventions and (Rationales)	Patient and Family Education

▪ Observe for signs and symptoms of infection. (Immunosuppressants increase the risk of infections, especially with opportunistic infections such as herpes, varicella, CMV, and fungal infections.)	▪ Teach the patient to report signs and symptoms of infection immediately such as: wounds with redness or drainage, increasing cough, increasing fatigue, white-patches on oral mucous membranes or white and itchy vaginal discharge, or itchy blister-like vesicles on skin.
	▪ Instruct the patient on infection control measures, including:
	  ▪ Frequent handwashing.
	  ▪ Avoiding large crowds, especially indoors.
	  ▪ Avoiding people with known infection or young children who have a higher risk of having an infection.
	  ▪ Cooking food thoroughly, allowing family or caregiver to prepare raw foods and to clean up afterwards. The patient should not consume raw fruits or vegetables.
	▪ Teach the patient to report any fever per parameters set by the health care provider, and symptoms of infection.

▪ Assess for changes in level of consciousness, disorientation or confusion, or tremors. (Neurologic changes may indicate adverse drug effects.)	▪ Instruct the patient to immediately report increasing lethargy, disorientation, confusion, changes in behavior or mood, slurred speech, or tremors or ataxia.
▪ Continue to monitor CBC, platelets, electrolytes, glucose, liver and renal function studies, and lipid levels. (Immunosuppressants may cause leukopenia, anemia, thrombocytopenia, hyperglycemia, and hyperkalemia.)	▪ Instruct the patient on the need to return frequently for follow-up lab work. ▪ Advise patient to carry a wallet identification card or wear medical identification jewelry indicating immunosuppressant therapy.
▪ Inspect oral mucous membranes and dental health. (Immunosuppression increases the risk of oral candidiasis and gingivitis. Oral antifungal rinses may be required.)	▪ Teach the patient to maintain excellent oral hygiene, inspecting the oral cavity daily. Keep regular dental visits and consult dentist about the frequency needed.
▪ Assess the patient's diet and consumption of grapefruit juice. (Grapefruit juice significantly increases cyclosporine levels and should be avoided while on immunosuppressant therapy.)	▪ Teach the patient to avoid or eliminate grapefruit and grapefruit juice while on the drug. Flavored beverages without juice are permissible.
▪ Assess for pregnancy. (Pregnancy should be avoided for up to 4 months after discontinuing immunosuppressive therapy. Women who become pregnant while on the drug should consult their health care provider.)	▪ Discuss pregnancy and family planning with women of child-bearing age. Explain the effect of medications on pregnancy and breast-feeding and the need to discuss any pregnancy plans with the health care provider. Discuss the need for additional forms of contraception, including barrier methods, with patients taking immunosuppressants.
▪ Assess for the development of hirsutism or alopecia. (Hirsutism is reversible when the drug is discontinued. Alopecia may indicate significant immunosuppression.)	▪ Advise the patient to notify the provider of changes to hair growth or texture.
Patient understanding of drug therapy: ▪ Use opportunities during administration of medications and during assessments to discuss rationale for drug therapy, desired therapeutic outcomes, most common adverse effects, parameters for when to call the health care provider, and any necessary monitoring or precautions. (Using time during nursing care helps to optimize and reinforce key teaching areas.)	▪ The patient, family, or caregiver should be able to state the reason for the drug; appropriate dose and scheduling; what adverse effects to observe for and when to report; and the anticipated length of medication therapy.

Patient self-administration of drug therapy:
▪ When administering medications, instruct the patient, family, or caregiver in proper self-administration techniques followed by return demonstration. (Proper administration will increase the effectiveness of the drug.).
	▪ Teach the patient to take the medication as follows:
	  ▪ Use enclosed equipment to measure or mix drug.
	  ▪ Use glass and not paper or plastic cups unless package directions indicate they are to be used.
	  ▪ Mix drug with milk, chocolate milk, or orange juice, stirring well. After taking the drug, rinse the cup with additional liquid to ensure the entire dose is taken.

Evaluation of Outcome Criteria

Evaluate the effectiveness of drug therapy by confirming that patient goals and expected outcomes have been met (see "Planning").

See Table 32.4 for a list of drugs to which these nursing actions apply.

Chapter REVIEW

KEY CONCEPTS

The numbered key concepts provide a succinct summary of the important points from the corresponding numbered section within each chapter. If any of these points are not clear, refer to the numbered section within the chapter for review.

32.1 Nonspecific defenses deny entrance of pathogens to the body by providing general responses that are not specific to a particular threat. Specific body defenses are activated by specific antigens, and each is effective against one particular microbe species.

32.2 Antibody-mediated, or humoral, immunity involves the production of antibodies by plasma cells, which neutralize the foreign agent or mark it for destruction by other defense cells.

32.3 Vaccines are biologic agents used to prevent illness by boosting antibody production and producing active immunity. Passive immunity is obtained through the administration of antibodies.

32.4 Cell-mediated immunity involves the activation of specific T cells and the secretion of cytokines such as interferons and interleukins that enhance the immune response and rid the body of the foreign agent.

32.5 Immunostimulants are biologic response modifiers, including interferons and interleukins, that boost the patient's immune system. They are used to treat certain viral infections, immunodeficiencies, and specific cancers.

32.6 Immunosuppressants inhibit the patient's immune system and are used to treat severe autoimmune disease and to prevent tissue rejection following organ transplantation.

NCLEX-RN® REVIEW QUESTIONS

1 A 55-year-old female patient is receiving cyclosporine (Neoral, Sandimmune) after a heart transplant. The patient exhibits a white blood cell count of 12,000 cells/mm^3, a sore throat, fatigue, and a low-grade fever. The nurse suspects:
1. transplant rejection.
2. heart failure.
3. dehydration.
4. infection.

2 Which of the following statements by a patient taking cyclosporine (Neoral, Sandimmune) would indicate the need for more teaching by the nurse?
1. "I will report any reduction in urine output to my physician."
2. "I will wash my hands frequently."
3. "I will take my blood pressure at home every day."
4. "I will take my cyclosporine at breakfast with a glass of grapefruit juice."

3 The nurse should monitor a transplant patient for the major adverse effect of cyclosporine (Neoral, Sandimmune) therapy by assessing which lab test?
1. CBC
2. Serum creatinine
3. Liver enzymes
4. Electrolytes

4 The nurse would question an order for immunostimulant therapy if the patient had which of the following conditions? (Select all that apply.)
1. Pregnancy
2. Renal disease
3. Infection
4. Liver disease
5. Metastatic cancer

5 The type of immunity achieved through the administration of a vaccine is called:
1. active immunity.
2. passive immunity.
3. titer.
4. vaccine.

6 A 5-year-old child is due for prekindergarten immunizations. After interviewing her mother, which of the following responses may indicate a possible contraindication for giving this preschooler a live vaccine (e.g., MMR) at this visit and would require further exploration by the nurse?
1. Her cousin has the flu.
2. The mother has just finished her series of hepatitis B vaccines.
3. Her arm got really sore after her last tetanus shot.
4. They are caring for her grandmother who has just finished her second chemotherapy treatment for breast cancer.

CRITICAL THINKING QUESTIONS

1. A patient is taking sirolimus (Rapamune) following a liver transplant. On the most recent CBC, the nurse notes a marked 50% decrease in platelets and leukocytes. During the physical assessment, what signs and symptoms should the nurse look for? What are appropriate nursing interventions?

2. A patient has been exposed to hepatitis A and has been referred for an injection of gamma globulin. The patient is hesitant to get a "shot" and says that his immune system is fine. How should the nurse respond?

3. A patient had a renal transplant 6 months ago and is taking cyclosporine (Neoral, Sandimmune) daily. Identify three precautions that the nurse should be aware of when caring for this patient.

See Appendix D for answers and rationales for all activities.

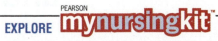

EXPLORE PEARSON **mynursingkit**™

MyNursingKit is your one stop for online chapter review materials and resources. Prepare for success with additional NCLEX®-style practice questions, interactive assignments and activities, web links, animations and videos, and more!

Register your access code from the front of your book at
www.mynursingkit.com.

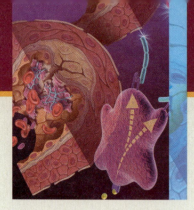

Chapter 33

Drugs for Inflammation and Fever

LEARNING OUTCOMES

After reading this chapter, the student should be able to:

1. Explain the pathophysiology of inflammation and fever.
2. Outline the basic steps in the acute inflammatory response.
3. Explain the role of chemical mediators in the inflammatory response.
4. Outline the general strategies for treating inflammation.
5. Compare and contrast the actions and adverse effects of the different nonsteroidal anti-inflammatory drugs (NSAIDs).
6. Explain the role of glucocorticoids in the pharmacologic management of inflammation.
7. For each of the classes listed in Drugs at a Glance, know representative drugs, and explain their mechanisms of drug action, primary actions related to inflammation and fever, and important adverse effects.
8. Use the nursing process to care for patients receiving drug therapy for inflammation and fever.

KEY TERMS

The pain and redness of inflammation following minor abrasions and cuts is something everyone has experienced. Although there is discomfort from such scrapes, inflammation is a normal and expected part of our body's defense against injury. For some diseases, however, inflammation can rage out of control, producing severe pain, fever, and other distressing symptoms. It is these sorts of conditions for which pharmacotherapy may be needed.

INFLAMMATION

Inflammation is a nonspecific defense system of the body. Through the process of inflammation, a large number of potentially damaging chemicals and microorganisms may be neutralized.

33.1 The Function of Inflammation

The human body has developed many complex ways to defend against physical injury and invasion by microorganisms. Inflammation is one of these defense mechanisms. **Inflammation** occurs in response to many different stimuli, including physical injury, exposure to toxic chemicals, extreme heat, invading microorganisms, or death of cells. It is considered a *nonspecific* defense mechanism because inflammation proceeds in the same manner, regardless of the cause that triggered it. The *specific* immune defenses of the body were presented in chapter 32.

The central purpose of inflammation is to contain the injury or destroy the microorganism. By neutralizing the foreign agent and removing cellular debris and dead cells, repair of the injured area can proceed at a faster pace. Signs of inflammation include swelling, pain, warmth, and redness of the affected area.

Inflammation may be classified as *acute* or *chronic*. Acute inflammation has an immediate onset and lasts 1 to 2 weeks. During acute inflammation, such as that caused by minor physical injury, 8 to 10 days are normally needed for the symptoms to resolve and for repair to begin. If the body cannot contain or neutralize the damaging agent, inflammation may continue for long periods and become chronic.

In chronic autoimmune disorders such as lupus and rheumatoid arthritis, inflammation may persist for years, with symptoms becoming progressively worse over time. Other chronic disorders such as seasonal allergy arise at predictable times during each year, and inflammation may produce only minor, annoying symptoms.

33.2 The Role of Chemical Mediators in Inflammation

Whether the injury is due to pathogens, chemicals, or physical trauma, the damaged tissue releases a number of chemical mediators that act as "alarms" to notify the surrounding area of the injury. Chemical mediators of inflammation include histamine, leukotrienes, bradykinin, complement, and prostaglandins. Table 33.1 describes the sources and actions of these mediators.

Histamine is a key chemical mediator of inflammation. It is stored primarily within **mast cells** located in tissue spaces under epithelial membranes such as the skin, bronchial tree, digestive tract, and along blood vessels. Mast cells detect foreign agents or injury and respond by releasing histamine, which initiates the inflammatory response within seconds. Drugs that act as specific antagonists histamine receptors are in widespread therapeutic use for the treatment of allergic rhinitis (chapter 38).

When released at an injury site, histamine dilates nearby blood vessels, causing capillaries to become more permeable. Plasma, complement proteins, and phagocytes can then enter the area to neutralize foreign agents. The affected area may become congested with blood, which can lead to

TABLE 33.1	Chemical Mediators of Inflammation
Mediator	**Description**
Bradykinin	Present in an inactive form in plasma and mast cells; vasodilator that causes pain; effects are similar to those of histamine
Complement	Series of at least 20 proteins that combine in a cascade fashion to neutralize or destroy an antigen
Histamine	Stored and released by mast cells; causes dilation of blood vessels, smooth-muscle constriction, tissue swelling, and itching
Leukotrienes	Stored and released by mast cells; effects are similar to those of histamine
Prostaglandins	Present in most tissues and stored and released by mast cells; increase capillary permeability, attract white blood cells to site of inflammation, and cause pain

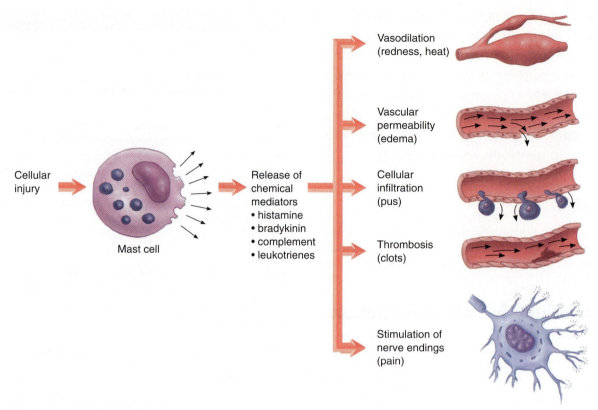

➤ **Figure 33.1** Steps in acute inflammation
Source: Pearson Education/PM College.

significant swelling and pain. ➤ Figure 33.1 illustrates the fundamental steps in acute inflammation.

Rapid release of the chemical mediators of inflammation on a large scale throughout the body is responsible for **anaphylaxis,** a life-threatening allergic response that may result in shock and death. A number of chemicals, insect stings, foods, and some therapeutic drugs can cause this widespread release of histamine from mast cells if the person has an allergy to these substances. The pharmacotherapy of anaphylaxis was presented in chapter 29∞.

33.3 General Strategies for Treating Inflammation

Because inflammation is a nonspecific process and may be caused by such a variety of etiologies, it may occur in virtually any tissue or organ system. When treating inflammation, the following general principles apply:

- Inflammation is not a disease, but a symptom of an underlying disorder. Whenever possible, the *cause* of the inflammation should be identified and treated.

- Inflammation is a natural process for ridding the body of antigens, and it is usually self-limiting. For mild symptoms, nonpharmacologic treatments such as ice packs and rest should be used whenever applicable.

- Topical drugs should be used when applicable because they cause fewer adverse effects. Inflammation of the skin and mucous membranes of the mouth, nose,

rectum, and vagina are best treated with topical drugs. These include antiinflammatory creams, ointments, patches, suppositories, and intranasal sprays. Many of these are available over the counter (OTC).

The goal of pharmacotherapy with anti-inflammatory drugs is to prevent or decrease the intensity of the inflammatory response and reduce fever, if present. Most anti-inflammatory agents are nonspecific; the drug will exhibit the same inhibitory actions regardless of the cause of the inflammation. Common diseases that benefit from anti-inflammatory agents include allergic rhinitis, anaphylaxis, ankylosing spondylitis, contact dermatitis, Crohn's disease, glomerulonephritis, Hashimoto's thyroiditis, peptic ulcer disease, rheumatoid arthritis, systemic lupus erythematosus, and ulcerative colitis.

The two primary drug classes used for inflammation are the nonsteroidal anti-inflammatory drugs (NSAIDs) and the glucocorticoids (also called corticosteroids). For mild to moderate pain, inflammation, and fever, NSAIDs are the drugs of choice. Should inflammation become severe or disabling, corticosteroid therapy is begun. Due to their serious long-term adverse effects, corticosteroids are usually used for only 1 to 3 weeks to bring inflammation under control, then the patient is switched to NSAIDs.

A few anti-inflammatory drug classes are *specific* for certain disorders. For example, sulfasalazine (Azulfidine) is specific to treating inflammatory bowel disease, and colchicine and allopurinol (Zyloprim) are used for gouty arthritis.

NONSTEROIDAL ANTI-INFLAMMATORY DRUGS

Nonsteroidal anti-inflammatory drugs (NSAIDs) such as aspirin and ibuprofen have analgesic, antipyretic, and anti-inflammatory properties. They are widely prescribed for mild to moderate inflammation. Doses for these agents are listed in Table 33.2.

33.4 Treating Inflammation with NSAIDs

Because of their relatively high safety margin and availability as over-the-counter (OTC) drugs, the NSAIDs are drugs of choice for the treatment of mild to moderate inflammation. The NSAID class includes some of the most frequently used drugs in medicine, including aspirin and ibuprofen. All NSAIDs have approximately the same efficacy, although the adverse-effect profiles vary among the different drugs. The NSAIDs also exhibit analgesic and antipyretic actions. Although acetaminophen shares the analgesic and antipyretic properties of these other drugs, it has no anti-inflammatory action and is not classified as an NSAID.

NSAIDs act by inhibiting the synthesis of prostaglandins. **Prostaglandins** are lipids found in all tissues that have potent physiologic effects, in addition to promoting inflammation, depending on the tissue in which they are found. The NSAIDs block inflammation by inhibiting **cyclooxygenase (COX)**, the key enzyme in the biosynthesis of prostaglandins. This inhibition is illustrated in ➤ Figure 33.2.

There are two forms of COX, cyclooxygenase-1 (COX-1) and cyclooxygenase-2 (COX-2). COX-1 is present in all tissues and serves *protective* functions such as reducing gastric

TABLE 33.2	Selected Nonsteroidal Anti-Inflammatory Drugs	
Drug	**Route and Adult Dose (max dose where indicated)**	**Adverse Effects**
aspirin (ASA and others) (see page 228 for the Prototype Drug box ∞)	PO; 350–650 mg every 4 h (max: 4 g/day) for pain or fever PO; 3.6–5.4 g/day in four to six divided doses for arthritic conditions PO; 80–325 mg/day for acute MI or prevention of thrombi	*Stomach pain, heartburn, nausea, vomiting, tinnitus, prolonged bleeding time* <u>Severe GI bleeding, bronchospasm, anaphylaxis, hemolytic anemia, Reye's syndrome in children, metabolic acidosis</u>
SELECTIVE COX-2 INHIBITOR		
celecoxib (Celebrex)	PO; 100–200 mg bid (max: 800 mg/day)	*Diarrhea, dyspepsia, headache, pharyngitis, rash* <u>No serious adverse effects, but cardiovascular risk is being investigated</u>
IBUPROFEN AND SIMILAR AGENTS		
diclofenac (Cataflam, Solaraze, Voltaren, others)	PO; 50 mg bid–qid (max: 200 mg/day)	*Nausea, diarrhea, vomiting, abdominal cramping, dyspepsia, dizziness* <u>Renal failure, GI bleeding, anaphylaxis, metabolic acidosis, hepatic impairment</u>
diflunisal	PO; 1000 mg followed by 500 mg every 8–12 hours (max: 1,500 mg/day)	
etodolac	PO; 200–400 mg tid–qid (max: 1,200 mg/day)	
fenoprofen (Nalfon)	PO; 300–600 mg tid–qid (max: 3,200 mg/day)	
flurbiprofen (Ansaid)	PO; 50–100 mg tid–qid (max: 300 mg/day)	
Pr ibuprofen (Advil, Motrin, others)	PO; 400–800 mg tid–qid (max: 3,200 mg/day)	
indomethacin (Indocin)	PO; 25–50 mg bid or tid (max: 200 mg/day) or 75 mg sustained-release one to two times/day	
ketoprofen	PO; 75 mg tid or 50 mg qid (max: 300 mg/day)	
meloxicam (Mobic)	PO; 7.5–15 mg once daily	
nabumetone	PO; 1,000 mg/day (max: 2,000 mg/day)	
naproxen (Aleve, Anaprox, Naprosyn, others)	PO; 250–500 mg bid (max: 1,000 mg/day)	
oxaprozin (Daypro)	PO; 600–1,200 mg/day (max: 1,800 mg/day)	
piroxicam (Feldene)	PO; 10–20 mg one to two times/day (max: 20 mg/day)	
tolmetin (Tolectin)	PO; 400 mg tid (max: 1,800 mg/day)	

Italics indicate common adverse effects; <u>underlining</u> indicates serious adverse effects.

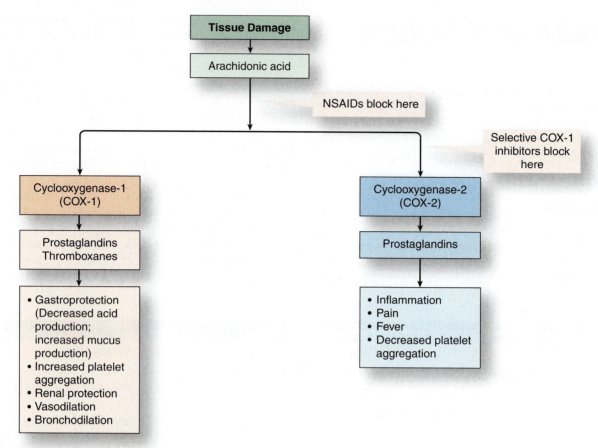

➤ **Figure 33.2** Inhibition of cyclooxygenase

acid secretion, promoting renal blood flow, and regulating smooth muscle tone in blood vessels and the bronchial tree. COX-2, on the other hand, is formed only after tissue injury and serves to promote inflammation. Thus, two nearly identical enzymes serve very different functions. The two forms of cyclooxygenase are compared in Table 33.3.

First-generation NSAIDs such as aspirin and ibuprofen block both COX-1 and COX-2. Although this inhibition reduces inflammation, the inhibition of COX-1 results in *undesirable* effects such as bleeding, gastric upset, and reduced kidney function. Most of the adverse effects of aspirin and ibuprofen are due to inhibition of COX-1, the protective form of the enzyme.

SALICYLATES

Aspirin belongs to the chemical family known as the **salicylates.** Since the discovery of salicylates in 1828, aspirin has become one of the most highly used drugs in the world. Aspirin binds to both COX-1 and COX-2 enzymes, changing their structures and preventing them from forming inflammatory prostaglandins. This inhibition of cyclooxygenase is particularly prolonged in platelets, where a single dose of aspirin may cause total inhibition for the entire 8- to 11-day life span of a platelet. Because it is readily available, inexpensive, and effective, aspirin is often a drug of choice for treating mild inflammation. Aspirin also has a protective effect on the cardiovascular system and is taken daily in small doses by millions of people to prevent abnormal

clot formation and strokes. The fundamental pharmacology and a drug prototype for aspirin were presented in chapter 18∞.

Unfortunately, the large doses of aspirin that are needed to suppress severe inflammation may result in a high incidence of adverse effects, especially on the digestive system. By increasing gastric acid secretion and irritating the stomach lining, aspirin may cause epigastric pain, heartburn, and even bleeding due to ulceration. Some aspirin formulations are buffered or given an enteric coating to minimize adverse GI effects. In some patients, however, even small doses may cause GI bleeding. Because aspirin also has a potent antiplatelet effect, the potential for bleeding must be carefully monitored. High doses may produce **salicylism,** a syndrome that includes symptoms such as tinnitus (ringing in the ears), dizziness, headache, and excessive sweating.

IBUPROFEN AND IBUPROFEN-LIKE NSAIDS

Ibuprofen (Motrin, Advil) and a large number of ibuprofen-like drugs are NSAIDs that were developed as alternatives to aspirin. Like aspirin, they exhibit their effects through inhibition of both COX-1 and COX-2, although the inhibition by these drugs is reversible. Sharing the same mechanism of action, all drugs in this class have similar efficacy for treating pain, fever, and inflammation. For some patients, the choice of NSAID is based on cost and availability: aspirin, ibuprofen, and naproxen (Aleve) are the only NSAIDs sold over the counter. NSAIDs differ in their duration of action,

TABLE 33.3	Forms of Cyclooxygenase	
	Cyclooxygenase-1	Cyclooxygenase-2
Location	Present in all tissues	Present at sites of tissue injury
Functions	Protects gastric mucosa, supports kidney function, promotes platelet aggregation	Mediates inflammation, sensitizes pain receptors, mediates fever in the brain
Inhibition by medications	Undesirable: increases risk of gastric bleeding and kidney failure	Desirable: results in suppression of inflammation

which may be important when patients are taking these drugs on an ongoing basis. Although drugs in this class have similar *overall* effectiveness, there is variability in response to NSAIDs, with some patients responding better to a particular drug. The choice of prescription NSAID is often based on the clinical experiences and preference of the prescriber.

Most ibuprofen-like NSAIDs share a low incidence of adverse effects. The most common side effects are nausea and vomiting. These agents have the potential to cause gastric ulceration and bleeding; however, the incidence is less than that of aspirin. Kidney toxicity is possible, and renal assessments should be conducted periodically. Patients with significant pre-existing renal impairment usually receive acetaminophen for pain or fever, rather than an NSAID. Ibuprofen-like NSAIDs affect platelet function and increase

the potential for bleeding, although this risk is lower than from aspirin. An FDA boxed warning states that ibuprofen and other NSAIDs are associated with an increased risk of thromboembolic events (including stroke and MI) and that the drugs may cause or worsen hypertension. For the occasional user who takes the medications at recommended doses and who has no risk factors, the drugs are safe and rarely produce any significant adverse effects.

SELECTIVE COX-2 INHIBITORS

Selective inhibition of COX-2 produces analgesic, anti-inflammatory, and antipyretic effects without causing some of the serious adverse effects of the older NSAIDs. Because they do not inhibit COX-1, these drugs do not produce adverse effects on the digestive system and lack any effect on blood coagulation. Upon their approval by the FDA, the

---

Pr Prototype Drug | Ibuprofen *(Advil, Motrin, others)*

Therapeutic Class: Analgesic, anti-inflammatory drug, antipyretic | **Pharmacologic Class:** NSAID

ACTIONS AND USES
Ibuprofen is an older drug that is prescribed for the treatment of mild to moderate pain, fever, and inflammation. Its effectiveness is equivalent to that of aspirin and other NSAIDs. Its actions are due to inhibition of prostaglandin synthesis. Common indications include pain associated with chronic musculoskeletal disorders such as rheumatoid and osteoarthritis, headache, dental pain, and dysmenorrhea. Chewable tablets, drops, and solutions are available in low doses for administration to children.

ADMINISTRATION ALERTS
- Give drug on an empty stomach as tolerated. If nausea, vomiting, or abdominal pain occurs, give with food.
- Be aware that patients with asthma or who have allergies to aspirin are more likely to exhibit a hypersensitivity reaction to ibuprofen.
- Pregnancy category B

PHARMACOKINETICS
Onset: 30–60 min
Peak: 1–2 h
Half-life: 2–4 h
Duration: 4–6 h

ADVERSE EFFECTS
Adverse effects of ibuprofen are generally mild and include nausea, heartburn, epigastric pain, and dizziness. GI ulceration with occult or gross bleeding may occur, especially in patients taking high doses for prolonged periods. Patients with active peptic ulcers should not take ibuprofen. Chronic use of ibuprofen may lead to renal impairment.

Contraindications: Ibuprofen has an FDA black box warning that its use is contraindicated for treatment of perioperative pain in the setting of coronary artery bypass graft surgery due to the potential for a stroke or MI. This drug is also contraindicated in patients with significant renal or hepatic impairment and in those who have a syndrome of nasal polyps, angioedema, or bronchospasm due to aspirin or other NSAID use. It should be used cautiously in patients who have heart failure, serious hypertension, or a history of stroke or MI.

INTERACTIONS
Drug–Drug: Because ibuprofen can affect platelet function, its use should be avoided when taking anticoagulants and other coagulation modifiers. Aspirin use can decrease the anti-inflammatory action of ibuprofen. Ibuprofen may increase plasma levels of lithium, causing lithium toxicity. The actions of certain diuretics may be diminished when taken concurrently with ibuprofen. Use with other NSAIDs, alcohol, or corticosteroids may cause serious adverse GI events.

Lab Tests: Ibuprofen may increase bleeding time, aspartate transaminase (AST), and alanine transaminase (ALT) levels. It may decrease hemoglobin and hematocrit.

Herbal/Food: Feverfew, garlic, ginger, or ginkgo may increase the risk of bleeding.

Treatment of Overdose: There is no specific treatment for overdose. Administration of an alkaline drug may increase the urinary excretion of ibuprofen.

Refer to MyNursingKit for a Nursing Process Focus specific to this drug.

selective COX-2 inhibitors quickly became the treatment of choice for moderate to severe inflammation.

However, in 2004, postmarketing data revealed that rofecoxib (Vioxx) doubled the risk of heart attack and stroke in patients taking the drug for extended periods. Based on these reports, the drug manufacturer voluntarily removed rofecoxib from the market. Shortly afterward, a second COX-2 inhibitor, valdecoxib (Bextra) was also voluntarily withdrawn, leaving celecoxib (Celebrex) the sole drug in this class. Other selective COX-2 inhibitors are still available outside the United States. In addition to its anti-inflammatory indications, celecoxib is used to reduce the number of colorectal polyps in adults with familial adenomatous polyposis (FAP). Patients with FAP have an inherited mutation in a gene that results in hundreds of polyps and an almost 100% risk of colon cancer.

GLUCOCORTICOIDS (CORTICOSTEROIDS)

Glucocorticoids have numerous therapeutic applications. One of their most useful properties is the ability to suppress severe inflammation. Because of potentially serious adverse effects, however, systemic glucocorticoids are reserved for the short-term treatment of severe disease. Glucocorticoids are often referred to as corticosteroids. These agents are listed in Table 33.4.

33.5 Treating Acute or Severe Inflammation with Glucocorticoids

Glucocorticoids are natural hormones released by the adrenal cortex that have powerful effects on nearly every cell in the body. When used as drugs to treat inflammatory disorders, the doses are many times higher than the amount naturally present in the blood. The uses of glucocorticoids include the treatment of neoplasia (chapter 37), asthma (chapter 39), arthritis (chapter 47), and corticosteroid deficiency (chapter 43).

Like the NSAIDs, glucocorticoids inhibit the biosynthesis of prostaglandins. Glucocorticoids, however, affect inflammation by multiple mechanisms. They have the ability to suppress histamine release and can inhibit certain functions of phagocytes and lymphocytes. These multiple actions markedly reduce inflammation, making glucocorticoids the most effective medications available for the treatment of severe inflammatory disorders.

When given by the oral or parenteral routes, glucocorticoids have a number of serious adverse effects that limit their therapeutic utility. These include suppression of the normal functions of the adrenal gland (adrenal insufficiency), hyperglycemia, mood changes, cataracts, peptic ulcers, electrolyte imbalances, and osteoporosis. Because of their effectiveness at reducing the signs and symptoms of inflammation, glucocorticoids can mask infections that may be present in the patient. This combination of masking signs of active infection and suppressing the immune response creates a potential for infections to grow rapidly and remain undetected. An active infection is usually a contraindication for glucocorticoid therapy.

Because the appearance of these adverse effects is a function of the dose and duration of therapy, treatment is often

TABLE 33.4	Selected Glucocorticoids for Severe Inflammation	
Drug	**Route and Adult Dose (max dose where indicated)**	**Adverse Effects**
betamethasone (Celestone)	PO; 0.6–7.2 mg/day	*Mood swings, weight gain, acne, facial flushing, nausea, insomnia, sodium and fluid retention, impaired wound healing, menstrual abnormalities*
cortisone	PO/IM; 20–300 mg/day in divided doses	
dexamethasone	PO; 0.25–4 mg bid–qid	
hydrocortisone (Cortef, Hydrocortone, others) (see page 673 for the Prototype Drug box)	PO; 10–320 mg/day in three to four divided doses	<u>Peptic ulcer, hypocalcemia, osteoporosis with possible bone fractures, loss of muscle mass, decreased growth in children, possible masking of infections</u>
	IV/IM; 15–800 mg/day in three to four divided doses (max: 2 g/day)	
methylprednisolone (Depo-Medrol, Medrol)	PO; 2–60 mg/day in divided doses	
prednisolone (Orapred, Prelone)	PO; 5–60 mg one to four times/day	
prednisone	PO; 5–60 mg one to four times/day	
triamcinolone (Aristospan, Kenalog)	PO; 4–48 mg one to four times/day	

Italics indicate common adverse effects; <u>underlining</u> indicates serious adverse effects.

Pr Prototype Drug | Prednisone

Therapeutic Class: Anti-inflammatory agent   **Pharmacologic Class:** Glucocorticoid

ACTIONS AND USES

Prednisone is a synthetic glucocorticoid. Its actions are the result of being metabolized to an active form, which is also available as a drug called prednisolone (Orapred, Prelone, others). When used for inflammation, duration of therapy is commonly limited to 4 to 10 days. For long-term therapy, alternate-day dosing is used. Prednisone is occasionally used to terminate acute bronchospasm in patients with asthma and as an antineoplastic agent for patients with certain cancers such as Hodgkin's disease, acute leukemia, and lymphomas. It is available in tablet and oral solution forms.

ADMINISTRATION ALERTS

- Administer IM injections deep into the muscle mass to avoid atrophy or abscesses.
- Do not use if signs of a systemic infection are present.
- When using the drug for more than 10 days, the dose must be slowly tapered.
- Pregnancy category C

PHARMACOKINETICS
Onset: Unknown
Peak: 1–2 h
Half-life: 3.5 h
Duration: 24–36 h

ADVERSE EFFECTS

When used for short-term therapy, prednisone has few serious adverse effects. Long-term therapy may result in Cushing's syndrome, a condition that includes hyperglycemia, fat redistribution to the shoulders and face, muscle weakness, bruising, and bones that easily fracture. Because gastric ulcers may occur with long-term therapy, an antiulcer medication may be prescribed prophylactically. Use with caution in patients with peptic ulcer, ulcerative colitis, or diverticulitis.

Contraindications: Patients with active viral, bacterial, fungal, or protozoan infections should not take prednisone.

INTERACTIONS

Drug–Drug: Because barbiturates, phenytoin, and rifampin increase prednisone metabolism, increased doses may be required. Concurrent use with amphotericin B or diuretics increases potassium loss, which may be serious for patients taking digoxin. Because prednisone can raise blood glucose levels, diabetic patients may require an adjustment in the doses of insulin or oral hypoglycemic agents.

Lab Tests: Prednisone may inhibit antibody response to toxoids and vaccines and may increase blood glucose. Serum calcium, potassium, and thyroxine may decrease.

Herbal/Food: Herbal supplements such as aloe, buckthorn, and senna may increase potassium loss. Licorice may potentiate the effect of glucocorticoids. St. John's wort may decrease prednisone levels.

Treatment of Overdose: There is no specific treatment for overdose.

Refer to MyNursingKit for a Nursing Process Focus specific to this drug.

---

limited to the short-term control of acute disease. When longer therapy is indicated, doses are kept as low as possible and alternate-day therapy is sometimes implemented; the medication is taken every other day to encourage the patient's adrenal glands to function on the days when no drug is given. During long-term therapy, the nurse must be alert for signs of overtreatment with glucocorticoids, a condition known as **Cushing's syndrome.** Because the body becomes accustomed to high doses of glucocorticoids, patients must discontinue these drugs gradually; abrupt withdrawal can result in acute lack of adrenal function.

FEVER

Like inflammation, fever is a natural defense mechanism for neutralizing foreign organisms. Many species of bacteria are killed by high fever. Often, the health care provider must determine whether the fever needs to be dealt with aggressively or allowed to run its course. Drugs used to treat fever are called **antipyretics.**

33.6 Treating Fever with Antipyretics

In most patients, fever is more of a discomfort than a life-threatening problem. Prolonged, high fever, however, can become dangerous, especially in young children in whom fever can stimulate febrile seizures. In adults, excessively high fever can break down body tissues, reduce mental acuity, and lead to delirium or coma, particularly among elderly patients. In rare instances, an elevated body temperature may be fatal.

The goal of antipyretic therapy is to lower body temperature while treating the underlying cause of the fever, usually an infection. Aspirin, ibuprofen, and acetaminophen are safe, inexpensive, and effective drugs for reducing fever. Many of these antipyretics are marketed for different age groups, including special, flavored brands for infants and children. For fast delivery and effectiveness, drugs may come in various forms including gels, caplets, enteric-coated tablets, and suspensions. Aspirin and acetaminophen are also available as suppositories. The antipyretics come in various dosages and concentrations, including extra strength.

Although most fevers are caused by infectious processes, drugs themselves may be the cause. When the etiology of fever cannot be diagnosed, the nurse should consider drugs as a possible source. In many cases, withdrawal of the agent causing the drug-induced fever will quickly return body temperature to normal. In rare cases, drug-induced fever may be lethal. It is important for the nurse to recognize drugs that are most likely to cause drug-induced fever, including those in the following list:

- *Anti-infectives:* Anti-infectives, especially those derived from microorganisms such as amphotericin B or penicillin G, may be seen as foreign by the body and

RESEARCH SHOWS

The Question: Is there any evidence to support the use of alternating doses of ibuprofen and acetaminophen for children with fever?

The Study: Many health care providers treat febrile children with alternating doses of ibuprofen and acetaminophen in the belief that this combination is more effective or safer than using either drug individually. A recent study found a lack of evidence to support this practice.

Nursing Implications: Nurses should not assume that using these two drugs is either more effective or safer than using the drugs individually. Nurses should be certain that parents understand the proper dosing schedules for the individual antipyretics and advise them not to combine or alternate medications without the approval of their health care provider.

HOME & COMMUNITY CONSIDERATIONS

Aspirin for Cardiovascular Event Risk Reduction

Current practice related to cardiovascular and neurovascular event prevention and treatment may include the use of aspirin therapy. The blood's clotting action is slowed by the administration of aspirin. This therapy has been recommended for men older than 40 years of age, postmenopausal women, and men younger than 40 years of age and premenopausal women who have high cholesterol, hypertension, diabetes, history of a clot-related stroke or transient ischemic attack, or a history of cigarette smoking. Even though the frequently used dose for this therapy—81 mg—is available over the counter, patients should be advised to consult their health care providers before initiating self-medication with aspirin.

produce fever. When antibiotics kill microorganisms, fever-producing chemicals known as *pyrogens* may be released. Anti-infectives are the most common drugs known to induce fever.

- *Selective serotonin reuptake inhibitors (SSRIs):* Use of SSRIs such as paroxetine (Paxil) for depression or other

mood disorders can result in a high fever accompanied by serious mental status and cardiovascular changes, known as *serotonin syndrome* (chapter 16∞).

- *Conventional antipsychotic drugs:* Drugs such as chlorpromazine (Thorazine) may produce an elevated temperature with serious cardiovascular and respiratory

---

Pr Prototype Drug | Acetaminophen *(Tylenol, others)*

Therapeutic Class: Antipyretic and analgesic   **Pharmacologic Class:** Centrally acting COX inhibitor

ACTIONS AND USES

Acetaminophen reduces fever by direct action at the level of the hypothalamus and dilation of peripheral blood vessels, which enables sweating and dissipation of heat. Acetaminophen, ibuprofen, and aspirin have equal efficacy in relieving pain and reducing fever.

Acetaminophen has no anti-inflammatory properties; therefore, it is not effective in treating arthritis or pain caused by tissue swelling following injury. The primary therapeutic usefulness of acetaminophen is for the treatment of fever in children and for relief of mild to moderate pain when aspirin is contraindicated. In the treatment of severe pain, acetaminophen may be combined with opioids. This allows the dose of opioid to be reduced, thus decreasing the risk of dependence and serious opioid toxicity. It is available as tablets, caplets, solutions, and suppositories.

ADMINISTRATION ALERT

- Liquid forms are available in varying concentrations. Use the appropriate strength product in children to avoid toxicity.
- Never administer to patients who consume alcohol regularly due to the potential for hepatotoxicity.
- Advise patients that acetaminophen is found in many OTC products and that extreme care must be taken to not duplicate doses by taking several of these products concurrently.
- Pregnancy category B

PHARMACOKINETICS
Onset: 30–60 min
Peak: 0.5–2 h
Half-life: 1–3 h
Duration: 1–3 h

ADVERSE EFFECTS

Acetaminophen is generally safe, and adverse effects are uncommon at therapeutic doses. Acetaminophen causes less gastric irritation than aspirin, and does not affect blood coagulation. It is not recommended in patients who are malnourished. In such cases, acute toxicity may result, leading to renal failure, which can be fatal. Other signs of acute toxicity include nausea, vomiting, chills, abdominal discomfort, and fatal hepatic necrosis.

A major concern with the use of high doses of acetaminophen is the risk for liver damage. The drug has caused liver failure in a number of patients, which has resulted in the FDA issuing warnings regarding the use of the drug. The risk is significantly greater in patients who consume alcohol.

Contraindications: Contraindications include hypersensitivity to acetaminophen or phenacetin and chronic alcoholism.

INTERACTIONS

Drug–Drug: Acetaminophen inhibits warfarin metabolism, causing the anticoagulant to accumulate to toxic levels. High-dose or long-term acetaminophen use may result in elevated warfarin levels and bleeding. Ingestion of this drug with alcohol, or other hepatotoxic drugs such as phenytoin or barbiturates, is not recommended because of the possibility of liver failure from hepatic necrosis.

Lab Tests: Acetaminophen may increase hepatic function test values such as serum bilirubin, aspartate aminotransferase (AST), and alanine aminotransferase (ALT). It may increase urinary 5-hydroxyindole acetic acid (5-HIAA) and serum uric acid.

Herbal/Food: The patient should avoid taking herbs that have the potential for liver toxicity, including comfrey, coltsfoot, and chaparral.

Treatment of Overdose: The specific treatment for overdose is the oral or IV administration of *N*-acetylcysteine (Acetadote) as soon as possible after the overdose. This drug protects the liver from toxic metabolites of acetaminophen.

Refer to MyNursingKit for a Nursing Process Focus specific to this drug.

distress, called *neuroleptic malignant syndrome (NMS)* (chapter 17∞).

- *Volatile anesthetics and depolarizing neuromuscular blockers:* Agents such as succinylcholine can cause life-threatening *malignant hyperthermia* (chapter 19∞).

- *Immunomodulators:* Interferons and monoclonal antibodies such as muromonab-CD3 may cause a flulike syndrome because they cause the release of fever-producing cytokines (chapter 32∞).

- *Cytotoxic drugs:* Certain drugs used in cancer chemotherapy and to prevent transplant rejection profoundly dampen the immune response and result in fevers due to secondary infections.

- *Neutropenic agents:* Drugs such as NSAIDs, phenothiazines, antithyroid drugs, and antipsychotic agents can cause neutropenia and a subsequent fever.

- *Other drugs:* Systemic hypersensitivity reactions can result in high fever and anaphylaxis.

TREATING THE DIVERSE PATIENT

Ethnic Differences in Acetaminophen Metabolism

Certain ethnic populations, including Asians, African Americans, and Saudis, have higher rates of an enzyme deficiency that affects how they metabolize certain drugs. More than 200 million people worldwide are believed to have a hereditary deficiency of the enzyme, glucose-6-phosphate dehydrogenase (G6PD). Patients with G6PD deficiency are at risk for developing hemolysis after ingestion of certain drugs, including acetaminophen. Conflicting data exist on whether therapeutic dosages of acetaminophen can cause hemolysis in these patients. However, because acetaminophen is one of the most common drugs ingested in intentional overdoses, health care providers should recommend that patients with G6PD deficiency avoid this drug.

NURSING PROCESS FOCUS   PATIENTS RECEIVING ANTI-INFLAMMATORY AND ANTIPYRETIC THERAPY

Assessment	Potential Nursing Diagnoses
Baseline assessment prior to administration: ■ Understand the reason the drug has been prescribed in order to assess for therapeutic effects. ■ Obtain a complete health history including hepatic, renal, respiratory, cardiovascular or neurologic disease, pregnancy, or breast-feeding. Obtain a drug history including allergies, current prescription and OTC drugs, herbal preparations, caffeine, nicotine, and alcohol use. Be alert to possible drug interactions. ■ Obtain baseline vital signs and weight. ■ Evaluate appropriate laboratory findings (e.g., CBC, coagulation panels, bleeding time, electrolytes, glucose, lipid profile, hepatic or renal function studies).	■ Pain (Acute or Chronic) ■ Hyperthermia ■ Fluid Volume Deficit (related to fever) ■ Risk for Injury (related to adverse drug effects) ■ Risk for Infections (related to adverse drug effects of glucocorticoids) ■ Risk for Impaired Skin Integrity (related to adverse drug effects of glucocorticoids)
Assessment throughout administration: ■ Assess for desired therapeutic effects (e.g., temperature returns to normal range, pain is decreased or absent, signs and symptoms of inflammation such as redness or swelling are decreased). ■ Continue periodic monitoring of CBC, coagulation studies, bleeding time, electrolytes, glucose, lipids, and hepatic and renal function studies. ■ Assess vital signs and weight periodically or if symptoms warrant. For patients on glucocorticoids, obtain weight daily and report any weight gain over 1 kg in a 24-hour period or more than 2 kg in 1 week. ■ Assess for and promptly report adverse effects: symptoms of GI bleeding (dark or "tarry" stools, hematemesis or coffee-ground emesis, blood in the stool), abdominal pain, severe tinnitus, dizziness, drowsiness, confusion, agitation, euphoria or depression, palpitations, tachycardia, hypertension, increased respiratory rate and depth, pulmonary congestion, or edema.	

Planning: Patient Goals and Expected Outcomes

The patient will:
- Experience therapeutic effects (e.g., diminished fever, decreased or absent pain, decreased signs and symptoms of inflammation).
- Be free from, or experience minimal, adverse effects.
- Verbalize an understanding of the drug's use, adverse effects, and required precautions.
- Demonstrate proper self-administration of the medication (e.g., dose, timing, when to notify provider).

(Continued)

NURSING PROCESS FOCUS **PATIENTS RECEIVING ANTI-INFLAMMATORY AND ANTIPYRETIC THERAPY** *(Continued)*

Implementation

Interventions and (Rationales)	Patient and Family Education
Ensuring therapeutic effects: ▪ Continue assessments as described earlier for therapeutic effects. (Diminished fever, pain, or signs and symptoms of infection should begin after taking the first dose and continue to improve. The health care provider should be notified if fever remains present after 3 days or if increasing signs of infection are present.)	▪ Teach the patient to supplement drug therapy with nonpharmacologic measures, e.g., "RICE": **R**est, **I**ce or cool compresses, **C**ompression bandage (e.g., ACE wrap), and **E**levation of inflamed joint or limb; increased fluid intake for fever; positioning for comfort; diversionary distractions (e.g., television or music); and rest for pain.
Minimizing adverse effects: ▪ Continue to monitor vital signs, especially temperature if fever is present, and blood pressure and pulse for patients on glucocorticoids. (Fever should begin to diminish within 1 to 3 hours after taking the drug. Glucocortocoids may cause increased blood pressure, hypertension, and tachycardia due to increased retention of fluids.)	▪ Teach the patient to immediately report fever that does not diminish below 100°F, or per parameters set by the health care provider, febrile seizures, changes in behavior or level of consciousness, tachycardia, palpitations, or increased BP to the health care provider. ▪ Teach the patient on glucocorticoids how to monitor pulse and blood pressure. Ensure the proper use and functioning of any home equipment obtained.
▪ Continue to monitor periodic lab work: hepatic and renal function tests, CBC, electrolytes, glucose, lipid levels, and coagulation studies or bleeding time. (Aspirin and salicylates affect platelet aggregation and should be monitored if used long-term or if excessive bleeding or bruising is noted. Acetaminophen can be hepatotoxic. Corticosteroids affect the CBC, and a wide range of electrolytes, glucose.)	▪ Instruct the patient on the need to return periodically for lab work. ▪ Advise the patient taking glucocorticoids long term to carry a wallet identification card or wear medical identification jewelry indicating glucocorticoid therapy. ▪ Teach the patient to abstain from alcohol while taking acetaminophen. Men who consume more than two alcoholic beverages per day or women who consume more than one alcoholic beverage per day should not take acetaminophen.
▪ Monitor for abdominal pain, black or tarry stools, blood in the stool, hematemesis or coffee-ground emesis, dizziness, and hypotension, especially if associated with tachycardia. (NSAIDs and glucocorticoids may cause GI bleeding.)	▪ Instruct the patient to immediately report any signs or symptoms of GI bleeding. ▪ Teach the patient to take the drug with food or milk to decrease GI irritation and to swallow enteric-coated tablets whole without crushing or breaking. Alcohol use should be avoided or eliminated.
▪ Monitor for tinnitus, difficulty hearing, light-headedness, or difficulty with balance and report promptly. (NSAIDs and salicylates may be ototoxic.)	▪ Instruct the patient to immediately report any signs or symptoms of ringing, humming, buzzing in ears, difficulty with balance, dizziness or vertigo, or nausea.
▪ Monitor urine output and renal function studies periodically. (NSAIDs and salicylates may be renal toxic during long-term or high-dose therapy.)	▪ Instruct the patient on NSAIDs and salicylates to promptly report changes in quantity of urine output, darkening of urine, or edema. ▪ Teach the patient on NSAIDs and salicylates to increase fluid intake, especially if fever is present.
▪ Monitor electrolyte, blood glucose, and lipid levels periodically in patients on corticosteroids. (Glucocorticoids may cause hyperglycemia, hypernatremia, hyperlipidemia, and hypokalemia. Diabetics may require a change in antidiabetic medication if glucose remains elevated.)	▪ Instruct the patient to return periodically for lab work as needed. ▪ Teach the diabetic patient to test the blood sugar more frequently and notify the health care provider if a consistent elevation is noted.
▪ Monitor for signs and symptoms of infection in patients on glucocorticoids. (Glucocorticoids suppress the body's normal immune and inflammatory response and may mask the signs and symptoms of infection.)	▪ Instruct the patient to immediately report any signs or symptoms of infections (e.g., increasing temperature or fever, sore throat, redness or swelling at site of injury, white patches in mouth, vesicular rash).
▪ Monitor for osteoporosis (e.g., bone density testing) periodically in patients on glucocorticoids. Encourage adequate calcium intake, avoidance of carbonated sodas, and weight-bearing exercise. (Glucocorticoids affect bone metabolism and may cause osteoporosis and fractures. Weight-bearing exercise stresses bone and encourages normal bone remodeling. Excessive or long-term consumption of carbonated sodas has been linked to an increased risk of osteoporosis.)	▪ Teach the patient to maintain adequate calcium in the diet, avoid carbonated sodas, and to do weight-bearing exercises at least three to four times per week. ▪ Teach the postmenopausal woman to consult with her provider about the need for additional drug therapy (e.g., bisphosphonates) for osteoporosis.
▪ Monitor for unusual changes in mood or affect in patients on corticosteroids. (Glucocorticoids may cause mood changes, euphoria, depression, or severe mental instability.)	▪ Teach the patient, family, or caregiver to promptly report excessive mood swings or unusual changes in mood.

NURSING PROCESS FOCUS   **PATIENTS RECEIVING ANTI-INFLAMMATORY AND ANTIPYRETIC THERAPY** *(Continued)*

Implementation

Interventions and (Rationales)	Patient and Family Education
▪ Weigh patient on glucocorticoids daily and report a weight gain of 1 kg or more in a 24-hour period or more than 2 kg per week or increasing peripheral edema. Measure intake and output in the hospitalized patient. (Daily weight is an accurate measure of fluid status and takes into account intake, output, and insensible losses. Patients on corticosteroids will experience some fluid retention.)	▪ Instruct the patient to weigh self daily, ideally at the same time of day. The patient should report significant weight gain or increasing peripheral edema.
▪ Monitor vision periodically in patients on glucocorticoids. (These drugs may cause increased intraocular pressure and an increased risk or glaucoma, and may cause cataracts.)	▪ Teach the patient on glucocorticoids to maintain eye exams twice yearly or more frequently as instructed by the health care provider. Report any eye pain, rainbow halos around lights, diminished vision, or blurring and inability to focus immediately.
▪ Avoid the use of aspirin or salicylates in children under 18 unless explicitly ordered by the health care provider. (Aspirin has been associated with an increased risk of Reye's syndrome in children under 18, particularly associated with the flu virus and varicella infections.)	▪ Instruct parents to use NSAIDs or acetaminophen in children under 18 for fever or pain control, unless otherwise ordered by the provider. ▪ Teach parents to read labels on all OTC medications and to avoid formulations with aspirin or salicylate on the label.
▪ Do not stop glucocorticoids abruptly. Drug must be tapered off if used longer than 1 or 2 weeks. (Adrenal insufficiency and crisis may occur with profound hypotension, tachycardia, and other adverse effects if the drug is stopped abruptly.)	▪ Teach the patient to not stop taking glucocorticoids abruptly and to notify the health care provider if unable to take medication for more than 1 day due to illness.
Patient understanding of drug therapy: ▪ Use opportunities during administration of medications and during assessments to discuss the rationale for drug therapy, desired therapeutic outcomes, most common adverse effects, parameters for when to call the health care provider, and any necessary monitoring or precautions. (Using time during nursing care helps to optimize and reinforce key teaching areas.)	▪ The patient, family, or caregiver should be able to state the reason for the drug; appropriate dose and scheduling; what adverse effects to observe for and when to report; and the anticipated length of medication therapy.
Patient self-administration of drug therapy: ▪ When administering the medication, instruct the patient, family, or caregiver in proper self-administration of drug, e.g., with food or milk. (Proper administration will increase the effectiveness of the drug. Household measuring devices such as teaspoons differ significantly in size and amount and should not be used for pediatric or liquid doses.)	▪ The patient, family, or caregiver are able to discuss appropriate dosing and administration needs, including: ▪ Glucocorticoids should be taken in the morning at the same time each day. ▪ NSAIDs and glucocorticoids should be taken with food or milk to decrease GI upset. ▪ Liquid doses of acetaminophen or NSAIDs should be measured with the enclosed dosage cup, dropper, or spoon. If that measuring device is no longer available, do NOT use a household spoon but obtain another calibrated measuring cup or dropper.

Evaluation of Outcome Criteria

Evaluate the effectiveness of drug therapy by confirming that patient goals and expected outcomes have been met (see "Planning").

See Table 33.2 for a list of the drugs to which these nursing actions apply. Acetaminophen is also covered in this Nursing Process Focus chart.

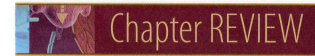

Chapter REVIEW

KEY CONCEPTS

The numbered key concepts provide a succinct summary of the important points from the corresponding numbered section within the chapter. If any of these points are not clear, refer to the numbered section within the chapter for review.

33.1 Inflammation is a natural, nonspecific body defense that limits the spread of invading microorganisms or injury. Acute inflammation occurs over several days, whereas chronic inflammation may continue for months or years.

33.2 Chemicals, pathogens, and physical trauma cause the release of chemical mediators that trigger the inflammatory response. Histamine is one of the key chemical mediators in inflammation. Release of histamine produces vasodilation, allowing capillaries to become leaky, thus causing tissue swelling.

33.3 Inflammation may be treated with nonpharmacologic and pharmacologic therapies. When possible, topical drugs are used because they produce fewer adverse effects than oral or parenteral drugs. The two primary drug classes used for inflammation are the NSAIDs and glucocorticoids.

33.4 Nonsteroidal anti-inflammatory drugs (NSAIDs) are the primary drugs for the treatment of mild to moderate inflammation. All drugs in this class have similar effectiveness in treating inflammation. The selective COX-2 inhibitors cause less GI distress but have significant cardiovascular side effects.

33.5 Systemic glucocorticoids are effective in treating acute or severe inflammation. Overtreatment with these drugs can cause a serious condition called Cushing's syndrome; thus, therapy for inflammation is generally short term.

33.6 Acetaminophen and NSAIDs are the primary agents used to treat fever. Certain medications may cause drug-induced fever, which may range from mild to life threatening.

NCLEX-RN® REVIEW QUESTIONS

1 On discharge of the patient, the nurse discusses types of over-the-counter NSAID medications that are available. The nurse knows that which of the following OTC medications is often used for pain and fever but is not classified as an NSAID?
1. Aspirin
2. Ibuprofen
3. Acetaminophen
4. Motrin

2 The patient has been taking aspirin for several days for headache. During the assessment, the nurse discovers the patient is experiencing ringing in the ears and dizziness. What is the most appropriate action by the nurse?
1. Question the patient about history of sinus infections.
2. Determine if the patient has mixed the aspirin with other medications.
3. Tell the patient not to take any more aspirin.
4. Tell the patient to take the aspirin with food or milk.

3 While educating the patient about glucocorticoids, the nurse would instruct the patient to contact the health care provider immediately if:
1. there is a decrease of 2 lb in weight.
2. there is an increase in appetite.
3. there is any diarrhea.
4. there is any difficulty breathing.

4 The nurse is admitting a patient with rheumatoid arthritis. The patient has been taking glucocorticoids for an extended period of time. During the assessment, the nurse observes that the patient has a very round moon-shaped face, bruising, and an abnormal contour of the shoulders. What does the nurse conclude based on these findings?
1. These are normal reactions with the illness.
2. These are probably birth defects.
3. These are symptoms of myasthenia gravis.
4. These are symptoms of adverse drug effects from the corticosteroids.

5 A 24-year-old patient reports taking acetaminophen (Tylenol) fairly regularly for headaches. The nurse knows that a patient who consumes excess acetaminophen per day or regularly consumes alcoholic beverages should be observed for:
1. hepatic toxicity.
2. renal damage.
3. thrombotic effects.
4. pulmonary damage.

6 The nurse is counseling a mother regarding antipyretic choices for her 8-year-old daughter. When asked why aspirin is not a good drug to use, the nurse bases her answer on her knowledge that aspirin:
1. is not as good an antipyretic as is acetaminophen.
2. may increase fever in children under age 10.
3. may produce nausea and vomiting.
4. increases the risk of Reye's syndrome in children under 18 with viral infections.

CRITICAL THINKING QUESTIONS

1. A 64-year-old diabetic patient is on prednisone for rheumatoid arthritis. The patient has recently been admitted to the hospital for stabilization of hyperglycemia. What are the nurse's primary concerns when caring for this patient?

2. A 44-year-old patient is requesting medication for a painful tendinitis of the elbow. This patient has mild hypertension, a history of alcohol abuse, and nutritional deficits. This patient has orders for acetaminophen (Tylenol), ibuprofen (Motrin), and celecoxib (Celebrex). Which one would the nurse give and why?

3. The mother of a 7-year-old child calls the health care provider's office stating that her daughter has a temperature of 101°F. She states the child is also complaining of being tired and "achy" all over. The mother asks how much aspirin she can giver her daughter for her temperature. How should the nurse respond?

See Appendix D for answers and rationales for all activities.

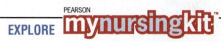

EXPLORE **mynursingkit**

MyNursingKit is your one stop for online chapter review materials and resources. Prepare for success with additional NCLEX®-style practice questions, interactive assignments and activities, web links, animations and videos, and more!

Register your access code from the front of your book at
www.mynursingkit.com.

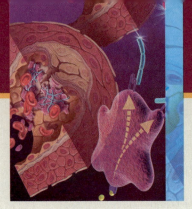

Chapter 34

Drugs for Bacterial Infections

LEARNING OUTCOMES

After reading this chapter, the student should be able to:

1. Distinguish between the terms pathogenicity and virulence.
2. Explain how bacteria are described and classified.
3. Compare and contrast the terms bacteriostatic and bacteriocidal.
4. Using a specific example, explain how resistance can develop to an anti-infective drug.
5. Describe the nurse's role in the pharmacologic management of bacterial infections.
6. Explain the importance of culture and sensitivity testing to anti-infective chemotherapy.
7. Identify the mechanism of development and symptoms of superinfections caused by anti-infective therapy.
8. For each of the drug classes listed in Drugs at a Glance, know representative drug examples, and explain their mechanism of action, primary actions, and important adverse effects.
9. Explain how the pharmacotherapy of tuberculosis differs from that of other infections.
10. Use the nursing process to care for patients who are receiving drug therapy for bacterial infections.

KEY TERMS

he human body has adapted quite well to living in a world teeming with microorganisms (microbes). Present in the air, water, food, and soil, microbes are an essential component of life on the planet. In some cases, such as with microorganisms in the colon, microbes play a beneficial role in human health. When in an unnatural environment or when present in unusually high numbers, however, microorganisms can cause a variety of ailments ranging from mildly annoying to fatal. The development of the first anti-infective drugs in the mid-1900s was a milestone in the field of medicine. In the last 50 years, pharmacologists have attempted to keep pace with microbes that rapidly become resistant to therapeutic agents. This chapter examines two groups of anti-infectives, the antibacterial agents and the specialized drugs used to treat tuberculosis.

34.1 Pathogenicity and Virulence

An organism that can cause disease is called a **pathogen.** Human pathogens include viruses, bacteria, fungi, unicellular organisms (protozoans), and multicellular animals. To infect humans, pathogens must bypass a number of elaborate body defenses, such as those described in chapters 32 and 33∞. Pathogens may enter through broken skin, or by ingestion, inhalation, or contact with a mucous membrane such as the nasal, urinary, or vaginal mucosa.

Some pathogens are extremely infectious and life threatening to humans, while others simply cause annoying symptoms or none at all. The ability of an organism to cause infection, or **pathogenicity,** depends on an organism's ability to evade or overcome body defenses. Fortunately for us, only a few dozen pathogens commonly cause disease in humans. Another common word used to describe a pathogen is

virulence. A highly virulent microbe is one that can produce disease when present in minute numbers.

After gaining entry, pathogens generally cause disease by one of two basic mechanisms: invasiveness or toxin production. **Invasiveness** is the ability of a pathogen to grow extremely rapidly and cause direct damage to surrounding tissues by their sheer numbers. Because a week or more may be needed to mount an immune response against the organism, this rapid growth can easily overwhelm body defenses. A second mechanism is the production of toxins. Even very small amounts of some bacterial toxins may disrupt normal cellular activity and, in extreme cases, result in death.

34.2 Describing and Classifying Bacteria

Because of the enormous number of different bacterial species, several descriptive systems have been developed to simplify their study. It is important for nurses to learn these classification schemes, because drugs that are effective against one organism in a class are likely to be effective against other pathogens in the same class. Common bacterial pathogens and the types of diseases that they cause are listed in Table 34.1.

One of the simplest methods of classifying bacteria is to examine them microscopically after a crystal violet Gram stain is applied. Some bacteria contain a thick cell wall and retain a purple color after staining. These are called **gram-positive bacteria** and include staphylococci, streptococci, and enterococci. Bacteria that have thinner cell walls will lose the violet stain and are called **gram-negative bacteria.** Examples of gram-negative bacteria include bacteroides, *Escherichia coli,* klebsiella, pseudomonas, and salmonella. The distinction between gram-positive and gram-negative bacteria is a profound one that reflects important biochemical and physiologic differences between the two groups. Some antibacterial agents are effective only against gram-positive bacteria, whereas others are used to treat gram-negative bacteria.

A second descriptive method is based on cellular shape. Bacteria assume several basic shapes that can be readily determined microscopically. Rod shapes are called *bacilli,* spherical shapes are called *cocci,* and spirals are called *spirilla.*

A third factor used to classify bacteria is based on their ability to use oxygen. Those that thrive in an oxygen-rich environment are called **aerobic;** those that grow best without oxygen are called **anaerobic.** Some organisms have the ability to change their metabolism and survive in *either* aerobic or anaerobic conditions, depending on their external environment. Antibacterial drugs differ in their effectiveness in treating aerobic versus anaerobic bacteria.

34.3 Classification of Anti-Infective Drugs

Anti-infective is a general term that applies to any drug that is effective against pathogens. In its broadest sense, an

---

PharmFacts

Bacterial Infections

- Infectious diseases are the third most common cause of death in the United States, and first in the world.
- Food-borne illness is responsible for 76,000,000 illnesses; 300,000 hospitalizations; and 5,000 deaths each year.
- Urinary tract infections (UTIs) are the most common infection acquired in hospitals, and nearly all are associated with the insertion of a urinary catheter.
- More than 2 million nosocomial infections are acquired each year. These infections add 1 day for UTIs, 7 to 8 days for surgical site infections, and 6 to 30 days for pneumonia.
- Up to 30% of all *S. pneumoniae* found in some areas of the United States are resistant to penicillin.
- Nearly all strains of *S. aureus* in the United States are resistant to penicillin.
- About 73,000 cases of *E. coli* poisoning are reported annually in the United States, with the most common source being ground beef.

TABLE 34.1   Common Bacterial Pathogens and Disorders

Name of Organism	Disease(s)	Description
Bacillus anthracis	Anthrax	Aerobe; appears in cutaneous and respiratory forms
Borrelia burgdorferi	Lyme disease	Acquired from tick bites
Chlamydia trachomatis	Venereal disease, eye infection	Most common cause of sexually transmitted disease in the United States
Escherichia coli	Traveler's diarrhea, UTI, bacteremia, meningitis in children	Part of host flora of the intestinal tract
Haemophilus	Pneumonia, meningitis in children, bacteremia, otitis media, sinusitis	Some species are part of the normal host flora of the upper respiratory tract
Klebsiella	Pneumonia, UTI	Common opportunistic microbe
Mycobacterium leprae	Leprosy	Most cases in the United States occur in immigrants from Africa or Asia
Mycobacterium tuberculosis	Tuberculosis	Incidence very high in HIV-infected patients
Mycoplasma pneumoniae	Pneumonia	Most common cause of pneumonia in patients age 5–35
Neisseria gonorrhoeae	Gonorrhea and other sexually transmitted diseases, endometriosis, neonatal eye infection	Some species are part of the normal host flora
Neisseria meningitidis	Meningitis in children	Some species are part of the normal host flora
Pneumococci	Pneumonia, otitis media, meningitis, bacteremia, endocarditis	Part of normal host flora in upper respiratory tract
Proteus mirabilis	UTI, skin infections	Part of normal host flora in GI tract
Pseudomonas aeruginosa	UTI, skin infections, septicemia	Common opportunistic microbe
Rickettsia rickettsii	Rocky Mountain spotted fever	Acquired from tick bites
Salmonella enteritidis	Food poisoning	Acquired from infected animal products; raw eggs, undercooked meat or chicken
Staphylococcus aureus	Pneumonia, food poisoning, impetigo, wounds, bacteremia, endocarditis, toxic shock syndrome, osteomyelitis, UTI	Some species are part of the normal host flora
Streptococcus	Pharyngitis, pneumonia, skin infections, septicemia, endocarditis, otitis media	Some species are part of the normal host flora

anti-infective drug may be used to treat bacterial, fungal, viral, or parasitic infections. The most frequent term used to describe an anti-infective drug is antibiotic. Technically, **antibiotic** refers to a natural substance produced by bacteria that can kill other bacteria. In clinical practice, however, the terms *antibacterial, anti-infective, antimicrobial,* and *antibiotic* are often used interchangeably.

With more than 300 anti-infective drugs available, it is helpful to group these drugs into classes that have similar properties. Two means of grouping are widely used: chemical classes and pharmacologic classes.

Chemical class names such as aminoglycosides, fluoroquinolones, and sulfonamides refer to the fundamental chemical structure of the anti-infectives. Anti-infectives belonging to the same chemical class usually share similar antibacterial properties and adverse effects. Although chemical names are often long and difficult to pronounce, placing drugs into chemical classes will assist the student in mentally organizing these drugs into distinct therapeutic groups.

Pharmacologic classes are used to group anti-infectives by their *mechanism of action*. Examples include cell wall inhibitors, protein synthesis inhibitors, folic acid inhibitors,

and reverse transcriptase inhibitors. These classifications are used in this textbook, where appropriate.

34.4 Actions of Anti-Infective Drugs

The primary goal of antimicrobial therapy is to assist the body's defenses in eliminating a pathogen. Medications that accomplish this goal by *killing* bacteria are called **bacteriocidal**. Some drugs do not kill the bacteria but instead slow their growth, allowing the body's natural defenses to eliminate the microorganisms. These *growth-slowing* drugs are called **bacteriostatic**.

Bacterial cells have distinct anatomic and physiologic differences compared to human cells. Bacteria have cell walls, use different biochemical pathways, and contain certain enzymes that human cells lack. Antibiotics exert *selective toxicity* on bacterial cells by targeting these unique differences. Through this selective action, pathogens can be killed or their growth severely hampered without major effects on human cells. Of course, there are limits to this selective toxicity, depending on the specific antibiotic and the dose employed, and adverse effects can be expected from all anti-infectives. The basic mechanisms of action of antimicrobial drugs are shown in ▶ Figure 34.1.

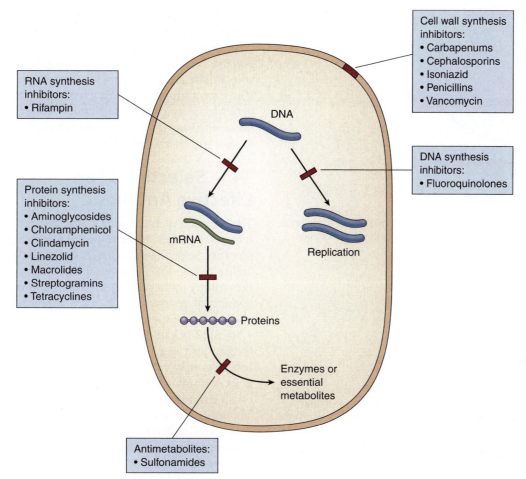

RNA synthesis
inhibitors:
• Rifampin

Cell wall synthesis
inhibitors:
• Carbapenums
• Cephalosporins
• Isoniazid
• Penicillins
• Vancomycin

DNA

DNA synthesis
inhibitors:
• Fluoroquinolones

Protein synthesis
inhibitors:
• Aminoglycosides
• Chloramphenicol
• Clindamycin
• Linezolid
• Macrolides
• Streptogramins
• Tetracyclines

mRNA

Replication

Proteins

Enzymes or
essential
metabolites

Antimetabolites:
• Sulfonamides

> **Figure 34.1** Mechanisms of action of antimicrobial drugs

34.5 Acquired Resistance

Microorganisms have the ability to replicate extremely rapidly. For example, under ideal conditions *E. coli* can produce a million cells every 20 minutes. During this rapid replication, bacteria make frequent errors while duplicating their genetic code. These **mutations** occur spontaneously and randomly throughout the bacterial chromosome. Although most mutations are harmful to the organism, mutations occasionally result in a bacterial cell that has reproductive advantages over its neighbors. The mutated bacterium may be able to survive in harsher conditions or perhaps grow faster than surrounding cells. Mutations that are of particular importance to medicine are those that confer drug resistance to a microorganism.

Antibiotics help promote the development of drug-resistant bacterial strains. Killing populations of bacteria that are sensitive to the drug leaves behind those microbes that possess mutations that made them insensitive to the effects of the antibiotic. These drug-resistant bacteria are then free to grow, unrestrained by their neighbors that were killed by the antibiotic, and the patient develops an infection that is resistant to conventional drug therapy. This phenomenon, **acquired resistance**, is illustrated in ➤ Figure 34.2. Bacteria may pass the resistance gene to other bacteria through *conjugation*, the transfer of small pieces of circular DNA called **plasmids.**

It is important to understand that the antibiotic did not *create* the mutation that caused bacteria to become resistant. The mutation occurred randomly. The role that the antibiotic plays in resistance is to kill the surrounding cells that were susceptible to the drug, leaving the mutated ones plenty of room to divide and infect the host. It is the bacteria that have become resistant, not the patient. An individual with an infection that is resistant to certain antibacterial agents can transmit the resistant bacteria to others.

The widespread and sometimes unwarranted use of antibiotics has led to a large number of resistant bacterial strains. At least 60% of *Staphylococcus aureus* infections are now resistant to penicillin, and resistant strains of *Enterococcus faecalis, Enterococcus faecium,* and *Pseudomonas aeruginosa* have become major clinical problems. The longer an antibiotic is used in the population and the more often it is prescribed, the larger the percentage of resistant strains. Infections acquired in a hospital or other health care setting, called **nosocomial infections,** are often resistant to common antibiotics. Resistant nosocomial infections are especially troublesome in critical care units, where seriously ill patients are often treated with high amounts of antibiotics. Two particularly serious resistant infections are those caused by methicillin-resistant *Staphylococcus aureus* (MRSA) and vancomycin-resistant enterococci (VRE).

MyNursingKit | Veterinary Antibiotics and Human Health

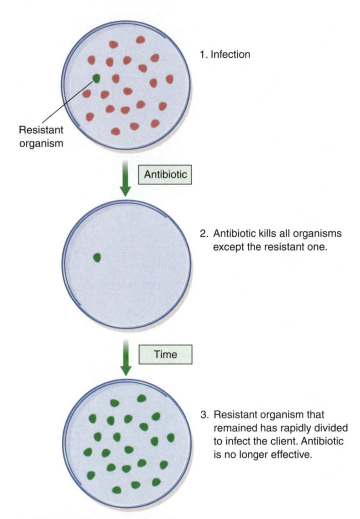

1. Infection

Resistant organism

Antibiotic

2. Antibiotic kills all organisms except the resistant one.

Time

3. Resistant organism that remained has rapidly divided to infect the client. Antibiotic is no longer effective.

➤ *Figure 34.2* Acquired resistance

Health care providers play important roles in delaying the emergence of resistance. The following are five principles recommended by the CDC:

- Prevent infections whenever possible. It is always easier to prevent an infection, than to treat one. This includes teaching the patient the importance of getting immunizations.

- Use the right drug for the infection. Infections should be cultured so that the offending organism can be identified and the correct drug chosen (see Section 34.6).

- Restrict the use of antibiotics to those conditions deemed medically necessary. Antibiotics should only be prescribed when there is a clear rationale for their use.

- Advise the patient to take anti-infectives for the full length of therapy, even if symptoms disappear before the regimen is finished. Prematurely stopping antibiotic therapy allows some pathogens to survive, thus promoting the development of resistant strains.

- Prevent transmission of the pathogen by using proper infection control procedures. This includes the use of standard precautions and teaching patients methods of proper hygiene for preventing transmission in the home and community settings.

In most cases, antibiotics are given when there is clear evidence of bacterial infection. Some patients, however, receive antibiotics to *prevent* an infection, a practice called *prophylactic* use, or *chemoprophylaxis*. Examples of patients who might receive prophylactic antibiotics include those who have a suppressed immune system, those who have experienced deep puncture wounds such as from dog bites, or those who have prosthetic heart valves and are about to have medical or dental procedures.

34.6 Selection of an Effective Antibiotic

The selection of an antibiotic that will be effective against a specific pathogen is an important task of the health care provider. Selecting an incorrect drug will delay proper treatment, giving the microorganisms more time to invade. Prescribing ineffective antibiotics also promotes the development of resistance, and may cause unnecessary adverse effects in the patient.

Ideally, laboratory tests should be conducted to identify the specific pathogen *prior to* beginning anti-infective therapy. Lab tests may include examination of urine, stool, spinal fluid, sputum, blood, or purulent drainage for microorganisms. Organisms isolated from the specimens are grown in the laboratory and identified. After identification, the laboratory tests several different antibiotics to determine which is most effective against the infecting microorganism. This process of growing the pathogen and identifying the most effective antibiotic is called **culture and sensitivity (C&S) testing.**

Because antibiotic therapy alters the composition of infected fluids, samples should be collected prior to starting pharmacotherapy. However, laboratory testing and identification may take several days and, in the case of viruses, several weeks. If the infection is severe, therapy is often begun with a **broad-spectrum antibiotic,** one that is effective against a wide variety of different microbial species. After laboratory testing is completed, the drug may be changed to a **narrow-spectrum antibiotic,** one that is effective against a smaller group of microbes or only the isolated species. In general, narrow-spectrum antibiotics have less effect on normal host flora, thus causing fewer side effects. For mild infections, laboratory identification is not always necessary; skilled health care providers are often able to make an accurate diagnosis based on patient signs and symptoms.

In most cases, antibacterial therapy is best conducted using a single drug. Combining two antibiotics may actually decrease each drug's efficacy, a phenomenon known as *antagonism*. If incorrect combinations are prescribed, the use of multiple antibiotics also has the potential to promote resistance. Multidrug therapy is warranted, however, if several different organisms are causing the patient's infection or if the infection is so severe that therapy must be started before laboratory tests have been completed. Multidrug therapy is clearly warranted in the treatment of tuberculosis or in patients infected with HIV.

One common adverse effect of anti-infective therapy is the appearance of secondary infections, known as **superinfections,** which occur when microorganisms normally present in the body are destroyed. These normal microorganisms, or **host flora,** inhabit the skin and the upper respiratory, genitourinary, and intestinal tracts. Some of these organisms serve a useful purpose by producing antibacterial substances and by competing with pathogenic organisms for space and nutrients. Removal of host flora by an antibiotic gives the remaining microorganisms an opportunity to grow, allowing for overgrowth of pathogenic microbes. Host flora themselves can cause disease if allowed to proliferate without control, or if they establish colonies in abnormal locations. For example *E. coli* is part of the host flora in the colon but can become a serious pathogen if it enters the urinary tract. Host flora may also become pathogenic if the patient's immune system becomes suppressed. Microbes that become pathogenic when the immune system is suppressed are called *opportunistic* organisms. Viruses such as the herpes virus, and fungi are examples of opportunistic organisms that exist on the human body but may become pathogenic if normal flora are suppressed.

Superinfection should be suspected if a new infection appears while the patient is receiving anti-infective therapy. Signs and symptoms of a superinfection commonly include diarrhea, bladder pain, painful urination, or abnormal vaginal discharges. Broad-spectrum antibiotics are more likely to cause superinfections because they kill so many different species of microorganisms.

34.7 Host Factors

The most important factor in selecting an appropriate antibiotic is to be certain that the microbe is sensitive to the effects of the drug. However, the nurse must also take into account certain host factors that can influence the success of antibacterial chemotherapy.

The primary goal of antibiotic therapy is to kill enough bacteria, or to slow the growth of the infection, so that natural body defenses can overcome the invading agent. Unless an infection is highly localized, the antibiotic alone may not be enough: The patient's immune system and phagocytic cells will be needed to completely rid the body of the infectious agent. Patients with suppressed immune systems may require aggressive antibiotic therapy with bacteriocidal agents. These patients include those with AIDS and those being treated with immunosuppressive or antineoplastic drugs. Because therapy is more successful when the number of microbes is small, antibiotics may be given on a prophylactic basis to patients whose white blood cell (WBC) count is extremely low.

Local conditions at the infection site should be considered when selecting an antibiotic because factors that hinder the drug from reaching microbes will limit therapeutic success. Infections of the central nervous system are particularly difficult to treat because many drugs cannot cross the blood–brain barrier. Injury or inflammation can cause tissues to become acidic or anaerobic and to have poor circulation. Excessive pus formation or hematomas can block drugs from reaching their targets. Although most bacteria are extracellular in nature, pathogens such as *Mycobacterium tuberculosis,* salmonella, toxoplasma, and

listeria may reside intracellularly and thus be difficult for anti-infectives to reach in high concentrations. Consideration of these factors may necessitate a change in the route of drug administration or the selection of a more effective antibiotic specific for the local conditions.

Severe allergic reactions to antibiotics, while not common, may be fatal. The nurse's initial patient assessment must include a thorough drug history and a description of any reactions to those drugs. A previous acute allergic incident is highly predictive of future hypersensitivity. If severe allergy to an anti-infective is established, it is best to avoid all drugs in the same chemical class. Because the patient may have been exposed to an antibiotic unknowingly, through food products or molds, allergic reactions can occur without previous incident. Penicillins are the class of antibacterials having the highest incidence of allergic reactions; between 0.7% and 4% of all patients who receive them exhibit some degree of hypersensitivity.

Other host factors to be considered are age, pregnancy status, and genetics. The very young and the very old are often unable to readily metabolize or excrete antibiotics; thus, doses are generally decreased. Some antibiotics cross the placenta. For example, tetracyclines taken by the mother can cause teeth discoloration in the newborn; aminoglycosides can affect the infant's hearing. The benefits of antibiotic use in pregnant or lactating women must be carefully weighed against the potential risks to the fetus and neonate. Lastly, some patients have a genetic absence of certain enzymes used to metabolize antibiotics. For example, patients with a deficiency of the enzyme glucose-6-phosphate dehydrogenase should not receive sulfonamides, chloramphenicol, or nalidixic acid because their erythrocytes may rupture.

ANTIBACTERIAL AGENTS

Antibacterial agents are derived from a large number of chemical classes. Although drugs within a class have similarities in their mechanisms and spectrum of activity, each is slightly different, and learning the differences and therapeutic applications among antibacterial agents can be challenging. Basic nursing assessments and interventions

TREATING THE DIVERSE PATIENT

Hispanic Cultural Beliefs and Antibacterials

Certain ethnic groups, such as Hispanics, believe that illness is caused by an imbalance in hot and cold. In a healthy individual, hot and cold are in balance; when an imbalance occurs, disease results.

Illnesses are classified as either hot or cold as well. For example, sore throat and diarrhea are considered hot diseases; colds, upper respiratory infections, arthritis, and rheumatism are considered cold diseases. Traditional treatment in such cultures is to restore the body's balance through the addition or subtraction of herbs, foods, or medications that are classified as either hot or cold. To treat a hot disease, medications or herbs considered cold are used. For example, penicillin is considered a hot medicine, but amoxicillin is less hot. Using acetaminophen with amoxicillin makes it cooler.

apply to all antibiotic therapies; however, the nurse should individualize the plan of care based on the patient's condition, the infection, and the antibacterial agent prescribed.

Penicillins

Although not the first anti-infective discovered, penicillin was the first mass-produced antibiotic. Isolated from the fungus *Penicillium* in 1941, the drug quickly became a miracle product by preventing thousands of deaths from infections. The penicillins are listed in Table 34.2.

34.8 Pharmacotherapy with Penicillins

Penicillins kill bacteria by disrupting their cell walls. Many bacterial cell walls contain a substance called **penicillin-binding protein** that serves as a receptor for penicillin. Upon binding, penicillin weakens the cell wall and allows water to enter, thus killing the organism. Human cells do not contain cell walls; therefore, the actions of the penicillins are specific to bacterial cells. Gram-positive bacteria are the most commonly affected by the penicillins, including streptococci and staphylococci. Penicillins are indicated for the treatment of

pneumonia; meningitis; skin, bone, and joint infections; stomach infections; blood and valve infections; gas gangrene; tetanus; anthrax; and sickle-cell anemia in infants.

The portion of the chemical structure of penicillin that is responsible for its antibacterial activity is called the **beta-lactam ring**. Some bacteria secrete an enzyme, called **beta-lactamase** or **penicillinase**, which splits the beta-lactam ring. This structural change allows these bacteria to become resistant to the effects of most penicillins. Since their discovery, large numbers of resistant bacterial strains have emerged that limit the therapeutic usefulness of the penicillins. The action of penicillinase is illustrated in ➤ Figure 34.3. Other classes of antibiotics also contain the beta-lactam ring, including the cephalosporins, carbapenems, and monobactams.

Chemical modifications to the natural penicillin molecule produced drugs offering several advantages. They include the following:

- *Penicillinase-resistant penicillins:* Oxacillin and cloxacillin (Cloxapen) are examples of drugs that are effective against penicillinase-producing bacteria. These are sometimes called antistaphylococcal penicillins.

- *Broad-spectrum penicillins:* Ampicillin (Principen) and amoxicillin (Amoxil, Trimox) are effective against a wide range of microorganisms and are called *broad-spectrum*

TABLE 34.2	Penicillins	
Drug	**Route and Adult Dose (max dose where indicated)**	**Adverse Effects**
NATURAL PENICILLINS		
penicillin G benzathine (Bicillin)	IM; 1.2 million units as a single dose (max: 2.4 million units/day)	*Rash, pruritus, diarrhea, nausea, fever, drowsiness*
penicillin G procaine (Wycillin)	IM; 600,000–1.2 million units/day (max: 4.8 million units/day)	
℞ penicillin G sodium/potassium	IM/IV; 2–24 million units divided every 4–6 h (max: 80 million units/day)	Anaphylaxis symptoms, including angioedema, circulatory collapse and cardiac arrest; nephrotoxicity
penicillin V (Pen-Vee K, Veetids, Vee-Cillin-K)	PO; 125–250 mg qid (max: 7.2 g/day)	
PENICILLINASE-RESISTANT		
cloxacillin (Cloxapen)	PO; 250–500 mg bid	
dicloxacillin	PO; 125–500 mg qid (max: 4 g/day)	
nafcillin	PO; 250 mg–1 g qid (max: 12 g/day)	
oxacillin	PO; 250 mg–1 g qid (max: 12 g/day)	
BROAD-SPECTRUM (AMINOPENICILLINS)		
amoxicillin (Amoxil, Trimox)	PO; 250–500 mg every 6 h (max: 1,750 mg/day)	
amoxicillin–clavulanate (Augmentin)	PO; 250 or 500 mg tablet (each with 125 mg clavulanic acid) every 8–12 h	
ampicillin (Principen)	PO/IV/IM; 250–500 mg every 6 h (max: 4 g/day PO or 14 g/day IV/IM)	
bacampicillin (Spectrobid)	PO; 400–800 mg bid	
EXTENDED-SPECTRUM (ANTIPSEUDOMONAL)		
carbenicillin (Geocillin)	PO; 382–764 mg qid	
piperacillin sodium	IM; 2–4 g tid–qid (max: 24 g/day)	
piperacillin tazobactam (Zosyn)	IV; 3.375 g qid over 30 min	
ticarcillin (Ticar)	IM; 1–2 g qid (max: 24 g/day)	

Italics indicate common adverse effects; underlining indicates serious adverse effects.

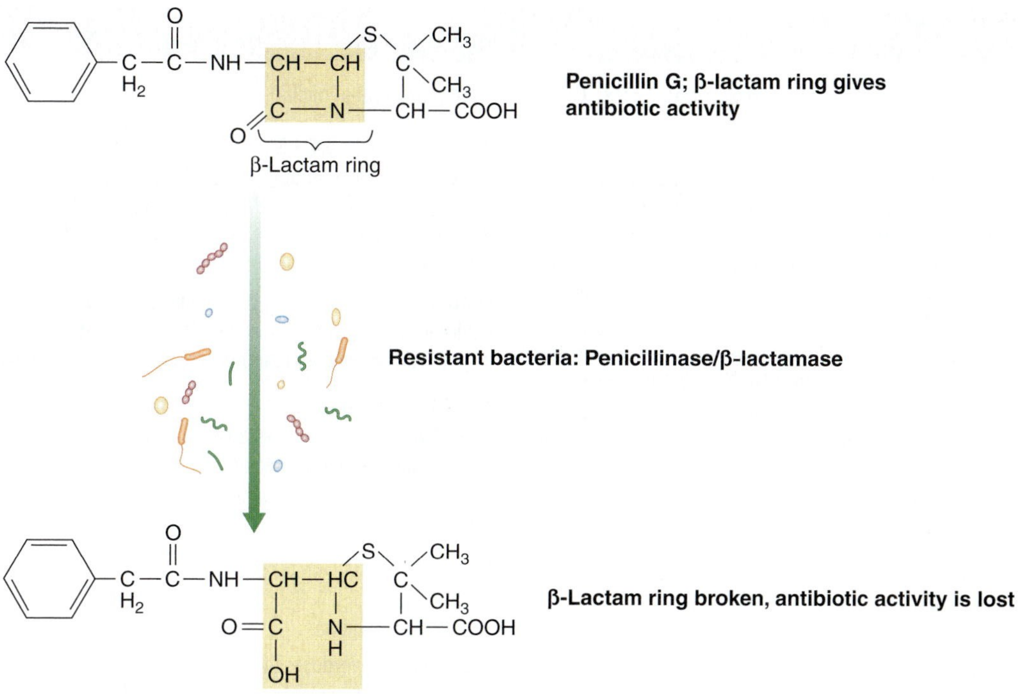

Penicillin G; β-lactam ring gives antibiotic activity

β-Lactam ring

Resistant bacteria: Penicillinase/β-lactamase

β-Lactam ring broken, antibiotic activity is lost

OH

> *Figure 34.3* Action of penicillinase

penicillins. These are sometimes referred to as aminopenicillins.

- *Extended-spectrum penicillins:* Carbenicillin (Geocillin) and piperacillin are effective against even more microbial species than the aminopenicillins, including *Pseudomonas, Enterobacter, Klebsiella,* and *Bacteroides fragilis.*

Several drugs are available that inhibit the bacterial beta-lactamase enzyme. When combined with a penicillin, these agents protect the penicillin molecule from destruction, extending its spectrum of activity. The three beta-lactamase inhibitors, clavulanate, sulbactam, and tazobactam, are available only in fixed-dose combinations with specific penicillins. These include Augmentin (amoxicillin plus clavulanate), Timentin (ticarcillin plus clavulanate), Unasyn (ampicillin plus sulbactam), and Zosyn (piperacillin plus tazobactam).

In general, the adverse effects of penicillins are minor; they are one of the safest classes of antibiotics. This has contributed to their widespread use for more than 60 years. Allergy to penicillin is the most common adverse effect. Common symptoms of penicillin allergy include rash, pruritus, and fever. Incidence of anaphylaxis ranges from 0.04% to 2%. Allergy to one penicillin increases the risk of allergy to other drugs in the same class. Other less common adverse effects of the penicillins include skin rashes and lowered red blood cell (RBC), WBC, or platelet counts.

See Nursing Process Focus: Patients Receiving Antibacterial Therapy on page 496 for the Nursing Process applied to all antibacterials.

Cephalosporins

Isolated shortly after the penicillins, the cephalosporins constitute the largest antibiotic class. The cephalosporins

act by essentially the same mechanism as the penicillins and have similar pharmacologic properties.

34.9 Pharmacotherapy with Cephalosporins

The primary therapeutic use of the cephalosporins is for gram-negative infections and for patients who cannot tolerate the less expensive penicillins. More than 20 cephalosporins are available, all having similar sounding names that can challenge even the best memory. Selection of a specific cephalosporin is first based on the sensitivity of the pathogen, and secondly on possible adverse effects. Doses for the cephalosporins are listed in Table 34.3.

Like the penicillins, many cephalosporins contain a beta-lactam ring that is responsible for their antimicrobial activity. The cephalosporins are bacteriocidal and act by attaching to penicillin-binding proteins to inhibit bacterial cell-wall synthesis. They are classified by their "generation," but there are not always clear distinctions among the generations. For example, cefdinir is considered either a third- or a fourth-generation drug, depending on the reference source. The following generalizations may be made regarding the generations:

- First-generation cephalosporins are the most effective drugs in this class against gram-positive organisms including staphylococci and streptococci. They are sometimes drugs of choice for these organisms. Bacteria that produce beta lactamase will usually be resistant to these drugs.

- Second-generation cephalosporins are more potent, are more resistant to beta lactamase, and exhibit a broader spectrum against gram-negative organisms than the

---

Pr Prototype Drug | Penicillin G Sodium/Potassium

Therapeutic Class: Antibacterial   **Pharmacologic Class:** Cell wall inhibitor; natural penicillin

ACTIONS AND USES

Similar to penicillin V, penicillin G is a drug of choice against streptococci, pneumococci, and staphylococci organisms that do not produce penicillinase and are shown to be susceptible by C&S testing. It is also a medication of choice for gonorrhea and syphilis caused by susceptible strains. Penicillin G is available as either a potassium or sodium salt; there is no difference therapeutically between the two salts.

Only 15–30% of an oral dose of penicillin G is absorbed. Because of its low oral absorption, penicillin G is often given by the IV or IM routes. Penicillin V and amoxicillin are more stable in acid and are used when oral penicillin therapy is desired. Penicillinase-producing organisms inactivate both penicillin G and penicillin V. Penicillin G benzathine (Bicillin) and penicillin G procaine (Wycillin) are longer acting parenteral salts of the drug.

ADMINISTRATION ALERTS

- After parenteral administration, observe for possible allergic reactions for 30 minutes, especially following the first dose.
- Do not mix penicillin and aminoglycosides in the same intravenous solution. Give IV medications 1 hour apart to prevent interactions.
- Pregnancy category B

> **PHARMACOKINETICS**
> **Onset:** Rapid
> **Peak:** 30–60 min PO; 15–30 min IM
> **Half-life:** 30–60 min
> **Duration:** 4–6 h

ADVERSE EFFECTS

Penicillin G has few serious adverse effects. Diarrhea, nausea, and vomiting are the most common adverse effects and can cause serious complications in children and older adults. Pain at the injection site may occur, and superinfections are possible. Anaphylaxis is the most serious adverse effect.

Contraindications: The only contraindication is hypersensitivity to a drug in the penicillin class. Because penicillin G is excreted extensively by the kidneys, the drug should be used with caution in patients with severe renal disease.

INTERACTIONS

Drug–Drug: Penicillin G may decrease the effectiveness of oral contraceptives. Colestipol taken with this medication will decrease the absorption of penicillin. Potassium-sparing diuretics may cause hyperkalemia when administered with penicillin G potassium.

Lab Tests: Penicillin G may give positive Coombs' test and false positive urinary or serum proteins.

Herbal/Food: Unknown

Treatment of Overdose: There is no specific treatment for overdose.

Refer to MyNursingKit for a Nursing Process Focus specific to this drug.

Pr Prototype Drug | Cefotaxime *(Claforan)*

Therapeutic Class: Antibacterial   **Pharmacologic Class:** Cell wall inhibitor; first-generation cephalosporin

ACTIONS AND USES

Cefotaxime is a third-generation cephalosporin with a broad spectrum of activity against gram-negative organisms. It is effective against many bacterial species that have developed resistance to earlier generation cephalosporins and to other classes of anti-infectives. Cefotaxime exhibits bactericidal activity by inhibiting cell-wall synthesis. It is prescribed for serious infections of the lower respiratory tract, central nervous system, genitourinary system, bones, and joints. It may also be used for blood infections such as bacteremia or septicemia. Like many other cephalosporins, cefotaxime is not absorbed from the GI tract and must be given by the IM or IV route.

ADMINISTRATION ALERTS

- Administer IM injections deep into a large muscle mass to prevent injury to surrounding tissues.
- Pregnancy category B

> **PHARMACOKINETICS**
> **Onset:** 30 min (IM); 5 min (IV)
> **Peak:** Unknown
> **Half-life:** 1 h
> **Duration:** Unknown

ADVERSE EFFECTS

For most patients, cefotaxime and the other cephalosporins are safe medications. Hypersensitivity is the most common adverse effect, although symptoms may include only a minor rash and itching. Anaphylaxis is possible. GI-related side effects such as diarrhea, vomiting, and nausea may occur. Some patients experience considerable pain at the injection site.

Contraindications: The only contraindication is hypersensitivity to a drug in the cephalosporin class. Because cefotaxime is excreted extensively by the kidneys, the drug should be used with caution in patients with severe renal disease.

INTERACTIONS

Drug–Drug: Probenecid causes decreased renal elimination of cefotaxime and may result in cephalosporin toxicity. Alcohol interacts with cefotaxime to produce a disulfiram-like reaction. Cefotaxime interacts with NSAIDs to cause an increase in platelet inhibition.

Lab Tests: Liver function test values may be increased; may give a positive Coombs' test and false elevations of serum or urinary creatinine levels.

Herbal/Food: Unknown

Treatment of Overdose: There is no specific treatment for overdose.

Refer to MyNursingKit for a Nursing Process Focus specific to this drug.

TABLE 34.3	**Cephalosporins**	
Drug	**Route and Adult Dose (max dose where indicated)**	**Adverse Effects**
FIRST-GENERATION		
cefadroxil (Duricef)	PO; 500 mg–1 g one to two times/day (max: 2 g/day)	*Diarrhea, abdominal cramping, nausea, fatigue, rash, pruritus, pain at injection sites, oral or vaginal candidiasis*
cefazolin (Ancef, Kefzol)	IV/IM; 250 mg–2 g tid (max: 12 g/day)	
cephalexin (Keflex)	PO; 250–500 mg qid	<u>Pseudomembranous colitis, nephrotoxicity, anaphylaxis</u>
cephradine (Velosef)	PO; 250–500 mg every 6 h or 500 mg–1 g every 12 h (max: 4 g/day)	
SECOND-GENERATION		
cefaclor (Ceclor)	PO; 250–500 mg tid (max: 2 g/day)	
cefotetan (Cefotan)	IV/IM; 1–2 g every 12 h (max: 6 g/day)	
cefoxitin (Mefoxin)	IV/IM; 1–2 g every 6–8 h (max: 12 g/day)	
cefprozil (Cefzil)	PO; 250–500 mg one to two times/day (max: 1 g/day)	
cefuroxime (Ceftin, Zinacef)	PO; 250–500 mg bid (max: 1 g/day)	
	IM/IV; 750 mg–1.5 g every 8 h (max: 9 g/day)	
THIRD-GENERATION		
cefdinir (Omnicef)	PO; 300 mg bid (max: 600 mg/day)	
cefditoren (Spectracef)	PO; 400 mg bid for 10 days (max: 800 mg/day)	
cefixime (Suprax)	PO; 400 mg/day or 200 mg bid (max: 800 mg/day)	
cefoperazone (Cefobid)	IV/IM; 1–2 g every 12 h; 16 g/day in two to four divided doses (max: 12 g/day)	
Ⓟ cefotaxime (Claforan)	IV/IM; 1–2 g bid–tid (max: 12 g/day)	
cefpodoxime (Vantin)	PO; 200 mg every 12 h for 10 days (max: 800 mg/day)	
ceftazidime (Fortaz, Tazicef)	IV/IM; 1–2 mg every 8–12 h (max: 6 g/day)	
ceftibuten (Cedax)	PO; 400 mg/day for 10 days (max: 400 mg/day)	
ceftizoxime (Cefizox)	IV/IM; 1–2 g every 8–12 h, up to 2 g every 4 h (max: 12 g/day)	
ceftriaxone (Rocephin)	IV/IM; 1–2 g every 12–24 h (max: 4 g/day)	
FOURTH-GENERATION		
cefepime (Maxipime)	IV/IM; 0.5–1.0 g every 12 h for 7–10 days (max: 6 g/day)	

Italics indicate common adverse effects; <u>underlining</u> indicates serious adverse effects.

first-generation drugs. The second-generation agents have largely been replaced by third-generation cephalosporins.

- Third-generation cephalosporins exhibit an even broader spectrum against gram-negative bacteria than the second-generation agents. They generally have a longer duration of action, and are resistant to beta lactamase. These cephalosporins are sometimes drugs of choice against infections by *Pseudomonas, Klebsiella, Neisseria, Salmonella, Proteus,* and *H. influenza.*

- Fourth-generation cephalosporins are effective against organisms that have developed resistance to earlier cephalosporins. Third- and fourth-generation agents are capable of entering the cerebrospinal fluid (CSF) to treat CNS infections.

In general, the cephalosporins are safe drugs, with adverse effects similar to those of the penicillins. Allergic reactions are the most frequent adverse effect. Skin rashes are a common sign of allergy, and may appear several days following the initiation of therapy. The nurse must be aware that 5% to 10% of the patients who are allergic to penicillin are also allergic to the cephalosporins. Cephalosporins are contraindicated for patients who have previously experienced a severe allergic reaction to a penicillin. Despite this incidence of cross hypersensitivity, the cephalosporins offer a reasonable alternative for many patients who are unable to take penicillin. In addition to allergy and rash, GI complaints are common adverse effects of cephalosporins. Earlier generation cephalosporins caused kidney toxicity, but this adverse effect is diminished with the newer drugs in this class.

See Nursing Process Focus: Patients Receiving Antibacterial Therapy on page 496 for the Nursing Process applied to all antibacterials.

Tetracyclines

The first tetracyclines were extracted from *Streptomyces* soil microorganisms in 1948. The five tetracyclines are effective

TABLE 34.4	Tetracyclines	
Drug	**Route and Adult Dose (max dose where indicated)**	**Adverse Effects**
demeclocycline (Declomycin)	PO; 150 mg every 6 h or 300 mg every 12 h (max: 2.4 g/day)	*Nausea, vomiting, abdominal cramping, flatulence, diarrhea, mild phototoxicity, rash, dizziness, stinging/burning with topical applications*
doxycycline (Vibramycin, others)	PO/IV; 100 mg bid on day 1, then 100 mg/day (max: 200 mg/day)	
minocycline (Minocin, others)	PO/IV; 200 mg as single dose followed by 100 mg bid	
ⓟ tetracycline (Sumycin, others)	PO; 250–500 mg bid–qid (max: 2 g/day)	<u>Anaphylaxis, secondary infections, hepatotoxicity, exfoliative dermatitis</u>
tigecycline (Tygacil)	IV; 100 mg, followed by 50 mg every 12 h	

Italics indicate common adverse effects; <u>underlining</u> indicates serious adverse effects.

against a large number of different gram-negative and gram-positive organisms and have one of the broadest spectrums of any class of antibiotics. The tetracyclines are listed in Table 34.4.

34.10 Pharmacotherapy with Tetracyclines

Tetracyclines act by inhibiting bacterial protein synthesis. By binding to the bacterial ribosome, which differs in structure from a human ribosome, the tetracyclines slow microbial growth and exert a bacteriostatic effect. All tetracyclines have the same spectrum of activity and exhibit similar adverse effects. Doxycycline (Vibramycin, others) and minocy-

cline (Minocin, others) have longer durations of actions and are more lipid soluble, permitting them to enter the CSF.

The widespread use of tetracyclines in the 1950s and 1960s resulted in the emergence of a large number of resistant bacterial strains that now limit their therapeutic utility. They are drugs of choice for only a few diseases: Rocky Mountain spotted fever, typhus, cholera, Lyme disease, peptic ulcers caused by *Helicobacter pylori*, and chlamydial infections. Drugs in this class are occasionally used for the treatment of acne vulgaris, for which they are given topically or PO at low doses.

Tetracyclines exhibit few serious adverse effects. Gastric distress is relatively common with tetracyclines, however, and patients will tend to take tetracyclines *with* food. Because these drugs bind metal ions such as calcium and iron,

---

ⓟ Prototype Drug | Tetracycline *(Sumycin, others)*

Therapeutic Class: Antibacterial   **Pharmacologic Class:** Tetracycline; protein synthesis inhibitor

ACTIONS AND USES
Tetracycline is effective against a broad range of gram-positive and gram-negative organisms, including *Chlamydia*, *Rickettsiae*, and *Mycoplasma*. Its use has increased over the past decade due to its effectiveness against *H. pylori* in the treatment of peptic ulcer disease. Tetracycline is given orally, though it has a short half-life that may require administration four times per day. Topical and oral preparations are available for treating acne. An IM preparation is available; injections may cause local irritation and be extremely painful.

ADMINISTRATION ALERTS
- Administer oral drug with full glass of water to decrease esophageal and GI irritation.
- Administer antacids and tetracycline 1 to 3 hours apart.
- Administer antilipidemic agents at least 2 hours before or after tetracycline.
- Pregnancy category D

PHARMACOKINETICS
Onset: 1–2 h
Peak: 2–4 h
Half-life: 6–12 h
Duration: 12 h

ADVERSE EFFECTS
Being a broad-spectrum antibiotic, tetracycline has a tendency to affect vaginal, oral, and intestinal flora and cause superinfections. Tetracycline irritates the GI mucosa and may cause nausea, vomiting, epigastric burning, and diarrhea. Diarrhea may be severe enough to cause discontinuation of therapy. Other common side effects include discoloration of the teeth and photosensitivity.

Contraindications: Tetracycline is contraindicated in patients with hypersensitivity to drugs in this class. The drug should not be used during the second half of pregnancy, in children 8 years or younger, and in patients with severe renal or hepatic impairment.

INTERACTIONS
Drug–Drug: Milk products, iron supplements, magnesium-containing laxatives, and antacids reduce the absorption and serum levels of tetracyclines. Tetracycline binds with the lipid-lowering drugs colestipol and cholestyramine, thereby decreasing the antibiotic's absorption. This drug decreases the effectiveness of oral contraceptives.

Lab Tests: May increase the following lab values: blood urea nitrogen (BUN), aspartate aminotransferase (AST), alanine aminotransferase (ALT), amylase, bilirubin, and alkaline phosphatase.

Herbal/Food: Dairy products interfere with tetracycline absorption.

Treatment of Overdose: There is no specific treatment for overdose.

Refer to MyNursingKit for a Nursing Process Focus specific to this drug.

tetracyclines should not be taken with milk or iron supplements. Calcium and iron can decrease the drug's absorption by as much as 50%. Direct exposure to sunlight can result in severe photosensitivity during therapy. Unless suffering from a life-threatening infection, patients younger than 8 years of age are not given tetracyclines because these drugs may cause permanent yellow-brown discoloration of the permanent teeth in young children. Tetracyclines also affect fetal bone growth and teeth development and are pregnancy category D agents; therefore, they should be avoided during pregnancy. Because of the drugs' broad spectrum, the risk for superinfection is relatively high and the nurse should be observant for signs of a secondary infection. When administered parenterally or in high doses, certain tetracyclines can cause hepatotoxicity, especially in patients with pre-existing liver disease. Because outdated tetracycline may deteriorate and become nephrotoxic, unused prescriptions should be discarded promptly.

The newest of the tetracyclines is tigecycline (Tygacil), approved in 2005. Tigecycline is indicated for drug-resistant intra-abdominal infections and complicated skin and skin-structure infections, especially those caused by MRSA. Nausea and vomiting may be severe with this drug. Tigecycline is available by IV infusion.

See Nursing Process Focus: Patients Receiving Antibacterial Therapy on page 496 for the Nursing Process applied to all antibacterials.

Macrolides

Erythromycin (E-mycin, Erythrocin), the first macrolide antibiotic, was isolated from *Streptomyces* in a soil sample in 1952. Macrolides are considered safe alternatives to penicillin, although they are drugs of choice for relatively few infections.

34.11 Pharmacotherapy with Macrolides

The macrolides inhibit protein synthesis by binding to the bacterial ribosome. At low doses, this inhibition produces a bacteriostatic effect. At higher doses, and in susceptible species, macrolides may be bacteriocidal. Macrolides are effective against most gram-positive bacteria and many gram-negative species. Common indications include the treatment of whooping cough, Legionnaires' disease, and infections by streptococcus, *H. influenza,* and *Mycoplasma pneumoniae.* Drugs in this class are used against bacteria re-

siding *inside* host cells, such as *Listeria, Chlamydia, Neisseria,* and *Legionella.* Clarithromycin is one of several antibiotics used to treat peptic ulcer disease, due to its activity against *H. pylori* (chapter 40∞). The macrolides are listed in Table 34.5.

The newer macrolides are synthesized from erythromycin. Although their spectrums of activity are similar, these drugs have longer half-lives and cause less gastric irritation than erythromycin. For example, azithromycin (Zithromax, Z-Pak) has such an extended half-life that it is administered for only 5 days, rather than the 10 days required for most antibiotics. The shorter duration of therapy is thought to increase patient adherence.

The macrolides exhibit few serious adverse effects. Mild GI upset, diarrhea, and abdominal pain are the most frequent adverse effects. Because macrolides are broad-spectrum agents, superinfections may occur. Like most of the older antibiotics, macrolide-resistant strains are becoming more common. Other than prior allergic reactions to macrolides, there are no contraindications to therapy.

See Nursing Process Focus: Patients Receiving Antibacterial Therapy on page 496 for the Nursing Process applied to all antibacterials.

Aminoglycosides

The first aminoglycoside, streptomycin, was named after *Streptomyces griseus,* the soil organism from which it was isolated in 1942. Although more toxic than other antibiotic classes, aminoglycosides have important therapeutic applications for the treatment of aerobic gram-negative bacteria, mycobacteria, and some protozoans. The aminoglycosides are listed in Table 34.6.

AVOIDING MEDICATION ERRORS

Mr. Johnson is admitted for a severe upper respiratory infection and dehydration. During the nurse's initial assessment, Mr. Johnson is questioned about allergies and reports being allergic to peanuts, aspirin, sulfa, and ragweed. Following a history and physical examination, the primary care physician orders trimethoprim–sulfamethoxazole (Bactrim) DS. When the medication arrives from the pharmacy, it is in a unit-dose package. It is a large tablet containing 160 mg of trimethoprim and 800 mg of sulfamethoxazole. The nurse breaks the tablet in half, for easier swallowing, and gives Mr. Johnson his first dose with a large glass of water. What should the nurse have done differently?

See Appendix D for the suggested answer.

TABLE 34.5	Macrolides	
Drug	Route and Adult Dose (max dose where indicated)	Adverse Effects
azithromycin (Zithromax, Z-Pak)	PO; 500 mg for one dose, then 250 mg/day for 4 days	*Nausea, vomiting, diarrhea, abdominal cramping, dry skin or burning (topical route)*
clarithromycin (Biaxin)	PO; 250–500 mg bid	
dirithromycin (Dynabac)	PO; 500 mg/day	Anaphylaxis, ototoxicity, pseudomembranous colitis, hepatotoxicity, superinfections, dysrhythmias
erythromycin (E-Mycin, Erythrocin)	PO; 250–500 mg bid or 333 mg tid	

Pr Prototype Drug | Erythromycin *(E-Mycin, Erythrocin)*

Therapeutic Class: Antibacterial   **Pharmacologic Class:** Macrolide; protein synthesis inhibitor

ACTIONS AND USES

Erythromycin is inactivated by stomach acid and is thus formulated as coated, acid-resistant tablets or capsules that dissolve in the small intestine. Its main application is for patients who are unable to tolerate penicillins or who may have a penicillin-resistant infection. It has a spectrum similar to that of the penicillins and is effective against most gram-positive bacteria. It is often a preferred drug for infections by *Bordetella pertussis* (whooping cough) and *Corynebacterium diphtheriae*.

ADMINISTRATION ALERTS

- Administer oral drug on an empty stomach with a full glass of water.
- For suspensions, shake the bottle thoroughly to ensure the drug is well mixed.
- Do not give with or immediately before or after fruit juices.
- Pregnancy category B

PHARMACOKINETICS
Onset: 1 h
Peak: 1–4 h
Half-life: 1.5–2 h
Duration: Unknown

ADVERSE EFFECTS

The most frequent adverse effects from erythromycin are nausea, abdominal cramping, and vomiting, although these are rarely serious enough to cause discontinuation of therapy. Concurrent administration with food reduces these symptoms. The most severe adverse effect is hepatotoxicity caused by the estolate salt (Ilosone) of the drug. Hearing loss, vertigo, and dizziness may be experienced when using high doses, particularly in older adults and in those with impaired hepatic or renal excretion.

Contraindications: Erythromycin is contraindicated in patients with hypersensitivity to drugs in the macrolide class, and for those taking terfenadine, astemizole, or cisapride.

INTERACTIONS

Drug–Drug: Anesthetics, azole antifungals and anticonvulsants may interact to cause serum drug levels of erythromycin to rise and result in toxicity. This drug interacts with cyclosporine, increasing the risk for nephrotoxicity. It may increase the effects of warfarin. The concurrent use of erythromycin with lovastatin or simvastatin is not recommended because it may increase the risk of muscle toxicity. Ethanol use may decrease the absorption of erythromycin.

Lab Tests: Erythromycin may interfere with AST and give false urinary catecholamine values.

Herbal/Food: St. John's wort may decrease the effectiveness of erythromycin.

Treatment of Overdose: There is no specific treatment for overdose.

Refer to MyNursingKit for a Nursing Process Focus specific to this drug.

TABLE 34.6 Aminoglycosides

Drug	Route and Adult Dose (max dose where indicated)	Adverse Effects
amikacin (Amikin)	IM; 5.0–7.5 mg/kg as a loading dose, then 7.5 mg/kg bid	*Pain or inflammation at injection site, rash, fever, nausea, diarrhea, dizziness, tinnitus*
gentamicin (Garamycin, others)	IM; 1.5–2.0 mg/kg as a loading dose, then 1–2 mg/kg bid–tid	
kanamycin (Kantrex)	IM; 5.0–7.5 mg/kg bid–tid	<u>Anaphylaxis, nephrotoxicity, irreversible ototoxicity, superinfections</u>
neomycin	PO; 4–12 g/day in divided doses	
paromomycin (Humatin)	PO; 7.5–12.5 mg/kg in three doses	
streptomycin	IM; 15 mg/kg up to 1 g as a single dose	
tobramycin (Nebcin)	IM/IM; 1 mg/kg tid (max: 5 mg/kg/day)	

Italics indicate common adverse effects; <u>underlining</u> indicates serious adverse effects.

34.12 Pharmacotherapy with Aminoglycosides

Aminoglycosides are bacteriocidal and act by inhibiting bacterial protein synthesis. They are normally reserved for serious systemic infections caused by aerobic gram-negative organisms, including those caused by *E. coli, Serratia, Proteus, Klebsiella,* and *Pseudomonas.* They are sometimes administered concurrently with a penicillin, cephalosporin, or vancomycin for treatment of enterococcal infections. When used for systemic bacterial infections, aminoglycosides are given parenterally because they are poorly absorbed from the GI tract. They are occasionally given orally for their local effect on the GI tract to sterilize the bowel prior to intestinal surgery. Neomycin is available for topical infections of the skin, eyes, and ears. Paromomycin (Humatin) is given orally for the treatment of parasitic infections. Once widely used, streptomycin is now usually restricted to the treatment of tuberculosis because of the emergence of a large number of strains resistant to the antibiotic. The nurse should note the differences in spelling of some drugs—such as -mycin versus -micin—which reflect the different organisms from which the drugs were originally isolated.

Pr Prototype Drug | Gentamicin *(Garamycin, others)*

Therapeutic Class: Antibacterial   **Pharmacologic Class:** Aminoglycoside; protein synthesis inhibitor

ACTIONS AND USES

Gentamicin is a broad-spectrum, bacteriocidal antibiotic usually prescribed for serious urinary, respiratory, nervous, or GI infections when less toxic antibiotics are contraindicated. Activity includes *Enterobacter, E. Coli, Klebsiella, Citrobacter, Pseudomonas, and Serratia.* Gentamicin is effective against a few gram-positive bacteria, including some strains of methicillin-resistant *Staphylococcus aureus* (MRSA). It is often used in combination with other antibiotics. A topical formulation (Genoptic) is available for infections of the external eye.

ADMINISTRATION ALERTS

- For IM administration, give deep into a large muscle.
- Use only IM and IV drug solutions that are clear and colorless or slightly yellow. Discard discolored solutions or those that contain particulate matter.
- Withhold the drug if the peak serum level lies above the normal range of 5–10 mcg/mL.
- Pregnancy category C

PHARMACOKINETICS
Onset: Rapid
Peak: 1–2 h
Half-life: 3–4 h
Duration: 8–12 h

ADVERSE EFFECTS

Rash, nausea, vomiting, and fatigue are the most frequent adverse effects. As with other aminoglycosides, certain adverse effects may be severe. Ototoxicity can produce a loss of hearing or balance, which may become permanent with continued use. Tinnitus, vertigo, and persistent headaches are early signs of ototoxicity. Nephrotoxicity is of particular concern to patients with pre-existing kidney impairment, and may limit pharmacotherapy. Signs of reduced kidney function include oliguria, proteinuria, and elevated BUN and creatinine levels. Resistance to gentamicin is increasing, and some cross resistance among aminoglycosides has been reported.

Contraindications: Gentamicin is contraindicated in patients with hypersensitivity to drugs in the aminoglycoside class. Drug therapy must be monitored carefully in patients with impaired renal function, or those with pre-existing hearing loss.

INTERACTIONS

Drug–Drug: The risk of ototoxicity increases if the patient is currently taking amphotericin B, furosemide, aspirin, bumetanide, ethacrynic acid, cisplatin, or paromomycin. Concurrent use with amphotericin B, capreomycin, cisplatin, polymyxin B, or vancomycin increases the risk of nephrotoxicity.

Lab Tests: Gentamicin may increase values of the following: serum bilirubin, serum creatinine, serum lactate dehydrogenase (LDH), BUN, AST, or ALT; may decrease values for the following: serum calcium, sodium, or potassium.

Herbal/Food: Unknown

Treatment of Overdose: There is no specific treatment for overdose.

Refer to MyNursingKit for a Nursing Process Focus specific to this drug.

The clinical applications of the aminoglycosides are limited by their potential to cause serious adverse effects. The degree and types of potential toxicity are similar for all drugs in this class. Of greatest concern are their effects on the inner ear and the kidneys. Damage to the inner ear, or ototoxicity, is recognized by hearing impairment, dizziness, loss of balance, persistent headache, and ringing in the ears. Because permanent deafness may occur, aminoglycosides are usually discontinued when symptoms of hearing impairment first appear. Aminoglycoside nephrotoxicity may be severe, affecting up to 26% of patients receiving these antibiotics. Nephrotoxicity is recognized by abnormal urinary function tests, such as elevated serum creatinine or BUN. Nephrotoxicity is usually reversible.

See Nursing Process Focus: Patients Receiving Antibacterial Therapy on page 496 for the Nursing Process applied to all antibacterials.

Fluoroquinolones

Fluoroquinolones were once reserved only for UTIs because of their toxicity. Development of safer drugs in this class began in the late 1980s and has continued to the present day. Newer fluoroquinolones have a broad spectrum of activity and are used for a variety of infections. The fluoroquinolones are listed in Table 34.7.

34.13 Pharmacotherapy with Fluoroquinolones

Although the first drug in this class, nalidixic acid (NegGram), was approved by the FDA in 1962, it had a narrow spectrum of activity, and its use was restricted to UTIs. Nalidixic acid is still used for the pharmacotherapy of UTI, although it is not a preferred drug for this infection. Since then, four generations of fluoroquinolones have become available. All fluoroquinolones have activity against gram-negative pathogens; the newer ones are significantly more effective against gram-positive microbes, such as staphylococci, streptococci, and enterococci.

The fluoroquinolones are bacteriocidal and affect DNA synthesis by inhibiting two bacterial enzymes: DNA gyrase and topoisomerase IV. These antibiotics are infrequently first-line drugs, although they are extensively used as alternatives to other antibiotics. Clinical applications include infections of the respiratory, GI, and genitourinary tracts, and some skin and soft-tissue infections. The most widely used drug in this class, ciprofloxacin (Cipro), is an agent of choice for the postexposure prophylaxis of *Bacillus anthracis*, the organism responsible for causing anthrax. Moxifloxacin (Avelox) is a newer drug that is highly effective against anaerobes. Recent studies suggest that some fluoroquinolones may be effective against *M. tuberculosis*.

TABLE 34.7	Fluoroquinolones	
Drug	Route and Adult Dose (max dose where indicated)	Adverse Effects
FIRST GENERATION		
cinoxacin (Cinobac)	PO; 250–500 mg bid–qid	*Nausea, diarrhea, vomiting, rash, headache, restlessness, pain and inflammation at injection site, local burning, stinging and corneal irritation (ophthalmic)*
nalidixic acid (NegGram)	PO; Acute therapy: 1 g qid	
	PO; Chronic therapy: 500 mg qid	
SECOND GENERATION		<u>Anaphylaxis, tendon rupture, superinfections, photosensitivity, pseudomembranous colitis, seizure, peripheral neuropathy, hepatotoxicity</u>
ⓟ ciprofloxacin (Cipro)	PO; 250–750 mg bid	
norfloxacin (Noroxin)	PO; 400 mg bid or 800 mg once daily	
ofloxacin (Floxin)	PO; 200–400 mg bid (max: 800 mg/day)	
THIRD GENERATION		
gatifloxacin (Zymar)	Drops (0.3% ophthalmic solution); On days 1 and 2, one drop in each affected eye every 2 hours; on days 3–7, one drop in each affected eye up to four times/day	
levofloxacin (Levaquin)	PO; 250–500 mg/day (max: 750 mg/day)	
FOURTH GENERATION		
gemifloxacin (Factive)	PO; 320 mg/day (max: 320 mg/day)	
moxifloxacin (Avelox)	PO/IV; 400 mg/day (max: 400 mg/day)	
Italics indicate common adverse effects; <u>underlining</u> indicates serious adverse effects.		

A major advantage of the fluoroquinolones is that most are well absorbed orally and may be administered either once or twice a day. Although they may be taken with food, they should not be taken concurrently with multivitamins or mineral supplements because calcium, magnesium, iron, or zinc ions can reduce the absorption of some fluoroquinolones by as much as 90%.

Fluoroquinolones are well tolerated by most patients, with nausea, vomiting, and diarrhea being the most common adverse effects. The most serious adverse effects are dysrhythmias (gatifloxacin and moxifloxacin) and potential hepatotoxicity. Central nervous system effects such as dizziness, headache, and sleep disturbances affect 1% to 8% of patients. Most recently, fluoroquinolones have been associated with an increased risk of tendonitis and tendon rupture, particularly of the Achilles tendon. The risk of tendon rupture is increased in patients over age 60 and those receiving concurrent corticosteroids. Because animal studies have suggested that fluoroquinolones affect cartilage development, these drugs are not approved for children under age 18. Use in pregnancy or in lactating patients should be avoided.

See Nursing Process Focus: Patients Receiving Antibacterial Therapy on page 496 for the Nursing Process applied to all antibacterials.

Sulfonamides

Sulfonamides are older drugs that have been prescribed for a variety of infections over the past 70 years. Although their use has declined, sulfonamides are still useful in treating susceptible UTIs. The sulfonamides are listed in Table 34.8.

34.14 Pharmacotherapy with Sulfonamides

The discovery of the sulfonamides in the 1930s heralded a new era in the treatment of infectious disease. With their wide spectrum of activity against both gram-positive and gram-negative bacteria, the sulfonamides significantly reduced mortality from susceptible microbes and earned their discoverer a Nobel Prize in Medicine. Sulfonamides are bacteriostatic and active against a broad spectrum of microorganisms.

Sulfonamides suppress bacterial growth by inhibiting the synthesis of folic acid, or folate. These drugs are sometimes referred to as *folic acid inhibitors*. In human physiology, folic acid is a B-complex vitamin that is essential during periods of rapid growth, especially during childhood and pregnancy. Bacteria also require this substance during periods of rapid cell division and growth.

Although initially very effective, several factors led to a significant decline in the use of sulfonamides. Their widespread availability for over 60 years resulted in a substantial number of resistant strains. The discovery of the penicillins, cephalosporins, and macrolides gave physicians larger choices of safer agents. Approval of the combination antibiotic sulfamethoxazole–trimethoprim (Bactrim, Septra, TMP-SMZ) marked a resurgence in the use of sulfonamides in treating UTIs. In communities with high resistance rates, however, TMP-SMZ is no longer a drug of first choice, unless C&S testing determines it to be the most effective drug for the specific pathogen. Sulfonamides are also prescribed for the treatment of *Pneumocystis carinii* pneumonia and shigella infections of the small bowel. Sulfasalazine (Azulfidine) is a

Pr Prototype Drug | Ciprofloxacin (Cipro)

Therapeutic Class: Antibacterial   **Pharmacologic Class:** Fluoroquinolone; bacterial DNA synthesis inhibitor

ACTIONS AND USES
Ciprofloxacin, a second-generation fluoroquinolone, was approved in 1987 and is the most widely prescribed drug in this class. By inhibiting bacterial DNA gyrase, ciprofloxacin affects bacterial replication and DNA repair. More effective against gram-negative than gram-positive organisms, it is prescribed for UTI, sinusitis, pneumonia, skin, bone and joint infections, infectious diarrhea, and certain eye infections. As of 2007, the FDA recommended that ciprofloxacin no longer be used to treat gonorrhea. The drug is rapidly absorbed after oral administration and is distributed to most body tissues. Oral, intravenous, ophthalmic, and otic formulations are available. An extended release form of the drug, Proquin XR, is administered for only 3 days and is approved for bladder infections.

ADMINISTRATION ALERTS
- Administer at least 4 hours before antacids and ferrous sulfate.
- Pregnancy category C

PHARMACOKINETICS
Onset: Rapid
Peak: 1–2 h
Half-life: 1–4 h
Duration: 12 h

ADVERSE EFFECTS
Ciprofloxacin is well tolerated by most patients, and serious adverse effects are uncommon. Nausea, vomiting, and diarrhea may occur in as many as 20% of patients. Ciprofloxacin may be administered with food to diminish adverse GI effects. The patient should not, however, take this drug with antacids or mineral supplements, since drug absorption will be diminished. Some patients report phototoxicity, headache, and dizziness. The FDA has issued a black box warning that ciprofloxacin may cause tendon inflammation or rupture. Any complaints of difficulty with walking or pain in the foot or leg should be reported immediately.

Contraindications: Ciprofloxacin is contraindicated in patients with hypersensitivity to drugs in the fluoroquinolone class. The drug should be discontinued if the patient experiences pain or inflammation of a tendon, as tendon ruptures have been reported.

INTERACTIONS
Drug–Drug: Concurrent administration with warfarin may increase anticoagulant effects and result in bleeding. This drug may increase theophylline levels 15–30%. Antacids, ferrous sulfate, and sucralfate decrease the absorption of ciprofloxacin.

Lab Tests: Ciprofloxacin may increase values of ALT, AST, serum creatinine, and BUN.

Herbal/Food: Ciprofloxacin can increase serum levels of caffeine; caffeine consumption should be restricted to prevent excessive nervousness, anxiety, or tachycardia. Dairy products or calcium-fortified drinks can decrease the absorption of ciprofloxacin.

Treatment of Overdose: There is no specific treatment for overdose.

Refer to MyNursingKit for a Nursing Process Focus specific to this drug.

TABLE 34.8	Sulfonamides	
Drug	**Route and Adult Dose (max dose where indicated)**	**Adverse Effects**
sulfacetamide (Cetamide, others)	Ophthalmic; 1–3 drops of 10%, 15%, or 30% solution into lower conjunctival sac every 2–3 h	*Nausea, vomiting, anorexia, rash, photosensitivity, crystalluria*
sulfadiazine (Microsulfon)	PO; Loading dose: 2–4 g	<u>Anaphylaxis, Stevens–Johnson syndrome, blood dyscrasias, fulminant hepatic necrosis</u>
	Maintenance dose: 2–4 g/day in four to six divided doses	
sulfadoxine–pyrimethamine (Fansidar)	PO; 1 tablet weekly (500 mg sulfadoxine, 25 mg pyrimethamine)	
sulfasalazine (Azulfidine)	PO; 1–2 g/day in four divided doses (max: 8 g/day)	
sulfisoxazole (Gantrisin)	PO; 2–4 g initially, followed by 1–2 g qid (max: 12 g/day)	
Pr trimethoprim–sulfamethoxazole (Bactrim, Septra)	PO; 160 mg TMP, 800 mg SMZ bid	

Italics indicate common adverse effects; <u>underlining</u> indicates serious adverse effects.

sulfonamide with anti-inflammatory properties that is prescribed for rheumatoid arthritis and ulcerative colitis.

Sulfonamides are classified by their route of administration: systemic or topical. Systemic agents, such as sulfisoxazole (Gantrisin) and TMP-SMZ, are readily absorbed when given orally and excreted rapidly by the kidneys. Other sulfonamides, including sulfadiazine (Microsulfon), are used only for topical infections. The topical sulfonamides are not preferred drugs because many patients are allergic to substances containing sulfur. One drug in this class, sulfadoxine–pyrimethamine (Fansidar) has an excep-

tionally long half-life and is occasionally prescribed for malarial prophylaxis.

In general, the sulfonamides are safe drugs; however, some adverse effects may be serious. Adverse effects include the formation of crystals in the urine, hypersensitivity reactions, nausea, and vomiting. Although not common, potentially fatal blood abnormalities, such as aplastic anemia, acute hemolytic anemia, and agranulocytosis can occur.

See Nursing Process Focus: Patients Receiving Antibacterial Therapy on page 496 for the Nursing Process applied to all antibacterials.

Pr Prototype Drug | Trimethoprim–Sulfamethoxazole *(Bactrim, Septra)*

Therapeutic Class: Antibacterial   **Pharmacologic Class:** Sulfonamide; folic acid inhibitor

ACTIONS AND USES

The fixed-dose combination of sulfamethoxazole (SMZ) with the anti-infective trimethoprim (TMP) is most frequently prescribed for the pharmacotherapy of urinary tract infections. It is also approved for the treatment of *Pneumocystis carinii* pneumonia, shigella infections of the small bowel, and for acute episodes of chronic bronchitis. Oral and IV preparations are available.

Both SMZ and TMP are inhibitors of the bacterial metabolism of folic acid. Their action is synergistic: A greater bacterial kill is achieved by the fixed combination than would be achieved with either drug used separately. Because humans obtain the precursors of folate in their diets and can use preformed folate, these medications are selective for *bacterial* metabolism. Another advantage of the combination is that development of resistance is lower than is observed when either of the agents is used alone.

ADMINISTRATION ALERTS

- Administer oral dosages with a full glass of water.
- Pregnancy category C

PHARMACOKINETICS
Onset: 30–60 min
Peak: 1–4 h
Half-life: 8–12 h
Duration: Unknown

ADVERSE EFFECTS

Nausea and vomiting are the most frequent adverse effects of TMP-SMZ therapy. Hypersensitivity is relatively common and usually manifests as skin rash, itching, and fever. This medication should be used cautiously in patients with pre-existing kidney disease, since crystalluria, oliguria, and renal failure have been reported. Periodic laboratory evaluation of the blood is usually performed to identify early signs of agranulocytosis or thrombocytopenia. Due to the potential for photosensitivity, the patient should avoid direct sunlight during therapy.

Contraindications: TMP-SMZ is contraindicated in patients with hypersensitivity to drugs in the sulfonamide class. Patients with documented megaloblastic anemia due to folate deficiency should not receive this drug. Pregnant women at term and nursing mothers should not take this drug because sulfonamides may cross the placenta and are excreted in milk and may cause kernicterus. Trimethoprim decreases potassium excretion and is contraindicated in patients with hyperkalemia.

INTERACTIONS

Drug–Drug: TMP-SMZ may enhance the effects of oral anticoagulants. These drugs may also increase methotrexate toxicity. By decreasing the hepatic metabolism of phenytoin, TMP-SMZ may cause phenytoin toxicity. TMP-SMZ exerts a potassium-sparing effect on the nephron and should be used with caution with diuretics such as spironolactone (Aldactone) to prevent hyperkalemia.

Lab Tests: Unknown

Herbal/Food: Potassium supplements should not be taken during therapy, unless directed by the health care provider.

Treatment of Overdose: The renal elimination of trimethoprim can be increased by acidification of the urine. If signs of bone marrow suppression occur during high-dose therapy, 5 to 15 mg of leucovorin should be given daily.

Refer to MyNursingKit for a Nursing Process Focus specific to this drug.

34.15 Miscellaneous Antibacterials

Some anti-infectives cannot be grouped into classes, or the class is too small to warrant separate discussion. That is not to diminish their importance in medicine, because some of the miscellaneous anti-infectives are critical drugs for specific infections. The miscellaneous antibiotics are listed in Table 34.9.

Clindamycin (Cleocin) is effective against both gram-positive and gram-negative bacteria and is considered to be appropriate treatment when less toxic alternatives are not effective options. Susceptible bacteria include *Fusobacterium* and *Clostridium perfringens*. Clindamycin is sometimes the drug of choice for oral infections caused by *bacteroides*. It is contraindicated in patients with a history of hypersensitivity to clindamycin or lincomycin, regional enteritis, or ulcerative colitis. Indications for clindamycin are limited because some patients develop antibiotic-associated pseudomembranous colitis (AAPMC), the most severe adverse effect of this drug. Serious adverse effects such as diarrhea, rashes, difficulty breathing, itching, or difficulty swallowing should be reported to the health care provider immediately.

Metronidazole (Flagyl) is another older anti-infective that is effective against anaerobes that are common causes of abscesses, gangrene, diabetic skin ulcers, and deep-wound infections. A relatively new use is for the treatment of *H. pylori* infections of the stomach associated with peptic ulcer disease (chapter 40 ∞). Metronidazole is one of only a few drugs that have dual activity against both bacteria and multicellular parasites; it is a prototype for the antiprotozoal medications in chapter 35 ∞. When metronidazole is given orally, adverse effects are generally minor, the most common being nausea, dry mouth, and headache. High doses can produce neurotoxicity.

Quinupristin/dalfopristin (Synercid) is a combination drug that is the first in a newer class of antibiotics called *streptogramins*. This drug is primarily indicated for treatment of vancomycin-resistant *Enterococcus faecium* infections. It is contraindicated in patients with hypersensitivity to the drug and should be used cautiously in patients with renal or hepatic dysfunction. Hepatotoxicity is the most serious adverse effect of this drug. The patient should be advised to report significant adverse effects immediately, including irritation, pain, or burning at the IV infusion site, joint and muscle pain, rash, diarrhea, or vomiting.

Linezolid (Zyvox) is significant as the first drug in a newer class of antibiotics called the *oxazolidinones*. This drug is as

TABLE 34.9 Selected Miscellaneous Antibacterials

Drug	Route and Adult Dose (max dose where indicated)	Adverse Effects
aztreonam (Azactam)	IV/IM; 0.5–2.0 g bid–qid (max: 8 g/day)	*Nausea, vomiting, diarrhea, rash, fever, insomnia, cough* <u>Anaphylaxis, superinfections</u>
chloramphenicol	PO/IV; 50 mg/kg qid	*Nausea, vomiting, diarrhea* <u>Anaphylaxis, superinfections, pancytopenia, bone marrow depression, aplastic anemia</u>
clindamycin (Cleocin)	PO; 150–450 mg qid	*Nausea, vomiting, diarrhea, rash* <u>Anaphylaxis, superinfections, cardiac arrest, pseudomembranous colitis, blood dyscrasias</u>
daptomycin (Cubicin)	IV; 4 mg/kg once every 24 h for 7–14 days	*Nausea, diarrhea, constipation, headache* <u>Anaphylaxis, superinfections, myopathy, pseudomembranous colitis</u>
ertapenem (Invanz)	IV/IM; 1 g/day	*Nausea, diarrhea, headache* <u>Anaphylaxis, superinfections, pseudomembranous colitis, seizures</u>
fosfomycin (Monurol)	PO; 3-g sachet dissolved in 3–4 oz of water as a single dose	*Nausea, diarrhea, back pain, headache* <u>Anaphylaxis, superinfections</u>
imipenem-cilastatin (Primaxin)	IV; 250–500 mg tid–qid (max: 4 g/day)	*Nausea, vomiting, diarrhea, pain at injection site, headache* <u>Anaphylaxis, superinfections, pseudomembranous colitis</u>
lincomycin (Lincocin)	PO; 500 mg tid–qid (max: 8 g/day)	*Nausea, vomiting, diarrhea* <u>Anaphylaxis, superinfections, cardiac arrest, pseudomembranous colitis, blood dyscrasias</u>
linezolid (Zyvox)	PO; 600 mg bid (max: 1,200 mg/day)	*Nausea, diarrhea, headache* <u>Anaphylaxis, superinfections, pseudomembranous colitis, blood dyscrasias</u>
meropenem (Merrem IV)	IV; 1–2 g tid	*Nausea, vomiting, diarrhea, pain at injection site, headache* <u>Anaphylaxis, superinfections, pseudomembranous colitis, seizures</u>
methenamine (Mandelamine, Hiprex, Urex)	PO; 1 g bid (Hiprex) or qid (Mandelamine)	*Nausea, vomiting, diarrhea, increased urinary urgency* <u>Anaphylaxis, crystalluria</u>
metronidazole (Flagyl)	PO; 7.5 mg/kg every 6 h (max: 4 g/day) IV loading dose; 15 mg/kg IV maintenance dose; 7.5 mg/kg every 6 h (max: 4 g/day)	*Dizziness, headache, anorexia, abdominal pain, metallic taste and nausea, Candida infections* <u>Seizures, peripheral neuropathy, leukopenia</u>
nitrofurantoin (Furadantin, Macrobid, Macrodantin)	PO; 50–100 mg qid (max: 7 mg/kg/day)	*Nausea, vomiting, anorexia, dark urine* <u>Anaphylaxis, superinfections, hepatic necrosis, interstitial pneumonitis, Stevens–Johnson syndrome</u>
quinupristin–dalfopristin (Synercid)	IV; 7.5 mg/kg infused over 60 min every 8 h	*Pain and inflammation at injection site, myalgia, arthralgia, diarrhea* <u>Superinfections, pseudomembranous colitis</u>
telithromycin (Ketek)	PO; 800 mg/day	*Nausea, vomiting, diarrhea* <u>Visual disturbances, hepatotoxicity, dysrhythmias</u>
vancomycin (Vancocin, others)	IV; 500 mg qid or 1 g bid PO; 125–500 mg every 6 h	*Nausea, vomiting* <u>Anaphylaxis, superinfections, nephrotoxicity, ototoxicity, red-man syndrome</u>

Italics indicate common adverse effects; <u>underlining</u> indicates serious adverse effects.

NURSING PROCESS FOCUS   PATIENTS RECEIVING ANTIBACTERIAL THERAPY

Assessment	Potential Nursing Diagnoses
Baseline assessment prior to administration: ■ Understand the reason the drug has been prescribed in order to assess for therapeutic effects. ■ Obtain a complete health history including neurologic, cardiovascular, respiratory, hepatic or renal disease, and the possibility of pregnancy. Obtain a drug history including allergies, including specific reactions to drugs, current prescription and OTC drugs, herbal preparations, and alcohol use. Be alert to possible drug interactions. ■ Assess signs and symptoms of current infection noting location, characteristics, presence or absence of drainage and character of drainage, duration, and presence or absence of fever or pain. ■ Evaluate appropriate laboratory findings (e.g., CBC, C&S, hepatic and renal function studies).	■ Infection ■ Pain (related to infection) ■ Hyperthermia ■ Deficient Knowledge (drug therapy) ■ Risk for Injury (related to adverse drug effects) ■ Risk for Deficient Fluid Volume (related to fever, diarrhea caused by adverse drug effects) ■ Risk for Noncompliance (related to adverse drug effects, deficient knowledge, or cost of medication)
Assessment throughout administration: ■ Assess for desired therapeutic effects (e.g., diminished signs and symptoms of infection and fever). ■ Continue periodic monitoring of CBC, hepatic and renal function, urinalysis, C&S, peak and trough drug levels. ■ Assess for adverse effects: nausea, vomiting, abdominal cramping, diarrhea, drowsiness, dizziness, and photosensitivity. Severe diarrhea, especially containing mucus, blood, or pus; yellowing of sclera or skin; and decreased urine output or darkened urine should be reported immediately.	

Planning: Patient Goals and Expected Outcomes

The patient will:
■ Experience therapeutic effects (e.g., diminished signs and symptoms of infection, decreased fever).
■ Be free from, or experience minimal, adverse effects.
■ Verbalize an understanding of the drug's use, adverse effects, and required precautions.
■ Demonstrate proper self-administration of the medication (e.g., dose, timing, when to notify provider).

Implementation

Interventions and (Rationales)	Patient and Family Education
Ensuring therapeutic effects: ■ Continue assessments as described earlier for therapeutic effects. (Diminished fever, pain, or signs and symptoms of infection should begin after taking the first dose and continue to improve. The health care provider should be notified if fever and signs of infection remain after 3 days or if entire course of the drug has been taken and signs of infection are still present.)	■ Teach the patient to report a fever that does not diminish below 100°F within 3 days; increasing signs and symptoms of infection; or symptoms that remain present after taking the entire course of the drug. ■ Teach the patient to not stop antibacterial when "feeling better" but to take the entire course of antibacterial; do not share doses with other family members with similar symptoms; and return to the health care provider if symptoms have not resolved after entire course of therapy.
Minimizing adverse effects: ■ Continue to monitor vital signs. Immediately report undiminished fever, changes in level of consciousness (LOC), or febrile seizures to the health care provider. (Fever should begin to diminish within 1 to 3 days after starting the drug. A continued fever may be a sign of worsening infection, adverse drug effects, or antibiotic resistance.)	■ Teach the patient to immediately report a fever that does not diminish below 100°F; febrile seizures; and changes in behavior or LOC to the health care provider.
■ Continue to monitor periodic lab work: hepatic and renal function tests, CBC, urinalysis, C&S, and peak and trough drug levels. (Many antibacterials are hepatic and/or renal toxic. Periodic C&S tests may be ordered if infections are severe or are slow to resolve to confirm appropriate therapy. Drug levels will be monitored with drugs with known severe adverse effects.)	■ Instruct the patient on the need for periodic lab work.

NURSING PROCESS FOCUS   **PATIENTS RECEIVING ANTIBACTERIAL THERAPY** *(Continued)*

Implementation

Interventions and (Rationales)	Patient and Family Education
▪ Monitor for hypersensitivity and allergic reactions, especially with the first dose of any antibacterial. Continue to monitor for up to 2 weeks after completing antibacterial therapy. (Anaphylactic reactions are possible, particularly with the first dose of an antibacterial. Post-use, residual drug levels, dependent on length of half-life, may cause delayed reactions.)	▪ Teach the patient to immediately report any itching; rashes; swelling, particularly of face, tongue, or lips; urticaria; flushing; dizziness; syncope; wheezing; throat tightness; or difficulty breathing. ▪ Instruct the patient with known antibacterial allergies to carry a wallet identification card or wear medical identification jewelry indicating allergy.
▪ Continue to monitor for hepatic, renal, and/or ototoxicity. (Antibacterials that are hepatic, renal, or ototoxic require frequent monitoring to prevent adverse effects. Increasing fluid intake will prevent drug accumulation in kidneys.)	▪ Teach the patient to immediately report any nausea; vomiting; yellowing of skin or sclera; abdominal pain; light or clay-colored stools; diminished urine output or darkening of urine; ringing, humming, or buzzing in ears; and dizziness or vertigo. ▪ Advise the patient to increase fluid intake to 2 to 3 L per day.
▪ Continue to monitor for dermatologic effects including red or purplish skin rash, blisters, and sunburning. Immediately report severe rashes, especially associated with blistering. (Tetracyclines, sulfonamides, and fluoroquinolones may cause significant dermatologic effects including Stevens–Johnson syndrome. Sunscreens and protective clothing should be used for antibacterials that cause photosensitivity.)	▪ Teach the patient to wear sunscreens and protective clothing for sun exposure and to avoid tanning beds. Immediately report any severe sunburn or rashes.
▪ Monitor for severe diarrhea. (Severe diarrhea may indicate the presence of antibiotic-associated pseudomembranous colitis, or AAPMC, a superinfection caused by *Clostridium difficile*.)	▪ Instruct the patient to report any diarrhea that increases in frequency, amount, or contains mucus, blood, or pus. ▪ Instruct the patient to consult the health care provider before taking antidiarrheal drugs, which could cause retention of harmful bacteria. ▪ Teach the patient to increase the intake of dairy products with live active cultures such as kefir, yogurt, or buttermilk, to help restore and maintain normal intestinal flora.
▪ Monitor for development of superinfections, e.g., AAPMC, or fungal or yeast infections. (Superinfections with opportunistic organisms may occur when normal host flora are diminished or killed by the antibacterial.)	▪ Teach the patient to observe for changes in stool, white patches in mouth, whitish thick vaginal discharge, itching in urogenital area, blistering itchy rash, and to immediately report severe diarrhea as described earlier. ▪ Teach the patient infection control measures such as frequent hand washing, allowing for adequate drying after bathing, and to increase intake of live-culture–rich dairy foods.
▪ Monitor for significant GI effects, including nausea, vomiting, and abdominal pain or cramping. Give the drug with food or milk to decrease adverse GI effects. (Many antibiotics are associated with significant GI effects. Food or milk may impair absorption of some antibiotics such as macrolides, but if patient compliance with drug regimen can be ensured with lessened GI effects, give with a snack and continue to monitor for therapeutic effects.)	▪ Teach the patient to take drug with food or milk but to avoid acidic foods and beverages or carbonated drinks. ▪ Teach the patient to observe for continuing signs of improvement in infection.
▪ Monitor for signs and symptoms of neurotoxicity, e.g., dizziness, drowsiness, severe headache, changes in LOC, and seizures. (Penicillins, cephalosporins, sulfonamides, aminoglycosides, and fluoroquinolones have an increased risk of neurotoxicity. Previous seizure disorders or head injuries may increase this risk.)	▪ Instruct the patient to immediately report increasing headache, dizziness, drowsiness, changes in behavior or LOC, or seizures. ▪ Caution the patient that drowsiness may occur and to be cautious with driving or other activities requiring mental alertness until the effects of the drug are known.
▪ Monitor for signs and symptoms of blood dyscrasias, e.g., low-grade fevers, bleeding, bruising, and significant fatigue. (Penicillins, aminoglycosides, and fluoroquinolones may cause blood dyscrasias with resulting decreases in RBCs, WBCs, and/or platelets. Periodic monitoring of CBC may be required.)	▪ Teach the patient to report any low-grade fever, sore throat, rashes, bruising or increased bleeding, and unusual fatigue or shortness of breath, especially after taking an antibiotic for a prolonged period.

(Continued)

NURSING PROCESS FOCUS   PATIENTS RECEIVING ANTIBACTERIAL THERAPY *(Continued)*

Implementation

Interventions and (Rationales)	Patient and Family Education
■ Monitor for development of red-man syndrome in patients receiving vancomycin. Report any significantly large area of reddening such as trunk, head or neck, limbs, or gluteal area especially if associated with decreased blood pressure or tachycardia. (Vancomycin hypersensitivity may cause the release of large amounts of histamine. If a significant area is involved, vasodilation from histamine may cause hypotension and reflex tachycardia. Giving IV drip more slowly may prevent or decrease the effects of the syndrome.)	■ Instruct the patient to immediately report unusual flushing, especially involving a large body area; dizziness; dyspnea; or palpitations.
■ Monitor electrolytes, pulse, and ECG if indicated in patients on penicillins. (Some preparations of penicillin may be based in sodium or potassium salts and may cause hypernatremia and hyperkalemia.)	■ Teach the patient to promptly report any palpitations or dizziness.
■ Monitor patients on fluoroquinolones for leg or heel pain, or difficulty walking. (Fluoroquinolones have been associated with tendinitis and tendon rupture, especially of the Achilles tendon.)	■ Instruct the patient to immediately report any significant or increasing heel, lower leg or calf pain, or difficulty walking to the provider.
■ Assess for the possibility of pregnancy or breast-feeding in patients prescribed tetracycline antibiotics. (Tetracyclines affect fetal bone growth and teeth development, causing permanent yellowish-brown staining of teeth.)	■ Advise women who are pregnant, breast-feeding, or attempting to become pregnant to advise their health care provider before receiving any tetracycline antibiotic.
■ Women of child-bearing age taking penicillin antibiotics should use an alternative form of birth control to prevent pregnancy. (Penicillins may reduce the effectiveness of oral contraceptives.)	■ Teach women of child-bearing age on oral contraceptives to consult their health care provider about birth control alternatives if penicillin antibiotics are used.
Patient understanding of drug therapy: ■ Use opportunities during administration of medications and during assessments to discuss the rationale for drug therapy, desired therapeutic outcomes, most common adverse effects, parameters for when to call the health care provider, and any necessary monitoring or precautions. (Using time during nursing care helps to optimize and reinforce key teaching areas.)	■ The patient, family, or caregiver should be able to state the reason for the drug; appropriate dose and scheduling; what adverse effects to observe for and when to report; and the anticipated length of medication therapy.

Patient self-administration of drug therapy:
■ When administering medications, instruct the patient, family, or caregiver in proper self-administration techniques followed by return demonstration. (Proper administration increases the effectiveness of the drug.)
	■ Teach the patient to take the medication as follows:
	  ■ Complete the entire course of therapy unless otherwise instructed.
	  ■ Avoid or eliminate alcohol. Some antibiotics (e.g., cephalosporins) cause significant reactions when taken with alcohol and alcohol increases adverse GI effects of the antibacterial.
	  ■ Take the drug with food or milk but avoid acidic beverages. If instructed to take the drug on an empty stomach, take with a full glass of water.
	  ■ Take the medication as evenly spaced throughout each day as feasible.
	  ■ Do not take tetracycline with milk products, iron-containing preparations such as multivitamins, or with antacids.
	  ■ Increase overall fluid intake while taking the antibacterial drug.
	  ■ Discard outdated medications or those no longer in use. Review medicine cabinet twice a year for old medications.

Evaluation of Outcome Criteria

Evaluate the effectiveness of drug therapy by confirming that patient goals and expected outcomes have been met (see "Planning").

See Tables 34.2 through 34.9 for lists of drugs to which these nursing actions apply.

effective as vancomycin against MRSA infections. Linezolid is administered intravenously or orally. Most patients can be converted from IV to oral routes in about 5 days. Linezolid is contraindicated in patients with hypersensitivity to the drug and in pregnancy, and should be used with caution in patients who have hypertension. Cautious use is also necessary in patients taking serotonin reuptake inhibitors, because the drugs can interact, causing a hypertensive crisis. Linezolid can cause thrombocytopenia. The patient should be advised to report serious adverse effects such as bleeding, diarrhea, headache, nausea, vomiting, rash, dizziness, or fever to the health care provider immediately.

Vancomycin (Vancocin) is an antibiotic usually reserved for severe infections from gram-positive organisms such as *S. aureus* and *Streptococcus pneumoniae*. It is often used after bacteria have become resistant to other, safer antibiotics. Vancomycin is the most effective drug for treating MRSA infections. Because of the drug's ototoxicity, hearing must be evaluated frequently throughout the course of therapy. Vancomycin can also cause nephrotoxicity, leading to uremia. Peak and trough levels are drawn after three doses have been administered. A reaction that can occur with rapid IV administration is known as **red-man syndrome** and results as large amounts of histamine are released in the body. Symptoms include hypotension with flushing and a red rash most often of the face, neck, trunk, or upper body. Other significant side effects include superinfections, generalized tingling after IV administration, chills, fever, skin rash, hives, hearing loss, and nausea.

Daptomycin (Cubicin) is the first in a newer class of antibiotics called the cyclic lipopeptides. It is approved for the treatment of serious skin and skin-structure infections such as major abscesses, postsurgical skin-wound infections, and infected ulcers caused by *S. aureus*, *Streptococcus pyogenes*, *Streptococcus agalactiae*, and *E. faecalis*. The most frequent adverse effects are GI distress, injection site reactions, fever, headache, dizziness, insomnia, and rash.

Imipenem-cilastatin (Primaxin), ertapenem (Invanz), and meropenem (Merrem IV) belong to a newer class of antibiotics called *carbapenems*. These drugs are bacteriocidal and have some of the broadest antimicrobial spectrums of any class of antibiotics. Of the three carbapenems, imipenem has the broadest antimicrobial spectrum and is the most widely prescribed drug in this small class. Imipenem is always administered in a fixed-dose combination with cilastatin, which increases the serum levels of the antibiotic. Meropenem is approved only for peritonitis and bacterial meningitis. Ertapenem has a narrower spectrum but longer half-life than the other carbapenems. It is approved for the treatment of serious abdominopelvic and skin infections, community-acquired pneumonia, and complicated UTI. All the carbapenems exhibit a low incidence of adverse effects. Diarrhea, nausea, rashes, and thrombophlebitis at injection sites are the most frequent adverse effects.

In 2004, the FDA approved telithromycin (Ketek), the first in a class of antibiotics known as the *ketolides*, for respiratory infections. Its indications include acute bacterial exacerbation of chronic bronchitis, acute bacterial sinusitis, and community-acquired pneumonia due to *S. pneumoniae*. Telithromycin is an oral drug, and its most common adverse effects are diarrhea, nausea, and headache. Because of the drug's recent approval, resistance is not yet a clinical problem.

TUBERCULOSIS

Tuberculosis (TB) is a highly contagious infection caused by the organism *Mycobacterium tuberculosis*. The incidence is staggering: More than 1.8 billion people, or 32% of the world population, are believed to be infected. It is treated with multiple anti-infectives for a prolonged period. The antitubercular agents are listed in Table 34.10.

34.16 Pharmacotherapy of Tuberculosis

Although *M. tuberculosis* typically invades the lung, it may travel to other body systems, particularly bone, via the blood or lymphatic system. *M. tuberculosis* activates the body's immune defenses, which attempt to isolate the pathogens by creating a wall around them. The slow-growing mycobacteria usually become dormant, existing inside cavities called **tubercles.** They may remain dormant during an entire lifetime, or become reactivated if the patient's immune response becomes suppressed. Because of the immune suppression characteristic of AIDS, the incidence of TB greatly increased from 1985 to 1992; as many as 20% of all AIDS patients develop active tuberculosis infections. The overall incidence of TB, however, has been declining in the United States since 1992, due to the improved pharmacotherapy of HIV-AIDS.

Drug therapy of TB differs from that of most other infections. Mycobacteria have a cell wall that is resistant to penetration by anti-infective drugs. For medications to reach the microorganisms isolated in the tubercles, therapy must continue for 6 to 12 months. Although the patient may not be infectious this entire time and may have no symptoms, it is critical that therapy continue for the entire period. Some patients develop multidrug-resistant infections and require therapy for as long as 24 months.

A second distinguishing feature of pharmacotherapy for tuberculosis is that at least two, and sometimes four or more, antibiotics are administered concurrently. During the 6- to 24-month treatment period, different combinations of drugs may be used. Multiple drug therapy is necessary because the mycobacteria grow slowly, and resistance is common. Using multiple drugs in different combinations during the long treatment period lowers the potential for resistance and increases therapeutic success. Although many different drug combinations are used, a typical regimen for patients with no complicating factors includes the following:

- *Initial phase:* 2 months of daily therapy with isoniazid, rifampin (Rifadin, Rimactane), pyrazinamide (PZA), and ethambutol (Myambutol). If laboratory test results show that the strain is sensitive to the first three drugs, ethambutol is dropped from the regimen.

TABLE 34.10	Antituberculosis Drugs	
Drug	Route and Adult Dose (max dose where indicated)	Adverse Effects
FIRST-LINE AGENTS		
ethambutol (Myambutol)	PO; 15–25 mg/kg/day (max: 1,600 mg for daily therapy)	*Nausea, vomiting, headache, dizziness* <u>Anaphylaxis, optic neuritis</u>
℞ isoniazid (INH, Nydrazid)	**Latent TB** PO; 300 mg/day or 900 mg twice weekly for 6–9 months **Active TB** PO; daily therapy 5 mg/kg/day or 300 mg/day; if given by DOT, 15 mg/kg or 900 mg twice weekly	*Nausea, vomiting, diarrhea, epigastric pain* <u>Anaphylaxis, peripheral neuropathy, optic neuritis, hepatotoxicity, blood dyscrasias</u>
pyrazinamide (PZA)	PO; 5–15 mg/kg tid–qid (max: 2 g/day)	*Gouty arthritis, increase in serum uric acid, rash* <u>Anaphylaxis, hepatotoxicity, fatal hemoptysis, hemolytic anemia</u>
rifabutin (Mycobutin) rifampin (Rifadin, Rimactane) rifapentine (Priftin)	PO; 300 mg once daily (for prophylaxis) or 5 mg/kg/day (for active TB) (max: 300 mg/day) PO/IV; 600 mg/day as a single dose or 900 mg twice weekly for 4 months PO; 600 mg twice a week for 2 mo; then once a week for 4 mo	*Nausea, vomiting, heartburn, epigastric pain, anorexia flatulence, diarrhea, cramping, orange discoloration of urine, sweat, and tears* <u>Pseudomembranous colitis, acute renal failure, hepatotoxicity, hyperuricemia, blood dycrasias</u>
Rifater: combination of pyrazinamide with isoniazid and rifampin	PO; 6 tablets/day (for patients weighing 121 lb or more)	(See individual drugs)
SECOND-LINE AGENTS		
amikacin (Amikin)	IV/IM; 5–7.5 mg/kg as a loading dose; then 7.5 mg/kg bid	(See Table 34.6)
aminosalicylic acid (Paser)	PO; 150 mg/kg/day in 3–4 equally divided doses	*GI intolerance, anorexia, diarrhea, fever* <u>Hypersensitivity, inhibition of vitamin B$_{12}$ absorption, hepatotoxicity</u>
capreomycin (Capastat Sulfate)	IM; 1 g/day (not to exceed 20 mg/kg/day) for 60–120 days, then 1 g two to three times/wk	*Rash, pain and inflammation at injection site* <u>Blood dyscrasias, nephrotoxicity, ototoxicity</u>
ciprofloxacin (Cipro)	PO/IV; 250–750 mg bid	(See Table 34.7)
cycloserine (Seromycin)	PO; 250 mg every 12 h for 2 wk; may increase to 500 mg every 12 h (max 1 g/day)	*Drowsiness, headache, lethargy* <u>Convulsions, psychosis, confusion</u>
ethionamide (Trecator-SC)	PO; 0.5–1.0 g/day divided every 8–12 h (max: 1 gram given in three to four divided doses)	*Nausea, vomiting, epigastric pain, diarrhea* <u>Convulsions, hallucinations, mental depression</u>
kanamycin (Kantrex)	IM; 5–7.5 mg/kg bid–tid	(See Table 34.6)
ofloxacin (Floxin)	PO; 200–400 mg bid	(See Table 34.7)
streptomycin	IM; 15 mg/kg up to 1 g/day as a single dose	*Nausea, vomiting, pain at injection site, drowsiness headache* <u>Anaphylaxis, ototoxicity, profound CNS depression in infants, respiratory depression, exfoliative dermatitis, nephrotoxicity</u>

Italics indicate common adverse effects; <u>underlining</u> indicates serious adverse effects.

Pr Prototype Drug | Isoniazid *(INH)*

Therapeutic Class: Antituberculosis drug   **Pharmacologic Class:** Mycolic acid inhibitor

ACTIONS AND USES

Isoniazid is a drug of choice for the treatment of *M. tuberculosis* because decades of experience have shown it to have a superior safety profile and to be the most effective, single drug for the infection. The drug acts by inhibiting the synthesis of mycolic acids, which are essential components of mycobacterial cell walls. It is bactericidal for actively growing organisms but bacteriostatic for dormant mycobacteria. It is selective for *M. tuberculosis*. Isoniazid may be used alone for chemoprophylaxis, or in combination with other antituberculosis drugs for treating active disease.

ADMINISTRATION ALERTS

- Give on an empty stomach, 1 hour after or 2 hours before meals.
- For IM administration, administer deep IM, and rotate sites.
- Pregnancy category C

PHARMACOKINETICS
Onset: 30 min
Peak: 1–2 h
Half-life: 1–4 h
Duration: 6–8 h

ADVERSE EFFECTS

The most common adverse effects of isoniazid are numbness of the hands and feet, rash, and fever. An FDA black box warning for isoniazid states that severe and sometimes fatal hepatitis has been reported with this drug. Although rare, hepatotoxicity usually occurs in the first 1 to 3 months of therapy but may present at any time during treatment. The nurse should be alert for signs of jaundice, fatigue, elevated hepatic enzymes, or loss of appetite. Hepatic enzyme tests are usually performed monthly during therapy to identify early hepatotoxicity.

Contraindications: Isoniazid is contraindicated in patients with hypersensitivity to the drug and in patients with severe hepatic impairment.

INTERACTIONS

Drug–Drug: Aluminum-containing antacids should not be administered concurrently because they can decrease the absorption of isoniazid. When disulfiram is taken with INH, lack of coordination or psychotic reactions may result. Drinking alcohol with INH increases the risk of hepatotoxicity. Isoniazid may increase serum levels of phenytoin and carbamazepine.

Lab Tests: Isoniazid may increase values of AST and ALT.

Herbal/Food: Food interferes with the absorption of isoniazid. Foods containing tyramine may increase isoniazid toxicity.

Treatment of Overdose: Isoniazid overdose may be fatal. Treatment is mostly symptomatic. Pyridoxine (vitamin B_6) may be infused in a dose equal to that of the isoniazid overdose to prevent seizures and to correct metabolic acidosis. The dose may be repeated several times until the patient regains consciousness.

Refer to MyNursingKit for a Nursing Process Focus specific to this drug.

- *Continuation phase:* 4 months of therapy with isoniazid and rifampin, two to three times per week.

There are two broad categories of antitubercular agents. One category consists of primary, first-line drugs, which are generally the most effective and best tolerated by patients. Secondary (second-line) drugs, more toxic and less effective than the first-line agents, are used when resistance develops. Infections due to multidrug-resistant *M. tuberculosis* can be rapidly fatal and can cause serious public health problems in some communities.

A third feature of antitubercular therapy is that drugs are extensively used for *preventing* the disease in addition to treating it. Chemoprophylaxis is initiated for close contacts of recently infected tuberculosis patients or for those who are susceptible to infections because they are immunosuppressed. Therapy usually begins immediately after a patient receives a positive tuberculin test. Patients with immunosuppression, such as those with AIDS or those receiving immunosuppressant drugs, may receive chemoprophylaxis with antituberculosis drugs. A short-term therapy of 2 months, consisting of a combination treatment with isoniazid (INH) and pyrazinamide (PZA), is approved for tuberculosis prophylaxis in HIV-positive patients.

Two other types of mycobacteria infect humans. *Mycobacterium leprae* is responsible for leprosy, a disease rarely seen in the United States. *M. leprae* is treated with multiple drugs, usually beginning with dapsone (DDS). *Mycobacterium avium complex* (MAC) causes an infection of the lungs, most commonly observed in AIDS patients. The most effective drugs against MAC are the macrolides azithromycin (Zithromax) and clarithromycin (Biaxin).

See Nursing Process Focus: Patients Receiving Antituberculosis Drugs on page 502 for specific teaching points.

COMPLEMENTARY AND ALTERNATIVE THERAPIES

Antibacterial Properties of Goldenseal

Goldenseal *(Hydrastis canadensis)* was once a common plant found in woods in the eastern and midwestern United States. American Indians used the root for a variety of medicinal applications, including wound healing, diuresis, and washes for inflamed eyes. In recent years, the plant has been harvested to near extinction. In particular, goldenseal was reported to mask the appearance of drugs in the urine of patients wanting to hide drug abuse. This claim has since been proved false.

The roots and leaves of goldenseal are dried and available as capsules, tablets, salves, and tinctures. One of the primary active ingredients in goldenseal is hydrastine, which is reported to have antibacterial and antifungal properties. When used topically or locally, goldenseal is claimed to be of value in treating bacterial and fungal skin infections and oral conditions such as gingivitis and thrush. As an eyewash, it can soothe inflamed eyes. Considered safe for most people, it is contraindicated in pregnancy and hypertension.

NURSING PROCESS FOCUS   PATIENTS RECEIVING ANTITUBERCULOSIS DRUGS

Assessment	Potential Nursing Diagnoses
Baseline assessment prior to administration: ■ Understand the reason the drug has been prescribed in order to assess for therapeutic effects. ■ Obtain a complete health history including neurologic, cardiovascular, respiratory, gastrointestinal hepatic or renal disease, and the possibility of pregnancy. Obtain a drug history including allergies, including specific reactions to drugs, current prescription and OTC drugs, herbal preparations, and alcohol use. Be alert to possible drug interactions. ■ Assess signs and symptoms of current infection noting symptoms, duration, or any recent changes. Assess for concurrent infections, particularly HIV. ■ Evaluate appropriate laboratory findings (e.g., CBC, AFB C&S, hepatic and renal function studies).	■ Infection ■ Fatigue ■ Imbalanced Nutrition, Less than Body Requirements (related to fatigue, adverse drug effects) ■ Deficient Knowledge (drug therapy, infection control measures) ■ Risk for Noncompliance (related to adverse drug effects, deficient knowledge, length of treatment required, or cost of medication) ■ Risk for Social Isolation (related to disease, length of treatment)
Assessment throughout administration: ■ Assess for desired therapeutic effects (e.g., diminished signs and symptoms of infection, fever, night-sweating, increasing ease of breathing, decreased sputum production, improved radiographic evidence of improving infection). ■ Continue periodic monitoring of CBC, and hepatic and renal function. ■ Assess for adverse effects: nausea, vomiting, abdominal cramping, diarrhea, drowsiness, dizziness, paresthesias, tinnitus, vertigo, blurred vision, changes in visual color sense, and increasing fatigue. Eye pain, acute vision change, sudden or increasing numbness or tingling in extremities, decreased hearing or significant tinnitus, and increase in bruising or bleeding should be immediately reported.	

Planning: Patient Goals and Expected Outcomes

The patient will:
■ Experience therapeutic effects (e.g., diminished signs and symptoms of infection, decreased fever and fatigue, increased appetite).
■ Be free from, or experience minimal, adverse effects.
■ Verbalize an understanding of the drug's use, adverse effects, and required precautions.
■ Demonstrate proper self-administration of the medication (e.g., dose, timing, when to notify provider).

Implementation

Interventions and (Rationales)	Patient Education/Discharge Planning
Ensuring therapeutic effects: ■ Continue assessments as described earlier for therapeutic effects. (Diminished fever, cough, sputum, and other signs and symptoms of infection should be noted.) ■ Recognize that tuberculosis treatment requires long-term compliance and many reasons exist for noncompliance. (Noncompliance may increase the risk to the patient's health, family and community health, and promotes the development of resistant organisms. Monitoring of drug administration may be required to ensure therapy is continued.)	■ Teach the patient to not stop drugs when "feeling better" but to continue prescribed course of therapy; do not share doses with other family members with similar symptoms; and return to provider if adverse effects develop to ensure drug therapy is maintained. ■ Discuss with the patient concerns about cost, family members who have similar symptoms or may need prophylactic treatment, and how to manage adverse effects to help encourage compliance.
Minimizing adverse effects: ■ Continue to monitor vital signs, breath sounds, and sputum production and quality. Immediately report undiminished fever, increases in sputum production, hemoptysis, or increase in adventitious breath sounds to the health care provider. (Increasing signs of infection may signify drug resistance or significant noncompliance with drug regimen.)	■ Teach the patient to promptly report a fever that does not diminish below 100°F; continued symptoms of disease (e.g., night sweating, fatigue); or increase in sputum production to the health care provider.
■ Continue to monitor periodic lab work: hepatic and renal function tests, CBC, and sputum culture for AFB. (Antituberculosis drugs are hepatic and/or renal toxic. Periodic C&S tests may be ordered if infections are severe or are slow to resolve to confirm appropriate therapy. Drug levels will be monitored on drugs with known severe adverse effects.)	■ Instruct the patient on the need for periodic lab work.

NURSING PROCESS FOCUS   PATIENTS RECEIVING ANTITUBERCULOSIS DRUGS *(Continued)*

Implementation

Interventions and (Rationales)	Patient Education/Discharge Planning
▪ Continue to monitor for hepatic, renal, and/or ototoxicity. (Antituberculosis drugs that are hepatic, renal, or ototoxic require frequent monitoring to prevent adverse effects. Increasing fluid intake will prevent drug accumulation in kidneys.)	▪ Teach the patient to report any nausea, vomiting, yellowing of skin or sclera, abdominal pain, light or clay-colored stools, diminished urine output, darkening of urine, ringing, humming, or buzzing in ears, and dizziness or vertigo immediately. ▪ Advise the patient to increase fluid intake to 2 to 3 L per day and to eliminate all alcohol use.
▪ Monitor for signs and symptoms of neurotoxicity, particularly peripheral and optic neuropathy. (Neurotoxicity and peripheral neuritis are adverse effects of antituberculosis drugs. Vitamin B_6 may be ordered to decrease the risk of peripheral neuropathy.)	▪ Instruct the patient to report drowsiness, dizziness, numbness or tingling in peripheral extremities, and vision changes. Eye pain, acute blurring of vision or loss of color sense, and sudden or increasing numbness or tingling in extremities should be reported immediately. ▪ Encourage the patient to increase the intake of vitamin B_6 rich foods (e.g., fortified cereals, baked potato with skin on, bananas, lean meats, garbanzo beans) and discuss vitamin B_6 supplements with the health care provider.
▪ Monitor blood glucose in patients taking isoniazid. (Isoniazid may increase glucose levels. Diabetic patients may require a change in their antidiabetic drug routine.)	▪ Teach the diabetic patient to test glucose more frequently, reporting any consistent elevations to the health care provider.
▪ Monitor dietary routine in patients taking isoniazid. (Foods high in tyramine can interact with the drug and cause palpitations, flushing, and hypertension.)	▪ Advise the patient taking isoniazid to avoid foods containing tyramine, such as aged cheese, smoked and pickled fish, beer and red wine, bananas, and chocolate and to report headache, palpitations, tachycardia, or fever immediately.
▪ Patients taking rifampin should be cautioned that drug may turn body fluids (tears, sweat, saliva, urine) reddish-orange. (Effect is harmless but may stain soft, hydrophilic contact lenses or clothing.)	▪ Teach the patient to consult with the eye care provider before using hydrophilic contact lenses. Consider wearing nonwhite clothing or use undergarments if sweating is excessive.
▪ Encourage infection control measures based on the extent of disease condition, and follow established protocol in hospitalized patients. (Infection control measures prevent disease transmission. Specific isolation precautions or use of specialized masks may be required for hospitalized patient.)	▪ Teach the patient adequate infection control and hygiene measures such as frequent hand washing, covering the mouth when coughing or sneezing, and proper disposal of soiled tissues.
Patient understanding of drug therapy: ▪ Use opportunities during administration of medications and during assessments to discuss rationale for drug therapy, desired therapeutic outcomes, most commonly observed adverse effects, parameters for when to call the health care provider, and any necessary monitoring or precautions. (Using time during nursing care helps to optimize and reinforce key teaching areas.)	▪ The patient, family, or caregiver should be able to state the reason for the drug; appropriate dose and scheduling; what adverse effects to observe for and when to report; and the anticipated length of medication therapy.

Patient self-administration of drug therapy:
▪ When administering medications, instruct the patient, family, or caregiver in proper self-administration techniques followed by return demonstration. (Proper administration will increase the effectiveness of the drug.)
	▪ Teach the patient to take the medication as follows:
	  ▪ Complete the entire course of therapy unless otherwise instructed. The duration of the required therapy may be quite lengthy but it is necessary to prevent active infection.
	  ▪ Eliminate alcohol while on these medications. These drugs cause significant reactions when taken with alcohol.
	  ▪ Take the drug with food or milk but avoid acidic beverages. If instructed to take the drug on an empty stomach, take with a full glass of water.
	  ▪ Take the medication as evenly spaced throughout each day as feasible.
	  ▪ Increase overall fluid intake while taking these drugs.

Evaluation of Outcome Criteria

Evaluate the effectiveness of drug therapy by confirming that patient goals and expected outcomes have been met (see "Planning").

See Table 34.10 for a list of drugs to which these nursing actions apply.

Chapter REVIEW

KEY CONCEPTS

The numbered key concepts provide a succinct summary of the important points from the corresponding numbered section within the chapter. If any of these points are not clear, refer to the numbered section within the chapter for review.

34.1 Pathogens are organisms that cause disease due to their ability to divide rapidly or secrete toxins.

34.2 Bacteria are described by their shape (bacilli, cocci, or spirilla), their ability to utilize oxygen (aerobic or anaerobic), and by their staining characteristics (gram positive or gram negative).

34.3 Anti-infective drugs are classified by their chemical structures (e.g., aminoglycoside, fluoroquinolone) or by their mechanism of action (e.g., cell-wall inhibitor, folic acid inhibitor).

34.4 Anti-infective drugs act by affecting the target organism's unique structure, metabolism, or life cycle and may be bacteriocidal or bacteriostatic.

34.5 Acquired resistance occurs when a pathogen acquires a gene for bacterial resistance, either through mutation or from another microbe. Resistance results in loss of antibiotic effectiveness and is worsened by the overprescribing of these agents.

34.6 Careful selection of the correct antibiotic, through the use of culture and sensitivity testing, is essential for effective pharmacotherapy and to limit adverse effects. Superinfections may occur during antibiotic therapy if too many host flora are killed.

34.7 Host factors such as immune system status, local conditions at the infection site, allergic reactions, age, and genetics influence the choice of antibiotic.

34.8 Penicillins, which kill bacteria by disrupting the cell wall, are most effective against gram-positive bacteria. Allergies occur most frequently with the penicillins.

34.9 The cephalosporins are similar in structure and function to the penicillins and are one of the most widely prescribed anti-infective classes. Cross sensitivity may exist with the penicillins in some patients.

34.10 Tetracyclines have some of the broadest spectrums of any antibiotic class. They are drugs of choice for Rocky Mountain spotted fever, typhus, cholera, Lyme disease, peptic ulcers caused by *Helicobacter pylori,* and chlamydial infections.

34.11 The macrolides are safe alternatives to penicillin. They are effective against most gram-positive bacteria and many gram-negative species.

34.12 The aminoglycosides are narrow-spectrum drugs, most commonly prescribed for infections by aerobic, gram-negative bacteria. They have the potential to cause serious adverse effects such as ototoxicity, nephrotoxicity, and neuromuscular blockade.

34.13 The use of fluoroquinolones has expanded far beyond their initial role in treating urinary tract infections. All fluoroquinolones have activity against gram-negative pathogens, and newer drugs in the class have activity against gram-positive microbes.

34.14 Resistance has limited the usefulness of once widely prescribed sulfonamides to urinary tract infections and a few other specific infections.

34.15 A number of miscellaneous antibacterials have specific indications, distinct antibacterial mechanisms, and related nursing care.

34.16 Multiple drug therapies are needed in the treatment of tuberculosis, since the complex microbes are slow growing and commonly develop drug resistance.

NCLEX-RN® REVIEW QUESTIONS

1 Superinfections are an adverse effect common to all antibiotic therapy. The best description of a superinfection is:
1. an initial infection so overwhelming that it requires multiple antimicrobial agents to treat successfully.
2. bacterial resistance that creates infections difficult to treat and often resistant to multiple drugs.
3. infections requiring high-dose antimicrobial therapy with increased chance of organ toxicity.
4. the overgrowth of normal body flora or of opportunistic organisms no longer held in check by normal, beneficial flora.

2 A patient has been discharged with a prescription for penicillin. Discharge instructions include that:
1. penicillins can be taken while breast-feeding.
2. the entire prescription must be finished.
3. all penicillins can be taken without regard to eating.
4. some possible side effects include abdominal pain and constipation.

3 A patient has been prescribed tetracycline. When providing information regarding this drug, the nurse would be correct in stating that tetracycline:
1. is classified as a narrow-spectrum antibiotic and only treats a few infections.
2. is used to treat a wide variety of disease processes.
3. has been identified to be safe during pregnancy.
4. is contraindicated in children younger than 8 years.

4 Important information to include in the patient's education regarding taking fluoroquinolones is that:
1. the drug can cause discoloration of teeth.
2. fluid intake should be decreased to prevent urine retention.
3. this drug is primarily given orally because it is absorbed in the GI tract.
4. a serious side effect is hearing loss.

5 A patient has been diagnosed with tuberculosis. While his medicine is being administered, he asks questions regarding his treatment. What teaching should the nurse supply to this patient? (Select all that apply.)
1. "It is critical to continue therapy for at least 6 to 12 months."
2. "Two or more drugs may be used to prevent resistance."
3. "These drugs may be used to prevent tuberculosis also."
4. "No special precautions are required."
5. "After 1 month of treatment, the medication will be discontinued."

6 A 32-year-old female has been started on ampicillin for a severe UTI. Before sending her home with this prescription, the nurse will:
1. teach her to wear sunscreens.
2. ask her about oral contraceptive use and recommend an alternative method for the duration of the ampicillin course.
3. assess for hearing loss.
4. recommend taking the pill with some antacid to prevent GI upset.

CRITICAL THINKING QUESTIONS

1. An 18-year-old woman comes to a clinic for prenatal care. She is 8 weeks pregnant. She is healthy and takes no other medication other than low-dose tetracycline for acne. What is a priority of care for this patient?

2. A 32-year-old patient has a diagnosis of otitis external and the health care provider has ordered erythromycin PO. This patient has a history of hepatitis B, allergies to sulfa and penicillin, and mild hypertension. Should the nurse give the erythromycin?

3. A 66-year-old hospitalized patient has MRSA in a cellulitis of the lower extremity and is on gentamicin IV. What is a priority for the nurse to monitor in this patient?

See Appendix D for answers and rationales for all activities.

PEARSON
EXPLORE mynursingkit

MyNursingKit is your one stop for online chapter review materials and resources. Prepare for success with additional NCLEX®-style practice questions, interactive assignments and activities, web links, animations and videos, and more!

Register your access code from the front of your book at
www.mynursingkit.com.

NURSING PROCESS FOCUS — PATIENTS RECEIVING ANTIFUNGAL DRUGS

Assessment	Potential Nursing Diagnoses
Baseline assessment prior to administration: • Understand the reason the drug has been prescribed in order to assess for therapeutic effects. • Obtain a complete health history including neurologic, cardiovascular, respiratory, hepatic or renal disease, and the possibility of pregnancy. Obtain a drug history including allergies, including specific reactions to drugs, current prescription and OTC drugs, herbal preparations, and alcohol use. Be alert to possible drug interactions. • Assess signs and symptoms of current infection noting location, characteristics, presence or absence of drainage and character of drainage, duration, and presence or absence of fever or pain. • Evaluate appropriate laboratory findings (e.g., CBC, electrolytes, urinalysis, culture and sensitivity (C&S), hepatic and renal function studies). • Obtain baseline weight and vital signs, especially blood pressure and pulse.	• Infection (current or risk for concurrent bacterial infection) • Pain (related to infection) • Hyperthermia • Deficient Knowledge (drug therapy) • Risk for Injury (related to adverse drug effects) • Risk for Deficient Fluid Volume (related to fever, diarrhea caused by adverse drug effects) • Risk for Decreased Cardiac Output, Ineffective Tissue Perfusion (related to adverse effects of IV antifungals) • Risk for Noncompliance (related to adverse drug effects, deficient knowledge, or length of therapy)
Assessment throughout administration: • Assess for desired therapeutic effects (e.g., diminished signs and symptoms of infection and fever). • Continue periodic monitoring of CBC, electrolytes, hepatic and renal function, and C&S. • Continue to monitor vital signs, especially blood pressure and pulse, in patients on IV antifungals. • Assess for adverse effects: nausea, vomiting, abdominal cramping, diarrhea, malaise, muscle cramping or pain, chills, drowsiness, dizziness, headache, tinnitus, vertigo, flushing, skin rash, urticaria, seizures, hypotension, and electrolyte imbalances (e.g., hypokalemia, hypomagnesemia). Hypotension, tachycardia, dysrhythmias, changes in level of consciousness (LOC), diminished urine output, or seizures should be reported immediately.	

Planning: Patient Goals and Expected Outcomes

The patient will:
• Experience therapeutic effects (e.g., diminished signs and symptoms of infection, decreased fever).
• Be free from, or experience minimal, adverse effects.
• Verbalize an understanding of the drug's use, adverse effects, and required precautions.
• Demonstrate proper self-administration of the medication (e.g., dose, timing, when to notify provider).

Implementation

Interventions and (Rationales)	Patient and Family Education
Ensuring therapeutic effects: • Continue assessments as described earlier for therapeutic effects. (Diminished fever, pain, or signs and symptoms of infection should be noted.)	• Teach the patient on oral antifungals that several months of treatment may be required. Teach the patient on topical antifungals to complete the entire course of therapy and notify the health care provider if symptoms have not resolved.
Minimizing adverse effects: • Continue frequent monitoring of vital signs, especially blood pressure and pulse, and respiratory rate and depth in patients on IV antifungals. Immediately report dysrhythmias, increasing pulmonary congestion, hypotension, or tachycardia. (Cardiovascular abnormalities are possible adverse effects of IV antifungals. Cardiac and respiratory assessment must be monitored closely to observe for adverse effects.)	• Instruct the patient on the need for frequent monitoring. Explain the rationale for all monitoring equipment used.

NURSING PROCESS FOCUS   PATIENTS RECEIVING ANTIFUNGAL DRUGS *(Continued)*

Implementation

Interventions and (Rationales)	Patient and Family Education
■ Continue to monitor periodic lab work: hepatic and renal function tests, CBC, urinalysis, culture and sensitivity, and electrolyte levels. (Antifungals are hepatic and renal toxic and labs should be monitored frequently. Periodic C&S tests may be ordered if infections are severe or are slow to resolve to confirm appropriate therapy is being delivered. Antifungals, particularly when given IV, may cause electrolyte imbalances, especially hypokalemia and hypomagnesemia, and electrolyte replacement may be needed.)	■ Teach the patient about the need for frequent lab testing. If on oral antifungals at home, instruct the patient on the need for periodic lab work.
■ Weigh the patient daily and report a weight gain of 1 kg or more in a 24-hour period. Measure intake and output in the hospitalized patient. (Daily weight is an accurate measure of fluid status and takes into account intake, output, and insensible losses. Excessive weight gain or edema may indicate renal dysfunction.)	■ Have the patient taking oral antifungal drugs at home weigh self daily, ideally at the same time of day, and record weight along with blood pressure and pulse measurements. Have the patient report significant weight gain.
■ Monitor for hypersensitivity and allergic reactions, especially with the first dose of IV antifungal. Continue to monitor the patient throughout therapy. (Anaphylactic reactions are possible and are most common with the first IV infusion. A test-dose of a small amount given slowly may be given before main infusion. Premedication, including antipyretics, antihistamines, and antiemetics may be necessary to prevent reactions.)	■ Instruct the patient to promptly report any chills, nausea, tremors, or headache.
■ Ensure adequate hydration in patients on oral or IV antifungals. (Antifungal drugs are renal toxic and adequate hydration helps to prevent adverse renal effects.)	■ Teach the patient to increase fluid intake to 2 L per day if on oral antifungals. Explain the rationale for increased IV fluid hydration in patients on IV antifungals.
■ Continue to monitor for signs of ototoxicity. (Antifungals may cause ototoxicity and require frequent monitoring to prevent adverse effects.)	■ Teach the patient to immediately report any ringing, humming, or buzzing in ears, and dizziness or vertigo.
■ Continue to monitor for hepatic toxicity; e.g., jaundice, RUQ pain, darkened urine, diminished urine output, tinnitus, vertigo, in patients on IV or oral antifungal therapy. (Antifungals may cause hepatic toxicity and require frequent monitoring to prevent adverse effects.)	■ Teach the patient to immediately report any nausea, vomiting, yellowing of skin or sclera, abdominal pain, light or clay-colored stools, or darkening of urine.
■ Monitor the IV site frequently for any signs of extravasation or thrombophlebitis. (IV antifungal medication is irritating to veins. Use a central line if possible or frequently monitor the IV site. Infusion pumps must be used to ensure the proper dosage rate and prevent excessive flow rate.)	■ Instruct the patient to immediately report any pain, burning, or redness at the site of the peripheral IV. Explain the rationale for all equipment used.
■ Monitor blood glucose in patients taking ketoconazole. (Ketoconazole may increase glucose levels. Diabetic patients may require a change in their antidiabetic drug routine.)	■ Teach the diabetic patient to test glucose more frequently, reporting any consistent elevations to the health care provider.
■ Monitor for significant GI effects, including nausea, vomiting, and abdominal pain or cramping. Give the drug with food or milk to decrease adverse GI effects. (Food or milk may decrease GI effects but an antiemetic may also be required if nausea is severe.)	■ Teach the patient to take the drug with food or milk but to avoid acidic foods and beverages or carbonated drinks.
■ Monitor for signs and symptoms of secondary infection in topical areas of fungal infection, e.g., athlete's foot. If systemic adverse effects are noted, check the drug dose or administration route the patient is using. (Intense itching with scratching may introduce bacteria into the area, resulting in a secondary bacterial infection that may require additional antibacterial therapy. Topical drug amounts are usually insufficiently absorbed to create systemic effects.)	■ Teach the patient to report any increasing redness, soreness or pain, or increasing drainage from affected site.

(Continued)

NURSING PROCESS FOCUS **PATIENTS RECEIVING ANTIFUNGAL DRUGS** *(Continued)*

Implementation

Interventions and (Rationales)	Patient and Family Education
Patient understanding of drug therapy: • Use opportunities during administration of medications and during assessments to discuss the rationale for drug therapy, desired therapeutic outcomes, most common adverse effects, parameters for when to call the health care provider, and any necessary monitoring or precautions. (Using time during nursing care helps to optimize and reinforce key teaching areas.)	• The patient, family, or caregiver should be able to state the reason for the drug; appropriate dose and scheduling; what adverse effects to observe for and when to report; and the anticipated length of medication therapy.

Patient self-administration of drug therapy:
 	
• When administering medications, instruct the patient, family, or caregiver in proper self-administration techniques. (Proper administration will increase the effectiveness of the drug.)
	• Teach the patient to take oral or topical antifungal medication as follows:
	  • Complete the entire course of therapy unless otherwise instructed. Several months of oral therapy may be required to adequately treat the infection.
	  • Avoid or eliminate alcohol while on oral antifungals to avoid hepatic complications.
	  • Dissolve oral antifungal lozenges (troches) in mouth or rinse with liquids after meals and at bedtime. If dentures are worn, remove them before using the drug and leave out overnight. Swish the liquid drug around mouth and hold in the mouth at least 2 minutes before expectorating. Do not swallow unless instructed to do so and do not rinse the mouth with water afterwards.
	  • Do not use occlusive dressings when topical antifungals are used. Apply a thin, even layer to the affected area.
	  • Allow affected skin areas to air dry and wear loose-fitting and "breathable" fabric clothes to allow adequate ventilation. Gently cleanse areas with mild soap and water and avoid vigorous scrubbing.

Evaluation of Outcome Criteria

Evaluate the effectiveness of drug therapy by confirming that patient goals and expected outcomes have been met (see "Planning").

See Tables 35.2, 35.3, and 35.4 for a list of drugs to which these nursing actions apply.

Although rarely used as monotherapy, flucytosine (Ancobon) is sometimes combined with amphotericin B in the pharmacotherapy of severe candidiasis. Flucytosine can cause immunosuppression and liver toxicity, and resistance has become a major problem.

A newer class of antifungals called *echinocandins* has been added to the treatment options for systemic mycoses. The first drug in this class, caspofungin, has become an important alternative to amphotericin B in the treatment of aspergillosis. Approved in 2006, anidulafungin (Eraxis) is approved for invasive candidiasis. The echinocandins are less nephrotoxic than amphotericin B and have fewer serious adverse effects.

AZOLES

The **azole** drugs consist of two different chemical classes, the imidazoles and the triazoles. Azole antifungal drugs interfere with the biosynthesis of ergosterol, which is essential for fungal cell membranes. Depleting fungal cells of ergosterol impairs their growth. The azole drugs are listed in Table 35.3.

35.5 Pharmacotherapy with the Azole Antifungals

The azole class is the largest and most versatile group of antifungals. These agents have a broad spectrum and are used to treat nearly any systemic, cutaneous, or superficial fungal infection. Fluconazole (Diflucan), itraconazole (Sporanox), ketoconazole (Nizoral), and voriconazole (Vfend) are used for both systemic and topical infections. The remainder of the azoles are prescribed for superficial infections.

Ketoconazole is available only orally, and is the most hepatotoxic of the azoles. Itraconazole has begun to replace ketoconazole in the therapy of systemic mycoses because it is less hepatotoxic and may be given either orally or intravenously. It also has a broader spectrum of activity than the other systemic azoles. Clotrimazole (Mycelex, others) is a preferred drug for superficial fungal infections of the skin, vagina, and mouth.

The *systemic* azole drugs have a spectrum of activity similar to that of amphotericin B, are considerably less toxic, and have the major advantage that they can be administered orally. Because of these characteristics, azoles have replaced amphotericin B in the pharmacotherapy of less

TABLE 35.3	Azole Antifungals	
Drug	**Route and Adult Dose (max dose where indicated)**	**Adverse Effects**
butoconazole (Femstat)	Topical; 1 applicator intravaginally at bedtime for 3 days	**Oral and parenteral routes:**
clotrimazole (FemCare, Gyne-Lotrimin, Mycelex, others)	Topical; apply bid for 4 wk; for vaginal mycoses, insert 1 applicator intravaginally at bedtime for 7 days	*Fever, chills, rash, dizziness, drowsiness, nausea, vomiting, diarrhea*
econazole (Spectazole)	Topical; apply bid for 4 wk	<u>Hepatotoxicity, anaphylaxis, blood dyscrasias</u>
(Pr) fluconazole (Diflucan)	PO/IV; 200–400 mg on day 1, then 100–200 mg/day for 2–4 wk	
itraconazole (Sporanox)	PO; 200 mg/day; may increase to 200 mg bid (max: 400 mg/day)	
ketoconazole (Nizoral)	PO; 200–400 mg/day	
	Topical; apply once or twice daily to affected area	**Topical route:**
miconazole (Micatin, Monistat, Cruex, others)	Topical; apply bid for 2–4 wk	*Drying of skin, stinging sensation at application site, pruritus, urticaria, contact dermatitis*
oxiconazole (Oxistat)	Topical; apply daily in the evening for 2 mo	
sertaconazole (Ertaczo)	Topical; 2% cream bid for 4 wk	<u>No serious adverse effects</u>
sulconazole nitrate (Exelderm)	Topical; apply once or twice daily for 2–6 wk	
terconazole (Terazol)	Topical; 1 applicator intravaginally at bedtime for 3–7 wk	
tioconazole (Vagistat)	Topical; 1 applicator intravaginally at bedtime for 1 day	
voriconazole (Vfend)	IV; 6 mg/kg every 12 h on day 1, then 4 mg/kg every 12 h; may reduce to 3 mg/kg every 12 h if not tolerated	

Italics indicate common adverse effects; <u>underlining</u> indicates serious adverse effects.

(Pr) **Prototype Drug | Fluconazole** *(Diflucan)*

Therapeutic Class: Antifungal   **Pharmacologic Class:** Inhibitor of fungal cell membrane synthesis; azole

ACTIONS AND USES
Like other azoles, fluconazole acts by interfering with the synthesis of ergosterol. Fluconazole, however, offers several advantages over other systemic antifungals. It is rapidly and completely absorbed when given orally, and it is particularly effective against *Candida albicans*. Unlike itraconazole (Sporanox) and ketoconazole (Nizoral), fluconazole is able to penetrate most body membranes to reach infections in the CNS, bone, eye, urinary tract, and respiratory tract.

A major disadvantage of fluconazole is its relatively narrow spectrum of activity. Although it is effective against *Candida albicans,* it may not be effective against non–*albicans Candida* species, which account for a significant percentage of opportunistic fungal infections.

ADMINISTRATION ALERTS
- Do not mix IV fluconazole with other drugs.
- Pregnancy category C

PHARMACOKINETICS
Onset: Unknown
Peak: 2 h
Half-life: 20–50 h
Duration: Unknown

ADVERSE EFFECTS
Fluconazole causes few serious adverse effects. Nausea, vomiting, and diarrhea are reported at high doses. Unlike ketoconazole, hepatotoxicity is rare with fluconazole, although patients with hepatic impairment should be monitored carefully. Stevens–Johnson syndrome has been reported in patients with immunosuppression.

Contraindications: Fluconazole is contraindicated in patients with hypersensitivity to the drug. Coadministration with cisapride is contraindicated. Because most of the drug is excreted by the kidneys, it should be used cautiously in patients with pre-existing kidney disease.

INTERACTIONS
Drug–Drug: Use of fluconazole with warfarin may cause increased risk for bleeding. Hypoglycemia may result if fluconazole is administered concurrently with certain oral hypoglycemics, including glyburide. Fluconazole levels may be decreased with concurrent rifampin or cimetidine use. The effects of fentanyl, alfentanil, or methadone may be prolonged with concurrent administration of fluconazole.

Lab Tests: Values for AST, ALT, and alkaline phosphatase may be increased.

Herbal/Food: Unknown

Treatment of Overdose: There is no specific treatment for overdose. Dialysis can be used to lower the serum drug level.

Refer to MyNursingKit for a Nursing Process Focus specific to this drug.

serious systemic fungal infections. Topical formulations are available for superficial mycoses, although they may also be given by the oral route for these infections.

The most common adverse effects of the systemic azoles are nausea and vomiting; severe nausea may require dose reduction or the concurrent administration of an antiemetic. Anaphylaxis and rash have been reported. Fatal drug-induced hepatitis has occurred with ketoconazole, though the incidence is rare and has not been reported with the other systemic azoles. Azoles may affect glycemic control in diabetic patients. Various reproductive abnormalities have been reported with systemic azoles, including menstrual irregularities, gynecomastia in men, and a decline in testosterone levels. Decreased libido and temporary sterility in men are other potential side effects. The azoles should be used with caution in pregnant patients.

DRUGS FOR SUPERFICIAL FUNGAL INFECTIONS

Superficial mycoses are generally not severe and patients are often treated with topical agents. Selected agents used to treat superficial mycoses are listed in Table 35.4.

35.6 Superficial Fungal Infections

Superficial fungal infections of the hair, scalp, nails, and the mucous membranes of the mouth and vagina are rarely medical emergencies. Infections of the nails and skin, for example, may be ongoing for months or even years before a patient seeks treatment. Unlike systemic fungal infections, superficial infections may occur in any patient, not just those who have suppressed immune systems. For example, about 75% of all adult women experience vulvovaginal candidiasis at least once in their lifetime. Athlete's foot (tinea pedis) and jock itch (tinea cruris) are two commonly experienced skin mycoses.

Antifungal drugs applied topically are much safer than their systemic counterparts because penetration into the deeper layers of the skin or mucous membranes is poor, and only small amounts are absorbed into the circulation. Adverse effects are generally minor and limited to the region being treated. Burning or stinging at the site of application, drying of the skin, rash, or contact dermatitis are the most frequent side effects from the topical agents.

Many medications for superficial mycoses are available as over-the-counter (OTC) creams, gels, powders, and ointments. If the infection has grown into the deeper skin layers, oral antifungal drug therapy may be indicated. Extensive superficial mycoses may be treated with both oral and topical antifungal agents to ensure that the infection is eliminated from deeper skin or mucous membrane layers.

Selection of a particular antifungal agent is based on the location of the infection and characteristics of the lesion. Griseofulvin (Fulvicin) is an inexpensive, older agent given by the oral route that is indicated for mycoses of the hair, skin, and nails that have not responded to conventional topical preparations. Itraconazole (Sporanox) and terbinafine (Lamisil) are oral preparations that have the advantage of accumulating in nail beds, allowing them to remain active many months after therapy is discontinued. Miconazole and

TABLE 35.4	Selected Drugs for Superficial Mycoses*	
Drug	**Route and Adult Dose (max dose where indicated)**	**Adverse Effects**
butenafine (Mentax)	Topical; apply daily for 4 wk for tineas	*Drying of skin, stinging sensation at application site, pruritus, urticaria, contact dermatitis*
ciclopirox cream, gel, shampoo (Loprox) or nail lacquer (Penlac)	Topical; apply cream bid × 4 weeks for tineas	
	Topical; apply lacquer to nail × 48 wks for onychomycoses	Granulocytopenia (griseofulvin), cholestatic hepatitis (oral terbinafine), neutropenia (oral terbinafine)
griseofulvin (Fulvicin)	PO; 500 mg microsize or 330–375 mg ultramicrosize daily for tineas and onychomycoses	
naftifine (Naftin)	Topical; apply cream daily or gel bid for 4 wk for tineas	
⊕ nystatin: topical powder (Mycostatin, Nystop); oral suspension (Nilstat); capsule (Bio-Statin); cream, ointment (Mycostatin, Nystex)	PO; 500,000–1,000,000 units tid	
	Intravaginal; 1–2 tablets daily for 2 wk	
terbinafine (Lamisil)	Topical; apply once daily or bid × 7 wk for tineas	
	PO; 250 mg daily × 6–12 wk for onychomycoses	
tolnaftate (Aftate, Tinactin)	Topical; apply bid for 4–6 wk	
undecylenic acid (Fungi-Nail, Gordochom, others)	Topical; apply once or twice daily	

*Azole antifungal drugs for superficial infections are included in Table 35.3.
Italics indicate common adverse effects; underlining indicates serious adverse effects.

Pr Prototype Drug | Nystatin *(Mycostatin, Nystop, others)*

Therapeutic Class: Topical antifungal   **Pharmacologic Class:** Polyene

ACTIONS AND USES

Nystatin binds to sterols in the fungal cell membrane, causing leakage of intracellular contents as the membrane becomes weakened. Although it belongs to the same chemical class as amphotericin B, the **polyenes,** nystatin is available in a wider variety of formulations, including cream, ointment, powder, tablet, and lozenge. Too toxic for parenteral administration, nystatin is primarily used topically for candida infections of the vagina, skin, and mouth. It may also be used orally to treat candidiasis of the intestine, because it travels through the GI tract without being absorbed.

ADMINISTRATION ALERTS

- Apply with a swab to the affected area in infants and children, as swishing is difficult or impossible.
- For oral candidiasis, the drug should be swished in the mouth for at least 2 minutes.
- Pregnancy category C (oral preparations) or A (topical preparations)

PHARMACOKINETICS
Onset: Rapid
Peak: Unknown
Half-life: Unknown
Duration: 6–12 h

ADVERSE EFFECTS

When given topically, nystatin produces few adverse effects other than minor skin irritation. There is a high incidence of contact dermatitis, related to the preservatives found in some of the formulations. When given orally, it may cause diarrhea, nausea, and vomiting.

Contraindications: The only contraindication is hypersensitivity to the drug.

INTERACTIONS
Drug–Drug: Unknown

Lab Tests: Unknown

Herbal/Food: Unknown

Treatment of Overdose: There is no specific treatment for overdose.

Refer to MyNursingKit for a Nursing Process Focus specific to this drug.

---

clotrimazole are OTC drugs of choice for vulvovaginal candida infections, although several other medications are equally effective. Some of the therapies for vulvovaginal candidiasis require only a single dose. Tolnaftate and undecylenic acid are frequently used to treat athlete's foot and jock itch.

PROTOZOAN INFECTIONS

Protozoa are single-celled organisms that inhabit water, soil, and animal hosts. Although only a few of the more than 20,000 species cause disease in humans, they cause significant morbidity and mortality in Africa, South America, Central America, and Asia. Travelers to these continents may acquire these infections overseas and bring them back to the United States and Canada. These parasites often thrive in conditions where sanitation and personal hygiene are poor and population density is high. In addition, protozoan infections often occur in patients who are immunocompromised, such as those in the advanced stages of AIDS or who are receiving antineoplastic drugs. Agents for malarial infections are listed in Table 35.5.

35.7 Pharmacotherapy of Malaria

Drug therapy of protozoan infections is difficult because of the parasites' complicated life cycles, during which they may change form and travel to infect distant organs. When faced with adverse conditions, protozoans can form cysts that allow the pathogen to survive in harsh environments, and infect other hosts. When cysts occur inside the host, the parasite is often resistant to pharmacotherapy. With few exceptions, antibiotic, antifungal, and antiviral drugs are ineffective against protozoans.

Malaria is caused by four species of the protozoan *Plasmodium.* Although rare in the United States and Canada, malaria is the second most common fatal infectious disease in the world, with 300 to 500 million cases occurring annually.

Malaria begins with a bite from an infected female *Anopheles* mosquito, which is the *carrier* for the parasite. Once inside the human host, *Plasmodium* multiplies in the liver and transforms into progeny called **merozoites.** About 14 to 25 days after the initial infection, the merozoites are released into the blood. The merozoites infect red blood cells, which eventually rupture, releasing more merozoites, and causing severe fever and chills. This phase is called the **erythrocytic stage** of the infection. *Plasmodium* can remain in a latent state in body tissues for extended periods. Relapses may occur months, or even years, after the initial infection. The life cycle of *Plasmodium* is shown in ➤ Figure 35.1.

Pharmacotherapy of malaria attempts to interrupt the complex life cycle of *Plasmodium.* Although successful early in the course of the disease, therapy becomes increasingly

TABLE 35.5	Selected Drugs for Malaria	
Drug	Route and Adult Dose (max dose where indicated)	Adverse Effects
artemether/lumefantrine (Coartem)	PO; 4 tablets twice daily for 3 days with food	*Headache, dizziness, anorexia, fever, arthralgia, myalgia, nausea* Hypersensitivity, QT prolongation
atovaquone and proguanil (Malarone)	PO for prophylaxis; 1 tablet/day starting 1–2 days before travel, and continuing until 7 days after return PO for treatment; 4 tablets/day for 3 days	*Nausea, vomiting, abdominal pain, diarrhea, headache, myalgia* Neutropenia, hypotension
Pr chloroquine (Aralen) hydroxychloroquine (Plaquenil) (see page 743 for the Prototype Drug box)∞	PO; 600 mg initial dose, then 300 mg/wk For acute attacks: PO; 620 mg initial dose, then 310 mg at 6, 18, and 28 h For prophylaxis: PO; 310 mg starting 2 wk before travel and continuing 4–6 wk following return	*Nausea, vomiting and diarrhea; visual changes, including blurred vision, photophobia and difficulty focusing* Hemolytic anemia in patients with G6PD deficiency; irreversible retinal damage
mefloquine (Lariam)	PO; Prevention: begin 250 mg once a week for 4 wk, then 250 mg every other week Treatment: 1,250 mg as a single dose	*Vomiting, nausea, diarrhea, myalgia, dizziness, anorexia, abdominal pain* AV block, bradycardia, tachycardia, psychosis
primaquine	For acute attacks: PO; 15 mg/day for 2 wk For prophylaxis: PO; 15 mg/day following return for 14 days	*Vomiting, nausea, diarrhea, myalgia, headache, anorexia, abdominal pain* Hemolytic anemia in patients with G6PD deficiency
pyrimethamine (Daraprim)	PO; 25 mg once a week for 10 wk	*Vomiting, nausea, diarrhea, myalgia, abdominal pain* Megaloblastic anemia, leukopenia, thrombocytopenia
quinine (Quinamm)	For acute attacks: PO; 650 mg tid × 3 days For prophylaxis: 325 mg bid × 6 wk	*Vomiting, nausea, diarrhea* Cinchonism (tinnitus, ototoxicity, vertigo, fever, visual impairment), hypothermia, coma, cardiovascular collapse, agranulocytosis

Italics indicate common adverse effects; underlining indicates serious adverse effects.

difficult as the parasite enters different stages of its life cycle. Goals of antimalarial therapy include the following:

- *Prevention of the disease:* Prevention of malaria is the best therapeutic option, because the disease is very difficult to treat after it has been acquired. The Centers for Disease Control and Prevention (CDC) recommends that travelers to infested areas receive prophylactic antimalarial drugs prior to and during their visit, and for 1 week after leaving. Chloroquine (Aralen) is the drug of choice, unless travel is to a region known to have a high incidence of chloroquine-resistant strains.

- *Treatment of acute attacks:* Drugs are used to interrupt the erythrocytic stage and eliminate the merozoites from red blood cells. Treatment is most successful if begun immediately after symptoms are recognized. Chloroquine (Aralen) is the classic antimalarial for treating the acute stage, although resistance has become a major clinical problem. Other medications are prescribed in regions of the world where chloroquine resistance is prevalent.

- *Prevention of relapse:* Drugs are given to eliminate the latent forms of *Plasmodium* residing in the liver. Primaquine phosphate is one of the few drugs able to eliminate hepatic cysts and achieve a total cure.

In 2009, the FDA approved the use of a fixed dose combination of artemether/lumefantrine (Coartem) to treat acute, uncomplicated malaria infections. Artemether is prepared from substances obtained from the Chinese herb *Artemisa annua*, which had been known to have antimalarial properties for over a thousand years. Lumefantrine extends the half-life of the combination drug. Coartem is significant because it is very effective and offers an additional option for treating chloroquine-resistant infections. This drug is approved for treatment, not prevention, of malaria.

35.8 Pharmacotherapy of Nonmalarial Protozoan Infections

Although infection by *Plasmodium* is the most significant protozoan disease worldwide, infections caused by other protozoans affect significant numbers of people in endemic

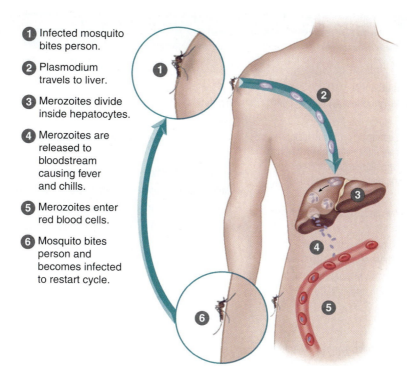

1. Infected mosquito bites person.

2. Plasmodium travels to liver.

3. Merozoites divide inside hepatocytes.

4. Merozoites are released to bloodstream causing fever and chills.

5. Merozoites enter red blood cells.

6. Mosquito bites person and becomes infected to restart cycle.

➤ **Figure 35.1** Life cycle of *Plasmodium*

TREATING THE DIVERSE PATIENT

G6PD Deficiency and Antimalarials

G6PD (glucose-6-phosphate dehydrogenase) deficiency is a genetic disorder found in approximately 10% of African Americans and in 5% to 10% of Sephardic Jews, Greeks, Iranians, Filipinos, and Chinese. It is the most common genetic enzyme defect, occurring in over 400 million people worldwide. It is believed that people with this deficiency in their red blood cells may have some natural immunity to malaria. Without G6PD, chloroquine and other antimalarial drugs impair the metabolism of red blood cells and may cause acute intravascular hemolysis. If this deficiency is suspected, the patient should be tested before treatment is initiated. Other drugs that should be avoided by patients with G6PD deficiency include the fluoroquinone antibiotics, sulfonamides, and phenytoin (Dilantin).

---

areas. These infections include amebiasis, toxoplasmosis, giardiasis, cryptosporidiosis, trichomoniasis, trypanosomiasis, and leishmaniasis. Protozoans can invade nearly any tissue in the body. For example, *Plasmodia* prefer erythrocytes, *Giardia* the colon, and *Entamoeba* travels to the liver.

Like *Plasmodium* infections, the nonmalarial protozoan infections occur more frequently in areas where public sanitation is poor and population density is high. Drinking water may not be disinfected before consumption and may be contaminated with pathogens from human waste. In such regions, parasitic infections are endemic and contribute significantly to mortality, especially in children, who are often more susceptible to the pathogens. Several of these infections occur in severely immunocompromised patients. Each of the organisms has unique differ-

ences in its distribution pattern and physiology. Descriptions of common nonmalarial protozoan infections are given in Table 35.6.

One such protozoan infection, amebiasis, affects more than 50 million people and causes 100,000 deaths worldwide. Caused by the protozoan *Entamoeba histolytica*, amebiasis is common in Africa, Latin America, and Asia. Although primarily a disease of the large intestine, where it causes ulcers, *E. histolytica* can invade the liver and create abscesses. The primary symptom of amebiasis is amebic **dysentery**, a severe form of diarrhea. Drugs used to treat amebiasis include those that act directly on amoebas in the intestine and those that are administered for their systemic effects on the liver and other organs. Drugs for amebiasis and other nonmalarial protozoan infections are listed in Table 35.7.

Although several treatment options are available, metronidazole (Flagyl) has been the traditional drug of choice for nonmalarial protozoan infections. In 2005, tinidazole (Tindamax) was approved by the FDA for treatment of trichomoniasis, giardiasis, and amebiasis. This drug is very similar to metronidazole but has a longer duration of action that allows for less frequent dosing.

DRUGS FOR HELMINTHIC INFECTIONS

Helminths consist of various species of parasitic worms, which have more complex anatomy, physiology, and life cycles than the protozoans. Diseases due to these pathogens affect more than 2 billion people worldwide, and are quite common in

NURSING PROCESS FOCUS
PATIENTS RECEIVING PHARMACOTHERAPY FOR PROTOZOAN OR HELMINTHIC INFECTIONS

Assessment	Potential Nursing Diagnoses
Baseline assessment prior to administration: ■ Understand the reason the drug has been prescribed in order to assess for therapeutic effects. ■ Obtain a complete health history including neurologic, cardiovascular, respiratory, hepatic or renal disease, and the possibility of pregnancy. Obtain a drug history including allergies, including specific reactions to drugs, current prescription and OTC drugs, herbal preparations, and alcohol use. Be alert to possible drug interactions. ■ Assess signs and symptoms of current infection and assess family members or others living in the home. ■ Obtain a travel history, noting dates of travel and note when current symptoms started in relation to travel (i.e., before, during, or after travel). ■ Evaluate appropriate laboratory and diagnostic test findings (e.g., CBC, C&S, fecal ova and parasites, hepatic and renal function studies, ECG as appropriate).	■ Diarrhea ■ Nausea ■ Deficient Fluid Volume (related to diarrhea, vomiting) ■ Fatigue ■ Imbalanced Nutrition, Less Than Body Requirements ■ Pain (related to diarrhea, abdominal cramping, muscle pain) ■ Impaired Skin Integrity (related to diarrhea) ■ Deficient Knowledge (related drug therapy)
Assessment throughout administration: ■ Assess for desired therapeutic effects (e.g., diminished diarrhea, chills, fever, muscle pain). ■ Continue periodic monitoring of CBC, hepatic and renal function, C&S, fecal ova and parasites, and ECG as appropriate. ■ Assess for adverse effects: nausea, vomiting, abdominal cramping, increasing diarrhea, drowsiness, dizziness, paresthesias, metallic taste, darkened urine, dysrhythmias, and palpitations. Severe diarrhea, especially containing mucus, blood, or pus; yellowing of sclera or skin; decreased urine output; numbness of extremities; seizures; dysrhythmias; hypotension; and tachycardia should be reported immediately.	

Planning: Patient Goals and Expected Outcomes

The patient will:
■ Experience therapeutic effects (e.g., diminished signs and symptoms of infection, decreased fever and malaise).
■ Be free from, or experience minimal, adverse effects.
■ Verbalize an understanding of the drug's use, adverse effects, and required precautions.
■ Demonstrate proper self-administration of the medication (e.g., dose, timing, when to notify provider).

Implementation

Interventions and Rationales	Patient and Family Education
Ensuring therapeutic effects: ■ Continue assessments as described earlier for therapeutic effects. (Diminished fever, pain, diarrhea, or signs of infection should begin soon after taking the first dose and continue to improve. The health care provider should be notified if signs of infection remain after 3 days or if the entire course of treatment has been taken and signs of infection are still present.)	■ Teach the patient to report a fever that does not diminish below 100°F within 3 days, increasing signs and symptoms of infection, or symptoms that remain present after taking the entire course of the drug. ■ Teach the patient to not stop the antibacterial when "feeling better" but to take the entire course of the antibacterial; do not share doses with other family members with similar symptoms; and return to the provider if symptoms have not resolved after the entire course of therapy.
Minimizing adverse effects: ■ Continue to monitor vital signs, especially temperature if fever is present. Report undiminished fever or changes in level of consciousness to the health care provider immediately. (Fever should begin to diminish within 1 to 3 days after starting the drug. Continued fever may be a sign of worsening infection, adverse drug effects, or antibiotic resistance.)	■ Teach the patient to immediately report a fever that does not diminish below 100°F, or per parameters, or changes in behavior or LOC to the health care provider.

NURSING PROCESS FOCUS	PATIENTS RECEIVING PHARMACOTHERAPY FOR PROTOZOAN OR HELMINTHIC INFECTIONS *(Continued)*

Implementation

Interventions and Rationales	Patient and Family Education
▪ Continue to monitor periodic lab work: hepatic and renal function tests, CBC, ECG, C&S, and fecal ova and parasites. (Hepatic and renal labs, particularly with IV therapy, should be monitored to prevent adverse effects. Periodic C&S tests or fecal ova and parasites tests may be ordered if infections are severe or are slow to resolve to confirm appropriate therapy. ECG monitoring may be required with some antimalarial drugs.)	▪ Instruct the patient on the need for periodic lab work. Provide a kit and instructions for home use if fecal specimens are required. ▪ Cultures are collected *before* drug therapy is started or if started in an emergency (e.g., overwhelming infection with significant body-wide symptoms), as soon as feasibly possible, and thereafter as ordered by the health care provider.
▪ Monitor for hypersensitivity and allergic reactions, especially with first few doses of any drug treatment. (Anaphylactic reactions are possible, particularly with the first dose. As parasites die, increasing diarrhea, abdominal pain, or chills may occur.)	▪ Teach the patient to immediately report any itching, rashes, swelling, particularly of face, tongue or face, urticaria, flushing, dizziness, syncope, wheezing, throat tightness, or difficulty breathing. Report significant increases in abdominal pain, diarrhea, chills, or fever to the health care provider.
▪ Continue to monitor for hepatic or renal toxicity. (Frequent monitoring is required to prevent adverse effects. Increasing fluid intake will prevent drug accumulation in kidneys.)	▪ Teach the patient to immediately report any nausea, vomiting, yellowing of skin or sclera, abdominal pain, light or clay-colored stools, diminished urine output, or darkening of urine,. ▪ Advise the patient to increase fluid intake to 2 to 3 L per day. Alcohol use should be avoided or eliminated.
▪ Monitor for significant GI effects, including nausea, vomiting, and abdominal pain or cramping. Give drug with food or milk to decrease adverse GI effects. (An antiemetic may be considered if nausea is severe. Alcohol use, especially in patients on metronidazole, may cause a disulfiram-like reaction with excessive nausea, vomiting, and possible hypotension.)	▪ Teach the patient to take the drug with food or milk but to avoid acidic foods, beverages or carbonated drinks, and alcohol use, especially in patients on metronidazole.
▪ Monitor for signs and symptoms of neurologic effects—e.g., dizziness, drowsiness, and headache—and ensure patient safety. Be cautious with the elderly who may be at increased risk for dizziness and falls. (Teach the patient to rise from lying or sitting to standing gradually if dizziness occurs.)	▪ Teach the patient to rise from lying or sitting to standing slowly to avoid dizziness or falls and to avoid driving or other activities requiring mental alertness or physical coordination until the effects of the drug are known. ▪ Instruct the hospitalized patient to call for assistance prior to getting out of bed or attempting to walk alone.
▪ Monitor pulse and ECG as indicated in patients on antimalarial treatment. (Some antimalarials may cause dysrhythmias and hypotension.)	▪ Teach the patient to promptly report any palpitations or dizziness.
▪ Monitor for signs and symptoms of bone marrow suppression and blood dyscrasias, e.g., low-grade fevers, bleeding, bruising, or significant fatigue. (Bone marrow suppression may cause blood dyscrasias with resulting decreases in RBCs, WBCs, and/or platelets. Periodic monitoring of CBC may be required.)	▪ Teach the patient to report any low-grade fevers, sore throat, rashes, bruising or increased bleeding, unusual fatigue, or shortness of breath, especially after taking drug therapy for a prolonged period.
▪ Assess the patient's sexual partners for infection and treat current partners to avoid reinfection. (The infection may be reintroduced by the nontreated sexual partner.)	▪ Have the patient notify sexual partners for assessment and treatment.
▪ Teach general hygiene measures to prevent reinfestation with parasites. (Families with young children should practice thorough handwashing, proper disposal of diapers, and notify daycare or childcare providers of infection. Assess for family pets who may carry infection and also require treatment. International travelers should practice scrupulous hygiene, especially in developing countries.)	▪ Teach the patient and family or caregiver hygiene measures and encourage veterinary assessment of family pets, even if asymptomatic.
Patient understanding of drug therapy: ▪ Use opportunities during administration of medications and during assessments to discuss the rationale for drug therapy, desired therapeutic outcomes, most commonly observed adverse effects, parameters for when to call the health care provider, and any necessary monitoring or precautions. (Using time during nursing care helps to optimize and reinforce key teaching areas.)	▪ The patient, family, or caregiver should be able to state the reason for the drug; appropriate dose and scheduling; what adverse effects to observe for and when to report; and the anticipated length of medication therapy.

(Continued)

NURSING PROCESS FOCUS   PATIENTS RECEIVING PHARMACOTHERAPY FOR PROTOZOAN OR HELMINTHIC INFECTIONS (Continued)

Implementation

Interventions and Rationales	Patient and Family Education

Patient self-administration of drug therapy:
 	
• When administering medications, instruct the patient, family, or caregiver in proper self-administration techniques followed by return demonstration. (Proper administration increases the effectiveness of the drug.)
	• Teach the patient to take the medication as follows:
	  ▪ Complete the entire course of therapy unless otherwise instructed.
	  ▪ Avoid or eliminate alcohol. Some medications (e.g., metronidazole) cause significant reactions when taken with alcohol and alcohol increases adverse GI effects of many drugs.
	  ▪ Take the drug with food or milk but avoid acidic beverages. If instructed to take the drug on an empty stomach, take with a full glass of water.
	  ▪ Take the medication as evenly spaced throughout each day as feasible.
	  ▪ Increase overall fluid intake while taking the antibacterial drug.
	  ▪ Discard outdated medications or those no longer in use. Review medicine cabinet twice a year for old medications.

Evaluation of Outcome Criteria

Evaluate the effectiveness of drug therapy by confirming that patient goals and expected outcomes have been met (see "Planning").

See Tables 35.5, 35.7, and 35.8 for a list of drugs to which these nursing actions apply.

Pr Prototype Drug | Chloroquine (Aralen)

Therapeutic Class: Antimalarial agent   **Pharmacologic Class:** Heme complexing agent

ACTIONS AND USES

Developed to counter the high incidence of malaria among American soldiers in the Pacific Islands during World War II, chloroquine has been the prototype medication for the prophylaxis and treatment of malaria for more than 60 years. It is effective in treating the erythrocytic stage, but has no activity against latent *Plasmodium*. Both chloroquine and the closely related hydroxychloroquine (Plaquenil) are also used off-label for the treatment of rheumatic and inflammatory disorders, including lupus erythematosus and rheumatoid arthritis.

Chloroquine concentrates in the food vacuoles of *Plasmodium* residing in red blood cells. Once in the vacuoles, it is believed to prevent the metabolism of heme, which then builds to toxic levels within the parasite.

Chloroquine can reduce the high fever of patients in the acute stage in less than 48 hours. It also is used to *prevent* malaria by being administered 2 weeks before the patient enters an endemic area and continuing 4 to 6 weeks after the patient leaves. Although chloroquine is a drug of choice, many other agents are available, as resistance to chloroquine is common.

ADMINISTRATION ALERTS

• Pediatric dosage should be monitored closely, because children are susceptible to overdose.

• If administrating IM, inject into a deep muscle and aspirate prior to injecting medication because of its irritating effects to the tissues.

• Pregnancy category C

PHARMACOKINETICS
Onset: 8–10 h

Peak: 3–4 h

Half-life: 1.5–2 days

Duration: Variable (several days to weeks)

ADVERSE EFFECTS

Chloroquine exhibits few serious adverse effects at low to moderate doses. Nausea and diarrhea may occur. At higher doses, CNS and cardiovascular toxicity may be observed. Symptoms include confusion, convulsions, reduced reflexes, hypotension, and dysrhythmias. Chloroquine can cause retinal toxicity, including, blurred vision, photophobia, and difficulty focusing.

Contraindications: Because chloroquine can cause retinal toxicity, it is contraindicated in patients with pre-existing retinal or visual field changes. It is also contraindicated in patients with renal impairment and in those with hypersensitivity to the drug.

INTERACTIONS

Drug–Drug: Antacids and laxatives containing aluminum and magnesium can decrease chloroquine absorption and must not be given within 4 hours of each other. Chloroquine may also interfere with the response to rabies vaccine.

Lab Tests: Unknown

Herbal/Food: Unknown

Treatment of Overdose: Overdose may be fatal. Symptomatic treatment may include anticonvulsants and vasopressors for shock. Ammonium chloride may be used to acidify the urine to hasten excretion of chloroquine.

Refer to MyNursingKit for a Nursing Process Focus specific to this drug.

TABLE 35.6	Selected Protozoan Infections	
Name of Disease and Protozoan Specie(s)	Description	Source of Infection
Amebiasis *Entamoeba histolytica*	Primarily infects the large intestine, causing severe diarrhea; commonly travels to the liver to form liver abscesses; rarely travels to other organs such as the brain, lungs, or kidney	Fecal-contaminated water
Cryptosporidiosis *Cryptosporidium parvum*	Infects the intestines, causing diarrhea; often seen in immunocompromised patients	Fecal-contaminated water; humans and other animals
Giardiasis *Giardia lamblia*	Infects the intestines, causing malabsorption, fatigue, and abdominal pain	Fecal-contaminated water
Malaria *Plasmodium* (various species)	Infects red blood cells to cause fever, chills, and fatigue; some *Plasmodia* invade the liver and other tissues.	Bite of female *Anopheles* mosquito
Toxoplasmosis *Toxoplasma gondii*	Can invade any organ; causes a fatal encephalitis in immunocompromised patients	Congenital transmission; cat feces
Trichomoniasis *Trichomonas vaginalis*	Common STD that causes vaginitis in females and urethritis in males	Transmission through sexual contact with infected fluids
Trypanosomiasis *Trypanosoma cruzi* (American) *Trypanosoma brucei* (African)	The American form (Chagas' disease) invades cardiac tissue and autonomic ganglia; the African form (sleeping sickness) causes fatigue and CNS depression	Bite of kissing bug (American) or tsetse fly (African)

areas lacking high standards of sanitation. Helminthic infections in the United States and Canada are neither common nor fatal, although drug therapy may be indicated. Drugs used to treat these infections, the anthelmintics, are listed in Table 35.8.

35.9 Pharmacotherapy of Helminthic Infections

Helminths are classified as roundworms (nematodes), flukes (trematodes), or tapeworms (cestodes). The most common

TABLE 35.7	Selected Drugs for Nonmalarial Protozoan Infections	
Drug	Route and Adult Dose (max dose where indicated)	Adverse Effects
iodoquinol (Yodoxin)	PO; 630–650 mg tid for 20 days (max: 2 g/day)	*Nausea, vomiting, headache, dizziness* Loss of vision, agranulocytosis, peripheral neuropathy
Pr metronidazole (Flagyl)	PO; 250–750 mg tid	*Dizziness, headache, anorexia, abdominal pain, metallic taste, nausea* Seizures, peripheral neuropathy, transient leukopenia
nifurtimox (Lampit)	PO; 8–10 mg/kg three to four times/day for 90–120 days	*Rash, dizziness, headache, nausea/vomiting* Seizures, paresthesia with myalgia, pneumonia
paromomycin (Humatin)	PO; 25–35 mg/kg in three divided doses for 5–10 days	*Nausea, vomiting, headache, diarrhea, abdominal cramps* Ototoxicity, nephrotoxicity
pentamidine (Pentam, NebuPent)	IV/IM; 4 mg/kg/day for 14–21 days; infuse over 60 min	*Cough, bronchospasm, nausea, anorexia* Leukopenia, hypoglycemia, abscess or pain at injection site, hypotension, nephrotoxicity
sodium stibogluconate (Pentostam)	IM; 20 mg/kg/day	*Nausea, vomiting, diarrhea, anorexia, cough, substernal pain* ECG changes, pneumonia, blood dyscrasias
tinidazole (Tindamax)	PO; giardiasis: 50 mg/kg in single dose (max: 2 g); amebiasis: 2 g/day for 3–5 days	*Anorexia, metallic taste, and nausea* Seizures, peripheral neuropathy, transient leukopenia

Italics indicate common adverse effects; underlining indicates serious adverse effects.

Pr Prototype Drug | Metronidazole *(Flagyl)*

Therapeutic Class: Anti-infective, antiprotozoan   **Pharmacologic Class:** Agent that disrupts nucleic acid synthesis

ACTIONS AND USES

Metronidazole is the prototype drug for most forms of amebiasis, being effective against both the intestinal and hepatic stages of the disease. Resistant forms of *E. histolytica* have not yet emerged as a clinical problem with metronidazole therapy. Metronidazole is a drug of choice for two other protozoan infections: giardiasis and trichomoniasis.

Metronidazole is unique among antiprotozoan drugs in that it also has antibiotic activity against anaerobic bacteria and thus is used to treat a number of respiratory, bone, skin, and CNS infections. Topical forms of metronidazole (MetroGel, MetroCream, MetroLotion) are used to treat rosacea, a disease characterized by skin reddening and hyperplasia of the sebaceous glands, particularly around the nose and face. Off-label uses include the pharmacotherapy of pseudomembranous colitis and Crohn's disease. Helidac is a combination drug containing metronidazole, bismuth, and tetracycline that is used to eradicate *H. pylori* infection associated with peptic ulcer disease.

ADMINISTRATION ALERTS

- The extended-release form must be swallowed whole and taken on an empty stomach.
- Contraindicated during the first trimester of pregnancy.
- Pregnancy category B

PHARMACOKINETICS (PO)
Onset: Rapid
Peak: 1–3 h
Half-life: 6–8 h
Duration: Unknown

ADVERSE EFFECTS

Although adverse effects occur relatively frequently, most are not serious enough to cause discontinuation of therapy. The most common adverse effects of metronidazole are anorexia, nausea, diarrhea, dizziness, and headache. Dryness of the mouth and an unpleasant metallic taste may be experienced. Although rare, metronidazole can cause bone marrow suppression.

Contraindications: Metronidazole is contraindicated in patients with trichomoniasis during the first trimester of pregnancy and those with hypersensitivity to the drug. Metronidazole can cause bone marrow suppression; thus, it is contraindicated for patients with blood dyscrasias.

INTERACTIONS

Drug–Drug: Metronidazole interacts with oral anticoagulants to potentiate hypoprothrombinemia. In combination with alcohol, or other medications that may contain alcohol, metronidazole may elicit a disulfiram reaction. In patients taking lithium, the drug may elevate lithium levels.

Lab Tests: Metronidazole may decrease values for AST and ALT.

Herbal/Food: Unknown

Treatment of Overdose: There is no specific treatment for overdose.

Refer to MyNursingKit for a Nursing Process Focus specific to this drug.

helminth disease worldwide is ascariasis, which is caused by the roundworm *Ascaris lumbricoides.* In the United States, this worm is most common in the Southeast, and primarily infects children aged 3 to 8 years, since this group is most likely to be exposed to contaminated soil without proper hand washing. Enteriobiasis, an infection by the pinworm *Enterobius vermicularis,* is the most common helminth infection in the United States. For ascariasis, oral mebendazole (Vermox) for 3 days is

TABLE 35.8	Selected Drugs for Helminthic Infections	
Drug	**Route and Adult Dose (max dose where indicated)**	**Adverse Effects**
albendazole (Albenza)	PO; 400 mg bid with meals (max: 800 mg/day)	*Abnormal liver function tests, abdominal pain, nausea, vomiting* <u>Agranulocytosis, leukopenia</u>
ivermectin (Stromectol)	PO; 150–200 mcg/kg as a single dose	*Fever, pruritus, dizziness, arthralgia, lymphadenopathy* <u>Acute allergic or inflammatory response</u>
Pr mebendazole (Vermox)	PO; 100 mg as a single dose, or 100 mg bid for 3 days	*Abdominal pain, diarrhea, rash* <u>Angioedema, convulsions</u>
praziquantel (Biltricide)	PO; 5 mg/kg as a single dose, or 25 mg/kg tid	*Headache, dizziness, malaise, fever, abdominal pain* <u>CSF reaction syndrome</u>
pyrantel (Antiminth, Ascarel, Pin-X, Pinworm Caplets)	PO; 11 mg/kg as a single dose (max: 1 g)	*Nausea, tenesmus, anorexia, diarrhea, fever* <u>No serious adverse effects</u>
Italics indicate common adverse effects; <u>underlining</u> indicates serious adverse effects.		

the standard treatment. Pharmacotherapy of enterobiasis includes a single dose of mebendazole, albendazole (Albenza) or pyrantel (Antiminth, Ascarel, Pin-X, Pinworm Caplets).

Like protozoans, helminths have several stages in their life cycle, which include immature and mature forms. Typically, the immature forms of helminths enter the body through the skin or the digestive tract. Most attach to the human intestinal tract, although some species form cysts in skeletal muscle or in organs such as the liver.

Not all helminthic infections require pharmacotherapy, because the adult parasites often die without reinfecting the host. When the infestation is severe or complications occur, pharmacotherapy is initiated. Complications caused by extensive infestations may include physical obstruction in the intestine, malabsorption, increased risk for secondary bacterial infections, and severe fatigue. Pharmacotherapy is targeted at killing the parasites locally in the intestine and systemically in the tissues and organs they have invaded. Some anthelmintics have a broad spectrum and are effective against multiple organisms, whereas others are specific for a certain species. Resistance has not yet become a clinical problem with anthelmintics.

LIFESPAN CONSIDERATIONS

Childhood Play Areas and Parasitic Infections

Pinworms and roundworms are more commonly seen in children because many of their hygiene and play habits contribute to the transmission and reinfestation of the worms. Instruct parents and family members about ways to prevent exposure to and spread of helminths. Teach children correct hand washing techniques, emphasizing cleansing under the nails and washing before eating and after using the toilet. Discourage placing hands in mouth and biting nails. Do not allow child to scratch the anal area. Make sure that children wear shoes when playing outside. Avoid use of sandboxes, which can be accessed by dogs or cats; keep sandboxes covered when not in use. Cleanse all fruits and vegetables before eating. Change diapers frequently and dispose of properly (out of children's reach). Do not allow children to swim in pools that allow diapered children. Discuss whole-family treatment, particularly in households with several young children, if one family member has an infection.

LIFESPAN CONSIDERATIONS

Parasitic Infections in Children

Many parasitic infections are common among children, with the national rates highest among children less than 5 years of age. In public health labs, the most commonly diagnosed intestinal parasite is *Giardia*. Giardiasis cases are associated with swimming in contaminated waterways or drinking contaminated ground well water, via contaminated diapers in child-care settings, and drinking water or consuming raw fruits or vegetables during international travel. *Giardia* infections may also be difficult to diagnose because stool specimens do not always contain the ova or parasites, although stool antigen testing specific to *Giardia* is available.

Children adopted from countries outside of the United States also have a high rate of parasitic infection. Up to 35% of foreign-born adopted children are reported to have *Giardia lamblia*. Environments in which these children have been living, particularly orphanages, often provide favorable conditions for infectious disease. The CDC recommends that internationally adopted children undergo examination of at least one stool sample, and three stool samples if GI symptoms are present. Unfortunately, evidence has shown that in communities where helminth infections are common, whether in the United States or overseas, poor nutritional status, anemia, and impaired growth and learning in children result.

Pr Prototype Drug | Mebendazole (Vermox)

Therapeutic Class: Drug for worm infections   **Pharmacologic Class:** Antihelmintic

ACTIONS AND USES

Mebendazole is the most widely prescribed anthelmintic in the United States. It is used in the treatment of a wide range of helminth infections, including those caused by roundworm (*Ascaris*) and pinworm (*Enterobiasis*). As a broad-spectrum drug, it is particularly valuable in mixed helminth infections, which are common in areas having poor sanitation. It is effective against both the adult and larval stages of these parasites. It is poorly absorbed after oral administration, which allows it to retain high concentrations in the intestine. For pinworm infections, a single dose is usually sufficient; other infections require 3 consecutive days of therapy.

ADMINISTRATION ALERTS

- The drug is most effective when chewed and taken with a fatty meal.
- Pregnancy category C

PHARMACOKINETICS

Onset: Unknown
Peak: 1–7 h
Half-life: 3–9 h
Duration: Unknown

ADVERSE EFFECTS

Because so little of the drug is absorbed, mebendazole does not generally cause serious systemic side effects. As the worms die, some abdominal pain, distension, and diarrhea may be experienced.

Contraindications: The only contraindication is hypersensitivity to the drug.

INTERACTIONS

Drug–Drug: Carbamazepine and phenytoin can increase the metabolism of mebendazole.

Lab Tests: Unknown

Herbal/Food: High-fat foods may increase the absorption of the drug.

Treatment of Overdose: There is no specific treatment for overdose.

Refer to MyNursingKit for a Nursing Process Focus specific to this drug.

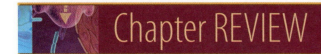

Chapter REVIEW

KEY CONCEPTS

The numbered key concepts provide a succinct summary of the important points from the corresponding numbered section within the chapter. If any of these points are not clear, refer to the numbered section within the chapter for review.

35.1 Fungi have more complex physiology than bacteria and are unaffected by most antibiotics. Most serious fungal infections occur in patients with suppressed immune defenses.

35.2 Fungal infections are classified as superficial (affecting hair, skin, nails, and mucous membranes) or systemic (affecting internal organs).

35.3 Antifungal medications act by disrupting aspects of growth or metabolism that are unique to these organisms.

35.4 Systemic mycoses affect internal organs and may require prolonged and aggressive drug therapy. Amphotericin B (Fungizone) is the traditional drug of choice for serious fungal infections.

35.5 The azole class of antifungal drugs has become widely used in the pharmacotherapy of both systemic and superficial mycoses owing to a favorable safety profile.

35.6 Antifungal drugs to treat superficial mycoses may be given topically or orally. They exhibit few serious side effects and are effective in treating infections of the skin, nails, and mucous membranes.

35.7 Malaria is the most common protozoan disease and requires multidrug therapy owing to the complicated life cycle of the parasite. Drugs may be administered for prophylaxis, and therapy for acute attacks and prevention of relapses.

35.8 Treatment of non-*Plasmodium* protozoan disease requires a different set of medications from those used for malaria. Other protozoan diseases that may be indications for pharmacotherapy include amebiasis, toxoplasmosis, giardiasis, cryptosporidiosis, trichomoniasis, trypanosomiasis, and leishmaniasis.

35.9 Helminths are parasitic worms that cause significant disease in certain regions of the world. The goals of pharmacotherapy are to kill the parasites locally and to disrupt their life cycle.

NCLEX-RN® REVIEW QUESTIONS

1 A patient has been diagnosed with a fungal nail infection. The health care provider has prescribed fluconazole (Diflucan). The nurse will include which of the following in her patient education?
1. Drug therapy will be for a very short time, probably 2 to 4 weeks.
2. Carefully inspect all intramuscular injection sites for bruising.
3. Notify the provider should you come down with symptoms of a bacterial infection.
4. Limit fluid intake to approximately 1,000 mL/day.

2 A patient is given a prescription for quinine (Quinamm) for treatment of malaria. Prior to beginning therapy, the patient will need to:
1. sign a consent form for taking this medication.
2. have an ECG done.
3. stop all other medications for 24 hours.
4. be admitted to an ICU for the first 24 hours of therapy.

3 A patient has returned from South America, where malaria was contracted. A drug the nurse expects to see used is:
1. proguanil (Paludrine).
2. penicillin (Ampicillin).
3. rizatriptan (Maxalt).
4. chloroquine (Aralen).

4 The nurse is providing community education about pinworms and roundworms. Which of the following should be included in this teaching? (Select all that apply.)
1. Hand washing is very important in preventing the spread of pinworms and roundworms.
2. Play habits contribute to the transmission of pinworms and roundworms.
3. It is important that children wear shoes when playing outside.
4. Children should not be allowed to play in open sandboxes.
5. Once the child has had worms, reinfestation cannot occur.

5 A patient, age 32, is started on metronidazole (Flagyl) for treatment of a trichomonas vaginal infection. While she is on this medication, she must avoid:
1. caffeine.
2. acidic juices.
3. antacids.
4. alcohol.

6 Metronidazole (Flagyl) is being used to treat a patient's *Giardia lamblia* infection, a protozoal infection of the intestines. Which of the following are appropriate to teach this patient? (Select all that apply.)
1. Metronidazole may leave a metallic taste in the mouth.
2. The urine may turn dark amber brown while on the medication.
3. The metronidazole may be discontinued once the diarrhea subsides, to minimize adverse effects.
4. Taking the metronidazole with food reduces GI upset.
5. Current sexual partners do not require treatment for this infection.

CRITICAL THINKING QUESTIONS

1. A nurse is caring for a severely immunosuppressed patient who is on IV amphotericin B (Fungizone). The nurse understands that this medication is highly toxic to the patient. What are three priority nursing assessment areas for patients on this medication?

2. A young female patient recently diagnosed with insulin-dependent diabetes has been given a prescription for metronidazole (Flagyl) for a vaginal yeast infection. Identify priority teaching for this patient.

3. A patient is traveling to Africa for 3 months and is requesting a prescription for Malarone to prevent malaria. What premedication assessment must be done for this patient?

See Appendix D for answers and rationales for all activities.

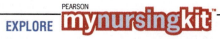

EXPLORE **PEARSON mynursingkit**

MyNursingKit is your one stop for online chapter review materials and resources. Prepare for success with additional NCLEX®-style practice questions, interactive assignments and activities, web links, animations and videos, and more!

Register your access code from the front of your book at
www.mynursingkit.com.

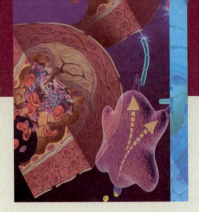

Chapter 36

Drugs for Viral Infections

LEARNING OUTCOMES

After reading this chapter, the student should be able to:

1. Describe the major structures of viruses.
2. Identify viral infections that benefit from pharmacotherapy.
3. Explain the purpose and expected outcomes of HIV pharmacotherapy.
4. Explain the advantages of HAART in the pharmacotherapy of HIV infection.
5. Describe the nurse's role in the pharmacologic management of patients receiving antiretroviral and antiviral drugs.
6. For each of the classes listed in Drugs at a Glance, know representative drugs, and explain the mechanism of drug action, primary actions, and important adverse effects.
7. Use the nursing process to care for patients receiving drug therapy for viral infections.

KEY TERMS

acquired immune deficiency syndrome (AIDS) *page 528*

antiretroviral *page 528*

capsid *page 527*

CD4 receptor *page 528*

hepatitis *page 540*

highly active antiretroviral therapy (HAART) *page 530*

HIV-AIDS *page 528*

human immunodeficiency virus (HIV) *page 528*

influenza *page 540*

intracellular parasite *page 527*

latent phase (of HIV infection) *page 529*

pegylation *page 541*

protease *page 528*

reverse transcriptase *page 528*

viral load *page 529*

virion *page 527*

virus *page 527*

Viruses are tiny infectious agents capable of causing disease in humans and other organisms. After infecting an organism, viruses use host enzymes and cellular structures to replicate. Although the number of antiviral drugs has increased dramatically in recent years because of research into the AIDS epidemic, antivirals remain the least effective of all the anti-infective drug classes.

36.1 Characteristics of Viruses

Viruses are *nonliving* agents that infect bacteria, plants, and animals. Viruses contain none of the cellular organelles necessary for self-survival that are present in living organisms. In fact, the structure of viruses is quite primitive compared with that of even the simplest cell. Surrounded by a protective protein coat, or **capsid,** a virus possesses only a few dozen genes, either in the form of ribonucleic acid (RNA) or deoxyribonucleic acid (DNA), that contain the necessary information needed for viral replication. Some viruses also have a lipid envelope that surrounds the capsid. The viral envelope contains glycoprotein and protein "spikes" that are recognized as foreign by the host's immune system, and trigger body defenses to remove the invader. A mature infective particle is called a **virion.** ➤ Figure 36.1 shows the basic structure of the human immunodeficiency virus (HIV).

Although nonliving and structurally simple, viruses are capable of remarkable feats. They infect their host by locating and entering a target cell and then using the machinery inside that cell to replicate. Thus, viruses are **intracellular parasites:** They must be inside a host cell to cause infection. Virions do, however, bring along a few enzymes that assist the pathogen in duplicating its genetic material, inserting its genes into the host's chromosome, and assembling newly formed virions. These unique viral enzymes sometimes serve as important targets for antiviral drug action.

The host organism and cell are often very specific; it may be a single species of plant, bacteria, or animal, or even a single type of cell within that species. Most often viruses infect only one species, although cases have been documented in which viruses mutated and crossed species, as is likely the case for HIV.

Many viral infections, such as the rhinoviruses that cause the common cold, are self-limiting and require no medical intervention. Although symptoms may be annoying, they resolve in 7 to 10 days, and the virus causes no permanent effects if the patient is otherwise healthy. Some viral infections, however, require drug therapy to prevent the infection or to alleviate symptoms. For example, HIV is uniformly fatal if left untreated. The hepatitis B virus can cause permanent liver damage and increase a patient's risk of hepatocellular carcinoma. Although not life threatening in most patients, herpesviruses can cause significant pain and, in the case of ocular herpes, permanent disability.

Antiviral pharmacotherapy can be extremely challenging because of the rapid mutation rate of viruses, which can quickly render drugs ineffective. Also complicating therapy is the intracellular nature of the virus, which makes it difficult to eliminate the pathogen without giving excessively high doses of drugs that injure normal cells. Antiviral drugs have narrow spectrums of activity, usually limited to one specific virus. The three basic strategies used for antiviral pharmacotherapy are as follows:

- Prevent viral infections through the administration of vaccines (chapter 32 ∞).
- Treat active infections with drugs such as acyclovir (Zovirax) that interrupt an aspect of the virus's replication cycle.
- For long-term infections, use drugs that boost the patient's immune response (immunostimulants) so that the virus remains in latency with the patient symptom free.

➤ **Figure 36.1** Structure of HIV

Labels: Glycoproteins, Protein coat, Reverse transcriptase, Core proteins, Envelope (lipid bilayer), Viral RNA

PHARMFACTS

Viral Infections

- Approximately 85% of adults have serologic evidence of infections by HSV-1.
- About 45 million Americans are infected with genital herpes—one of every five of the total adolescent and adult population.
- Genital herpes is more common in women than in men, and in African Americans than in other ethnic groups.
- About 900,000 Americans are currently living with HIV infections, and about 40,000 new infections occur each year.
- Roughly 70% of new HIV infections occur in men; the largest risk category is men who have sex with other men.
- Of the new HIV infections in women, 75% are acquired through heterosexual contact.
- Since the beginning of the AIDS epidemic, more than 20 million people worldwide, including 450,000 Americans, have died of this disease.

HIV-AIDS

Acquired immune deficiency syndrome (AIDS) is characterized by profound immunosuppression that leads to opportunistic infections and malignancies not commonly found in patients with healthy immune defenses. Antiretroviral drugs slow the growth of the causative agent for AIDS, the **human immunodeficiency virus (HIV)**, by several different mechanisms. Resistance to these drugs is a major clinical problem, and a pharmacologic cure for **HIV-AIDS** is not yet achievable.

36.2 Replication of HIV

Infection with HIV occurs by exposure to contaminated body fluids, most commonly blood or semen. Transmission may occur through sexual activity (oral, anal, or vaginal) or through contact of infected fluids with broken skin, mucous membranes, or needle sticks. Newborns can receive the virus during birth or from breast-feeding.

Shortly after entry into the body, the virus attaches to its preferred target—the **CD4 receptor** on T4 (helper) lymphocytes. During this early stage, structural proteins on the surface of HIV fuse with the CD4 receptor. The virus uncoats, and the genetic material of HIV, single-stranded RNA, enters the cell. After entering the host cell, the RNA strands are converted to DNA by the viral enzyme **reverse transcriptase**. The viral DNA enters the nucleus of the T4 lymphocyte, where it

becomes incorporated into the host's DNA. It may remain in the DNA for many years before it becomes activated to begin producing more viral particles. The new virions eventually bud from the host cell and enter the bloodstream. The new virions, however, are not yet infectious. As a final step, the viral enzyme **protease** cleaves some of the proteins associated with the HIV DNA, enabling the virion to infect other T4 lymphocytes. Once budding occurs, the immune system recognizes that the cell is infected and kills the T4 lymphocyte. Unfortunately, it is too late; an HIV-infected patient may produce as many as 10 billion new virions every day, and the patient's devastated immune system is unable to remove them. Knowledge of the replication cycle of HIV is critical to understanding the pharmacotherapy of HIV-AIDS, as shown in ➤ Figure 36.2.

Only a few viruses such as HIV are able to use reverse transcriptase to construct DNA from RNA; no bacteria, plants, or animals are able to perform this unique metabolic function. All living organisms make RNA from DNA. Because of their "backward" or reverse synthesis, these viruses are called retroviruses, and drugs used to treat HIV infections are called **antiretrovirals**. Progression of HIV to AIDS is characterized by gradual destruction of the immune system, as measured by the decline in the number of CD4 T-lymphocytes. Unfortunately, the CD4 T-lymphocyte is the primary cell coordinating the immune response. When the CD4 T-cell count falls below a certain level, the patient begins to expe-

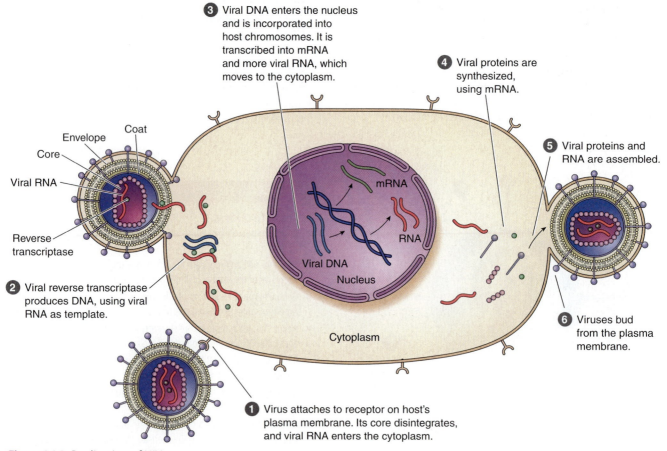

3 Viral DNA enters the nucleus and is incorporated into host chromosomes. It is transcribed into mRNA and more viral RNA, which moves to the cytoplasm.

4 Viral proteins are synthesized, using mRNA.

5 Viral proteins and RNA are assembled.

Envelope
Coat
Core
Viral RNA
Reverse transcriptase

mRNA
RNA
Viral DNA
Nucleus
Cytoplasm

6 Viruses bud from the plasma membrane.

2 Viral reverse transcriptase produces DNA, using viral RNA as template.

1 Virus attaches to receptor on host's plasma membrane. Its core disintegrates, and viral RNA enters the cytoplasm.

➤ *Figure 36.2* Replication of HIV

rience opportunistic bacterial, fungal, and viral infections, and certain malignancies. A point is reached at which the patient is unable to mount any immune defenses, and death ensues.

36.3 General Principles of HIV Pharmacotherapy

The widespread appearance of HIV infection in 1981 created enormous challenges for public health and an unprecedented need for the development of new antiviral drugs. HIV-AIDS is unlike any other infectious disease because it is most often sexually transmitted, is uniformly fatal, and demands a continuous supply of new drugs for patient survival. The challenges of HIV-AIDS have resulted in the development of about 20 new antiretroviral drugs. Unfortunately, the initial hopes of curing HIV-AIDS through antiretroviral therapy or vaccines have not been realized; none of these drugs produces a cure for this disease. Stopping antiretroviral therapy almost always results in a rapid rebound in HIV replication. HIV mutates extremely rapidly, and resistant strains develop so quickly that the creation of novel approaches to antiretroviral drug therapy must remain an ongoing process.

Although pharmacotherapy for HIV-AIDS has not produced a cure, it has resulted in a number of therapeutic successes. For example, many patients with HIV infection are able to live symptom free with the disease for a longer time because of medications. Furthermore, the transmission of the virus from an HIV-infected mother to her newborn has been reduced dramatically (see Section 36.7). Along with better patient education and prevention, successes in pharmacotherapy have produced a 70% decline in the death rate due to HIV-AIDS in the United States. Unfortunately, this decline has not been observed in African countries, where antiviral drugs are not as readily available, largely because of their high cost. It is estimated that as many as 25 million Africans have HIV-AIDS, including more than one third of the entire adult population in several nations.

After HIV incorporates its viral DNA into the nucleus of the T4 lymphocyte, it may remain dormant for several months to many years. During this chronic **latent phase**, patients are asymptomatic and may not even realize they are infected. Once diagnosis is established, however, a decision must be made as to when to begin pharmacotherapy. The advantage of beginning during the asymptomatic stage is that the viral load or burden can be reduced. Presumably, early treatment will delay the onset of acute symptoms and the development of AIDS. Early therapy is especially critical for infants younger than 12 months, because the progression to AIDS can be rapidly fatal for these children.

Unfortunately, the decision to begin treatment during the asymptomatic phase has some negative consequences. Drugs for HIV-AIDS are expensive; treatment with some of the newer agents costs more than $20,000 per year. These drugs produce a number of uncomfortable and potentially serious adverse effects that lower the quality of life for the patient. Therapy over many years promotes viral resistance; thus, when the acute stage eventually develops, the drugs

may no longer be effective. Because of these consequences, current protocols call for deferring treatment in adult asymptomatic patients who have CD4 T-cell counts greater than 350 cells/mcL.

The decision to begin therapy during the acute phase is much easier because the severe symptoms of AIDS can rapidly lead to death. Thus, therapy is nearly always initiated during this phase when the CD4 T-cell count falls below 200 cells/mcL or when AIDS-defining symptoms become apparent.

The therapeutic goals for the pharmacotherapy of HIV-AIDS include the following:

- Reduce HIV-related morbidity and prolong survival
- Improve the quality of life
- Restore and preserve immunologic function
- Promote maximum suppression of viral load
- Prevent the transmission from mother to child in HIV-infected pregnant patients

Two laboratory tests used to guide pharmacotherapy are absolute CD4 T-cell count and measurement of the amount of HIV RNA in the plasma. The number of CD4 T-cells is an important indicator of immune function and predicts the likelihood of opportunistic disease; however, it does not indicate how rapidly HIV is replicating. **Viral load** is determined by measuring the amount of HIV RNA in the blood. The HIV RNA level is an estimate how rapidly the virus is replicating and is considered a more accurate predictor of clinical outcome than CD4 cell counts. These tests are performed every 3 to 6 months to assess the degree of success of antiretroviral therapy.

At one point, physicians recommended the routine use of structured treatment interruptions (STIs): periods during which all antiretroviral drugs were withdrawn. This technique was believed to reduce adverse effects, increase the patient's quality of life, and diminish the potential for resistant HIV strains. Research studies, however, have questioned the effectiveness of STIs; indeed, some data suggest that this strategy actually *promotes* drug resistance and hastens disease progression. In all cases, viral load increases when drug therapy is discontinued.

MyNursingKit | HIV-AIDS Resources at the CDC

MyNursingKit | HIV-AIDS Resources at the NIH

RESEARCH SHOWS

The Question: What factors influence a person to be tested for HIV infection?

The Study: Researchers analyzed two recent studies that examined the timing of HIV testing and demographic variables associated with testing. The analysis showed that many people wait to be tested until late into the course of the infection, when treatment options are less effective. Factors associated with waiting included minority groups and men. In a high school study, approximately 23% of students who ever had sex had been tested for HIV.

Nursing Implications: Nurses should teach patients the importance of preventing HIV infection. For those who have had unprotected sex, the nurse is in a key role to recommend HIV testing, especially among adolescents.

Source: Morbidity Mortality Weekly Report CDC Surveillance Summary 2009, 58:661–668.

36.4 Classification of Drugs for HIV-AIDS

Antiretroviral drugs target specific phases of the HIV replication cycle. The standard pharmacotherapy for HIV-AIDS includes aggressive treatment with multiple drugs concurrently, a regimen called **highly active antiretroviral therapy (HAART)**. The goal of HAART is to reduce the plasma HIV RNA to its lowest possible level. It must be understood, however, that HIV is harbored in locations other than the blood, such as lymph nodes;

therefore, elimination of the virus from the blood is not a cure. The simultaneous use of drugs from several classes reduces the probability that HIV will become resistant to treatment. Antiretroviral therapy must be continued for the lifetime of the patient. These drugs are listed in Table 36.1.

HIV-AIDS antiretrovirals are classified into the following groups, based on their mechanisms of action:

- Nucleoside reverse transcriptase inhibitor (NRTI)
- Nonnucleoside reverse transcriptase inhibitor (NNRTI)

TABLE 36.1	**Antiretroviral Drugs for HIV-AIDS**	
Drug	Route and Adult Dose (max dose where indicated)	Adverse Effects
NONNUCLEOSIDE REVERSE TRANSCRIPTASE INHIBITORS		
delavirdine (Rescriptor)	PO; 400 mg tid (max: 1,200 mg/day)	*Rash, fever, nausea, diarrhea, headache, stomatitis*
ⓟ efavirenz (Sustiva)	PO; 600 mg/days (max: 600 mg/day)	Paresthesia, hepatotoxicity, Stevens–Johnson syndrome, CNS toxicity (efavirenz)
etravirine (Intelence)	PO; 200 mg bid (max: 400 mg/day)	
nevirapine (Viramune)	PO; 200 mg/day for 14 days; then increase to bid	
NUCLEOSIDE AND NUCLEOTIDE REVERSE TRANSCRIPTASE INHIBITORS		
abacavir (Ziagen)	PO; 300 mg bid (max: 600 mg/day)	*Fatigue, generalized weakness, myalgia, nausea, headache, abdominal pain, vomiting, anorexia, rash*
didanosine (Videx, DDI)	PO; 125–300 mg bid	Bone marrow suppression, neutropenia, anemia, granulocytopenia, lactic acidosis with steatorrhea, neurotoxicity, peripheral neuropathy (zalcitabine, stavudine), pancreatitis (lamivudine)
emtricitabine (Emtriva)	PO; 200 mg/day (max: 200 mg/day)	
lamivudine (Epivir, 3TC)	PO; 150 mg bid (max: 300 mg/day)	
stavudine (Zerit, D4T)	PO; 40 mg bid (max: 80 mg/day)	
tenofovir (Viread)	PO; 300 mg/day	
ⓟ zidovudine (AZT, Retrovir)	PO; 200 mg every 4 h (1,200 mg/day); after 1 mo may reduce to 100 mg every 4 h (600 mg/day) IV; 1–2 mg/kg every 4 h (1,200 mg/day)	
PROTEASE INHIBITORS		
atazanavir (Reyataz)	PO; 400 mg/day	*Nausea, vomiting, diarrhea, abdominal pain, headache*
darunavir (Prezista)	PO; 600 mg taken with ritonavir 100 mg bid	Anemia, leukopenia, deep vein thrombosis, pancreatitis, lymphadenopathy, hemorrhagic colitis, nephrolithiasis (indinavir), cardiac arrest (atazanavir), thrombocytopenia (saquinavir), pancytopenia (saquinavir)
fosamprenavir (Lexiva)	PO; 700–1,400 mg bid in combination with 100–200 mg ritonavir bid (max: 2,800 mg/day)	
indinavir (Crixivan)	PO; 800 mg tid	
ⓟ lopinavir/ritonavir (Kaletra)	PO; 400/100 mg (3 capsules or 5 mL of suspension) bid; increase dose to 533/133 mg (4 capsules or 6.5 mL) bid, with concurrent efavirenz or nevirapine	
nelfinavir (Viracept)	PO; 750 mg tid	
ritonavir (Norvir)	PO; 600 mg bid (max: 12,000 mg/day)	
saquinavir (Invirase)	PO; 1 g tid (max: 2 g/day)	
tipranavir (Aptivus)	PO; 500 mg taken with 200 mg of ritonavir bid	
FUSION AND INTEGRASE INHIBITORS		
enfuvirtide (Fuzeon)	Subcutaneous; 90 mg bid	*Pain and inflammation at injection site (enfuvirtide), nausea, diarrhea, fatigue, abdominal pain, cough, dizziness, musculoskeletal symptoms, pyrexia, rash, upper respiratory tract infections*
maraviroc (Selzentry)	PO; 150–600 mg bid (max: 1,200 mg/day)	Hepatotoxicity, myocardial infarction, hypersensitivity, neutropenia, thrombocytopenia, nephrotoxicity (enfuvirtide), myopathy (raltegravir)
raltegravir (Isentress)	PO; 400 mg bid (max: 800 mg/day)	

Italics indicate common adverse effects; <u>underlining</u> indicates serious adverse effects.

- Protease inhibitor (PI)
- Nucleotide reverse transcriptase inhibitor (NtRTI)
- Fusion (entry) inhibitor
- HIV integrase inhibitor

The last three classes include recently discovered agents that act by unique mechanisms. Tenofovir (Viread) is a NtRTI that is structurally similar to adenosine monophosphate (AMP). After metabolism, tenofovir is incorporated into viral DNA in a manner similar to the NRTIs. Enfuvirtide (Fuzeon) blocks the fusion of the HIV virion to the CD4 receptor. Raltegravir (Isentress) blocks HIV integrase and prevents HIV from inserting its genes into uninfected DNA.

Research into HIV-AIDS is constantly evolving as clinicians strive to determine the most effective combinations of antiretroviral agents. Pharmacotherapeutic regimens are often different for patients who are receiving these drugs for the first time (treatment *naïve*) versus patients who have been taking antiretrovirals for months or years (treatment *experienced*). Current clinical guidelines suggest that treatment-naïve patients receive one of the following therapies:

1. A ritonavir-boosted protease inhibitor plus two NRTIs or

2. A nonnucleoside reverse transcriptase inhibitor plus two NRTIs

Treatment failures commonly occur during antiretroviral therapy. The primary factors responsible for treatment failure are inability to tolerate the adverse effects of the medications, nonadherence to the complex drug therapy regimen, emergence of resistant HIV strains, and genetic variability among patients. Pharmacologic options available for patients with treatment failure are limited. Higher doses are generally not indicated, because they lead to an increased incidence of serious side effects. Ideally, the patient is switched to at least two drugs from different chemical classes that they have not yet received, but this option is not always possible because there are so few drug classes available to treat HIV-AIDS. The therapy of HIV is rapidly evolving; thus the nurse should consult current medical reference sources for the latest treatment guidelines.

Drug manufacturers have responded to the need for simpler treatment regimens by combining several medications into a single capsule or tablet. For example, one of the newer therapies combines three HIV-AIDS drugs, manufactured by two different companies. Atripla combines efavirenz, emtricitabine, and tenofovir into a fixed-dose tablet. Approved by

---

Pr Prototype Drug | Zidovudine *(Retrovir, AZT)*

Therapeutic Class: Antiretroviral   **Pharmacologic Class:** Nucleoside reverse transcriptase inhibitor (NRTI)

ACTIONS AND USES

Zidovudine was first discovered in the 1960s, and its antiviral activity was demonstrated prior to the AIDS epidemic. Structurally, it resembles thymidine, one of the four nucleoside building blocks of DNA. As the reverse transcriptase enzyme begins to synthesize viral DNA, it mistakenly uses zidovudine as one of the nucleosides, thus creating a defective DNA strand. Zidovudine is used in combination with other antiretrovirals for both symptomatic and asymptomatic HIV-infected patients, as well as for postexposure prophylaxis in HIV-exposed health care workers (see Section 36.6). An important indication is reduction of the risk of transmission rate of HIV from an HIV-positive mother to her fetus.

Because of the drugs' widespread use since the beginning of the AIDS epidemic, resistant HIV strains have become common. Most treatment guidelines do not include zidovudine as a drug of first choice due to the potential for resistance. Combination products containing zidovudine include Combivir (zidovudine and lamivudine) and Trizivir (zidovudine, lamivudine, and abacavir).

ADMINISTRATION ALERTS

- Administer on an empty stomach, with water only.
- Avoid administering with fruit juice.
- Pregnancy category C

PHARMACOKINETICS (PO)
Onset: Unknown
Peak: 1–2 h
Half-life: 1 h
Duration: Unknown

ADVERSE EFFECTS

Zidovudine has the potential for serious adverse effects and has several FDA black box warnings. The drug can cause severe hematologic toxicity at high doses; anemia and neutropenia are common and may limit therapy. Severe cases may require blood transfusions. Lactic acidosis and severe hepatomegaly with steatosis have been reported, including a few fatal cases. Prolonged use has been associated with myopathy and myositis. Many patients experience fatigue and generalized weakness, anorexia, nausea, and diarrhea. Headache will occur in the majority of patients taking zidovudine, and more serious CNS effects have been reported.

Contraindications: Hypersensitivity to the drug is the only contraindication. It should be used with caution in patients with pre-existing anemia or neutropenia.

INTERACTIONS

Drug-Drug: Zidovudine interacts with many drugs. Concurrent administration with other drugs that depress bone marrow function, such as ganciclovir, interferon alfa, dapsone, flucytosine, or vincristine should be avoided due to cumulative immunosuppression. The following drugs may increase the risk of AZT toxicity: atovaquone, amphotericin B, aspirin, doxorubicin, fluconazole, methadone, and valproic acid. Use with other antiretroviral agents may cause lactic acidosis and severe hepatomegaly with steatosis.

Lab Tests: Mean corpuscular volume may be increased during zidovudine therapy. WBC and Hgb may decrease due to neutropenia and anemia, respectively.

Herbal/Food: Use with caution with herbal supplements, such as St. John's wort, which may cause a decrease in antiretroviral activity.

Treatment of Overdose: There is no specific treatment for overdose.

Refer to MyNursingKit for a Nursing Process Focus specific to this drug.

the FDA in only 3 months, the once-daily tablet simplifies treatment and is expected to improve patient compliance.

REVERSE TRANSCRIPTASE INHIBITORS (NRTIs, NNRTIs, AND NtRTIs)

Reverse transcriptase inhibitors are drugs that are structurally similar to nucleosides, the building blocks of DNA. This class includes nonnucleoside reverse transcriptase inhibitors, which bind directly to the viral enzyme reverse transcriptase and inhibit its function, and nucleotide reverse transcriptase inhibitors.

36.5 Pharmacotherapy with Reverse Transcriptase Inhibitors

One of the early steps in HIV infection is the synthesis of viral DNA from the viral RNA inside the T4 lymphocyte using the enzyme reverse transcriptase. Because reverse transcriptase is a viral enzyme not found in human cells, it has been possible to design drugs capable of selectively inhibiting viral replication.

Viral DNA synthesis requires building blocks known as *nucleosides*. The NRTIs and NtRTIs chemically resemble naturally occurring nucleosides. Thus, as reverse transcriptase uses these drugs to build DNA, the viral DNA chain is prevented from lengthening. The "unfinished" viral DNA chain is unable to be inserted into the host chromosome and HIV is unable to continue its replication cycle.

A second mechanism for inhibiting reverse transcriptase targets the enzyme's function. Drugs in the NNRTI class act by binding near the active site, causing a structural change in the enzyme molecule. The enzyme can no longer bind nucleosides and is unable to construct viral DNA.

Although there are differences in their pharmacokinetic and toxicity profiles, no single NRTI or NNRTI offers a clear therapeutic advantage over any other. Choice of drugs depends on patient response and the experience of the clinician. Because some of these drugs, such as zidovudine (Retrovir, AZT), have been used consistently for more than 25 years, the potential for resistance must be considered when selecting the specific agent. There is a high degree of cross-resistance among the NRTIs. The NRTIs and NNRTIs are nearly always used in multidrug combinations in HAART.

As a class, the NRTIs are well tolerated, although nausea, vomiting, diarrhea, headache, and fatigue are common during the first few weeks of therapy. After prolonged therapy with NRTIs, inhibition of mitochondrial function can cause various organ abnormalities, blood disorders, lactic acidosis, and lipodystrophy, a disorder in which fat is redistributed in specific areas in the body. Areas such as the face, arms, and legs tend to lose fat, whereas the abdomen, breasts, and base of the neck (buffalo hump) accumulate excessive fat deposits.

The NNRTIs are also generally well tolerated and exhibit few serious adverse effects. The adverse effects from these

---

Pr Prototype Drug | Efavirenz *(Sustiva)*

Therapeutic Class: Antiretroviral   **Pharmacologic Class:** Nonnucleoside reverse transcriptase inhibitor (NNRTI)

ACTIONS AND USES

Efavirenz is given orally in combination with other antiretrovirals in the treatment of HIV infection. The drug acts by inhibiting reverse transcriptase. It has the advantage of once-daily dosing and penetration into CSF. Efavirenz is a preferred drug for the initial therapy of HIV infection.

Resistance can develop rapidly to NNRTIs and cross resistance among drugs in this class can occur. High-fat meals increase the absorption by as much as 50% and may cause toxicity. Atripla is a fixed-dose combination of three antiretroviral drugs: efavirenz, emtricitabine, and tenofovir.

ADMINISTRATION ALERTS

- Administer on an empty stomach.
- Administer at bedtime to limit adverse CNS effects.
- Pregnancy category C

PHARMACOKINETICS
Onset: Rapid
Peak: 3–5 h
Half-life: 52–76 h
Duration: 24 h

ADVERSE EFFECTS

CNS adverse effects are observed in at least 50% of the patients when first initiating therapy, including sleep disorders, nightmares, dizziness, reduced ability to concentrate, and delusions. These symptoms gradually diminish after 3–4 weeks of therapy. Like other drugs in this class, rash is common and must be monitored carefully to prevent the development of severe blistering or desquamation.

Contraindications: Efavirenz is a known teratogen in laboratory animals and must not be given to pregnant patients. Patients in the child-bearing years should be advised to use reliable methods of birth control to avoid pregnancy.

INTERACTIONS

Drug–Drug: Patients who are receiving antiepileptic medications metabolized by the liver—such as carbamazepine, phenytoin, and Phenobarbital—may require periodic monitoring of plasma levels because efavirenz may increase the incidence of seizures. Efavirenz can decrease serum levels of the following: statins, methadone, sertraline, and calcium channel blockers. The CNS adverse effects of efavirenz are worsened if the patient takes psychotropic drugs or consumes alcohol. Levels of warfarin may either increase or decrease.

Lab Tests: Efavirenz may give false-positive results for the presence of marijuana. It may increase serum lipid values.

Herbal/Food: St. John's wort may cause a decrease in antiretroviral activity.

Treatment of Overdose: There is no specific treatment for overdose.

Refer to MyNursingKit for a Nursing Process Focus specific to this drug.

drugs, however, are different from those of the NRTIs. Rash is common, and liver toxicity is possible, increasing the risk of drug–drug interactions. Efavirenz (Sustiva) exhibits a high incidence of CNS effects such as dizziness, sleep disor-ders, and fatigue, but these symptoms are rare in patients taking nevirapine (Viramune). Unlike some other anti-retrovirals that negatively affect lipid metabolism, nevirap-ine actually improves the lipid profiles of many patients by increasing HDL levels.

PROTEASE INHIBITORS

Drugs in the protease inhibitor class block the viral enzyme protease, which is responsible for the final assembly of the HIV virions. They have become key drugs in the pharma-cotherapy of HIV infection.

36.6 Pharmacotherapy with Protease Inhibitors

Near the end of its replication cycle, HIV has assembled all the necessary molecular components to create new virions. HIV RNA has been synthesized using the metabolic ma-chinery of the host cell, and the structural and regulatory proteins of HIV are ready to be packaged into a new virion.

Pr Prototype Drug | Lopinavir with Ritonavir *(Kaletra)*

Therapeutic Class: Antiretroviral   **Pharmacologic Class:** Protease inhibitor

ACTIONS AND USES

Kaletra is a combination drug containing two protease inhibitors: lopinavir and ritonavir. Lopinavir is considered the active component of the combination. The small amount of ritonavir inhibits the hepatic breakdown of lopinavir, thus per-mitting serum levels of lopinavir to increase by more than 100-fold. It has an ex-tended half-life that allows for once- or twice-daily dosing.

Resistance to lopinavir/ritonavir has been reported in patients treated with other protease inhibitors prior to Kaletra therapy. Kaletra is a drug of choice for the initial therapy of HIV infection.

ADMINISTRATION ALERTS

- The oral solution form should be taken with food to enhance absorption. Tablets may be taken with or without food.
- Pregnancy category C

PHARMACOKINETICS
Onset: Rapid
Peak: 3–4 h
Half-life: 5–6 h
Duration: 12 h

ADVERSE EFFECTS

Kaletra is well tolerated by most patients, and the most frequently reported problem is diarrhea. Headache and GI-related effects are common, including nausea, vomiting, dyspepsia, and abdominal pain. Hyperglycemia has been re-ported and Kaletra may cause or worsen symptoms of diabetes mellitus. A lipodystrophy syndrome may occur that is associated with hyperglycemia and fat redistribution. Pancreatitis is a rare, though potentially fatal, adverse event.

Contraindications: Patients with liver impairment, especially those with pre-existing viral hepatitis, should be carefully monitored. Hepatic enzyme levels should be regularly evaluated in these patients to prevent hepatic failure. Pa-tients with diabetes should be monitored regularly because Kaletra may exac-erbate this condition. Breast feeding is contraindicated due to the potential risk of transmitting HIV to the newborn.

INTERACTIONS

Drug–Drug: Lopinavir is extensively metabolized by hepatic enzymes, and drugs that undergo hepatic metabolism may interact with Kaletra. Drugs that may *reduce* the effectiveness of the antiretroviral include nevirapine, efavirenz, barbiturates, rifampin, rifabutin, phenytoin, and carbamazepine. Drugs that may *increase* levels of lopinavir include aldesleukin, ketoconazole, delavirdine, indinavir, and ritonavir. Statins should not be administered with Kaletra due to an increased risk for myopathy. Concurrent use of rifampin may lower the effectiveness of Kaletra. Potentially life-threatening dysrhythmias may occur if Kaletra is used concurrently with terfenadine, cisapride, pimozide, and many antidysrhythmic agents. Kaletra may increase adverse effects associated with selective serotonin reuptake inhibitors (SSRIs), tricyclic antidepressants, and phenothiazines.

Lab Tests: Total cholesterol and triglycerides may increase.

Herbal/Food: St. John's wort may cause a decrease in antiretroviral activity and is contraindicated.

Treatment of Overdose: There is no specific treatment for overdose.

Refer to MyNursingKit for a Nursing Process Focus specific to this drug.

NURSING PROCESS FOCUS   PATIENTS RECEIVING PHARMACOTHERAPY FOR HIV-AIDS

Assessment	Potential Nursing Diagnoses
Baseline assessment prior to administration: • Understand the reason the drug has been prescribed in order to assess for therapeutic effects. • Obtain a complete health history including neurologic, cardiovascular, respiratory, hepatic or renal disease, and the possibility of pregnancy. Obtain a drug history including allergies, including specific reactions to drugs, current prescription and OTC drugs, herbal preparations, and alcohol use. Be alert to possible drug interactions. • Assess signs and symptoms of current infection noting onset, duration, characteristics, and presence or absence of fever or pain. • Evaluate appropriate laboratory findings (e.g., CBC, CD4 count, HIV RNA assay, culture and sensitivity [C&S] for any concurrent infections, hepatic and renal function studies, lipid levels, serum amylase, and glucose).	• Infection • Activity Intolerance • Fatigue • Anxiety • Imbalanced Nutrition, Less Than Body Requirements • Deficient Fluid Volume • Diarrhea • Impaired Oral Mucus Membranes • Impaired Skin Integrity • Insomnia • Social Isolation • Confusion (acute or chronic) • Ineffective Therapeutic Regimen Management (related to complex medication regimen and disease treatment) • Deficient Knowledge (related to disease process, transmission, and drug therapy) • Hopelessness • Spiritual Distress • Risk for Injury, Risk for Falls (related to adverse drug effects or disease) • Risk for Caregiver Role Strain
Assessment throughout administration: • Assess for desired therapeutic effects (e.g., CD4 counts and HIV RNA assays remain within acceptable limits, able to attend to normal ADLs, absence of signs and symptoms of concurrent infections). • Continue periodic monitoring of CBC, hepatic and renal function, CD4 and HIV RNA assays, lipid levels, serum amylase, and glucose. • Assess for adverse effects: nausea, vomiting, anorexia, abdominal cramping, diarrhea, fatigue, drowsiness, dizziness, mental changes, insomnia, delusions, fever, muscle or joint pain, paresthesias, hypotension, syncope, and hyperglycemia. Severe diarrhea, jaundice, decreased urine output or darkened urine, purplish-red blistering rash on body or oral mucous membranes, acute abdominal pain, and increasing mental or behavioral changes or decreased level of consciousness (LOC) should be reported immediately.	

Planning: Patient Goals and Expected Outcomes

The patient will:
• Experience therapeutic effects (e.g., CD4 counts and HIV RNA assays within acceptable limits, absence of signs and symptoms of concurrent infection, able to maintain ADLs).
• Be free from, or experience minimal, adverse effects.
• Verbalize an understanding of the drug's use, adverse effects, and required precautions.
• Demonstrate proper self-administration of the medication (e.g., dose, timing, when to notify health care provider).

Implementation

Interventions and (Rationales)	Patient and Family Education
Ensuring therapeutic effects: • Continue assessments as described earlier for therapeutic effects: maintenance of normal or increasing appetite, increasing energy level and ability to maintain ADLs, CD4 counts and HIV RNA assays within acceptable limits and stabilized, and maintaining therapeutic regimen. (Drugs will be required long-term and have many potential adverse effects, making adherence to the medication regimen difficult. The health care provider should be notified if fever and signs and symptoms of concurrent infections increase, excessive fatigue is present, or adverse effects place adherence with drug therapy at risk.)	• Teach the patient to not stop the drug regimen when "feeling better" but to continue to take course of medications; do not share doses with others; and return to the provider if adverse effects make compliance with regimen difficult to continue.

NURSING PROCESS FOCUS   PATIENTS RECEIVING PHARMACOTHERAPY FOR HIV-AIDS *(Continued)*

Implementation

Interventions and (Rationales)	Patient and Family Education
Minimizing adverse effects:	
■ Continue to monitor vital signs, especially temperature if fever is present. Immediately report increasing fever, diarrhea or vomiting, dyspnea, tachycardia, dizziness, syncope, changes in behavior, and lethargy or LOC to the health care provider. (Increasing fever, especially when accompanied by worsening symptoms, may be a sign of worsening infection, adverse drug effects, or drug resistance.)	■ Teach the patient, family, or caregiver to immediately report fever that exceeds 101°F, or per parameters; changes in behavior or level of consciousness; shortness of breath; inability to maintain hydration or nutrition; or dizziness and fainting to the health care provider.
■ Continue to monitor periodic lab work: hepatic and renal function tests, CBC, CD4 counts, HIV RNA assays, lipid levels, serum amylase, C&S if concurrent infections are present, and glucose. (Drugs used for the treatment of HIV are hepatic and renal toxic. Bone marrow suppression and resulting blood dyscrasias, particularly anemia and leukopenia, are also adverse effects and will be monitored by CBC. Lipid levels and serum amylase will be monitored to assess for pancreatitis and glucose levels checked for hyperglycemia.)	■ Instruct the patient on the need for periodic lab work, correlating any symptoms with need for possible labs (e.g., serum amylase if the patient is having upper abdominal pain). Advise lab personnel of HIV status.
■ Monitor for hypersensitivity and allergic reactions, especially with the first dose of any antiretroviral or protease inhibitor. Continue to monitor the patient as needed based on the drug used or the patient's condition. (Anaphylactic reactions are possible, particularly with zalcitabine. Because reactions may not always be predictable, caution and frequent monitoring are essential to ensure prompt treatment.)	■ Teach the patient to immediately report any itching; rashes; swelling, particularly of face, tongue, or lips; urticaria; flushing; dizziness; syncope; wheezing; throat tightness; or difficulty breathing.
■ Continue to monitor for hepatic and renal toxicities. (Antiretrovirals and protease inhibitors may be hepatic and renal toxic and require frequent monitoring to prevent adverse effects. Increasing fluid intake will prevent drug accumulation in kidneys.)	■ Teach the patient to immediately report any nausea, vomiting, yellowing of skin or sclera, abdominal pain, light or clay-colored stools, and diminished urine output or darkening of urine.
	■ Advise the patient to increase fluid intake to 2 to 3 L per day.
■ Continue to monitor for dermatologic effects including red or purplish skin rash, blisters, or peeling skin, including oral mucous membranes. Assess oral mucous membranes for signs of stomatitis, as drug effects or immunosuppression may result in the overgrowth of oral flora. Immediately report severe rashes, especially associated with blistering. (These drugs may cause significant dermatologic effects including stomatitis, and Stevens–Johnson syndrome, a potentially fatal condition.)	■ Teach the patient to inspect oral cavity at least once a day and maintain regular dental exams. Maintain good oral hygiene and rinse mouth with plain water or solution as prescribed by the health care provider after eating. Use protective clothing for sun exposure and immediately report any significant rashes or sunburned appearance.
■ Monitor for signs and symptoms of neurotoxicity, e.g., drowsiness, dizziness, mental changes, insomnia, delusions, paresthesias, headache, changes in LOC, and seizures. (Many HIV-AIDS drugs cause peripheral neuropathy and have neurologic adverse effects.)	■ Instruct the patient or caregiver to immediately report increasing headache, dizziness, drowsiness, worsening insomnia, numbness of hands, feet or extremities, and changes in behavior or LOC.
	■ Caution patient that drowsiness may occur and to be cautious with driving or other activities requiring mental alertness until effects of drug are known.
	■ Caution patient to be cautious when in contact with heat or cold as numbness from peripheral neuropathy may make sensing accurate temperature more difficult.
	■ Encourage sleep hygiene measures, e.g., restful routines before bed and avoiding large meals within 1 or 2 hours of sleep. Have the patient consult with the health care provider if insomnia causes daytime sleepiness or continues.
■ Monitor for signs and symptoms of blood dyscrasias, e.g., low-grade fevers, bleeding, bruising, and significant fatigue. (Bone marrow suppression may occur and may cause blood dyscrasias with resulting decreases in RBCs, WBCs, and/or platelets. Periodic monitoring of CBC will be required.)	■ Teach the patient to report any low-grade fevers, sore throat, rashes, bruising or increased bleeding, and unusual fatigue or shortness of breath, especially after taking the drug for a prolonged period.

(Continued)

NURSING PROCESS FOCUS   **PATIENTS RECEIVING PHARMACOTHERAPY FOR HIV-AIDS** *(Continued)*

Implementation

Interventions and (Rationales)	Patient and Family Education
▪ Monitor for significant GI effects, including nausea, vomiting, abdominal pain or cramping, and diarrhea. Administer drugs as per guidelines: Some require administration on an empty stomach, some with food or milk. Additional pharmacologic treatment may be necessary to limit adverse GI effects. Ensure adequate nutrition and caloric intake. (Adverse GI effects are common to most antiretrovirals and protease inhibitors. Always check administration guidelines before administering with or without food or milk.)	▪ Teach the patient to take the drug with food or milk if appropriate or to take drug on an empty stomach with a full glass of water. Avoid acidic foods and beverages or carbonated drinks, which may cause stomach upset. ▪ Encourage the patient to try small, frequent meals, which may be better tolerated than fewer, larger meals. High-caloric foods and supplemental beverages (e.g., Boost or Ensure) may help add additional calories and supply additional fluids. Assist the patient in obtaining a dietary consultation as needed if nausea or diarrhea makes maintaining intake difficult.
▪ Monitor for symptoms of pancreatitis including severe abdominal pain, nausea, vomiting, and abdominal distention. (Some antiretroviral drugs such as didanosine may cause pancreatitis. Serum amylase and lipid levels should be monitored periodically.)	▪ Instruct the patient to report fever, severe abdominal pain, nausea, vomiting, and abdominal distention immediately.
▪ Monitor blood glucose in patients taking antiretrovirals. (These drugs may cause hyperglycemia. Diabetic patients may require a change in their antidiabetic drug routine.)	▪ Teach the diabetic patient to test glucose more frequently, reporting any consistent elevations to the health care provider.
▪ Encourage infection control and good hygiene measures based on the extent of disease condition, and follow established protocol in hospitalized patients. (These drugs decrease the level of HIV infection but do not cure the disease. Excellent hygiene measures will limit the chance for secondary infections in the immunocompromised patient.)	▪ Teach the patient adequate infection control and hygiene measures such as frequent hand washing, avoiding crowded indoor places, and adequate nutrition and rest, especially if currently immunocompromised. ▪ Practice abstinence or always use barrier protection during sexual activity. ▪ Do not share needles with others and do not donate blood.
▪ Provide resources for medical and emotional support. (Treatment requires a multidisciplinary approach.)	▪ Advise the patient about community resources and support groups. Assist the caregiver with respite care as needed.
Patient understanding of drug therapy: ▪ Use opportunities during administration of medications and during assessments to discuss rationale for drug therapy, desired therapeutic outcomes, most common adverse effects, and parameters for when to call the health care provider, and any necessary monitoring or precautions. (Using time during nursing care helps to optimize and reinforce key teaching areas.)	▪ The patient, family, or caregiver should be able to state the reason for the drug; appropriate dose and scheduling; what adverse effects to observe for and when to report; and the anticipated length of medication therapy.

Patient self-administration of drug therapy:
▪ When administering medications, instruct the patient, family, or caregiver in proper self-administration techniques followed by return demonstration. (Proper administration increases the effectiveness of the drug.)
	▪ Teach the patient to take the medication as follows:
	  ▪ Complete the entire course of therapy unless otherwise instructed. The duration of the required therapy may be quite lengthy but it is necessary to prevent active infection. Do not stop medication when starting to feel better.
	  ▪ Eliminate alcohol while on these medications. These drugs cause significant reactions when taken with alcohol.
	  ▪ Take the drug with food or milk but avoid acidic beverages. If instructed to take the drug on an empty stomach, take with a full glass of water.
	  ▪ Take the medication as evenly spaced throughout each day as feasible.
	  ▪ Increase overall fluid intake while taking these drugs.

Evaluation of Outcome Criteria

Evaluate the effectiveness of drug therapy by confirming that patient goals and expected outcomes have been met (see "Planning").

See Table 36.1 for a list of drugs to which these nursing actions apply.

As the newly formed virions bud from the host cell and are released into the surrounding extracellular fluid, one final step remains before the HIV is mature: A long polypeptide chain must be cleaved by the enzyme protease to produce the final HIV proteins. The enzyme performing this step is HIV protease.

The protease inhibitors (PIs) attach to the active site of HIV protease, thus preventing the final maturation of the virions. The virions are noninfectious without this final step. When combined with other antiretroviral drug classes, the PIs are capable of lowering plasma levels of HIV RNA to an undetectable range. Since their development in 1995, the protease inhibitors have become essential drugs in the treatment of HIV-AIDS.

The PIs are metabolized in the liver and have the potential to interact with many different drugs. In general, they are well tolerated, with GI complaints being the most common side effects. Various lipid abnormalities have been reported, including elevated cholesterol and triglyceride levels, and abdominal obesity. Cross resistance among the various PIs has been reported.

All PIs have equivalent effectiveness and exhibit a similar range of adverse effects. The Panel on Antiretroviral Guidelines for Adults and Adolescents recommends the use of atazanavir, fosamprenavir, or lopinavir as preferred drugs for the initial treatment of HIV. The initial choice of protease inhibitor usually includes low doses of ritonavir. Addition of small amounts of ritonavir allows less frequent dosing intervals and increases the plasma concentration of the primary protease inhibitor. This is known as ritonavir boosting.

36.7 Prevention of HIV Infection

Early in the history of the AIDS epidemic, scientists were optimistic that the spread of HIV infection would be prevented by the development of an effective vaccine. After all, scientists had totally eradicated the smallpox virus as a human threat and have essentially controlled major viral infections such as measles and mumps. Such a vaccine could be given in childhood, offering lifetime protection against the fatal disease.

After decades of research, scientists are still far from developing a vaccine to prevent AIDS. A few HIV vaccines are currently in clinical trials, but none is expected to cause a major impact on the HIV epidemic. At best, the HIV vaccines produced thus far only boost the immune response; they are unable to prevent the infection or its fatal consequences. Although the immune response boost may help a patient already infected with the virus to better control the disease, it does not prevent new infections.

PREVENTION OF PERINATAL TRANSMISSION OF HIV

One of the most tragic aspects of the AIDS epidemic is transmission of the virus from a mother to her child during pregnancy, delivery, or breast-feeding. Newborns with HIV may succumb to the infection within weeks, or symptoms may be delayed for months or years. The prognosis for these children is generally poor; thus, the best approach to dealing with HIV infections in neonates is prevention.

In 1994, clinical trials determined that perinatal transmission of HIV could be markedly reduced through pharmacotherapy. The risk of transmission may be reduced approximately 70% using the following regimen:

- Oral administration of zidovudine to the mother, beginning at week 14 of gestation and continuing to week 34 of gestation.

- Intravenous administration of zidovudine to the mother during labor.

- Oral administration of zidovudine to the newborn for 6 weeks following delivery. (HIV infection is established in infants by age 1 to 2 weeks; starting antiretroviral therapy more than 48 hours after birth is ineffective in preventing the infection.)

This original regimen to prevent perinatal transmission has been supported by subsequent research and remains essentially unchanged. The specific drugs chosen depend on whether the mother is treatment experienced prior to the pregnancy and on the results of resistance studies. To date, there does not appear to be an increased incidence of congenital abnormalities or malignancies among the children born to women receiving this regimen. If the HIV infection is diagnosed earlier than week 14 of pregnancy, the patient is usually placed on HAART combination therapy, with zidovudine as one of the drugs in the regimen.

POSTEXPOSURE PROPHYLAXIS OF HIV INFECTION FOLLOWING OCCUPATIONAL EXPOSURE

Since the start of the AIDS epidemic, nurses and other health care workers have been concerned about acquiring the infection from their HIV-AIDS patients. Fortunately, if proper precautions are observed, the disease is rarely transmitted from patient to caregiver. Accidents have occurred, however, in which health care workers have acquired the infection by exposure to the blood or body fluids of an HIV-infected patient. Approximately 56 cases of patient-to-health-care-worker transmission have been documented in the United States following occupational exposure. Although the risk is very small, the question remains, Can HIV transmission be prevented *after* accidental occupational exposure to HIV? The answer is a qualified yes.

The success of postexposure prophylaxis (PEP) therapy following HIV exposure is difficult to assess because of the lack of controlled studies and the small number of cases. Enough data have been accumulated, however, to demonstrate that PEP is successful in certain circumstances. For prevention to be most successful, PEP should be started within 24 to 36 hours after exposure to a patient who is *known* to be HIV positive. The exposed health care professional should receive a baseline HIV RNA level as soon as possible after exposure and subsequent follow-up testing as recommended.

If the HIV status of the patient is *unknown*, PEP is decided case by case, based on the type of exposure and the likelihood that the blood or body fluid contained HIV. In some cases, PEP is initiated for a few days, until the patient can be tested. PEP should be initiated only if the exposure was sufficiently severe and the source fluid is known, or strongly suspected, to contain HIV. Using PEP outside established guidelines is both expensive and dangerous; the antiretrovirals used for PEP therapy produce adverse effects in more than half the patients. The *basic* PEP treatment includes one of the following regimens, conducted over a 4-week period:

- Zidovudine and lamivudine or
- Zidovudine and emtricitabine or
- Lamivudine and tenofovir or
- Tenofovir and emtricitabine

If the accidental HIV exposure was particularly severe, and the source is a symptomatic HIV-infected person with a high viral load, a third drug may be added to the regimen (lopinavir boosted with ritonavir). Adding a third drug increases the risk for adverse effects and has not been proved to be more successful than a two-drug regimen.

HERPESVIRUSES

Herpes simplex viruses (HSVs) are a family of DNA viruses that cause repeated blister-like lesions on the skin, genitals, and other mucosal surfaces. Antiviral drugs can lower the frequency of acute herpes episodes and diminish the intensity of acute disease. These drugs are listed in Table 36.2.

36.8 Pharmacotherapy of Herpesvirus Infections

Herpesviruses are usually acquired through direct physical contact with an infected person, but they may also be trans-

mitted from infected mothers to their newborns, sometimes resulting in severe CNS disease. The herpesvirus family includes the following:

- HSV-1 primarily causes infections of the eye, mouth, and lips, although the incidence of genital infections is increasing.
- HSV-2 causes genital infections.

LIFESPAN CONSIDERATIONS

HIV in the Pediatric and Geriatric Populations

Children infected with the HIV virus appear to develop opportunistic conditions at a much more rapid rate than do adults. The younger the age at which the child acquires the HIV virus, the poorer the prognosis tends to be. Like adults, children are also treated with combination therapy, although not all antiretroviral medications can be used in pediatric patients. Prophylactic treatment against *P. carinii* pneumonia is also started early in the treatment regimen, because respiratory infections are often a cause of death in young children. The caregivers of the child must be able to handle the intense medication regimen and also must be aware of the early symptoms of opportunistic diseases.

The diagnosis of the geriatric patient may be delayed because HIV is often not suspected in this population. The geriatric patient who has become infected with the HIV virus may be less than willing to disclose activities that are considered high-risk behaviors. The geriatric patient's need for antiretroviral treatment depends on the CD4 count. The older adult may have greater difficulty handling the rigorous regimen of the treatment. The physiologic changes associated with aging increase the possibility of drug toxicity in this population. The social factors must also be considered, because these patients may be living alone or even be the primary caretaker of a disabled spouse. The ability of a patient to be sexually active is not determined by age; therefore, it is very important to stress sexual activity precautions to prevent spread of the HIV virus.

TABLE 36.2	Drugs for Herpesviruses	
Drug	Route and Adult Dose (max dose where indicated)	Adverse Effects
SYSTEMIC AGENTS		
acyclovir (Zovirax)	PO; 400 mg tid	*Nausea, vomiting, diarrhea, headache, pain and inflammation at injection sites (parenteral agents)*
	IV; 5–10 mg/kg every 8 h for 7–14 days	
cidofovir (Vistide)	IV; 5 mg/kg once weekly for 2 consecutive wk	<u>Thrombocytopenic purpura/hemolytic uremic syndrome, nephrotoxicity, seizures (foscarnet), electrolyte imbalances (foscarnet), hematologic toxicity/bone marrow suppression (ganciclovir)</u>
famciclovir (Famvir)	PO; 500 mg tid for 7 days (max: 1,500 mg/day)	
foscarnet (Foscavir)	IV; 40–60 mg/kg infused over 1–2 h tid (max: 180 mg/kg/day)	
ganciclovir (Cytovene)	PO; 1 g tid	
	IV; 5 mg/kg infused over 1 h bid	
valacyclovir (Valtrex)	PO; 1.0 g tid (max: 3 g/day)	
TOPICAL AGENTS		
docosanol (Abreva)	Topical; 10% cream applied to cold sore up to five times/day for 10 days	*Burning, irritation, or stinging at site of application, headache*
idoxuridine (Dendrid, Herplex)	Topical; 1 drop in each eye every hour during waking hours and every 2 hr during the night	<u>Photophobia, keratopathy, and edema of eyelids (ocular agents)</u>
penciclovir (Denavir)	Topical; apply every 2 h while awake for 4 days	
trifluridine (Viroptic)	Topical; 1 drop in each eye every 2 h during waking hours (max: 9 drops/day)	

Italics indicate common adverse effects; <u>underlining</u> indicates serious adverse effects.

- Cytomegalovirus (CMV) affects multiple body systems in immunosuppressed patients.
- Varicella-zoster virus (VZV) causes shingles (zoster) and chicken pox (varicella).
- Epstein–Barr virus (EBV) results in mononucleosis and a form of cancer known as Burkitt's lymphoma.
- Herpesvirus-6 causes roseola in children and hepatitis or encephalitis in immunosuppressed patients.

Following its initial entrance into the patient, HSV may remain in a latent, asymptomatic state in ganglia for many years. Immunosuppression, physical challenges, or emotional stress can promote active replication of the virus and appearance of the characteristic lesions. Complications include secondary infections of nongenital tissues.

The pharmacologic goals for the management of herpes infections are twofold: to *relieve acute symptoms* and to *prevent recurrences*. It should be noted that the antiviral drugs used to treat herpesviruses do not cure patients; the virus remains in patients for the remainder of their lives.

Initial HSV-1 and HSV-2 infections are usually treated with oral antiviral therapy for 5 to 10 days. The most commonly prescribed antivirals for HSV and VZV include acyclovir (Zovirax), famciclovir (Famvir), and valacyclovir (Valtrex). Topical forms of several antivirals are available for application to herpes lesions, although they are not as effective as the oral forms. In immunocompromised patients, IV acyclovir may be indicated.

Recurrent herpes lesions are usually mild and often require no drug treatment. If drug therapy is initiated within 24 hours after recurrent symptoms first appear, the length of the acute episode may be shortened. Patients who experience particularly severe or frequent recurrences (more than six episodes per year) may benefit from low doses of prophylactic antiviral therapy. Prophylactic therapy may also be of benefit to immunocompromised patients, such as those receiving antineoplastic therapy or those with AIDS.

Herpes of the eye is the most common infectious cause of corneal blindness in the United States. Ocular herpes causes a painful, inflamed lesion on the eyelid or surface of the eye. Prompt treatment with antiviral drugs prevents permanent tissue destruction. As with genital herpes, once patients acquire ocular herpes, they often experience recurrences, which may occur years after the initial symptoms. Ocular herpes is treated with local application of drops or ointment. Trifluridine (Viroptic), and idoxuridine (Dendrid, Herplex) are available in ophthalmic formulations. Oral acyclovir is used when topical drops or ointments are contraindicated. Uncomplicated ocular herpes usually resolves after 1 to 2 weeks of pharmacotherapy.

Pr Prototype Drug | Acyclovir (Zovirax)

Therapeutic Class: Antiviral for herpesviruses   **Pharmacologic Class:** Nucleoside analog

ACTIONS AND USES

Approved by the FDA in 1982 as one of the first antiviral drugs, acyclovir is limited to pharmacotherapy for herpesviruses, for which it is a drug of choice. It is most effective against HSV-1 and HSV-2, and effective only at high doses against CMV and varicella zoster. By preventing viral DNA synthesis, acyclovir decreases the duration and severity of acute herpes episodes. When given for prophylaxis, it may decrease the frequency of herpes appearance, but it does not cure the patient. It is available as a 5% ointment for application to active lesions, in oral form for prophylaxis, and as an IV for severe episodes. Because of its short half-life, acyclovir is sometimes administered orally up to five times a day.

ADMINISTRATION ALERTS

- When given IV, the drug may cause painful inflammation of vessels at the site of infusion.
- Administer around the clock, even if sleep is interrupted.
- Administer with food.
- Pregnancy category C

PHARMACOKINETICS (PO)
Onset: Unknown
Peak: 1.5–2 h
Half-life: 2.5–5 h
Duration: 4–8 h

ADVERSE EFFECTS

There are few adverse effects to acyclovir when it is administered topically or orally. Nephrotoxicity is possible when the medication is given IV. Resistance has developed to the drug, particularly in patients with HIV-AIDS.

Contraindications: Acyclovir is contraindicated in patients with hypersensitivity to drugs in this class.

INTERACTIONS

Drug–Drug: Concurrent use of acyclovir with nephrotoxic agents should be avoided. Probenecid decreases acyclovir elimination, and zidovudine may cause increased drowsiness and lethargy.

Lab Tests: Values for kidney function tests such as BUN and serum creatinine may increase.

Herbal/Food: Unknown

Treatment of Overdose: There is no specific treatment for overdose.

Refer to MyNursingKit for a Nursing Process Focus specific to this drug.

INFLUENZA

Influenza is a viral infection characterized by acute symptoms that include sore throat, sneezing, coughing, fever, and chills. The infectious viral particles are easily spread via airborne droplets. In immunosuppressed patients, an influenza infection may be fatal. In 1919, a worldwide outbreak of influenza killed an estimated 20 million people. Influenza viruses are designated with the letters A, B, or C. Type A has been responsible for several serious pandemics throughout history. The RNA-containing influenza viruses should not be confused with *Haemophilus influenzae*, which is a bacterium that causes respiratory disease.

36.9 Pharmacotherapy of Influenza

The best approach to influenza infection is *prevention* through annual vaccination. Those who benefit greatly from vaccinations include residents of long-term care facilities, those with chronic cardiopulmonary disease, children ages 5 and younger, pregnant women in their second or third trimester during the peak flu season, and healthy adults older than age 65. Influenza vaccination is also recommended for health care workers who are involved in the direct care of patients at high risk for acquiring influenza, including HIV-infected patients. Depending on the stage of the disease, HIV-positive patients may also benefit from vaccination. Adequate immunity is achieved about 2 weeks after vaccination and lasts for several months up to a year. Additional details on vaccines are presented in chapter 32∞.

Antivirals may be used to prevent influenza or decrease the severity of acute symptoms. Amantadine (Symmetrel) has been available to prevent and treat influenza for many years. Chemoprophylaxis with amantadine or rimantadine (Flumadine) is indicated for unvaccinated individuals during a confirmed outbreak of influenza type A. Therapy with these antivirals is sometimes started concurrently with vaccination; the antiviral offers protection during the 2 weeks before therapeutic antibody titers are achieved from the vaccine. Because of the expense and possible adverse effects of these drugs, they are generally reserved for patients who are at greatest risk for the severe complications of influenza. Antivirals for influenza are listed in Table 36.3.

The neuroaminidase inhibitors were introduced in 1999 to treat *active* influenza infections. If given within 48 hours of the onset of symptoms, oseltamivir (Tamiflu) and zanamivir (Relenza) are reported to shorten the normal 7-day duration of influenza symptoms to 5 days. Oseltamivir is given orally, whereas zanamivir is inhaled. Because these agents are expensive and produce only modest results, prevention through vaccination remains the best alternative.

It is important to understand that these antivirals are not effective against the common cold virus. About 200 different viruses, including rhinoviruses, cause symptoms identified with the common cold. Despite considerable attempts to develop drugs to prevent this annoying infection, success has not yet been achieved. There are drugs, however, that may relieve symptoms of the common cold, and these are presented in chapter 38∞.

VIRAL HEPATITIS

Viral **hepatitis** is a common infection caused by a number of different viruses. Although each virus has its own unique clinical features, all hepatitis viruses cause inflammation and necrosis of liver cells. Symptoms of hepatitis may be acute or chronic. Acute symptoms include fever, chills, fatigue, anorexia, nausea, and vomiting. Chronic hepatitis may result in prolonged fatigue, jaundice, liver cirrhosis, and ultimately hepatic failure.

36.10 Pharmacotherapy of Viral Hepatitis

HEPATITIS A

Hepatitis A virus (HAV) is spread by the oral–fecal route and causes epidemics in regions of the world having poor sanitation. Outbreaks in the United States are most often sporadic events caused by the consumption of contaminated food.

Although approximately 20% of HAV-infected patients require some hospitalization for symptoms related to the infection, most recover without pharmacotherapy and develop lifelong immunity to the virus. Fatalities due to chronic disease are rare, and only a small number of patients

TABLE 36.3	Drugs for Influenza	
Drug	Route and Adult Dose (max dose where indicated)	Adverse Effects
INFLUENZA PROPHYLAXIS		
amantadine (Symmetrel)	PO; 100 mg bid (max: 400 mg/day)	*Nausea, dizziness, nervousness, difficulty concentrating, insomnia*
rimantadine (Flumadine)	PO; 100 mg bid (max: 200 mg/day)	<u>Leukopenia, hallucinations, orthostatic hypotension, urinary retention</u>
INFLUENZA TREATMENT: NEUROAMINIDASE INHIBITORS		
oseltamivir (Tamiflu)	PO; 75 mg bid for 5 days	*Nausea, vomiting, diarrhea, dizziness*
zanamivir (Relenza)	Inhalation; 2 inhalations/day for 5 days	<u>Bronchitis</u>

Italics indicate common adverse effects; <u>underlining</u> indicates serious adverse effects.

develop severe liver failure. Thus, HAV is normally considered an acute disease, having no significant chronic form. This makes HAV very different from hepatitis B or C.

Like all forms of hepatitis, the best treatment for HAV is prevention. HAV vaccine (Havrix, VAQTA) has been available since 1995. It is indicated for children living in communities or states with high infection rates, travelers to countries with high HAV infection rates, men who have sex with men, and illegal drug users. When a booster is given 6 to 12 months after the initial dose, close to 100% immunity is obtained. The average length of protection is approximately 5 to 8 years, although protection may last 20 years or longer in some patients. The availability of the HAV vaccine has led to a dramatic drop in the rate of this infection in the United States.

Prophylaxis or postexposure treatment for a patient recently exposed to HAV includes hepatitis A immunoglobulins (HAIg), a concentrated solution of antibodies. HAIg is administered as prophylaxis for patients traveling to endemic areas and to close personal contacts of infected patients to prevent transmission of the virus. A single IM dose of HAIg can provide passive protection and prophylaxis for about 3 months. It is estimated that the immunoglobulins are 85% effective at preventing HAV in patients exposed to the virus.

Therapy for acute HAV infection is symptomatic. No specific drugs are indicated; in otherwise healthy adults, the infection is self-limiting.

HEPATITIS B

Hepatitis B virus (HBV) in the United States is transmitted primarily through exposure to contaminated blood and body fluids. Major risk factors for HBV infection include injected drug abuse, sex with an HBV-infected partner, and sex between men. Health care workers are at risk because of accidental exposure to HBV-contaminated needles or body fluids. In many regions of the world, the primary mode of transmission of HBV is by the perinatal route and from child to child.

Treatment of acute HBV infection is symptomatic, because no specific therapy is available. Ninety percent of acute HBV infections resolve with complete recovery and do not progress to chronic disease. Lifelong immunity to HBV is usually acquired following resolution of the infection.

Symptoms of chronic HBV may develop as long as 10 years following exposure. HBV has a much greater probability of progression to chronic hepatitis and a greater mortality rate than does HAV. The final stage of the infection is hepatic cirrhosis. In addition, chronic HBV infections are associated with an increased risk of hepatocellular carcinoma.

As with HAV, the best treatment for HBV infection is *prevention* through immunization. Traditionally, HBV vaccine (Recombivax HB, Engerix-B) has been indicated for health care workers and others routinely exposed to blood and body fluids. However, universal vaccination of all children is now recommended, and some states require HBV vaccination prior to entry into school. Three doses of the vaccine provide up to 90% of patients with protection against HBV following exposure to the virus. A combina-

tion vaccine is available that provides immunity to both HAV and HBV (Twinrix).

For someone who has been recently exposed to the HBV, therapy with hepatitis B immunoglobulins (HBIg) may be initiated. Indications for HBIg therapy include probable exposure to HBV through the perinatal, sexual, or parenteral routes, or exposure of an infant to a caregiver with HBV. HBIg is administered as soon as possible after suspected exposure to HBV.

Once chronic hepatitis becomes active, pharmacotherapy is indicated with drugs listed in Table 36.4. The two basic strategies for eliminating HBV are to give antivirals that stop viral replication, or to administer immunomodulators that boost body defenses. Three different therapies are approved for chronic HBV pharmacotherapy:

- *Interferon alfa:* Thirty percent to forty percent of patients respond to 4 months of therapy. Five to ten percent of these patients relapse after completion of therapy.
- *Lamivudine (Epivir):* Twenty-five percent to forty-five percent of patients respond to therapy, which lasts 1 year or longer. Emergence of resistant viral strains is becoming a clinical problem.
- *Adefovir (Hespera):* Approximately 50% of patients respond to 48 weeks of therapy. The drug is new, and long-term studies are in progress.

In 2005 the FDA approved entecavir (Baraclude) for chronic HBV. Early data suggest entecavir is as effective as or more effective than lamivudine. Tenofovir (Viread), a medication used to treat HIV, was approved in 2008 to treat chronic hepatitis B infections (see Table 36.1). Early results suggest that tenofovir may have equal or greater effectiveness as adefovir. Entecavir and tenofovir offer new treatment options for patients who have developed resistance to older medications.

HEPATITIS C AND OTHER HEPATITIS VIRUSES

The hepatitis C, D, E, and G viruses are sometimes referred to as non A–non B viruses. Of the non A–non B viruses, hepatitis C has the greatest clinical importance.

Transmitted primarily through exposure to infected blood or body fluids, hepatitis C virus (HCV) is more common than HBV. Approximately half of all HIV-AIDS patients are coinfected with HCV. About 70% of patients infected with HCV proceed to chronic hepatitis, and up to 30% may develop end-stage cirrhosis. HCV is the most common cause of liver transplants.

Unlike with HAV and HBV, no vaccine is available to prevent hepatitis C. In addition, postexposure prophylaxis of HAC with immunoglobulins is not recommended because its effectiveness has not been demonstrated.

Current pharmacotherapy for chronic HCV infection includes several types of interferon and the antiviral ribavirin. Combination therapy has been found to produce a more sustained viral suppression than monotherapy with either agent. Commercially available interferons for hepatitis include both the regular and pegylated formulations. **Pegylation** is a process

TABLE 36.4	**Drugs for Hepatitis**	
Drug	Route and Adult Dose (max dose where indicated)	Adverse Effects
INTERFERONS		
interferon alfacon-1 (Infergen)	Subcutaneous; 9 mcg three times/wk for 24 wk	*Flulike symptoms, myalgia, fatigue, headache, anorexia, diarrhea*
interferon alfa-n1 (Wellferon)	Subcutaneous/IM; 3 million units three times/wk for 48 wk	
Pr interferon alfa-2b (Intron A)	Subcutaneous/IM; 3 million units/m² three times/wk	<u>Myelosuppression, thrombocytopenia, suicide ideation</u>
peginterferon alfa-2a (Pegasys)	Subcutaneous; 180 mcg of 1 wk for 48 wk	
peginterferon alfa-2b (PEG-Intron)	Subcutaneous; 1 mcg/kg/wk for monotherapy; 1.5 g/kg/wk when given with ribavirin	
NONINTERFERONS/COMBINATIONS		
adefovir dipivoxil (Hepsera)	PO; 10 mg/day	*Asthenia, headache, nausea, dizziness, fatigue, nasal disturbances (lamivudine)*
entecavir (Baraclude)	PO; 0.5 mg/day; 1 mg/day as a single dose for patients with history of lamivudine resistance	
lamivudine (Epivir HBV)	PO; 150 mg bid	<u>Nephrotoxicity and lactic acidosis (adefovir, telbivudine), pancreatitis (lamivudine), hepatomegaly with steatorrhea (lamivudine, entecavir), cardiac arrest (ribavirin), hemolytic anemia (ribavirin), apnea (ribavirin), myopathy (telbivudine), peripheral neuropathy (telbivudine)</u>
ribavirin (Rebetrol)/interferon alfa-2b (Introl A): Combination is called Robetron	ribavirin: PO; five to six, 200-mg capsules daily	
	interferon alfa-2b: Subcutaneous; 3 million international units, three times/wk	
telbivudine (Tyzeka)	PO: 600 mg/day	
Italics indicate common adverse effects; <u>underlining</u> indicates serious adverse effects.		

that attaches polyethylene glycol (PEG) to an interferon to extend its duration of action, thus allowing it to be administered less frequently. Whereas standard interferon formulations must be administered three times per week, pegylated versions require only one dose per week. The PEG molecule is inert and does not influence antiviral activity. Additional information on interferons used for other indications may be found in chapter 32∞.

NURSING PROCESS FOCUS

PATIENTS RECEIVING ANTIVIRAL PHARMACOTHERAPY FOR HERPESVIRUS INFECTIONS

Assessment	Potential Nursing Diagnoses
Baseline assessment prior to administration: ■ Understand the reason the drug has been prescribed in order to assess for therapeutic effects. ■ Obtain a complete health history including immunizations, respiratory, neurologic, hepatic or renal disease, and the possibility of pregnancy. Obtain a drug history including allergies, including specific reactions to drugs, current prescription and OTC drugs, herbal preparations, and alcohol use. Be alert to possible drug interactions. ■ Assess signs and symptoms of current infection noting onset, duration, characteristics, and presence or absence of fever or pain. ■ Evaluate appropriate laboratory findings (e.g., CBC, hepatic and renal function studies, viral cultures).	■ Infection ■ Impaired Oral Mucous Membranes ■ Impaired Skin Integrity ■ Fatigue ■ Activity Intolerance ■ Social Isolation ■ Deficient Knowledge (related to disease process, transmission, and drug therapy) ■ Risk for Deficient Fluid Volume (related to disease process or adverse drug reactions) ■ Risk for Imbalanced Nutrition, Less Than Body Requirements (related to disease process or adverse drug reactions)
Assessment throughout administration: ■ Assess for desired therapeutic effects (e.g., diminished or absence of signs and symptoms of herpesvirus infection and without symptoms of concurrent infections). ■ Continue periodic monitoring of CBC, and hepatic and renal function. ■ Assess for adverse effects: nausea, vomiting, diarrhea, anorexia, fatigue, drowsiness, dizziness, and headache. Decreased urine output or darkened urine, increased bruising or bleeding, and increasing fever or symptoms of infections should be reported immediately.	

NURSING PROCESS FOCUS	**PATIENTS RECEIVING ANTIVIRAL PHARMACOTHERAPY FOR HERPESVIRUS INFECTIONS** *(Continued)*

Planning: Patient Goals and Expected Outcomes

The patient will:

- Experience therapeutic effects (e.g., diminished or absence of signs and symptoms of infection, able to maintain nutrition and hydration).
- Be free from, or experience minimal, adverse effects.
- Verbalize an understanding of the drug's use, adverse effects, and required precautions.
- Demonstrate proper self-administration of the medication (e.g., dose, timing, when to notify provider).

Implementation

Interventions and (Rationales)	Patient and Family Education
Ensuring therapeutic effects: - Continue assessments as described earlier for therapeutic effects: diminishing signs of original infection, maintenance of normal appetite and fluid intake, and increasing energy level. (Drug effects may not be immediately observable. Gradual improvement should be noted and the patient should be encouraged to continue taking medication.)	- Teach the patient to not discontinue drug regimen when "feeling better" and to take the full course of medication. - Encourage adequate nutrition, rest, and activity levels as improvement is noted.
Minimizing adverse effects: - Continue to monitor vital signs. Immediately report increasing fever, dizziness, headache, or diminished urine output to the health care provider. (Increasing fever, especially when accompanied by worsening symptoms, may be a sign of worsening infection or adverse drug effects.)	- Teach the patient, family, or caregiver to promptly report fever that exceeds 101°F, or per parameters; inability to maintain hydration or nutrition; or dizziness to the health care provider.
- Continue to monitor periodic lab work: CBC, hepatic and renal function tests, and viral cultures. (Antiviral drugs may be toxic to the liver and kidneys. Blood dyscrasias due to bone marrow suppression, particularly thrombocytopenia, is an adverse effect and is monitored by CBC.)	- Instruct the patient on the need for periodic lab work, correlating any symptoms with the need for possible labs (e.g., increased bruising or bleeding).
- Continue to monitor for hepatic and renal, toxicities. (Hepatic and renal toxicities may occur and require frequent monitoring to prevent adverse effects. Increasing fluid intake may prevent drug accumulation in kidneys.)	- Teach the patient to immediately report any nausea, vomiting, yellowing of skin or sclera, abdominal pain, light or clay-colored stools, or diminished urine output or darkening of urine. - Advise the patient to maintain fluid intake at 2 to 3 L per day.
- Monitor for signs and symptoms of neurotoxicity, particularly in patients on IV acyclovir, e.g., drowsiness, dizziness, tremors, headache, confusion, changes in LOC, and seizures. Ensure patient safety and have the patient rise slowly from lying or sitting to standing. (Acyclovir, especially when given IV, may be neurotoxic.)	- Instruct the patient, family, or caregiver to immediately report increasing headache, dizziness, drowsiness, tremors, confusion, or changes in LOC. - Caution the patient that drowsiness may occur and to be cautious with driving or other hazardous activities until the effects of the drug are known. - If dizziness occurs, rise from a lying or sitting position to standing slowly.
- Monitor for signs and symptoms of blood dyscrasias, e.g., bleeding, bruising, significant fatigue, and increasing signs of infection. (Bone marrow suppression may occur and cause decreases in RBCs, WBCs, and/or platelets. Periodic monitoring of CBC will be required.)	- Instruct the patient to report any low-grade fevers, sore throat, rashes, bruising or increased bleeding, or unusual fatigue or shortness of breath, especially if on drug therapy for a prolonged period.
- Monitor for significant GI effects, including nausea, vomiting, and diarrhea. Ensure adequate nutrition and caloric intake. (Adverse GI effects are common and the patient may also have disease-related effects, e.g., mouth sores. Maintaining adequate nutrition and fluids is essential to healing.)	- Teach the patient to avoid acidic foods and beverages, carbonated drinks, or excessively hot or cold foods and beverages, which may cause mouth irritation. - Encourage the patient to try small, frequent meals, which may be better tolerated than fewer, larger meals. High-caloric foods and supplemental beverages may help add additional calories and supply additional fluids. Assist the patient in obtaining a dietary consultation as needed if nausea or diarrhea makes maintaining intake difficult.

(Continued)

NURSING PROCESS FOCUS   PATIENTS RECEIVING ANTIVIRAL PHARMACOTHERAPY FOR HERPESVIRUS INFECTIONS *(Continued)*

Implementation

Interventions and (Rationales)	Patient and Family Education
■ Encourage infection control and good hygiene measures based on disease condition, and follow the established protocol in hospitalized patients. (Antiviral drugs decrease the level of infection but do not cure the disease. Excellent hygiene measures will limit the chance for secondary infections in the immunocompromised patient. Infection control measures prevent disease transmission.)	■ Teach the patient adequate infection control and hygiene measures such as frequent hand washing, appropriate disposal of dressing material, and adequate nutrition and rest, especially if currently immunocompromised. ■ The patient may need to be isolated in hospital or remain at home during peak transmission periods, leading to social isolation. Ascertain if the patient has assistance available if a prolonged period of homebound status is anticipated. ■ Teach the patient to practice abstinence or to use barrier protection during sexual activity even if genital lesions are not present. Genital HSV infections may be transmitted even in the asymptomatic period. Have the patient consult with their health care provider about suppressive therapy.
■ Maintain hydration during acyclovir therapy. Hydration may be ordered in the immediate pre- and postadministration periods. Monitor intake and output in the hospitalized patient. (Acyclovir may be nephrotoxic and adequate hydration is essential to prevent adverse renal effects.)	■ Teach the patient on oral acyclovir to increase oral intake prior to taking oral acyclovir and increase fluids to 2 L per day throughout therapy.
Patient understanding of drug therapy: ■ Use opportunities during administration of medications and during assessments to discuss rationale for drug therapy, desired therapeutic outcomes, most common adverse effects, parameters for when to call the health care provider, and any necessary monitoring or precautions. (Using time during nursing care helps to optimize and reinforce key teaching areas.)	■ The patient, family, or caregiver should be able to state the reason for the drug; appropriate dose and scheduling; what adverse effects to observe for and when to report; and the anticipated length of medication therapy.
Patient self-administration of drug therapy: ■ When administering medications, instruct the patient, family, or caregiver in the proper self-administration techniques followed by return demonstration. (Proper administration will improve the effectiveness of the drug.)	■ Teach the patient to: ■ Complete the entire course of therapy unless otherwise instructed. ■ Take the medication as evenly spaced throughout each day as feasible. ■ Increase overall fluid intake. ■ If using ointments or creams, wash hands well before applying and again after application. If family or caregivers administer the medicine, gloves should be worn.

Evaluation of Outcome Criteria

Evaluate the effectiveness of drug therapy by confirming that patient goals and expected outcomes have been met (see "Planning").

See Table 36.2 for a list of drugs to which these nursing actions apply.

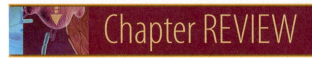

Chapter REVIEW

KEY CONCEPTS

The numbered key concepts provide a succinct summary of the important points from the corresponding numbered section within the chapter. If any of these points are not clear, refer to the numbered section within the chapter for review.

36.1 Viruses are nonliving intracellular parasites that require host organelles to replicate. Some viral infections are self-limiting, whereas others benefit from pharmacotherapy.

36.2 HIV targets the T4 lymphocyte, using reverse transcriptase to make viral DNA. The result is gradual destruction of the immune system.

36.3 Antiretroviral drugs used in the treatment of HIV-AIDS do not cure the disease, but they do help many patients live longer. Pharmacotherapy may be initiated in the acute (symptomatic) or chronic (asymptomatic) phase of HIV infection.

36.4 Drugs from five drug classes are used in various combinations in the pharmacotherapy of HIV-AIDS. The nucleotide reverse transcriptase inhibitors and the fusion inhibitors have recently been discovered.

36.5 The reverse transcriptase inhibitors block HIV replication at the level of the reverse transcriptase enzyme. These include the NRTIs, NNRTIs, and the NtRTIs.

36.6 The protease inhibitors inhibit the final assembly of the HIV virion. They are always used in combination with other antiretrovirals.

36.7 The risk of perinatal transmission of HIV can be markedly reduced by implementing drug therapy of the mother during pregnancy, and the newborn following birth. Postexposure prophylaxis of HIV infection is designed to prevent the accidental transmission of the virus to health care workers.

36.8 Pharmacotherapy can lessen the severity of acute herpes simplex infections and prolong the latent period of the disease.

36.9 Drugs are available to prevent and to treat influenza infections. Vaccination is the best choice, as drugs are relatively ineffective once influenza symptoms appear.

36.10 Hepatitis A and B are best treated through immunization. Newer drugs for HBV and HBC have led to therapies for chronic hepatitis.

NCLEX-RN® REVIEW QUESTIONS

1 When the patient is started on antiretroviral drugs for HIV, nursing education should include which of the following?
   1. This drug will cure the disease over time.
   2. This drug will not cure the disease but may extend the life expectancy.
   3. This type of drug will be used prior to vaccines.
   4. This drug is readily available all over the world for treatment.

2 The nurse understands that the laboratory tests that must be assessed while a patient is on drug therapy for HIV-AIDS are: (Select all that apply.)
   1. CBC.
   2. clotting factors.
   3. HIV RNA.
   4. CD4 lymphocyte count.
   5. BUN.

3 When providing patient and family education for the nucleoside reverse transcriptase inhibitor drugs for HIV-AIDS, the nurse would tell the patient to take the medication:
   1. on an empty stomach.
   2. on a full stomach.
   3. with apple juice to decrease the taste.
   4. with orange juice to increase absorption.

4 A patient is concerned about contracting influenza. The best response by the nurse would be:
   1. "After receiving the vaccination you will be protected in about 2 months."
   2. "If you have an exposure, two drugs, oseltamivir (Tamiflu) or zanamivir (Relenza) are now available to help prevent the disease or to shorten its duration."

   3. "You need to be vaccinated only if you are older than 50."
   4. "The infectious particles are not easily spread, and you can wait to be vaccinated until there is an increase in the population."

5 A patient is started on efavirenz (Sustiva), a nonnucleoside reverse transcriptase inhibitor (NNRTI) drug for HIV. The patient should be taught:
   1. this drug will cure the disease over time.
   2. there are few notable adverse effects of this drug but be cautious about taking it with citrus or milk-based beverages.
   3. nervous system effects such as dizziness, difficulty thinking clearly, or nightmares may occur but tend to improve after 3–4 weeks.
   4. the drug should be taken with a high-fat meal to delay absorption and prolong effect.

6 A patient has been diagnosed with herpes zoster and has been started on oral acyclovir (Zovirax). The nurse will be sure to include patient teaching instructions to: (Select all that apply.)
   1. increase fluid intake up to 2 L per day.
   2. report any dizziness, tremors, or confusion.
   3. decrease the amount of fluids taken so that the drug can be more concentrated.
   4. only take the drug when having the most itching or pain from the outbreak.

CRITICAL THINKING QUESTIONS

1. The patient is a 72-year-old woman who lives in an assisted living community. The nurse advises the patient of the importance of receiving an amantadine (Symmetrel) injection. What is the rationale supporting this recommendation? How could the nurse assist the patient in complying with this recommendation?

2. A newly diagnosed HIV-positive patient has been put on zidovudine (Retrovir). Identify priorities of nursing care for this patient.

3. A health care provider has ordered acyclovir (Zovirax) as an IV bolus to be infused over 15 minutes. The patient is seriously ill with a systemic herpesvirus infection, and the health care provider wants the patient to have immediate access to the medication. What is the nurse's best response?

See Appendix D for answers and rationales for all activities.

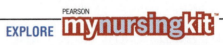

EXPLORE

MyNursingKit is your one stop for online chapter review materials and resources. Prepare for success with additional NCLEX®-style practice questions, interactive assignments and activities, web links, animations and videos, and more!

Register your access code from the front of your book at
www.mynursingkit.com.

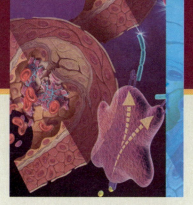

Chapter 37

Drugs for Neoplasia

LEARNING OUTCOMES

After reading this chapter, the student should be able to:

1. Explain differences between normal cells and cancer cells.
2. Identify factors associated with an increased risk of cancer.
3. Describe lifestyle factors associated with a reduced risk of acquiring cancer.
4. Identify the three primary therapies for cancer.
5. Explain the significance of growth fraction and the cell cycle to the success of chemotherapy.
6. Describe the nurse's role in the pharmacologic management of cancer.
7. Explain how combination therapy and special dosing protocols increase the effectiveness of chemotherapy.
8. Describe the general adverse effects of chemotherapeutic agents.
9. For each of the drug classes listed in Drugs at a Glance, know representative drugs, and explain their mechanism of drug action, primary actions, and important adverse effects.
10. Categorize anticancer drugs based on their classification and mechanism of action.
11. Use the nursing process to care for patients who are receiving antineoplastic medications as part of their treatment of cancer.

KEY TERMS

ancer is one of the most feared diseases in society for a number of valid reasons. It is often silent, producing no symptoms until it is far advanced. It sometimes requires painful and disfiguring surgery. It may strike at an early age, even during childhood, to deprive people of a normal life span. Perhaps worst of all, the medical treatment of cancer often cannot offer a cure, and progression to death is sometimes slow, painful, and psychologically difficult for patients and their loved ones.

Despite its feared status, many successes have been made in the diagnosis, understanding, and treatment of cancer. Some types of cancer are now curable, and therapies may provide the patient a longer, symptom-free life. This chapter examines the role of drugs in the treatment of cancer. Medications used to treat this disease are called *anticancer drugs, antineoplastics,* or *cancer chemotherapeutic agents.*

37.1 Characteristics of Cancer

Cancer, or **carcinoma,** is a disease characterized by abnormal, uncontrolled cell division. Cell division is a normal process occurring extensively in most body tissues from conception to late childhood. At some point in time, however, suppressor genes responsible for cell growth stop this rapid division. This may result in a total lack of replication, in the case of muscle cells and perhaps brain cells. In other cells, genes controlling replication can be turned on when it becomes necessary to replace worn-out cells, as in the case of blood cells and the mucosa of the digestive tract.

Cancer is thought to result from damage to the genes controlling cell growth. Once damaged, the cell is no longer responsive to normal chemical signals checking its growth. The cancer cells lose their normal functions, divide rapidly, and invade surrounding cells. The abnormal cells often travel to distant sites where they populate new tumors, a process called **metastasis.** ➤ Figure 37.1 illustrates some characteristics of cancer cells.

Tumor is defined as a swelling, abnormal enlargement, or mass. The word **neoplasm** is often used interchangeably with tumor. Tumors may be solid masses, such as lung or breast cancer, or they may be widely disseminated in the blood, such as leukemia. Tumors are named according to their tissue of origin, generally with the suffix *-oma.* Table 37.1 describes common types of tumors.

37.2 Causes of Cancer

Numerous factors have been found to cause cancer or to be associated with a higher risk for acquiring the disease. These factors are known as *carcinogens.*

Many chemical carcinogens have been identified. For example, chemicals in tobacco smoke are responsible for about one third of all cancer in the United States. Some chemicals, such as asbestos and benzene, have been associated with a higher incidence of cancer in the workplace. In

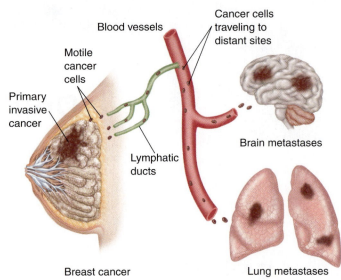

➤ **Figure 37.1** Invasion and metastasis by cancer cells

some cases, the site of the cancer may be distant from the entry location, as with bladder cancer caused by the inhalation of certain industrial chemicals. Some known chemical carcinogens are listed in Table 37.2.

A number of physical factors are also associated with cancer. For example, exposure to large amounts of x-rays is associated with a higher risk of leukemia. Ultraviolet (UV) light from the sun is a known cause of skin cancer.

It is estimated that viruses are associated with about 15% of all human cancers. Examples include herpes simplex types I and II, Epstein-Barr, human papillomavirus (HPV), cytomegalovirus, and human T-lymphotrophic viruses. Factors that suppress the immune system, such as HIV or drugs given after transplant surgery, may encourage the growth of cancer cells.

PHARMFACTS

Cancer

- It is estimated that more than 1,400,000 new cancer cases occur each year, with more than 565,000 deaths (over 1,500 people each day).
- Cancer is the chief cause of death by disease in children younger than age 15.
- Leukemia is the most common childhood cancer and is responsible for one fourth of all cancers occurring before age 20.
- Lung cancer has the highest mortality rate: It is responsible for 28% of all cancer deaths.
- Prostate cancer is the second leading cause of cancer death in men.
- The highest 5-year survival rates are for cancers of the prostate, testis, and thyroid. The lowest survival rates are for pancreatic and liver cancers.
- Among ethnic groups, African Americans have the highest incidence rates in many types of cancers, including those of the lung, breasts, and prostate; since 1990, this gap has been narrowing.
- Although breast cancer is predominant in women (second in cancer deaths), almost 2,000 men are diagnosed with the disease each year.

Source: Cancer Facts and Figures, American Cancer Society, 2008 (www.cancer.org).

TABLE 37.1	Classification and Naming of Tumors	
Name	Description	Examples
Benign tumor	Slow growing; does not metastasize and rarely requires drug treatment	Adenoma, papilloma and lipoma, osteoma, meningioma
Carcinoma	Cancer of epithelial tissue; most common type of malignant neoplasm; grows rapidly and metastasizes	Malignant melanoma, renal cell carcinoma, adenocarcinoma, hepatocellular carcinoma
Glioma	Cancer of glial (interstitial) cells in the brain, spinal cord, pineal gland, posterior pituitary gland, or retina	Telangiectatic glioma, brainstem glioma
Leukemia	Cancer of the blood-forming cells in bone marrow; may be acute or chronic	Myelocytic leukemia, lymphocytic leukemia
Lymphoma	Cancer of lymphoid tissue	Hodgkin's disease, lymphoblastic lymphoma
Malignant tumor	Grows rapidly, becomes resistant to treatment and results in death if untreated	Malignant melanoma
Sarcoma	Cancer of connective tissue; grows extremely rapidly and metastasizes early in the progression of the disease	Osteogenic sarcoma, fibrosarcoma, Kaposi's sarcoma, angiosarcoma

TABLE 37.2	Agents Associated with an Increased Risk of Cancer
Agent	Type of Cancer
Alcohol	Liver
Arsenic	Skin and lung
Asbestos	Lung
Benzene	Leukemia
Nickel	Lung and nasal
Polycyclic aromatic hydrocarbons	Lung and skin
Tobacco substances	Lung; head and neck
Vinyl chloride	Liver

COMPLEMENTARY AND ALTERNATIVE THERAPIES

Selenium's Role in Cancer Prevention

Selenium is an essential trace element that is necessary to maintain healthy immune function. It is a vital antioxidant, especially when combined with vitamin E. It protects the immune system by preventing the formation of free radicals, which can damage the body.

Selenium can be found in meat and grains, Brazil nuts, brewer's yeast, broccoli, brown rice, dairy products, garlic, molasses, and onions. The amount of selenium in food, however, has a direct correlation to the selenium content of the soil. The soil of much American farmland is low in selenium, resulting in selenium-deficient produce. Low dietary intake of selenium is associated with increased incidence of several cancers, including lung, colorectal, skin, and prostate. Selenium supplementation has resulted in increased natural killer cell activity, and studies show its promise as protection against prostate and colorectal cancers, especially among smokers.

Some cancers have a strong genetic component. The fact that close relatives may acquire the same type of cancer suggests that certain genes may predispose close relatives to the condition. These abnormal genes interact with chemical, physical, and biologic agents to promote cancer formation. Other genes, called *tumor suppressor genes,* may inhibit the formation of tumors. If these suppressor genes are damaged, cancer may result. Damage to the suppressor gene p53 is associated with cancers of the breast, lung, brain, colon, and bone.

Although the development of cancer has a genetic component, it is also greatly influenced by factors in the environment. Maintaining or adopting healthy lifestyle habits can reduce the risk of acquiring cancer. Following proper nutrition, avoiding chemical and physical risks, and maintaining a regular schedule of health checkups can help prevent cancer from developing into a fatal disease. The following are lifestyle factors regarding cancer prevention or diagnosis that should be used by the nurse when teaching patients about cancer prevention:

- Eliminate tobacco use and exposure to secondhand smoke.
- Limit or eliminate alcoholic beverage use.
- Maintain a healthy diet low in fat and high in fresh vegetables and fruit.
- Choose most foods from plant sources; increase fiber in the diet.

- Exercise regularly and maintain body weight within recommended guidelines.
- Self-examine your body monthly for abnormal lumps and skin lesions.
- Avoid chronic or prolonged exposure to direct sunlight and/or wearing protective clothing or sunscreen.
- Have periodic diagnostic testing performed at recommended intervals:
  - Women should have periodic mammograms, as directed by their health care provider.
  - Men should have annual prostate exams after age 50.
  - Both men and women should receive a screening colonoscopy, according to the schedule recommended by the health care provider.
  - Women who are sexually active or have reached age 18 should have an annual Pap test and pelvic examination.

37.3 Chemotherapy of Cancer: Cure, Control, and Palliation

Pharmacotherapy of cancer is sometimes simply referred to as **chemotherapy**. Because drugs are transported through the blood, chemotherapy has the potential to reach cancer cells in virtually any location. Certain drugs are able to cross the blood-brain barrier to reach brain tumors. Others are instilled directly into body cavities such as the urinary bladder to bring the highest dose possible to the cancer cells without producing systemic adverse effects. Chemotherapy has three general goals: cure, control, or palliation.

When diagnosed with cancer, the primary goal desired by most patients is to achieve a complete cure; permanent removal of all cancer cells from the body. The possibility for cure is much greater if a cancer is identified and treated in its early stages, when the tumor is small and localized to a well-defined region. Indeed, the 5-year survival rates for nearly all types of cancer has increased in the past two decades due to improved detection and more effective therapies. Examples in which chemotherapy has been used successfully as curative treatments include Hodgkin's lymphoma, certain leukemias, and choriocarcinoma.

When cancer has progressed and cure is not possible, a second goal of chemotherapy is to control or manage the disease. Although the cancer is not eliminated, preventing the growth and spread of the tumor may extend the patient's life. Essentially, the cancer is managed as a chronic disease, such as hypertension or diabetes.

In its advanced stages, cure or control of the cancer may not be achievable. For these patients, chemotherapy is used as **palliation.** Chemotherapy drugs are administered to reduce the size of the tumor, easing the severity of pain and other tumor symptoms, thus improving the quality of life. Examples of advanced cancers for which palliation is frequently used include osteosarcoma, pancreatic cancer, and Kaposi's sarcoma.

Chemotherapy may be used alone or in combination with other treatment modalities such as surgery or radiation ther-apy. Surgery is especially useful for removing solid tumors that are localized. Surgery lowers the number of cancer cells in the body so that radiation therapy and pharmacotherapy can be more successful. Surgery is not an option for tumors of blood cells or when it would not be expected to extend a patient's life span or to improve the quality of life.

Approximately 50% of patients with cancer receive radiation therapy as part of their treatment. Radiation therapy is most successful and produces the fewest adverse effects for cancers that are localized, when high doses of ionizing radiation can be aimed directly at the tumor and be confined to a small area. Radiation treatments are frequently prescribed postoperatively to kill cancer cells that may remain following an operation. Radiation is sometimes given as palliation for inoperable cancers to shrink the size of a tumor that may be pressing on vital organs, and to relieve pain, difficulty breathing, or difficulty swallowing.

Adjuvant chemotherapy is the administration of antineoplastic drugs *after* surgery or radiation therapy. The purpose of adjuvant chemotherapy is to rid the body of any cancerous cells that were not removed during the surgery or to treat any microscopic metastases that may be developing. In a few cases, drugs are given as *chemoprophylaxis* with the goal of preventing cancer from occurring in patients at high risk for developing tumors. For example, some patients who have had a primary breast cancer removed may receive tamoxifen, even if there is no evidence of metastases, because there is a high likelihood that the disease will recur. Chemoprophylaxis of cancer is uncommon, because most of these drugs have potentially serious adverse effects.

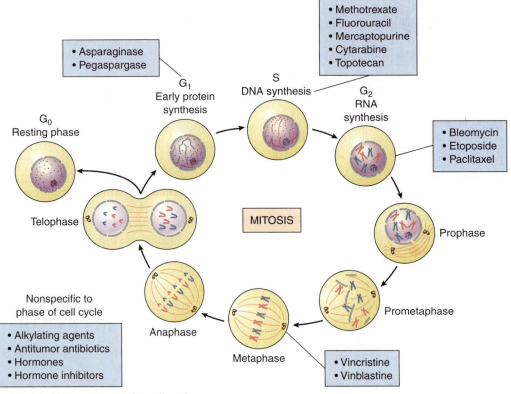

➤ *Figure 37.2* Antineoplastic agents and the cell cycle

37.4 Growth Fraction and Success of Chemotherapy

Although cancers grow rapidly, not all cells in a tumor are replicating at any given time. Because antineoplastic agents are generally more effective against cells that are replicating, the percentage of tumor cells dividing at the time of chemotherapy is critical.

Both normal and cancerous cells go through a sequence of events known as the *cell cycle,* illustrated in ➤ Figure 37.2. Cells spend most of their lifetime in the G_0 phase. Although sometimes called the *resting stage,* the G_0 is the phase during which cells conduct their everyday activities such as metabolism, impulse conduction, contraction, or secretion. If the cell receives a signal to divide, it leaves G_0 and enters the G_1 phase, during which it synthesizes the RNA, proteins, and other components needed to duplicate its DNA during the S phase. Following duplication of its DNA, the cell enters the premitotic phase, or G_2. Following mitosis in the M phase, the cell re-enters its resting G_0 phase, where it may remain for extended periods, depending on the specific tissue and surrounding cellular signals.

The actions of many of the antineoplastic agents are specific to certain phases of the cell cycle, whereas others are mostly independent of the cell cycle. For example, mitotic inhibitors such as vincristine (Oncovin) affect the M phase, which includes prophase, metaphase, anaphase, and telophase. Antimetabolites such as fluorouracil (5-FU, Adrucil, Carac, Efudex) are most effective during the S phase. The effects of alkylating agents such as cyclophosphamide (Cytoxan) are generally independent of the phases of the cell cycle. Some of these agents are shown in Figure 37.2.

The **growth fraction** is a measure of the number of cells undergoing mitosis in a tissue. It is a ratio of the number of *replicating* cells to the number of *resting* cells. Antineoplastic drugs are much more toxic to tissues and tumors with high growth fractions. For example, solid tumors such as breast and lung cancer generally have a *low* growth fraction; thus, they are less sensitive to antineoplastic agents. Certain leukemias and lymphomas have a *high* growth fraction and therefore have a greater antineoplastic success rate. Because certain normal tissues, such as hair follicles, bone marrow, and the gastrointestinal (GI) epithelium also have a high growth fraction, they are sensitive to the effects of the antineoplastics.

37.5 Achieving a Total Cancer Cure

To cure a patient, it is believed that every single cancer cell in a tumor must be eliminated from the body. Leaving even a single malignant cell could result in regrowth of the tumor. Eliminating every cancer cell, however, is a very difficult task.

As an example, consider that a small, 1-cm breast tumor may already contain 1 billion cancer cells before it can be detected on a manual examination. A drug that could kill 99% of these cells would be considered a very effective drug, indeed. Yet even with this fantastic achievement, 10 million cancer cells would remain, any one of which could poten-

tially cause the tumor to return and kill the patient. The relationship between cell kill and chemotherapy is shown in ➤ Figure 37.3.

It is likely that no antineoplastic drug (or combination of drugs) will kill 100% of the tumor cells. The large burden of cancer cells, however, may be lowered sufficiently to permit the patient's immune system to control or eliminate the remaining cancer cells. Because the immune system is able to eliminate only a relatively small number of cancer cells, it is imperative that as many cancerous cells as possible be eliminated during treatment. This example reinforces the need to diagnose and treat tumors at an *early* stage when the number of cancer cells is smaller.

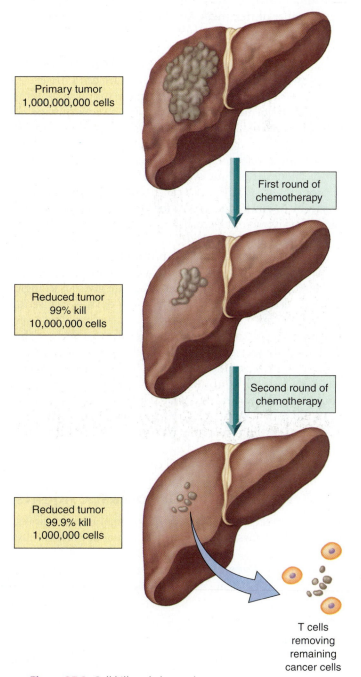

Primary tumor
1,000,000,000 cells

First round of chemotherapy

Reduced tumor
99% kill
10,000,000 cells

Second round of chemotherapy

Reduced tumor
99.9% kill
1,000,000 cells

T cells removing remaining cancer cells

➤ *Figure 37.3* Cell kill and chemotherapy

37.6 Special Pharmacotherapy Protocols and Strategies for Cancer Chemotherapy

Because of their rapid cell division, tumor cells express a high mutation rate. This causes the tumor to change and become more heterogenous as it grows, essentially becoming a mass of hundreds of different clones with different growth rates and physiologic properties. An antineoplastic drug may kill only a small portion of the tumor, leaving some clones unaffected. Complicating the chances for a cure is that cancer cells often develop resistance to antineoplastic drugs. Thus, a therapy that was very successful in reducing the tumor mass at the start of chemotherapy may become less effective over time. The tumor becomes "refractory" to treatment.

A number of treatment strategies have been found to increase the effectiveness of anticancer drugs. In most cases, multiple drugs from different antineoplastic classes are given during a course of chemotherapy. The use of multiple drugs affects different stages of the cancer cell's life cycle, and attacks the various clones within the tumor via several mechanisms of action, thus increasing the percentage of cell kill. Combination chemotherapy also allows lower dosages of each individual agent, thus reducing toxicity and slowing the development of resistance. Examples of combination therapies include cyclophosphamide-methotrexate-fluorouracil (CMF) for breast cancer and cyclophosphamide-doxorubicin-vincristine (CDV) for lung cancer. Each type of cancer has its own individual protocol, which is continually being refined and revised based on current research.

Specific dosing schedules, or protocols, have been found to increase the effectiveness of the antineoplastic agents. For example, some of the anticancer drugs are given as a single dose or perhaps several doses over a few days. A few weeks may pass before the next series of doses begins. This gives normal cells time to recover from the adverse effects of the drugs and allows tumor cells that may not have been replicating at the time of the first dose to begin dividing and become more sensitive to the next round of chemotherapy. Sometimes the optimum dosing schedule must be delayed until the patient sufficiently recovers from the drug toxicities, especially bone marrow suppression. The specific dosing schedule depends on the type of tumor, stage of the disease, and the patient's overall condition.

37.7 Toxicity of Antineoplastic Agents

Although cancer cells are clearly abnormal in many ways, much of their physiology is identical to that of normal cells.

Because it is difficult to kill cancer cells *selectively* without profoundly affecting normal cells, all anticancer drugs have the potential to cause serious toxicity. These drugs are often pushed to their maximum possible dosages, so that the greatest tumor kill can be obtained. Such high dosages always result in adverse effects in the patient. Table 37.3 lists typical adverse effects of anticancer drugs.

Normal cells that are replicating are most susceptible to adverse effects. Hair follicles are damaged, resulting in hair loss or **alopecia.** The epithelial lining of the digestive tract commonly becomes inflamed, a condition known as **mucositis.** Consequences of mucositis include painful ulcerations, difficulty eating or swallowing, GI bleeding, intestinal infections, or severe diarrhea. The vomiting center in the medulla is triggered by many antineoplastics, resulting in significant nausea and vomiting. Because of this effect, antineoplastics are sometimes classified by their **emetic potential.** Before starting therapy with the highest emetic potential agents, patients may be pretreated with antiemetic drugs such as odansetron (Zofran), prochlorperazine (Compazine), metoclopramide (Reglan, others), or lorazepam (Ativan) (chapter 41∞).

Stem cells in the bone marrow may be destroyed by antineoplastics, causing anemia, leukopenia, and thrombocytopenia. These adverse effects are dose limiting and the ones that most often cause discontinuation or delays of chemotherapy. Severe bone marrow suppression is a contraindication to therapy with most antineoplastics. Efforts to minimize bone marrow toxicity may include bone marrow transplantation, platelet infusions, or therapy with growth factors such as epoetin alfa or granulocyte colony-stimulating factor (G-CSF), filgrastim (Neupogen), or sargramostim (Leukine) (chapter 28∞). The administration of G-CSFs often prevents or shortens the time period of neutropenia, thus lowering the risk of opportunistic infections and allowing the patient to maintain an optimum dosing schedule.

Each antineoplastic drug has a documented **nadir,** the lowest point to which the erythrocyte, neutrophil, or platelet count is depressed by the drug. Although chemotherapy decreases all types of white blood cells (leukopenia), neutrophils are the type most affected. The nurse can calculate the absolute neutrophil count (ANC) by multiplying the white blood cell count by the percentage of neutrophils. This value can be obtained by reading the patient's complete blood count (CBC) with differential. If the ANC falls below 500/mm³, the risk of infection increases. Many times, patients who are significantly neutropenic will be placed in reverse isolation to protect them from exposure

TABLE 37.3 Adverse Effects of Antineoplastic Drugs		
Blood Toxicity	**GI Toxicity**	**Other Effects**
Anemia (low red blood cell count)	Anorexia	Alopecia
Leukopenia or neutropenia (low white blood cell count)	Bleeding	Fatigue
Thrombocytopenia (low platelet count)	Diarrhea, extreme nausea and vomiting	Fetal death/birth defects, opportunistic infections, ulceration and bleeding of the lips and gums

to an infection from family members or health care providers. If a neutropenic patient develops a fever, antibiotics are indicated.

When possible, antineoplastics are given locally by topical application or through direct instillation into a tumor site to minimize systemic toxicity. Most antineoplastics, however, must be administered intravenously. Many antineoplastics are classified as **vesicants,** agents that can cause serious tissue injury if they escape from an artery or vein during an infusion or injection. Extravasation from an injection site can produce severe tissue, and nerve damage, local infection, and even loss of a limb. Rapid treatment of extravasation is necessary to limit tissue damage, and certain antineoplastics have specific antidotes. For example, extravasation of carmustine (BiCNU, Gliadel) is treated with injections of equal parts of sodium bicarbonate and normal saline into the extravasation site. Before administering intravenous antineoplastic agents, the nurse should know the emergency treatment for extravasation. Central lines (subclavian vein) should be used with vesicants whenever possible. Antineoplastics with the strongest vesicant activity include busulfan, carmustine, dacarbazine, dactinomycin, daunorubicin, idarubicin, mechlorethamine, mitomycin, plicamycin, streptozocin, vinblastine, vincristine, and vinorelbine.

Cancer survivors face several possible long-term consequences from chemotherapy. Some antineoplastics, particularly the alkylating agents, affect the gonads and have been associated with infertility in both male and female patients. A second concern for long-term survivors is the induction of secondary malignancies caused by the antineoplastic agents. These secondary tumors may occur decades after the chemotherapy was administered. Although many different secondary malignancies have been reported, the most common is acute nonlymphocytic leukemia. In most cases, the immediate benefits of using antineoplastics to cure a cancer far outweigh the small risk of developing a secondary malignancy.

37.8 Classification of Antineoplastic Drugs

Drugs used in cancer chemotherapy come from diverse pharmacologic and chemical classes. Antineoplastics have been extracted from plants and bacteria, as well as created entirely in the laboratory. Some of the drug classes attack cellular macromolecules, such as DNA and proteins, whereas others poison vital metabolic pathways of rapidly growing cells. The common theme among all the antineoplastic agents is that they kill or at least stop the growth of cancer cells.

Classification of the various antineoplastics is quite variable because some of these drugs kill cancer cells by several different mechanisms and have characteristics from more than one class. Furthermore, the mechanisms by which some antineoplastics act are not completely understood. A simple method of classifying this complex group of drugs includes the following six categories:

- Alkylating agents
- Antimetabolites
- Antitumor antibiotics
- Hormones and hormone antagonists
- Natural products
- Biologic response modifiers and monoclonal antibodies
- Miscellaneous antineoplastic drugs

ALKYLATING AGENTS

The first alkylating agents, the nitrogen mustards, were developed in secrecy as chemical warfare agents during World War II. Although the drugs in this class have quite different chemical structures, all share the common characteristic of forming bonds or linkages with DNA, a process called **alkylation.** ➤ Figure 37.4 illustrates the process of alkylation.

37.9 Pharmacotherapy with Alkylating Agents

Alkylation changes the shape of the DNA double helix and prevents the nucleic acid from completing normal cell division. Each alkylating agent attaches to DNA in a different manner; however, collectively the alkylating agents have the effect of inducing cell death, or at least slowing the replication of tumor cells. Although the process of alkylation occurs independently of the cell cycle, the killing action does not occur until the affected cell attempts to divide. The alkylating agents have a broad spectrum and are used against many types of malignancies. They are some of the most widely prescribed antineoplastic drugs. These agents are listed in Table 37.4.

Blood cells are particularly sensitive to alkylating agents, and bone marrow suppression is the primary dose-limiting adverse effect of drugs in this class. Within days after administration, the numbers of erythrocytes, leukocytes, and platelets begin to decline, reaching a nadir at 6 to 10 days. Epithelial cells lining the GI tract are also damaged, resulting in nausea, vomiting, and diarrhea. Alopecia is expected from most of the alkylating agents. The nitrosoureas and mechlorethamine are strong vesicants. Approximately 5% of the patients treated with alkylating agents develop acute nonlymphocytic leukemia 4 years or more after chemotherapy has been completed.

ANTIMETABOLITES

Antimetabolites are antineoplastic drugs that chemically resemble essential building blocks of cells. These drugs interfere with aspects of the nutrient or nucleic acid metabolism of rapidly growing tumor cells.

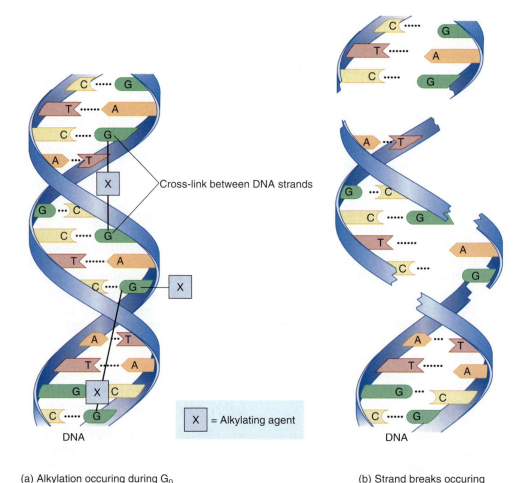

Cross-link between DNA strands

X = Alkylating agent

DNA

DNA

(a) Alkylation occuring during G_0
(resting) phase of cell cycle

(b) Strand breaks occuring
when DNA replicates
during S phase of cell cycle

➤ **Figure 37.4** Mechanism of action of the alkylating agents

37.10 Pharmacotherapy with Antimetabolites

Rapidly growing cancer cells require large quantities of nutrients to construct cellular proteins and nucleic acids. Antimetabolite drugs are structurally similar to these nutrients, but they do not perform the same functions as their natural counterparts. When cancer cells attempt to synthesize proteins, RNA, or DNA using the antimetabolites, metabolic pathways are disrupted and the cancer cells die or their growth is slowed. The three classes of antimetabolites are the folic acid analogs, the purine analogs, and the pyrimidine analogs. These agents are prescribed for leukemias and solid tumors and are listed in Table 37.5.

The purine and pyrimidine analogs are structurally similar to the natural building blocks of DNA and RNA. For example, the pyrimidine analog fluorouracil (5-FU, Adrucil, Carac, Efudex) is able to block the formation of thymidylate, an essential chemical needed to make DNA, and is used in treating various solid tumors. After becoming activated and incorporated into DNA, cytarabine (Cytosar, Cytosine arabinoside, Depot-Cyt) blocks DNA synthesis and is an important drug in treating acute myelocytic leukemia. Approved in 2005 clofarabine (Clolar) is a purine antimetabolite that was the first new drug approved for pediatric acute leukemia in over a decade. Methotrexate (Rheumatrex, Trexall) and the newer drugs pemetrexed (Alimta) and pralatrexate (Folotyn) resemble folic acid, a natural B vitamin. ➤ Figure 37.5 illustrates the structural similarities of some of these antimetabolites to their natural counterparts.

Bone marrow toxicity is the principal dose-limiting adverse effect of many drugs in this class. Some also cause serious GI toxicity, including ulcerations of the mucosa. Mercaptopurine and thioguanine can cause hepatotoxicity, including cholestatic jaundice.

ANTITUMOR ANTIBIOTICS

Antitumor antibiotics are drugs obtained from bacteria that have the ability to kill cancer cells. Although not widely used, they are very effective against certain tumors. The antitumor antibiotics are listed in Table 37.6.

TABLE 37.4 Alkylating Agents

Drug	Route and Adult Dose (max dose where indicated)	Adverse Effects
NITROGEN MUSTARDS		
bendamustine (Treanda)	IV; 90–120 mg/m² (variable schedule)	*Nausea, vomiting, stomatitis, anorexia, rash, headache, alopecia, fluid retention*
chlorambucil (Leukeran)	PO; Initial dose: 0.1–0.2 mg/kg/day; Maintenance dose: 4–10 mg/day	
℗ cyclophosphamide (Cytoxan)	PO; Initial dose: 1–5 mg/day; Maintenance dose: 1–5 mg/kg every 7–10 days	Bone marrow suppression (neutropenia, anemia, thrombocytopenia), severe nausea and vomiting, diarrhea, Stevens–Johnson syndrome, hemorrhagic cystitis, pulmonary toxicity, neurotoxicity (carboplatin, cisplatin, oxaliplatin), ototoxicity (cisplatin), hypersensitivity reactions (including anaphylaxis), nephrotoxicity
estramustine (Emcyt)	PO; 14 mg/kg/day in three to four divided doses	
ifosfamide (Ifex)	IV; 1.2 g/m²/day for 5 consecutive days	
mechlorethamine (Mustargen)	IV; 6 mg/m² on days 1 and 8 of a 28-day cycle	
melphalan (Alkeran)	PO; 6 mg/day for 2–3 wk	
NITROSOUREAS		
carmustine (BiCNU, Gliadel)	IV; 200 mg/m² every 6 wk	
lomustine (CeeNU, CCNU)	PO; 130 mg/m² as a single dose	
streptozocin (Zanosar)	IV; 500 mg/m² for 5 consecutive days	
MISCELLANEOUS ALKYLATING AGENTS		
busulfan (Myleran)	PO; 4–8 mg/day	
carboplatin (Paraplatin)	IV; 360 mg/m² once every 4 wk	
cisplatin (Platinol)	IV; 20 mg/m²/day for 5 days	
dacarbazine (DTIC-Dome)	IV; 2–4.5 mg/kg/day for 10 days	
oxaliplatin (Eloxatin)	IV; 85 mg/m² for 2 h for 2 wk	
procarbazine (Matulane)	PO; 2–4 mg/kg/day for 1 wk	
temozolomide (Temodar)	PO; 150 mg/m²/day for 5 consecutive days	
thiotepa (Thioplex, TSPA)	IV; 0.3–0.4 mg/kg every 1–4 wk	

Italics indicate common adverse effects; <u>underlining</u> indicates serious adverse effects.

TABLE 37.5 Antimetabolites

Drug	Route and Adult Dose (max dose where indicated)	Adverse Effects
FOLIC ACID ANTAGONISTS		
℗ methotrexate (Rheumatrex, Trexall)	PO; 10–30 mg/day for 5 days	*Nausea, vomiting, stomatitis, anorexia, rash, headache, alopecia*
pemetrexed (Alimta)	IV; 500 mg/m² on day 1 of each 21-day cycle	
pralatrexate (Folotyn)	30 mg/m² administered over 3–5 minutes	Bone marrow suppression (neutropenia, anemia, thrombocytopenia), severe nausea, vomiting and diarrhea, hepatotoxicity, mucositis, pulmonary toxicity, hypersensitivity reactions (including anaphylaxis), neurotoxicity (cytarabine, fluorouracil, fludarabine, cladribine)
PYRIMIDINE ANALOGS		
capecitabine (Xeloda)	PO; 2,500 mg/m²/day for 2 wk	
cytarabine (Cytosar, Cytosine arabinoside, Depot-Cyt)	IV; 200 mg/m² as a continuous infusion over 24 h	
floxuridine (FUDR)	Intra-arterial: 0.1–0.6 mg/kg/day as a continuous infusion	
fluorouracil (5-FU, Adrucil, Carac, Efudex)	IV; 12 mg/kg/day for 4 consecutive days	
gemcitabine (Gemzar)	IV; 1,000 mg/m² every 1 wk for 7 wk	
PURINE ANALOGS		
cladribine (Leustatin)	IV; 0.09 mg/m²/day as a continuous infusion	
clofarabine (Clolar)	IV; 52 mg/m²/day over 2 hours for 5 days	
fludarabine (Fludara)	IV; 25 mg/m²/day for 5 consecutive days	
mercaptopurine (6-MP, Purinethol)	PO; 2.5 mg/kg/day	
nelarabine (Arranon)	IV; 1,500 mg/m² on days 1, 3, and 5, repeated every 21 days	
pentostatin (Nipent)	IV; 4 mg/m² every other week	
thioguanine (6-TG, Tabloid)	PO; 2 mg/kg/day	

Italics indicate common adverse effects; <u>underlining</u> indicates serious adverse effects.

Pr Prototype Drug | Cyclophosphamide *(Cytoxan)*

Therapeutic Class: Antineoplastic   **Pharmacologic Class:** Alkylating agent; nitrogen mustard

ACTIONS AND USES

Cyclophosphamide is a commonly prescribed nitrogen mustard. It is used alone, or in combination with other drugs, against a wide variety of cancers, including Hodgkin's disease, lymphoma, multiple myeloma, breast cancer, and ovarian cancer. Cyclophosphamide acts by attaching to DNA and disrupting replication, particularly in rapidly dividing cells. It is one of only a few anticancer drugs that are well absorbed when given orally.

Cyclophosphamide is a powerful immunosuppressant. While this is considered an adverse effect during cancer chemotherapy, the drug is used to *intentionally* cause immunosuppression for the prophylaxis of organ transplant rejection and to treat severe rheumatoid arthritis and systemic lupus erythematosus (SLE).

ADMINISTRATION ALERTS

- Dilute prior to IV administration.
- Monitor platelet count prior to IM administration; if low, hold dose.
- To avoid GI upset, take with meals or divide doses.
- Pregnancy category C

PHARMACOKINETICS (PO)

Onset: Unknown

Peak: 1 h

Half-life: 3–12 h

Duration: Unknown

ADVERSE EFFECTS

Bone marrow suppression is a potentially life-threatening adverse reaction that occurs during days 9–14 of therapy; the patient is at dangerous risk for severe infection and sepsis during this period. Thrombocytopenia is common, though less severe than with many other alkylating agents. Nausea, vomiting, anorexia, and diarrhea are frequently experienced. Cyclophosphamide causes reversible alopecia, although the hair may regrow with a different color or texture. Several metabolites of cyclophosphamide may cause hemorrhagic cystitis if the urine becomes concentrated; patients should be advised to maintain high fluid intake during therapy. The drug may cause permanent sterility in some patients. Unlike other nitrogen mustards, cyclophosphamide exhibits little neurotoxicity.

Contraindications: Cyclophosphamide is contraindicated in patients with hypersensitivity to the drug and for those who have active infections or severely suppressed bone marrow.

INTERACTIONS

Drug–Drug: Immunosuppressant agents used concurrently with cyclophosphamide will increase the risk of infections and further development of neoplasms. There is an increased chance of bone marrow toxicity if cyclophosphamide is used concurrently with allopurinol. There is an increased risk of bleeding if given with anticoagulants.

If used concurrently with digoxin, decreased serum levels of digoxin occur. Use with insulin may lead to hypoglycemia. Phenobarbital, phenytoin, or glucocorticoids used concurrently may lead to an increased rate of cyclophosphamide metabolism by the liver. Thiazide diuretics increase the possibility of leukopenia.

Lab Tests: Serum uric acid levels may increase. Blood cell counts will diminish due to bone marrow suppression. Positive reactions to *Candida*, mumps, and tuberculin skin tests (PPD) are suppressed. PAP smears may give false positives.

Herbal/Food: St. John's wort may increase the toxic effects of cyclophosphamide.

Treatment of Overdose: There is no specific treatment for overdose.

Refer to MyNursingKit for a Nursing Process Focus specific to this drug.

Normal metabolite

Folic acid   Guanine   Uracil

Antimetabolite

Methotrexate   Thioguanine   Fluorouracil

➤ *Figure 37.5* Structural similarities between antimetabolites and their natural counterparts

Pr Prototype Drug | Methotrexate *(Rheumatrex, Trexall)*

Therapeutic Class: Antineoplastic   **Pharmacologic Class:** Antimetabolite, folic acid analog

ACTIONS AND USES

Methotrexate is an antimetabolite available by the oral, parenteral, and intrathecal routes. By blocking the synthesis of folic acid (vitamin B$_9$), methotrexate inhibits replication, particularly in rapidly dividing cells. It is prescribed alone or in combination with other drugs for choriocarcinoma, osteogenic sarcoma, leukemias, head and neck cancers, breast carcinoma, and lung carcinoma. In addition to its role as an antimetabolite, methotrexate has powerful immunosuppressant that can be used to treat severe rheumatoid arthritis, ulcerative colitis, lupus, and psoriasis that are unresponsive to safer medications.

ADMINISTRATION ALERTS

- Avoid skin exposure to drug.
- Avoid inhaling drug particles.
- Dilute prior to IV administration.
- Pregnancy category X

PHARMACOKINETICS

Onset: Variable
Peak: 1–4 h PO; 0.5–2 h IM/IV
Half-life: 1–4 h
Duration: Unknown

ADVERSE EFFECTS

Methotrexate has many adverse effects, some of which can be life threatening. The FDA has issued 13 black box warnings regarding the use of methotrexate. The drug can cause fatal bone marrow toxicity at high doses. Hemorrhage and bruising are often observed due to low platelet counts. Nausea, vomiting, and anorexia are common, and GI ulceration may result in serious intestinal bleeding. Severe and potentially fatal dermatologic reactions include Stevens–Johnson syndrome and exfoliative dermatitis. Although rare, pulmonary toxicity including life-threatening pneumonitis has been reported.

Contraindications: The use of methotrexate as an antineoplastic is contraindicated in thrombocytopenia, anemia, leukopenia, concurrent administration of hepatotoxic drugs and hematopoietic suppressants, alcoholism, or lactation. Methotrexate is teratogenic and is contraindicated in pregnant patients. Patients with alcoholism or other chronic liver disease should not receive methotrexate. Immunosuppressed patients or those with blood dyscrasias should not receive methotrexate.

INTERACTIONS

Drug–Drug: Bone marrow suppressants such as chemotherapy agents or radiation therapy may cause increased effects; the patient will require a lower dose of methotrexate. Concurrent use with NSAIDs may lead to severe methotrexate toxicity. Aspirin may interfere with excretion of methotrexate, leading to increased serum levels and toxicity. Concurrent administration with live oral vaccine may result in decreased antibody response and increased adverse reactions to the vaccine.

Lab Tests: Serum uric acid levels may increase. Blood cell counts will diminish due to bone marrow suppression.

Herbal/Food: Food delays the oral absorption of methotrexate. Echinacea may increase the risk of hepatotoxicity.

Treatment of Overdose: Leucovorin (folinic acid), a reduced form of folic acid, is sometimes administered with methotrexate to "rescue" normal cells, or to protect against severe bone marrow damage. It is most effective if administered as soon as possible after the overdose is discovered. In addition, the urine may be alkalinized to protect the kidneys from methotrexate toxicity.

Refer to MyNursingKit for a Nursing Process Focus specific to this drug.

TABLE 37.6	**Antitumor Antibiotics**	
Drug	**Route and Adult Dose (max dose where indicated)**	**Adverse Effects**
bleomycin (Blenoxane)	IV; 0.25–0.5 unit/kg every 4–7 days	*Nausea, vomiting, stomatitis, anorexia, rash, headache, alopecia*
dactinomycin (Actinomycin-D, Cosmegen)	IV; 500 mcg/day for a maximum of 5 days	
daunorubicin (Cerubidine)	IV; 30–60 mg/m²/day for 3–5 days	<u>Bone marrow suppression (neutropenia, anemia, thrombocytopenia), severe nausea and vomiting, diarrhea, cardiotoxicity, tissue necrosis due to extravasation, mucositis, pulmonary toxicity, hypersensitivity reactions (including anaphylaxis)</u>
daunorubicin liposomal (DaunoXome)	IV; 40 mg/m² every 2 wk	
🔵 doxorubicin (Adriamycin)	IV; 60–75 mg/m² as a single dose at 21-day intervals, or 30 mg/m² on each of 3 consecutive days (max: total cumulative dose 550 mg/m²)	
doxorubicin liposomal (Doxil, Evacet)	IV; 20 mg/m² every 3 wk	
epirubicin (Ellence)	IV; 100–120 mg/m² as a single dose	
idarubicin (Idamycin)	IV; 8–12 mg/m²/day for 3 days	
mitomycin (Mutamycin)	IV; 2 mg/m² as a single dose	
mitoxantrone (Novantrone)	IV; 12 mg/m²/day for 3 days	

Italics indicate common adverse effects; <u>underlining</u> indicates serious adverse effects.

37.11 Pharmacotherapy with Antitumor Antibiotics

A number of substances isolated from microorganisms have been found to possess antitumor properties. These chemicals are more cytotoxic than traditional antibiotics, and their use is limited to treating a few specific types of cancer. For example, the only indication for idarubicin (Idamycin) is acute myelogenous leukemia. Breast carcinoma is the only approved use for epirubicin (Ellence).

The antitumor antibiotics bind to DNA and affect its function by a mechanism similar to that of the alkylating agents. Thus, their general actions and side effects are similar to those of the alkylating agents. Unlike the alkylating agents, however, all the antitumor antibiotics must be administered intravenously or through direct instillation via a catheter into a body cavity.

As with other antineoplastics, a major dose-limiting adverse effect of drugs in this class is bone marrow suppression.

Doxorubicin, daunorubicin, epirubicin, and idarubicin are all closely related in structure, and cardiac toxicity is a major limiting adverse effect. Cardiotoxicity may occur within minutes of administration, or be delayed for months or years after chemotherapy has been completed.

NATURAL PRODUCTS (PLANT EXTRACTS AND ALKALOIDS)

Plants have been a valuable source for antineoplastic drugs. These natural products act by preventing the division of cancer cells.

37.12 Pharmacotherapy with Natural Products

Agents with antineoplastic activity have been isolated from a number of plants, including the common periwinkle

---

Pr Prototype Drug | Doxorubicin *(Adriamycin)*

Therapeutic Class: Antineoplastic   **Pharmacologic Class:** Antitumor antibiotic

ACTIONS AND USES

Doxorubicin attaches to DNA, distorting its double helical structure and preventing normal DNA and RNA synthesis. It is administered only by IV infusion. Doxorubicin is a broad-spectrum cytotoxic antibiotic, prescribed for solid tumors of the lung, breast, ovary, and bladder, and for various leukemias and lymphomas. It is structurally similar to daunorubicin. Doxorubicin is one of the most effective single agents against solid tumors.

A novel delivery method has been developed for both doxorubicin and daunorubicin. The drug is enclosed in small lipid sacs, or vesicles, called *liposomes*. The liposomal vesicle is designed to open and release the antitumor antibiotic when it reaches a cancer cell. The goal is to deliver a higher concentration of drug to the cancer cells, thus sparing normal cells. An additional advantage is that doxorubicin liposomal has a half-life of 50 to 60 hours, which is about twice that of regular doxorubicin. Doxorubicin liposomal is approved for use in patients with Kaposi's sarcoma, refractory ovarian tumors, and relapsed multiple myeloma.

ADMINISTRATION ALERTS

- Extravasation can cause severe pain and extensive tissue damage. Skin contact or extravasation should be treated immediately with local ice packs to reduce absorption of the drug.

- For infants and children, verify concentration and rate of IV infusion with the health care provider.

- Avoid skin contact with drug. If exposure occurs, wash thoroughly with soap and water.

- Pregnancy category D

PHARMACOKINETICS
Onset: Rapid

Peak: Unknown

Half-life: 17–32 h

Duration: Unknown

ADVERSE EFFECTS

The most serious dose-limiting adverse effect of doxorubicin is cardiotoxicity. Acute effects include dysrhythmias; delayed effects may include irreversible heart failure. Like many of the anticancer drugs, doxorubicin may profoundly lower blood cell counts. Acute nausea and vomiting are common and often require antiemetic therapy. Complete, though reversible, hair loss occurs in most patients. Secondary malignancies, especially acute myelogenous leukemia, may occur 1–3 years following therapy.

Contraindications: Doxorubicin is contraindicated in patients who are immunosuppressed or who have hypersensitivity to the drug.

INTERACTIONS

Drug–Drug: If digoxin is taken concurrently, patient serum digoxin levels will decrease. Use with phenobarbital may lead to increased plasma clearance of doxorubicin and decreased effectiveness. Use with phenytoin may lead to decreased phenytoin level, and possible seizure activity. Hepatotoxicity may occur if mercaptopurine is taken concurrently. Use with verapamil may increase serum doxorubicin levels, leading to doxorubicin toxicity.

Lab Tests: Serum uric acid and aspartate aminotransferase (AST) levels may increase. Blood cell counts will diminish due to bone marrow suppression.

Herbal/Food: Green tea may enhance the antitumor activity of doxorubicin. St. John's wort may decrease the effectiveness of doxorubicin.

Treatment of Overdose: The primary result of doxorubicin overdosage is immunosuppression. Treatment includes prophylactic antimicrobials, platelet transfusions, symptomatic treatment of mucositis, and possibly hemopoietic growth factor (G-CSF, GM-CSF).

Refer to MyNursingKit for a Nursing Process Focus specific to this drug.

(*Vinca rosea*), Pacific yew (*Taxus baccata*), mandrake (May apple), and the shrub *Camptotheca acuminata*. Although structurally very different, medications in this class have the common ability to affect cell division; thus, some of them are called *mitotic inhibitors*. The plant extracts, or natural products, are listed in Table 37.7.

The **vinca alkaloids,** vincristine (Oncovin) and vinblastine (Velban), are two older drugs derived from more than 100 alkaloids isolated from the periwinkle plant. The medicinal properties of this plant were described in folklore in several regions of the world long before their antineoplastic properties were discovered. Despite being derived from the same plant, vincristine, vinblastine, and the semisynthetic vinorelbine (Navelbine) exhibit different effects and toxicity profiles. Vincristine is a common component of regimens for treating pediatric leukemias, lymphomas, and solid tumors. The use of vinblastine has declined because of the development of newer and more effective agents, but it has traditionally been used to treat Hodgkin's disease and testicular tumors.

The **taxanes,** which include paclitaxel (Taxol) and docetaxel (Taxotere), were originally isolated from the bark of the Pacific yew, an evergreen found in forests throughout the western United States. More than 19 different taxane alkaloids have been isolated from the yew tree, and several others are being investigated for potential antineoplastic activity. Like the vinca alkaloids, the taxanes are mitotic inhibitors. Paclitaxel is approved for metastatic ovarian and breast cancer and for Kaposi's sarcoma; however, off-label uses include many other cancers. A semisynthetic product of paclitaxel, docetaxel, is claimed to have greater antitumor properties with lower toxicity. Bone marrow toxicity is usually the dose-limiting factor for the taxanes.

American Indians described uses of the May apple or wild mandrake (*Podophyllum peltatum*) long before pharmacologists isolated podophyllotoxin, the primary active ingredient in the plant. As a botanical, podophyllum has been used as an antidote for snakebites, as a cathartic, and as a topical treatment for warts. Teniposide (Vumon) and etoposide (VePesid) are semisynthetic products of podophyllotoxin. These agents act by inhibiting **topoisomerase I,** an enzyme that helps repair DNA damage. By binding in a complex with topoisomerase and DNA, these antineoplastics cause strand breaks that accumulate and permanently damage the tumor DNA. Etoposide is approved for refractory testicular carcinoma, small-cell carcinoma of the lung, and choriocarcinoma. Teniposide is approved only for refractory acute lymphoblastic leukemia in children. Bone marrow toxicity is the primary dose-limiting adverse effect.

More recently, isolated topoisomerase I inhibitors include topotecan (Hycamtin) and irinotecan (Camptosar). These agents are called **camptothecins** because they were first isolated from *Camptotheca acuminata,* a tree native to China. The camptothecins are administered only intravenously, and their indications are limited. Topotecan is approved for metastatic ovarian cancer and small-cell lung cancer after failure of initial chemotherapy. Irinotecan is indicated for metastatic cancer of the colon or rectum. As with many other cytotoxic natural products, bone marrow suppression is the dose-limiting toxicity for the camptothecins.

HORMONES AND HORMONE ANTAGONISTS

Use of hormones or their antagonists as antineoplastic agents is a strategy used to slow the growth of hormone-dependent tumors. Endocrine, or hormonal therapy, is limited to treating hormone-sensitive tumors of the breast or prostate.

37.13 Pharmacotherapy with Hormones and Hormone Antagonists

A number of hormones are used in cancer chemotherapy, including glucocorticoids, progestins, estrogens, and androgens. In addition, several hormone antagonists have been

TABLE 37.7	Natural Products with Antineoplastic Activity		
Drug	**Route and Adult Dose (max dose where indicated)**		**Adverse Effects**
VINCA ALKALOIDS			
vinblastine (Velban)	IV; 3.7–18.5 mg/m² every 1 wk		*Nausea, vomiting, asthenia, stomatitis, anorexia, rash, alopecia*
(Pr) vincristine (Oncovin)	IV; 1.4 mg/m² every 1 wk (max: 2 mg/m²)		Bone marrow suppression (neutropenia, anemia, thrombocytopenia), severe nausea and vomiting, diarrhea, cardiotoxicity, mucositis, pulmonary toxicity, hypersensitivity reactions, (including anaphylaxis), neurotoxicity (docetaxel, vincristine), nephrotoxicity (vincristine)
vinorelbine (Navelbine)	IV; 30 mg/m² every 1 wk		
TAXANES			
docetaxel (Taxotere)	IV; 60–100 mg/m² every 3 wk		
paclitaxel (Taxol)	IV; 135–175 mg/m² every 3 wk		
TOPOISOMERASE INHIBITORS			
etoposide (VePesid)	IV; 50–100 mg/m²/day for 5 days		
irinotecan (Camptosar)	IV; 125 mg/m² every 1 wk for 4 wk		
teniposide (Vumon)	IV; 165 mg/m² every 3–4 days for 4 wk		
topotecan (Hycamtin)	IV; 1.5 mg/m²/day for 5 days		
Italics indicate common adverse effects; underlining indicates serious adverse effects.			

Pr Prototype Drug | Vincristine *(Oncovin)*

Therapeutic Class: Antineoplastic   **Pharmacologic Class:** Vinca alkaloid, mitotic inhibitor, natural product

ACTIONS AND USES

Vincristine is a cell-cycle-specific (M-phase) agent that kills cancer cells by preventing their ability to complete mitosis. It exerts this action by inhibiting microtubule formation in the mitotic spindle. Although vincristine must be given intravenously, its major advantage is that it causes minimal immunosuppression. It has a wider spectrum of clinical activity than vinblastine, and is usually prescribed in combination with other antineoplastics for the treatment of Hodgkin's and non-Hodgkin's lymphomas, leukemias, Kaposi's sarcoma, Wilms' tumor, bladder carcinoma, and breast carcinoma.

ADMINISTRATION ALERTS

- Extravasation may result in serious tissue damage. Stop injection immediately if extravasation occurs and apply local heat and inject hyaluronidase as ordered. Observe site for sloughing.
- Avoid eye contact, which can cause severe irritation and corneal changes.
- Pregnancy category D

PHARMACOKINETICS
Onset: Unknown
Peak: Unknown
Half-life: 10–155 h
Duration: 7 days

ADVERSE EFFECTS

The most serious dose-limiting adverse effects of vincristine relate to nervous system toxicity. Children are particularly susceptible. Symptoms include numbness and tingling in the limbs, muscular weakness, loss of neural reflexes, and pain. Severe constipation is common and paralytic ileus may occur in young children. Reversible alopecia occurs in most patients.

Contraindications: Vincristine is contraindicated during pregnancy and lactation. Caution should be used when treating patients with hepatic impairment or obstructive jaundice.

INTERACTIONS

Drug–Drug: Asparaginase used concurrently with or before vincristine may cause increased neurotoxicity secondary to decreased hepatic clearance of vincristine. Doxorubicin or prednisone may increase bone marrow toxicity. Calcium channel blockers may increase vincristine accumulation in cells. Concurrent use with digoxin may decrease digoxin levels. When vincristine is given with methotrexate, the patient may need lower doses of methotrexate. Vincristine may decrease serum phenytoin levels, leading to increased seizure activity.

Lab Tests: Serum uric acid levels may increase.

Herbal/Food: Unknown

Treatment of Overdose: Overdose with vincristine may cause life-threatening symptoms or death. Symptoms are extensions of the drugs adverse effects. Supportive treatment may include administration of leucovorin (folinic acid).

Refer to MyNursingKit for a Nursing Process Focus specific to this drug.

---

found to exhibit antitumor activity. The mechanism of hormone antineoplastic activity is largely unknown. It is likely, however, that these antitumor properties are independent of their normal hormone mechanisms because the doses utilized in cancer chemotherapy are magnitudes larger than the amount normally present in the body. Only the antitumor properties of these hormones are discussed in this section; for other indications and actions, the student should refer to other chapters in this text. The antitumor hormones and hormone antagonists are listed in Table 37.8.

In general, the hormones and hormone antagonists act by blocking substances essential for tumor growth. Because these agents are not cytotoxic, they produce few of the debilitating adverse effects seen with other antineoplastics. They can, however, produce significant adverse effects when given at high doses for prolonged periods. Because they rarely produce cancer cures when used singly, these agents are normally given for palliation.

GLUCOCORTICOIDS (CORTICOSTEROIDS)

The primary glucocorticoids used in chemotherapy are dexamethasone and prednisone (Deltasone, others). Because of the natural ability of glucocorticoids to suppress cell division in lymphocytes, the principal value of these agents is in the treatment of lymphomas, Hodgkin's disease, and leukemias. They are sometimes given as adjuncts to chemotherapy to

reduce nausea, weight loss, and tissue inflammation caused by other antineoplastics. Prolonged use can result in symptoms of Cushing's disease (chapter 43 ∞).

GONADAL HORMONES

Gonadal hormones are used to treat tumors that contain specific hormone receptors. Two androgens, fluoxymesterone (Halotestin) and testolactone (Teslac), are used for palliative therapy for advanced breast cancer in postmenopausal women. The estrogens ethinyl estradiol and diethylstilbestrol (DES) are used to treat metastatic breast cancer and prostate cancer. The progestins medroxyprogesterone and megestrol (Megace) are used to treat advanced endometrial cancer. Leuprolide (Lupron) is similar to gonadotropin releasing hormone (GnRH), and is used for advanced prostate cancer when other therapies have failed. Also similar to GnRH is histrelin (Vantas), a drug approved in 2006. Approved for advanced prostate cancer, histrelin is an implant that is inserted subcutaneously in the inner aspect of the upper arm to release the hormone over 12 months.

ANTIESTROGENS

The antiestrogens are used to treat tumors that are dependent on estrogen for their growth. Tamoxifen (Soltamox),

TABLE 37.8 Hormone and Hormone Antagonists Used for Neoplasia

Drug	Route and Adult Dose (max dose where indicated)	Adverse Effects
HORMONES		
dexamethasone (Decadron, others)	PO; 0.25 bid–qid	*Weight gain, insomnia, abdominal distension, sweating, flushing, diarrhea, nervousness, gynecomastia, hirsutism (testosterone, testolactone)* Thrombophlebitis, muscle wasting (prednisone, dexamethasone), osteoporosis, hepatotoxicity (testosterone, testolactone)
diethylstilbestrol (DES, Stilbestrol)	PO; for treatment of prostate cancer, 500 mg tid; for palliation 1–15 mg/day	
ethinyl estradiol (Estinyl, others)	PO; for treatment of breast cancer, 1 mg tid for 2–3 months; for palliation of prostate cancer, 0.15–3 mg/day	
fluoxymesterone (Halotestin)	PO; 10 mg tid	
medroxyprogesterone (Provera, Depo-Provera) (see page 706 for the Prototype Drug box∞)	IM; 400–1,000 mg q1 wk	
megestrol (Megace)	PO; 40–160 mg bid–qid	
prednisone (Deltasone, others) (see page 471 for the Prototype Drug box∞)	PO; 20–100 mg/m²/day	
testolactone (Teslac)	PO; 250 mg qid	
testosterone (Andro, Histerone, Testred, Delatest, others) (see page 719 for the Prototype Drug box∞)	IM; 200–400 mg every 2–4 wk	
HORMONE ANTAGONISTS		
anastrozole (Arimidex)	PO; 1 mg/day	*Hot flashes, insomnia, breast enlargement/pain, headache, diarrhea, asthenia, nausea* Hypersensitivity reactions (including anaphylaxis), thrombophlebitis, CHF (bicalutamide, goserelin), hepatotoxicity (flutamide), sexual dysfunction (goserelin, nilutamide, tamoxifen), ocular toxicity (toremifene)
bicalutamide (Casodex)	PO; 50 mg/day	
degarelix (Firmagon)	Subcutaneous; 240 mg loading dose followed by 80 mg every 28 days	
exemestane (Aromasin)	PO; 25 mg/day after a meal	
flutamide (Eulexin)	PO; 250 mg tid	
fulvestrant (Faslodex)	IM; 250 mg once	
goserelin (Zoladex)	Subcutaneously; 3.6 mg every 28 days	
histrelin (Vantas)	Implant; 1 implant every 12 mo (50 mg)	
letrozole (Femara)	PO; 2.5 mg/day	
leuprolide (Eligard, Lupron, Viadur)	Subcutaneously; 1 mg/day	
nilutamide (Nilandron)	PO; 300 mg/day for 30 days; then 150 mg/day	
raloxifene (Evista)	PO; 60 mg once daily	
Ⓟ tamoxifen	PO; 10–20 mg one to two times/day (morning and evening)	
toremifene (Fareston)	PO; 60 mg/day	
triptorelin (Trelstar)	IM; 3.75 mg once monthly	

Italics indicate common adverse effects; underlining indicates serious adverse effects.

which is the most widely used drug for breast cancer, toremifene (Fareston), and raloxifene (Evista) are called selective estrogen-receptor modifiers (SERMs). These drugs *block* estrogen receptors on breast cancer cells but have an estrogen-*stimulating* effect on some nonbreast tissues. The progestogenic effects have positive actions on bone mineral density and improve lipid profiles (increase HDL and lower LDL).

The antiestrogen class also includes anastrozole (Arimidex), letrozole (Femara), and exemestane (Aromasin), which are called **aromatase inhibitors**. These antiestrogens block the enzyme aromatase, which normally converts adrenal androgen to estradiol. Aromatase inhibitors can reduce plasma estrogen levels by as much as 95% and are used in postmenopausal women with advanced breast cancer whose disease has progressed beyond tamoxifen therapy.

ANDROGEN ANTAGONISTS

Hormone inhibitors also include the antiandrogens bicalutamide (Casodex), nilutamide (Nilandron), and flutamide (Eulexin). These agents are prescribed for advanced prostate cancer, which is strongly dependent on androgens for growth.

Chemotherapy in Elderly Patients

The older adult population has a higher incidence of most types of cancer as a result of a greater accumulation of carcinogenic effects over time and age-related reduction in immune system function. Studies show that hepatic drug enzyme activity (P-450) is decreased by 30% in healthy older adults, resulting in decreased metabolism of drugs. The glomerular filtration rate also decreases, resulting in decreased excretion of drugs from the kidneys. Reduced hematopoietic stem cell mass and reduced ability to mobilize these cells from the bone marrow may slow recovery (Chatta et al., 1994). Myelosuppression is more common and more severe in older adults.

Include the following points when teaching older adults and their caregivers about chemotherapy:

- Older adults receiving chemotherapy drugs may experience greater toxicity from normal doses. Instruct the patient to monitor and report bleeding or bruising and to avoid aspirin products.
- Because older adults often have deficient nutritional intake, teach the patient and caregivers about healthy food choices, and assess the patient's ability to swallow foods and medications. Nutritional supplements may be required.
- Constipation may occur due to a decrease in elimination. Encourage the patient to drink adequate fluids and to increase dietary fiber by using grains and leafy vegetables.

BIOLOGIC RESPONSE MODIFIERS

Biologic response modifiers (BRMs) alter body defenses to enhance the destruction of cancer cells. BRMs include interferons, interleukins, and certain other cytokines. Some of the BRMs are immunostimulants.

37.14 Pharmacotherapy with Biologic Response Modifiers, Immune Therapies, and Miscellaneous Antineoplastics

Biologic response modifiers and immune therapies are medications that stimulate the body's immune system to rid the body of tumor cells. The immunostimulants are less toxic than most other classes of antineoplastics. These agents, along with some miscellaneous antineoplastics, are listed in Table 37.9. Types of drugs within this subclass include the following:

- *Interferons:* Natural proteins produced by T cells in response to viral infection and other biologic stimuli. Interferons bind to specific receptors on cancer cell membranes and suppress cell division, enhance the phagocytic activity of macrophages, and promote the cytotoxic activity of T lymphocytes. Peginterferon alfa-2a (Pegasys) and interferon alfa-2b (Intron-A) are approved to treat hairy cell leukemia, chronic

---

Pr Prototype Drug | Tamoxifen

Therapeutic Class: Antineoplastic   **Pharmacologic Class:** Hormonal agent, estrogen receptor blocker

ACTIONS AND USES

Tamoxifen is an oral antiestrogen that is a preferred drug for treating metastatic breast cancer. It is effective against breast tumor cells that require estrogen for their growth, which are known as estrogen receptor (ER) positive cells. It blocks estrogen receptors on breast cancer cells, but tamoxifen actually activates estrogen receptors in other parts of the body, resulting in typical estrogen-like effects such as reduced LDL levels and increased mineral density of bone.

A unique feature of tamoxifen is that it is the only antineoplastic that is approved for prophylaxis of breast cancer, for high-risk patients who are at risk of developing the disease. In addition, it is approved as adjunctive therapy in women following mastectomy to decrease the potential for cancer in the opposite breast.

ADMINISTRATION ALERTS

- Give with food or fluids to decrease GI irritation.
- Do not crush or chew drug.
- Avoid antacids for 1–2 h following PO dosage of tamoxifen.
- Pregnancy category D

PHARMACOKINETICS

Onset: Unknown

Peak: 3–6 h

Half-life: 7 days

Duration: Unknown

ADVERSE EFFECTS

Other than nausea and vomiting, tamoxifen produces little serious toxicity. Of concern, however, is the association of tamoxifen therapy with an increased risk of endometrial cancer and thromboembolic disease, including strokes and pulmonary emboli. Hot flashes, fluid retention, and vaginal discharges are relatively common. Tamoxifen causes initial "tumor flare"—an idiosyncratic increase in tumor size, but this is an expected therapeutic event. Hypertension and edema occur in about 10% of patients taking the drug

Contraindications: Contraindications to the use of tamoxifen include anticoagulant therapy, pre-existing endometrial hyperplasia, history of thromboembolic disease, pregnancy, and lactation. Precautions should be observed in patients with blood disorders, visual disturbances, cataracts, hypercalcemia, and hypercholesterolemia.

INTERACTIONS

Drug–Drug: Anticoagulants taken concurrently with tamoxifen may increase the risk of bleeding. Concurrent use with cytotoxic agents may increase the risk of thromboembolism. Estrogens will decrease the effectiveness of tamoxifen.

Lab Tests: Serum calcium levels may increase.

Herbal/Food: Unknown

Treatment of Overdose: Seizures, neurotoxicity, and dysrhythmias may occur with overdose. The patient is treated symptomatically.

Refer to MyNursingKit for a Nursing Process Focus specific to this drug.

myelogenous leukemia, Kapsoi's sarcoma, and chronic hepatitis B or C.

- *Interleukin-2:* Activates cytotoxic T lymphocytes and promotes other actions of the immune response. Marketed as aldesleukin (Proleukin), this drug is indicated for metastatic renal cell carcinoma.

- *Monoclonal antibodies (MABs):* Engineered to attack only one *specific* type of tumor cell, unlike interferons and interleukins, which are considered *general* immunostimulants. Once the MAB binds to its target cell, the cancer cell dies, or is marked for destruction by other cells of the immune response. For example, trastuzumab

TABLE 37.9	Selected Biologic Response Modifiers and Miscellaneous Antineoplastics	
Drug	**Route and Adult Dose (max dose where indicated)**	**Adverse Effects**
altretamine (Hexalen)	PO; 65 mg/m²/day	*Nausea, vomiting, asthenia, stomatitis anorexia, rash, alopecia, hyperlipidemia (bexarotene)*
arsenic trioxide (Trisenox)	IV; 0.15 mg/kg/day (max: 60 doses)	
asparaginase (Elspar)	IV; 200 international units/kg/day	Bone marrow suppression (neutropenia, anemia, thrombocytopenia), severe nausea and vomiting, diarrhea, pulmonary toxicity, hypersensitivity reactions, (including anaphylaxis), pancreatitis (asparaginase, bexarotene, pegaspargase), hypothyroidism (bexarotene), hepatotoxicity (asparaginase, pegaspargase), brain damage (mitotane)
bexarotene (Targretin)	PO; 100–400 mg/m²/day; topical; 1% gel applied to lesion one to four times/day	
hydroxyurea (Hydrea)	PO; 20–30 mg/kg/day	
interferon alfa-2 (Roferon-A, Intron A) (see page 454 for the Prototype Drug box∞)	Subcutaneous/IM; 2–3 million units/day for leukemia; increase to 36 million units/day for Kaposi's sarcoma	
ixabepilone (Ixempra)	IV; 40 mg/m² infused over 3 h every 3 wk	
levamisole (Ergamisol)	PO; 50 mg tid for 3 days	
mitotane (Lysodren)	PO; 1–6 g/day given in three to four divided doses; may be increased to 9–10 g/day, as tolerated	
pegaspargase (Oncaspar, PEG-L-asparaginase)	IV; 2,500 international units/m² every 14 days	
romidepsin (Istodax)	IV; 14 mg/m² administered over 4 hr on days 1, 8, and 15	
vorinostat (Zolinza)	PO; 400 mg once daily	
zoledronic acid (Zometa)	IV; 4 mg over at least 15 min	
MONOCLONAL ANTIBODIES		
alemtuzumab (Campath)	IV; 3–30 mg/day	*Nausea, vomiting, asthenia, tremors (alemtuzumab), anorexia, rash, diarrhea, stomatitis, fever, chills*
bevacizumab (Avastin)	IV; 5 mg/kg every 14 days	
bortezomib (Velcade)	IV; 1.3 mg/m² as a bolus twice weekly for 2 wk	Bone marrow suppression (neutropenia, anemia, thrombocytopenia), severe nausea and vomiting, diarrhea, pulmonary toxicity, pulmonary toxicity, CHF (bevacizumab, trastuzumab), hypersensitivity reactions (including anaphylaxis), dysrhythmias (rituximab), severe fluid retention (imatinib), progressive multifocal leukoencephalopathy (ofatumumab), hepatotoxicity (pazopanib)
cetuximab (Erbitux)	IV; 400 mg/m² over 2 h; then continue with 250 mg/m² over 1 h weekly	
erlotinib (Tarceva)	PO; 150 mg/day	
gefitinib (Iressa)	PO; 250–500 mg/day	
gemtuzumab ozogamicin (Mylotarg)	IV; 9 mg/m² for 2 h	
ibritumomab tiuxetan (Zevalin)	IV; 250 mg/m² of rituximab is infused followed by 5 mCi of Zevalin in a 10-min IV push	
imatinib mesylate (Gleevec)	PO; 400–600 mg/day	
lapatinib (Tykerb)	PO; 1,250 mg (5 tablets) once daily on days 1 to 21 continuously in combination with capecitabine	
ofatumumab (Arzerra)	IV; 300 mg initial dose followed by 2,000 mg weekly for 7 doses	
pazopanib (Votrient)	PO; 800 mg once daily	
rituximab (Rituxan)	IV; 375 mg/m²/day as a continuous infusion	
scinitinib (Sutent)	PO; 50 mg once daily for 4 weeks followed by 2 weeks off	
sorafenib (Nexavar)	PO; 400 mg bid	
tositumomab (Bexxar)	IV; 450 mg over 60 min	
trastuzumab (Herceptin)	IV; 4 mg/kg as a single dose; then 2 mg/kg every 1 wk	

Italics indicate common adverse effects; underlining indicates serious adverse effects.

(Herceptin) binds to specific proteins on breast cancer cells (called *HER2* proteins) and induces cell death. Alemtuzumab (Campath) binds to a protein known as *CD52*, which is present on the surface of B and T lymphocytes, monocytes, and other white blood cells, and is used to treat chronic lymphocytic leukemia. The key point about MABs is that the tumor cells must possess the specific protein receptor; otherwise, the MAB will be ineffective. This is illustrated in Pharmacotherapy Illustrated 37.1. In the treatment of rheumatoid arthritis and severe psoriasis, MABs are used to dampen overactive inflammatory cells.

When given concurrently with other antineoplastics, biologic response modifiers help limit the severe immunosuppressive effects caused by other agents. Additional information on the biologic response modifiers, a drug pro-

totype for interferon alfa-2b, and nursing considerations for this class of drugs can be found in chapter 32∞.

Certain anticancer drugs act through mechanisms other than those previously described. For example, asparaginase (Elspar) deprives cancer cells of asparagine, an essential amino acid. It is used to treat acute lymphocytic leukemia. Mitotane (Lysodren), similar to the insecticide DDT, poisons cancer cells by forming links to proteins, and is used for advanced adrenocortical cancer. Two of the newer antineoplastics, imatinib (Gleevec) and sorafenib (Nexavar), inhibit the enzyme tyrosine kinase in tumor cells. Lenalidomide (Revlimid) is an angiogenesis inhibitor that prevents the formation of new blood vessels that are vital to the growth of new tumors. Approved in late 2008, plerixafor (Mozobil) is classified as a hematopoietic stem cell mobilizer. The mobilized stem cells are then collected from the blood for subsequent autologous transplantation in patients with non-Hodgkin's lymphoma and multiple myeloma.

PHARMACOTHERAPY ILLUSTRATED

37.1 Monoclonal Antibodies and Cancer Cells

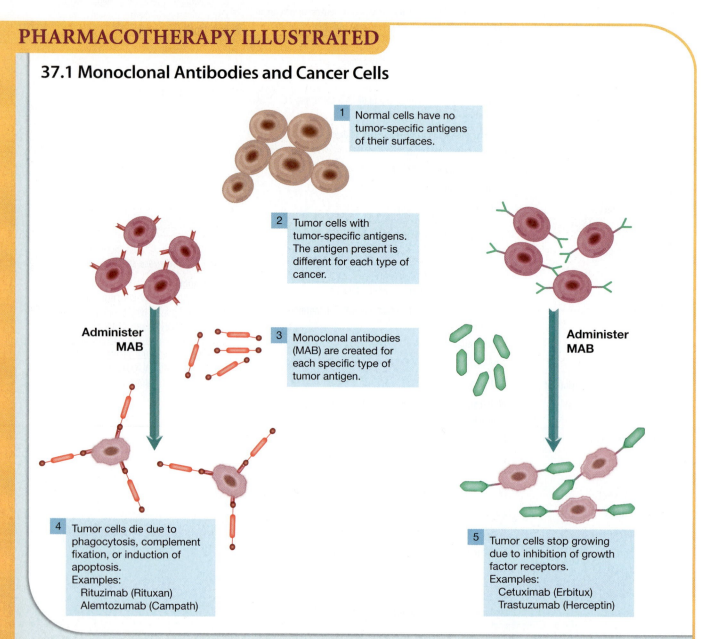

1 Normal cells have no tumor-specific antigens of their surfaces.

2 Tumor cells with tumor-specific antigens. The antigen present is different for each type of cancer.

3 Monoclonal antibodies (MAB) are created for each specific type of tumor antigen.

Administer MAB

4 Tumor cells die due to phagocytosis, complement fixation, or induction of apoptosis.
Examples:
   Rituzimab (Rituxan)
   Alemtozumab (Campath)

Administer MAB

5 Tumor cells stop growing due to inhibition of growth factor receptors.
Examples:
   Cetuximab (Erbitux)
   Trastuzumab (Herceptin)

NURSING PROCESS FOCUS   PATIENTS RECEIVING ANTINEOPLASTIC THERAPY

Assessment	Potential Nursing Diagnoses
Baseline assessment prior to administration: • Understand the reason the drug has been prescribed in order to assess for therapeutic effects. • Obtain a complete health history including neurologic, cardiovascular, respiratory, hepatic or renal disease, and the possibility of pregnancy. Obtain a drug history including allergies, including specific reactions to drugs, current prescription and OTC drugs, herbal preparations, and alcohol use. Be alert to possible drug interactions. • Assess signs and symptoms of current infections and for history of herpes zoster or chicken pox. • Obtain an immunization history, especially recent vaccinations with live vaccines, particularly varicella. • Evaluate appropriate laboratory findings (e.g., CBC, platelet count, urinalysis, hepatic and renal function studies, uric acid, electrolytes, glucose). • Assess findings from other diagnostic tests specific to the planned type of antineoplastic therapy (e.g., audiology, cardiac testing, ECG, EMG). • Obtain baseline weight and vital signs. Assess the level of fatigue and the presence of pain. Assess deep tendon reflexes (DTRs).	• Infection • Activity Intolerance • Fatigue • Anxiety • Imbalanced Nutrition, Less Than Body Requirements • Deficient Fluid Volume • Diarrhea • Impaired Oral Mucous Membranes • Impaired Skin Integrity • Pain (acute or chronic) • Social Isolation • Ineffective Therapeutic Regimen Management (related to complex medication regimen and disease treatment) • Deficient Knowledge (related to disease process and drug therapy) • Hopelessness • Spiritual Distress • Risk for Decreased Cardiac Output (related to adverse drug effects) • Risk for Injury, Risk for Falls (related to adverse drug effects or disease) • Risk for Caregiver Role Strain
Assessment throughout administration: • Assess for desired therapeutic effects (e.g., indicators of treatment success or palliation such as slowed growth in solid tumors, organ/body-specific MRI/CT scan demonstrates diminished tumor load without metastasis, able to attend to normal ADLs, absence of signs of concurrent infections). • Continue frequent monitoring of lab work (e.g., CBC, absolute neutrophil count [ANC], platelet count, urinalysis, hepatic and renal function studies, uric acid, electrolytes, glucose). (ANC = Total WBC count multiplied by the total percentage of neutrophils [segs plus bands]; e.g., WBC 5000 × [0.45 segmented neutrophils + 0.05 banded neutrophils] = 5000 × 0.5 = ANC of 2500.) • Continue to monitor findings from diagnostic tests specific to the planned type of antineoplastic therapy (e.g., audiology, cardiac testing, ECG, EMG). • Assess for the presence of nausea or pain. • Assess DTRs, and ECG as specific to the type of antineoplastic drugs given. • Continue daily weights and report any weight gain or loss of more than 1 kg in 24 hours. • Assess for adverse effects: nausea, vomiting, anorexia, abdominal cramping, diarrhea, constipation, fever, fatigue, dizziness, dysrhythmias, angina, dyspnea, muscle or joint pain, paresthesias, diminished or absent deep tendon reflexes, hypotension, hyperglycemia, bruising, and bleeding. Fever exceeding parameters established by the provider, severe diarrhea, jaundice, decreased urine output or hematuria, excessive bruising or bleeding, respiratory distress, and dysrhythmias or angina should be reported immediately.	

Planning: Patient Goals and Expected Outcomes

The patient will:
• Experience therapeutic effects (e.g., reduction in tumor mass or decreased progression of abnormal cell growth, absence of signs and symptoms of concurrent infection, able to maintain ADLs).
• Be free from, or experience minimal, adverse effects.
• Verbalize an understanding of the drug's use, adverse effects, and required precautions.
• Demonstrate proper self-administration of the medication (e.g., dose, timing, when to notify provider).

(Continued)

NURSING PROCESS FOCUS   **PATIENTS RECEIVING ANTINEOPLASTIC THERAPY** *(Continued)*

Implementation

Interventions and (Rationales)	Patient and Family Education
Ensuring therapeutic effects: ■ Continue assessments as described earlier for therapeutic effects: radiographic evidence of diminished tumor mass, decreased production of abnormal cell growth, absence of signs of infection, maintenance of appetite and food and fluid intake, nausea and vomiting controlled, and able to maintain acceptable levels of ADLs. (Antineoplastic drugs do not have immediately observable results and results will be measured over time. These drugs have many potential adverse effects.)	■ Provide explanations for all testing and treatments used. Provide general information on the expected course of chemotherapy: requirements for invasive lines (e.g., peripheral versus central access ports), initial infusion or dosing, frequency of expected treatments, nausea control, hydration and nutrition needs, frequent lab testing, onset of alopecia, techniques for managing fatigue, nutrition and fluid needs, follow-up appointments, in-hospital versus outpatient clinic locations, and how to reach oncology team, especially during off-hours. Involve the family and caregiver in information sessions.
Minimizing adverse effects: *General Care* ■ Continue to monitor vital signs. Report increasing temperature that exceeds parameters (e.g., three temperatures over 100.5°F or any temperature over 101°F) to the oncology provider. Avoid taking rectal temperatures. (Increasing fever, even low-grade temperatures may be sign of infection. Immunosuppression may cause infections to occur and disseminate rapidly. GI endothelial cells are affected by chemotherapy and rectal mucosa may be damaged if rectal temperatures are used.)	■ Teach the patient to take temperature every 4 hours if symptoms indicate a need (e.g., increased body warmth, general malaise, lethargy). Include instructions on when to call the oncology team if parameters are exceeded. ■ Instruct the patient that antipyretics are not to be used unless explicitly approved by the oncology provider. (Antipyretics may mask the symptoms of an infection, allowing rapid dissemination of the infection.)
■ Continue to monitor frequent lab work: CBC, ANC, platelet count, hepatic and renal function tests, electrolytes, glucose, and urinalysis. (Bone marrow suppression with resulting blood dyscrasias is an expected adverse effect and will be monitored by ANC, CBC, and platelet counts.)	■ Teach the patient of the need for frequent lab work. Have the patient alert lab personnel of chemotherapy use. ■ If peripheral veins are used for phlebotomy, scrupulous cleansing of the site prior to stick and prolonged pressure may be required. If a central line access is used, scrupulous cleansing of the port is required.
■ Continue to monitor nutritional and fluid intake. (Nausea and vomiting are common adverse effects and usually require antiemetic therapy to manage. Dietary consultation may be required to maintain optimum nutrition.)	■ Provide antiemetic therapy during administration of drugs with high and moderate emetic potential. If the patient has had previous treatment with the chemotherapy regimen, assess the extent of nausea and vomiting and which antiemetics had the most success in preventing nausea. ■ Encourage increased fluid intake, up to 2 L per day, taken in frequent small amounts. ■ Encourage small, high-calorie, nutrient-dense meals rather than large, infrequent meals. Nutritional supplements such as Un*jury*, Boost, or Ensure may help boost caloric intake. ■ Avoid spicy, highly scented foods, and excessively hot or cold foods during periods of nausea. Small sips of carbonated beverages, especially ginger ale, may provide relief. If GI effects predominate (e.g., diarrhea), avoid high-roughage foods. ■ Encourage frequent oral hygiene: rinse mouth, especially after eating; use lip balm; and avoid alcohol-based mouthwash, which can be drying to the mucosa.
■ Continue to assess for the presence of pain and provide for adequate pain medication. (Pain may result from advanced disease or adverse drug effects. In advanced disease, pain medication is not withheld. Assess possible drug-related causes for pain and treat the cause when possible.)	■ Encourage the patient to seek pain relief when needed. Teach the patient, family, and caregiver that absence of pain is a goal in the treatment of advanced disease and pain medication should not be withheld.
■ Provide for adequate rest. (Fatigue related to anemia and adverse drug effects is common, especially around the nadir and immediately after. Fatigue may continue after cell counts return to normal and may persist for several years after chemotherapy.)	■ Teach the patient the importance of spacing daily routines throughout the day. Encourage rest whenever fatigue occurs. ■ Assess transportation needs if fatigue affects ability to drive. Provide referral to social services as needed.

NURSING PROCESS FOCUS   PATIENTS RECEIVING ANTINEOPLASTIC THERAPY (Continued)

Implementation

Interventions and (Rationales)	Patient and Family Education
■ Protect the patient from infection: e.g., frequent hand washing before patient care; maintaining scrupulous infection control measures for all IV lines or venous punctures; encouraging the patient to maintain daily hygiene measures to limit external flora; and assessing for symptoms of opportunistic infections and acquiring early treatment or prophylaxis. (Immunosuppression places patients at high risk for infection. Prophylactic therapy with antifungal and antibacterial mouth rinses, and protective isolation may be required.)	■ Teach the patient, family, and caregiver infection control measures as follows: 　■ Avoid crowded indoor places. 　■ Avoid people with known infections or young children who have a higher risk of having an infection. 　■ Cook food thoroughly, allowing the family or caregiver to prepare raw foods and to clean up; patient should not consume raw fruits or vegetables. 　■ Report any fever and symptoms of infection such as: wounds with redness or drainage, increasing cough, increasing fatigue, white patches on oral mucous membranes or white and itchy vaginal discharge, or itchy blister-like vesicles on skin.
■ Provide for emotional support for the patient, family, and caregiver. (Cancer results in profound emotional reactions from all involved. Encourage discussion of concerns, appropriate referrals for social support or spiritual assistance, and assess the patient or family for distress that may require mental health referral.)	■ Encourage the patient, family, and caregiver to discuss concerns or questions and to seek appropriate spiritual or social support as desired. ■ Assess financial concerns and provide appropriate social service referral as needed.
Minimizing adverse effects: *Specific to Drug Therapy* ■ Monitor DTRs, neurologic status, and level of consciousness (LOC). (*Alkylating agents* such as cyclophosphamide and *natural product antineoplastics* such as vincristine have neurologic adverse effects. Changes may occur in DTRs that are not noticeable to the patient in early stages but may affect dexterity or steadiness when walking.)	■ Teach the patient to be cautious when walking or performing manual tasks requiring extra dexterity. Promptly report any significant difficulty with dexterity, or clumsiness when carrying out ADLs or when walking. ■ Encourage the increased intake of fluids and moderate fiber in the diet if constipation is an effect related to decreased peristalsis. Drug therapy may be required if constipation is severe to prevent straining during defecation.
■ Monitor cardiovascular status including ECG, heart and breath sounds, presence of edema, and angina or chest-wall pain. (*Alkylating agents* such as cyclophosphamide, *antitumor antibodies* such as doxorubicin, *natural product antineoplastics* such as vincristine, and *hormone and hormone antagonists* such as tamoxifen have cardiovascular adverse effects such as pericarditis and effects on the cardiac conduction system.)	■ Teach the patient about the need for frequent monitoring of cardiac status. Immediately report any chest-wall pain, angina, palpitations, dyspnea, lung congestion, or dizziness.
■ Monitor respiratory status including breath sounds and pulmonary function tests. (*Alkylating agents* such as cyclophosphamide, *antimetabolites* such as methotrexate, *antitumor antibodies* such as doxorubicin, *natural product antineoplastics* such as vincristine, and *biologic response modifiers* such as interferon alpha-2 have respiratory adverse effects such as interstitial pneumonitis.)	■ Teach the patient about the need for frequent monitoring of respiratory status. Immediately report any chest pain, dyspnea, lung congestion, or dizziness. ■ Teach the patient pulmonary hygiene measures such as increasing fluid intake to moisten respiratory tract, avoiding crowded indoor places and people with known respiratory disease, and avoiding use of room or body sprays, which may be an irritation to the respiratory tract.
■ Monitor hepatic and renal status and for urinary tract dysfunction. (Antineoplastic drugs may cause significant hepatic and renal toxicity. *Alkylating agents* such as cyclophosphamide may cause hemorrhagic cystitis.)	■ Teach the patient to immediately report any nausea, vomiting, yellowing of skin or sclera, abdominal pain, light or clay-colored stools, diminished urine output, darkening of urine, or suprapubic pain or blood in the urine. ■ Advise the patient to increase fluid intake to 2 to 3 L per day.
■ Monitor for ototoxicity. (*Alkylating agents* such as cyclophosphamide and *antimetabolites* such as methotrexate may cause otoxicity, affecting hearing, balance, or both.)	■ Teach the patient about the need for periodic monitoring of hearing. Immediately report any dizziness, vertigo, nausea related to motion, buzzing, ringing, or humming in ears.
■ Monitor for ocular toxicity. (*Hormone and hormone antagonists* such as tamoxifen may cause ocular toxicity.)	■ Teach the patient about the need for periodic eye exams. Immediately report any blurred vision, eye pain, or halos or other visual disturbances immediately. ■ Encourage the patient to wear sunglasses when in bright light.

(Continued)

NURSING PROCESS FOCUS   **PATIENTS RECEIVING ANTINEOPLASTIC THERAPY** *(Continued)*

Implementation

Interventions and (Rationales)	Patient and Family Education
▪ Monitor for dermatologic toxicity. (*Alkylating agents* such as cyclophosphamide may cause significant skin reactions including Stevens–Johnson syndrome.)	▪ Teach the patient to immediately report any unusual changes to skin, rashes, or sunburn-like appearance promptly. Report any purplish-red, blistering rash, or peeling skin.
▪ Monitor for mucositis. (Antineoplastic drugs may cause significant mucositis related to effects on rapidly dividing GI endothelial cells.)	▪ Teach the patient to inspect mouth at least once daily and maintain regular dental exams. Maintain good oral hygiene and rinse mouth with plain water or solution after eating. Use antibacterial and antifungal mouth rinses and do not rinse mouth with water after using. Avoid excessively hot or cold foods.
	▪ Teach the patient to avoid high-roughage foods, spicy foods, carbonated and acidic beverages, alcohol, and caffeine. If diarrhea is severe, drug therapy may be required. Immediately report any excessive diarrhea, especially if it contains mucus or blood.
▪ Monitor for hypersensitivity and allergic reactions. (Antineoplastic drugs may cause significant hypersensitivity and allergic responses, including anaphylaxis. Because reactions may not always be predictable, caution and frequent monitoring are essential to ensure prompt treatment.)	▪ Teach the patient to immediately report any itching, rashes, or swelling, particularly of face, tongue, or lips; urticaria; flushing; dizziness; syncope; wheezing; throat tightness; or difficulty breathing.
▪ Be aware of agency-specific policies and procedures related to antineoplastic administration, spill management, and required coursework before working with or giving chemotherapy. All IV infusions will be given via monitored pump. IV push drugs may utilize a push–pull technique. All spills will be managed via OSHA and agency protocols. Larger spills may require HAZMAT intervention. (Intensive education programs are required prior to administering vesicants and other chemotherapy drugs. Protection of the nurse, pharmacy personnel, and others involved in the preparation and administration of chemotherapy is essential.)	▪ Provide the patient, family, and caregiver education and support when giving chemotherapy.
Patient understanding of drug therapy:	
▪ Use opportunities during administration of medications and during assessments to discuss rationale for drug therapy, desired therapeutic outcomes, most common adverse effects, parameters for when to call the health care provider, and any necessary monitoring or precautions. (Using time during nursing care helps to optimize and reinforce key teaching areas.)	▪ The patient, family, or caregiver should be able to state the reason for the drug; appropriate dose and scheduling; what adverse effects to observe for and when to report; and the anticipated length of medication therapy.
Patient self-administration of drug therapy:	
▪ When administering medications, instruct the patient, family, or caregiver in proper self-administration techniques followed by return demonstration as needed. (Proper administration will increase the effectiveness of the drugs.)	▪ Provide explicit instructions for the patient, family, or caregiver on the routine to follow for any antineoplastic drugs used at home. Encourage the use of calendars for recording drugs and doses used; and provide information on handling a liquid spill and on proper disposal of any unused drug. (Consult local pharmacies, as many will accept unused drugs for proper disposal. Chemotherapy should never be flushed down the toilet, poured in a drain, or thrown away in the trash.)

Evaluation of Outcome Criteria

Evaluate the effectiveness of drug therapy by confirming that patient goals and expected outcomes have been met (see "Planning").

See Tables 37.2 through 37.8 for lists of drugs to which these nursing actions apply.

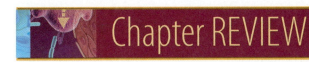

Chapter REVIEW

KEY CONCEPTS

The numbered key concepts provide a succinct summary of the important points from the corresponding numbered section within the chapter. If any of these points are not clear, refer to the numbered section within the chapter for review.

37.1 Cancer is characterized by rapid, uncontrolled growth of cells that eventually invade normal tissues and metastasize.

37.2 The causes of cancer may be chemical, physical, or biologic. Many environmental and lifestyle factors are associated with a higher risk of cancer.

37.3 Cancer may be treated using surgery, radiation therapy, and drugs. Chemotherapy may be used for cure, palliation, or prophylaxis.

37.4 The growth fraction, the percentage of cancer cells undergoing mitosis at any given time, is a major factor determining success of chemotherapy. Antineoplastics are more effective against cells that are rapidly dividing.

37.5 To achieve a total cure, every malignant cell must be removed or killed through surgery, radiation, or drugs, or by the patient's immune system.

37.6 Use of multiple drugs and special dosing protocols are strategies that allow for lower doses, fewer side effects, and greater success of chemotherapy.

37.7 Serious toxicity, including bone marrow suppression, severe nausea, vomiting, and diarrhea, limits therapy with most antineoplastic agents. Long-term consequences of chemotherapy include possible infertility and an increased risk for secondary tumors.

37.8 Classes of antineoplastic drugs include alkylating agents, antimetabolites, hormones/hormone antagonists, natu-

ral products, biologic response modifiers, and miscellaneous antineoplastics.

37.9 Alkylating agents have a broad spectrum of activity and act by changing the structure of DNA in cancer cells. Their use is limited because they can cause significant bone marrow suppression.

37.10 Antimetabolites act by disrupting critical pathways in cancer cells, such as folate metabolism or DNA synthesis. The three types of antimetabolites are purine analogs, pyrimidine analogs, and folate inhibitors.

37.11 Due to their cytotoxicity, a few antibiotics are used to treat cancer by inhibiting cell growth. They have a narrow spectrum of clinical activity.

37.12 Some plant extracts have been isolated that kill cancer cells by preventing cell division. These include the vinca alkaloids, taxanes, topoisomerase inhibitors, and camptothecins.

37.13 Some hormones and hormone antagonists are antineoplastic agents that are effective against reproductive-related tumors such as those of the breast, prostate, or uterus. They are less cytotoxic than other antineoplastics.

37.14 Biologic response modifiers and some additional antineoplastic drugs have been found to be effective against tumors by stimulating or assisting the patient's immune system. These include interferons, interleukins, and monoclonal antibodies.

NCLEX-RN® REVIEW QUESTIONS

1 A patient undergoing cancer chemotherapy asks the nurse why she is taking three different antineoplastics. What is the nurse's best response?
1. "Your cancer was very advanced and therefore requires more medications."
2. "Each drug attacks the cancer cells in a different way, increasing the effectiveness of the therapy."
3. "Several drugs are prescribed to find the right drug for your cancer."
4. "One drug will cancel out the side effects of the other."

2 The nurse understands the effective treatment method for the nausea and vomiting that accompany chemotherapy is to:
1. administer an oral antiemetic when the patient complains of nausea and vomiting.

2. administer an antiemetic by IM injection when the patient complains of nausea and vomiting.
3. administer an antiemetic prior to the antineoplastic medication.
4. push fluids prior to administering the antineoplastic medication.

3 Which of the following statements by a patient undergoing antineoplastic therapy would be of concern to the nurse? (Select all that apply.)
1. "I have attended a meeting of a cancer support group."
2. "My husband and I are planning a short trip next week."
3. "I am eating six small meals plus two protein shakes a day."
4. "I am taking my 15-month-old granddaughter to the pediatrician next week for her baby shots."
5. "I am going to go shopping at the mall next week."

4 To monitor for the presence of bone marrow suppression, the nurse evaluates the results of the:
1. BUN and serum creatinine.
2. serum electrolytes.
3. CBC.
4. bone scan.

5 A 2-year-old patient is receiving vincristine (Oncovin) for Wilms' tumor. Which of the following symptoms should be reported to the health care provider?
1. Diarrhea
2. Diminished bowel sounds
3. Stomatitis
4. Anorexia

6 The nurse notes that the patient has reached his "nadir." This means that:
1. the patient is receiving the highest dose possible of the chemotherapy.
2. the patient is experiencing bone marrow suppression and his blood counts are at their lowest point.
3. the patient has peaked on his chemotherapy level and should be going home in a few days.
4. the patient is experiencing extreme depression and will be having a psychiatric consult.

CRITICAL THINKING QUESTIONS

1. A patient is newly diagnosed with cancer and is about to start chemotherapy. Identify the teaching priorities for this patient.

2. Chemotherapy medications often cause neutropenia in cancer patients. What would be a priority for the nurse to teach a patient who is receiving chemotherapy at home?

3. A nurse is taking chemotherapy IV medication to a patient's room and the IV bag suddenly leaks solution (approximately 50 mL) on the floor. What action should the nurse take?

See Appendix D for answers and rationales for all activities.

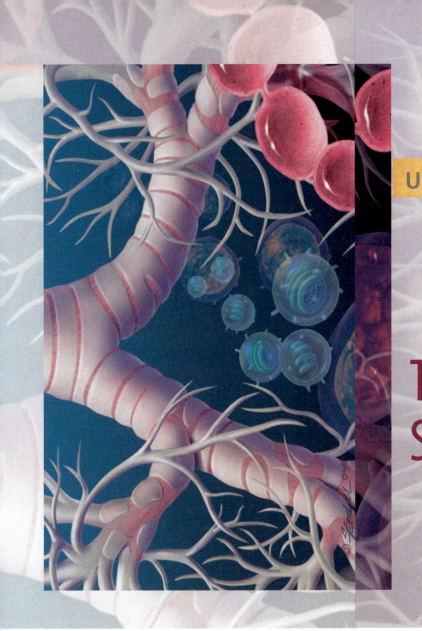

The Respiratory System

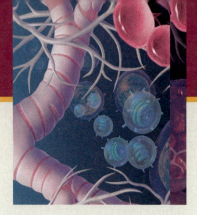

Chapter 38

Drugs for Allergic Rhinitis and the Common Cold

LEARNING OUTCOMES

After reading this chapter, the student should be able to:

1. Identify major functions of the upper respiratory tract.
2. Describe common causes and symptoms of allergic rhinitis.
3. Differentiate between H₁ and H₂ histamine receptors.
4. Compare and contrast the oral and intranasal decongestants.
5. Discuss the pharmacotherapy of cough.
6. Describe the role of expectorants and mucolytics in treating bronchial congestion.
7. For each of the classes listed in Drugs at a Glance, know representative drugs, and explain their mechanism of drug action, primary actions on the respiratory system, and important adverse effects.
8. Use the nursing process to care for patients who are receiving pharmacotherapy for allergic rhinitis and the common cold.

The respiratory system is one of the most important organ systems; a mere 5 to 6 minutes without breathing may result in death. When functioning properly, this system provides the body with the oxygen critical for all cells to carry on normal activities. The respiratory system also provides a means by which the body can rid itself of excess acids and bases, a topic presented in chapter 31∞. This chapter examines drugs used to treat conditions associated with the *upper* respiratory tract: allergic rhinitis, nasal congestion, and cough. Chapter 39∞ presents the pharmacotherapy of asthma and chronic obstructive pulmonary disease, conditions that affect the *lower* respiratory tract.

38.1 Physiology of the Upper Respiratory Tract

Knowledge of the basic anatomy and physiology of the upper respiratory tract (URT) is necessary to understand the pharmacotherapy of conditions affecting that region. The URT consists of the nose, nasal cavity, pharynx, and paranasal sinuses. These passageways warm, humidify, and clean the air before it enters the lungs. This process is sometimes referred to as the "air conditioning" function of the respiratory system. The basic structures of the upper respiratory tract are shown in ➤ Figure 38.1.

The URT traps particulate matter and many pathogens, preventing them from being carried to bronchioles and alveoli, where they could access the capillaries of the systemic circulation. The mucous membrane of the URT is lined with ciliated epithelium, which traps and "sweeps" the pathogens and particulate matter posteriorly, where it is swallowed when the person coughs or clears the throat.

The nasal mucosa is a dynamic structure, richly supplied with vascular tissue that is under the control of the autonomic nervous system. Activation of the sympathetic nervous system constricts arterioles in the nose, reducing the thickness of the mucosal layer. This serves to widen the airway and allow more air to enter. Parasympathetic activation has the opposite effect: arterioles dilate and more mucus is produced. This difference becomes important for drugs that affect the autonomic nervous system. For example, administration of a sympathomimetic will shrink the nasal mucosa, relieving the nasal stuffiness associated with the common cold (Section 38.5). Parasympathetic agents will cause increased blood flow to the nose, with increased nasal stuffiness and a runny nose as side effects.

The nasal mucosa is a first line of immune defense. Up to a quart of nasal mucus is produced daily, and this fluid is rich with immunoglobulins that are able to neutralize airborne pathogens. The mucosa also contains various body defense cells that can activate complement or engulf microbes. Mast cells, which contain histamine, also line the nasal mucosa, and these play a major role in causing the symptoms of allergic rhinitis.

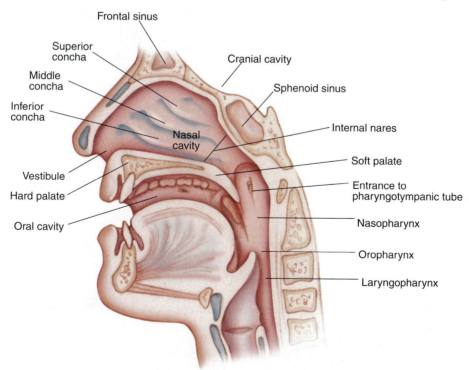

➤ *Figure 38.1* The respiratory system

Source: Rice, Medical Terminology with Human Anatomy, *5th ed., p. 292, © 2005. Reprinted by permission of Pearson Education, Inc., Upper Saddle River, NJ.*

ALLERGIC RHINITIS

Allergic rhinitis, or *hay fever*, is inflammation of the nasal mucosa due to exposure to allergens. Although not life threatening, allergic rhinitis is a condition affecting millions of patients, and pharmacotherapy is frequently necessary to control symptoms and to prevent secondary complications.

38.2 Pharmacotherapy of Allergic Rhinitis

Symptoms of allergic rhinitis resemble those of the common cold: tearing eyes, sneezing, nasal congestion, postnasal drip, and itching of the throat. In addition to the acute symptoms, potential complications of allergic rhinitis include loss of taste or smell, sinusitis, chronic cough, hoarseness, and middle ear infections in children.

As with other allergies, the cause of allergic rhinitis is exposure to an antigen. An antigen, also called an **allergen,** may be defined as anything that is recognized as foreign by the body's immune defenses. The specific allergen responsible for a patient's allergic rhinitis is often difficult to pinpoint; however, the most common agents are pollens from weeds, grasses, and trees; mold spores; dust mites; certain foods; and animal dander. Chemical fumes, tobacco smoke, or air pollutants such as ozone are nonallergenic factors that may worsen symptoms. In addition, there is a strong genetic predisposition to allergic rhinitis.

Some patients experience symptoms of allergic rhinitis only at specific times of the year, when pollen levels are at high levels in the environment. These periods are typically in the spring and fall when plants and trees are blooming, thus the name *seasonal* allergic rhinitis. Obviously, the "blooming" season changes with the geographic location, and with each species of plant. These patients may need pharmacotherapy for only a few months during the year.

Other patients, however, are afflicted with allergic rhinitis throughout the year because they are continuously exposed to indoor allergens, such as dust mites, animal dander, or mold. This variation is called *perennial* allergic rhinitis. These patients may require continuous pharmacotherapy.

It is often not clear whether a person is experiencing seasonal or perennial allergic rhinitis. Patients with seasonal allergies may also be sensitive to some of the perennial allergens. It is also common for one allergen to "sensitize" the patient to another. For example, during ragweed season, a patient may become hyper-responsive to other allergens such as mold spores or animal dander. The body's response and the symptoms of allergic rhinitis are the same, however, regardless of the specific allergen(s). Allergy testing can help to pinpoint the specific allergens producing the symptoms.

The fundamental pathophysiology responsible for allergic rhinitis is inflammation of the mucous membranes in the nose, throat, and airways. The nasal mucosa is rich with mast cells (a type of connective tissue cell) and basophils (a type of leukocyte), which recognize environmental agents as they try to enter the body. Patients with allergic rhinitis contain greater numbers of mast cells. An *immediate* hypersensitivity response releases histamine and other inflammatory mediators from the mast cells and basophils, producing sneezing, itchy nasal membranes, and watery eyes. A *delayed* hypersensitivity reaction also occurs 4 to 8 hours after the initial exposure, causing continuous inflammation of the mucosa and adding to the chronic nasal congestion experienced by these patients. Because histamine is released during an allergic response, many signs and symptoms of allergy are similar to those of inflammation (chapter 33∞). The pathophysiology of allergic rhinitis is illustrated in ➤ Figure 38.2.

The therapeutic goals of treating allergic rhinitis are to prevent its occurrence and to relieve symptoms. Thus, drugs used to treat allergic rhinitis may thus be grouped into two basic categories: preventers and relievers. *Preventers* are used for prophylaxis and include antihistamines, intranasal corticosteroids, and mast cell stabilizers. *Relievers* are used to provide immediate, though temporary, relief for acute allergy symptoms once they have occurred. Relievers include the oral and intranasal decongestants, usually drugs from the sympathomimetic class. In addition to treating allergic rhinitis with drugs, the nurse should help patients identify sources of the allergy and recommend appropriate interventions. These may include removing pets from the home

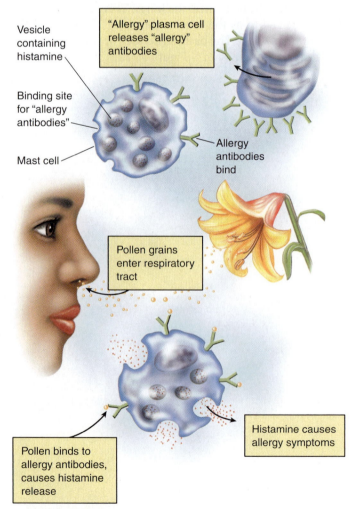

➤ *Figure 38.2* Allergic rhinitis

environment, cleaning moldy surfaces, using microfilters on air conditioning units, and cleaning dust mites out of bedding, carpet, or couches.

H$_1$-Receptor Antagonists/Antihistamines

Antihistamines block the actions of histamine at the H$_1$ receptor. They are widely used as over-the-counter (OTC) remedies for relief of allergy symptoms, motion sickness, and insomnia. These agents are listed in Table 38.1.

38.3 Treating Allergic Rhinitis with H$_1$-Receptor Antagonists

Histamine is a chemical mediator of inflammation that is responsible for many of the symptoms of allergic rhinitis. When released from mast cells and basophils, histamine reaches its receptors to cause itching, increased mucus secretion, and nasal congestion. In more severe allergic states, histamine release may cause bronchoconstriction, edema, hypotension, and other symptoms of anaphylaxis. The histamine receptors responsible for allergic symptoms are called **H$_1$ receptors.** The other major histamine receptor, H$_2$, is found in the gastric mucosa and is responsible for peptic ulcers (chapter 40 ∞).

Antihistamines are drugs that selectively block the actions of histamine at the H$_1$ receptor, thus alleviating allergic symptoms. Because the term *antihistamine* is nonspecific and does not indicate which of the two histamine receptors are affected, H$_1$-receptor antagonist is a more accurate name. In clinical practice, as well as in this text, the two terms are used interchangeably.

The most frequent therapeutic use of antihistamines is for the treatment of allergies. These medications provide symptomatic relief from the characteristic sneezing, runny nose, and itching of the eyes, nose, and throat of allergic rhinitis. Antihistamines are often combined with decongestants and antitussives in OTC cold and sinus medicines. Common OTC antihistamine combinations used to treat allergies are listed in Table 38.2. Antihistamines are most effective when taken prophylactically to *prevent* allergic symptoms; their effectiveness in *reversing* allergic symptoms is limited. Their effectiveness may diminish with long-term use.

In addition to producing their antihistamine effects, these drugs also cause typical anticholinergic effects. Anticholinergic effects are responsible for certain beneficial effects of the antihistamines, such as drying of mucous membranes, which results in less nasal congestion and tearing.

A large number of H$_1$-receptor antagonists are available as medications. They all have the same basic mechanism of action and are equally effective in treating allergic rhinitis and other mild allergies. Adverse effects are similar but

MyNursingKit | Pollen and Allergic Rhinitis

TABLE 38.1	H$_1$-Receptor Antagonists	
Drug	**Route and Adult Dose (max dose where indicated)**	**Adverse Effects**
FIRST-GENERATION AGENTS		
azelastine (Astelin)	Intranasal; 2 sprays per nostril bid	*Dry mouth, headache, dizziness, urinary retention, thickening of bronchial secretions, nausea, vomiting*
brompheniramine (Dimetapp, others)	PO; 4–8 mg tid–qid (max: 40 mg/day)	
chlorpheniramine (Chlor-Trimeton, others)	PO; 2–4 mg tid–qid (max: 24 mg/day)	
clemastine (Tavist)	PO; 1.34–2.68 mg bid (max: 8.04 mg/day)	Paradoxical excitation, sedation, hypersensitivity reactions, hypotension, extrapyramidal symptoms (promethazine), agranulocytosis (brompheniramine, promethazine), respiratory depression
cyproheptadine	PO; 4–20 mg tid or qid (max: 0.5 mg/kg/day)	
dexbrompheniramine (Drixoral)	PO; 6 mg bid	
dexchlorpheniramine (Dexchlor, Poladex, Polaramine)	PO; 2 mg every 4–6 h (max: 12 mg/day)	
dimenhydrinate (Dramamine)	PO; 50–100 mg every 4–6 hr	
diphenhydramine (Benadryl, others)	PO; 25–50 mg three to four times daily (max: 300 mg/day)	
promethazine (Phenergan)	PO; 12.5–25 mg/day (max: 100 mg/day)	
triprolidine (Zymine)	PO; 2.5 mg bid or tid (max: 10 mg/day)	
SECOND-GENERATION AGENTS		
cetirizine (Zyrtec)	PO; 5–10 mg/day (max: 10 mg/day)	*Dry mouth, headache, dizziness, urinary retention, nausea*
desloratadine (Clarinex)	PO; 5 mg/day (max: 5 mg/day)	
fexofenadine (Allegra)	PO; 60 mg bid or 180 mg once daily	Paradoxical excitation, hypersensitivity reactions, hypotension
levocetirizine (Xyzal)	PO; 5 mg (1 tablet or 2 teaspoons) once daily	
loratadine (Claritin)	PO; 10 mg/day	
olopatadine (Patanase)	Intranasal; 2 sprays per nostril bid	
Italics indicate common adverse effects; underlining indicates serious adverse effects.		

TABLE 38.2	Selected OTC Antihistamine Combinations		
Brand Name	Antihistamine	Decongestant	Analgesic
Actifed Cold and Allergy tablets	chlorpheniramine	phenylephrine	_____
Actifed Cold and Allergy	chlorpheniramine	phenylephrine	_____
Benadryl Allergy/Cold caplets	diphenhydramine	phenylephrine	acetaminophen
Chlor-Trimeton Allergy/Decongestant tablets	chlorpheniramine	pseudoephedrine	_____
Dimetapp Children's Cold and Allergy	brompheniramine	phenylephrine	_____
Sudafed PE Sinus and Allergy tablets	chlorpheniramine	phenylephrine	_____
Sudafed PE Nighttime Cold	diphenhydramine	phenylephrine	acetaminophen
Tavist Allergy tablets	clemastine	_____	_____
Triaminic Cold/Allergy	chlorpheniramine	phenylephrine	_____
Tylenol Allergy Sinus caplets	chlorpheniramine	phenylephrine	acetaminophen
Tylenol PM Gelcaps	diphenhydramine	_____	acetaminophen

differ in intensity among the various antihistamines. The older, first-generation drugs have the potential to cause significant drowsiness, which can be a limiting adverse effect in some patients. After a few doses, tolerance generally develops to this sedative action. The newer, second-generation agents have less tendency to cause sedation. Alcohol and other CNS depressants should be used with caution when taking antihistamines, because their sedating effects may be additive, even for the second-generation agents. Some patients exhibit CNS *stimulation,* which can cause insomnia, nervousness, and tremors.

Anticholinergic adverse effects are also common in some patients. These include excessive drying of mucous membranes, which can lead to dry mouth, and urinary hesitancy, an effect that is troublesome for patients with prostatic hypertrophy. Some antihistamines produce more pronounced anticholinergic effects than others. Diphenhydramine and clemastine produce the greatest incidence of anticholinergic

Pr Prototype Drug | Diphenhydramine (Benadryl, others)

Therapeutic Class: Drug to treat allergies | **Pharmacologic Class:** H_1-receptor antagonist; antihistamine

ACTIONS AND USES

Diphenhydramine is a first-generation H_1-receptor antagonist whose primary use is to treat minor symptoms of allergy and the common cold such as sneezing, runny nose, and tearing of the eyes. Diphenhydramine is often combined with an analgesic, decongestant, or expectorant in OTC cold and flu products. Diphenhydramine is also administered topically to treat rashes, and IM/IV forms are available for severe allergic reactions. Other indications for diphenhydramine include Parkinson's disease, motion sickness, and insomnia.

ADMINISTRATION ALERTS

- There is an increased risk of anaphylactic shock when this drug is administered parenterally.
- When administering IV, inject at a rate of 25 mg/min to reduce the risk of shock.
- When administering IM, inject deep into a large muscle to minimize tissue irritation.
- Pregnancy category C

PHARMACOKINETICS

Onset: 15–30 min

Peak: 1–4 h

Half-life: 3–7 h

Duration: 4–7 h

ADVERSE EFFECTS

First-generation H_1-receptor antagonists such as diphenhydramine cause significant drowsiness, although this usually diminishes with long-term use. Occasionally, paradoxical CNS stimulation and excitability will be observed, rather than drowsiness. Excitation is more frequent in children than adults. Anticholinergic effects such as dry mouth, tachycardia, and mild hypotension occur in some patients. Diphenhydramine may cause photosensitivity.

Contraindications: Hypersensitivity to the drug, prostatic hypertrophy, narrow-angle glaucoma, and GI obstruction are contraindications of use. The drug should be used cautiously in patients with asthma or hyperthyroidism.

INTERACTIONS

Drug–Drug: Use with CNS depressants such as alcohol or opioids will cause increased sedation. Other OTC cold preparations may increase anticholinergic side effects. MAO inhibitors may cause a hypertensive crisis.

Lab Tests: Drug should be discontinued at least 4 days prior to skin allergy tests; otherwise, false-negative tests may result.

Herbal/Food: Henbane may cause increased anticholinergic effects.

Treatment of Overdose: Overdose may cause either CNS depression or excitation. There is no specific treatment for overdose.

Refer to MyNursingKit for a Nursing Process Focus specific to this drug.

side effects, whereas the second-generation agents—loratadine, desloratadine, and fexofenadine—produce the least.

Although most antihistamines are given orally, two are available by the intranasal route. Azelastine (Astelin) is approved for nonallergic rhinitis and is as safe and effective as the oral antihistamines. Although a first-generation agent, azelastine causes less drowsiness than others in its class because it is applied locally to the nasal mucosa, and limited systemic absorption occurs. Olopatadine (Patanase) is a second-generation antihistamine approved in 2008 for allergic rhinitis.

In addition to allergic rhinitis, antihistamines have been used to treat a number of other disorders. These include the following:

- *Vertigo and motion sickness:* Nausea resulting from vertigo or motion sickness responds well to antihistamines. These drugs act by suppressing the vomiting center in the medulla and depressing neurons of the vestibular apparatus of the inner ear. To be effective, they must be taken prior to the onset of symptoms. Meclizine (Antivert) and dimenhydrinate (Dramamine) are two common antihistamines used for this purpose. The pharmacotherapy of nausea is discussed in chapter 41∞.

- *Parkinson's disease:* Drugs with significant anticholinergic actions are used to treat mild forms of Parkinson's disease. They are also used to treat the tremor and certain other adverse effects of conventional antipsychotic drugs. Because diphenhydramine exhibits greater anticholinergic action, it is sometimes used to treat these conditions. The pharmacotherapy of Parkinson's disease is discussed in chapter 20∞.

- *Insomnia:* Many patients become drowsy after taking first-generation antihistamines. OTC sleep aids usually include antihistamines such as diphenhydramine and doxylamine (Unisom Sleep Tabs). After a few days, patients will become tolerant to the drowsiness produced by these drugs; thus, they should be used for 2 weeks or less.

- *Urticaria and other skin rashes:* Urticaria or hives is often caused by the release of histamine; thus, the condition responds well to H_1-receptor antagonists. Symptomatic treatment may include any of the first- or second-generation agents, either using oral drugs or topical creams or lotions.

Intranasal Corticosteroids

Corticosteroids, also known as glucocorticoids, may be applied directly to the nasal mucosa to prevent symptoms of allergic rhinitis. They have largely replaced antihistamines as preferred drugs for the treatment of perennial allergic rhinitis. These drugs are listed in Table 38.3.

38.4 Treating Allergic Rhinitis with Intranasal Corticosteroids

The importance of the corticosteroids in treating severe inflammation was presented in chapter 33∞. Although corticosteroids are very effective, their use as *systemic* therapy is limited by potentially serious adverse effects. *Intranasal* corticosteroids, however, produce virtually no serious adverse effects. Because of their effectiveness and safety, the intranasal corticosteroids are often first-line drugs in the treatment of allergic rhinitis. Some of the corticosteroids are

---

Pr Prototype Drug | Fluticasone *(Flonase, Veramyst, others)*

Therapeutic Class: Drug for allergic rhinitis   **Pharmacologic Class:** Intranasal corticosteroid

ACTIONS AND USES
Fluticasone is typical of the intranasal corticosteroids used to treat seasonal allergic rhinitis. Therapy usually begins with two sprays in each nostril, twice daily, and decreases to one dose per day. Fluticasone acts to decrease local inflammation in the nasal passages, thus reducing nasal stuffiness.

ADMINISTRATION ALERTS
- Instruct the patient to carefully follow the directions for use provided by the manufacturer.
- Pregnancy category C

PHARMACOKINETICS
Onset: Unknown

Peak: Unknown

Half-life: 3 h

Duration: 12–24 h

ADVERSE EFFECTS
Adverse effects of fluticasone are rare. Swallowing large amounts increases the potential for systemic corticosteroid adverse effects. Nasal irritation and epistaxis occur in a small number of patients.

Contraindications: The only contraindication to fluticasone is prior hypersensitivity to the drug. Because corticosteroids can mask signs of infection, patients with known bacterial, viral, fungal, or parasitic infections (especially of the respiratory tract) should not receive intranasal corticosteroids.

INTERACTIONS
Drug–Drug: Concomitant use of an intranasal decongestant increases the risk of nasal irritation or bleeding. Use with ritonavir should be avoided, as this drug significantly increases plasma fluticasone levels.

Lab Tests: Unknown

Herbal/Food: Use with caution with licorice, which may potentiate the effects of corticosteroids.

Treatment of Overdose: There is no specific treatment for overdose.

Refer to MyNursingKit for a Nursing Process Focus specific to this drug.

NURSING PROCESS FOCUS   PATIENTS RECEIVING ANTIHISTAMINE THERAPY

Assessment	Potential Nursing Diagnoses
Baseline assessment prior to administration: • Understand the reason the drug has been prescribed in order to assess for therapeutic effects. • Obtain a complete health history including previous history of symptoms and association to seasons, foods, or environmental exposures; existing cardiovascular, respiratory, hepatic, renal, or neurologic disease; glaucoma; prostatic hypertrophy or difficulty with urination; presence of fever or active infections; pregnancy or breast-feeding; alcohol use; or smoking. Obtain a drug history, noting the type of adverse reaction or allergy experienced to any medications. • If allergy symptoms are of new onset, assess for any recent changes in diet, soaps, cosmetics, lotions, environment, or recent carpet cleaning, particularly in infants and young children. • Obtain baseline vital signs. An ECG may be ordered for patients with a history of cardiac conditions. • Evaluate appropriate laboratory findings (e.g., CBC, hepatic and renal labs).	• Ineffective Airway Clearance • Ineffective Breathing Pattern • Disturbed Sleep Pattern (related to adverse drug effects) • Fatigue • Deficient Knowledge (drug therapy) • Risk for Injury, Risk for Falls (related to adverse drug effects)
Assessment throughout administration: • Assess for desired therapeutic effects (e.g., decreased nasal congestion and drainage, decreased eye watering or itching). • Continue periodic monitoring of CBC, and liver and renal function studies as appropriate. • Assess vital signs, especially pulse rate and rhythm. • Assess for adverse effects: dizziness, drowsiness, dry mouth, blurred vision, or headache. Report immediately any increasing fever, confusion, muscle weakness, tachycardia, palpitations, hypotension, syncope, dyspnea, pulmonary congestion, urinary retention, and sudden severe eye pain or rainbow halos around lights.	

Planning: Patient Goals and Expected Outcomes

The patient will:
- Experience therapeutic effects (e.g., decreased nasal congestion and drainage, decreased eye watering and itching).
- Be free from, or experience minimal, adverse effects.
- Verbalize an understanding of the drug's use, adverse effects, and required precautions.
- Demonstrate proper self-administration of the medication (e.g., dose, timing, when to notify provider).

Implementation

Interventions and (Rationales)	Patient and Family Education
Ensuring therapeutic effects: • Continue assessments as described earlier for therapeutic effects. (Improvement in symptoms of allergy should begin after taking the first dose and continue to improve. The health care provider should be notified if symptoms continue to increase, especially if respiratory involvement worsens.)	• Teach the patient to supplement drug therapy with nonpharmacologic measures such as increased fluid intake to liquefy and assist to mobilize mucus and to reduce exposure to allergens where possible. • Advise the patient to carry a wallet identification card or wear medical identification jewelry indicating any significant allergies or anaphylyaxis.
• For treatment of seasonal allergies, drug therapy should be started *before* the beginning of the allergy season and appearance of symptoms. (Beginning drug therapy before the circulating histamine increases will result in greater therapeutic effects. Starting drug therapy after allergy symptoms are severe will require several doses before marked improvement of symptoms is noted.)	• Teach the patient to begin taking the drug before allergy season begins or at the earliest possible appearance of symptoms for best effects.
Minimizing adverse effects: • Ensure patient safety, especially in older adults. Observe for dizziness. Monitor ambulation until the effects of the drug are known. (Drowsiness or dizziness from orthostatic hypotension may occur and increases the risk of falls. Drowsiness tends to diminish over several doses.)	• Instruct the patient to call for assistance prior to getting out of bed or attempting to walk alone, and to avoid driving or other activities requiring mental alertness or physical coordination until the effects of the drug are known.

NURSING PROCESS FOCUS   PATIENTS RECEIVING ANTIHISTAMINE THERAPY *(Continued)*

Implementation

Interventions and (Rationales)	Patient and Family Education
■ Continue to monitor vital signs, especially pulse rate and rhythm for patients with existing cardiac disease. ECGs may be ordered periodically for patients with history of dysrhythmias. (Histamine plays a role in cardiac conduction and when blocked by antihistamines, may cause dysrhythmias in patients with history of cardiac disease.)	■ Instruct the patient to immediately report dizziness, palpitations, or syncope. ■ Teach the patient, family, or caregiver how to monitor pulse and blood pressure as appropriate. Ensure the proper use and functioning of any home equipment obtained.
■ Continue to monitor periodic hepatic and renal function labs, especially in patients on long-term antihistamine use or those with a previous history of hepatic or renal impairment. (Hepatic toxicity is a potential adverse effect of antihistamines. Impaired renal function will inhibit drug excretion and prolong effects.)	■ Instruct the patient on the need to return periodically for lab work.
■ Monitor for persistent dry cough, increasing cough severity, increasing congestion, or dyspnea. (Antihistamines are used with extreme caution in patients with existing respiratory disease, including COPD. Thickened mucus is a potential adverse drug effect. A change in the severity of the cough may indicate increasing allergic response, worsening disease process, or respiratory infection and should be reported immediately.)	■ Instruct the patient to promptly report any change in the severity or frequency of cough. Any cough accompanied by a shortness of breath, increasing congestion, fever, or chest pain should be reported immediately. ■ Encourage the patient to increase fluid intake to assist in liquifying mucous secretions and to ease dry mouth effects.
■ Assess for CNS effects including restlessness, nervousness, insomnia, headache, tremors, fatigue, or weakness. Report severe symptoms or any disorientation or confusion immediately. (CNS depressant effects such as drowsiness, fatigue, or mild weakness are common. Paradoxical excitement such as restlessness, nervousness, or insomnia may occur, especially in children. Alcohol consumption increases the CNS depressant effects and should be avoided.)	■ Instruct the patient, family, or caregiver to report increasing lethargy, disorientation, confusion, changes in behavior or mood, agitation or aggression, slurred speech, or ataxia immediately. ■ Instruct the patient to avoid or eliminate alcohol consumption while on antihistamines.
■ If used for sleep, ensure patient safety on awakening. Avoid using antihistamines for sleep for more than 2 weeks and consult the health care provider if insomnia continues. (Morning or daytime drowsiness, a "hangover" effect, may occur in some patients taking antihistamines for sleep and may impair normal acitivities. Patients may become tolerant to drowsiness-inducing effects within 2 weeks.)	■ Caution the patient about possible morning or daytime sleepiness and to exercise caution with activities requiring mental alertness or physical coordination until daytime effects of the drug are known. Do not keep the medication at the bedside to prevent overdosage from occurring if additional doses are taken when drowsy. Do not take the medication concurrently with alcohol.
■ Assess for changes in visual acuity, blurred vision, loss of peripheral vision, seeing rainbow halos around lights, acute eye pain, or any of these symptoms accompanied by nausea and vomiting and report immediately. (Increased intraocular pressure in patients with narrow-angle glaucoma may occur with antihistamines.)	■ Instruct the patient to report any visual changes or eye pain immediately.
■ Assess for urinary retention, especially in males over 40 or with a history of prostatic hypertrophy. (Antihistamines may cause urinary retention.)	■ Instruct the patient to immediately report inability to void, and increasing bladder pressure or pain.
■ Monitor for GI effects. (Nausea, vomiting, epigastric distress, anorexia, constipation, or diarrhea may occur and are treated symptomatically.)	■ Teach the patient to take the medication with food or milk. Report any significant GI symptoms (e.g., nausea with vomiting, diarrhea) to the health care provider.
■ Monitor for anticholinergic-related adverse effects including dry mouth, thickened mucus, nasal dryness, slightly blurred vision, and headache. (Mild anticholinergic effects are common and are treated symptomatically. Significant symptoms as listed previously are reported immediately.)	■ Teach the patient to increase fluid intake or suck on hard candy to relieve mouth and respiratory tract dryness. Exercise caution if blurred vision impairs normal activities and report significant visual disturbances as listed previously.
Patient understanding of drug therapy: ■ Use opportunities during administration of medications and during assessments to discuss the rationale for drug therapy, desired therapeutic outcomes, most common adverse effects, parameters for when to call the health care provider, and any necessary monitoring or precautions. (Using time during nursing care helps to optimize and reinforce key teaching areas.)	■ The patient should be able to state the reason for the drug, appropriate dose and scheduling, what adverse effects to observe for, and when to report them.

(Continued)

NURSING PROCESS FOCUS   PATIENTS RECEIVING ANTIHISTAMINE THERAPY *(Continued)*

Implementation

Interventions and (Rationales)	Patient and Family Education
Patient self-administration of drug therapy: ■ When administering the medication, instruct the patient, family, or caregiver in the proper self-administration of drug, e.g., take the drug before allergy season or before symptoms are severe. (Proper administration will increase the effectiveness of the drug.)	■ The patient and family or caregiver should be able to discuss appropriate dosing and administration needs.

Evaluation of Outcome Criteria

Evaluate the effectiveness of drug therapy by confirming that patient goals and expected outcomes have been met (see "Planning").

See Table 38.1 for a list of drugs to which these nursing actions apply.

TABLE 38.3	Intranasal Corticosteroids	
Drug	**Route and Adult Dose (max dose where indicated)**	**Adverse Effects**
beclomethasone (Beconase AQ, Qvar) (see page 600 for the Prototype Drug box∞)	Intranasal; 1 spray in each nostril bid–qid	*Transient nasal irritation, burning, sneezing, or dryness* <u>Hypercorticism (only if large amounts are swallowed)</u>
budesonide (Rhinocort Aqua)	Intranasal; 2 sprays in each nostril bid	
ciclesonide (Omnaris)	Intranasal: 2 sprays once daily (max 200 mcg/day)	
flunisolide (Nasalide, Nasarel)	Intranasal; 2 sprays in each nostril bid; may increase to tid if needed	
℗ fluticasone (Flonase, Veramyst, others)	Intranasal; 1 spray in each nostril once (Veramyst) or twice (Flonase) daily	
mometasone (Nasonex)	Intranasal; 2 sprays in each nostril/day	
triamcinolone acetonide (Nasacort AQ)	Intranasal; 2 sprays in each nostril daily	

Italics indicate common adverse effects; <u>underlining</u> indicates serious adverse effects.

also administered by inhaler for the treatment of asthma (chapter 39∞).

When sprayed onto the nasal mucosa, corticosteroids decrease the secretion of inflammatory mediators, reduce tissue edema, and cause a mild vasoconstriction. They are administered with a metered-spray device that delivers a consistent dose of drug per spray. All have equal effectiveness. Unlike with the sympathomimetics (Section 38.5), benefits are not immediate; 2 to 3 weeks may be required to achieve peak response. Because of this delayed effect, intranasal corticosteroids are most effective when taken in advance of the allergen exposure.

When corticosteroids are administered correctly, their action is limited to the nasal passages. The most frequently reported adverse effect is an intense burning sensation in the nose that occurs immediately after spraying. Excessive drying of the nasal mucosa may occur, leading to epistaxis.

For patients who do not respond to intranasal corticosteroids, intranasal cromolyn (NasalCrom) is an alternative. Because it inhibits the release of histamine from mast cells, cromolyn is called a *mast cell stabilizer*. Most effective when given prior to allergen exposure, cromolyn has few adverse effects, and was recently approved as an OTC drug for the treat-

ment of allergy and cold symptoms. Further discussion on the mast cell stabilizers is presented in chapter 39∞, because asthma is a second indication for drugs in this class. Other alternatives to the intranasal corticosteroids in treating allergies include montelukast (Singulair) and omalizumab (Xolair).

Decongestants

Decongestants are drugs that relieve nasal congestion. They are administered by either the oral or intranasal routes and are often combined with antihistamines in the pharmacotherapy of allergies or the common cold. Doses for the nasal decongestants are listed in Table 38.4.

38.5 Treating Nasal Congestion with Decongestants

Most decongestants are sympathomimetics: agents that activate the sympathetic nervous system. Sympathomimetics with alpha-adrenergic activity are effective at relieving the nasal congestion associated with the common cold or allergic rhinitis when given by either the oral or intranasal route. The intranasal preparations such as oxymetazoline (Afrin,

TABLE 38.4	Nasal Decongestants	
Drug	**Route and Adult Dose (max dose where indicated)**	**Adverse Effects**
SYMPATHOMIMETICS		
ephedrine (Pretz-D)	Intranasal (0.25%); 2–3 sprays/nostril, not more frequently than every 4 hrs	*Intranasal: transient nasal irritation, burning, sneezing, or dryness, headache*
naphazoline (Privine)	Intranasal; 2 drops each nostril every 3–6 h	*PO: nervousness, insomnia, headache, dry mouth*
oxymetazoline (Afrin 12 Hour, Neo-Synephrine 12 Hour, others)	Intranasal (0.05%); 2–3 sprays each nostril bid for up to 3–5 days	Intranasal: rebound congestion
phenylephrine (Afrin 4–6 Hour, Neo-Synephrine 4–6 Hour, others)	Intranasal (0.1%); 2–3 drops or sprays each nostril every 3–4 h, as needed	CNS excitation, tremors, dysrhythmias, tachycardia, difficulty in voiding, severe vasoconstriction
pseudoephedrine (Actifed, Sudafed, others)	PO; 60 mg 4–6h (max: 240 mg/day)	
tetrahydrozoline (Tyzine)	Intranasal; 2–4 drops or sprays each nostril every 3 h	
xylometazoline (Otrivin)	Intranasal (0.1%); 1–2 sprays each nostril bid (max: three doses/day)	
ANTICHOLINERGIC		
ipratropium bromide (Atrovent, Combivent)	Nasal spray; 2 sprays in each nostril three to four times/day up to 4 days	*Transient nasal irritation, burning, sneezing, or dryness, cough, headache*
		Urinary retention, worsening of narrow-angle glaucoma

Italics indicate common adverse effects; underlining indicates serious adverse effects.

others) are available OTC as sprays or drops, and produce an effective response within minutes.

Intranasal sympathomimetics produce few systemic effects because almost none of the drug is absorbed into the circulation. The most serious, limiting side effect of the intranasal preparations is **rebound congestion,** a condition characterized by hypersecretion of mucus and worsening nasal congestion once the drug effects wear off. This can lead to a cycle of increased drug use as the condition worsens. Because of this rebound congestion, intranasal sympathomimetics should be used for no longer than 3 to 5 days. Patients with allergic rhinitis who develop tolerance to the effects of decongestants should be gradually switched to intranasal corticosteroids because they do not cause rebound congestion.

When administered *orally,* sympathomimetics do not produce rebound congestion. Their onset of action by this route, however, is much slower than when administered intranasally, and they are less effective at relieving severe congestion. The possibility of systemic adverse effects is also greater with the oral drugs. Potential adverse effects include hypertension and CNS stimulation that may lead to insomnia and anxiety.

Prior to 2000, pseudoephedrine was the most common decongestant included in oral OTC cold and allergy medicines. Pseudoephedrine, however, is the starting chemical for the illegal synthesis of methamphetamine by drug traffickers. Although still OTC, pharmacists are required to monitor distribution of pseudoephedrine by keeping a log of patient names and address, checking the photo identification of the buyer, and limiting the quantities of the drug that are sold at one time. It should be noted that these precautions are not being taken because pseudoephedrine itself is a dangerous drug, but to limit the availability of the drug to illicit makers of methamphetamine. Manufacturers have reformulated their OTC cold medicines to contain phenylephrine rather than pseudoephedrine. A drug prototype feature for phenylephrine is included in chapter 13∞.

Because the sympathomimetics relieve only nasal congestion, they are often combined with antihistamines to control sneezing and tearing. It is interesting to note that some OTC drugs having the same basic name (Neo-Synephrine, Afrin, and Vicks) may contain different sympathomimetics. For example, Neo-Synephrine decongestants with 12-hour duration contain the drug oxymetazoline; Neo-Synephrine preparations that last 4 to 6 hours contain phenylephrine.

One anticholinergic, ipratropium (Atrovent), is used as a decongestant. Given by the intranasal route, ipratropium has no serious adverse effects. Its actions are limited to decreasing rhinorrhea; it does not stop the sneezing, postnasal drip, or itchy throat or eyes characteristic of allergic rhinitis or the common cold. A more common indication for ipratropium is in the pharmacotherapy of asthma, and a prototype feature for this drug may be found in chapter 39∞.

Pr Prototype Drug | Oxymetazoline (Afrin, others)

Therapeutic Class: Nasal decongestant   **Pharmacologic Class:** Sympathomimetic

ACTIONS AND USES

Oxymetazoline activates alpha-adrenergic receptors in the sympathetic nervous system. This causes arterioles in the nasal passages to constrict, thus drying the mucous membranes. Relief from nasal congestion occurs within minutes and lasts for 10 or more hours. Oxymetazoline is administered with a metered spray device or by nasal drops.

Oxymetazoline (Visine LR) is also available as eye drops. It causes vasoconstriction of vessels in the eye and is used to relieve redness and provide relief from dryness and minor eye irritations.

ADMINISTRATION ALERTS

- Wash hands carefully after administration to prevent anisocoria (blurred vision and inequality of pupil size).
- Pregnancy category C

PHARMACOKINETICS

Onset: 5–10 min

Peak: Unknown

Half-life: Unknown

Duration: 6–10 h

ADVERSE EFFECTS

Rebound congestion is common when oxymetazoline is used for longer than 3 to 5 days. Minor stinging and dryness in the nasal mucosa may be experienced. Systemic adverse effects are unlikely, unless a large amount of the medicine is swallowed.

Contraindications: Patients with thyroid disorders, hypertension, diabetes, or heart disease should use sympathomimetics only on the direction of their health care provider.

INTERACTIONS

Drug–Drug: No clinically important interactions occur, because absorption of oxymetazoline is limited.

Lab Tests: Unknown

Herbal/Food: Use with caution with herbal supplements such as St. John's wort that have properties of monoamine oxidase inhibitors.

Treatment of Overdose: There is no specific treatment for overdose.

Refer to MyNursingKit for a Nursing Process Focus specific to this drug.

HOME & COMMUNITY CONSIDERATIONS

Dextromethorphan and Drug Abuse

Dextromethorphan (DXM), a nonnarcotic cough suppressant available OTC has also gained the reputation and popularity as a hallucinogenic drug that is abused for the psychotropic effects it provides. It is known by names such as "DXM," "DM," "Robo," and "Velvet." Dissociative anesthesia effects, where the user experiences feeling "out of body," are similar to ketamine (chapter 19∞) and the illegal substance PCP. These effects are experienced by users after larger-than-normal doses are taken and may last up to 6 hours. Extra-strength cough syrups with dextromethorphan are the most frequently abused.

OTC cough medications are widely available and when taken in recommended doses, dextromethorphan is a safe and effective cough suppressant. The nurse should be aware of the potential for abuse of DXM and should counsel patients to avoid exceeding the recommended dose. Of particular concern are cough medications containing DXM and antihistamines or decongestants. While users may take extra-large doses to experience the psychotropic effects of DXM, additional antihistamine or decongestant doses may significantly increase the risks of dextromethorphan abuse. Nurses play a vital role in providing patients with accurate information about the dangers of abusing medications, including those available OTC.

AVOIDING MEDICATION ERRORS

A 42-year-old woman is admitted to the medical floor for observation after suffering several fractured ribs and dyspnea, secondary to severe coughing from acute bronchitis. Benzonatate (Tessalon Perles) 100 mg tid is ordered. The nurse brings in the medication and the patient states "I don't think I can take that. My coughing is so bad, I don't think I can swallow it." The nurse punctures the perle with a sterile needle to enable the patient to swallow the liquid inside. The patient experiences significant respiratory distress after swallowing the medication and the nurse calls for the emergency response team. What error did the nurse make and what should have been done differently?

See Appendix D for the suggested answer.

same drugs classes used for allergic rhinitis, including antihistamines and decongestants. A few additional drugs, such as those that suppress cough and loosen bronchial secretions, are used for symptomatic treatment.

COMMON COLD

The common cold is a viral infection of the upper respiratory tract that produces a characteristic array of annoying symptoms. It is fortunate that the disorder is self-limiting, because there is no cure or effective prevention for colds. Therapies used to relieve symptoms include some of the

Antitussives

Antitussives are drugs used to dampen the cough reflex. They are of value in treating coughs due to allergies or the common cold.

38.6 Pharmacotherapy with Antitussives

Cough is a natural reflex mechanism that serves to forcibly remove excess secretions and foreign material from the respiratory system. In diseases such as emphysema and bronchitis, or when liquids have been aspirated into the bronchi, it is not desirable to suppress the normal cough reflex. Dry, hacking, nonproductive cough, however, can be irritating to the membranes of the throat and can deprive a patient of much-needed rest. It is these types of conditions in which therapy with medications that control cough, known as **antitussives,** may be warranted. Antitussives are classified as opioid or nonopioid and are listed in Table 38.5.

Opioids, the most effective antitussives, act by raising the cough threshold in the CNS. Codeine and hydrocodone are the most frequently used opioid antitussives. Doses needed to suppress the cough reflex are very low; thus, there is minimal potential for dependence. Most opioid cough mixtures are classified as Schedule III, IV, or V drugs, and are reserved for more serious cough conditions. Though not common, overdose from opioid cough remedies may cause significant respiratory depression. Care must be taken when using these medications in patients with asthma, because bronchoconstriction may occur. Opioids may be combined with other agents such as antihistamines, decongestants, and nonopioid antitussives in the therapy of severe cold or flu symptoms. Some of these combinations are listed in Table 38.6.

TABLE 38.5	Selected Antitussives and Expectorants	
Drug	**Route and Adult Dose (max dose where indicated)**	**Adverse Effects**
ANTITUSSIVES: OPIOIDS		
codeine	PO; 10–20 mg every 4–6 h prn (max: 120 mg/24 h)	*Nausea, vomiting, constipation, confusion, dizziness, sedation*
hydrocodone combined with homatropine (Hycodan, others)	PO; 1 tablet or 5 mL every 4–6 h as needed (max: 30 mL/day or 6 tablets/day)	<u>Hypotension, seizures, bradycardia, respiratory depression, severe somnolence</u>
ANTITUSSIVES: NONOPIOIDS		
benzonatate (Tessalon)	PO; 100 mg tid prn (max: 600 mg/day)	*Drowsiness, constipation, GI upset*
		<u>Paradoxical excitation, tremors, euphoria, insomnia</u>
Pr dextromethorphan (Delsym, Robitussin, others)	PO; 10–20 mg every 4 h or 30 mg every 6–8 h (max: 120 mg/day)	*Drowsiness, headache, GI upset*
		<u>CNS depression, paradoxical excitation, respiratory depression</u>
EXPECTORANT		
guaifenesin (Mucinex, Robitussin, others)	PO; 200–400 mg every 4 h (max: 2.4 g/day) Extended release PO; 600–1,200 mg every 12 h (max: 2,400 mg/day)	*Drowsiness, headache, GI upset*
		<u>No serious adverse effects</u>
MUCOLYTIC		
acetylcysteine (Acetadote, Mucomyst)	MDI; Inhalation: 1–10 mL of 20% solution every 4–6 h or 2–20 mL of 10% solution every 4–6 h	*Unpleasant odor, nausea*
		<u>Severe nausea and vomiting, bronchospasm</u>

TABLE 38.6	Selected Opioid Combination Drugs for Severe Cold Symptoms	
Trade Name	**Opioid**	**Nonopioid Active Ingredients**
Ambenyl Cough Syrup	codeine	bromodiphenhydramine
Calcidrine Syrup	codeine	calcium iodide
Codamine Syrup	hydrocodone	phenylpropanolamine
Codiclear DH Syrup	hydrocodone	guaifenesin
Codimal DH	hydrocodone	phenylephrine, pyrilamine
Hycodan	hydrocodone	homatropine
Hycomine Compound	hydrocodone	phenylephrine, chlorpheniramine, acetaminophen
Hycotuss Expectorant	hydrocodone	guaifenesin
Novahistine DH	codeine	pseudoephedrine, chlorpheniramine
Phenergan with Codeine	codeine	promethazine
Robitussin A-C	codeine	guaifenesin
Tega-Tussin Syrup	hydrocodone	phenylephrine, chlorpheniramine
Tussionex	hydrocodone	chlorpheniramine

The most frequently used nonopioid antitussive is dextromethorphan, which is available in OTC cold and flu medications. Dextromethorphan is chemically similar to the opioids, and also acts on the CNS to raise the cough threshold. Though it does not have the same level of abuse potential as the opioids, in large amounts dextromethorphan symptoms of abuse include slurred speech, dizziness, drowsiness, euphoria, and lack of motor coordination.

Benzonatate (Tessalon) is a nonopioid antitussive that acts by a different mechanism. Chemically related to the local anesthetic tetracaine (Pontocaine), benzonatate suppresses the cough reflex by anesthetizing stretch receptors in the lungs. If chewed, the drug can cause the side effect of numbing the mouth and pharynx. Adverse effects are uncommon, but may include sedation, nausea, headache, and dizziness.

COMPLEMENTARY AND ALTERNATIVE THERAPIES

Horehound for Respiratory Disorders

Horehound has been used as an herbal remedy since the ancient Egyptians and was popular with American Indians. In folklore, it was reported to aid in a number of respiratory disorders including asthma, bronchitis, whooping cough, and infections such as tuberculosis. Nonrespiratory uses include bowel disorders, jaundice, and wound healing.

Active ingredients of horehound are found throughout the flowering plant. The chief constituent is a bitter substance called *marrubium* that stimulates secretions. Formulations include tea, dried or fresh leaves, and liquid extracts. Horehound has an expectorant action when treating colds and is also available as cough drops. It is claimed to restore normal secretions to the lung and other organs.

Expectorants and Mucolytics

Several drugs are available to control excess mucus production. Expectorants increase bronchial secretions, and mucolytics help loosen thick bronchial secretions. These agents are listed in Table 38.5.

38.7 Pharmacotherapy with Expectorants and Mucolytics

Expectorants are drugs that reduce the thickness or viscosity of bronchial secretions, thus increasing mucus flow that can then be removed more easily by coughing. The most effective OTC expectorant is guaifenesin (Mucinex, Robitussin,

RESEARCH SHOWS

The Question: Are medications effective in treating children with chronic cough?

The Study: Researchers examined the existing databases for evidence that antitussives, antihistamines, or other medications could reduce nonspecific cough in pediatric patients under age 15. The study found no evidence for using medications for the symptomatic relief of cough in this population. The authors stressed that if medications are used, the health care provider should follow up and stop the medications if there is no effect on the cough within a designated time frame.

Nursing Implications: Nurses should teach patients to obtain the advice of their pediatrician before treating their children with OTC cold and flu drugs for nonspecific cough symptoms.

Source: Chang, A.B. & Glomb, W.B. (2006). Guidelines for Evaluating Chronic Cough in Pediatrics ACCP Evidence-Based Clinical Practice Guidelines. Chest. 129(1 suppl) 260S-283S.

Pr Prototype Drug | Dextromethorphan *(Delsym, Robitussin, others)*

Therapeutic Class: Cough suppressant   **Pharmacologic Class:** Drug for increasing cough threshold

ACTIONS AND USES

Dextromethorphan is a nonopioid drug that is a component in many OTC severe cold and flu preparations. It is available in a large variety of formulations, including tablets, liquid-filled capsules, lozenges, and liquids. It has a rapid onset of action, usually within 15 to 30 minutes. Like codeine, it acts in the medulla, though it lacks the analgesic and euphoric effects of the opioids and does not produce dependence. Patients whose cough is not relieved by dextromethorphan after several days of therapy should see their health care provider.

ADMINISTRATION ALERTS

- Avoid pulmonary irritants, such as smoking or other fumes, because these agents may decrease drug effectiveness.
- Pregnancy category C

PHARMACOKINETICS

Onset: 15–30 min

Peak: Unknown

Half-life: Unknown

Duration: 3–6 h

ADVERSE EFFECTS

At therapeutic doses, adverse effects due to dextromethorphan are rare. Dizziness, drowsiness, and GI upset occur in some patients. In abuse situations, the drug can cause CNS toxicity with a wide variety of symptoms, including slurred speech, ataxia, hyperexcitability, stupor, respiratory depression, seizures, coma, and toxic psychosis.

Contraindications: Dextromethorphan is contraindicated in the treatment of chronic cough due to excessive bronchial secretions, such as in asthma, smoking, and emphysema. Suppressing the cough reflex is not desirable in these patients.

INTERACTIONS

Drug–Drug: Drug interactions with dextromethorphan include excitation, hypotension, and hyperpyrexia when used concurrently with MAO inhibitors. Use with alcohol, opioids, or other CNS depressants may result in sedation.

Lab Tests: Unknown

Herbal/Food: Grapefruit juice can raise serum levels of dextromethorphan and cause toxicity.

Treatment of Overdose: There is no specific treatment for overdose.

Refer to MyNursingKit for a Nursing Process Focus specific to this drug.

others). Like dextromethorphan, guaifenesin produces few adverse effects and is a common ingredient in many OTC multisymptom cold and flu preparations. It is most effective in treating dry, nonproductive cough, but may also be of benefit for patients with productive cough. *Nonprescription cough and cold products (including those containing guaifenesin) should not be used in children under 4 years of age.*

Acetylcysteine (Mucomyst) is one of the few drugs available to *directly* loosen thick, viscous bronchial secretions. Drugs of this type, which are called **mucolytics,** break down the chemical structure of mucus molecules. The mucus becomes thinner, and can be removed more easily by coughing. Acetylcysteine is delivered by the inhalation route and is

not available OTC. It is used in patients who have cystic fibrosis, chronic bronchitis, or other diseases that produce large amounts of thick bronchial secretions. Mucomyst can trigger brochospasm and has an offensive odor resembling rotten eggs. A second mucolytic, dornase alfa (Pulmozyme), is approved for maintenance therapy in the management of thick bronchial secretions. Dornase alfa breaks down DNA molecules in the mucus, causing it to become less viscous.

Acetylcysteine (Acetadote) is also administered by the oral or IV route to patients who have received an overdose of acetaminophen. Its use in the pharmacotherapy of acetaminophen toxicity is presented in chapter 33∞.

NURSING PROCESS FOCUS	PATIENTS RECEIVING SYMPTOMATIC COLD RELIEF: ANTITUSSIVE, NASAL DECONGESTANT, AND EXPECTORANT THERAPY

Assessment	Potential Nursing Diagnoses
Baseline assessment prior to administration: • Understand the reason the drug has been prescribed in order to assess for therapeutic effects. • Obtain a complete health history including previous history and length of symptoms; existing cardiovascular, respiratory, hepatic, or renal disease; presence of fever; pregnancy or breast-feeding; alcohol use; or smoking. Obtain a drug history, including allergies, current prescription and OTC drugs, herbal preparations, caffeine, nicotine, and alcohol use. Be alert to possible drug interactions. • Obtain baseline vital signs. • Evaluate appropriate laboratory findings (e.g., CBC, hepatic and renal labs).	• Ineffective Airway Clearance • Ineffective Breathing Pattern • Disturbed Sleep Pattern (related to adverse drug effects) • Deficient Knowledge (drug therapy) • Risk for Injury (related to adverse drug effects)
Assessment throughout administration: • Assess for desired therapeutic effects (e.g., decreased cough, increased ease in expectorating mucus, clearer nasal passages). • Assess vital signs, especially pulse rate and rhythm in patients with existing cardiac disease. • Assess for adverse effects: dizziness, drowsiness, blurred vision, headache, and epistaxis. Report immediately any increasing fever, tachycardia, palpitations, syncope, dyspnea, pulmonary congestion, or confusion.	

Planning: Patient Goals and Expected Outcomes

The patient will:
• Experience therapeutic effects (e.g., decreased nasal congestion and drainage, increased ease in expectorating mucus, thinner secretions).
• Be free from, or experience minimal, adverse effects.
• Verbalize an understanding of the drug's use, adverse effects, and required precautions.
• Demonstrate proper self-administration of the medication (e.g., dose, timing, when to notify provider).

Implementation

Interventions and (Rationales)	Patient and Family Education
Ensuring therapeutic effects: • Continue assessments as described earlier for therapeutic effects. (Cough is diminished, secretions are thinner and expectoration ease is increased, nasal passages are clear, and breath sounds are clear. Improvement in other signs and symptoms of the common cold should begin after taking the first dose. The health care provider should be notified if symptoms increase, especially if respiratory involvement worsens or if fever is present.)	• Teach the patient to supplement drug therapy with nonpharmacologic measures such as increased fluid intake to liquefy and assist to mobilize mucus and to moisten the respiratory tract. • Instruct the patient to contact the health care provider if symptoms worsen or if fever is present or increasing.

(Continued)

NURSING PROCESS FOCUS PATIENTS RECEIVING SYMPTOMATIC COLD RELIEF: ANTITUSSIVE, NASAL DECONGESTANT, AND EXPECTORANT THERAPY *(Continued)*

Implementation

Interventions and (Rationales)	Patient and Family Education
Minimizing adverse effects:	
■ Ensure patient safety, especially for older adults. Observe for dizziness. (Drowsiness or dizziness may occur, increasing risk of falls, especially in older adults.)	■ Instruct the patient to call for assistance prior to getting out of bed or attempting to walk alone, and to avoid driving or other activities requiring mental alertness or physical coordination until the effects of the drug are known.
■ Continue to monitor vital signs, especially pulse rate and rhythm for patients taking decongestants, including nasal decongestants. (Sympathomimetic decongestants may cause tachycardia and dysrhythmias in patients with history of cardiac disease.)	■ Instruct the patient to immediately report dizziness, palpitations, or syncope. ■ Teach the patient, family, or caregiver how to monitor pulse and blood pressure as appropriate. Ensure the proper use and functioning of any home equipment obtained.
■ Monitor for persistent dry cough, increasing cough severity, increasing congestion, or dyspnea. (Some of these drugs are used with caution or are contraindicated in patients with existing respiratory disease, including COPD. A change in the severity of the cough may indicate worsening disease process or a more serious respiratory infection and should be reported immediately.)	■ Instruct the patient to report promptly any change in the severity or frequency of cough. Any cough accompanied by shortness of breath, increasing congestion, fever, or chest pain should be reported immediately. ■ Encourage the patient to increase fluid intake to assist in liquifying mucous secretions and to moisten the upper respiratory tract.
■ Assess the color and consistency of any expectorated sputum. (Increasing thickness, color, hemoptysis, or quantity of sputum may indicate a serious respiratory infection and should be reported immediately.)	■ Instruct the patient to report any significant change in the color, consistency, or quantity of expectorated mucus to the health care provider.
■ Monitor for GI effects. Encourage the patient to take tablets or capsules with a full glass of water. (Taking the drug with additional fluids or food may decrease GI adverse effects.)	■ Teach the patient to take the medication with additional fluid or food. Report any significant GI symptoms (e.g., nausea with vomiting, diarrhea) to the health care provider.
■ Have the patient clear nose before using decongestant nasal sprays and to wait 5 minutes before using a second spray if ordered. If nasal corticosteroids or mast cell stabilizers are also ordered, use a decongestant nasal spray first, followed in 5 to 10 minutes by the glucocorticoid. Spit out any excess liquid drug that may drain into the mouth. (Clearing the nasal passages before administering the nasal spray and allowing the first of two sprays' time to constrict local vessels and mucosa will allow the spray to reach higher into passages. Using decongestant spray before other sprays will open nasal mucosa, allowing the other drug to reach more nasal mucosa. Swallowing additional drug may increase risk of systemic adverse effects.)	■ Teach the patient to clear nasal passages, then administer the decongestant spray. After a waiting period of 5 to 10 minutes, use additional spray if ordered or follow with additional nasal sprays as ordered. Any excess that drains into the mouth should be spit out and not swallowed. ■ Teach the patient to limit use of decongestant nasal sprays to 3 to 5 days, unless otherwise ordered by the provider, to avoid rebound congestion.
■ Encourage the use of single-symptom drug preparations when possible. (Multisystem formulations increase the risk of adverse effects. Additional drugs not needed in multiuse preparations should be avoided.)	■ Teach the patient to consider symptoms when selecting OTC cold remedies and choose preparations based on current symptoms. ■ Instruct the patient that multiuse cold remedies containing acetaminophen must be taken in prescribed doses to avoid acetaminophen overdose and potential liver damage.
Patient understanding of drug therapy:	
■ Use opportunities during administration of medications and during assessments to discuss the rationale for drug therapy, desired therapeutic outcomes, most common adverse effects, parameters for when to call the health care provider, and any necessary monitoring or precautions. (Using time during nursing care helps to optimize and reinforce key teaching areas.)	■ The patient should be able to state the reason for the drug, appropriate dose and scheduling, and what adverse effects to observe for and when to report them.

NURSING PROCESS FOCUS	PATIENTS RECEIVING SYMPTOMATIC COLD RELIEF: ANTITUSSIVE, NASAL DECONGESTANT, AND EXPECTORANT THERAPY (Continued)

Implementation

Interventions and (Rationales)	Patient and Family Education
Patient self-administration of drug therapy: ■ When administering the medication, instruct the patient, family, or caregiver in the proper self-administration of the drug, e.g., take the drug before allergy season or before symptoms are severe. (Proper administration will increase the effectiveness of the drug.)	■ The patient and family or caregiver are able to discuss appropriate dosing and administration needs, including: ■ *Cough suppressants:* Cough syrups should be swallowed without water and allowed to coat the throat for soothing effects, followed by increased fluid intake 30 to 60 minutes later. ■ *Expectorants:* Syrups should be taken with a full glass of liquid and increased fluid intake throughout the day to assist in thinning mucus for ease of expectoration. ■ *Nasal decongestants:* Nasal passages should be cleared by blowing, followed by the nasal spray.

Evaluation of Outcome Criteria

Evaluate the effectiveness of drug therapy by confirming that patient goals and expected outcomes have been met (see "Planning").

See Tables 38.3, 38.4, 38.5, and 38.6 for a list of drugs to which these nursing actions apply.

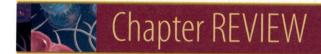

Chapter REVIEW

KEY CONCEPTS

The numbered key concepts provide a succinct summary of the important points from the corresponding numbered section within the chapter. If any of these points are not clear, refer to the numbered section within the chapter for review.

38.1 The upper respiratory tract humidifies and cleans incoming air. The nasal mucosa is richly supplied with vascular tissue and is the first line of immunologic defense.

38.2 Allergic rhinitis is a disorder characterized by sneezing, watery eyes, and nasal congestion. Pharmacotherapy is targeted at preventing the disorder, or relieving its symptoms.

38.3 Antihistamines, or H_1-receptor antagonists, can provide relief from the symptoms of allergic rhinitis. Major side effects include drowsiness and anticholinergic effects such as dry mouth. Newer drugs in this class are nonsedating.

38.4 Intranasal corticosteroids have become drugs of choice in treating allergic rhinitis due to their high efficacy and wide margin of safety. For maximum effectiveness, they must be administered 2 to 3 weeks prior to allergen exposure.

38.5 The most commonly used decongestants are oral and intranasal sympathomimetics that alleviate the nasal congestion associated with allergic rhinitis and the common cold. Intranasal drugs are more efficacious but should be used for only 3 to 5 days due to rebound congestion.

38.6 Antitussives are effective at relieving cough due to the common cold. Opioids are used for severe cough. Nonopioids such as dextromethorphan are used for mild or moderate cough.

38.7 Expectorants promote mucus secretion, making it thinner and easier to remove by coughing. Mucolytics directly break down mucus molecules.

NCLEX-RN® REVIEW QUESTIONS

1 The patient has been prescribed oxymetazoline (Afrin). The nurse understands that:
1. the most serious side effect is rebound congestion.
2. the average use is for 10 days.
3. this drug should not be used in conjunction with antihistamines.
4. this is an OTC drug and may be used as needed for congestion.

2 A patient is prescribed an intranasal corticosteroid for allergic rhinitis. The nurse's teaching would include: (Select all that apply.)
1. there are no known side effects.
2. the spray is a consistent dose.
3. it could take 2 to 4 weeks before improvement in symptoms is noticed.
4. it is contraindicated to use saline nasal sprays with this medicine.
5. the medication can be used any time symptoms increase.

3 A patient's history includes taking a first-generation H_1-receptor antagonist. Considering this history, the nurse assesses for which of the following findings?
1. A history of heart disease
2. Any recent weight gain
3. A history of respiratory illnesses
4. A history of peptic ulcer

4 When teaching patients how to self-administer intranasal corticosteroids, which of the following must be included? (Select all that apply.)
1. Prime device prior to initial use.
2. Clear nose before administration.
3. Clear nose after administration.
4. Swallow any excess that drains into the mouth.
5. Spit out any excess that drains into the mouth.

5 Prior to administration of antihistamines, the nurse assesses for:
1. prostatic hypertrophy.
2. itching.
3. dry skin.
4. increased restlessness.

6 Which of the following is the <u>best</u> advice that the nurse can give a patient with viral rhinitis who intends to purchase an OTC combination cold remedy?
1. Dosages in these remedies provide precise dosing for each symptom that you are experiencing.
2. These agents are best used in conjunction with an antibiotic.
3. It is safer to use a single-agent preparation if you are only experiencing one symptom.
4. Since these agents are available over the counter, it is safe to use any of them as long as needed.

CRITICAL THINKING QUESTIONS

1. A 74-year-old male patient informs the nurse that he is taking diphendydramine (Benadryl) to reduce seasonal allergy symptoms. This patient has a history of an enlarged prostate and mild glaucoma (controlled by medication). What is the nurse's response?

2. A 65-year-old patient has bronchitis and has been coughing for several days. Of the two antitussive medications, dextromethorphan and codeine, which is the drug of choice for this patient? Why?

3. A 67-year-old patient has allergic rhinitis and always carries a handkerchief in his pocket because he has nasal discharge nearly every day. Sometimes his nose is stuffy and dry. The health care provider prescribes fluticasone (Flonase). He is to take one spray intranasally at bedtime. The patient starts to take fluticasone and a week later calls the provider's office and talks to the nurse. He says, "This Flonase is not helping me." What is the nurse's best response?

See Appendix D for answers and rationales for all activities.

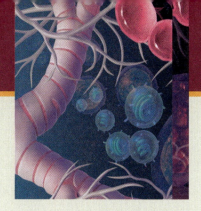

Chapter 39

Drugs for Asthma and Other Pulmonary Disorders

LEARNING OUTCOMES

After reading this chapter, the student should be able to:

1. Identify anatomical structures associated with the lower respiratory tract and their functions.

2. Explain how the autonomic nervous system regulates airflow in the lower respiratory tract, and how this process can be modified with drugs.

3. Compare the advantages and disadvantages of using the inhalation route of administration for pulmonary drugs.

4. Describe the types of devices used to deliver aerosol therapies via the inhalation route.

5. Compare and contrast the pharmacotherapy of acute and chronic asthma.

6. Describe the nurse's role in the pharmacologic treatment of lower respiratory tract disorders.

7. For each of the classes listed in Drugs at a Glance, know representative drugs, and explain their mechanism of drug action, primary actions on the respiratory system, and important adverse effects.

8. Use the nursing process to care for patients who are receiving pharmacotherapy for lower respiratory tract disorders.

KEY TERMS

The flow of oxygen, carbon dioxide, and other gases in and out of the human body is dynamic and in constant flux. Minute-by-minute control of the airways is necessary to bring an abundant supply of essential gases to the pulmonary capillaries and to rid the body of some of its most toxic waste products. Any restriction in this dynamic flow, even for brief periods, may result in serious consequences. This chapter examines drugs used in the pharmacotherapy of two primary pulmonary disorders—asthma and chronic obstructive pulmonary disease.

39.1 Physiology of the Lower Respiratory Tract

The primary function of the respiratory system is to bring oxygen into the body and to remove carbon dioxide. The process by which gases are exchanged is called *respiration*. The basic structures of the lower respiratory tract are shown in ➤ Figure 39.1.

Ventilation is the process of moving air into and out of the lungs. As the diaphragm contracts and lowers in position, it creates a negative pressure that draws air into the lungs, and inspiration occurs. During expiration, the diaphragm relaxes and air leaves the lungs passively, with no energy expenditure required. Ventilation is a purely mechanical process that occurs approximately 12 to 18 times per minute in adults, a rate determined by neurons in the brainstem. This rate may be modified by a number of factors, including emotions, fever, stress, the pH of the blood, and certain medications.

The bronchial tree ends in dilated sacs called *alveoli*, which have no smooth muscle but are abundantly rich in capillaries. An extremely thin membrane in the alveoli separates the airway from the pulmonary capillaries, allowing gases to readily move between the internal environment of the blood and the inspired air. As oxygen crosses this membrane, it is exchanged for carbon dioxide, a cellular waste product that travels from the blood to the air. The lung is richly supplied with blood. Blood flow through the lungs is called **perfusion**. The process of gas exchange is shown in Figure 39.1.

39.2 Bronchiolar Smooth Muscle

Bronchioles are muscular, elastic structures whose diameter, or lumen, varies with the contraction or relaxation of smooth muscle. Bronchodilation opens the lumen, allowing air to enter the lungs more freely, thus increasing the supply of oxygen to the body's tissues. Bronchoconstriction closes the lumen, resulting in less airflow. Bronchodilation and bronchoconstriction are largely regulated by the two branches of the autonomic nervous system.

- The *sympathetic branch* activates beta$_2$-adrenergic receptors, which causes bronchiolar smooth muscle to relax, the airway diameter to increase, and *bronchodilation* to occur.

- The *parasympathetic branch* causes bronchiolar smooth muscle to contract, the airway diameter to narrow, and *bronchoconstriction* to occur.

Drugs that enhance bronchodilation will cause the patient to breathe easier. Drugs that stimulate beta$_2$-adrenergic receptors, commonly called *bronchodilators*, are some of the most frequently prescribed drugs for treating pulmonary disorders. On the other hand, drugs that cause bronchoconstriction may cause breathing to become labored and the patient to become short of breath.

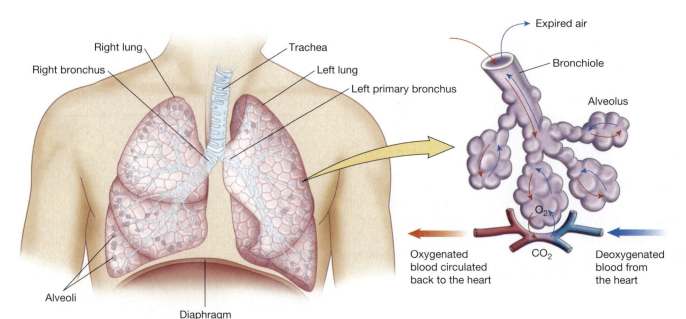

➤ *Figure 39.1* The lower respiratory tract

39.3 Administration of Pulmonary Drugs via Inhalation

The respiratory system offers a rapid and efficient mechanism for delivering drugs. The enormous surface area of the bronchioles and alveoli, and the rich blood supply to these areas, results in an almost instantaneous onset of action for inhaled substances.

Medications are delivered to the respiratory system by aerosol therapy. An **aerosol** is a suspension of minute liquid droplets or fine solid particles suspended in a gas. The major advantage of aerosol therapy is that it delivers pulmonary drugs to their immediate site of action, thus reducing systemic side effects. To produce an equivalent therapeutic action, an oral drug would have to be given at higher doses, and be distributed to all body tissues. Aerosol therapy can give immediate relief for **bronchospasm,** an acute condition during which the bronchiolar smooth muscle rapidly contracts, leaving the patient gasping for breath. Drugs may also be given to loosen viscous mucus in the bronchial tree.

It should be clearly understood that agents delivered by inhalation have the potential to produce *systemic* effects because of absorption across the pulmonary capillaries. For example, anesthetics such as nitrous oxide and halothane (Fluothane) are delivered via the inhalation route and are rapidly distributed to cause CNS depression (chapter 19∞). Solvents such as paint thinners and glues are sometimes intentionally inhaled and can cause serious adverse effects on the nervous system and even death. In general, however, drugs administered by the inhalation route for respiratory conditions produce minimal systemic toxicity.

Several devices are used to deliver drugs via the inhalation route. **Nebulizers** are small machines that vaporize a liquid medication into a fine mist that can be inhaled, using a face mask or handheld device. If the drug is a solid, it may be administered using a **dry powder inhaler (DPI).** A DPI is a small device that is activated by the process of inhalation to deliver a fine powder directly to the bronchial tree. Turbuhaler and Rotahaler are types of DPIs. **Metered-dose inhalers (MDIs)** are a

third type of device commonly used to deliver respiratory drugs. MDIs use a propellant to deliver a measured dose of drugs to the lungs during each breath. The patient times the inhalation to the puffs of drug emitted from the MDI.

There are disadvantages to administering aerosol therapy. The precise dose received by the patient is difficult to measure because it depends on the patient's breathing pattern and the correct use of the inhaler device. Even under optimal conditions, only 10% to 50% of the drug actually reaches the lower respiratory tract. Patients must be carefully instructed on the correct use of these devices. Swallowing medication that has been deposited in the oral cavity may cause systemic adverse effects if the drug is absorbed in the GI tract. In addition, patients should rinse their mouth thoroughly following drug use to reduce the potential for absorption of the drug across the oral mucosa. Three devices used to deliver respiratory drugs are shown in ➤ Figure 39.2.

ASTHMA

Asthma is a chronic pulmonary disease with inflammatory and bronchospasm components. Drugs may be given to decrease the frequency of asthmatic attacks or to terminate attacks in progress.

PharmFacts

Asthma

- Asthma is responsible for more than 1.5 million emergency department visits and more than 500,000 hospitalizations each year.
- More than 5,500 patients die of asthma each year.
- The incidence of asthma has been dramatically increasing each year since 1980 in all age, gender, and ethnic groups. The highest rate of increase has been among African Americans.
- The highest incidence of asthma is in patients younger than age 18; from 7% to 10% of children have the disease.
- In adults, asthma is 35% more common in women than in men. In children, however, the disease affects twice as many boys as girls.

MyNursingKit | Metered-Dose Inhaler

MyNursingKit | Dry Powder Inhaler

MyNursingKit | Small-Volume Nebulizer

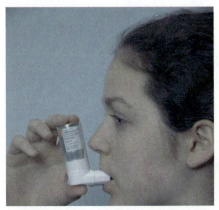
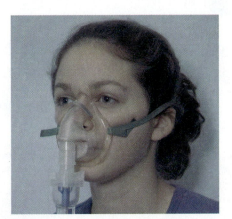
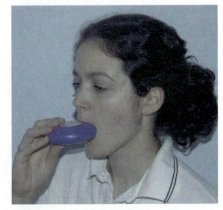

➤ **Figure 39.2** Devices used to deliver respiratory drugs: (a) metered-dose inhaler; (b) nebulizer with face mask; (c) dry powder inhaler

Source: Pearson Education/PH College.

39.4 Pathophysiology of Asthma

Asthma is one of the most common chronic conditions in the United States, affecting 20 million Americans. Although the disorder can affect a person of any age, asthma is often considered a pediatric disease. Characterized by acute bronchospasm, asthma can cause intense breathlessness, coughing, and gasping for air. Along with bronchoconstriction, an acute inflammatory response stimulates histamine secretion, which increases mucus and edema in the airways. As in allergic rhinitis, the airway becomes hyper-responsive to allergens. Both bronchospasm and inflammation contribute to airway obstruction, as illustrated in ➤ Figure 39.3.

The patient with asthma can present with acute or chronic symptoms. Intervals between symptoms may vary from days to weeks to months. Some patients experience asthma when exposed to specific triggers, such as those listed in Table 39.1. Others experience the disorder on exertion, a condition called *exercise-induced asthma*. **Status asthmaticus** is a severe, prolonged form of asthma unresponsive to drug treatment that may lead to respiratory failure.

Because asthma has both a bronchoconstriction component and an inflammation component, pharmacotherapy of the disease focuses on one or both of these mechanisms. The goals of drug therapy are twofold: to *terminate* acute bronchospasms in progress and to *reduce the frequency* of asthma attacks. Different medications are needed to achieve each of these goals.

Beta-Adrenergic Agonists

Beta$_2$-adrenergic agonists (or simply beta agonists) are effective bronchodilators for the management of asthma and other pulmonary diseases. They are drugs of choice for the treatment of *acute* bronchoconstriction. These drugs are listed in Table 39.2.

39.5 Treating Acute Asthma with Beta-Adrenergic Agonists

Beta-adrenergic agonists are drugs that activate the sympathetic nervous system, which relaxes bronchial smooth muscle resulting in bronchodilation. Beta-agonist medications may act on either beta$_1$ receptors, which are located primarily in the heart, or on beta$_2$ receptors, which are located in smooth muscle of the lung, uterus, and other organs. Beta agonists that activate both beta$_1$ and beta$_2$ receptors are called nonselective bronchodilators. Beta agonists that activate only the beta$_2$ receptors are called selective agents. The selective beta$_2$-adrenergic agonists have largely replaced the older, nonselective agents such as epinephrine

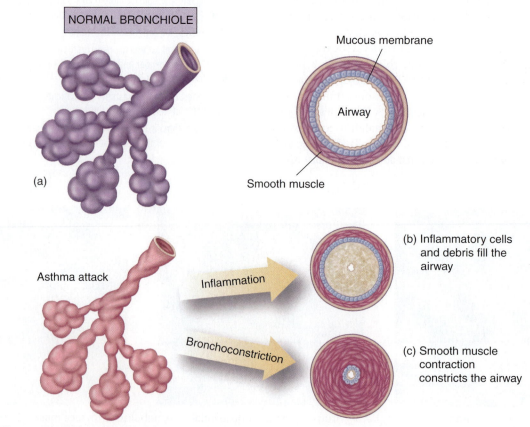

➤ *Figure 39.3* Changes in the bronchioles during an asthma attack: (a) Normal bronchiole; (b) the inflammatory component plugs the airway; (c) bronchoconstriction narrows the airway

TABLE 39.1	Common Triggers of Asthma
Cause	Sources
Air pollutants	Tobacco smoke
	Ozone
	Nitrous and sulfur oxides
	Fumes from cleaning fluids or solvents
	Burning leaves
Allergens	Pollen from trees, grasses, and weeds
	Animal dander
	Household dust
	Mold
Chemicals and food	Drugs, including aspirin, ibuprofen, and beta blockers
	Sulfite preservatives
	Food and condiments, including nuts, monosodium glutamate (MSG), shellfish, and dairy products
Respiratory infections	Bacterial, fungal, and viral
Stress	Emotional stress/anxiety
	Exercise in dry, cold climates

and isoproterenol (Isuprel) for asthma pharmacotherapy because they produce fewer cardiac side effects.

Beta agonists are bronchodilators that relax bronchial smooth muscle, thus widening the airway and making breathing easier for the patient. Although quite effective at relieving bronchospasm, beta agonists have no anti-inflammatory properties; thus, other drug classes are required to control the inflammatory component of *chronic* asthma.

A practical method for classifying beta-adrenergic agonists for asthma is by their duration of action. Short-acting agents such as pirbuterol (Maxair) have a rapid onset of action, usually several minutes. Short-acting beta agonists are the most frequently prescribed drugs for aborting or terminating an acute asthma attack. For this reason, they are sometimes referred to as *rescue agents*. Their effects, however, last only 2 to 6 hours so the use of short-acting agents is generally limited to as-needed (prn) management of acute episodes.

Intermediate duration beta agonists such as albuterol (Proventil) and levalbuterol (Xopenex) have therapeutic effects that last approximately 8 hours, while long-acting agents such as salmeterol (Serevent) last up to 12 hours. These agents have a relatively slow onset of action. The intermediate and long-acting agents are used in combination with inhaled corticosteroids for the prophylaxis of moderate to severe, persistent asthma. The specific drug chosen for pharmacotherapy is dependent on the pattern of symptoms experienced by the patient.

In 2005, the U.S. Food and Drug Administration (USDA) issued a public health advisory regarding an in-

crease in deaths among persons taking long-acting beta$_2$ agonists (LABAs). Because LABAs are not indicated to abort an asthma attack, taking a LABA instead of a short-acting beta agonist could result in unrelieved bronchospasm and subsequent death. The LABAs are also delivered via handheld inhalers and patients may assume they have the same actions as the short-acting agents. Patients must be warned of the inherent dangers of taking LABAs during an acute episode.

Beta-adrenergic agonists are available in oral, inhaled, and parenteral formulations. When taken for respiratory conditions, inhalation is by far the most common route. Inhaled beta agonists produce minimal systemic toxicity because only small amounts of the drugs are absorbed. When given orally, a longer duration of action is achieved, but systemic adverse effects are more frequently experienced. Systemic effects may include some activation of beta$_1$ receptors in the heart, which could cause an angina attack or a dysrhythmia in patients with cardiac impairment. With chronic use, tolerance may develop to the bronchodilation effect and the duration of action will become shorter. Should this occur, the dose of beta$_2$ agonist may need to be increased, or a second drug may be added to the therapeutic regimen. Increased use of a beta agonist over a period of hours or days is an indication that the patient's condition is rapidly deteriorating, and medical attention should be sought immediately.

See Nursing Process Focus: Patients Receiving Adrenergic (Sympathomimetic) Therapy, page 134 in chapter 13∞, for the complete Nursing Process applied to caring for patients receiving beta-adrenergic agonists (sympathomimetics).

HOME & COMMUNITY CONSIDERATIONS

Asthma Management in the Schools

Approximately 9 million children younger than age 18 have asthma. Researchers suggest that asthma accounts for 14 million missed school days each year and potential missed workdays for parents, making this disease one of the most common causes for school and work absenteeism. In a typical class of 30 children, two students suffer from asthmatic attacks each year while at school. Children cannot learn while experiencing wheezing, coughing, and shortness of breath.

Assisting schools to develop asthma management programs has become the focus of several federal agencies and dozens of professional and patient advocacy groups. Many schools are adopting asthma management plans as part of a coordinated school health program. Schools with these programs have established "asthma-friendly" policies, such as allowing students to carry and administer quick-relief asthma medications. Additionally, the schools routinely maintain a copy of the student's asthma action plan from the caregiver or health care provider. The role of the school nurse is to review the plan, determine the student's specific needs, and be sure that the student has immediate access to quick-relief asthma medications. The optimal plan for each student is determined case by case, with input from the student, parents, health care provider, and school nurse. Typically, older students are permitted to carry the inhaler and self-administer as needed. The nurse often keeps a backup supply of the student's medication. For younger children, a supervised health assistant may be delegated to administer the medication.

TABLE 39.2	Bronchodilators	
Drug	**Route and Adult Dose (max dose where indicated)**	**Adverse Effects**
BETA AGONISTS/SYMPATHOMIMETICS		
albuterol (Proventil, Ventolin, VoSpire)	MDI; 2 inhalations every 4–6 h as needed (max: 12 inhalations/day) Nebulizer: 1.25–5 mg every 4–8 h as needed PO; 2–4 mg tid–qid (max: 32 mg/day) Extended release tabs: 8 mg every 12 h (max: 32 mg/day divided)	*Headache, dizziness, tremor, nervousness, throat irritation, drug tolerance* <u>Tachycardia, dysrhythmias, hypokalemia, hyperglycemia, paradoxical bronchoconstriction</u>
arformoterol (Brovan)	Nebulizer; 15 mcg twice daily (max: 30 mcg/day)	
formoterol (Foradil, Perforomist)	DPI; 12 mcg inhalation capsule every 12 h (max: 24 mcg/day) Nebulizer: 20 mcg bid (max: 40 mcg/day)	
levalbuterol (Xopenex)	Nebulizer; 0.63 mg tid–qid MDI; 2 inhalations q 4–6 h	
pirbuterol (Maxair)	MDI; 2 inhalations qid (max: 12 inhalations/day)	
⊙ salmeterol (Serevent)	DPI; 2 aerosol inhalations bid or 1 powder diskus bid	
terbutaline (Brethine)	PO; 2.5–5 mg tid (max: 15 mg/day) Subcutaneous; 250 mcg (may be repeated in 15 min) Inhalation; 2 inhalations (200 mcg/spray) every 4–6 h	
ANTICHOLINERGICS		
⊙ ipratropium (Atrovent, Combivent)	MDI; 2 inhalations qid (max: 12 inhalations/day) Nebulizer: 500 mcg every 6–8 h as needed	*Headache, cough, dry mouth, bad taste* <u>Pharyngitis</u>
tiotropium (Spiriva)	DPI; 1 capsule inhaled/day	
METHYLXANTHINES		
aminophylline (Truphylline)	PO; 380 mg/day in divided doses every 6–8 h (max: 928 mg/day)	*Nervousness, tremors, dizziness, headache, nausea, vomiting, anorexia*
theophylline (Theo-Dur, others)	PO; 300–600 mg/day in divided doses (max: 900 mg/day)	<u>Tachycardia, dysrhythmias, hypotension, seizures, circulatory failure, respiratory arrest</u>

Italics indicate common adverse effects; <u>underlining</u> indicates serious adverse effects.

Anticholinergics

Although beta agonists are drugs of choice for treating acute asthma, anticholinergics are alternative bronchodilators. Only two anticholinergics are commonly used for pulmonary disease, and these agents are listed in Table 39.2.

39.6 Treating Chronic Asthma with Anticholinergics

Although short-acting beta agonists are drugs of choice for treating acute bronchospasm, anticholinergics (also called cholinergic blockers or antagonists) are alternative bronchodilators. Anticholinergics block the parasympathetic nervous system. Because the parasympathetic response is largely the opposite of the sympathetic response, blocking the parasympathetic nervous system results in actions similar to those of stimulating the sympathetic nervous system (chapter 13 ∞). It is predictable, then, that anticholinergic drugs would cause bronchodilation and have potential applications in the pharmacotherapy of asthma and COPD.

Although anticholinergics such as atropine have been available for many decades, drugs in this class exhibit many adverse effects when administered by the oral or parenteral routes. However, the relatively recent discovery of anticholinergics that can be delivered by inhalation led to the approval of two important drugs in this class for asthma: ipratropium (Atrovent) and tiotropium (Spiriva).

Ipratropium (Atrovent) is the most common anticholinergic prescribed for the pharmacotherapy of chronic obstructive pulmonary disease (COPD) and asthma. It has a slower onset of action than most beta agonists and produces a less intense bronchodilation. However, combining ipratropium with a beta agonist produces a greater and more prolonged bronchodilation than using either drug separately. Taking advantage of this increased effect, Combivent is a mixture of ipratropium and albuterol in a single MDI canister. Tiotropium (Spiriva) is a newer anticholinergic for COPD that has a longer duration of action than ipratropium.

The inhaled anticholinergics are safe medications. The wide range of anticholinergic adverse effects observed when drugs in this class are administered systemically rarely occur by inhalation. Dry mouth, gastrointestinal (GI) distress, headache, and anxiety are the most common patient complaints.

Pr Prototype Drug | Salmeterol *(Serevent)*

Therapeutic Class: Bronchodilator   **Pharmacologic Class:** Beta$_2$-adrenergic agonist

ACTIONS AND USES

Salmeterol is a LABA that acts by selectively binding to beta$_2$-adrenergic receptors in bronchial smooth muscle to cause bronchodilation. Its 12-hour duration of action is longer than that of many other bronchodilators, thus making it best suited for the management of chronic asthma. When taken 30–60 minutes prior to physical activity, it can prevent exercise-induced bronchospasm. Salmeterol is also approved for reducing bronchospasm in patients with COPD. Because salmeterol takes 15–25 minutes to act, it should never be used to terminate acute bronchospasm.

ADMINISTRATION ALERTS

- The proper use of the metered-dose inhaler is important to the effective delivery of the drug. Observe and instruct the patient in proper use.
- Pregnancy category C

PHARMACOKINETICS

Onset: 10–20 min

Peak: 2 h

Half-life: 3–4 h

Duration: Up to 12 h

ADVERSE EFFECTS

Serious adverse effects from salmeterol are uncommon. Some patients experience headaches, throat irritation, tremor, nervousness, and restlessness. Because of its potential to cause tachycardia, patients with heart disease should be monitored regularly. Salmeterol has a black box warning that LABAs may increase the risk of asthma-related deaths.

Contraindications: Salmeterol use is contraindicated in patients with hypersensitivity to the drug and in patients experiencing acute bronchospasm (a shorter-acting drug should be used). Caution should be used when treating patients with dysrhythmias, hypertension, heart failure, or seizures.

INTERACTIONS

Drug–Drug: Concurrent use with beta blockers will inhibit the bronchodilation effect of salmeterol.

Lab Tests: Salmeterol may cause hypokalemia.

Herbal/Food: Products containing caffeine such as coffee and tea may cause nervousness, tremor, or palpitations.

Treatment of Overdose: Overdose results in an exaggerated sympathetic activation, causing dysrhythmias, hypokalemia, and hyperglycemia. In severe cases, administration of a cardioselective beta-adrenergic antagonist may be necessary.

Refer to MyNursingKit for a Nursing Process Focus specific to this drug.

The complete nursing process applied to patients receiving anticholinergics is presented in Nursing Process Focus: Patients Receiving Anticholinergic Therapy, on page 145 in chapter 13∞.

For additional nursing considerations, please refer to Nursing Process Focus: Patients Receiving Bronchodilator Therapy, on page 597.

Methylxanthines

The methylxanthines were considered drugs of choice for treating asthma 30 years ago. Now they are primarily reserved for the long-term management of persistent asthma that is unresponsive to beta agonists or inhaled corticosteroids. These agents are shown in Table 39.2.

39.7 Treating Chronic Asthma with Methylxanthines

The **methylxanthines**, theophylline (Theo-Dur, others) and aminophylline (Truphylline), are bronchodilators chemically related to caffeine. The methylxanthines are infrequently prescribed because they have a narrow safety margin, especially with prolonged use. Adverse effects such as nausea, vomiting, and CNS stimulation occur frequently, and dysrhythmias may be observed at high doses. Like caffeine, methylxanthines can cause nervousness and insomnia. These drugs also have significant interactions with numerous other drugs.

Methylxanthines are administered by the PO or IV routes, rather than by inhalation. Having been largely re-

placed by safer and more effective drugs, theophylline is currently used primarily for the long-term oral prophylaxis of asthma that is unresponsive to beta agonists or inhaled corticosteroids.

Corticosteroids

Inhaled corticosteroids (ICS) are used for the long-term prevention of asthmatic attacks. Oral corticosteroids may be used for the short-term management of acute severe asthma. These drugs are listed in Table 39.3.

39.8 Prophylaxis of Asthma with Corticosteroids

Corticosteroids, also known as glucocorticoids, are the most potent natural anti-inflammatory substances known. Because asthma has a major inflammatory component, it should not be surprising that drugs in this class play a major role in the management of this disorder. Corticosteroids dampen the activation of inflammatory cells and increase the production of anti-inflammatory mediators. Mucus production and edema is diminished, thus reducing airway obstruction. Although corticosteroids are not bronchodilators, they sensitize the bronchial smooth muscle to be more responsive to beta-agonist stimulation. In addition, they reduce the bronchial hyper-responsiveness to allergens that is responsible for triggering some asthma attacks. In the pharmacotherapy of asthma, corticosteroids may be given systemically or by inhalation.

Therapeutic Class: Bronchodilator   **Pharmacologic Class:** Anticholinergic

ACTIONS AND USES

Ipratropium is an anticholinergic agent that is delivered by the inhalation and intranasal routes. The inhalation form is approved to relieve and prevent the bronchospasm that is characteristic of asthma and COPD. When combined with albuterol (Combivent), it is a preferred drug for treating bronchospasms due to COPD, including bronchitis and emphysema. Although it has not received FDA approval for the treatment of asthma, it is prescribed off-label for the disorder. Ipratropium is an alternative to short-acting beta agonists, and for patients experiencing severe asthma exacerbations. It is sometimes combined with beta agonists or corticosteroids to provide additive bronchodilation.

When administered via inhalation, ipratropium can relieve acute bronchospasm within minutes after administration, although peak effects may take 1–2 hours. Bronchodilation action may continue for up to 6 hours.

The nasal spray formulation of ipratropium is approved for the relief of runny nose associated with the common cold and allergic rhinitis. The drug inhibits nasal secretions but does not have decongestant action. Treatment is limited to 3 weeks.

ADMINISTRATION ALERTS

- The proper use of the metered-dose inhaler (MDI) is important to the effective delivery of drug. Observe and instruct the patient in proper use.
- Wait 2–3 minutes between dosages.
- Avoid contact with eyes; otherwise, blurred vision may occur.
- Pregnancy category B

PHARMACOKINETICS
Onset: 5–15 min   **Half-life:** 1.5–2 h
Peak: 1.5–2 h   **Duration:** 3–6 h

ADVERSE EFFECTS

Because very little is absorbed from the lungs, ipratropium produces few systemic adverse effects. Irritation of the upper respiratory tract may result in cough, drying of the nasal mucosa, or hoarseness. It produces a bitter taste, which may be relieved by rinsing the mouth after use.

Contraindications: Ipratropium is contraindicated in patients with hypersensitivity to soya lecithin or related food products such as soybean and peanut. Soya lecithin is used as a propellant in the inhaler.

INTERACTIONS

Drug–Drug: Use with other drugs in this class such as atropine may lead to additive anticholinergic side effects.

Lab Tests: Unknown

Herbal/Food: Unknown

Treatment of Overdose: Overdose with ipratropium does not occur because very little of the drug is absorbed when given by aerosol.

Refer to MyNursingKit for a Nursing Process Focus specific to this drug.

TABLE 39.3	**Anti-Inflammatory Drugs for Asthma**	
Drug	Route and Adult Dose (max dose where indicated)	Adverse Effects
INHALED CORTICOSTEROIDS*		
Pr beclomethasone (Beconase AQ, Qvar)	MDI; 1–2 inhalations tid–qid (max: 20 inhalations/day)	*Hoarseness, dry mouth, cough, sore throat*
budesonide (Pulmicort)	DPI; 1–2 inhalations (200 mcg/inhalation) qid (max: 800 mcg/day)	<u>Oropharyngeal candidiasis, hypercorticism, hypersensitivity reactions</u>
ciclesonide (Alvesco)	Inhalation; 1–2 inhalations/day (320–640 mcg)	
flunisolide (AeroBid)	MDI; 2–3 inhalations bid–tid (max: 12 inhalations/day)	
fluticasone (Flovent) (see page 577 for the Prototype Drug box∞)	MDI (44 mcg); 2 inhalations bid (max: 10 inhalations/day)	
mometasone (Asmanex)	DPI; 1 inhalation daily (max: 2 inhalations daily)	
triamcinolone (Azmacort)	MDI; 2 inhalations tid–qid (max: 16 inhalations/day)	
MAST CELL STABILIZERS		
cromolyn (Intal)	MDI; 1 inhalation qid	*Nausea, sneezing, nasal stinging, throat irritation, unpleasant taste*
nedocromil sodium (Tilade)	MDI; 2 inhalations qid	<u>Anaphylaxis, angioedema, bronchospasm</u>
LEUKOTRIENE MODIFIERS		
montelukast (Singulair)	PO; 10 mg/day in evening	*Headache, nausea, diarrhea*
Pr zafirlukast (Accolate)	PO; 20 mg bid 1 h before or 2 h after meals	<u>Liver toxicity (zileuton), increased AST</u>
zileuton (Zyflo)	PO; 1,200 mg bid	

*For doses of systemic corticosteroids, refer to chapter 43∞.
Italics indicate common adverse effects; <u>underlining</u> indicates serious adverse effects.

NURSING PROCESS FOCUS PATIENTS RECEIVING BRONCHODILATOR THERAPY

Assessment	Potential Nursing Diagnoses
Baseline assessment prior to administration: ■ Understand the reason the drug has been prescribed in order to assess for therapeutic effects. ■ Obtain a complete health history including previous history of symptoms and association to seasons, foods, or environmental exposures; existing cardiovascular, respiratory, hepatic, renal, or neurologic disease; glaucoma; prostatic hypertrophy or difficulty with urination; presence of fever or active infections; pregnancy or breast-feeding; alcohol use; or smoking. Obtain a drug history, noting the type of adverse reaction experienced to any medications. ■ If asthma symptoms are of new onset, assess for any recent changes in diet, soaps including laundry detergent or softener, cosmetics, lotions, environment, or recent carpet cleaning (particularly in young children) that may correlate with onset of symptoms. ■ Obtain baseline vital signs, noting respiratory rate and depth. ■ Assess pulmonary function with pulse oximeter, peak expiratory flow meter, and/or arterial blood gases to establish baseline levels. ■ Evaluate appropriate laboratory findings (e.g., CBC, hepatic and renal labs). ■ Assess symptom-related effects on eating, sleep, and activity level.	■ Impaired Gas Exchange ■ Ineffective Tissue Perfusion ■ Anxiety (related to difficulty in breathing) ■ Disturbed Sleep Pattern (related to adverse drug effects) ■ Activity Intolerance (related to disease or ineffective drug therapy) ■ Deficient Knowledge (drug therapy)
Assessment throughout administration: ■ Assess for desired therapeutic effects (e.g., increased ease of breathing, improvement in pulmonary function studies, improved signs of peripheral oxygenation and increased activity levels, maintenance of normal eating and sleep periods). ■ Continue periodic monitoring of pulmonary function with pulse oximeter, peak expiratory flow meter, and/or arterial blood gases as appropriate. ■ Assess vital signs, especially respiratory rate and depth. Assess breath sounds, noting presence of adventitious sounds, and any mucus production. ■ Assess for adverse effects: dizziness, tachycardia, palpitations, blurred vision, or headache. Report immediately any fever, confusion, tachycardia, palpitations, hypotension, syncope, dyspnea, or increasing pulmonary congestion.	

Planning: Patient Goals and Expected Outcomes

The patient will:
■ Experience therapeutic effects (e.g., increased ease of breathing, improvement in pulmonary function studies, able to experience normal sleep and eating periods, and to carry out ADLs to a level appropriate for condition).
■ Be free from, or experience minimal, adverse effects.
■ Verbalize an understanding of the drug's use, adverse effects, and required precautions.
■ Demonstrate proper self-administration of the medication (e.g., dose, timing, when to notify provider).

Implementation

Interventions and (Rationales)	Patient and Family Education
Ensuring therapeutic effects: ■ Continue assessments as described earlier for therapeutic effects. (Increased ease of breathing; lessened adventitious breath sounds; improved signs of tissue oxygenation; and normal appetite, eating, and sleep patterns should occur. The health care provider should be notified if symptoms worsen, especially if respiratory involvement increases or fever is present.)	■ Teach the patient to supplement drug therapy with nonpharmacologic measures such as increased fluid intake to liquefy and assist to mobilize mucus and to reduce exposure to allergens where possible. ■ Advise the patient to carry a wallet identification card or wear medical identification jewelry indicating the presence of asthma or respiratory condition, any significant allergies or anaphylaxis, and use of inhaler therapy.

(Continued)

NURSING PROCESS FOCUS   PATIENTS RECEIVING BRONCHODILATOR THERAPY *(Continued)*

Implementation

Interventions and (Rationales)	Patient and Family Education
• Monitor pulmonary function periodically with pulse oximeter, peak expiratory flow meter, and/or arterial blood gases. (Periodic monitoring is necessary to assess drug effectiveness.)	• Teach the patient the use of the peak expiratory flow meter or other equipment ordered to monitor pulmonary function. • Instruct the patient to immediately report symptoms of deteriorating respiratory status such as increased dyspnea, breathlessness with speech, increased anxiety, and/or orthopnea.
• To abort an acute asthmatic attack, inhaler therapy should be started at the first sign of respiratory difficulty. For preventative therapy, long-term bronchodilation by inhaler or orally will be used. *Long-acting beta$_2$ agonists (LABAs) and long-acting bronchodilators are not to be used to abort an acute attack.* (Acute asthmatic attacks are managed with quick-acting bronchodilation such as beta$_2$ agonists. For preventing attacks, LABAs, anticholinergics, mast cell stabilizers, and corticosteroid therapy may be used. It is crucial to know and recognize the difference in quick-acting and long-acting inhalers.)	• Provide explicit instructions on the use of quick-acting versus long-acting inhalers. Teach the patient to use quick-acting inhalers at the earliest possible appearance of symptoms. Long-acting inhalers or oral therapy may be used to maintain bronchodilation but do not discard quick-acting inhalers if on long-term maintenance therapy. They may still be needed for periodic acute attacks.
Minimizing adverse effects: • Continue to monitor respirations, rate, depth, breath sounds, mucus production, increasing dyspnea, adventitious breath sounds, signs of tissue hypoxia, anxiety, confusion, and decreasing pulmonary functions studies. (Increasing dyspnea, adventitious breath sounds, diminished oxygenation, or increasing anxiety or confusion may indicate inadequate drug therapy, worsening disease process, or respiratory infection and should be reported immediately.)	• Instruct the patient to immediately report symptoms of deteriorating respiratory status such as increased dyspnea, breathlessness with speech, increased anxiety, or orthopnea.

• Monitor eating and sleep patterns and the ability to maintain functional ADLs. Provide for calorie-rich, nutrient-dense foods, frequent rest periods between eating or activity, and a cool room for sleeping. (Respiratory difficulty and fatigue associated with hypoxia and the work of breathing may affect appetite, and the ability to eat during dyspnea and maintain required ADLs. Maintaining adequate nutrition, fluids, rest, and sleep are essential to support optimal health.)	• Teach the patient to supplement drug therapy with nonpharmacologic measures including:
	  • Increased fluid intake to liquefy and assist to mobilize mucus
	  • Small, frequent meals of calorie- and nutrient-dense foods to prevent fatigue and maintain normal nutrition
	  • Adequate rest periods between eating and activities
	  • Decrease room temperature for ease of breathing during sleep.
	  • Reduce exposure to allergens where possible.
	• Instruct the patient to immediately report any significant change in appetite, an inability to maintain normal intake, inadequate sleep periods, or an inability to carry out required ADLs.

• Eliminate smoking, limit exposure to secondhand smoke, and limit caffeine intake, especially if taking methylxanthines. (Cigarette smoke irritates respiratory mucous membranes, increasing the risk of adverse effects and increasing bronchoconstriction. Caffeine may increase the risk of tachycardia.)	• Teach the patient about smoking cessation programs, to avoid environments with secondhand smoke, and to limit or eliminate caffeine intake while taking bronchodilator therapy.
• Maintain consistent dosing of long-acting bronchodilators. (Regular, consistent dosing with LABAs, anticholinergics, mast-cell stabilizers, and corticosteroids is used to prevent or limit acute bronchoconstrictive attacks.)	• Teach the patient the importance of consistent administration of bronchodilation therapy to prevent acute attacks.
• Utilize appropriate spacer between inhaler and mouth as appropriate and rinse mouth after using inhaler, especially after corticosteroids. (Spacers between metered-dose inhalers assist in the coordination and timing of inhalation and prevent medication being delivered to the back of the pharynx. Rinsing the mouth after the use of inhalers prevents systemic absorption or localized reactions to the drug such as ulceration.)	• Instruct the patient in the proper use of spacers if ordered, followed by return-demonstration. • Teach the patient to rinse the mouth after each use of the inhaler and to spit out after rinsing.
Patient understanding of drug therapy: • Use opportunities during the administration of medications and during assessments to discuss the rationale for drug therapy, desired therapeutic outcomes, most commonly observed adverse effects, parameters for when to call the health care provider, and any necessary monitoring or precautions. (Using time during nursing care helps to optimize and reinforce key teaching areas.)	• The patient should be able to state the reason for the drug, appropriate dose and scheduling, and what adverse effects to observe for and when to report them.

NURSING PROCESS FOCUS PATIENTS RECEIVING BRONCHODILATOR THERAPY *(Continued)*

Implementation

Interventions and (Rationales)	Patient and Family Education

Patient self-administration of drug therapy:
 	
• When administering the medication, instruct the patient, family, or caregiver in the proper self-administration of the drug, e.g., take the drug at the first appearance of symptoms before symptoms are severe. (Proper administration increases the effectiveness of the drugs.)
	• The patient recognizes the difference between quick-acting and long-acting inhalers and knows when each is to be used.
	• Instruct the patient in proper administration techniques for inhalers, followed by return-demonstration, including:
	  ▪ Use a spacer if instructed between the metered-dose inhaler and mouth.
	  ▪ Shake the inhaler or load inhaler with tablet or powder as instructed.
	  ▪ If using bronchodilator and corticosteroid inhalers, use the bronchodilator first, wait 5 minutes, then use the corticosteroid to ensure that the drug reaches deeper into the bronchi.
	  ▪ Rinse the mouth after using any inhaler.

Evaluation of Outcome Criteria

Evaluate the effectiveness of drug therapy by confirming that patient goals and expected outcomes have been met (see "Planning").

See Tables 39.2 and 39.3 for a list of drugs to which these nursing actions apply.

Inhaled corticosteroids are the preferred therapy for *preventing* asthma attacks. When inhaled on a daily schedule, corticosteroids suppress inflammation without producing major adverse effects. Although symptoms will improve in the first 1 to 2 weeks of therapy, 4 to 8 weeks may be required for maximum benefit. For patients with persistent asthma, a long-acting beta₂-adrenergic agonist may be prescribed along with the inhaled corticosteroid to obtain an additive effect. Inhaled corticosteroids must be taken daily to produce their therapeutic effect and these drugs are not effective at terminating acute asthmatic episodes in progress. Most patients with asthma carry an inhaler containing a rapid-acting beta agonist to terminate acute attacks if they occur.

For severe, unstable asthma that is unresponsive to other treatments, systemic corticosteroids such as oral prednisone may be prescribed. Treatment time is limited to the shortest length possible, usually 5 to 7 days. At the end of the brief treatment period, patients are switched to inhaled corticosteroids for long-term management.

Inhaled corticosteroids are absorbed into the circulation so slowly that systemic adverse effects are rarely observed. Local side effects include hoarseness and oropharyngeal candidiasis. If taken for longer than 10 days, *systemic* corticosteroids can produce significant adverse effects, including adrenal gland atrophy, peptic ulcers, osteoporosis, and hyperglycemia. Because asthma most commonly occurs in children, growth retardation is a concern with the use of these drugs. Because these effects are all dose and time dependent, they can be avoided by limiting systemic therapy to less than 10 days. Other uses and adverse effects of corticosteroids are presented in chapters 33 and 43∞.

See Nursing Process Focus: Patients Receiving Systemic Corticosteroid Therapy, on page 674 in chapter 43∞, for the complete nursing process applied to caring for patients receiving corticosteroids.

Leukotriene Modifiers

The leukotriene modifiers are relatively new drugs used to reduce inflammation and ease bronchoconstriction. Leukotriene modifiers are used as alternative drugs in the management of asthma symptoms. These drugs are listed in Table 39.3.

39.9 Prophylaxis of Asthma with Leukotriene Modifiers

Leukotrienes are mediators of the immune response that are involved in allergic and asthmatic reactions. Although the prefix *leuko-* implies white blood cells, these mediators are synthesized by mast cells, as well as neutrophils, basophils, and eosinophils. When released in the airway, leukotrienes promote edema, inflammation, and bronchoconstriction.

There are currently three drugs that modify leukotriene function. Zileuton (Zyflo) acts by blocking lipoxygenase, the enzyme used to synthesize leukotrienes. The remaining two agents in this class, zafirlukast (Accolate) and montelukast (Singulair), act by blocking leukotriene receptors. All three reduce inflammation. They are not considered bronchodilators like the beta₂ agonists, although they do reduce bronchoconstriction indirectly.

The leukotriene modifiers are oral medications approved for the prophylaxis of chronic asthma. Zileuton has a more rapid onset of action (2 hours) than the other two leukotriene modifiers, which take as long as 1 week to produce optimum therapeutic benefit. Because of their delayed onset, leukotriene modifiers are ineffective in terminating

Pr Prototype Drug | Beclomethasone *(Beconase AQ, Qvar)*

Therapeutic Class: Anti-inflammatory drug for asthma and allergic rhinitis

Pharmacologic Class: Inhaled corticosteroid

ACTIONS AND USES

Beclomethasone is a corticosteroid available through aerosol inhalation for asthma (Qvar) or as a nasal spray (Beconase AQ) for allergic rhinitis. Beclomethasone and other drugs in this class are preferred drugs for the long-term management of persistent asthma in both children and adults. For asthma, two inhalations, two to three times per day, usually provide adequate prophylaxis. Beclomethasone acts by reducing inflammation, thus decreasing the frequency of asthma attacks. It is not a bronchodilator and should not be used to terminate asthma attacks in progress.

ADMINISTRATION ALERTS

- Do not use if the patient is experiencing an acute asthma attack.
- Oral inhalation products and nasal spray products are not to be used interchangeably.
- Pregnancy category C

PHARMACOKINETICS

Onset: 1–4 wks

Peak: 30–70 min

Half-life: 15 h

Duration: Unknown

ADVERSE EFFECTS

Inhaled beclomethasone produces few systemic adverse effects. Because small amounts may be swallowed with each dose, the patient should be observed for signs of corticosteroid toxicity when taking the drug for prolonged periods. Local effects may include hoarseness, dry mouth, and changes in taste.

As with all corticosteroids, the anti-inflammatory properties of beclomethasone can mask signs of infections, and the drug is contraindicated if an active infection is present. A significant percentage of patients taking beclomethasone on a long-term basis will develop oropharyngeal candidiasis, a fungal infection in the throat, due to the constant deposits of drug in the oral cavity.

Contraindications: Beclomethasone is contraindicated in those with hypersensitivity to the drug. The growth of pediatric patients should be monitored carefully because inhaled corticosteroids may reduce growth velocity in some children.

INTERACTIONS

Drug–Drug: Unknown

Lab Tests: Unknown

Herbal/Food: Unknown

Treatment of Overdose: Overdose does not occur when the drug is given by the inhalation route.

Refer to MyNursingKit for a Nursing Process Focus specific to this drug.

---

acute asthma attacks. The current role of leukotriene modifiers in the management of asthma is for persistent asthma that cannot be controlled with inhaled corticosteroids or short-acting beta agonists.

Few serious adverse effects are associated with the leukotriene modifiers. Headache, cough, nasal congestion, or GI upset may occur. Patients older than age 65 have been found to experience an increased frequency of infections when taking leukotriene modifiers. These drugs may be contraindicated in patients with significant hepatic dysfunction or in chronic alcoholics, because they are extensively metabolized by the liver.

Mast Cell Stabilizers

Two mast cell stabilizers serve limited, though important, roles in the prophylaxis of asthma. These drugs act by inhibiting the release of histamine from mast cells, and their doses are listed in Table 39.3.

39.10 Prophylaxis of Asthma with Mast Cell Stabilizers

Cromolyn (Intal) and nedocromil (Tilade) are classified as mast cell stabilizers because their action serves to inhibit mast cells from releasing histamine and other chemical mediators of inflammation. By reducing inflammation, they are able to prevent asthma attacks. Like the corticosteroids, these agents should be taken on a daily basis because they are not effective for terminating acute attacks. Maximum

therapeutic benefit may take several weeks. Both cromolyn and nedocromil are pregnancy category B and exhibit no serious toxicity. The mast cell stabilizers are less effective in preventing chronic asthma than the inhaled corticosteroids.

Cromolyn (Intal) was the first mast stabilizer discovered. The drug is administered via an MDI or a nebulizer, and an intranasal form (Nasalcrom) is used in the treatment of seasonal allergic rhinitis (chapter 38∞). Adverse effects include stinging or burning of the nasal mucosa, irritation of the throat, and nasal congestion. Although not common, bronchospasm and anaphylaxis have been reported. Because of its short half-life (80 minutes), cromolyn must be inhaled four to six times per day.

Nedocromil (Tilade) is a newer mast cell stabilizer that has actions and uses similar to those of cromolyn. Administered with an MDI, the drug produces adverse effects similar to those of cromolyn, although the longer half-life of nedocromil allows less-frequent dosing. Patients often experience a bitter, unpleasant taste, which is a common cause for discontinuation of therapy.

CHRONIC OBSTRUCTIVE PULMONARY DISEASE

Chronic obstructive pulmonary disease (COPD), is a progressive pulmonary disorder characterized by chronic and recurrent obstruction of airflow. The two most common examples of conditions causing chronic pulmonary obstruction are chronic bronchitis and emphysema.

Pr Prototype Drug | Zafirlukast *(Accolate)*

Therapeutic Class: Anti-inflammatory drug for asthma prophylaxis

Pharmacologic Class: Leukotriene modifier

ACTIONS AND USES

Zafirlukast is used for the prophylaxis of persistent, chronic asthma. It prevents airway edema and inflammation by blocking leukotriene receptors in the airways. An advantage of the drug is that it is given by the oral route. Its relatively long onset of action makes it unsuitable for termination of acute bronchospasm. It is less effective than inhaled corticosteroids at asthma prophylaxis.

ADMINISTRATION ALERTS

- Do not use to terminate acute asthma attacks.
- Pregnancy category B

PHARMACOKINETICS
Onset: 1 wk

Peak: 3 h

Half-life: 10 h

Duration: Unknown

ADVERSE EFFECTS

Zafirlukast produces few serious adverse effects. Headache is the most common complaint, and nausea and diarrhea are reported by some patients.

Contraindications: The only contraindication is hypersensitivity to the drug. Because a few rare cases of hepatic failure have been reported in patients taking zafirlukast, those with pre-existing hepatic impairment should be treated with caution.

INTERACTIONS

Drug–Drug: Use with warfarin may increase prothrombin time. Erythromycin may decrease serum levels of zafirlukast.

Lab Tests: Zafirlukast may increase serum ALT values.

Herbal/Food: Food can reduce the bioavailability; thus, the drug should be taken on an empty stomach.

Treatment of Overdose: There is no specific treatment for overdose.

Refer to MyNursingKit for a Nursing Process Focus specific to this drug.

HOME & COMMUNITY CONSIDERATIONS

Helping Patients Manage Asthma

One noninvasive, inexpensive, and easy-to-use tool that can assist a patient with managing asthma is the peak-flow meter. The meter measures lung capacity and gives a reading. The result can then be categorized on a chart to determine if the patient is having any changes, even early breathing changes. This will allow the patient to select which level of treatment, if any, may be needed prior to visiting the health care provider. It can give an early warning and possibly help the patient avoid an acute attack with early intervention. The categories can be set up with the health care provider and individualized for the patient.

39.11 Pharmacotherapy of COPD

COPD is a major cause of death and disability. The three specific COPD conditions are asthma, chronic bronchitis, and emphysema. Chronic bronchitis and emphysema are strongly associated with smoking tobacco products (cigarette smoking accounts for 85% to 90% of all cases of nonasthmatic COPD) and, secondarily, breathing air pollutants. In **chronic bronchitis,** excess mucus is produced in the lower respiratory tract due to the inflammation and irritation from cigarette smoke or pollutants. The airway becomes partially obstructed with mucus, thus resulting in the classic signs of dyspnea and coughing. An early sign of bronchitis is often a productive cough on awakening. Gas exchange may be impaired; thus, wheezing and decreased exercise tolerance are additional clinical signs. Microbes thrive in the mucus-rich environment, and pulmonary infections are common. Because most patients with COPD are lifelong tobacco users, they often have serious comorbid cardiovascular conditions such as heart failure and hypertension.

COPD is progressive, with the terminal stage being **emphysema.** After years of chronic inflammation, the bronchioles lose their elasticity, and the alveoli dilate to maximum size to allow more air into the lungs. The patient suffers extreme dyspnea from even the slightest physical activity. The clinical distinction between chronic bronchitis and emphysema is sometimes unclear, because patients may exhibit symptoms of both conditions concurrently.

The goals of pharmacotherapy of COPD are to relieve symptoms and avoid complications of the condition. Various classes of drugs are used to treat infections, control cough, and relieve bronchospasm. Most patients receive bronchodilators such as ipratropium (Atrovent), beta$_2$ agonists, or inhaled corticosteroids. Both short-acting and long-acting bronchodilators are prescribed. Mucolytics and expectorants (chapter 38 ∞) are sometimes used to reduce

LIFESPAN CONSIDERATIONS

Respiratory Distress Syndrome

Respiratory distress syndrome (RDS) is a condition, primarily occurring in premature babies, in which the lungs are not producing surfactant. Surfactant forms a thin layer on the inner surface of the alveoli to raise the surface tension, thereby preventing the alveoli from collapsing during expiration. If birth occurs before the pneumocytes in the lung are mature enough to secrete surfactant, the alveoli collapse and RDS results.

Surfactant medications can be delivered to the newborn, either as prophylactic therapy or as rescue therapy after symptoms develop. The two natural surfactant agents used for RDS are calfactant (Infasurf) and beractant (Survanta). Calfactant is harvested from calf lungs, and beractant from mature cattle lungs. These drugs are administered intratracheally every 4 to 6 hours, until the patient's condition improves. The only synthetic surfactant, colfosceril (Exosurf), is no longer used in the United States because it is less effective than the natural surfactants.

the viscosity of the bronchial mucus and to aid in its removal. Long-term oxygen therapy assists breathing and has been shown to decrease mortality in patients with advanced COPD. Antibiotics may be prescribed for patients who experience multiple bouts of pulmonary infections.

Patients with COPD should not receive drugs that have beta-adrenergic antagonist activity or otherwise cause bronchoconstriction. Respiratory depressants such as opi-oids and barbiturates should be avoided. It is important to note that none of the pharmacotherapies offer a cure for COPD; they only treat the symptoms of a progressively worsening disease. The most important teaching point for the nurse is to strongly encourage smoking cessation in these patients. Smoking cessation has been shown to slow the progression of COPD and to result in fewer respiratory symptoms.

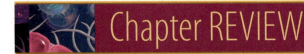

Chapter REVIEW

KEY CONCEPTS

The numbered key concepts provide a succinct summary of the important points from the corresponding numbered section within the chapter. If any of these points are not clear, refer to the numbered section within the chapter for review.

39.1 The physiology of the respiratory system involves two main processes. Ventilation moves air into and out of the lungs, and perfusion allows for gas exchange across capillaries.

39.2 Bronchioles are lined with smooth muscle that controls the amount of air entering the lungs. Dilation and constriction of the airways are controlled by the autonomic nervous system.

39.3 Inhalation is a common route of administration for pulmonary drugs because it delivers drugs directly to the sites of action. Nebulizers, MDIs, and DPIs are devices used for aerosol therapies.

39.4 Asthma is a chronic disease that has both inflammatory and bronchospasm components. Drugs are used to prevent asthmatic attacks and to terminate an attack in progress.

39.5 Beta-adrenergic agonists are the most effective drugs for relieving acute bronchospasm. These agents act by activating beta$_2$ receptors in bronchial smooth muscle to cause bronchodilation.

39.6 The anticholinergic ipratropium is a bronchodilator occasionally used as an alternative to the beta agonists in asthma therapy.

39.7 Methylxanthines such as theophylline were once the mainstay of chronic asthma pharmacotherapy. They are less effective and produce more side effects than the beta agonists.

39.8 Inhaled corticosteroids are often drugs of choice for the long-term prophylaxis of asthma. Oral corticosteroids are used for the short-term therapy of severe, acute asthma.

39.9 The leukotriene modifiers, primarily used for asthma prophylaxis, act by reducing the inflammatory component of asthma.

39.10 Mast cell stabilizers are safe drugs for the prophylaxis of asthma. They are less effective than the inhaled corticosteroids and are ineffective at relieving acute bronchospasm.

39.11 Chronic obstructive pulmonary disease (COPD) is a progressive disorder treated with multiple pulmonary drugs. Bronchodilators, expectorants, mucolytics, antibiotics, and oxygen may offer symptomatic relief.

NCLEX-RN® REVIEW QUESTIONS

1 The patient receives treatment for a respiratory condition through aerosol therapy. The nurse explains that the major advantage of this type of therapy is that:
1. it has no systemic side effects.
2. it delivers the medication to the site of action.
3. it requires no skill to use it.
4. it is safe for all patients.

2 The patient is using a beta-adrenergic agonist for treatment of asthma. The nurse teaches that the action of this drug is:
1. reducing mucus production.
2. relaxing bronchiole smooth muscle, thereby causing bronchodilation.
3. liquefying mucus.
4. reducing cough.

3 Patient teaching for patients on long-term therapy with beta-adrenergic agonists for treatment of asthma should include:
   1. discontinuing the drug if the heart rate increases.
   2. monitoring intake and output.
   3. reducing the dosage of the drug if insomnia occurs.
   4. notifying the health care provider if the drug no longer seems effective.

4 A 65-year-old male is prescribed ipratropium (Atrovent) for the treatment of asthma. An appropriate nursing intervention includes:
   1. teaching the patient to avoid caffeine in the diet.
   2. assessing for an enlarged liver.
   3. teaching the patient to report an inability to urinate.
   4. monitoring for development of diarrhea.

5 Nursing assessment for a patient on long-term oral corticosteroids would include: (Select all that apply.)
   1. assessing liver function tests.
   2. assessing cardiac dysrhythmias.
   3. assessing for signs of peptic ulcers.
   4. monitoring blood glucose for hyperglycemia.
   5. assessing for changes in level of consciousness.

6 Which of the following agents is most immediately helpful in treating a severe acute asthma attack?
   1. Beclomethasone (Qvar)
   2. Zileuton (Zyflo)
   3. Albuterol (Proventil, Ventolin)
   4. Salmeterol (Serevent)

CRITICAL THINKING QUESTIONS

1. A 72-year-old male patient has recently been started on an ipratropium (Atrovent) inhaler. What teaching is important for the nurse to provide?

2. A 45-year-old patient with chronic asthma is on corticosteroids. What must the nurse monitor when caring for this patient?

3. A 7-year-old boy with a history of asthma goes to the health room at his elementary school and states that he has increased shortness of breath and chest tightness. On assessment, the school nurse notes scattered expiratory wheezes throughout his upper and middle lung fields and a decreased peak meter flow. The current therapeutic regimen for this child includes salmeterol (Serevent) two puffs every 12 h, montelukast (Singulair) 5 mg/day PO in the evening, triamcinolone (Azmacort) two puffs tid, and albuterol (Proventil) two puffs every 4 h prn. After observing the child's technique in using the metered-dose inhaler (MDI), the school nurse wishes to reinforce the child's education as it relates to the administration technique of his inhalants. What areas should be emphasized?

See Appendix D for answers and rationales for all activities.

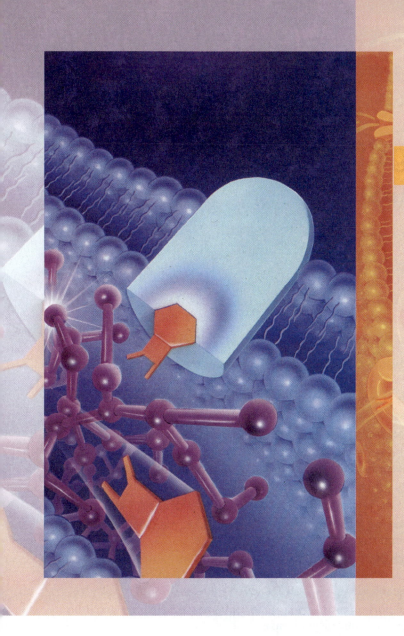

The Gastrointestinal System

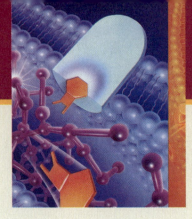

Chapter 40

Drugs for Peptic Ulcer Disease

DRUGS AT A GLANCE

LEARNING OUTCOMES

After reading this chapter, the student should be able to:

1. Describe the major anatomic structures of the upper gastrointestinal tract.
2. Identify common causes, signs, and symptoms of peptic ulcer disease and gastroesophageal reflux disease.
3. Compare and contrast duodenal ulcers and gastric ulcers.
4. Describe treatment goals for the pharmacotherapy of gastroesophageal reflux disease.
5. Identify the classification of drugs used to treat peptic ulcer disease.
6. Explain the pharmacologic strategies for eradicating *Helicobacter pylori*.
7. Describe the nurse's role in the pharmacologic management of patients with peptic ulcer disease.
8. For each of the classes listed in Drugs at a Glance, know representative drugs, and explain their mechanism of drug action, describe primary actions, and identify important adverse effects.
9. Use the nursing process to care for patients who are receiving drug therapy for peptic ulcer disease.

KEY TERMS

Very little of the food we eat is directly available to body cells. Food must be broken down, absorbed, and chemically modified before it is in a useful form. The digestive system performs these functions, and more. Some disorders of the digestive system are mechanical in nature, providing for the transit of substances through the gastrointestinal tract. Others are metabolic, involving the secretion of digestive enzymes and fluids, or the absorption of essential nutrients. Many signs and symptoms of digestive disorders are nonspecific and may be caused by any number of different pathologies. This chapter examines the pharmacotherapy of two common disorders of the upper digestive system: peptic ulcer disease (PUD) and gastroesophageal reflux disease (GERD).

40.1 Normal Digestive Processes

The digestive system consists of two basic anatomic divisions: the alimentary canal and the accessory organs. The alimentary canal, or gastrointestinal (GI) tract, is a long, continuous, hollow tube that extends from the mouth to the anus. The accessory organs of digestion include the salivary glands, liver, gallbladder, and pancreas. Major structures of the digestive system are illustrated in ➤ Figure 40.1.

The inner lining of the alimentary canal is the **mucosa layer**, which provides a surface area for the various acids, bases, mucus, and enzymes to break down food. In many parts of the alimentary canal, the mucosa is folded and contains deep grooves and pits. The small intestine is lined with tiny projections called *villi* and *microvilli*, which provide a huge surface area for the absorption of food and medications.

Substances are propelled along the GI tract by **peristalsis**, rhythmic contractions of layers of smooth muscle. The speed at which substances move through the GI tract is critical to the absorption of nutrients and water and for the removal of wastes. If peristalsis is too fast, nutrients and drugs will not have sufficient contact with the mucosa to be absorbed. In addition, the large intestine will not have enough time to absorb water, and diarrhea may result. Abnormally

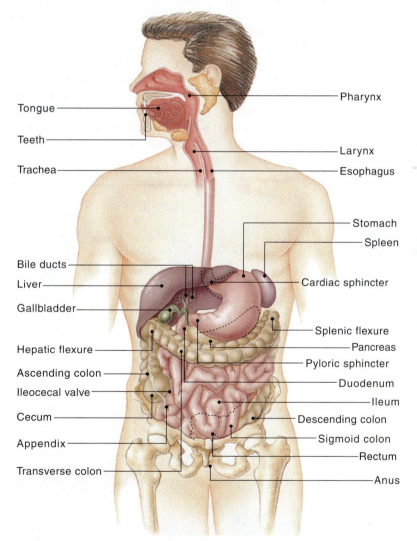

➤ *Figure 40.1* The digestive system

Source: Mulvihill et al., Human Diseases: A Systemic Approach, *6th edition, © 2006, p. 276. Reprinted by permission of Pearson Education, Inc., Upper Saddle River, NJ.*

slow transit may result in constipation or even obstructions in the small or large intestine. Disorders of the lower digestive tract are discussed in chapter 41∞.

To chemically break down ingested food, a large number of enzymes and other substances are required. Digestive enzymes are secreted by the salivary glands, stomach, small intestine, and pancreas. The liver makes bile, which is stored in the gallbladder, until needed for lipid digestion. Because these digestive substances are not common targets for drug therapy, their discussion in this chapter is limited, and the student should refer to anatomy and physiology texts for additional information.

40.2 Acid Production by the Stomach

Food passes from the esophagus to the stomach by traveling through the lower esophageal (cardiac) sphincter. This ring of smooth muscle usually prevents the stomach contents from moving backward, a condition known as **esophageal reflux**. A second ring of smooth muscle, the pyloric sphincter, is located at the entrance to the small intestine. This sphincter regulates the flow of substances leaving the stomach.

The stomach thoroughly mixes ingested food and secretes substances that promote the processes of chemical digestion. Gastric glands extending deep into the mucosa of the stomach contain several cell types critical to digestion and important to the pharmacotherapy of digestive disorders. **Chief cells** secrete pepsinogen, an inactive form of the enzyme pepsin that chemically breaks down proteins. **Parietal cells** secrete 1 to 3 L of hydrochloric acid each day. This strong acid

helps break down food, activates pepsinogen, and kills microbes that may have been ingested. Parietal cells also secrete **intrinsic factor,** which is essential for the absorption of vitamin B$_{12}$ (chapter 42∞). Parietal cells are targets for the classes of antiulcer drugs that limit acid secretion.

The combined secretion of the chief and parietal cells, gastric juice, is the most acidic fluid in the body, having a pH of 1.5 to 3.5. A number of natural defenses protect the stomach mucosa against this extremely acidic fluid. Certain cells lining the surface of the stomach secrete a thick mucous layer and bicarbonate ion to neutralize the acid. These form such an effective protective layer that the pH at the mucosal surface is nearly neutral. Once they reach the duodenum, the stomach contents are further neutralized by bicarbonate from pancreatic and biliary secretions. These natural defenses are shown in ➤ Figure 40.2.

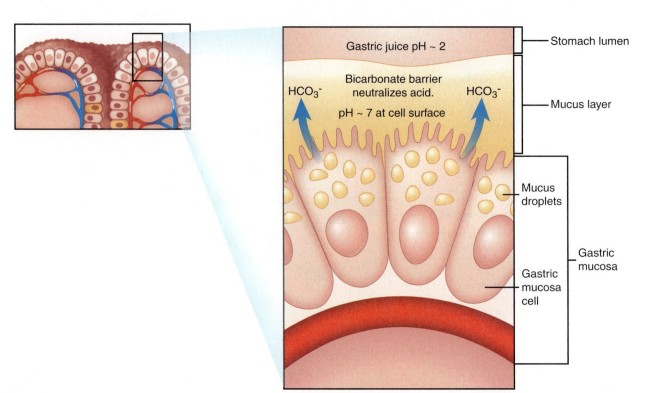

➤ **Figure 40.2** Natural defenses against stomach acid

40.3 Pathogenesis of Peptic Ulcer Disease

An *ulcer* is an erosion of the mucosa layer of the GI tract, usually associated with acute inflammation. Although ulcers may occur in any portion of the alimentary canal, the duodenum is the most common site. The term **peptic ulcer** refers to a lesion located in either the stomach (gastric) or small intestine (duodenal). Peptic ulcer disease is associated with the following risk factors:

- Close family history of PUD
- Blood group O
- Smoking tobacco
- Beverages and food containing caffeine
- Drugs, particularly corticosteroids and nonsteroidal anti-inflammatory drugs (NSAIDs), including aspirin
- Excessive psychologic stress
- Infection with *Helicobacter pylori*

The primary cause of PUD is infection by the gram-negative bacterium **Helicobacter pylori**. Approximately 50% of the population has *H. pylori* present in their stomach and proximal small intestine. In *noninfected* patients, the most common cause of PUD is drug therapy with NSAIDs. Secondary factors that *contribute* to ulcer formation and subsequent inflammation include secretion of excess gastric acid and hyposecretion of adequate mucous protection.

The characteristic symptom of *duodenal* ulcer is a gnawing or burning, upper abdominal pain that occurs 1 to 3 hours after a meal. The pain is worse when the stomach is empty and often disappears on ingestion of food. Night-time pain, nausea, and vomiting are uncommon. If the erosion progresses deeper into the mucosa, bleeding occurs and may be evident as either bright red blood in vomit or black, tarry stools. Many duodenal ulcers heal spontaneously, although they frequently recur after months of remission. Long-term medical follow-up is usually not necessary.

Gastric ulcers are less common than the duodenal type and have different symptoms. Although relieved by food, pain may continue even after a meal. Loss of appetite, known as anorexia, as well as weight loss and vomiting are more common. Remissions may be infrequent or absent. Medical follow-up of gastric ulcers should continue for several years, because a small percentage of the erosions become cancerous. The most severe ulcers may penetrate the wall of the stomach and cause death. Whereas duodenal ulcers occur most frequently in males in the 30- to 50-year age group, gastric ulcers are more common in women over age 60.

Ulceration in the distal small intestine is known as *Crohn's disease,* and erosions in the large intestine are called *ulcerative colitis*. These diseases, together categorized as inflammatory bowel disease, are discussed in chapter 41∞.

40.4 Pathogenesis of Gastroesophageal Reflux Disease

Gastroesophageal reflux disease (GERD) is a common condition in which the acidic contents of the stomach move upward into the esophagus. This causes an intense burning (heartburn) sometimes accompanied by belching. In severe cases, untreated GERD can lead to complications such as esophagitis, or esophageal ulcers or strictures. Although most often thought a disease of people older than age 40, GERD also occurs in a significant percentage of infants.

The cause of GERD is usually a weakening of the lower esophageal sphincter. The sphincter may no longer close tightly, allowing the contents of the stomach to move upward when the stomach contracts. GERD is associated with obesity, and losing weight may eliminate the symptoms. Other lifestyle changes that can improve GERD symptoms include elevating the head of the bed, avoiding fatty or acidic foods, eating smaller meals at least 3 hours before sleep, and eliminating tobacco and alcohol use.

Because patients often self-treat this disorder with OTC drugs, a thorough medication history may give clues to the presence of GERD. Many of the drugs prescribed for peptic ulcers are also used to treat GERD, with the primary goal being to reduce gastric acid secretion. Drug classes include antacids, H_2-receptor antagonists, and proton pump inhibitors. Because drugs provide only symptomatic relief, surgery may become necessary to eliminate the cause of GERD in patients with persistent disease.

40.5 Pharmacotherapy of Peptic Ulcer Disease

Before initiating pharmacotherapy, patients are usually advised to change lifestyle factors contributing to the severity of PUD or GERD. For example, eliminating tobacco and alcohol use and reducing stress promote healing of the ulcer and may cause it to go into remission. Avoiding certain foods and beverages can lessen the severity of symptoms.

The goals of PUD pharmacotherapy are to provide immediate relief from symptoms, promote healing of the ulcer, and prevent future recurrence of the disease. A wide variety of both prescription and OTC drugs are available. These drugs fall into four primary classes, plus a miscellaneous group. The mechanisms of action of the four major drug classes for PUD are shown in Pharmacotherapy Illustrated 40.1:

- H_2-receptor antagonists
- Proton pump inhibitors
- Antacids
- Antibiotics
- Miscellaneous drugs

For patients on NSAIDs, the initial approach to PUD is to switch the patient to an alternative medication, such as acetaminophen or a selective COX-2 inhibitor. This is not always possible, because NSAIDs are drugs of choice for treating

PHARMACOTHERAPY ILLUSTRATED

40.1 Mechanisms of Action of Antiulcer Drugs

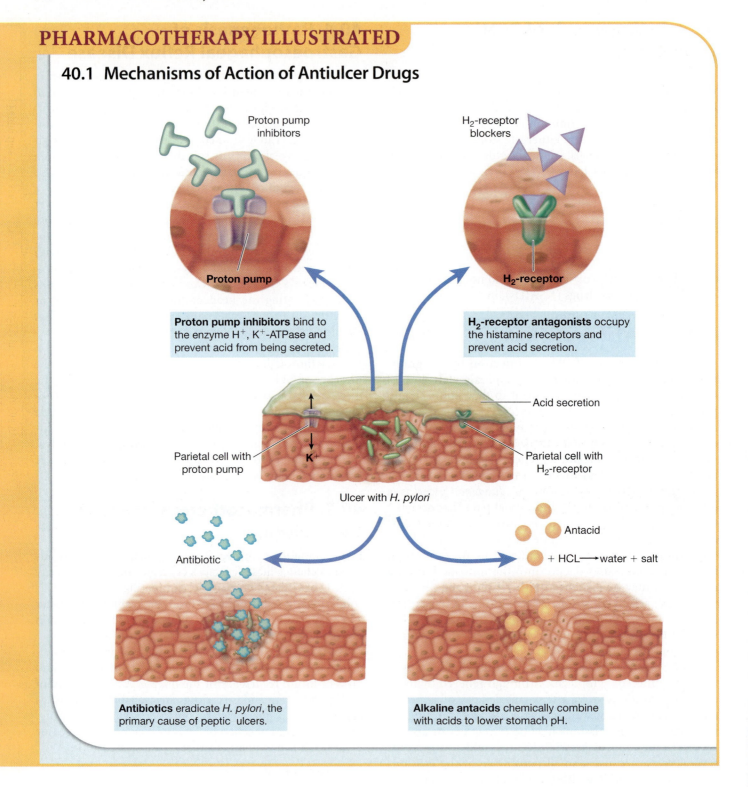

Proton pump inhibitors

Proton pump

Proton pump inhibitors bind to the enzyme H^+, K^+-ATPase and prevent acid from being secreted.

H_2-receptor blockers

H_2-receptor

H_2-receptor antagonists occupy the histamine receptors and prevent acid secretion.

Acid secretion

Parietal cell with proton pump

K^+

Parietal cell with H_2-receptor

Ulcer with *H. pylori*

Antibiotic

Antibiotics eradicate *H. pylori*, the primary cause of peptic ulcers.

Antacid

+ HCL ⟶ water + salt

Alkaline antacids chemically combine with acids to lower stomach pH.

chronic arthritis and other disorders associated with pain and inflammation. If discontinuation of the NSAID is not possible, or if symptoms persist after the NSAID has been withdrawn, antiulcer medications are indicated.

For patients with *H. pylori* infection, eradication of the bacteria with antibiotics is the primary goal of pharmacotherapy (see Section 40.9). Treatment using only antiulcer drugs *without* eradicating *H. pylori* results in a very high recurrence rate of PUD.

PROTON PUMP INHIBITORS

Proton pump inhibitors act by blocking the enzyme responsible for secreting hydrochloric acid in the stomach. They are drugs of choice for the short-term therapy of PUD and GERD. These agents are listed in Table 40.1.

TABLE 40.1	Proton Pump Inhibitors		
Drug	**Route and Adult Dose (max dose where indicated)**		**Adverse Effects**
esomeprazole (Nexium)	PO; 20–40 mg/day		*Headache, diarrhea, nausea, rash, dizziness*
lansoprazole (Prevacid)	PO; 15–60 mg/day		<u>Serious adverse effects are rare</u>
Pr omeprazole (Prilosec)	PO; 20–60 mg one to two times/day		
pantoprazole (Protonix)	PO; 40 mg/day		
rabeprazole (AcipHex)	PO; 20 mg/day		

Italics indicate common adverse effects; <u>underlining</u> indicates serious adverse effects.

40.6 Pharmacotherapy with Proton Pump Inhibitors

Proton pump inhibitors reduce acid secretion in the stomach by binding irreversibly to the enzyme **H+, K+-ATPase**. In the parietal cells of the stomach, this enzyme acts as a pump to release acid (also called H+, or protons) onto the surface of the GI mucosa. The proton pump inhibitors reduce acid secretion to a greater extent than the H$_2$-receptor antagonists and have a longer duration of action. PPIs heal more than 90% of duodenal ulcers within 4 weeks and about 90% of gastric ulcers in 6 to 8 weeks.

Several days of proton pump inhibitor therapy may be needed before patients gain relief from ulcer pain. Beneficial effects continue for 3 to 5 days after the drugs have been stopped. These drugs are used only for the short-term control of peptic ulcers and GERD: The typical length of therapy is 4 weeks. Omeprazole and lansoprazole are used concurrently with antibiotics to eradicate *H. pylori*. The newer agents esomeprazole (Nexium) and pantoprazole (Protonix) offer the convenience of once-a-day dosing.

All proton pump inhibitors have similar efficacy and adverse effects. Serious adverse effects from drugs in this class are uncommon. Headache, abdominal pain, diarrhea, nausea, and vomiting are the most frequently reported effects.

H$_2$-RECEPTOR ANTAGONISTS

The discovery of the H$_2$-receptor antagonists in the 1970s marked a major breakthrough in the treatment of PUD. They have since become available OTC and are widely used

---

Pr Prototype Drug | Omeprazole *(Prilosec)*

Therapeutic Class: Antiulcer drug   **Pharmacologic Class:** Proton pump inhibitor

ACTIONS AND USES
Omeprazole was the first proton pump inhibitor to be approved for PUD: Both prescription and OTC forms are available. It reduces acid secretion in the stomach by binding irreversibly to the enzyme H+, K+-ATPase. Although this agent can take 2 hours to reach therapeutic levels, its effects last up to 72 hours. It is used for the short-term, 4- to 8-week therapy of active peptic ulcers and GERD. Most patients are symptom free after 2 weeks of therapy. It is used for longer periods in patients who have chronic hypersecretion of gastric acid, a condition known as **Zollinger–Ellison syndrome.** It is the most effective drug for this syndrome. Omeprazole is available only in oral form. Zegerid is a combination drug containing omeprazole and the antacid sodium bicarbonate.

ADMINISTRATION ALERTS
- If possible, administer before breakfast on an empty stomach.
- It may be administered with antacids.
- Capsules and tablets should not be chewed, divided, or crushed.
- Pregnancy category C

PHARMACOKINETICS
Onset: 0.5–3.5 h
Peak: 5 days
Half-life: 0.5–1.5 h
Duration: 3–4 days

ADVERSE EFFECTS
Adverse effects are generally minor and include headache, nausea, diarrhea, rash, and abdominal pain. The main concern with proton pump inhibitors is that long-term use has been associated with an increased risk of gastric cancer in laboratory animals. Because of this possibility, therapy is generally limited to 2 months.

Contraindications: The only contraindication is hypersensitivity to the drug. OTC use is not approved for patients under 18 years of age.

INTERACTIONS
Drug–Drug: Concurrent use with diazepam, phenytoin, and CNS depressants may cause increased blood levels of these drugs. Concurrent use with warfarin may increase the likelihood of bleeding. Alcohol can aggravate the stomach mucosa and decrease the effectiveness of omeprazole.

Lab Tests: Omeprazole may increase values for ALT, AST, and serum alkaline phosphatase.

Herbal/Food: Ginkgo and St. John's wort may decrease the plasma concentration of omeprazole.

Treatment of Overdose: There is no specific treatment for overdose.

Refer to MyNursingKit for a Nursing Process Focus specific to this drug.

TABLE 40.2	H₂-Receptor Antagonists	
Drug	**Route and Adult Dose (max dose where indicated)**	**Adverse Effects**
cimetidine (Tagamet)	PO; 300 mg every 6 h or 800 mg at bedtime or 400 mg bid with food	*Diarrhea, constipation, headache, fatigue, nausea, gynecomastia* Rare: Hepatitis, blood dyscrasias, anaphylaxis, dysrhythmias, skin reactions, galactorrhea, confusion or psychoses
famotidine (Pepcid, Mylanta AP) nizatidine (Axid) Ⓟ ranitidine (Zantac)	PO; 20 mg bid or 40 mg at bedtime PO; 150–300 mg at bedtime PO; 100–150 mg bid or 300 mg at bedtime	*Headache, nausea, dry mouth* Rare: Musculoskeletal pain, tachycardia, blood dyscrasia, blurred vision
Italics indicate common adverse effects; underlining indicates serious adverse effects.		

in the treatment of hyperacidity disorders of the GI tract. These agents are listed in Table 40.2.

40.7 Pharmacotherapy with H₂-Receptor Antagonists

Histamine has two types of receptors: H₁ and H₂. Activation of H₁ receptors produces the classic symptoms of inflammation and allergy, whereas the H₂ receptors are responsible for increasing acid secretion in the stomach. The **H₂-receptor antagonists** are effective at suppressing the volume and acidity of parietal cell secretions. These drugs are used to treat the symptoms of both PUD and GERD.

All H₂-receptor antagonists have similar safety profiles: Adverse effects are minor and rarely cause discontinuation of therapy. Patients taking high doses, or those with renal or hepatic disease may experience confusion, restlessness, hallucinations, or depression. The first drug in this class, cimetidine (Tagamet), is used less frequently than other H₂-receptor antagonists because of numerous drug–drug interactions (it inhibits hepatic drug-metabolizing enzymes) and because it must be taken up to four times a day. Antacids should not be taken at the same time because the absorption of the H₂-receptor antagonist will be diminished.

ANTACIDS

Antacids are alkaline substances that have been used to neutralize stomach acid for hundreds of years. These agents, listed in Table 40.3, are readily available as OTC drugs.

Ⓟ Prototype Drug | Ranitidine (Zantac)

Therapeutic Class: Antiulcer drug **Pharmacologic Class:** H₂-receptor antagonist

ACTIONS AND USES
Ranitidine acts by blocking H₂ receptors in the stomach to decrease acid production. It has a higher potency than cimetidine, which allows it to be administered once daily, usually at bedtime. Adequate healing of the ulcer takes approximately 4 to 8 weeks, although those at high risk for PUD may continue on drug maintenance for prolonged periods to prevent recurrence. Gastric ulcers require longer therapy for healing to occur. IV and IM forms are available for the treatment of acute, stress-induced bleeding ulcers. Tritec is a combination drug with ranitidine and bismuth citrate. Ranitidine is available in a dissolving tablet form (EFFERdose) for treating GERD in children and infants older than 1 month of age.

ADMINISTRATION ALERT
- Administer after meals and monitor liver and renal function.
- Pregnancy category B

PHARMACOKINETICS
Onset: Unknown
Peak: 2–3 h
Half-life: 2–3 h
Duration: 8–12 h

ADVERSE EFFECTS
Adverse effects are uncommon and mild. Ranitidine does not cross the blood–brain barrier to any appreciable extent, so it does not cause the confusion and CNS depression observed with cimetidine. Although rare, severe reductions in the number of red and white blood cells and platelets are possible; thus, periodic blood counts may be performed. High doses may result in impotence or loss of libido in men.

Contraindications: Contraindications include hypersensitivity to H₂-receptor antagonists, acute porphyria, and OTC administration in children less than 12 years of age.

INTERACTIONS
Drug–Drug: Ranitidine has fewer drug–drug interactions than cimetidine. Ranitidine may reduce the absorption of cefpodoxime, ketoconazole, and itraconazole. Antacids should not be given within 1 hour of H₂-receptor antagonists because the effectiveness may be decreased due to reduced absorption. Smoking decreases the effectiveness of ranitidine.

Lab Tests: Ranitidine may increase the values of serum creatinine, AST, ALT, LDH, alkaline phosphatase, and bilirubin. It may produce false positives for urine protein.

Herbal/Food: Absorption of vitamin B₁₂ depends on an acidic environment; thus, deficiency may occur. Iron is also better absorbed in an acidic environment.

Treatment of Overdose: There is no specific treatment for overdose.

Refer to MyNursingKit for a Nursing Process Focus specific to this drug.

| NURSING PROCESS FOCUS | PATIENTS RECEIVING DRUG THERAPY FOR PEPTIC ULCER (PUD) AND GASTROESOPHAGEAL REFLUX DISEASE (GERD) |

Assessment	Potential Nursing Diagnoses
Baseline assessment prior to administration: ■ Understand the reason the drug has been prescribed in order to assess for therapeutic effects. ■ Obtain a complete health history including GI, hepatic, renal, respiratory, or cardiovascular disease; pregnancy; or breast-feeding. Obtain a drug history including allergies, current prescription and OTC drugs, herbal preparations, caffeine, nicotine, and alcohol use. Be alert to possible drug interactions. ■ Obtain a history of past and current symptoms, noting any correlations between the onset or presence of any pain related to meals, sleep, positioning, or associated with other medications. Also note what measures have been successful to relieve the pain (e.g., eating). ■ Obtain baseline vital signs and weight. ■ Evaluate appropriate laboratory findings (e.g., CBC, platelets, electrolytes, hepatic or renal function studies).	■ Acute Pain ■ Altered Nutrition, Less Than Body Requirements ■ Deficient Knowledge (drug therapy) ■ Risk for Ineffective Health Maintenance (Individual or Family; dietary and lifestyle changes)
Assessment throughout administration: ■ Assess for desired therapeutic effects (e.g., diminished gastric area pain, lessened bloating or belching). ■ Continue periodic monitoring of CBC, electrolytes, and hepatic and renal function labs. Testing for *H. pylori* may be needed if symptoms fail to resolve. ■ Assess for adverse effects: nausea, vomiting, diarrhea, headache, drowsiness, and dizziness. Severe abdominal pain, vomiting, coffee-ground or bloody vomiting, or blood in stool or tarry stools should be reported immediately.	

Planning: Patient Goals and Expected Outcomes

The patient will:

■ Experience therapeutic effects (e.g., diminished or absent gastric pain, absence of related symptoms such as bloating or belching).

■ Be free from, or experience minimal, adverse effects.

■ Verbalize an understanding of the drug's use, adverse effects, and required precautions.

■ Demonstrate proper self-administration of the medication (e.g., dose, timing, when to notify provider).

Implementation	
Interventions and (Rationales)	**Patient and Family Education**
Ensuring therapeutic effects: ■ Encourage appropriate lifestyle changes, including an increased intake of yogurt and *acidophilus*-containing foods. Have the patient keep a food diary noting correlations between discomfort or pain and meals or activities. (Smoking and alcohol use increase gastric acid and irritation and should be eliminated. Correlating symptoms with dietary habits may help to eliminate a triggering factor.)	■ Encourage the patient to adopt a healthy lifestyle of low-fat food choices and increased exercise, and to eliminate alcohol consumption and smoking. Provide for dietitian consultation or information on smoking cessation programs as needed.
Minimizing adverse effects: ■ Continue to monitor the presence of gastric area pain. (Continued symptoms may indicate ineffectiveness of current drug therapy or the need for testing for *H. pylori*.)	■ Teach the patient that full drug effects may take several days to weeks or longer. Consistent drug therapy will provide the best results. If gastric discomfort or pain continue or worsen after several weeks of therapy, the health care provider should be notified.
■ Monitor for any severe abdominal pain, vomiting, coffee-ground or bloody vomiting, or blood in stool or tarry stools and report immediately. (Drugs used to treat PUD and GERD decrease gastric acidity, making the gastric environment less favorable for ulcer development but they do not heal existing ulcers. Severe abdominal pain or blood in emesis or stools may indicate a worsening of disease or more serious conditions and should be reported immediately.)	■ Teach the patient that severe abdominal pain or any blood in emesis or stools should be reported immediately to the health care provider.

(Continued)

NURSING PROCESS FOCUS — PATIENTS RECEIVING DRUG THERAPY FOR PEPTIC ULCER (PUD) AND GASTROESOPHAGEAL REFLUX DISEASE (GERD) (Continued)

Implementation

Interventions and (Rationales)	Patient and Family Education
• Continue to monitor periodic hepatic and renal function tests and CBC, platelets, and electrolyte levels. (Abnormal liver function tests may indicate drug-induced adverse hepatic effects. Decreased RBC, WBC, or platelets have been noted with long-term H_2-receptor blocker therapy and decreases should be reported to the health care provider. Excessive use of antacids may affect electrolyte levels.)	• Instruct the patient on the need to return periodically for lab work.
• Ensure patient safety, especially in older adults. Observe for dizziness and monitor ambulation until the effects of the drug are known. (Drowsiness or dizziness from H_2-receptor blockers may occur, which increases the risk of falls. Continued dizziness or drowsiness may require a change in drug therapy.)	• Instruct the patient to call for assistance prior to getting out of bed or attempting to walk alone, and to avoid driving or other activities requiring mental alertness or physical coordination until the effects of the drug are known.
Patient understanding of drug therapy: • Use opportunities during administration of medications and during assessments to discuss the rationale for drug therapy, desired therapeutic outcomes, most common adverse effects, parameters for when to call the health care provider, and any necessary monitoring or precautions. (Using time during nursing care helps to optimize and reinforce key teaching areas.)	• The patient, family, or caregiver should be able to state the reason for the drug; appropriate dose and scheduling; what adverse effects to observe for and when to report; and the anticipated length of medication therapy.
Patient self-administration of drug therapy: • When administering the medication, instruct the patient, family, or caregiver in the proper self-administration of the drug, e.g., during evening meal. (Proper administration improves the effectiveness of the drugs.)	• Teach the patient to take the drug according to appropriate guidelines as follows: • H_2-receptor blockers: Take the drug after meals. Do not take concurrently with antacids unless the drug is available in a combination product such as Pepcid-Complete. • Proton pump inhibitors: Take 30 minutes before meals. If once-a-day dosing is ordered, take the drug in the morning before breakfast. Antacids may be used concurrently. Do not continue taking the drug beyond 3 to 4 months unless directed by the health care provider. • Antacids: Take 2 hours before or after meals with a full glass of water. Do not take other medications concurrently unless available as a combination product or directed to do so by the health care provider.

Evaluation of Outcome Criteria

Evaluate the effectiveness of drug therapy by confirming that patient goals and expected outcomes have been met (see "Planning").

See Tables 40.1, 40.2, and 40.3 for a list of drugs to which these nursing actions apply.

LIFESPAN CONSIDERATIONS

H_2 Receptors and Vitamin B_{12} in Older Adults

H_2-receptor blockers decrease the secretion of hydrochloric acid in the stomach. Unfortunately, gastric acid is essential for releasing vitamin B_{12} in foods, which is bound in a protein matrix. By affecting stomach acidity, these drugs can affect the absorption of this essential vitamin.

H_2-receptor blockers are frequently prescribed for older adults, who are more likely to have pre-existing lower vitamin B_{12} reserves or even deficiencies. With aging, the ability to produce adequate amounts of hydrochloric acid, intrinsic factor, and digestive enzymes progressively diminishes. These losses can lead to lower absorption rates, depletion of reserves, and eventually B_{12} deficiency. The nurse must educate older adults taking these drugs as to the importance of including plenty of foods rich in vitamin B_{12} in their diets, including red meat, poultry, fish, and eggs.

HOME & COMMUNITY CONSIDERATIONS

Over-the-Counter Medications for GI Disorders

Many patients purchase OTC medications based on information obtained from the media. Antacids, H_2-receptor agonists, and proton pump inhibitors are available as OTC medications. Although every OTC medication includes an information sheet, many people do not read them. Some do not read them because they feel that all OTC medications are safe, and others have difficulty reading the small print on the information sheets. Still others may not realize that they are taking an OTC that may interact with a prescribed medication. It is important to stress to patients that OTC medications may result in drug–drug interactions and produce adverse effects. Patients should be instructed to check with their health care provider if their digestive symptoms worsen or are not relieved by OTC products.

TABLE 40.3	Antacids	
Drug	**Route and Adult Dose (max dose where indicated)**	**Adverse Effects**
⊕ aluminum hydroxide (AlternaGEL, others)	PO; 600 mg tid–qid	*Constipation, nausea, stomach cramps* <u>Fecal impaction, hypophosphatemia</u>
calcium carbonate (Titralac, Tums) calcium carbonate with magnesium hydroxide (Mylanta Gel-caps, Rolaids)	PO; 1–2 g bid–tid PO; 2–4 capsules or tablets prn (max: 12 tablets/day)	*Constipation, flatulence* <u>Fecal impaction, metabolic alkalosis, hypercalcemia, renal calculi</u>
magaldrate (Riopan) magnesium hydroxide (Milk of Magnesia) magnesium hydroxide with aluminum hydroxide (Maalox) magnesium hydroxide with aluminum hydroxide with simethicone (Mylanta, Maalox Plus, others)	PO; 540–1,080 mg (5–10 mL suspension or 1–2 tablets) daily (max: 20 tablets or 100 mL/day) PO; 5–15 mL or 2–4 tablets as needed up to four times daily PO; 2–4 tablets prn (max: 16 tablets/day) PO; 10–20 mL prn (max: 120 mL/day) or 2–4 tablets prn (max: 24 tablets/day)	*Diarrhea, nausea, vomiting, abdominal cramping* <u>Hypermagnesemia, dysrhythmias (when given parenterally)</u>
sodium bicarbonate (Alka-Seltzer, baking soda) (see page 441 for the Prototype Drug box ∞)	PO; 325 mg–2 g one to four times/day	*Abdominal distention, belching, flatulence* <u>Metabolic alkalosis, fluid retention, edema, hypernatremia</u>

Italics indicate common adverse effects; <u>underlining</u> indicates serious adverse effects.

40.8 Pharmacotherapy with Antacids

Prior to the development of H$_2$-receptor antagonists and proton pump inhibitors, **antacids** were the mainstays of peptic ulcer and GERD pharmacotherapy. Indeed, many patients still use these inexpensive and readily available OTC drugs. Although antacids may provide temporary relief from heartburn or indigestion, they are no longer recommended as the primary drug class for PUD. This is because antacids do not promote healing of the ulcer, nor do they help to eradicate *H. pylori*.

Antacids are alkaline, inorganic compounds of aluminum, magnesium, sodium, or calcium. Combinations of aluminum hydroxide and magnesium hydroxide, the most common type, are capable of rapidly neutralizing stomach acid. Chewable tablets and liquid formulations are available. A few products combine antacids and H$_2$-receptor blockers into a single tablet; for example, Pepcid Complete contains calcium carbonate, magnesium hydroxide, and famotidine.

Simethicone is sometimes added to antacid preparations, because it reduces gas bubbles that cause bloating and discomfort. For example, Mylanta contains simethicone, aluminum hydroxide, and magnesium hydroxide. Simethicone is classified as an **antiflatulent,** because it reduces gas. It also is available by itself in OTC products such as Gas-X and Mylanta Gas.

Self-medication with antacids is safe, when taken in doses directed on the labels. Although antacids act within 10 to 15 minutes, their duration of action is only 2 hours; thus, they must be taken often during the day. Antacids containing sodium, calcium, or magnesium can result in absorption of these minerals to the general circulation. Absorption of antacids is clinically unimportant unless the patient is on a sodium-restricted diet or has diminished renal function that could result in accumulation of these minerals. In fact, some manufacturers advertise their calcium-based antacid products as mineral supplements. Patients should follow the label instructions carefully and keep within the recommended dosage range.

Antacids containing calcium can cause constipation and may cause or aggravate kidney stones. Administering calcium carbonate antacids with milk or any items with vitamin D can cause **milk–alkali syndrome** to occur. Early symptoms are those of hypercalcemia and include headache, urinary frequency, anorexia, nausea, and fatigue. Milk–alkali syndrome may result in permanent renal damage if the drug is continued at high doses.

ANTIBIOTICS FOR *H. PYLORI*

The gram-negative bacterium *H. pylori* is associated with 80% of patients with duodenal ulcers and 70% of those with gastric ulcers. It is also strongly associated with gastric cancer. To more rapidly and completely heal peptic ulcers, combination therapy with several antibiotics is used to eradicate this bacterium.

40.9 Pharmacotherapy with Combination Antibiotic Therapy

H. pylori has adapted well as a human pathogen by devising ways to neutralize the high acidity surrounding it and by making chemicals called *adhesins* that allow it to stick tightly to the GI mucosa. *H. pylori* infections can remain active for life, if not treated appropriately. Elimination of this organism

Pr　Prototype Drug ┃ Aluminum Hydroxide (AlternaGEL, others)

Therapeutic Class: Antiheartburn agent　　**Pharmacologic Class:** Antacid

ACTIONS AND USES

Aluminum hydroxide is an inorganic agent used alone or in combination with other antacids. Combining aluminum compounds with magnesium (Maalox, Mylanta) increases their effectiveness and reduces the potential for constipation. Unlike calcium-based antacids that can be absorbed and cause systemic effects, aluminum compounds are minimally absorbed. Their primary action is to neutralize stomach acid by raising the pH of the stomach contents. Unlike H_2-receptor antagonists and proton pump inhibitors, aluminum antacids do not reduce the volume of acid secretion. They are most effectively used in combination with other antiulcer agents for the symptomatic relief of heartburn due to PUD or GERD. A second aluminum salt, aluminum carbonate (Basaljel), is also available to treat heartburn.

ADMINISTRATION ALERTS

- Administer aluminum antacids at least 2 hours before or after other drugs because absorption could be affected.
- Pregnancy category C

PHARMACOKINETICS

Onset: 20–40 min

Peak: 30 min

Half-life: Unknown

Duration: 2 h when taken with food, 3 h when taken 1 h after food

ADVERSE EFFECTS

Aluminum antacids frequently cause constipation. At high doses, aluminum products bind with phosphate in the GI tract and long-term use can result in phosphate depletion. Those at risk include those malnourished, alcoholics, and those with renal disease.

Contraindications: This drug should not be used in patients with suspected bowel obstruction.

INTERACTIONS

Drug–Drug: Aluminum compounds should not be taken with other medications, as they may interfere with their absorption. Use with sodium polystyrene sulfonate may cause systemic alkalosis.

Lab Tests: Values for serum gastrin and urinary pH may increase. Serum phosphate values may decrease.

Herbal/Food: Aluminum antacids may inhibit the absorption of dietary iron.

Treatment of Overdose: There is no specific treatment for overdose.

Refer to MyNursingKit for a Nursing Process Focus specific to this drug.

---

allows ulcers to heal more rapidly and remain in remission longer. The following antibiotics are commonly used for this purpose:

- amoxicillin (Amoxil, others)
- clarithromycin (Biaxin)
- metronidazole (Flagyl)
- tetracycline (Achromycin, others)
- bismuth subsalicylate (Pepto-Bismol) or ranitidine bismuth citrate (Tritec)

Two or more antibiotics are given concurrently to increase the effectiveness of therapy and to lower the potential for bacterial resistance. The antibiotics are also combined with a proton pump inhibitor or an H_2-receptor antagonist. Bismuth compounds (Pepto-Bismol, Tritec) are sometimes added to the antibiotic regimen. Although technically not antibiotics, bismuth compounds inhibit bacterial growth and prevent *H. pylori* from adhering to the gastric mucosa. Antibiotic therapy generally continues for 7 to 14 days. Additional information on anti-infectives can be found in chapters 21 and 22∞.

40.10 Miscellaneous Drugs for Peptic Ulcer Disease

Several additional drugs are beneficial in treating PUD. Sucralfate (Carafate) consists of sucrose (a sugar) plus alu-

COMPLEMENTARY AND ALTERNATIVE THERAPIES

Ginger's Tonic Effects on the GI Tract

The use of ginger (*Zingiber officinalis*) for medicinal purposes dates to antiquity in India and China. The active ingredients of ginger, and those that create its spicy flavor and pungent odor, are located in its roots or rhizomes. It is sometimes standardized according to its active substances, gingerols and shogaols. It is sold in pharmacies as dried ginger root powder, at a dose of 250 to 1,000 mg, and is readily available at most grocery stores for home cooking. Ginger is one of the best studied herbs, and it appears to be useful for a number of digestive-related conditions. Perhaps its widest use is for treating nausea, including that caused by motion sickness, pregnancy morning sickness, and postoperative procedures. It has been shown to stimulate appetite, promote gastric secretions, and increase peristalsis. Newer research has shown that ginger may inhibit the effects of *H. pylori* and may help heal peptic ulcers. Its effects appear to stem from direct action on the GI tract, rather than on the CNS. Ginger has no toxicity when used at recommended doses. Adverse effects include abdominal discomfort and diarrhea. Overdoses may lead to CNS depression, inhibition of platelet aggregation, and cardiotonic effects (Chaiyakunapruk, Nathisuwan, Leeprakoffoon, & Leetasettagool, 2006; Padein, 2007).

minum hydroxide (an antacid). The drug produces a thick, gel-like substance that coats the ulcer, protecting it against further erosion and promoting healing. It does not affect the secretion of gastric acid. Other than constipation, adverse effects are minimal, because little of the drug is absorbed from the GI tract. A major disadvantage of sucralfate is that it must be taken four times daily.

Misoprostol (Cytotec) inhibits gastric acid secretion and stimulates the production of protective mucus. Its primary use is for the prevention of peptic ulcers in patients taking high doses of NSAIDs or corticosteroids. Diarrhea and abdominal cramping are relatively common adverse effects. Classified as a pregnancy category X drug, misoprostol is contraindicated during pregnancy. In fact, misoprostol is sometimes used to terminate pregnancies, as discussed in chapter 45∞.

Metoclopramide (Reglan) is occasionally used for the short-term therapy of symptomatic, PUD in patients who fail to respond to first-line agents. It is more commonly prescribed to treat nausea/vomiting associated with surgery or cancer chemotherapy. Metoclopramide is available by the oral, IM, or IV routes. It causes muscles in the upper intestine to contract, resulting in faster emptying of the stomach. It also blocks food from re-entering the esophagus from the stomach, which is of benefit in patients with GERD. Adverse CNS effects such as drowsiness, fatigue, confusion, and insomnia occur in a significant number of patients.

Chapter REVIEW

KEY CONCEPTS

The numbered key concepts provide a succinct summary of the important points from the corresponding numbered section within the chapter. If any of these points are not clear, refer to the numbered section within the chapter for review.

40.1 The digestive system is responsible for breaking down food, absorbing nutrients, and eliminating wastes.

40.2 The stomach secretes enzymes and hydrochloric acid that accelerate the process of chemical digestion. A thick mucus layer and bicarbonate ions protect the stomach mucosa from the damaging effects of the acid.

40.3 Peptic ulcer disease (PUD) is caused by an erosion of the mucosal layer of the stomach or duodenum. Gastric ulcers are more commonly associated with cancer and require longer follow-up.

40.4 Gastroesophageal reflux disease (GERD) results when acidic stomach contents enter the esophagus. GERD and PUD are treated with similar medications.

40.5 Peptic ulcer disease is best treated by a combination of lifestyle changes and pharmacotherapy. Treatment goals are to eliminate infection by *H. pylori*, promote ulcer healing, and prevent recurrence of symptoms.

40.6 Proton pump inhibitors block the enzyme H^+, K^+-ATPase and are effective at reducing gastric acid secretion.

40.7 H_2-receptor blockers slow acid secretion by the stomach and are often drugs of choice in treating PUD and GERD.

40.8 Antacids are effective at neutralizing stomach acid and are inexpensive OTC therapy for PUD and GERD. Although they relieve symptoms, antacids do not promote ulcer healing.

40.9 Combinations of antibiotics are administered to treat *H. pylori* infections of the GI tract, the cause of many peptic ulcers. A proton pump inhibitor and bismuth compounds are often included in the regimen.

40.10 Several miscellaneous drugs, including sucralfate, misoprostol, and pirenzepine are also beneficial in treating PUD.

NCLEX-RN® REVIEW QUESTIONS

1 A woman has been using OTC antacids for relief of gastric upset. She is on renal dialysis three times a week. The nurse should carefully monitor the patient for the development of what condition?
  1. Hypomagnesemia
  2. Hyperkalemia
  3. Hypermagnesemia
  4. Hyponatremia

2 In the treatment of *H. pylori,* the nurse must recognize that the use of two or more antibiotics is essential for what reason?
  1. To lower the potential for bacterial resistance
  2. To decrease the chances of development of duodenal ulcers

  3. To increase the likelihood of eliminating redevelopment of gastric ulcers
  4. To decrease the cost of future drug therapies

3 Simethicone (Gas-X, Mylicon) may be added to some medications or given plain in order to:
  1. decrease the amount of gas associated with GI disorders.
  2. increase the acid-fighting ability of some medications.
  3. prevent constipation associated with GI drugs.
  4. prevent diarrhea associated with GI drugs.

4 In addition to multiple antibiotics, what compound should the nurse anticipate will be added to the regimen for treatment of *H. pylori*?
1. Antacids
2. H$_2$-receptor antagonists
3. Bismuth compounds
4. Vitamin E compounds

5 The nurse assesses for which of the following risk factors associated with PUD? (Select all that apply.)
1. Smoking tobacco
2. Blood group O
3. Excessive psychologic stress levels
4. Type II diabetes mellitus
5. Caffeine use

6 In taking a new patient's history, the nurse notices that he has been taking omeprazole (Prilosec), consistently over the past 6 months for treatment of epigastric pain. The nurse will recommend:
1. switching to a different form of the drug.
2. trying a drug like cimetidine (Tagamet) or famotidine (Pepcid).
3. taking the drug after meals instead of before meals.
4. checking with his health care provider about his continued discomfort.

CRITICAL THINKING QUESTIONS

1. A patient with chronic hyperacidity of the stomach takes aluminum hydroxide (Amphojel) on a regular basis. The patient presents to the clinic with complaints of increasing weakness. What may be the cause of this increasing weakness?

2. Identify why nurses who work at night are at higher risk for developing PUD.

3. A patient who is on ranitidine (Zantac) for PUD smokes and drinks alcohol daily. What education will the nurse provide to this patient?

See Appendix D for answers and rationales for all activities.

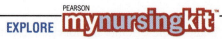

EXPLORE **mynursingkit**™   PEARSON

MyNursingKit is your one stop for online chapter review materials and resources. Prepare for success with additional NCLEX®-style practice questions, interactive assignments and activities, web links, animations and videos, and more!

Register your access code from the front of your book at **www.mynursingkit.com**.

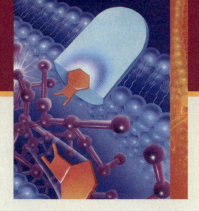

Chapter 41

Drugs for Bowel Disorders and Other Gastrointestinal Conditions

DRUGS AT A GLANCE

LEARNING OUTCOMES

After reading this chapter, the student should be able to:

1. Identify major anatomic structures of the lower gastrointestinal tract.
2. Explain the pathogenesis of constipation and diarrhea.
3. Discuss conditions in which the pharmacotherapy of bowel disorders is indicated.
4. Explain conditions in which the pharmacotherapy of nausea and vomiting is indicated.
5. Describe the types of drugs used in the short-term management of obesity.
6. Explain the use of pancreatic enzyme replacement in the pharmacotherapy of pancreatitis.
7. Describe the nurse's role in the pharmacologic management of bowel disorders, nausea and vomiting, and other GI conditions.
8. For each of the drug classes listed in Drugs at a Glance, know representative drugs, and explain the mechanism of drug action, describe primary actions, and identify important adverse effects.
9. Use the nursing process to care for patients who are receiving drug therapy for bowel disorders, nausea and vomiting, and other GI conditions.

KEY TERMS

owel disorders, nausea, and vomiting are among the most common complaints for which patients seek medical assistance. These nonspecific symptoms may be caused by a large number of infectious, metabolic, inflammatory, neoplastic, and neuropsychologic disorders. In addition, nausea, vomiting, constipation, and diarrhea are the most common adverse effects of oral medications. Although symptoms often resolve without the need for pharmacotherapy, when severe or prolonged, these conditions may lead to serious consequences unless drug therapy is initiated. This chapter examines the pharmacotherapy of these and other conditions associated with the gastrointestinal (GI) tract.

41.1 Normal Function of the Lower Digestive Tract

The lower portion of the GI tract consists of the small and large intestines, as shown in ➤ Figure 41.1. The first 10 inches of the small intestine, the duodenum, is the site where partially digested food from the stomach, known as chyme, mixes with bile from the gallbladder and digestive enzymes from the pancreas. It is sometimes considered part of the upper GI tract because of its close proximity to the stomach. The most common disorder of the duodenum, peptic ulcer, was discussed in chapter 40∞.

The remainder of the small intestine consists of the jejunum and ileum. The jejunum is the site where most nutrient absorption occurs. The ileum empties its contents into the large intestine through the ileocecal valve. Peristalsis through the intestines is controlled by the autonomic nervous system. Activation of the parasympathetic division will increase peristalsis and speed materials through the intestine; the sympathetic division has the opposite effect. Travel time for chyme through the entire small intestine varies from 3 to 6 hours.

The large intestine, or colon, receives chyme from the ileum in a fluid state. The major functions of the colon are to reabsorb water from the waste material and to excrete the remaining fecal material from the body. The colon harbors a substantial number of bacteria and fungi, the host flora, which serve a useful purpose by synthesizing B-complex vitamins and vitamin K. Disruption of the host flora in the colon can lead to diarrhea. With few exceptions, little reabsorption of nutrients occurs during the 12- to 24-hour journey through the colon.

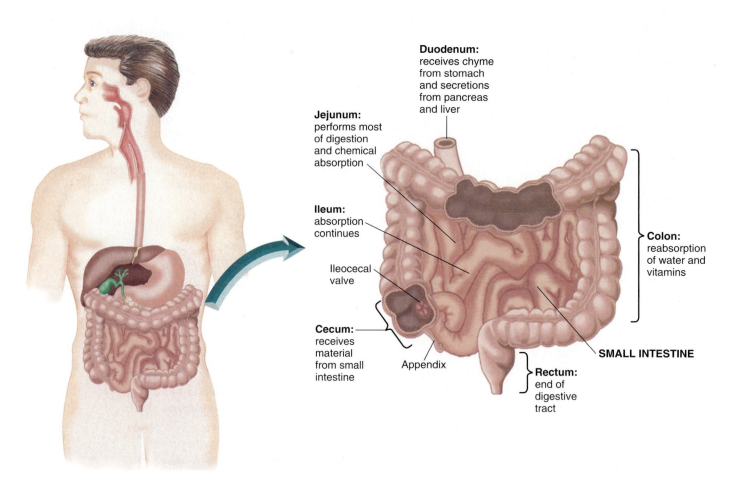

➤ **Figure 41.1** The digestive system: functions of the small intestine and large intestine (colon)
Source: Pearson Education/PH College.

PharmFacts

Gastrointestinal Disorders

- Ulcerative colitis has a peak onset from ages 15 to 30 and another from ages 60 to 80.
- As many as 40% of those aged 65 and older report recurrent constipation.
- Irritable bowel syndrome affects 10% to 20% of adults.
- Americans spend more than $33 billion annually on weight-reduction products and services.
- The incidence of motion sickness peaks from ages 4 to 10, and then begins to decline.
- Gallstones account for 90% of all cases of acute pancreatitis, whereas alcohol consumption is associated with 70% of all chronic pancreatitis.
- About 25% of Americans (more than 1 million adults) who are using weight-loss supplements are not overweight.

CONSTIPATION

Constipation is a decrease in the frequency of bowel movements. Stools may become dry, hard, and difficult to evacuate from the rectum without straining.

41.2 Pathophysiology of Constipation

As waste material travels through the large intestine, water is reabsorbed. Reabsorption of the proper amount of water results in stools of a normal, soft-formed consistency. If the waste material remains in the colon for an extended period, however, too much water will be reabsorbed, leading to small, hard stools. Constipation may cause abdominal distention and discomfort, and flatulence.

Constipation is not a disease, but a symptom of an underlying disorder. The etiology of constipation may be related to a lack of exercise; insufficient food intake, especially insoluble dietary fiber; diminished fluid intake; or a medication regimen that includes drugs that reduce intestinal motility. Opioids, anticholinergics, antihistamines, certain antacids, and iron supplements are just some of the medications that promote constipation. Foods that can cause constipation include alcoholic beverages, products with a high content of refined white flour, dairy products, and chocolate. In addition, certain diseases such as hypothyroidism, diabetes, and irritable bowel syndrome (IBS) can cause constipation.

The normal frequency of bowel movements varies widely among individuals, from two to three per day, to as few as one per week. Patients should understand that variations in frequency are normal, and that a daily bowel movement is not a requirement for good health.

Occasional constipation is self-limiting and does not require drug therapy. Lifestyle modifications that incorporate increased dietary fiber, fluid intake, and physical activity should be considered before drugs are utilized for constipation. Chronic, infrequent, and painful bowel movements, accompanied by severe straining, may justify initiation of treatment. In its most severe form, constipation can lead to a fecal impaction and complete obstruction of the bowel. Constipation occurs more frequently in older adults, because fecal transit time through the colon slows with aging; this population also exercises less and has a higher frequency of chronic disorders that cause constipation.

Laxatives

Laxatives are drugs that promote bowel movements. Many are available over the counter (OTC) for the self-treatment of simple constipation. Doses of laxatives are identified in Table 41.1.

41.3 Pharmacotherapy with Laxatives

Laxatives promote the evacuation of the bowel, or defecation, and are widely used to prevent and treat constipation. **Cathartic** is a related term that implies a stronger and more complete bowel emptying. A variety of prescription and OTC products are available, including tablet, liquid, and suppository formulations.

Prophylactic laxative pharmacotherapy is appropriate following abdominal surgeries. Such treatment reduces straining or bearing down during defecation—a situation that has the potential to precipitate increased intra-abdominal, intraocular, or blood pressure. In addition, laxatives, in conjunction with enemas, are often given to cleanse the bowel prior to diagnostic or surgical procedures of the colon or genitourinary tract. Cathartics are usually the drug of choice preceding diagnostic procedures of the colon, such as colonoscopy or barium enema.

The two most frequently reported adverse effects of laxatives are abdominal distension and cramping. Diarrhea may result from excessive use. When cleansing the bowel prior to colonoscopy or purging the bowel of toxic substances or parasites, forceful, frequent bowel movements are *expected* outcomes. Care must be taken to rule out acute abdominal pathology such as bowel obstruction prior to administration because the drugs will increase colon pressure and possibly cause bowel perforation.

When taken in prescribed amounts, laxatives have few adverse effects. These drugs are often classified into five primary groups and a miscellaneous category:

- *Bulk-forming* laxatives absorb water, thus adding size to the fecal mass. These are preferred drugs for the treatment and prevention of chronic constipation, and may be taken on a regular basis without ill effects. Because of their slow onset of action, they are not used when a rapid and complete bowel evacuation is necessary.

- *Stool softeners* or *surfactant* laxatives cause more water and fat to be absorbed into the stools. They are most often used to *prevent* constipation, especially in patients who have undergone recent surgery.

- *Stimulant* laxatives promote peristalsis by irritating the bowel mucosa. They are rapid acting and more likely to

TABLE 41.1 Laxatives and Cathartics

Drug	Route and Adult Dose (max dose where indicated)	Adverse Effects
BULK FORMING		
calcium polycarbophil (Equalactin, FiberCon, others)	PO; 1 g/day prn	*Abdominal fullness or cramping, fainting*
methylcellulose (Citrucel)	PO; 1 tbsp tid in 8–10 oz water	Esophageal or GI obstruction if taken with insufficient fluid
🅟 psyllium mucilloid (Metamucil, Naturacil, others)	PO; 1–2 tsp in 8 oz water daily prn	
SALINE AND OSMOTIC		
magnesium hydroxide (Milk of Magnesia)	PO; 20–60 mL/day prn	*Diarrhea, abdominal cramping*
polyethylene glycol (MiraLax)	PO; 17 g in 8 oz of liquid daily for 2–4 days	Hypermagnesemia with magnesium hydroxide (dysrhythmias, respiratory failure)
sodium biphosphate (Fleet Phospho-Soda)	PO; 15–30 mL mixed in water daily prn	
STIMULANT		
bisacodyl (Correctol, Dulcolax, others)	PO; 10–15 mg/day prn	*Abdominal cramping, nausea, fainting, diarrhea*
castor oil (Emulsoil, Neoloid, Purge)	PO; 15–60 mL/day prn	Fluid and electrolyte loss
STOOL SOFTENER/SURFACTANT		
docusate (Colace)	PO; 50–500 mg/day	*Abdominal cramping, diarrhea*
		No serious adverse effects
HERBAL AGENT		
senna/sennosides (Ex-Lax, Senokot, others)	PO; 8.6–17.2 mg/day	*Abdominal cramping, diarrhea*
		No serious adverse effects
MISCELLANEOUS AGENTS		
lubiprostone (Amitiza)	PO; 24 mcg bid	*Nausea, diarrhea, headache, dysphea*
		Allergic reactions
mineral oil	PO; 15–30 mL bid	*Diarrhea, nausea*
		Nutritional deficiencies, aspiration pneumonia

Italics indicate common adverse effects; <u>underlining</u> indicates serious adverse effects.

cause diarrhea and cramping than the bulk-forming type of laxatives. They should only be used occasionally because they may cause laxative dependence and depletion of fluid and electrolytes.

- *Saline cathartics,* also called osmotic laxatives, are not absorbed in the intestine; they pull water into the fecal mass to create a more watery stool. These agents can produce a bowel movement very quickly and should not be used on a regular basis because of the possibility of fluid and electrolyte depletion.

- *Herbal agents* are natural products available OTC that are widely used for self-treatment of constipation. The most commonly used herbal laxative is senna, a potent herb that irritates the bowel and increases peristalsis. Other natural laxatives include rhubarb, cascara sagrada, aloe, flaxseed, and dandelion.

- *Miscellaneous agents* include mineral oil, which acts by lubricating the stool and the colon mucosa. The use of mineral oil should be discouraged, because it may

interfere with the absorption of fat-soluble vitamins and can cause other potentially serious adverse effects. Lubiprostone (Amitiza) is a newer drug that increases the secretion of intestinal fluid by activating chloride channels in the mucosa of the large bowel. This drug is approved for chronic idiopathic constipation and for the constipation phase of irritable bowel syndrome.

DIARRHEA

When the large intestine does not reabsorb enough water from the fecal mass, stools become watery. **Diarrhea** is an increase in the frequency and fluidity of bowel movements. Diarrhea is not a disease but a symptom of an underlying disorder.

41.4 Pathophysiology of Diarrhea

Like constipation, occasional diarrhea is often a self-limiting disorder that does not warrant drug therapy. Indeed, diar-

Pr Prototype Drug | Psyllium Mucilloid *(Metamucil, others)*

Therapeutic Class: Bulk-type laxative   **Pharmacologic Class:** Natural product

ACTIONS AND USES

Psyllium is derived from a natural product, the seeds of the plantain plant. Like other bulk-forming laxatives, psyllium is an insoluble fiber that is indigestible and not absorbed from the GI tract. When taken with a sufficient quantity of water, psyllium swells and increases the size of the fecal mass. The larger the size of the fecal mass, the more the defecation reflex will be stimulated, thus promoting the passage of stool. Several doses of psyllium may be needed over 1 to 3 days to produce a therapeutic effect. The drug may be taken daily as a fiber supplement.

Frequent use of psyllium (7 g/day) may cause a small reduction in blood cholesterol level. Because of this effect, psyllium may be used as part of a regiment to reduce the risk of coronary heart disease.

ADMINISTRATION ALERTS

- Mix with at least 8 oz of water, fruit juice, or milk, and administer immediately. Follow each dose with an additional 8 oz of liquid.
- Observe older adults closely for possible aspiration.
- Pregnancy category C

> **PHARMACOKINETICS**
> **Onset:** 12–24 h
> **Peak:** 1–3 days
> **Half-life:** Unknown
> **Duration:** Unknown

ADVERSE EFFECTS

Psyllium is a safe laxative and rarely produces adverse effects. It causes less cramping than stimulant-type laxatives and results in a more natural bowel movement. If taken with insufficient water, it may cause obstructions in the esophagus or intestine.

Contraindications: Psyllium should not be administered to patients with undiagnosed abdominal pain, intestinal obstruction, or fecal impaction.

INTERACTIONS

Drug-Drug: Psyllium may decrease the absorption and effects of warfarin, digoxin, nitrofurantoin, antibiotics, and salicylates.

Lab Tests: Psyllium may increase the serum glucose level.

Herbal/Food: Unknown

Treatment of Overdose: Overdose from psyllium is unlikely.

Refer to MyNursingKit for a Nursing Process Focus specific to this drug.

---

rhea may be considered a type of body defense, rapidly and completely eliminating the body of toxins and pathogens. When prolonged or severe, especially in children, diarrhea can result in significant loss of body fluids, and pharmacotherapy is indicated. Prolonged diarrhea may lead to fluid, acid–base, or electrolyte disorders (chapter 31 ∞).

Diarrhea may be caused by certain medications, infections of the bowel, and substances such as lactose. Inflammatory

COMPLEMENTARY AND ALTERNATIVE THERAPIES

Acidophilus for Diarrhea

Lactobacillus acidophilus is a probiotic bacterium normally found in the human alimentary canal and vagina. It is considered to be protective flora, inhibiting the growth of potentially pathogenic species such as *Escherichia coli, Candida albicans, H. pylori,* and *Gardnerella vaginalis*. One mechanism used by *L. acidophilus* to limit the growth of other bacterial species is the generation of hydrogen peroxide, which is toxic to most cells.

The primary use of *L. acidophilus* is to restore the normal flora of the intestine following diarrhea, particularly from antibiotic therapy. It has also been shown to be effective at shortening episodes of acute infectious diarrhea (Teitelbaum, 2005). *L. acidophilus* may be obtained by drinking acidophilus milk or by eating yogurt or kefir containing live (or active) cultures. Those wishing to obtain *L. acidophilus* from yogurt should read the labels carefully, because not all products contain active cultures; frozen yogurt contains no active cultures. Supplements include capsules, tablets, and granules. Doses are not standardized, and tablet doses range from 50 to 500 mg.

disorders such as ulcerative colitis, Crohn's disease, and irritable bowel syndrome can cause episodes of intense diarrhea. Antibiotics often cause diarrhea by killing normal intestinal flora, thus allowing an overgrowth of opportunistic pathogenic organisms. The primary goal in treating diarrhea is to assess and treat the underlying condition causing the diarrhea. Assessing the patient's recent travels, dietary habits, immune system competence, and recent drug history may provide information about its etiology. Critically ill patients with a reduced immune response who are exposed to many antibiotics may have diarrhea related to pseudomembranous colitis, a condition that may lead to shock and death.

Antidiarrheals

For mild diarrhea, OTC products are effective at returning elimination patterns to normal. For chronic or severe cases, the opioids are the most effective of the antidiarrheal agents. The antidiarrheals are listed in Table 41.2.

41.5 Pharmacotherapy with Antidiarrheals

Pharmacotherapy related to diarrhea depends on the severity of the condition and any identifiable etiologic factors. If the cause is an infectious disease, then an antibiotic or antiparasitic drug is indicated. If the cause is inflammatory in

TABLE 41.2 **Antidiarrheals**

Drug	Route and Adult Dose (max dose where indicated)	Adverse Effects
OPIOIDS		
camphorated opium tincture (Paregoric)	PO; 5–10 mL every 2 h qid prn	*Drowsiness, light-headedness, nausea, dizziness, dry mouth (from atropine), constipation*
difenoxin with atropine (Motofen)	PO; 1–2 mg after each diarrhea episode (max: 8 mg/day)	
🅟 diphenoxylate with atropine (Lomotil)	PO; 1–2 tabs or 5–10 mL tid–qid	<u>Paralytic ileus with toxic megacolon, respiratory depression, CNS depression</u>
loperamide (Imodium)	PO; 4 mg as a single dose, then 2 mg after each diarrhea episode (max: 16 mg/day)	
MISCELLANEOUS AGENTS		
bismuth salts (Pepto-Bismol)	PO; 2 tabs or 30 mL prn	*Constipation, nausea, tinnitus*
		<u>Impaction, Reye's syndrome</u>
octreotide (Sandostatin)	SC/IV; 100–600 mcg/day in two to four divided doses	*Nausea, diarrhea, abdominal pain*
		<u>Changes in serum glucose, gallstones, cholestatic hepatitis</u>

Italics indicate common adverse effects; <u>underlining</u> indicates serious adverse effects.

nature, anti-inflammatory drugs are warranted. When the diarrhea appears to be an adverse effect of pharmacotherapy, the health care provider may discontinue the offending medication, lower the dose, or substitute an alternative drug.

The most effective drugs for the symptomatic treatment of diarrhea are the opioids, which can dramatically slow peristalsis in the colon. The most common opioid antidiarrheals are codeine and diphenoxylate with atropine (Lomotil). Diphenoxylate is a Schedule V agent that acts directly on the intestine to slow peristalsis, thereby allowing more fluid and electrolyte absorption in the large intestine. The opioids cause CNS depression at high doses, and are generally reserved for the short-term therapy of acute diarrhea because of the potential for dependence. Details on indications and adverse effects of opioids may be found in chapter 18∞.

OTC drugs for diarrhea act by a number of different mechanisms. Loperamide (Imodium) is similar to meperidine but it has no narcotic effects and is not classified as a controlled substance. Low-dose loperamide is available OTC; higher

---

🅟 Prototype Drug | Diphenoxylate with Atropine *(Lomotil)*

Therapeutic Class: Antidiarrheal   **Pharmacologic Class:** Opioid

ACTIONS AND USES

The primary antidiarrheal ingredient in Lomotil is diphenoxylate. Like other opioids, diphenoxylate slows peristalsis, allowing time for additional water reabsorption from the colon and more solid stools. It acts within 45 to 60 minutes. It is effective for moderate to severe diarrhea, but is not recommended for children. The atropine in Lomotil is not added for its anticholinergic effect, but to discourage patients from taking too much of the drug. At higher doses, the anticholinergic effects of atropine may be observed, which include drowsiness, dry mouth, and tachycardia. Diphenoxylate is discontinued as soon as the diarrhea symptoms resolve.

ADMINISTRATION ALERT

- If administering to young children, measure the drug accurately by using the dropper packaged with the liquid form of the drug.
- Pregnancy category C

PHARMACOKINETICS
Onset: 45–60 min
Peak: 2 h
Half-life: 4.4 h
Duration: 3–4 h

ADVERSE EFFECTS

Unlike most opioids, diphenoxylate has no analgesic properties and has an extremely low potential for abuse. The drug is well tolerated at normal doses. Some patients experience dizziness or drowsiness, and they should not drive or operate machinery until the effects of the drug are known.

Contraindications: Contraindications include hypersensitivity to the drug, severe liver disease, obstructive jaundice, severe dehydration or electrolyte imbalance, narrow angle glaucoma, and diarrhea associated with pseudomembranous colitis.

INTERACTIONS

Drug-Drug: Diphenoxylate with atropine interacts with other CNS depressants, including alcohol, to produce additive sedation. When taken with MAO inhibitors, diphenoxylate may cause hypertensive crisis.

Lab Tests: Diphenoxylate with atropine may increase serum amylase.

Herbal/Food: Unknown

Treatment of Overdose: Overdose with Lomotil may be serious. Narcotic antagonists such as naloxone may be administered parenterally to reverse respiratory depression within minutes.

Refer to MyNursingKit for a Nursing Process Focus specific to this drug.

TREATING THE DIVERSE PATIENT

Cultural Remedies for Diarrhea

Because diarrhea is an age-old malady that affects all populations, different cultures have adopted tried-and-true symptomatic remedies for the condition. One preparation used by people in many regions of the world is cornstarch (a heaping teaspoonful) in a glass of tepid water. For centuries, mothers have boiled rice and given the diluted rice water to babies to treat diarrhea. The rationale behind these two therapies is that they work by absorbing excess water in the intestines, thus stopping the diarrhea. Although a rationale was not specified in earlier times, people of many cultures found that eating grated apple that had turned brown alleviated symptoms. These practices apparently evolved into what today is known as the ABC of diarrhea treatment: apples, bananas (just barely ripe), and carrots. The underlying principle is that the pectin present in these foods is oxidized, producing the same ingredient found in many OTC diarrhea medicines.

doses are available by prescription. Other OTC treatments include bismuth subsalicylate (Pepto-Bismol), which acts by binding and absorbing toxins. Psyllium preparations may also slow diarrhea, because they absorb large amounts of fluid, which helps form bulkier stools. Probiotic supplements containing *Lactobacillus*, a normal inhabitant of the human gut and vagina, are sometimes taken to correct the altered GI flora following a serious diarrhea episode.

41.6 Pharmacotherapy of Inflammatory Bowel Disease and Irritable Bowel Syndrome

Inflammatory bowel disease (IBD) is characterized by the presence of ulcers in the distal portion of the small intestine (**Crohn's disease**) or mucosal erosions in the large intestine (**ulcerative colitis**). IBD is treated with medications from several classifications. Over 1 million Americans are estimated to have IBD.

Symptoms of IBD range from mild to acute, and the condition is often characterized by alternating periods of remission and exacerbation. The most common clinical presentation of ulcerative colitis is abdominal cramping with frequent bowel movements. Severe disease may result in weight loss, bloody diarrhea, high fever, and dehydration. The patient with Crohn's disease also presents with abdominal pain, cramping, and diarrhea, which may have been present for years before the patient sought treatment. Symptoms of Crohn's are sometimes similar to those of ulcerative colitis.

Mild-to-moderate IBD is treated with 5-aminosalicylic acid (5-ASA) agents. These include the sulfonamide sulfasalazine (Azulfidine), olsalazine (Dipentum), and mesalamine (Asacol, Pentasa, others). Corticosteroids such as prednisone, methylprednisolone, or hydrocortisone are used in more persistent cases. Particularly severe disease may require immunosuppressant drugs such as azathioprine (Imuran) or methotrexate (MTX). Infliximab (Remicade) is a monoclonal antibody approved for Crohn's disease and ulcerative colitis. A single infusion of infliximab can cause remission in 65% of patients with moderate to severe Crohn's disease that may last up to 12 weeks.

Budesonide (Entocort-EC) is a corticosteroid with interesting properties that allow it to be used as a first-line therapy for IBD. Entocort-EC is encapsulated to prevent significant absorption in the stomach or duodenum. The drug is released slowly and reaches a high concentration in the terminal ileum and proximal colon, the two most frequently affected sites for IBD. Thus, the drug is in direct contact with the GI mucosa and, in effect, it produces a *topical* anti-inflammatory effect. In addition, when it is absorbed, budesonide is almost entirely removed by first-pass metabolism in the liver. Thus, this drug shows few of the adverse effects seen with the long-term use of other corticosteroids. It is approved for mild to moderate Crohn's disease.

The introduction of biologic therapies in the late 1990s gave clinicians another valuable tool in the pharmacotherapy of IBD. The tumor necrosis factor (TNF) inhibitor infliximab (Remicade) has been shown to effectively reduce acute symptoms and provide maintenance therapy for both Crohn's disease and ulcerative colitis. A second anti-TNF drug, adalimumab (Humira), was approved in 2007 for Crohn's disease. Recently, a pegylated TNF inhibitor, certolizumab pegol (Cimzia), was approved that offers dosing at 2- to 4-week intervals. Natalizumab (Tysabri), a drug previously approved for multiple sclerosis, was approved for treating Crohn's disease in 2008. The biologic therapies are expensive and patients experience a much higher rate of serious infections due to their immunosuppressive actions. Biologic therapies are currently recommended only when corticosteroid therapy is unable to control symptoms.

Irritable bowel syndrome (IBS), also known as *spastic colon* or *mucous colitis,* is a common disorder of the lower GI tract. Symptoms include abdominal pain, bloating, excessive gas, and colicky cramping. Bowel habits are altered, with diarrhea alternating with constipation, and there may be mucus in the stool. IBS is considered a functional bowel disorder, meaning that the normal operation of the digestive tract is impaired without the presence of detectable organic disease. It is not a precursor of more serious disease. Stress is often a precipitating factor along with dietary factors.

Drugs used to treat IBS do not alter the course of the disease and, in some cases, they may actually worsen patient symptoms. Research has not demonstrated that drugs are any more effective than nonpharmacologic treatments such as IBS support groups, relaxation therapy, or dietary changes. There is not prototype drug for this condition. Drugs that provide symptomatic relief for some patients include alosetron (Lotronex), dicyclomine (Bentyl), and hyoscyamine (Anaspaz, others). Tegaserod (Zelnorm) was once considered a prototype drug for IBS but the United States and Canada have suspended marketing of the drug due to the potential for adverse cardiovascular events. Drug therapy of IBS is targeted at symptomatic treatment, depending on whether constipation or diarrhea is the predominant symptom.

NAUSEA AND VOMITING

Nausea is an unpleasant, subjective sensation that is accompanied by weakness, diaphoresis, and hyperproduction of saliva. It is sometimes accompanied by dizziness. Intense nausea often leads to vomiting, or **emesis**.

Assessment	Potential Nursing Diagnoses
Baseline assessment prior to administration: - Understand the reason the drug has been prescribed in order to assess for therapeutic effects. - Obtain a complete health history including GI, cardiovascular, hepatic, or renal disease; pregnancy; or breast-feeding. Obtain a drug history including allergies, current prescription and OTC drugs, herbal preparations, caffeine, nicotine, and alcohol use. Be alert to possible drug interactions. - Obtain a history of past and current symptoms, noting what measures have been successful at relieving the symptoms (e.g., increased fluids, fiber, dietary changes). - Obtain baseline weight and vital signs. - Evaluate appropriate laboratory findings (e.g., CBC, electrolytes, hepatic or renal function studies). - Obtain an abdominal assessment (e.g., bowel sounds, firmness, distention, presence of tenderness).	- Constipation (related to medication, diet, inadequate toileting, etc.) - Diarrhea (related to medication, diet, infections, etc.) - Deficient Knowledge (drug therapy) - Risk for Deficient Fluid Volume (related to diarrhea, overuse of laxatives)
Assessment throughout administration: - Assess for desired therapeutic effects (e.g., adequate pattern of elimination, normal stool consistency and volume). - Continue periodic monitoring of abdominal assessment findings, especially bowel sounds. - Continue periodic monitoring of CBC, electrolytes, and hepatic and renal function labs as appropriate. - Assess for adverse effects: nausea, vomiting, diarrhea, constipation, headache, drowsiness, and dizziness. Severe abdominal pain, coffee-ground or bloody vomiting, or blood in stool or tarry stools should be reported immediately.	

Planning: Patient Goals and Expected Outcomes

The patient will:
- Experience therapeutic effects (e.g., return to more normal pattern of elimination, normal stool volume and consistency).
- Be free from, or experience minimal, adverse effects.
- Verbalize an understanding of the drug's use, adverse effects, and required precautions.
- Demonstrate proper self-administration of the medication (e.g., dose, timing, when to notify provider).

Implementation

Interventions and (Rationales)	Patient and Family Education
Ensuring therapeutic effects: - If a definitive cause for the current symptoms can be identified (e.g., infection, food poisoning, inadequate fluid intake), correct the cause where possible. (Constipation and diarrhea are usually symptoms of other underlying conditions such as infections, inadequate fluid or fiber intake, stress, or sedentary lifestyle.)	- For recurrent constipation or diarrhea, encourage the patient to maintain a diary of correlations between symptoms, foods, beverages, stress, or medications to help identify causative factors.
- Encourage appropriate lifestyle changes. Have the patient keep a diary noting correlations between symptoms and foods, beverages, stress, or medications. (Ensuring adequate amounts of daily fluids and dietary fiber, and increasing activity levels assists in encouraging normal peristaltic activity. Smoking and alcohol use alter normal peristalsis and should be limited or eliminated. Correlating symptoms with medications or stress may help to identify a triggering factor. Overall healthy lifestyle changes will support and minimize the need for drug therapy.)	- Encourage the patient to adopt a healthy lifestyle of increased dietary fiber and fluid intake, increased intake of yogurt and *acidophilus*-containing foods, stress management techniques, increased exercise, and limited or eliminated alcohol consumption and smoking. Provide for dietitian consultation or information on smoking cessation programs as needed.
- Follow appropriate administration guidelines. Do not administer laxatives if bowel obstruction is possible. Do not administer antidiarrheal drugs if infection is possible. (Guidelines for exact mixing, fluid intake, or administering with meals should be followed. If bowel sounds are hypoactive or absent, consult the health care provider before administering the drug. If infection is possible cause of diarrhea, consult with the health care provider before giving antidiarrheal drugs because decreased peristalsis may give the infection the opportunity to increase and spread.)	- Teach the patient to take the drug following appropriate guidelines or label directions, particularly for any additional fluid intake required, for best results. - Instruct the patient that diarrhea or constipation associated with increasing nausea or vomiting, especially if accompanied by abdominal pain, should be reported to the health care provider before taking drug.

NURSING PROCESS FOCUS   **PATIENTS RECEIVING DRUG THERAPY FOR BOWEL DISORDERS (CONSTIPATION, DIARRHEA, IRRITABLE BOWEL SYNDROME)** *(Continued)*

Implementation

Interventions and (Rationales)	Patient and Family Education
Minimizing adverse effects:	
■ Continue to monitor abdominal assessment findings. Any significant increase or decrease in bowel sounds, or new onset or increase in discomfort or pain should be reported promptly. (Any significant change in bowel sound activity or increased discomfort or pain may signal the development of worsening bowel disease or of adverse drug effects.)	■ Teach the patient that some easing of discomfort related to constipation or diarrhea may be noticed soon after beginning drug therapy but the full effects may take several days or longer. If gastric discomfort or pain continue or worsen, the health care provider should be notified.
■ Monitor for any severe abdominal pain, vomiting, coffee-ground or bloody emesis, or blood in stool or tarry stools. (Severe abdominal pain or blood in emesis or stools may indicate a worsening of disease or more serious conditions and should be reported immediately.)	■ Teach the patient that severe abdominal pain or any blood in emesis or stools should be reported immediately to the health care provider.
■ Ensure patient safety, especially in older adults. Observe for dizziness and monitor ambulation until the effects of the drug are known. Obtain electrolyte levels if dizziness continues. (Drowsiness or dizziness from opioid-based or related antidiarrheals may occur and increases the risk of falls. Continued dizziness may indicate electrolyte imbalance.)	■ Instruct the patient to call for assistance prior to getting out of bed or attempting to walk alone if dizziness or drowsiness occur. Provide commode or bedpan nearby. For home use, avoid driving or other activities requiring mental alertness or physical coordination until the effects of the drug are known.
■ Continue to monitor periodic hepatic and renal function tests, and electrolyte levels as needed. (Abnormal liver function tests may indicate drug-induced adverse hepatic effects. Excessive use of laxatives or continued diarrhea may affect electrolyte levels.)	■ Instruct the patient on the need to return periodically for lab work.
■ Monitor vital signs, particularly respiratory rate and depth, on patients taking opioid or opioid-related drugs. (Opioids may decrease respiratory rate and depth. Intervention with narcotic-antagonists may be needed if overdose occurs.)	■ Teach the patient to take the drug as ordered and not to increase the dose or frequency unless instructed to do so by the health care provider. Any drowsiness, dizziness, or disorientation should be promptly reported to the provider.
Patient understanding of drug therapy:	
■ Use opportunities during administration of medications and during assessments to discuss the rationale for drug therapy, desired therapeutic outcomes, most common adverse effects, parameters for when to call the health care provider, and any necessary monitoring or precautions. (Using time during nursing care helps to optimize and reinforce key teaching areas.)	■ The patient, family, or caregiver should be able to state the reason for the drug; appropriate dose and scheduling; what adverse effects to observe for and when to report; and the anticipated length of medication therapy.
Patient self-administration of drug therapy:	
■ When administering the medication, instruct the patient, family, or caregiver in the proper self-administration of the drug, e.g., taken with additional fluids. (Proper administration increases the effectiveness of the drug.)	■ Teach the patient on laxatives to take the drug according to appropriate guidelines, as follows:
	■ All laxative drugs: Take the drug with additional fluids and increase fluid intake throughout the day. Increase the intake of dietary fiber. Exceeding recommended dose or frequent laxative use increases the risk of adverse and decreases normal peristalsis over time, resulting in "laxative dependence."
	■ Bulk-forming laxatives: Take other medications 1 hour before or 2 hours after the laxative. Powdered formulations should be mixed with a full glass of liquid and immediately taken, followed by an additional full glass of liquid. Powders should *never* be swallowed dry or esophageal obstruction may result.
	■ Mineral oil laxatives: Do not take if nausea is present and do not take at bedtime to avoid the possibility of aspiration.

Evaluation of Outcome Criteria

Evaluate the effectiveness of drug therapy by confirming that the patient goals and expected outcomes have been met (see "Planning").

See Tables 41.1 and 41.2 for a list of drugs to which these nursing actions apply.

Pr Prototype Drug | Sulfasalazine (Azulfidine)

Therapeutic Class: Drug for inflammatory bowel disease   **Pharmacologic Class:** 5-aminosalicylate, sulfonamide

ACTIONS AND USES

Sulfasalazine is an oral drug with anti-inflammatory properties that is approved to treat mild to moderate symptoms of ulcerative colitis. Sulfasalazine is used off-label to treat Crohn's disease. It is approved as an alternate drug in the pharmacotherapy of rheumatoid arthritis and is classified as a disease-modifying antirheumatic drug (DMARD) (chapter 47 ∞).

Sulfasalazine inhibits mediators of inflammation in the colon such as prostaglandins and leukotrienes. Colon bacteria metabolize sulfasalazine to active metabolites. One of these metabolites, mesalamine (Asacol, Canasa, others), is available as an IBS drug.

ADMINISTRATION ALERTS

- Do not administer this drug to patients who have allergies to sulfonamide antibiotics or furosemide (Lasix).
- Not approved for children under age 2.
- Do not crush or chew extended-release tablets.
- Pregnancy category B

PHARMACOKINETICS
Onset: Poorly absorbed

Peak: 1.5–6 h

Half-life: 5–10 h

Duration: 5–10 h

ADVERSE EFFECTS

The most frequent adverse effects of sulfasalazine are GI-related: nausea, vomiting, diarrhea, dyspepsia, and abdominal pain. Dividing the total daily dose evenly throughout the day and using the enteric-coated tablets may improve adherence. Headache is common. Blood dyscrasias occur infrequently during therapy. Skin rashes are relatively common and may be a sign of a more serious adverse effect such as Stevens–Johnson syndrome. The drug may impair male fertility, which reverses when the drug is discontinued. Sulfasalazine can cause photosensitivity.

Contraindications: Sulfasalazine is contraindicated in patients with sulfonamide or salicylate (aspirin or 5-ASA) hypersensitivity. Patients with pre-existing anemia, folate, or other hematologic disorders should use the drug with caution because it may worsen blood dyscrasias. Sulfasalazine should be used with caution in patients with hepatic impairment because the drug can cause hepatotoxicity. The drug is contraindicated in patients with urinary obstruction and should be used with caution in dehydrated patients because it may cause crystalluria. Patients with diabetes or hypoglycemia should use sulfasalazine with caution because the drug can increase insulin secretion and worsen hypoglycemia.

INTERACTIONS

Drug-Drug: Sulfasalazine may worsen bone marrow suppression caused by methotrexate and also result in additive hepatotoxicity. Absorption of digoxin may be decreased. Sulfasalazine can displace warfarin from its protein binding sites, causing increased anticoagulant effects.

Lab Tests: Unknown

Herbal/Food: Sulfasalazine may decrease the absorption of iron and folic acid.

Treatment of Overdose: Overdose will cause abdominal pain, anuria, drowsiness, gastric distress, nausea, seizures, and vomiting. Treatment is supportive.

Refer to MyNursingKit for a Nursing Process Focus specific to this drug.

41.7 Pathophysiology of Nausea and Vomiting

Vomiting is a defense mechanism used by the body to rid itself of toxic substances. Vomiting is a reflex primarily controlled by the vomiting center of the medulla of the brain, which receives sensory signals from the digestive tract, the inner ear, and the **chemoreceptor trigger zone (CTZ)** in the cerebral cortex. Interestingly, the CTZ is not protected by the blood–brain barrier, as is the vast majority of the brain; thus, these neurons can directly sense the presence of toxic substances in the blood. Once the vomiting reflex is triggered, wavelike contractions of the stomach quickly propel its contents upward and out of the body.

The treatment outcomes for nausea or vomiting should focus on removal of the cause, whenever feasible. Nausea and vomiting are common symptoms associated with a wide variety of conditions such as GI infections, food poisoning, nervousness, emotional imbalances, changes in body position (motion sickness), and extreme pain. Other conditions that promote nausea and vomiting are general anesthetic agents, migraine headache, trauma to the head or abdominal organs, inner ear disorders, and diabetes. Psychologic factors play a significant role, as patients often become nauseated during periods of extreme stress or when confronted with unpleasant sights, smells, or sounds.

The nausea and vomiting experienced by many women during the first trimester of pregnancy is referred to as *morning sickness*. If this condition becomes acute, with continual vomiting, it may lead to *hyperemesis gravidarum*, a situation in which the health and safety of the mother and developing baby can become compromised. Pharmacotherapy is initiated after other antinausea measures have proved ineffective.

Nausea and vomiting are the most frequently listed adverse effects for oral medications. The nurse should remember that because the vomiting center lies in the brain, nausea and vomiting may occur with parenteral formulations as well as with oral drugs. The most extreme example of this occurs with the antineoplastic drugs, most of which cause intense nausea and vomiting regardless of the route they are administered. The capacity of a chemotherapeutic drug to cause vomiting is called its **emetogenic potential**. Nausea and vomiting is a common reason for patients' lack of adherence to the therapeutic regimen and for discontinuation of drug therapy.

When large amounts of fluids are vomited, dehydration and significant weight loss may occur. Because the contents lost from the stomach are strongly acidic, vomiting may cause a change in the pH of the blood, resulting in metabolic alkalosis. With excessive loss, severe acid–base disturbances can lead to vascular collapse, resulting in death if medical intervention is not initiated. Dehydration is especially dangerous for infants, small children, and older adults, and is evidenced by dry mouth, sticky saliva, and reduced urine output that is dark yellow-orange to brown.

Antiemetics

Drugs from at least eight different classes are used to prevent nausea and vomiting. Many of these act by inhibiting dopamine or serotonin receptors in the brain. The antiemetics are listed in Table 41.3.

41.8 Pharmacotherapy with Antiemetics

A large number of **antiemetics** are available to treat nausea and vomiting. Selection of a particular agent depends on the experience of the health care provider and the cause of the nausea and vomiting. Patients seeking self-treatment can find several options available OTC. For example, simple nausea and vomiting is sometimes relieved by antacids or diphenhydramine (Benadryl). Herbal options include peppermint and ginger, the most popular herbal therapy for nausea and vomiting. Relief of serious nausea or vomiting, however, requires prescription medications. Patients receiving antineoplastic drugs may receive three or more antiemetics concurrently to reduce the nausea and vomiting from chemotherapy. In fact, therapy with antineoplastic drugs is one of the most common reasons for prescribing antiemetic drugs.

Serotonin (5-HT$_3$) Antagonists

The serotonin antagonists include dolasetron (Anzemet), granisetron (Kytril, Sancuso), ondansetron (Zofran), and palonosetron (Aloxi). These agents are preferred drugs for the pharmacotherapy of serious nausea and vomiting due to antineoplastic therapy, radiation therapy, or surgical procedures. They are usually given prophylactically, just prior to antineoplastic therapy. IV, oral, and transdermal patch forms are available.

Antihistamines and Anticholinergics

These agents are effective for treating simple nausea, with some being available OTC. For example, nausea due to motion sickness is effectively treated with anticholinergics or antihistamines. Motion sickness is a disorder affecting a portion of the inner ear that is associated with significant nausea. The most common drug used for motion sickness is scopolamine (Transderm Scop), which is usually administered as a transdermal patch. Antihistamines such as dimenhydrinate (Dramamine) and meclizine (Antivert) are also effective, but may cause significant drowsiness in some patients. Drugs used to treat motion sickness are most effective when taken 20 to 60 minutes before travel is expected.

Antipsychotic Drugs

The major indication for phenothiazines relates to treating psychoses (chapter 17 ∞), but they are also very effective antiemetics. The serious nausea and vomiting associated with antineoplastic therapy is sometimes treated with the phenothiazines. To prevent loss of the antiemetic medication due to vomiting, some of these agents are available through the IM, IV, and/or suppository routes. Nonphenothiazine antipsychotics that have high antiemetic activity include haloperidol (Haldol) and droperidol (Inapsine).

Corticosteroids

Dexamethasone (Decadron) and methylprednisolone (Solu-Medrol) are used to prevent chemotherapy-induced and postsurgical nausea and vomiting. They are reserved for the short-term therapy of acute cases because of the potential for serious adverse effects.

Other Antiemetics

Aprepitant (Emend) is the first of a new class of antiemetics, the neurokinin receptor antagonists, used to prevent nausea and vomiting following antineoplastic therapy. The benzodiazepine lorazepam (Ativan) has the advantage of promoting relaxation along with having antiemetic properties. Cannabinoids are drugs that contain the same active ingredient as marijuana. Dronabinol (Marinol) and nabilone (Cesamet) are given orally to produce antiemetic effects and relaxation without the euphoria produced by marijuana. Dronabinol and nabilone are Schedule II controlled drugs.

On some occasions, it is desirable to *stimulate* the vomiting reflex with drugs called **emetics**. Indications for emetics include ingestion of poisons and overdoses of oral drugs. Ipecac syrup, given orally, or apomorphine, given subcutaneously, will induce vomiting in about 15 minutes.

OBESITY

Obesity is a growing epidemic in the United States: It is estimated that 95 million adults are overweight or obese. This represents 34% of the adult population over age 20. Obesity is closely associated with increased health risks that include premature death, hypertension, hyperlipidemia, diabetes mellitus, heart disease, sleep apnea, and osteoarthritis.

TABLE 41.3	Selected Antiemetics	
Drug	**Route and Adult Dose (max dose where indicated)**	**Adverse Effects**
ANTICHOLINERGICS AND ANTIHISTAMINES		
cyclizine (Marezine)	PO; 50 mg every 4–6 h (max: 200 mg/day)	*Drowsiness, dry mouth, blurred vision (scopolamine)*
dimenhydrinate (Dramamine, others)	PO; 50–100 mg every 4–6 h (max: 400 mg/day)	
diphenhydramine (Benadryl, others) (see page 576 for the Prototype Drug box∞)	PO; 25–50 mg tid–qid (max: 300 mg/day)	<u>Hypersensitivity reaction, sedation, tremors, seizures, hallucinations, paradoxical excitation (more common in children), hypotension</u>
hydroxyzine (Atarax, Vistaril)	PO; 25–100 mg tid–qid	
meclizine (Antivert, Bonine, others)	PO; 25–50 mg/day, taken 1 h before travel (max: 50 mg/day)	
scopolamine (Hyoscine, Transderm-Scop)	Transdermal patch; 0.5 mg every 72 h	
BENZODIAZEPINE		
lorazepam (Ativan) (see page 158 for the Prototype Drug box∞)	IV; 1–1.5 mg prior to chemotherapy	*Dizziness, drowsiness, ataxia, fatigue, slurred speech* <u>Paradoxical excitation (more common in children), seizures (if abruptly discontinued), coma</u>
CANNABINOIDS		
dronabinol (Marinol)	PO; 5 mg/m^2 1–3 h before administration of chemotherapy (max: 15 mg/m^2)	*Dizziness, drowsiness, euphoria, confusion, ataxia, asthenia, increased sensory awareness*
nabilone (Cesamet)	PO; 1–2 mg bid	<u>Paranoia, decreased motor coordination, hypotension</u>
CORTICOSTEROIDS		
dexamethasone (Decadron)	PO; 0.25–4 mg bid–qid	*Mood swings, weight gain, acne, facial flushing, nausea, insomnia, sodium and fluid retention, impaired wound healing, menstrual abnormalities, insomnia*
methylprednisolone (Medrol, Solu-Medrol, others)	PO; 4–48 mg/day in divided doses	<u>Peptic ulcer, hypocalcemia, osteoporosis with possible bone fractures, loss of muscle mass, decreased growth in children, possible masking of infections</u>
NEUROKININ RECEPTOR ANTAGONIST		
aprepitant (Emend)	PO; 125 mg 1 h prior to chemotherapy	*Fatigue, constipation, diarrhea, anorexia, nausea, hiccup* <u>Dehydration, peripheral neuropathy, blood dyscrasias, pneumonia</u>
PHENOTHIAZINE AND PHENOTHIAZINE-LIKE		
metoclopramide (Reglan, others)	PO; 2 mg/kg 1 h prior to chemotherapy	*Dry eyes, blurred vision, dry mouth, constipation, drowsiness, photosensitivity*
perphenazine (Phenazine, Trilafon)	PO; 8–16 mg bid–qid	
🔵 prochlorperazine (Compazine)	PO; 5–10 mg tid–qid	<u>Extrapyramidal symptoms, neuroleptic malignant syndrome, agranulocytosis</u>
promethazine (Phenergan, others)	PO; 12.5–25 mg every 4 h qid	
SEROTONIN RECEPTOR ANTAGONISTS		
dolasetron (Anzemet)	PO; 100 mg 1 h prior to chemotherapy	*Headache, drowsiness, fatigue, constipation, diarrhea*
granisetron (Kytril, Sancuso)	PO; 2 mg/day 1 h prior to chemotherapy	
	IV; 10 mcg/kg 30 min prior to chemotherapy	<u>Dysrhythmias, extrapyramidal symptoms</u>
	Transdermal patch: 1 patch 24–48 h prior to chemotherapy	
ondansetron (Zofran)	PO; 4 mg tid prn	
	IV; 32 mg single dose or three 0.15 mg/kg doses 30 minutes prior to chemotherapy	
palonosetron (Aloxi)	PO; 0.5 mg single dose 1 h prior to chemotherapy	
	IV; 0.25 mg 30 min prior to chemotherapy	

Italics indicate common adverse effects; <u>underlining</u> indicates serious adverse effects.

Pr Prototype Drug | Prochlorperazine *(Compazine)*

Therapeutic Class: Antiemetic   **Pharmacologic Class:** Phenothiazine antipsychotic

ACTIONS AND USES

Prochlorperazine is a phenothiazine, a class of drugs usually prescribed for psychoses. The phenothiazines are the largest group of drugs prescribed for severe nausea and vomiting, and prochlorperazine is the most frequently prescribed antiemetic in its class. Prochlorperazine acts by blocking dopamine receptors in the brain, which inhibits signals to the vomiting center in the medulla. As an antiemetic, it is frequently given by the rectal route, where absorption is rapid. It is also available in tablet, extended-release capsule, and IM formulations.

ADMINISTRATION ALERTS

- Administer 2 hours before or after antacids and antidiarrheals.
- Pregnancy category C

> #### PHARMACOKINETICS
> **Onset:** 30–40 min PO; 60 min rectal
> **Peak:** Unknown
> **Half-life:** Unknown
> **Duration:** 3–4 h PO or rectal

ADVERSE EFFECTS

Prochlorperazine produces dose-related anticholinergic side effects such as dry mouth, sedation, constipation, orthostatic hypotension, and tachycardia. When used for prolonged periods at higher doses, extrapyramidal symptoms resembling those of Parkinson's disease are a serious concern.

Contraindications: This drug should not be used in patients with hypersensitivity to phenothiazines, in comatose patients, or in the presence of profound CNS depression. It is also contraindicated in children younger than age 2 or weighing less than 20 lb. Patients with narrow-angle glaucoma, bone marrow suppression, or severe hepatic or cardiac impairment should not take this drug.

INTERACTIONS

Drug-Drug: Prochlorperazine interacts with alcohol and other CNS depressants to cause additive sedation. Antacids and antidiarrheals inhibit the absorption of prochlorperazine. When taken with phenobarbital, metabolism of prochlorperazine is increased. Use with tricyclic antidepressants may produce increased anticholinergic and hypotensive effects.

Lab Tests: Unknown

Herbal/Food: Unknown

Treatment of Overdose: Overdose may result in serious CNS depression and extrapyramidal signs. Patients may be treated with antiparkinsonism drugs (for extrapyramidal symptoms) and possibly a CNS stimulant such as dextroamphetamine.

Refer to MyNursingKit for a Nursing Process Focus specific to this drug.

41.9 Etiology of Obesity

Obesity may be simply defined as being more than 20% above the ideal body weight. Clinically, obesity is commonly measured by the **body mass index (BMI)**. BMI is determined by dividing body weight (in kilograms) by the square of height (in meters).

The etiology of obesity is a complex combination of genetic, lifestyle, and physiologic factors. In a few cases, weight gain can be attributed to medical conditions, the most common being hypothyroidism. Certain rare disorders of the hypothalamus can also cause overeating. Drugs such as corticosteroids are clearly causes of weight gain.

Lifestyle choices play a key role in the development of obesity, the two most obvious factors being diet and physical activity. The fundamental shift in obesity levels in the past three decades has likely been due to high-fat, calorie-dense diets combined with less physically active lifestyles.

Despite an ongoing debate on the "best" diet, the fact remains that body weight is determined by energy (calorie) balance. Simply stated, if the number of calories *consumed* equals the number of calories *expended*, body weight will be maintained (balanced) at the current level. Changes in weight are due to an energy *imbalance*. For example, an imbalance of as little as 10 surplus calories per day can lead to a 1 lb weight gain each year. While this seems insignificant, if the imbalance persists over several decades it can lead to obesity in older adults. Of course, this calculation holds true for losing weight, but few are patient enough to wait an entire year to lose a single pound.

Therefore, to lose weight one has to expend more calories than one consumes. Although nutritionists disagree, in terms of weight loss, the *source* of the calories (carbohydrates, proteins, or lipids) does not matter. Of course, the source is indeed important in terms of overall health and wellness.

Hunger occurs when the hypothalamus recognizes the levels of certain chemicals (glucose) or hormones (insulin) in the blood. Hunger is a normal physiologic response that drives people to seek nourishment. Appetite is somewhat different than hunger. Appetite is a *psychologic* response that drives food intake based on associations and memory. For example, people often eat not because they are experiencing hunger but because it is a particular time of day, or because they find the act of eating pleasurable or social. This is a key concept because blocking hunger sensations with drugs does not guarantee that a person will have less appetite or consume fewer calories.

Nonpharmacologic strategies should always be attempted before initiating drug therapy for obesity. This is true for two reasons. First, drugs for treating obesity produce only modest results and should be taken for only a few months. For someone who needs to lose 25 or more pounds, nonpharmacologic strategies *must* be employed. Secondly, maintaining an optimum weight cannot be accomplished by drugs alone: Smart lifestyle choices are required. A sustainable, healthy diet and an appropriate exercise program are essential to losing weight and maintaining optimum weight.

NURSING PROCESS FOCUS — PATIENTS RECEIVING ANTIEMETIC DRUG THERAPY

Assessment	Potential Nursing Diagnoses
Baseline assessment prior to administration: ■ Understand the reason the drug has been prescribed in order to assess for therapeutic effects. ■ Obtain a complete health history including GI, cardiovascular, hepatic, or renal disease; pregnancy; or breast-feeding. Obtain a drug history including allergies, current prescription and OTC drugs, herbal preparations, caffeine, nicotine, and alcohol use. Be alert to possible drug interactions. ■ Obtain baseline weight and vital signs, especially blood pressure and pulse. ■ Evaluate appropriate laboratory findings (e.g., electrolytes, glucose, CBC, hepatic or renal function studies). ■ Obtain an abdominal assessment (e.g., bowel sounds, firmness, distention, presence of tenderness). ■ Assess emesis for amount, color, and presence of blood.	■ Deficient Fluid Volume (related to vomiting) ■ Deficient Knowledge (drug therapy) ■ Risk for Injury, Falls (related to dizziness, adverse drug effects)
Assessment throughout administration: ■ Assess for desired therapeutic effects (e.g., nausea is decreased, no vomiting present, able to tolerate fluids and increasing solids). ■ Continue to monitor and measure any emesis. Assess urine output and maintain intake and output measurements in the hospitalized patient. ■ Monitor vital signs, especially blood pressure and pulse, and report any hypotension or tachycardia to the health care provider. ■ Continue periodic monitoring of abdominal assessment findings, especially bowel sounds. ■ Continue periodic monitoring of electrolytes, glucose, CBC, and hepatic and renal function labs as appropriate. ■ Assess for adverse effects: headache, drowsiness, dizziness, dry mouth, blurred vision, and fatigue. Continued vomiting, severe nausea, emesis with blood present or coffee-ground appearance, hypotension, tachycardia, or confusion should be reported immediately.	

Planning: Patient Goals and Expected Outcomes

The patient will:
■ Experience therapeutic effects (e.g., decreased or absence of nausea, vomiting, ability to take fluids and food).
■ Be free from, or experience minimal, adverse effects.
■ Verbalize an understanding of the drug's use, adverse effects, and required precautions.
■ Demonstrate proper self-administration of the medication (e.g., dose, timing, when to notify provider).

Implementation

Interventions and (Rationales)	Patient and Family Education
Ensuring therapeutic effects: ■ If a definitive cause for the current symptoms can be identified (e.g., infection, adverse drug effects), correct the cause where possible. (Nausea and vomiting are often symptoms of other underlying conditions such as adverse drug effects or infections.)	■ Review medications, foods, and the possibility of illness with the patient, family, or caregiver to help identify causative factors. ■ Decrease noxious stimuli (e.g., strong odors, rapid changes in position) that may increase nausea or vomiting.
■ Encourage a small amount of fluids or ice chips and decreasing activity level while nauseated; eliminating alcohol intake, smoking cessation, and increasing intake of yogurt and *acidophilus*-containing foods after nausea has ceased. (These interventions may help ease symptoms during the acute phase. Ensuring adequate amounts of fluids, including intravenous fluids if necessary, will help maintain a normal fluid balance. Smoking and alcohol use cause gastric irritation.)	■ Encourage the patient to limit physical movement or activity during periods of acute nausea or vomiting. Encourage increasing fluid intake gradually, with ice chips or small sips of water. Ginger ale may act as a natural antinausea beverage and may be palatable for some patients.
■ Administer antiemetics 30 to 60 minutes before anticipated nausea-inducing travel or drug administration (e.g., chemotherapy). Ensure adequate hydration prior to the onset of anticipated nausea. (Antiemetics are most effective when taken before nausea occurs. Ensuring adequate prehydration decreases the risk of dehydration should vomiting occur.)	■ Teach the patient to take the antiemetic before travel if nausea is anticipated. If drowsiness or dizziness may occur, encourage the patient to consider a "trial run" with the medication taken in evening before bedtime to ascertain effects prior to taking if driving is required. ■ Teach the patient on at-home chemotherapy to take antiemetics prior to chemotherapy dose or routinely as ordered by the health care provider.

Implementation

Interventions and (Rationales)	Patient and Family Education
Minimizing adverse effects:	
■ Monitor vital signs, particularly blood pressure and pulse. Take blood pressure lying, sitting, and standing to detect orthostatic hypotension. Be cautious with older adults who are at an increased risk for hypotension. Report any hypotension, especially associated with tachycardia, immediately. (Excessive vomiting may cause dehydration and decreased blood pressure or hypotension. Anticholinergics, antihistamines, and phenothiazine or phenothiazine-like drugs may also decrease blood pressure.)	■ Teach the patient to rise from lying or sitting to standing slowly to avoid dizziness or falls.
■ Continue to monitor abdominal assessment findings. Immediately report any significant increase or decrease in bowel sounds, distention, new onset or increase in discomfort or pain, severe abdominal pain, or vomiting that is coffee-ground in consistency or contains blood. (Increasing or severe abdominal pain or blood in emesis may indicate a worsening of disease.)	■ Teach the patient to report any increasing gastric discomfort or pain. ■ Instruct the patient that severe abdominal pain or any blood in emesis should be reported immediately to the health care provider.
■ Ensure patient safety, especially in older adults. Observe for dizziness and monitor ambulation until the effects of the drug are known. Obtain electrolyte levels if dizziness continues. (Drowsiness or dizziness from dehydration or from adverse drug effects may occur and increases the risk of falls. Continued dizziness may indicate electrolyte imbalance and electrolyte levels should be assessed.)	■ Instruct the patient to call for assistance prior to getting out of bed or attempting to walk alone if dizziness or drowsiness occur. Provide an emesis basin nearby. For home use, avoid driving or other activities requiring mental alertness or physical coordination until the effects of the drug are known.
■ Continue to monitor periodic electrolyte, glucose levels, and hepatic and renal function tests as needed. (Loss of electrolytes may occur with severe vomiting. Abnormal liver function tests may indicate drug-induced adverse hepatic effects.)	■ Instruct the patient on the need for lab work.
■ Monitor intake and output in the hospitalized patient. Initiate IV fluid replacement when indicated. Hold oral fluids until acute vomiting has ceased and then gradually increase fluid intake, beginning with small sips of water or ice chips. (Continuing oral intake may worsen nausea and vomiting. Gradually resuming fluids will allow for hydration without stimulating nausea. IV fluid replacement may be required if fluid loss has been severe and dehydration present.)	■ Instruct the patient on the need to withhold fluids and food until vomiting has ceased. Initiate incremental increases in intake beginning with small sips of water and clear fluids. ■ Explain the rationale for any IV hydration required and any equipment used.
■ If pregnancy is suspected or confirmed, hold the antiemetic until consulting with the health care provider. (Alternative antinausea measures should be used to ease nausea when possible. The drug's pregnancy class and pregnancy trimester will be considered by the health care provider before prescribing.)	■ If the patient is pregnant, or if pregnancy is suspected, teach the patient to consult with the health care provider before taking any antiemetic drug for morning sickness. ■ Encourage the use of nondrug measures such as dry and unsweetened cereals or crackers taken in small amounts, avoiding noxious stimuli during periods of nausea, or ginger ale may aid in diminishing nausea.
Patient understanding of drug therapy:	
■ Use opportunities during the administration of medications and during assessments to discuss the rationale for drug therapy, desired therapeutic outcomes, most common adverse effects, parameters for when to call the health care provider, and any necessary monitoring or precautions. (Using time during nursing care helps to optimize and reinforce key teaching areas.)	■ The patient, family, or caregiver should be able to state the reason for the drug; appropriate dose and scheduling; what adverse effects to observe for and when to report; and the anticipated length of medication therapy.
Patient self-administration of drug therapy:	
■ When administering the medication, instruct the patient, family, or caregiver in the proper self-administration of the drug, e.g., taken with small sips of fluid. (Proper administration increases the effectiveness of the drugs.)	■ The patient and family or caregiver are able to discuss appropriate dosing and administration needs.

Evaluation of Outcome Criteria

Evaluate the effectiveness of drug therapy by confirming that the patient goals and expected outcomes have been met (see "Planning").

See Table 41.3 for a list of drugs to which these nursing actions apply.

Drugs for Obesity

Despite the public's desire for effective drugs to promote weight loss, however, there are few such drugs on the market. The approved agents produce only modest results.

41.10 Pharmacotherapy of Obesity

Because of the prevalence of obesity in society and the difficulty most patients experience when following weight reduction plans for extended periods, drug manufacturers have long sought to develop safe drugs that induce rapid and sustained weight loss. In the 1970s, amphetamine and dextroamphetamine (Dexedrine) were widely prescribed to reduce appetite; however, these drugs are addictive and rarely prescribed for this purpose today. In the 1990s, the combination of fenfluramine and phentermine (fen-phen) was widely prescribed, until fenfluramine was removed from the market for causing heart valve defects. An OTC appetite suppressant, phenylpropanolamine, was removed from the market in 2000 due to an increased incidence of strokes and adverse cardiac events. Until 2004, natural alternative weight-loss products contained ephedra alkaloids, but these have been removed from the market because of an increased incidence of adverse cardiovascular events. The quest to produce a "magic pill" to lose weight has indeed been elusive.

Current pharmacologic strategies for weight management focus on two sites of action. One strategy to reduce weight is to block the absorption of dietary fats using drugs called **lipase inhibitors**. Orlistat (Xenical) blocks lipid absorption in the GI tract. Unfortunately, orlistat may also decrease absorption of other substances, including fat-soluble vitamins and warfarin (Coumadin). To avoid having severe GI effects such as flatus with discharge, oily stool, abdominal pain, and discomfort, patients should restrict their fat intake when taking this drug. GI effects often diminish after 4 weeks of therapy. This drug produces only a very small decrease in weight compared with placebos.

A second strategy to reduce weight is to block parts of the nervous system responsible for hunger with **anorexiants**, also called appetite suppressants. Sibutramine (Meridia), a selective serotonin reuptake inhibitor (SSRI), is the most widely prescribed appetite suppressant for the short-term control of obesity. Two other SSRIs, fluoxetine (Prozac) and sertraline (Zoloft), produce a similar loss in weight, although they are not FDA approved for this purpose. Phentermine, once part of the now-banned combination of fen-phen, is still available as monotherapy, although it produces only a small, transient weight loss.

All the anorexiants have the potential to produce serious side effects; thus, their use is limited to short-term therapy. Anorexiants are prescribed for patients with a body mass index (BMI) of at least 30 or greater, or a BMI of 27 or greater, with other risk factors for disease such as hypertension, hyperlipidemia, or diabetes.

PANCREATIC ENZYMES

The pancreas secretes essential digestive enzymes: Pancreatic juice contains carboxypeptidase, chymotrypsin, and trypsin, which are converted to their active forms once they

---

Pr Prototype Drug | Sibutramine *(Meridia)*

Therapeutic Class: Antiobesity agent; appetite suppressant   **Pharmacologic Class:** Anorexiant; SSRI

ACTIONS AND USES
Sibutramine is only approved for the treatment of obesity when combined with a reduced-calorie diet and increased physical activity. The drug is able to produce a 5% to 10% loss of body weight within 6–12 months of treatment. Patients who have not lost at least 4 lb after the first month of therapy require an increase in dose or discontinuation of therapy. Sibutramine therapy is not recommended for longer than 1 year.

ADMINISTRATION ALERTS
- Allow at least 2 weeks between discontinuing MAO inhibitors and starting sibutramine.
- This drug is not approved for use in patients under age 16.
- Pregnancy category C

PHARMACOKINETICS
Onset: Unknown
Peak: 1.2 h
Half-life: 14–16 h
Duration: Unknown

ADVERSE EFFECTS
Sibutramine is generally well tolerated and serious adverse effects are uncommon. Headache, constipation, insomnia, and xerostomia are the most common complaints reported during sibutramine therapy. Weight gain may occur after sibutramine is discontinued. It is a Schedule IV drug with low potential for dependence.

Contraindications: Sibutramine is contraindicated in patients with eating disorders (anorexia nervosa or bulimia) and those taking MAO inhibitors. The drug should be used with care in patients with heart disease, dysrhythmias, or stroke because it may cause tachycardia and raise blood pressure.

INTERACTIONS
Drug–Drug: Use with decongestants, cough, and allergy medications may cause elevated blood pressure. Ketoconazole and erythromycin may inhibit the metabolism of sibutramine. Concurrent use with a monoamine oxidase inhibitor (MAOI) or selective serotonin reuptake inhibitor (SSRI) may cause serotonin syndrome.

Lab Tests: Unknown

Herbal/Food: Unknown

Treatment of Overdose: Tachycardia and hypertension may result from overdose. Beta-adrenergic blockers may be administered.

Refer to MyNursingKit for a Nursing Process Focus specific to this drug.

RESEARCH SHOWS

The Question: What are the most effective strategies for producing sustained weight loss?

The Study: The authors conducted systematic review to determine types of weight-loss interventions that contribute to the most successful outcomes. Eight types of weight-loss interventions were reviewed: diet alone, diet plus exercise, exercise alone, meal replacements, very-low-energy diets, weight-loss medications (orlistat and sibutramine), and advice alone. The most successful interventions were a reduced-energy diet and/or weight-loss medications. During the first 6 months, an average weight loss of 5 to 8.5 kg (5% to 9%) was observed. In studies extending to 48 months, a mean 3 to 6 kg (3% to 6%) of weight loss was maintained. Advice-only and exercise-alone groups experienced minimal weight loss. The authors concluded that the addition of weight-loss medications somewhat enhances weight-loss maintenance.

Nursing Implications: Nurses should teach patients that drugs can be used to enhance weight loss, but they must be combined with a low-energy diet to be most effective.

M. Franz, J. VanWormer, A. Crain, J. Boucher, T. Histon, W. Caplan, J. Bowman, N. Pronk (2007). Weight-Loss Outcomes: A Systematic Review and Meta-Analysis of Weight-Loss Clinical Trials with a Minimum 1-Year Follow-Up. Journal of the American Dietetic Association, 107(10), 1755–1767.

reach the small intestine. Three other pancreatic enzymes—lipase, amylase, and nuclease—are secreted in their active form but require the presence of bile for optimum activity. Because lack of secretion will result in malabsorption disorders, replacement therapy is sometimes warranted.

41.11 Pharmacotherapy of Pancreatitis

Pancreatitis results when amylase and lipase remain in the pancreas rather than being released into the duodenum. The enzymes escape into the surrounding tissue, causing inflammation in the pancreas. Pancreatitis can be either acute or chronic.

Acute pancreatitis usually occurs in middle-aged adults and is often associated with gallstones in women and alcoholism in men. Symptoms of acute pancreatitis present suddenly, often after eating a fatty meal or consuming excessive amounts of alcohol. The most common symptom is a continuous severe pain in the epigastric area that often radiates to the back. The patient usually recovers from the illness and regains normal function of the pancreas. Some patients with acute pancreatitis have recurring attacks and progress to chronic pancreatitis.

Many patients with acute pancreatitis require only bed rest and withholding food and fluids by mouth for a few days for the symptoms to subside. For patients with acute pain, meperidine (Demerol) brings effective relief. To reduce or neutralize gastric secretions, H_2-receptor blockers such as cimetidine (Tagamet) or proton pump inhibitors such as omeprazole (Prilosec) may be prescribed. To decrease the amount of pancreatic enzymes secreted, carbonic anhydrase inhibitors such as acetazolamide (Diamox) or

antispasmodics such as dicyclomine (Bentyl) may be used. In particularly severe cases, IV fluids and total parenteral nutrition may be necessary.

The majority of chronic pancreatitis is associated with alcoholism. Alcohol is thought to promote the formation of insoluble proteins that occlude the pancreatic duct. Pancreatic juice is prevented from flowing into the duodenum and remains in the pancreas to damage cells and cause inflammation. Symptoms include chronic epigastric or left upper quadrant pain, anorexia, nausea, vomiting, and weight loss. **Steatorrhea**, the passing of bulky, foul-smelling fatty stools, occurs late in the course of the disease. Chronic pancreatitis eventually leads to pancreatic insufficiency that may necessitate insulin therapy as well as replacement of pancreatic enzymes.

Drugs prescribed for the treatment of acute pancreatitis may also be used for patients with chronic pancreatitis. Opioid analgesics, IV fluids, insulin, and antiemetics may be necessary. Oral pancreatic enzyme supplementation is often used in patients with chronic pancreatitis. Pancreatic enzyme supplements such as pancrelipase (Cotazym, Pancrease, others) or pancreatin (Ku-Zyme, Kutrase) help to digest fats, and prevent steatorrhea.

LIFESPAN CONSIDERATIONS

Psychosocial and Community Impacts of Alcohol-Related Pancreatitis

Patients with acute pancreatitis are most often middle aged, and those with chronic pancreatitis are most often in their 50s or 60s. Patients whose pancreatitis is associated with gallstones may receive a different type and amount of support from significant others, the community, and even from nurses as compared with those who have pancreatitis associated with alcoholism. Nurses will need to examine their feelings and attitudes related to alcoholism in general and to patients with alcoholism-associated pancreatitis in particular, and will need to adopt attitudes to help the patient attain treatment goals.

Patients who abuse alcohol often need referral to community agencies to manage their addiction and/or remain in recovery. Family members may also need referral to community agencies for help in dealing with altered family processes due to the patient's drinking and any role they may have played in enabling the patient to abuse alcohol.

HOME & COMMUNITY CONSIDERATIONS

Educating Patients About OTC Medications for Bowel Disorders, Nausea, and Vomiting

Bowel disorders, nausea, and vomiting are among the most common complaints for which patients seek medical consultation; therefore, they are also the most common complaints treated with OTC medications. Many patients, especially older adults, do not understand that these OTC medications have the potential to cause severe drug–drug interactions and adverse effects. Most of these OTC medications interfere with the metabolism of prescription medications and should be used with caution in patients with enlarged prostates because they can cause life-threatening reactions. Patients also need to be aware that these OTCs can cause drowsiness and hypotension. Careful education is required so that patients understand that continued use of these medications may mask a more severe health disorder.

Pr Prototype Drug | Pancrelipase *(Cotazym, Pancrease, others)*

Therapeutic Class: Pancreatic enzymes   **Pharmacologic Class:** None

ACTIONS AND USES

Pancrelipase contains lipase, protease, and amylase of pork origin and is used as replacement therapy for patients with insufficient pancreatic exocrine secretions, including those with pancreatitis and cystic fibrosis. Given orally, the capsule dissolves in the alkaline environment of the duodenum and releases its enzymes. The enzymes act locally in the GI tract and are not absorbed. Pancrelipase is available in powder, tablet, and delayed-release capsule formulations.

On an equal-eight basis, pancrelipase is more potent than pancreatin, with 12 times the enzyme activity. It also contains at least four times as much trypsin and amylase.

ADMINISTRATION ALERTS

- Do not crush or open enteric-coated tablets.
- Powder formulations may be sprinkled on food.
- Give the drug 1–2 h before or with meals, or as directed by the health care provider.
- Pregnancy category C

PHARMACOKINETICS
Onset: Immediate

Peak: Unknown

Half-life: Unknown

Duration: Unknown

ADVERSE EFFECTS

Adverse effects of pancrelipase are uncommon, since the enzymes are not absorbed. The most frequent adverse effects are GI symptoms of nausea, vomiting, and diarrhea. Very high doses are associated with a risk for hyperuricemia.

Contraindications: Pancrelipase is contraindicated in patients allergic to the drug or to pork products. The delayed-release products should not be given to patients with acute pancreatitis.

INTERACTIONS

Drug–Drug: Pancrelipase interacts with iron, which may result in decreased absorption of iron. Antacids may decrease the effect of pancrelipase.

Lab Tests: Pancrelipase may increase serum or urinary levels of uric acid.

Herbal/Food: Unknown

Treatment of Overdose: High levels of uric acid may occur with overdose. Patients are treated symptomatically.

Refer to MyNursingKit for a Nursing Process Focus specific to this drug.

Chapter REVIEW

KEY CONCEPTS

The numbered key concepts provide a succinct summary of the important points from the corresponding numbered section within the chapter. If any of these points are not clear, refer to the numbered section within the chapter for review.

41.1 The small intestine is the location for most nutrient and drug absorption. The large intestine is responsible for the reabsorption of water.

41.2 Constipation, the infrequent passage of hard, small stools, is a common condition caused by insufficient dietary fiber and slow motility of waste material through the large intestine.

41.3 Laxatives and cathartics are drugs given to promote emptying of the large intestine by stimulating peristalsis, lubricating the fecal mass, or adding more bulk or water to the colon contents.

41.4 Diarrhea is an increase in the frequency and fluidity of bowel movements that occurs when the colon fails to reabsorb enough water.

41.5 For simple diarrhea, OTC medications such as loperamide or bismuth compounds are effective. Opioids are the most effective drugs for controlling severe diarrhea.

41.6 Inflammatory bowel disease includes ulcerative colitis and Crohn's disease. Treatment includes 5-aminosalicylic acid (5-ASA) agents or corticosteroids. Drugs for irritable bowel syndrome are targeted at symptomatic treatment, depending on whether constipation or diarrhea is the predominant symptom.

41.7 Vomiting is a defense mechanism used by the body to rid itself of toxic substances. Nausea is an uncomfortable feeling that may precede vomiting. Many drugs can cause nausea and vomiting as side effects.

41.8 Symptomatic treatment of nausea and vomiting includes drugs from many different classes, including phenothiazines, antihistamines, anticholinergics, cannabinoids, corticosteroids, benzodiazepines, and serotonin receptor antagonists.

41.9 Obesity has become widespread in the United States and is associated with multiple chronic diseases such as hypertension and heart disease. The etiology of obesity is a combination of genetic, lifestyle, and physiologic factors. A sustainable diet and exercise program should be implemented before pharmacotherapy is considered.

41.10 The pharmacotherapy of obesity includes the anorexiants sibutramine and the lipase inhibitor orlistat. Both

drugs are used for the short-term management of obesity but produce only modest effects.

41.11 Pancreatitis results when pancreatic enzymes are trapped in the pancreas and not released into the duodenum. Pharmacotherapy includes replacement enzymes and supportive drugs for reduction of pain and gastric acid secretion.

NCLEX-RN® REVIEW QUESTIONS

1 In a patient with a prolonged episode of vomiting, the nurse must assess for the development of what problem?
1. Acid–base disturbances
2. Intractable diarrhea
3. Esophageal tears
4. Hypoventilation

2 The nurse should educate patients to take diphenhydrinate (Dramamine) how long before they board an airplane for a trip?
1. 20 to 60 minutes
2. 15 minutes
3. 2 hours
4. 6 hours

3 The nurse assesses for one of the major precipitating factors in the development IBS, which is:
1. stress.
2. peptic ulcers.
3. gastroesophageal reflux disease (GERD).
4. *Helicobacter pylori.*

4 The patient has been given a drug for treatment of nausea and vomiting and is now complaining of dry mouth, constipation, and a rapid heart rate. What drug would cause these side effects? (Select all that apply.)

1. Loperamide (Immodium, Kaopectate)
2. Prochlorperazine (Compazine)
3. Peppermint
4. Diphenoxylate with atropine (Lomotil)
5. Promethazine (Phenergan)

5 The patient has been prescribed sibutramine (Meridia) for obesity. The nurse assesses for what as a possible contraindication? (Select all that apply.)
1. Uncontrolled hypertension
2. Hepatic impairment
3. Renal impairment
4. Coronary artery disease (CAD)
5. Bowel obstruction

6 The nurse has administered prochlorperazine (Compazine) to a patient for postoperative nausea. Before administering this medication, it is essential to check the patient's:
1. pulse.
2. blood pressure.
3. lung sounds.
4. temperature.

CRITICAL THINKING QUESTIONS

1. The patient has been taking diphenoxylate with atropine (Lomotil) for diarrhea for the past 3 days. The patient has had diarrhea five times today. Identify the priorities of nursing care.

2. The health care provider has ordered morphine and prochlorperazine (Compazine) for a patient with postoperative pain. The patient insists that she is "needle phobic" and wants all the medication in one syringe. What is the nurse's response?

3. A patient comes to the clinic complaining of no bowel movement for 4 days (other than small amounts of liquid stool). The patient has been taking psyllium mucilloid (Metamucil) for his constipation and wants to know why this is not working. What is the nurse's response?

See Appendix D for answers and rationales for all activities.

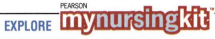

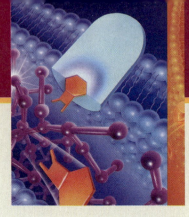

Drugs for Nutritional Disorders

LEARNING OUTCOMES

After reading this chapter, the student should be able to:

1. Identify characteristics that differentiate vitamins from other nutrients.
2. Describe the functions of vitamins and minerals.
3. Compare and contrast the properties of water-soluble and fat-soluble vitamins.
4. Identify diseases and conditions that may benefit from vitamin or mineral pharmacotherapy.
5. Describe the nurse's role in the pharmacologic management of nutritional disorders.
6. Compare and contrast the properties of macrominerals and trace minerals.
7. Identify differences among oligomeric, polymeric, modular, and specialized formulations for enteral nutrition.
8. Compare and contrast enteral and parenteral methods of providing nutrition.
9. For each of the drug classes listed in Drug at a Glance, know representative drugs, and explain the mechanism of drug action, describe primary actions, and identify important adverse effects.
10. Use the nursing process to care for patients who are receiving drug therapy for nutritional disorders.

KEY TERMS

The nutritional supplement business is a multibillion-dollar industry. Although clever marketing often leads people to believe that vitamin and dietary supplements are essential to maintain health, most people obtain all the necessary nutrients through a balanced diet. Once the body has obtained the amounts of vitamins, minerals, or nutrients it needs to carry on metabolism, the excess is simply excreted or stored. In certain conditions, however, dietary supplementation is necessary and benefits the patient's health. This chapter focuses on these conditions and explores the role of vitamins, minerals, and nutritional supplements in pharmacology.

VITAMINS

Vitamins are essential substances needed to maintain optimum wellness. Patients having a low or unbalanced dietary intake, those who are pregnant, or those experiencing a chronic disease may benefit from vitamin therapy.

42.1 Role of Vitamins in Maintaining Health

Vitamins are organic compounds required by the body in small amounts for growth and for the maintenance of normal metabolic processes. Since the discovery of thiamine in 1911, more than a dozen vitamins have been identified. Because scientists did not know the chemical structures of the vitamins when they were discovered, they assigned letters and numbers such as A, B_{12}, and C. These names are still widely used today.

An important characteristic of vitamins is that, with the exception of vitamin D, human cells cannot synthesize them. They, or their precursors known as **provitamins**, must be supplied in the diet. A second important characteristic is that if the vitamin is not present in adequate amounts, then the body's metabolism will be disrupted and disease will result. However, the symptoms of the deficiency can be reversed by administering the missing vitamin.

Vitamins serve diverse and important roles. For example, the B-complex vitamins are coenzymes essential to many metabolic pathways. Vitamin A is a precursor of retinal, a pigment needed for vision. Calcium metabolism is regulated by a hormone that is derived from vitamin D. Without vitamin K, abnormal prothrombin is produced, and blood clotting is affected.

42.2 Classification of Vitamins

A simple way to classify vitamins is by their ability to mix with water. Those that dissolve easily in water are called *water-soluble* vitamins. Examples include vitamin C and the B vitamins. Those that dissolve in lipids are called *fat-* or *lipid-soluble* and include vitamins A, D, E, and K.

The difference in solubility affects the way the vitamins are absorbed by the gastrointestinal (GI) tract and stored in the body. The water-soluble vitamins are absorbed with water in the digestive tract and readily dissolve in blood and body fluids. When excess water-soluble vitamins are absorbed, they cannot be stored for later use and are simply excreted in the urine. Because they are not stored to any significant degree, they must be ingested daily; otherwise, deficiencies will quickly develop.

Fat-soluble vitamins, on the other hand, cannot be absorbed in sufficient quantity in the small intestine unless they are ingested with other lipids. These vitamins can be stored in large quantities in the liver and adipose tissue. Should the patient not ingest sufficient amounts, fat-soluble vitamins are removed from storage depots in the body, as needed. Unfortunately, storage may lead to dangerously high levels of these vitamins if they are taken in excessive amounts.

42.3 Recommended Dietary Allowances

Based on scientific research on humans and animals, the Food and Nutrition Board of the National Academy of Sciences has established levels for the dietary intake of vitamins and minerals called **Recommended Dietary Allowances (RDAs)**. The RDA values represent the *minimum* amount of vitamin or mineral needed to prevent a deficiency in a healthy adult. The RDAs are revised periodically to reflect the latest scientific research. Current RDAs for vitamins are listed in Table 42.1. A newer standard, the Dietary Reference Intake (DRI) is sometimes used to represent the *optimal* level of nutrient needed to ensure wellness.

Vitamin, mineral, or herbal supplements should never substitute for a balanced diet. Sufficient intake of proteins, carbohydrates, and lipids is needed for proper health. Furthermore, although the label on a vitamin supplement may indicate that it contains 100% of the RDA for a particular

---

PHARMFACTS

Vitamins, Minerals, and Nutritional Supplements

- About 40% of Americans take vitamin supplements daily.
- There is no difference between the chemical structure of a natural vitamin and a synthetic vitamin, yet consumers pay much more for the natural type.
- Vitamin B_{12} is present only in animal products. Vegetarians may find adequate amounts in fortified cereals, nutritional supplements, or yeast.
- Administration of folic acid during pregnancy has been found to reduce birth defects in the nervous system of the baby.
- Patients who never receive sun exposure may need vitamin D supplements.
- Vitamins technically cannot increase a patient's energy level. Energy can be provided only by adding calories from carbohydrates, proteins, and lipids.

TABLE 42.1	Vitamins				
		RDA			
Vitamin	Function(s)	Men	Women	Common Cause(s) of Deficiency	
A	Visual pigments, epithelial cells	1,000 mg RE*	800 mg RE	Prolonged dietary deprivation, particularly when rice is the main food source; pancreatic disease; cirrhosis	
B complex: biotin	Coenzyme in metabolic reactions	30 mcg	30 mcg	Deficiencies are rare	
cyanocobalamin (B$_{12}$)	Coenzyme in nucleic acid metabolism	2 mcg	2 mcg	Lack of intrinsic factor, inadequate intake of foods from animal origin	
folic acid/folate (B$_9$)	Coenzyme in amino acid and nucleic acid metabolism	200 mcg	160–180 mcg	Pregnancy, alcoholism, cancer, oral contraceptive use	
niacin (B$_3$)	Coenzyme in oxidation–reduction reactions	15–20 mg	13–15 mg	Prolonged dietary deprivation, particularly when Indian corn (maize) or millet is the main food source; chronic diarrhea; liver disease; alcoholism	
pantothenic acid (B$_5$)	Coenzyme in metabolic reactions	5 mg	5 mg	Deficiencies are rare	
pyridoxine (B$_6$)	Coenzyme in amino acid metabolism, RBC production	2 mg	1.5–1.6 mg	Alcoholism, oral contraceptive use, malabsorption diseases	
riboflavin (B$_2$)	Coenzyme in oxidation–reduction reactions	1.4–1.8 mg	1.2–1.3 mg	Inadequate consumption of milk or animal products, chronic diarrhea, liver disease, alcoholism	
thiamine (B$_1$)	Coenzyme in metabolic reactions, RBC formation	1.2–1.5 mg	1.0–1.1 mg	Prolonged dietary deprivation, particularly when rice is the main food source; hyperthyroidism; pregnancy; liver disease; alcoholism	
C (ascorbic acid)	Coenzyme and antioxidant	60 mg	60 mg	Inadequate intake of fruits and vegetables, pregnancy, chronic inflammatory disease, burns, diarrhea, alcoholism	
D	Calcium and phosphate metabolism	5–10 mg	5–10 mg	Low dietary intake, inadequate exposure to sunlight	
E	Antioxidant	10 TE**	8 mg TE	Prematurity, malabsorption diseases	
K	Cofactor in blood clotting	65–80 mcg	55–65 mcg	Newborns, liver disease, long-term parenteral nutrition, certain drugs such as cephalosporins and salicylates	

*RE = retinoid equivalents; **TE = alpha-tocopherol equivalents

vitamin, the body may absorb as little as 10% to 15% of the amount ingested. With the exception of vitamins A and D, it is not harmful for most patients to consume two to three times the recommended levels of vitamins. In cases where dietary needs are increased, the RDAs will need adjustment and supplements are indicated to achieve optimum wellness.

42.4 Indications for Vitamin Pharmacotherapy

Most people who eat a normal, balanced diet obtain all the necessary nutrients without vitamin supplementation. Indeed, megavitamin therapy is not only expensive but also harmful to health if taken for long periods. **Hypervitaminosis,** or toxic levels of vitamins, has been reported for vitamins A, C, D, E, B$_6$, niacin, and folic acid. In the United States, it is actually more common to observe syndromes of vitamin *excess* than of vitamin *deficiency*. Most patients are unaware that taking too much of a vitamin or mineral can cause serious adverse effects.

Vitamin deficiencies follow certain patterns. The following are general characteristics of vitamin deficiency disorders:

- Patients more commonly present with *multiple* vitamin deficiencies than with a single vitamin deficiency.
- Symptoms of deficiency are *nonspecific,* and often do not appear until the deficiency has been present for a long time.
- Deficiencies in the United States are most often the result of poverty, fad diets, chronic alcohol or drug abuse, or prolonged parenteral feeding.

Certain patients and conditions require higher levels of vitamins. Infancy and childhood are times of potential deficiency due to the high growth demands placed on the body. In addition, requirements for all nutrients are increased during pregnancy and lactation. With normal aging, the absorption of food diminishes and the quantity of ingested food is often reduced, leading to a higher risk of vitamin deficiencies in older adults. Men and women can have different vitamin and mineral needs as do persons who participate in vigorous exercise. Vitamin deficiencies in patients with chronic liver and kidney disease are well documented.

Certain drugs have the potential to affect vitamin metabolism. Alcohol is known for its ability to inhibit the absorption of thiamine and folic acid: Alcohol abuse is the most common cause of thiamine deficiency in the United States. Folic acid levels may be reduced in patients taking phenothiazines, oral contraceptives, phenytoin (Dilantin), or barbiturates. Vitamin D deficiency can be caused by therapy with certain anticonvulsants. Inhibition of vitamin B_{12} absorption has been reported with a number of drugs, including trifluoperazine (Stelazine), alcohol, and oral contraceptives. The nurse must be aware of these drug interactions and recommend vitamin therapy when appropriate.

Lipid-Soluble Vitamins

The lipid- or fat-soluble vitamins are abundant in both plant and animal foods, and are relatively stable during cooking. Because the body stores them, it is not necessary to ingest the recommended amounts on a daily basis.

42.5 Pharmacotherapy with Lipid-Soluble Vitamins

Lipid-soluble vitamins are absorbed from the intestine with dietary lipids and are stored primarily in the liver. When consumed in high amounts, these vitamins can accumulate to toxic levels and produce hypervitaminosis. Because these are available OTC, patients must be advised to carefully follow the instructions of the health care provider, or the label directions, for proper dosage. It is not unusual to find over-the-counter (OTC) preparations that contain 200% to 400% of the RDA. Medications containing lipid-soluble vitamins, and their recommended doses, are listed in Table 42.2.

Vitamin A, also known as *retinol*, is obtained from foods containing **carotenes.** Carotenes are precursors to vitamin A that are converted to retinol in the wall of the small intestine when absorbed. The most abundant and biologically active carotene is beta carotene. During metabolism, each molecule of beta carotene yields two molecules of vitamin A. Good sources of dietary vitamin A include yellow and dark leafy vegetables, butter, eggs, whole milk, and liver. Vitamin A is used as replacement therapy for conditions affecting absorption, mobilization, or storage of vitamin A, such as steatorrhea, severe biliary obstruction, liver cirrhosis, or total gastrectomy.

Vitamin D is actually a group of chemicals sharing similar activity. Vitamin D_2, also known as **ergocalciferol,** is obtained from fortified milk, margarine, and other dairy products. Vitamin D_3 is formed in the skin by a chemical reaction requiring ultraviolet radiation. Vitamin D is used to treat skeletal diseases that weaken the bones such as rickets, osteomalacia (adult rickets), osteoporosis, and hypocalcemia. Sometimes vitamin D is helpful in treating psoriasis, rheumatoid arthritis, and lupus vulgaris. The pharmacology of the D vitamins and a drug prototype for the active form of vitamin D are detailed in chapter 46∞.

Vitamin E consists of about eight chemicals, called **tocopherols,** having similar activity. Alpha tocopherol constitutes 90% of the tocopherols, and is the only one of pharmacologic importance. Dosage of vitamin E is sometimes reported as milligrams of alpha-tocopherol equivalents (TE). Vitamin E is found in plant-seed oils, whole-grain cereals, eggs, and certain organ meats such as liver, pancreas, and heart. It is considered a primary antioxidant, preventing the formation of free radicals that damage plasma membranes and other cellular structures. Deficiency in adults has been observed only with severe malabsorption disorders; however, deficiency in premature neonates may lead to hemolytic anemia. Patients often self-administer vitamin E because it is thought to be useful in preventing heart disease and increasing sexual prowess, although research has not

TABLE 42.2	Lipid-Soluble Vitamins for Treating Nutritional Disorders	
Drug	Route and Adult Dose (max dose where indicated)	Adverse Effects
🅟 vitamin A (Aquasol A, others)	PO; 500,000 units/day for 3 days, followed by 50,000 units/day for 2 wk; then 10,000–20,000 units/day for 2 mo IM; 100,000 units/day for 3 days followed by 50,000 units/day for 2 wk	*Adverse effects are uncommon at recommended doses* High doses: nausea, vomiting, fatigue, irritability, night sweats, alopecia, dry skin
🅟 vitamin D: calcitriol (Calcijex, Rocaltrol) (see page 735 for the Prototype Drug box ∞)	PO; 0.25 mcg/day; may be increased by 0.25 mcg/day every 4–8 wk for dialysis patients or every 2–4 wk for hypoparathyroid patients, if necessary IV; 0.5 mcg three times/wk at the end of dialysis; may need up to 3 mcg three times/wk	*Adverse effects are uncommon at recommended doses, metallic taste* High doses: nausea, vomiting, fatigue, headache, polyuria, weight loss, hallucinations, dysrhythmias, muscle and bone pain
vitamin E: tocopherol (Aquasol E, Vita-Plus E, others)	PO/IM; 60–75 units/day	*Adverse effects are uncommon at recommended doses* High doses: nausea, vomiting, fatigue, headache, blurred vision
vitamin K: phytonadione (AquaMEPHYTON)	PO/IM/subcutaneous; 2.5–10 mg (up to 25 mg), may be repeated after 6–8 h if needed	*Facial flushing, pain at injection site* IV route may result in dyspnea, hypotension, shock, cardiac arrest

Italics indicate common adverse effects; underlining indicates serious adverse effects.

Pr **Prototype Drug | Vitamin A** *(Aquasol A, others)*

Therapeutic Class: Lipid-soluble vitamin   **Pharmacologic Class:** Retinoid

ACTIONS AND USES

Vitamin A is essential for general growth and development, particularly of the bones, teeth, and epithelial membranes. It is necessary for proper wound healing, is essential for the biosynthesis of steroids, and is one of the pigments required for night vision. Vitamin A is indicated in deficiency states and during periods of increased need such as pregnancy, lactation, or undernutrition. Night blindness and slow wound healing can be effectively treated with as little as 30,000 units of vitamin A given daily over a week. It is also prescribed for GI disorders, when absorption in the small intestine is diminished or absent. Topical forms are available for acne, psoriasis, and other skin disorders. Doses of vitamin A are sometimes measured in retinoid equivalents (RE). In severe deficiency states, up to 500,000 units may be given per day for 3 days, gradually tapering off to 10,000–20,000 units/day.

ADMINISTRATION ALERTS

- Pregnancy category A at low doses
- Pregnancy category X at doses above the RDA

> **PHARMACOKINETICS**
> **Onset:** Unknown
> **Peak:** Unknown
> **Half-life:** Unknown
> **Duration:** Unknown

ADVERSE EFFECTS

Adverse effects are not observed with normal doses of vitamin A. Acute ingestion, however, produces serious CNS toxicity, including headache, irritability, drowsiness, delirium, and possible coma. Long-term ingestion of high amounts causes drying and scaling of the skin, alopecia, fatigue, anorexia, vomiting, and leukopenia.

Contraindications: Vitamin A in excess of the RDA is contraindicated in pregnant patients, or those who may become pregnant. Fetal harm may result.

INTERACTIONS

Drug–Drug: People taking vitamin A should avoid taking mineral oil and cholestyramine, because both may decrease the absorption of vitamin A. Concurrent use with isotretinoin may result in additive toxicity.

Lab Tests: Vitamin A may increase serum calcium and BUN.

Herbal/Food: Unknown

Treatment of Overdose: There is no specific treatment for overdose.

Refer to MyNursingKit for a Nursing Process Focus specific to this vitamin.

---

always supported these claims. In addition to oral and IM preparations, a topical form is available to treat dry, cracked skin.

Vitamin K is also a mixture of several chemicals. Vitamin K_1 is found in plant sources, particularly green leafy vegetables, tomatoes, and cauliflower; and in egg yolks, liver, and cheeses. Vitamin K_2 is synthesized by microbial flora in the colon. Deficiency states, caused by inadequate

intake or by antibiotic destruction of normal intestinal flora, may result in delayed hemostasis. The body does not have large stores of vitamin K, and a deficiency may occur in only 1 to 2 weeks. Blood clotting factors II, VII, IX, and X depend upon vitamin K for their biosynthesis. Vitamin K is used as a treatment for patients with clotting disorders and is the antidote for warfarin (Coumadin) overdose. It is also given to infants at birth to promote blood clotting. Administration of vitamin K completely reverses deficiency symptoms.

Water-Soluble Vitamins

The water-soluble vitamins consist of the B-complex vitamins and vitamin C. These vitamins must be consumed on a daily basis because they are not stored in the body.

42.6 Pharmacotherapy with Water-Soluble Vitamins

The B-complex group of vitamins is comprised of 12 different substances that are grouped together because they were originally derived from yeast and foods that counteracted the disease beriberi. They have very different chemical structures and serve various metabolic functions. The B vitamins are known by their chemical names as well as their vitamin number. For example, vitamin B_{12} is also called *cyanocobalamin*. Medications containing water-soluble vitamins, and their doses, are listed in Table 42.3.

TREATING THE DIVERSE PATIENT

Vitamin D and Diabetes Risk

Emerging studies and meta analyses have suggested a link between the development of Type I diabetes and vitamin D deficiency. Vitamin D deficiency has also been suggested as a potential factor in the development of other chronic conditions such as heart disease, high blood pressure, cancer, Type II diabetes, and autoimmune disorders. Multiple studies are being conducted to confirm these links in the general population and in special populations such as older adults and in different ethnic groups.

People with dark skin have greater amounts of the pigment melanin and have a reduced ability to produce vitamin D from sun exposure. In a study by the USDA Human Research Nutrition Center, African Americans were found to have the highest rates of vitamin D deficiency when compared with other Americans. And research by the American Diabetes Association has suggested that African Americans are almost two times more likely to have Type I diabetes than non-Latino whites. With strong evidence emerging that maintaining adequate amounts of vitamin D may prevent chronic illness, including Type I diabetes, vitamin D supplementation may be a low-cost, low-risk prevention option for Type I diabetes, especially in people with a high risk of developing the disease.

TABLE 42.3	**Water-Soluble Vitamins for Treating Nutritional Disorders**	
Drug	Route and Adult Dose (max dose where indicated)	Adverse Effects
vitamin B₁: thiamine	IV/IM; 50–100 mg tid PO; 5–30 mg/day	*Pain at injection site* <u>IV route may result in angioedema, cyanosis, pulmonary edema, GI bleeding, and cardiovascular collapse</u>
vitamin B₂: riboflavin	PO; 5–10 mg/day	*Adverse effects have not been reported*
vitamin B₃: niacin (Nicobid, Nicolar, others)	PO; 10–20 mg/day IV/IM/subcutaneous; 25–100 mg two to five times/day	*Adverse effects are uncommon at doses used for vitamin therapy* <u>High doses: dysrhythmias</u>
vitamin B₆: pyridoxine (Hexa-Betalin, Nestrex, others)	PO/IM/IV; 2.5–10 mg/day for 3 wk; then may reduce to 2.5–5 mg/day	*Pain at injection site* <u>High doses: neuropathy, ataxia, seizures</u>
⊕ vitamin B₉: folic acid (Folacin)	PO/IM/IV/subcutaneous; 0.4–1 mg/day	*Adverse effects are uncommon at recommended doses* <u>Parenteral routes: allergic hypersensitivity</u>
vitamin B₁₂: cyanocobalamin (Betalin 12, Cobex, Cynapin, others) (see page 400 for the Prototype Drug box ∞)	IM/deep subcutaneous; 30 mcg/day for 5–10 day; then 100–200 mcg/mo	*Rash, diarrhea* <u>High doses: thrombosis, hypokalemia, pulmonary edema, heart failure</u>
vitamin C: ascorbic acid (Ascorbicap, Cebid, Vita-C, others)	PO/IV/IM/subcutaneous; 150–500 mg/day in one to two doses	*Adverse effects are uncommon at recommended doses* <u>High doses: deep vein thrombosis (IV route), crystalluria</u>
Italics indicate common adverse effects; <u>underlining</u> indicates serious adverse effects.		

Vitamin B₁, or *thiamine,* is a precursor of an enzyme responsible for several steps in the oxidation of carbohydrates. It is abundant in both plant and animal products, especially whole-grain foods, dried beans, and peanuts. Because of the vitamin's abundance, thiamine deficiency in the United States is not common, except in alcoholics and in patients with chronic liver disease. Thiamine deficiency, or **beriberi,** is characterized by neurologic signs such as paresthesia, neuralgia, and progressive loss of feeling and reflexes. With pharmacotherapy, symptoms can be completely reversed in the early stages of the disease; however, permanent disability can result in patients with prolonged deficiency.

Vitamin B₂, or *riboflavin,* is a component of coenzymes that participate in a number of different oxidation–reduction reactions. Riboflavin is abundantly found in plant and meat products, including wheat germ, eggs, cheese, fish, nuts, and leafy vegetables. As with thiamine, deficiency of riboflavin is most commonly observed in alcoholics. Signs of deficiency include corneal vascularization and anemia, as well as skin abnormalities such as dermatitis and cheilosis. Most symptoms resolve by administering 25 to 100 mg/day of the vitamin until improvement is observed.

Vitamin B₃, or *niacin,* is a key component of coenzymes essential for oxidative metabolism. Niacin is synthesized from the amino acid tryptophan and is widely distributed in both animal and plant foodstuffs, including beans, wheat germ, meats, nuts, and whole-grain breads. Niacin deficiency, or **pellagra,** is most commonly seen in alcoholics, and in those areas of the world where corn is the primary food source. Early symptoms include fatigue, anorexia, and drying of the skin. Advanced symptoms include three classic signs: dermatitis, diarrhea, and dementia. Deficiency is treated with niacin at dosages ranging from 10 to 25 mg/day. When used to treat hyperlipidemia, niacin is given as nicotinic acid, and doses are much higher—up to 3 g/day (chapter 22∞).

COMPLEMENTARY AND ALTERNATIVE THERAPIES

Sea Vegetables

Sea vegetables, or seaweeds, are a form of marine algae that grow in the upper levels of the ocean, where sunlight can penetrate. Examples of these edible seaweeds include spirulina, kelp, chlorella, arame, and nori, many of which are used in Asian cooking. Sea vegetables are found in coastal locations throughout the world. Kelp, or Laminaria, is found in the cold waters of the North Atlantic and Pacific Oceans.

Sea vegetables contain a multitude of vitamins, as well as protein. Their most notable nutritional aspect, however, is their mineral content. Plants from the sea contain more minerals than most other food sources, including calcium, magnesium, phosphorous, iron, potassium, and all essential trace elements. Because they are so rich in minerals, seaweeds act as alkalizers for the blood, helping to rid the body of acid conditions (acidosis). Spirulina, kelp, and chlorella are available in capsule or tablet form, or as part of a "greens" mix containing other nutritional ingredients.

Pr **Prototype Drug** | Folic Acid *(Folacin)*

Therapeutic Class: Water-soluble vitamin   **Pharmacologic Class:** None

ACTIONS AND USES

Folic acid is administered to reverse symptoms of deficiency, which most commonly occurs in patients with inadequate intake, such as with chronic alcohol abuse. Because this vitamin is destroyed at high temperatures, people who overcook their food may experience folate deficiency. Pregnancy markedly increases the need for dietary folic acid; folic acid is given during pregnancy to promote normal fetal growth. Because insufficient vitamin B_{12} creates a lack of activated folic acid, deficiency symptoms resemble those of vitamin B_{12} deficiency. The megaloblastic anemia observed in folate-deficient patients, however, does not include the severe nervous system symptoms seen in patients with B_{12} deficiency. Administration of 1 mg/day of oral folic acid often reverses the deficiency symptoms within 5 to 7 days.

ADMINISTRATION ALERTS

- Pregnancy category A (category C when taken in doses above the RDA)

PHARMACOKINETICS
Onset: Unknown

Peak: 30–60 min

Half-life: Unknown

Duration: Unknown

ADVERSE EFFECTS

Adverse effects during folic acid therapy are uncommon. Patients may feel flushed following IV injections. Allergic hypersensitivity to folic acid by the IV route is possible.

Contraindications: Folic acid is contraindicated in anemias other than those caused by folate deficiency.

INTERACTIONS

Drug–Drug: Phenytoin, trimethoprim–sulfasoxazole, and other medications may interfere with the absorption of folic acid. Chloramphenicol may antagonize effects of folate therapy. Oral contraceptives, alcohol, barbiturates, methotrexate, and primidone may cause folate deficiency.

Lab Tests: Folic acid may decrease serum levels of vitamin B_{12}.

Herbal/Food: Unknown

Treatment of Overdose: There is no specific treatment for overdose.

HOME & COMMUNITY CONSIDERATIONS

Vitamin B_9 and Neural Tube Defects

It is now well documented that low vitamin B_9 (folic acid) levels in pregnant women may contribute to the formation of neural tube defects in the fetus. Women's health care providers are now suggesting that young women begin taking folic acid prior to attempting pregnancy. It has not been determined how long a woman must take folic acid prior to conception, but it is now being suggested that young women begin taking the supplement as soon as menstruation begins. To avoid possible overdoses, most health care providers recommend taking a daily multivitamin that contains folic acid.

Vitamin B_6, or *pyridoxine,* consists of several closely related compounds, including pyridoxine itself, pyridoxal, and pyridoxamine. Vitamin B_6 is essential for the synthesis of heme, and is a primary coenzyme involved in the metabolism of amino acids. Deficiency states can result from alcoholism, uremia, hypothyroidism, or heart failure. Certain drugs can also cause vitamin B_6 deficiency, including isoniazid (INH), cycloserine (Seromycin), hydralazine (Apresoline), oral contraceptives, and pyrazinamide (PZA). Patients receiving these drugs may routinely receive B_6 supplements. Deficiency symptoms include skin abnormalities, cheilosis, fatigue, and irritability. Symptoms reverse after administration of about 10 to 20 mg/day for several weeks.

Vitamin B_9, more commonly known as *folate* or *folic acid,* is metabolized to tetrahydrofolate, which is essential for normal DNA synthesis and for red blood cell production. Folic acid is widely distributed in plant products, especially green leafy vegetables and citrus fruits. This vitamin is highlighted as a drug prototype in this chapter.

Vitamin B_{12}, or *cyanocobalamin,* is a cobalt-containing vitamin that is a required coenzyme for a number of metabolic pathways. It also has important roles in cell replication, erythrocyte maturation, and myelin synthesis. Sources include lean meat, seafood, liver, and milk. Deficiency of vitamin B_{12} results in **pernicious (megaloblastic) anemia.** This vitamin is featured as a prototype drug in chapter 28 ∞.

Vitamin C, or *ascorbic acid,* is the most commonly purchased OTC vitamin. It is a potent antioxidant, and serves many functions including collagen synthesis, tissue healing, and maintenance of bone, teeth, and epithelial tissue. Many consumers purchase the vitamin for its ability to prevent the common cold, a function that has not been definitively proved. Deficiency of vitamin C, or **scurvy,** is caused by diets lacking fruits and vegetables. Alcoholics, cigarette smokers, cancer patients, and those with renal failure are at highest risk for vitamin C deficiency. Symptoms include fatigue, bleeding gums and other hemorrhages, gingivitis, and poor wound healing. Symptoms can normally be reversed by the administration of 300 to 1,000 mg/day of vitamin C for several weeks.

MINERALS

Minerals are inorganic substances needed in small amounts to maintain homeostasis. Minerals are classified as macrominerals or microminerals; the macrominerals must be ingested in larger amounts. A normal, balanced diet will

NURSING PROCESS FOCUS   PATIENTS RECEIVING VITAMIN AND MINERAL PHARMACOTHERAPY

Assessment	Potential Nursing Diagnoses
Baseline assessment prior to administration: ■ Understand the reason the drug has been prescribed in order to assess for therapeutic effects (e.g., replacement therapy for deficiencies, preventative health maintenance). ■ Obtain a complete health history including cardiovascular, neurologic, endocrine, hepatic, or renal disease. Obtain a drug history including allergies, current prescription and OTC drugs, and herbal preparations, alcohol use or smoking. Be alert to possible drug interactions. ■ Obtain a history of any current symptoms that may indicate vitamin deficiencies or hypervitaminosis (e.g., dry itchy skin, alopecia, sore and reddened gums or tongue, tendency to bleed easily or excessive bruising, nausea or vomiting, excessive fatigue). ■ Obtain a dietary history noting adequacy of essential vitamins, minerals, and nutrients obtained through food sources. ■ Note sunscreen use and the amount of sun exposure. ■ Obtain baseline weight and vital signs. ■ Evaluate appropriate laboratory findings (e.g., CBC, electrolytes, hepatic and renal function studies, ferritin and iron levels).	■ Imbalanced Nutrition: Less Than Body Requirements ■ Impaired Health Maintenance (related to dietary habits, deficient knowledge) ■ Readiness for Enhanced Therapeutic Regimen Management ■ Deficient Knowledge (drug therapy) ■ Risk for Injury (related to adverse drug effects, hypervitaminosis)
Assessment throughout administration: ■ Assess for desired therapeutic effects dependent on the reason for the drug (symptoms of deficiency are diminished or absent). ■ Continue monitoring of vital signs, and periodic lab values as appropriate. ■ Assess for and promptly report adverse effects: nausea, vomiting, excessive fatigue, tachycardia, palpitations, hypotension, constipation, drowsiness, dizziness, disorientation, hyper-reflexia, and electrolyte imbalances.	

Planning: Patient Goals and Expected Outcomes

The patient will:
■ Experience therapeutic effects (e.g., maintenance of overall health, symptoms of previous deficiency are absent).
■ Be free from, or experience minimal, adverse effects.
■ Verbalize an understanding of the drug's use, adverse effects, and required precautions.
■ Demonstrate proper self-administration of the medication (e.g., dose, timing, when to notify provider).

Implementation

Interventions and (Rationales)	Patient and Family Education
Ensuring therapeutic effects: ■ If a definitive cause of vitamin or mineral deficiency is identified, correct the deficiency using dietary sources of the nutrient where possible. (The dietary history can assist in determining the cause of the symptoms and the adequacy of the patient's current diet. Natural food sources provide additional nutrients, fiber, and essential requirements not found in vitamin and mineral supplementation.)	■ Review the dietary history with the patient and discuss food source options for correcting any deficiencies. Encourage the patient to adopt a healthy lifestyle of increased variety in the diet. Provide for dietitian consultation as needed. ■ Assist the patient and family or caregiver to become "educated consumers," aware of marketing of supplements that may not be required if the diet is adequate. Provide educational materials or web-based references to reputable sources as needed (e.g., NIH Office of Dietary Supplements at http://ods.od.nih.gov).
Minimizing adverse effects: ■ Review the dietary and supplement history to correct any existing possibility for hypervitaminosis and adverse drug effects. (Excessive intake of vitamins A, C, D, E, B_6, niacin, and folic acid may lead to toxic effects.)	■ Discuss the need for nutritional supplements if the normal diet is unable to supply these or if disease conditions (e.g., pernicious anemia) prevent absorption or utilization. ■ Discourage the overuse of supplementation and provide information on adverse effects and symptoms related to hypervitaminosis.

(Continued)

NURSING PROCESS FOCUS — **PATIENTS RECEIVING VITAMIN AND MINERAL PHARMACOTHERAPY** *(Continued)*

Implementation

Interventions and (Rationales)	Patient and Family Education
▪ Continue to monitor periodic lab work as needed. (Lab tests appropriate to condition [e.g., pernicious anemia and Hgb and Hct levels] will help to ensure therapeutic effects are met. With mineral replacement, electrolytes should return to normal levels.)	▪ Instruct the patient on the need to return periodically for lab work.
▪ Monitor the use of fat-soluble vitamins. Excessive intake may lead to toxic effects. (Fat-soluble vitamins are stored in the body and may accumulate and result in toxic levels. Monitor liver function studies and for symptoms such as nausea, vomiting, headache, fatigue, dry and itchy skin, blurred vision, or palpitations. Report any symptoms immediately.)	▪ Instruct the patient not to take large amounts of fat-soluble vitamins unless instructed by the health care provider. ▪ Encourage obtaining fat-soluble vitamins from natural sources such as: ▪ Vitamin A: carrots, pumpkin, winter squash, dark green leafy vegetables, apricots, meats, fish, and liver. ▪ Vitamin D: milk and other dairy products fortified with vitamin D, oily fish (e.g., salmon, sardines), adequate sun exposure. ▪ Vitamin E: vegetable oils and margarines made from vegetable oils, fruits and vegetables, grains, nuts, seeds, and fortified cereals. ▪ Vitamin K: green vegetables such as turnip greens, spinach, cauliflower, cabbage and broccoli, and certain vegetable oils including soybean oil, cottonseed oil, canola oil, and olive oil.
▪ Assess for pregnancy. Assess storage availability for any prenatal vitamins kept in the house. (Folic acid supplementation reduces the incidence of neurologic birth defects. Excessive vitamin intake may have deleterious effects on the developing fetus and prenatal vitamin use should be monitored. Poisonings with vitamins and iron are common in children.)	▪ Teach women of child-bearing age about folic acid and its usefulness in preventing neurologic-related birth defects. Encourage the adequate intake of vitamin and folic acid–rich foods *prior* to conception. ▪ Instruct the patient to keep prenatal vitamins in a secure location if young children are in the household to prevent accidental poisoning.
▪ Ensure adequate hydration if large doses of water-soluble vitamins are taken. (Water-soluble vitamins are not stored in the body but are excreted. Large doses of vitamin C may cause renal calculi.)	▪ Encourage the patient to increase fluid intake to 2 L of fluid per day, divided throughout the day.
Patient understanding of drug therapy: ▪ Use opportunities during administration of medications and during assessments to discuss the rationale for drug therapy, desired therapeutic outcomes, most common adverse effects, parameters for when to call the health care provider, and any necessary monitoring or precautions. (Using time during nursing care helps to optimize and reinforce key teaching areas.)	▪ The patient should be able to state the reason for the drug; appropriate dose and scheduling; what adverse effects to observe for and when to report; and the anticipated length of medication therapy.
Patient self-administration of drug therapy: ▪ When administering the medication, instruct the patient, family, or caregiver in the proper self-administration of the drug, e.g., taken with additional fluids. (Proper administration will increase the effectiveness of the drug.)	▪ The patient is able to discuss appropriate dosing and administration needs.

Evaluation of Outcome Criteria

Evaluate the effectiveness of drug therapy by confirming that patient goals and expected outcomes have been met (see "Planning").

See Tables 42.1, 42.2, 42.3, & 42.4 for a list of drugs to which these nursing actions apply.

provide the proper amounts of the required minerals in most people. The primary minerals used in pharmacotherapy are listed in Table 42.4.

42.7 Pharmacotherapy with Minerals

Minerals are essential substances that constitute about 4% of the body weight and serve many diverse functions. Some are essential ions or electrolytes in body fluids; others are bound to organic molecules such as hemoglobin, phospholipids, or metabolic enzymes. Those minerals that function as critical electrolytes in the body, most notably sodium and potassium, are covered in more detail in chapter 31∞. Sodium chloride and potassium chloride are featured as drug prototypes in that chapter.

Because minerals are needed in very small amounts for human metabolism, a balanced diet will supply the necessary quantities for most patients. As with vitamins, patients should be advised not to exceed recommended doses because excess

TABLE 42.4	Selected Minerals for Treating Nutritional and Electrolyte Disorders	
Drug	**Route and Adult Dose (max dose where indicated)**	**Adverse Effects**
potassium chloride (K-Dur, Micro-K, Klor-Con, others) (see page 439 for the Prototype Drug box ∞)	PO; 10–100 mEq/h in divided doses IV; 10–40 mEq/h diluted to at least 10–20 mEq/100 mL of solution (max: 200–400 mEq/day)	*Nausea, vomiting, diarrhea, abdominal cramping* <u>Hyperkalemia, hypotension, confusion, dysrhythmias</u>
sodium bicarbonate (see page 441 for the Prototype Drug box ∞)	PO; 0.3–2.0 g/day–qid or 1 tsp of powder in a glass of water	*Headache, weakness, belching, flatulence* <u>Hypernatremia, hypertension, muscle twitching, dysrhythmias, pulmonary edema, peripheral edema</u>
CALCIUM SALTS		
calcium acetate (PhosLo) calcium carbonate (Rolaids, Tums, OsCal, others) calcium chloride calcium citrate (Citracal) calcium gluconate (Kalcinate) calcium lactate (Cal-Lac) calcium phosphate tribasic (Posture)	PO; 2–4 tablets with each meal (each tablet contains 169 mg) PO; 1–2 g bid–tid IV; 0.5–1.0 g/q3days PO; 1–2 g bid–tid PO; 1–2 g bid–qid PO; 325 mg–1.3 g tid with meals PO; 1–2 g bid–tid	*Parenteral route: flushing, nausea, vomiting, pain at injection site* *Oral route: abdominal pain, loss of appetite, nausea, vomiting, constipation, dry mouth, increased thirst/urination.* <u>Hypercalcemia, hypotension, constipation, fatigue, anorexia, confusion, dysrhythmias</u>
IRON SALTS		
ferrous fumarate (Feostat, others) ferrous gluconate (Fergon, others) ferrous sulfate (Feosol, others) (see page 401 for the Prototype Drug box ∞) iron dextran (Dexferrum, others)	PO; 200 mg tid–qid PO; 325–600 mg qid; may be gradually increased to 650 mg qid as needed and tolerated PO; 750–1,500 mg/day in single dose or two to three divided doses IM/IV; dose is individualized and determined from a table of correlations between patient's weight and hemoglobin (max: 100 mg (2 mL) of iron dextran within 24 h)	*Nausea, constipation or diarrhea, abdominal pain, leg cramps (iron sucrose)* <u>Anaphylaxis (iron dextran), hypovolemia, hematemesis, hepatotoxicity, metabolic acidosis</u>
MAGNESIUM		
magnesium chloride (Chloromag, Slo-Mag) magnesium hydroxide (Milk of Magnesia) magnesium oxide (Mag-Ox, Maox, others) Pr magnesium sulfate (Epsom salts)	PO; 270–400 mg/day PO; 5–15 mL or 2–4 tablets up to four times/day PO; 400–1,200 mg/day in divided doses IV/IM; 0.5–3.0 g/day	*Nausea, vomiting, diarrhea, flushing* <u>Cardiotoxicity, respiratory failure, hypotension, deep tendon reflex reduction, facial paresthesias, weakness</u>
PHOSPHORUS/PHOSPHATE		
potassium/sodium phosphates (K-Phos original, K-Phos MF, K-Phos neutral, Neutra-Phos-K, Uro-KP neutral)	PO; 250–1,000 mg /day	*Nausea, vomiting, diarrhea* <u>Hyperphosphatemia, bone pain, fractures, muscle weakness, confusion</u>
ZINC		
zinc acetate (Galzin) zinc gluconate zinc sulfate (Orazinc, Zincate, others)	PO; 50 mg tid PO; 20–100 mg (20 mg lozenges may be taken to a max of six lozenges/day) PO; 15–220 mg/day	*Adverse effects are uncommon at recommended doses* <u>High doses: nausea, vomiting, fever, immunosuppression, anemia</u>

Italics indicate common adverse effects; <u>underlining</u> indicates serious adverse effects.

amounts of minerals can lead to toxicity. Mineral supplements are, however, indicated for certain disorders. Iron-deficiency anemia is the most common nutritional deficiency in the world and is a common indication for iron supplements.

Women at high risk for osteoporosis are advised to consume extra calcium, either in their diet or as a dietary supplement.

Certain drugs affect normal mineral metabolism. For example, loop or thiazide diuretics can cause significant urinary potassium loss. Corticosteroids and oral contraceptives are among several classes of drugs that can promote sodium retention. The uptake of iodine by the thyroid gland can be impaired by certain oral hypoglycemics and lithium carbonate (Eskalith). Oral contraceptives have been reported to lower the plasma levels of zinc and to increase those of copper. The nurse must be aware of drug-related mineral interactions, and recommend changes to mineral intake when appropriate.

42.8 Pharmacotherapy with Macrominerals

Macrominerals (major minerals) are inorganic substances that must be consumed daily in amounts of 100 mg or higher. The macrominerals include calcium, chlorine, magnesium, phosphorus, potassium, sodium, and sulfur. Approximately 75% of the total mineral content in the body consists of calcium and phosphorus salts in bony matrix. Recommended daily allowances have been established for each of the macrominerals except sulfur, as listed in Table 42.5.

Calcium is essential for nerve conduction, muscular contraction, construction of bony matrix, and hemostasis. Hypocalcemia occurs when serum calcium falls below 4.5 mEq/L and may be caused by inadequate intake of calcium-containing foods, lack of vitamin D, chronic diarrhea, or decreased secretion of parathyroid hormone. Symptoms of hypocalcemia involve the nervous and muscular systems. The patient often becomes irritable and restless, and muscular twitches, cramps, spasms, and cardiac abnormalities are common. Prolonged hypocalcemia may lead to fractures. Pharmacotherapy includes calcium compounds, which are available in many oral salts such as calcium carbonate, calcium citrate, calcium gluconate, or calcium lactate. In severe cases, IV preparations are administered. Calcium gluconate is featured as a prototype drug for hypocalcemia and osteoporosis in chapter 47∞.

Phosphorus is an essential mineral, 85% of which is bound to calcium in the form of calcium phosphate in bones. In addition to playing a role in bone structure, phosphorus is a component of proteins, adenosine triphosphate (ATP), and nucleic acids. Phosphate (PO_4^{3-}) is an important buffer in the blood. Because phosphorus is a primary component of phosphate, phosphorus balance is normally considered the same as phosphate balance. Hypophosphatemia is most often observed in patients with serious medical illnesses, especially those with kidney disorders that cause excess phosphorus loss in the urine. Because of its abundance in food, the patient must be suffering from severe malnutrition or an intestinal malabsorption disorder to experience a dietary deficiency. Symptoms of hypophosphatemia include weakness, muscle tremor, anorexia, weak pulse, and bleeding abnormalities. When serum phosphorus levels fall below 1.5 mEq/L, phosphate supplements are usually administered. Sodium phosphate and potassium phosphate are available for treating phosphorus deficiencies.

Magnesium is the second most abundant intracellular cation and, like potassium, it is essential for proper neuromuscular function. Magnesium also serves a metabolic role in activating certain enzymes in the breakdown of carbohydrates and proteins. Because it produces few symptoms until serum levels fall below 1.0 mEq/L, hypomagnesemia is sometimes called the most common undiagnosed electrolyte abnormality. Patients may experience general weakness, dysrhythmias, hypertension, loss of deep tendon reflexes, and respiratory depression—signs and symptoms that are sometimes mistaken for hypokalemia. Pharmacotherapy with magnesium sulfate can quickly reverse the symptoms of hypomagnesemia. Magnesium sulfate is a CNS depressant and is sometimes given to prevent or terminate seizures associated with eclampsia. Magnesium salts have additional applications as cathartics or antacids (magnesium citrate, magnesium hydroxide, and magnesium oxide) and as analgesics (magnesium salicylate).

42.9 Pharmacotherapy with Microminerals

The nine **microminerals**, commonly called **trace minerals**, are required daily in amounts of 20 mg or less. The fact that they are needed in such small amounts does not diminish their key role in human health; deficiencies in some of the trace minerals can result in profound illness. The functions of some of the trace minerals, such as iron and iodine, are well

TABLE 42.5	Macrominerals	
Mineral	RDA	Function
calcium	800–1,200 mg	Forms bony matrix; regulates nerve conduction and muscle contraction
chloride	750 mg	Major anion in body fluids; part of gastric acid (HCl)
magnesium	Men: 350–400 mg Women: 280–300 mg	Cofactor for many enzymes; necessary for normal nerve conduction and muscle contraction
phosphorus	700 mg	Forms bony matrix; part of ATP and nucleic acids
potassium	2.0 g	Necessary for normal nerve conduction and muscle contraction; principal cation in intracellular fluid; essential for acid–base and electrolyte balance
sodium	500 mg	Necessary for normal nerve conduction and muscle contraction; principal cation in extracellular fluid; essential for acid–base and electrolyte balance
sulfur	not established	Component of proteins, B vitamins, and other critical molecules

Pr Prototype Drug | Magnesium Sulfate (MgSO₄)

Therapeutic Class: Magnesium supplement   **Pharmacologic Class:** Electrolyte

ACTIONS AND USES

Severe hypomagnesemia can be rapidly reversed by the administration of IM or IV magnesium sulfate. Parenteral formulations include 4%, 8%, 12.5%, and 50% solutions. Hypomagnesemia has a number of causes, including the loss of body fluids due to diarrhea, diuretic therapy, or nasogastric suctioning; and prolonged parenteral feeding with magnesium-free solutions.

After administration, magnesium sulfate is distributed throughout the body, and therapeutic effects are observed within 30–60 minutes. Oral forms of magnesium sulfate are used as cathartics, when complete evacuation of the colon is desired. Its action as a CNS depressant has led to its occasional use as an anticonvulsant.

ADMINISTRATION ALERTS

- Continuously monitor the patient during IV infusion for early signs of decreased cardiac function.
- Monitor serum magnesium levels every 6 h during parenteral infusion.
- When giving IV infusion, give required dose over 4 h.
- Pregnancy category A

PHARMACOKINETICS
Onset: 1–2 h PO; 1 h IM
Peak: Unknown
Half-life: Unknown
Duration: 3–4 h PO; 30 min IV

ADVERSE EFFECTS

Patients receiving IV infusions of magnesium sulfate require careful observation to prevent toxicity. Early signs of magnesium overdose include flushing of the skin, sedation, confusion, intense thirst, and muscle weakness. Extreme levels cause neuromuscular blockade with resultant respiratory paralysis, heart block, and circulatory collapse. Plasma magnesium levels should be monitored frequently. Because of these potentially fatal adverse effects, the use of magnesium sulfate is restricted to severe magnesium deficiency: Mild-to-moderate hypomagnesemia is treated with oral forms of magnesium such as magnesium gluconate or magnesium hydroxide.

Contraindications: Magnesium is contraindicated in patients with serious cardiac disease. Oral administration is contraindicated in patients with undiagnosed abdominal pain, intestinal obstruction, or fecal impaction. The drug should be used cautiously in patients with renal impairment because the drug may rapidly rise to toxic levels.

INTERACTIONS

Drug–Drug: Use with neuromuscular blockers may increase respiratory depression and apnea. Concurrent use of magnesium with alcohol or other CNS depressants may lead to increased sedation. Magnesium salts may decrease the absorption of certain anti-infectives such as tetracycline.

Lab Tests: Unknown

Herbal/Food: Magnesium salts may decrease the absorption of certain anti-infectives such as tetracycline.

Treatment of Overdose: Serious respiratory and cardiac suppression may result from overdose. Calcium gluconate or gluceptate may be administered IV as an antidote.

Refer to MyNursingKit for a Nursing Process Focus specific to this mineral.

TABLE 42.6	Microminerals	
Trace Mineral	**RDA**	**Function**
chromium	0.05–2.0 mg	Potentiates insulin and is necessary for proper glucose metabolism
cobalt	0.1 mcg	Cofactor for vitamin B₁₂ and several oxidative enzymes
copper	1.5–3.0 mg	Cofactor for hemoglobin synthesis
fluorine	1.5–4.0 mg	Influences tooth structure and possibly affects growth
iodine	150 mcg	Component of thyroid hormone
iron	Men: 10–12 mg Women: 10–15 mg	Component of hemoglobin and some enzymes of oxidative phosphorylation
manganese	2–5 mg	Cofactor in some enzymes of lipid, carbohydrate, and protein metabolism
molybdenum	75–250 mg	Cofactor for certain enzymes
selenium	Men: 50–70 mcg Women: 50–55 mcg	Antioxidant cofactor for certain enzymes
zinc	12–15 mg	Cofactor for certain enzymes, including carbonic anhydrase; needed for proper protein structure, normal growth, and wound healing

established; the role of others are less completely understood. The RDA for each of the microminerals is listed in Table 42.6.

Iron is an essential micromineral that is most closely associated with hemoglobin. Excellent sources of dietary iron include meat, shellfish, nuts, and legumes. Excess iron in the body results in hemochromatosis, whereas lack of iron re-sults in iron-deficiency anemia. The pharmacology of iron supplements is presented in chapter 28∞, where ferrous sulfate is featured as a drug prototype for anemia.

Iodine is a trace mineral needed to synthesize thyroid hormone. The most common source of dietary iodine is iodized salt. When dietary intake of iodine is low, hypothyroidism occurs and enlargement of the thyroid gland (goiter) results. At high concentrations, iodine suppresses thyroid function. *Lugol's solution*, a mixture containing 5% elemental iodine and 10% potassium iodide, is given to hyperthyroid patients prior to thyroidectomy or during a thyrotoxic crisis. Sodium iodide acts by rapidly suppressing the secretion of thyroid hormone and is indicated for patients having an acute thyroid crisis. Radioactive iodine (I-131) is given to destroy overactive thyroid glands. Pharmacotherapeutic uses of iodine as a drug extend beyond the treatment of thyroid disease. Iodine is an effective topical antiseptic that can be found in creams, tinctures, and solutions. Iodine salts such as iothalamate and diatrizoate are very dense and serve as diagnostic contrast agents in radiologic procedures of the urinary and cardiovascular systems. The role of potassium iodide in protecting the thyroid gland during acute radiation exposure is discussed in chapter 3 ∞.

Fluorine is a trace mineral found abundantly in nature and is best known for its beneficial effects on bones and teeth. Research has validated that adding fluoride to the water supply in very small amounts (1 part per billion) can reduce the incidence of dental caries. This effect is more pronounced in children, because fluoride is incorporated into the enamel of growing teeth. Concentrated fluoride solutions can also be applied to the teeth topically by dental professionals. Sodium fluoride and stannous fluoride are components of most toothpastes and oral rinses. Because high amounts of fluoride can be quite toxic, the use of fluoride-containing products should be closely monitored in children.

Zinc is a component of at least 100 enzymes, including alcohol dehydrogenase, carbonic anhydrase, and alkaline phosphatase. This trace mineral has a regulatory function in enzymes controlling nucleic acid synthesis and is believed to have roles in wound healing, male fertility, bone formation, and cell-mediated immunity. Because symptoms of zinc deficiency are often nonspecific, diagnosis is usually confirmed by a serum zinc level of less than 70 mcg/dL. Zinc sulfate, zinc acetate, and zinc gluconate are available to prevent and treat deficiency states, at doses of 60 to 120 mg/day. In addition, lozenges containing zinc are available OTC for treating sore throats and symptoms of the common cold.

NUTRITIONAL SUPPLEMENTS

The nurse will encounter many patients who are undernourished. Major goals in resolving nutritional deficiencies are to identify the specific type of deficiency and supply the missing nutrients. Nutritional supplements may be needed for short-term therapy or for the remainder of a patient's life.

42.10 Etiology of Undernutrition

Undernutrition is the ingestion or absorption of fewer nutrients than required for normal body growth and maintenance. Successful pharmacotherapy of this condition relies on the skills of the nurse in identifying the symptoms and causes of the patient's undernutrition.

Causes of undernutrition range from the simple to the complex, and include the following:

- Advanced age
- HIV-AIDS
- Alcoholism
- Burns
- Cancer
- Chronic inflammatory bowel disease (IBD)
- Eating disorders
- GI disorders
- Chronic neurologic disease such as progressive dysphagia and multiple sclerosis
- Surgery
- Trauma

The most obvious cause for undernutrition is low dietary intake, although reasons for the inadequate intake must be assessed. Patients may have no resources to purchase food and may be suffering from starvation. Clinical depression leads many patients to shun food. Older adult patients may have poorly fitting dentures or difficulty chewing or swallowing after a stroke. In terminal disease, patients may be comatose or otherwise unable to take food orally. Although the etiologies differ, patients with insufficient intake exhibit a similar pattern of general weakness, muscle wasting, and loss of subcutaneous fat.

When the undernutrition is caused by lack of one specific nutrient, vitamin, or mineral, the disorder is more difficult to diagnose. Patients may be on a fad diet lacking only protein or fat in their intake. Certain digestive disorders may lead to malabsorption of specific nutrients or vitamins. Patients may simply avoid certain foods such as green leafy vegetables, dairy products, or meat products, which can lead to specific nutritional deficiencies. Proper pharmacotherapy requires the expert knowledge and assessment skills of the nurse, and sometimes a nutritional consult, so that the correct treatment can be administered.

42.11 Enteral Nutrition

Numerous nutritional supplements are available, and a common method of classifying these agents is by their *route of administration*. Products that are administered via the GI tract, either orally or through a feeding tube, are classified as **enteral nutrition**. Those that are administered by means of IV infusion are called **parenteral nutrition**.

When the patient's condition permits, enteral nutrition is best provided by oral consumption. Oral feeding allows natural digestive processes to occur and requires less intense nursing care. It does, however, rely on patient cooperation, because it is not feasible for the health care provider to observe the patient at every meal.

Tube feeding, or enteral tube alimentation, is necessary when the patient has difficulty swallowing or is otherwise unable to take meals orally. An advantage of tube feeding is that the amount of enteral nutrition the patient receives can be precisely measured and recorded. Various tube feeding routes are possible, including nasogastric (nose to stomach), nasoduodenal (nose to duodenum), nasojejunal (nose to jejunum), gastrostomy, or jejunostomy (tube is placed directly into the stomach or jejunum, respectively, through a surgical incision). A nasogastric tube may be inserted by a registered nurse or licensed practical nurse. The nasoduodenal and nasojejunal tubes are usually inserted by a radiologist or other physician. The gastrostomy and jejunostomy tubes are placed by a surgeon or a gastroenterologist.

The particular enteral product is chosen to address the specific nutritional needs of the patient. Because of the wide diversity in their formulas, it is difficult to categorize enteral products, and several different methods are used. A simple method is to classify enteral products as oligomeric, polymeric, modular, or specialized formulations.

- *Oligomeric formulas* contain basic forms of free amino acids and peptide combinations that require little or no digestion, and are easily absorbed into the body. They are usually low in fat, which allows for rapid gastric emptying, and many of these preparations are designed for administration directly into the intestines. Indications include partial bowel obstruction, irritable bowel syndrome, radiation enteritis, bowel fistulas, and short-bowel syndrome. Sample products include Vivonex T.E.N., and Peptamen Liquid.

- *Polymeric* formulas are the most common enteral preparations. These products contain various mixtures of proteins, carbohydrates, and lipids. These formulas are used in patients who are generally undernourished, but have a fully functioning GI tract. Sample products include Compleat regular, Sustacal Powder, and Ensure-Plus.

- *Modular* formulas contain a single nutrient, protein, lipid, or carbohydrate. While not designed to serve as a sole source of nutrition, they can be added to other products to meet a specific nutrient deficiency. For example, protein modules can be utilized to meet the extra nitrogen needs of patients with burns or severe trauma. Sample products include Casec, Polycose, Microlipid, and MCT Oil.

- *Specialized* formulations are products that contain a specific nutrient combination for a particular condition. Indications include a specific disease state such as hepatic failure, renal failure, or a specific genetic enzyme deficiency. Sample products include Amin-Aid, Hepatic-Aid II, and Pulmocare.

42.12 Total Parenteral Nutrition

When a patient's metabolic needs are unable to be met through enteral nutrition, **total parenteral nutrition (TPN)**, or hyperalimentation, is indicated. For short-term therapy, peripheral vein TPN may be used. Because of the risk of phlebitis, however, long-term therapy often requires central vein TPN. Patients who have undergone major surgery or trauma and those who are severely undernourished are candidates for central vein TPN. Because the GI tract is not being utilized, patients with severe malabsorption disease may be treated successfully with TPN.

TPN is able to provide all of a patient's nutritional needs in a hypertonic solution containing amino acids, lipid emulsions, carbohydrates (as dextrose), electrolytes, vitamins, and minerals. The particular formulation may be specific to the disease state, such as renal failure or hepatic failure. TPN should be administered through an infusion pump, so that nutrition delivery can be precisely monitored. Patients in various settings such as acute care, long-term care, and home health care often benefit from TPN therapy.

NURSING PROCESS FOCUS	PATIENTS RECEIVING ENTERAL AND PARENTERAL NUTRITION
Assessment	**Potential Nursing Diagnoses**
Baseline assessment prior to administration: - Understand the reason the drug has been prescribed in order to assess for therapeutic effects (e.g., short- or long-term therapy, underlying health disorders). - Obtain a complete health history including cardiovascular, neurologic, endocrine, hepatic, or renal disease. Obtain a drug history including allergies, current prescription and OTC drugs, herbal preparations, alcohol use, or smoking. Be alert to possible drug interactions. - Obtain a dietary history noting the ability to eat and take adequate fluids. - Obtain baseline height, weight, and vital signs. - Evaluate appropriate laboratory findings (e.g., CBC, electrolytes, glucose, BUN, hepatic and renal function studies, total protein, serum albumin, lipid profile, serum iron levels).	- Imbalanced Nutrition: Less Than Body Requirements - Deficient Knowledge (drug therapy) - Risk for Imbalanced Fluid Volume - Risk for Infection

(Continued)

NURSING PROCESS FOCUS **PATIENTS RECEIVING ENTERAL AND PARENTERAL NUTRITION** *(Continued)*

Assessment	Potential Nursing Diagnoses
Assessment throughout administration: ■ Assess for desired therapeutic effects dependent on the reason for the drug (e.g., weight is maintained, electrolytes, glucose, proteins, lipid levels remain within normal limits). ■ Continue monitoring of vital signs, and periodic lab values as appropriate. ■ Weigh daily at the same time each day and record. ■ Assess for and promptly report adverse effects: fever, nausea, vomiting, tachycardia, palpitations, hypotension, dyspnea, drowsiness, dizziness, disorientation, hypo- or hyperglycemia, and electrolyte imbalances.	

Planning: Patient Goals and Expected Outcomes

The patient will:
■ Experience therapeutic effects (e.g., maintenance or improvement of overall health and nutritional status).
■ Be free from, or experience minimal, adverse effects.
■ Verbalize an understanding of the drug's use, adverse effects, and required precautions.
■ Demonstrate proper self-administration of the medication (e.g., dose, timing, when to notify provider).

Implementation

Interventions and (Rationales)	Patient and Family Education
Ensuring therapeutic effects: ■ Assess the patient's ability to take oral nutrition and encourage small oral feedings if allowed. (Supplementation with oral feedings may be allowed if enteral or parenteral nutrition will be used short term. Encouraging small amounts of oral intake will maintain normal salivation and ADLs during the time of replacement nutrition.)	■ If allowed, encourage the patient to maintain small, frequent oral intake or have a caregiver assist with oral nutrition and hydration.
Minimizing adverse effects: ■ Monitor vital signs, particularly temperature, throughout nutrition replacement. Assess all access sites (e.g., gastric tube site, IV or port sites) frequently for redness, streaking, swelling, or drainage. Report any fever, chills, malaise, or changes in mental status immediately. (Enteral and parenteral nutritional replacement contains high glucose, protein, and lipid sources that may serve as a reservoir for infection. Access sites may also serve as a point-of-entry for infection.)	■ Instruct the patient, family, or caregiver to immediately report any fever, chills, unusual changes to the access site, or changes in the level of consciousness to the health care provider.
■ Use strict aseptic technique with all IV tubing or bag changes, and site dressing changes. Refrigerate the TPN solution until 30 minutes before using and store extra enteral formula in the refrigerator after opening. (Infusion and access sites are at high risk for development of infection and must be monitored frequently. Solutions and extra formula must be refrigerated to inhibit bacterial growth.)	■ Explain the rationale for all dressing and equipment monitoring and changes. ■ Teach appropriate technique (aseptic or clean) to the family or caregiver if nutrition is to be continued at home, followed by return demonstration until the family is comfortable with the routine.
■ Monitor blood glucose levels. Observe for signs of hyperglycemia or hypoglycemia and obtain capillary glucose levels as ordered. (Blood glucose levels may be affected if TPN or enteral feeding is stopped, the rate is reduced, or is dependent on other medications the patient is taking. Supplemental insulin, subcutaneously or added to the IV solution, may be required.)	■ Instruct the patient on the need for frequent glucose monitoring. Teach the patient, family, or caregiver to report signs of hyperglycemia (excessive thirst, copious urination, and insatiable hunger) or hypoglycemia (nervousness, irritability, and dizziness) promptly. ■ Instruct the patient, family, or caregiver in the technique to monitor capillary glucose, followed by return-demonstration, if the patient will be on nutrition replacement at home.
■ Monitor for signs of fluid overload. (TPN is a hypertonic solution and can create intravascular shifting of extracellular fluid with resulting increase in intravascular fluid. Monitoring for increased pulse rate and quality, increasing blood pressure, dyspnea, or edema will assist in quickly noting adverse effects.)	■ Instruct the patient, family, or caregiver to immediately report shortness of breath, heart palpitations, swelling, decreased urine output, disorientation, or confusion.

NURSING PROCESS FOCUS   PATIENTS RECEIVING ENTERAL AND PARENTERAL NUTRITION *(Continued)*

Implementation

Interventions and (Rationales)	Patient and Family Education
■ Monitor renal status. (Intake and output ratio, daily weight, and laboratory studies such as serum creatinine and BUN should be monitored.)	■ Instruct the patient on home therapy to weigh self daily at the same time each day and record. An increase or loss in weight of over 1 kg per 24 hours should be reported to the health care provider. Report any edema or dyspnea immediately.
■ Maintain accurate enteral feeding or TPN infusion rate with infusion pump; make rate changes gradually; and avoid abruptly discontinuing TPN feeding. (The use of infusion pumps allows precise control over enteral feeding rate or TPN infusion. Abrupt discontinuation may cause hypoglycemia, and a sudden change in parenteral flow rate can cause fluctuations in blood glucose levels.)	■ Teach the patient about the rationale for all equipment used and the need for frequent monitoring. If using home equipment, ensure the proper functioning of equipment and the proper use by the patient, family, or caregiver.
■ Assess for appropriate enteral tube placement before administering any feeding. (Proper tube insertion should be confirmed radiographically before any feeding is initiated. Confirmation of placement by observing the characteristics of the gastric aspirate or pH may be used to confirm placement.)	■ Explain the rationale for checking tube placement prior to each feeding to the patient, family, or caregiver. If home enteral therapy is ordered, teach the patient, family, or caregiver the appropriate methods for checking placement prior to feeding.
Patient understanding of drug therapy: ■ Use opportunities during administration of medications and during assessments to discuss the rationale for drug therapy, desired therapeutic outcomes, most common adverse effects, parameters for when to call the health care provider, and any necessary monitoring or precautions. (Using time during nursing care helps to optimize and reinforce key teaching areas.)	■ The patient, family, or caregiver should be able to state the reason for the drug; appropriate dose and scheduling; what adverse effects to observe for and when to report; and the anticipated length of medication therapy.
Patient self-administration of drug therapy: ■ When administering the medication, instruct the patient, family, or caregiver in the proper self-administration of the drug, e.g., taken with additional fluids. (Proper administration can improve the effectiveness of the drugs.)	■ The patient and family or caregiver are able to discuss appropriate dosing and administration needs. ■ The patient, family, or caregiver is able to return-demonstrate appropriate dosing, and administration and care of access sites and tubes prior to home use.

Evaluation of Outcome Criteria

Evaluate the effectiveness of drug therapy by confirming that patient goals and expected outcomes have been met (see "Planning").

Chapter REVIEW

KEY CONCEPTS

The numbered key concepts provide a succinct summary of the important points from the corresponding numbered section within the chapter. If any of these points are not clear, refer to the numbered section within the chapter for review.

42.1   Vitamins are organic substances needed in small amounts to promote growth and maintain health. Deficiency of a vitamin will result in disease.

42.2   Vitamins are classified as lipid soluble (A, D, E, and K) or water soluble (C and B complex). Excess quantities of lipid-soluble vitamins are stored in the liver and adipose tissue.

42.3   Failure to meet the Recommended Dietary Allowances (RDAs) for vitamins may result in deficiency disorders. The RDA is the amount of a vitamin needed to prevent symptoms of deficiency.

42.4   Vitamin therapy is indicated for conditions such as poor nutritional intake, pregnancy, and chronic disease states. Symptoms of deficiency are usually nonspecific and occur over a prolonged period.

42.5   Deficiencies of vitamins A, D, E, or K are indications for pharmacotherapy with lipid-soluble vitamins.

42.6   Deficiencies of vitamins C, thiamine, niacin, riboflavin, folic acid, cyanocobalamin, or pyridoxine are indications for pharmacotherapy with water-soluble vitamins.

42.7 Minerals are inorganic substances needed in very small amounts to maintain normal body metabolism.

42.8 Pharmacotherapy with macrominerals includes agents containing calcium, magnesium, potassium, or phosphorus.

42.9 Pharmacotherapy with microminerals includes agents containing iron, iodine, fluorine, or zinc.

42.10 Undernutrition may be caused by low dietary intake, malabsorption disorders, fad diets, or wasting disorders such as cancer or AIDS.

42.11 Enteral nutrition, provided orally or through a feeding tube, is a means of meeting a patient's complete nutritional needs.

42.12 Total parenteral nutrition (TPN) is a means of supplying nutrition to patients via a peripheral vein (short term) or central vein (long term).

NCLEX-RN® REVIEW QUESTIONS

1 An older adult has been diagnosed with pernicious anemia and replacement therapy is ordered. The nurse will anticipate administering which vitamin, and by what technique?
1. B_6, orally in liquid form
2. K, via intramuscular injection
3. D, by light-box therapy or increased sun exposure
4. B_{12}, by intramuscular injection

2 The nurse is preparing to administer magnesium sulfate intravenously. The nurse should assess for which of the following adverse affects? (Select all that apply.)
1. Decreased liver function
2. Respiratory failure
3. Complete heart block
4. Circulatory collapse
5. Increase in peripheral edema

3 The nurse is assessing a patient who is exhibiting generalized weakness, cardiac dysrhythmias, hypertension, loss of deep tendon reflexes, and respiratory distress. What could be the possible cause of these symptoms?
1. Hypocalcemia
2. Hypercalcemia
3. Hypomagnesemia
4. Hypermagnesemia

4 The patient is a long-time alcoholic. The nurse understands that alcoholism is the most common cause of which vitamin deficiency?
1. Vitamin E
2. Vitamin A
3. Vitamin D
4. Thiamine

5 The patient is a 12-year-old child with hemophilia. The nurse is aware that this patient will require administration of which vitamin to improve the function of clotting factors?
1. Folic acid
2. Riboflavin
3. Vitamin K
4. Vitamin A

6 Total parenteral nutrition (TPN) has been ordered for a patient with gastric cancer who is no longer able to maintain oral intake. The nurse notes that the patient has a temperature of 100.4° F. What should the nurse assess *first*?
1. The date the TPN was ordered
2. The patient's last electrolyte levels, particularly glucose
3. The intravenous access site and all IV equipment and TPN bag
4. The patient's last chest x-ray report

CRITICAL THINKING QUESTIONS

1. A patient has been self-medicating with vitamin B_3 (niacin) for an elevated cholesterol level. The patient comes to the clinic with a severe case of redness and flushing and is concerned about an allergic reaction. What is the nurse's best response?

2. A patient complains of a constant headache for the past several days. The only supplements the patient has been taking are megadoses of vitamins A, C, and E. What would be a priority for the nurse with this patient?

3. A patient presents to the health care provider with complaints of severe flank pain. This patient has a history of renal calculi. The only medication the patient takes is a daily multivitamin as well as vitamin C. The nurse should assess for what potential problem?

See Appendix D for answers and rationales for all activities.

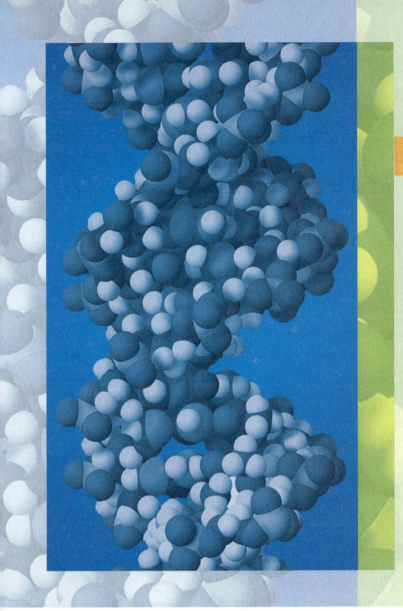

The Endocrine System

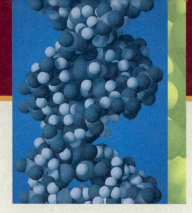

Chapter 43

Drugs for Pituitary, Thyroid, and Adrenal Disorders

DRUGS AT A GLANCE

LEARNING OUTCOMES

After reading this chapter, the student should be able to:

1. Describe the general structure and functions of the endocrine system.
2. Through the use of a specific example, explain the concept of negative feedback in the endocrine system.
3. Describe the clinical applications of the hypothalamic and pituitary hormones.
4. Explain the pharmacotherapy of diabetes insipidus.
5. Identify the signs and symptoms of hypothyroidism and hyperthyroidism.
6. Explain the pharmacotherapy of thyroid disorders.
7. Describe the signs and symptoms of Addison's disease and Cushing's syndrome.
8. Explain the pharmacotherapy of adrenal gland disorders.
9. Describe the nurse's role in the pharmacologic management of pituitary, thyroid, and adrenal disorders.
10. For each of the classes listed in Drugs at a Glance, know representative drugs, and explain the mechanisms of drug action, primary actions, and important adverse effects.
11. Use the nursing process to care for patients who are receiving drug therapy for pituitary, thyroid, and adrenal disorders.

KEY TERMS

Like the nervous system, the endocrine system is a major controller of homeostasis. Whereas a nerve exerts instantaneous control over a single muscle fiber or gland, a hormone from the endocrine system may affect thousands of cells and take as long as several days to produce an optimum response. Hormonal balance is kept within a narrow range: Too little or too much of a hormone produces profound physiologic changes. This chapter examines common endocrine disorders and their pharmacotherapy. The reproductive hormones are covered in chapters 45 and 46∞.

43.1 The Endocrine System and Homeostasis

The endocrine system consists of various glands that secrete **hormones,** chemical messengers released in response to a change in the body's internal environment. The role of hormones is to maintain the body in homeostasis. For example, when the level of glucose in the blood rises above normal, the pancreas secretes insulin to return glucose levels to normal. The various endocrine glands and their hormones are illustrated in ➤ Figure 43.1.

After secretion from an endocrine gland, hormones enter the blood and are transported throughout the body. Some, such as insulin and thyroid hormone, have receptors on nearly every cell in the body; thus, these hormones have widespread effects. Others, such as parathyroid hormone (PTH) and oxytocin, have receptors on only a few specific types of cells.

In the endocrine system, it is common for one hormone to control the secretion of another hormone. In addition, it is common for the last hormone or action in the pathway to provide feedback to turn off the secretion of the first hormone. For example, as serum calcium levels fall, PTH is released; PTH causes an increase in serum calcium, which provides feedback to the parathyroid glands to shut off PTH secretion. This characteristic feature of endocrine homeostasis is known as negative feedback. Negative feedback helps to prevent excessive secretion of hormones thereby limiting their physiologic responses. It is important to understand that when a hormone is administered as pharmacotherapy, it provides negative feedback in the same manner as the normal, endogenous hormone.

43.2 The Hypothalamus and Pituitary Gland

Two endocrine structures in the brain, the hypothalamus and the pituitary gland, deserve special recognition because they control many other endocrine glands. The hypothalamus secretes **releasing hormones** that travel via blood vessels a short distance to the pituitary gland. These releasing hormones specify which hormone is to be released by the pituitary. After secretion, the pituitary hormone travels to its target tissues to cause its biologic effects. For example, the hypothalamus secretes thyrotropin-releasing hormone (TRH)

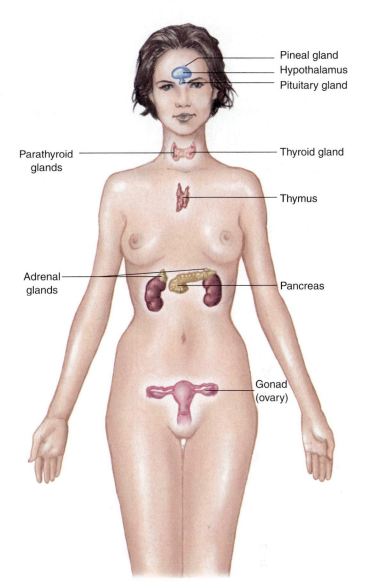

➤ **Figure 43.1** The endocrine system
Source: Pearson Education/PH College.

that travels to the pituitary gland with the message to secrete thyroid-stimulating hormone (TSH). TSH then travels to its target organ, the thyroid gland, to stimulate the release of thyroid hormone. Although the pituitary is often called the master gland, the pituitary and hypothalamus are best visualized as an integrated unit.

The pituitary gland comprises two distinct regions. The anterior pituitary, or **adenohypophysis,** consists of *glandular tissue* and secretes adrenocorticotropic hormone (ACTH), thyroid-stimulating hormone (TSH), growth hormone, prolactin, follicle-stimulating hormone (FSH), and leuteinizing hormone (LH). The posterior pituitary, or **neurohypophysis,** contains *nervous tissue* rather than glandular tissue. Neurons in the posterior pituitary store antidiuretic hormone (ADH) and oxytocin, which are released in response to nerve impulses from the hypothalamus. Those hormones that affect the female reproductive tract are presented in chapter 45∞. Selected hormones associated with the hypothalamus and pituitary gland are shown in ➤ Figure 43.2.

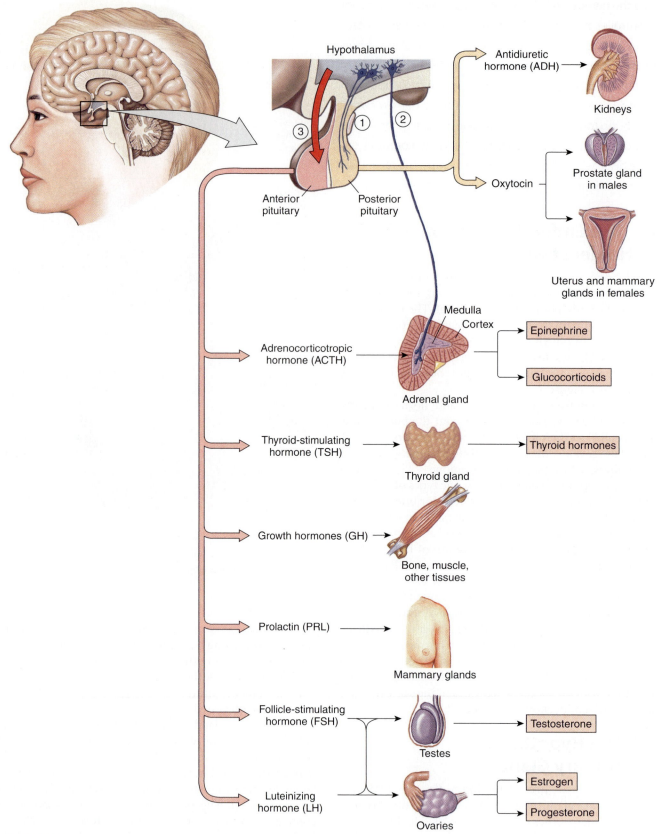

Hypothalamus

Antidiuretic hormone (ADH) → Kidneys

③ ① ②

Anterior pituitary   Posterior pituitary

Oxytocin → Prostate gland in males

Uterus and mammary glands in females

Medulla
Cortex

Adrenocorticotropic hormone (ACTH) → Adrenal gland → Epinephrine

Glucocorticoids

Thyroid-stimulating hormone (TSH) → Thyroid gland → Thyroid hormones

Growth hormones (GH) → Bone, muscle, other tissues

Prolactin (PRL) → Mammary glands

Follicle-stimulating hormone (FSH) → Testes → Testosterone

Luteinizing hormone (LH) → Ovaries → Estrogen

Progesterone

➤ **Figure 43.2** Hormones associated with the hypothalamus and the pituitary gland
Source: Pearson Education/PH College.

43.3 Indications for Hormone Pharmacotherapy

The goals of hormone pharmacotherapy vary widely. In many cases, a hormone is administered as simple replacement therapy for patients who are unable to secrete sufficient quantities of their own endogenous hormones. Examples of replacement therapy include the administration of thyroid hormone after the thyroid gland has been surgically removed, or supplying insulin to patients whose pancreas is not functioning. Replacement therapy supplies the same physiologic, low-level amounts of the hormone that would normally be present in the body. Selected endocrine disorders and their drug therapy are summarized in Table 43.1.

Some hormones are used in cancer chemotherapy to shrink the size of hormone-sensitive tumors. Examples include testosterone for breast cancer and estrogen for testicular cancer. Exactly how these hormones produce their antineoplastic action is largely unknown. When hormones are used as antineoplastics, their doses far exceed normal physiologic levels. Hormones are always used in combination with other antineoplastic medications, as discussed in chapter 37.

Another goal of hormonal pharmacotherapy may be to produce an *exaggerated response* that is part of the normal action of the hormone. Administering hydrocortisone to suppress inflammation takes advantage of the normal action of the glucocorticoids, but to a greater extent than would normally occur in the body. Supplying estrogen or progesterone at specific times during the menstrual cycle can prevent ovulation and pregnancy. In this example, the patient is given natural hormones; however, they are taken at a time when levels in the body are normally low.

Endocrine pharmacotherapy also involves the use of "antihormones." These hormone antagonists block the actions of endogenous hormones. For example, propylthiouracil

(PTU) is given to block the effects of an overactive thyroid gland (Section 43.7). Tamoxifen (Nolvadex) is given to block the actions of estrogen in estrogen-dependent breast cancers (chapter 37).

43.4 Pharmacotherapy with Pituitary and Hypothalamic Hormones

Of the 15 different hormones secreted by the pituitary and the hypothalamus, only a few are used in pharmacotherapy, as listed in Table 43.2. There are valid reasons why they are not widely used. Some of these hormones can be obtained only from natural sources (human brains) and can be quite expensive when used in therapeutic quantities. Furthermore, it is usually more effective to give drugs that *directly* affect secretion at the target organs.

The only hypothalamic hormone used clinically is gonadotropin-releasing hormone (GnRH). Leuprolide (Lupron), goserelin (Zoladex), and nafarelin (Synarel) are analogs of GnRH that are used to treat endometriosis, a common cause of infertility (chapter 45). Leuprolide and goserelin are also used for the palliative treatment of advanced prostate cancer. Two pituitary hormones, prolactin and oxytocin, affect the female reproductive system and are discussed in chapter 45. Corticotropin affects the adrenal gland, and is discussed later in this chapter. Of the remaining, growth hormone and antidiuretic hormone have the most clinical utility.

GROWTH HORMONE (GH) Growth hormone, or **somatotropin**, stimulates the growth and metabolism of nearly every cell in the body. Deficiency of this hormone in children can cause **short stature**, a condition characterized by significantly decreased physical height compared with the norm of a specific age group. Severe deficiency results in dwarfism. Short stature is caused by many conditions other than GH deficiency, and often a specific cause cannot be identified.

Prior to 1985, all GH was obtained by extracting the hormone from human pituitary glands, which severely limited the amount available for pharmacotherapy. Human GH, somatotropin (Accretropin, Genotropin, Humatrope, others) is now available by the subcutaneous route in large quantities through recombinant DNA technology. If therapy is begun early in life, as much as 6 inches of growth may be achieved. GH therapy is contraindicated in patients after the epiphyses

TABLE 43.1	Selected Endocrine Disorders and Their Pharmacotherapy		
Gland	Hormone(s)	Disorder	Drug Therapy
Adrenal cortex	Glucocorticoids	Hypersecretion: Cushing's syndrome	Antiadrenal agents
		Hyposecretion: Addison's disease	Glucocorticoids
Pituitary	Growth hormone	Hyposecretion: small stature	Somatrem (Protropin) and somatotropin (Genotropin)
		Hypersecretion: acromegaly (adults)	Octreotide (Sandostatin)
	Antidiuretic hormone	Hyposecretion: diabetes insipidus	Vasopressin, desmopressin, and lypressin
Thyroid	Thyroid hormone (T₃ and T₄)	Hypersecretion: Graves' disease	Propylthiouracil (PTU), methimazole (Tapazole), and I-131
		Hyposecretion: myxedema (adults)	Thyroid hormone, levothyroxine (T₄)

TABLE 43.2	Selected Hypothalamic and Pituitary Agents*	
Drug	**Route and Adult Dose (max dose where indicated)**	**Adverse Effects**
HYPOTHALAMIC AGENTS		
octreotide (Sandostatin)	Subcutaneous; 100–600 mcg/day in two to four divided doses; may switch to IM depot injection after 2 wk at 20 mg every 4 wk for 2 mo	*Nausea, vomiting, diarrhea, headache, flushing, injection site pain, cholelithiasis* <u>Dysrhythmias, congestive heart failure, sinus bradycardia</u>
pegvisomant (Somavert)	Subcutaneous; 40-mg loading dose, then 10 mg/day (max: 30 mg/day)	*Nausea, diarrhea, injection site pain, flulike symptoms* <u>Liver damage, elevated transaminase levels</u>
ANTERIOR PITUITARY AGENTS		
corticotropin (ACTH)	IV; 10–25 international units in 500 mL D5W infused over 8 h	*Sodium and water retention*
cosyntropin (Cortrosyn)	IM/IV; 0.25 mg injected over 2 min	<u>Cushing's syndrome</u>
mecasermin (Increlex, Iplex)	Subcutaneous (≥3 yrs and older): 0.5 mg/kg once daily, up to 1–2 mg/kg/day, given once daily	*Injection site reaction, iron deficency anemia, goiter, antibody development, headache, hypertrophy of adenoids and tonsils* <u>Hypoglycemia, increased intracranial pressure</u>
somatotropin (Accretropin, Genotropin, Humatrope, Norditropin, Nutropin, Serostim, Saizen, Zorbtive)	Subcutaneous; doses are highly individualized, based on a child's growth rate	*Pain at injection site, hyperglycemia, arthalgia, myalgia, abdominal pain, otitis media, headache, bronchitis, hypothyroidism, hypertension, flulike symptoms* <u>Severe respiratory impairment in severely obese patients with Prader-Willi Syndrome, diabetes, pancreatitis, scoliosis of the spine, papilledema, intracranial tumor</u>
thyrotropin (thyrogen, thyroid-stimulating hormone (TSH)	IM/subcutaneous; 10 international units/day for 1–3 days	*Nausea, headache, asthenia* <u>No serious adverse reactions</u>
POSTERIOR PITUITARY AGENTS		
🅟 desmopressin (DDAVP, Stimate)	Intranasal; 0.1–0.4 mL (10–40 mcg) in one to three divided doses IV/Subcutaneous; 2–4 mcg in two divided doses PO; 0.2–0.4 mg/day	*Headache, nasal congestion or irritation, nausea* <u>Water intoxication, coma, thromboembolic disorder, hyponatremia</u>
vasopressin	IM/subcutaneous; 5–10 units aqueous solution two to four times/day IV; 0.2–0.4 units/min up to 1 unit/min	*Tremor, pallor, vomiting, water retention* <u>Angina, MI, gangrene, anaphylaxis</u>

*Hypothalamic and pituitary agents used for conditions of the female reproductive system are presented in chapter 45 ∞ .
Italics indicate common adverse effects; <u>underlining</u> indicates serious adverse effects.

have closed. GH agents are usually well tolerated, although patients must undergo regular assessments of glucose tolerance and thyroid function during pharmacotherapy.

Mecasermin (Increlex, Iplex) is a newer agent, approved in 2005, that has the same actions as growth hormone. Mecasermin is indicated for the long-term treatment of growth failure in children with severe deficiency of insulin-like growth factor (IGF) or for those who have developed neutralizing antibodies to GH. It is administered once daily by the subcutaneous route. Adverse effects include hypoglycemia, headache, dizziness, vomiting, and tonsillar hypertrophy.

Prior to 2003, growth hormone therapy was approved only for treating short stature in children who had deficiencies in GH. The FDA, however, has now approved growth hormone therapy to treat children with short stature who have *normal* levels of GH. The height criterion for treatment is defined as

an expected adult height of less than 5 feet 3 inches for men and 4 feet 11 inches for women. GH therapy in children with normal growth hormone levels may add 1 to 3 inches in height to children after 4 to 6 years of pharmacotherapy. The annual cost of $30,000 to $40,000 may discourage many parents from seeking this therapy for their children.

Excess secretion of growth hormone in adults is known as *acromegaly*. A rare disease nearly always caused by a pituitary tumor, acromegaly sometimes requires pharmacotherapy. Octreotide (Sandostatin) is a synthetic growth hormone *antagonist* structurally related to growth hormone–inhibiting hormone (somatostatin). In addition to inhibiting growth hormone, octreotide promotes fluid and electrolyte reabsorption from the GI tract and prolongs intestinal transit time. It has limited applications in treating acromegaly in adults and in treating the severe diarrhea sometimes associated with metastatic carcinoid tumors. Acromegaly may also be treated with pegvisomant (Somavert), a growth hormone–receptor antagonist.

ANTIDIURETIC HORMONE It is essential that the concentration of fluids in the body be maintained within narrow limits. Loss of large amounts of water leads to dehydration, whereas too much body fluid leads to congestion, edema, and water intoxication. **Antidiuretic hormone (ADH)** is one of the most important means the body uses to maintain fluid homeostasis.

As its name implies, ADH conserves water in the body. ADH is secreted from the posterior pituitary gland when the hypothalamus senses that plasma volume has decreased, or that the osmolality of the blood has become too high. ADH acts on the collecting ducts in the kidneys to increase water reabsorption. The increased amount of water in the body reduces serum osmolality to normal levels and ADH secretion stops. ADH is also called *vasopressin*, because it has the ability to constrict blood vessels and raise blood pressure.

A deficiency in ADH results in **diabetes insipidus (DI)**, a rare condition characterized by the production of large volumes of very dilute urine, usually accompanied by increased thirst. Two ADH preparations are available for the treatment of diabetes insipidus: vasopressin and desmopressin (DDAVP, Stimate).

Vasopressin is a synthetic hormone that has a structure identical with that of human ADH. It acts on the renal collecting tubules to increase their permeability to water, thus enhancing water reabsorption. Although it acts within minutes, vasopressin has a short half-life that requires it to be administered three to four times per day. Vasopressin tannate is formulated in peanut oil to increase its duration of action. Vasopressin is usually given IM or IV, although an intranasal form is available for mild diabetes insipidus.

Desmopressin is the most common form of antidiuretic hormone in use. Details regarding this drug may be found in the Prototype Drug feature.

43.5 Normal Function of the Thyroid Gland

The thyroid gland secretes hormones that affect nearly every cell in the body. Thyroid hormone increases **basal metabolic rate**, the baseline speed at which cells perform their functions. By increasing cellular metabolism, this hormone increases body temperature. Adequate secretion of thyroid hormone is also necessary for the normal growth and development in infants and children, including mental development and attainment of sexual maturity. The thyroid strongly affects cardiovascular, respiratory, gastrointestinal (GI), and neuromuscular function.

The thyroid gland has two basic types of cells, which secrete different hormones. **Parafollicular cells** secrete calcitonin, a

---

Pr Prototype Drug | Desmopressin *(DDAVP, Stimate)*

Therapeutic Class: Antidiuretic hormone replacement   **Pharmacologic Class:** Vasopressin analog

ACTIONS AND USES

Desmopressin is a synthetic analog of human ADH that acts on the kidneys to increase the reabsorption of water. It is used to control the acute symptoms of diabetes insipidus in patients who have insufficient ADH secretion. The oral route is preferred, although intranasal, rhinal tube, nasal spray, and parenteral forms are available. It has a duration of action of up to 20 hours, whereas vasopressin (Pitressin) has a duration of only 2–8 hours.

Desmopressin causes contraction of smooth muscle in the vascular system, uterus, and GI tract. It also produces an increase in clotting factor VIII and von Willebrand's factor, and is thus indicated for the management of bleeding in patients with hemophilia A and von Willebrand's disease (type I). An off-label use for this drug is to control enuresis (bed-wetting) among children.

ADMINISTRATION ALERTS

- When administered IV for diabetes insipidus, desmopressin is given undiluted over 1 minute.
- Following an IV injection, fluids must be restricted and carefully monitored to prevent serious water intoxication.
- Pregnancy category B

PHARMACOKINETICS
Onset: Immediate IV; 1 h PO
Peak: 15–30 min IV; 4–7 h PO
Half-life: 75 min
Duration: 3 h IV; 8–20 h PO

ADVERSE EFFECTS

Desmopressin can cause symptoms of water intoxication: drowsiness, headache, and listlessness, progressing to convulsions and coma. Other adverse effects include transient headache, nausea, mild abdominal pain and cramping, facial flushing, hypertension, pain, or swelling at injection site. Intranasal forms can cause nasal congestion, rhinitis, and epistaxis. Tolerance develops to the effects of desmopressin when it is administered more frequently than every 48 hours, or by the IV route.

Contraindications: Desmopressin is contraindicated in patients with diabetes insipidus that is caused by kidney disease because the drug can worsen fluid retention and overload. It is used with caution in patients with coronary artery disease, hypertension, and in patients at risk for hyponatremia or thrombi. Young children and the older adults should be treated with caution because these patients are more prone to water intoxication and hyponatremia.

INTERACTIONS

Drug–Drug: Increased antidiuretic action can occur with carbamazepine, chlorpropamide, clofibrate, and nonsteroidal anti-inflammatory drugs (NSAIDs). Decreased antidiuretic action can occur with lithium, alcohol, heparin, and epinephrine.

Lab Tests: Unknown

Herbal/Food: Unknown

Treatment of Overdose: Overdose may cause severe water intoxication. Treatment includes water restriction and osmotic diuretics.

Refer to MyNursingKit for a Nursing Process Focus specific to this drug.

hormone that is involved with calcium homeostasis (chapter 47 ∞). **Follicular cells** in the gland secrete thyroid hormone, which actually consist of two different hormones: thyroxine (T_4) and triiodothyronine (T_3). Iodine is essential for the synthesis of these hormones, and is provided through the dietary intake of common iodized salt. The names of these hormones refer to the number of bound iodine atoms in each molecule, either three (T_3) or four (T_4). Thyroxine is the major hormone secreted by the thyroid gland, however, it is converted to T_3 before it enters its target cells. T_3 is three to five times more biologically active than T_4.

As it travels through the blood, thyroid hormone is attached to a carrier protein, **thyroxine-binding globulin (TBG)**, which protects it from degradation. Any condition that causes decreased amounts of plasma proteins, such as protein malnutrition or liver impairment, can lead to a larger percentage of *free* thyroid hormone, with subsequent symptoms of hyperthyroidism.

The secretion of thyroid hormone is regulated by the hypothalamus and anterior pituitary gland by way of a negative feedback loop, as shown in ➤ Figure 43.3. When blood levels of thyroid hormone are low, the hypothalamus secretes thyrotropin-releasing hormone (TRH). Secretion of TRH stimulates the anterior pituitary to secrete thyroid stimulating hormone (TSH). TSH, then, stimulates the thyroid to produce and secrete T_3 and T_4. As blood levels of thyroid hormone increases, negative feedback suppresses the secretion of TSH and TRH. High levels of iodine can also cause a temporary decrease in thyroid activity that can last for several weeks. One of the strongest stimuli for increased thyroid hormone production is exposure to cold.

THYROID AGENTS

Thyroid disorders are common and drug therapy is often indicated. The correct dose of thyroid drug is highly individualized and requires careful, periodic adjustment. The medications used to treat thyroid disease are listed in Table 43.3.

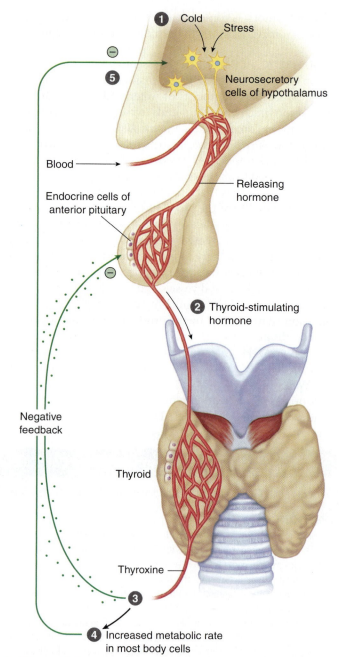

➤ **Figure 43.3** Feedback mechanisms of the thyroid gland: (1) stimulus; (2) release of TSH; (3) release of thyroid hormone; (4) increased BMR; (5) negative feedback

43.6 Pharmacotherapy of Hypothyroidism

Hypothyroidism may result from either a poorly functioning thyroid gland or low secretion of TSH by the pituitary gland. The most common cause of hypothyroidism in the United States is destruction of the thyroid gland due to chronic autoimmune thyroiditis, a condition known as *Hashimoto's thyroiditis.* Early symptoms of hypothyroidism in adults, or **myxedema**, include general weakness, muscle cramps, and dry skin. More severe symptoms include slurred speech, bradycardia, weight gain, decreased sense of taste and smell, and intolerance to cold environments. Lab

---

PHARMFACTS

Thyroid Disorders
- Hypothyroidism is 10 times more common in women; hyperthyroidism is 5 to 10 times more common in women.
- The two most common thyroid diseases, Graves' disease and Hashimoto's thyroiditis, are autoimmune diseases and may have a genetic link.
- One of every 4,000 babies is born without a working thyroid gland.
- About 15,000 new cases of thyroid cancer are diagnosed each year.
- One of every five women older than 75 years has Hashimoto's thyroiditis.
- Postpartum thyroiditis occurs in 5% to 9% of women and may recur in future pregnancies.
- Both hyperthyroidism and hypothyroidism can affect a woman's ability to become pregnant and can cause miscarriages.

TABLE 43.3	**Thyroid and Antithyroid Drugs**	
Drug	Route and Adult Dose (max dose where indicated)	Adverse Effects
THYROID AGENTS		
desiccated thyroid (Armour, Bio-Thyroid, Thyroid USP, others)	PO; 60–180 mg/day	*Weight loss, headache, tremors, nervousness, heat intolerance, insomnia, menstrual irregularities*
℞ levothyroxine (Levothroid, Synthroid, others)	PO; 100–400 mcg/day	
liothyronine (Cytomel, Triostat)	PO; 25–75 mcg/day	<u>Dysrhythmias, hypertension, palpitations</u>
	IV; 25–100 mcg/day	
liotrix (Thyrolar)	PO; 12.5–30 mcg/day	
ANTITHYROID AGENTS		
methimazole (Tapazole)	PO; 5–15 mg tid	*Nausea, rash, pruritus, weight gain, headache, fever, numbness in fingers, leukopenia, diarrhea*
potassium iodide and iodine (Lugol's Solution, Pima, SSKI, Thyro-Block)	PO; 250 mg tid	
℞ propylthiouracil (PTU)	PO; 300–450 mg tid	<u>Agranulocytosis, bradycardia, hepatotoxicity (methimazole)</u>
radioactive iodide (I-131, Iodotope)	PO; 0.8–150 mCi (a Ci or curie is a unit of radioactivity)	

Italics indicate common adverse effects; <u>underlining</u> indicates serious adverse effects.

results generally reveal elevated TSH with diminished T_3 and T_4 levels. The etiology of myxedema may include autoimmune disease, surgical removal of the thyroid gland, or aggressive treatment with antithyroid drugs. At high doses, the antidysrhythmic drug amiodarone (Cordarone) can induce hypothyroidism in patients due to its high iodine content. Enlargement of the thyroid gland, or goiter, may be absent or present, depending on the cause of the disease.

Hypothyroidism is treated by replacement therapy with T_3 or T_4. The standard replacement regimen consists of levothyroxine (T_4), although combined therapy with levothyroxine plus liothyronine (T_3) is an option. Desiccated thyroid gland from beef, pork, or sheep sources (Thyroid USP) is an inexpensive option, although it is rarely used because of the possibility of allergic reactions to animal protein. Liothyronine sodium is a short-acting synthetic form of thyroid hormone that can be administered IV to individuals with myxedema coma. The short duration of action allows for a rapid response to critically ill patients.

Serum TSH levels are used to evaluate the progress of therapy. Because small changes in drug bioavailability can affect thyroid function, patients should avoid switching brands of medication once their condition has stabilized. When initiating therapy in older adults, the precaution is to "go low and go slow," because there is a risk for inducing acute coronary syndromes in susceptible individuals. Replacement therapy for most patients is continued lifelong.

ANTITHYROID AGENTS

Medications are often used to treat the cause of hyperthyroidism or to relieve its distressing symptoms. The goal of antithyroid therapy is to lower the activity of the thyroid gland.

43.7 Pharmacotherapy of Hyperthyroidism

Hypersecretion of thyroid hormone results in symptoms that are the opposite of those caused by hypothyroidism: increased body metabolism, tachycardia, weight loss, elevated body temperature, and anxiety. The most common type of hyperthyroidism is called **Graves' disease**. Considered an autoimmune disease in which the body develops antibodies against its own thyroid gland, Graves' disease is four to eight times more common in women, and most often occurs between the ages of 30 and 40. Other causes of hyperthyroidism are adenomas of the thyroid, pituitary tumors, and pregnancy. If the cause of the hypersecretion is found to be a tumor, or if the disease cannot be controlled through pharmacotherapy, surgical removal of the thyroid gland is indicated.

LIFESPAN CONSIDERATIONS

Shift Workers, Hypothyroidism, and Drug Compliance

Many body processes such as temperature, blood pressure, levels of certain hormones, biochemical processes, and alertness fluctuate on a 24-hour schedule known as the *circadian rhythm*. Circadian processes are thought to be regulated by daylight. Normal circadian cycles may be interrupted in those people who work varied shifts. Therefore, medications that must be given at a specified time to enhance their potential effect can be a concern for shift workers.

For example, thyroid medication is best given at the same time each day, usually on awakening, because it can disrupt sleep if taken later in the day. But for shift workers who rotate shifts, and therefore awaken at different times, this consistent dosing schedule can be a challenge. Advise patients of this challenge, and have them work with the health care provider to reach a medication schedule that allows optimization of the drug effects.

Pr Prototype Drug | Levothyroxine *(Levothroid, Synthroid, others)*

Therapeutic Class: Thyroid hormone   **Pharmacologic Class:** Thyroid hormone replacement

ACTIONS AND USES

Levothyroxine is a synthetic form of T_4 that is a drug of choice for replacement therapy in patients with low thyroid function. Actions are those of endogenous thyroid hormone, and include loss of weight, improved tolerance to environmental temperature, increased activity, and increased pulse rate.

To avoid adverse effects, doses of levothyroxine are highly individualized for each patient. When given by the oral route, 1–3 weeks may be required to obtain full therapeutic benefits. Doses for patients with pre-existing cardiac disease are usually increased at 4–6 week intervals to avoid triggering dysrhythmias or angina attacks. Serum TSH levels are regularly monitored to determine whether the patient is receiving sufficient levothyroxine—high TSH levels usually indicate that the dosage of T_4 needs to be increased.

ADMINISTRATION ALERTS

- Administer the medication at the same time every day, preferably in the morning to decrease the potential for insomnia.
- Pregnancy category A

PHARMACOKINETICS

Onset: 3–5 hr (oral), 24 h (IV)

Peak: 3–4 wk

Half-life: 6–7 days

Duration: 1–3 wk

ADVERSE EFFECTS

At therapeutic doses, adverse effects of levothyroxine therapy are rare, although care must be taken to avoid overtreatment. Adverse effects are those of hyperthyroidism and include palpitations, dysrhythmias, anxiety, insomnia, weight loss, and heat intolerance. Menstrual irregularities may occur in females, and long-term use of levothyroxine has been associated with osteoporosis in women.

Contraindications: Levothyroxine is contraindicated if the patient is hypersensitive to the drug, is experiencing thyrotoxicosis, or has severe cardiovascular conditions or acute myocardial infarction (MI). If given to patients with adrenal insufficiency, thyroid hormone may cause a serious adrenal crisis; thus, the insufficiency should be corrected prior to administration of levothyroxine. It should be used with caution in patients with cardiac disease, hypertension, older adults, and impaired kidney function. Symptoms of diabetes mellitus may be worsened with administration of thyroid hormone and doses of antidiabetic drugs may require adjustment. Levothyroxine has a black box warning that it is ineffective for weight reduction and can be potentially toxic when used with anorectic drugs.

INTERACTIONS

Drug–Drug: Cholestyramine and colestipol decrease the absorption of levothyroxine. Concurrent administration of epinephrine and norepinephrine increases the risk of cardiac insufficiency. Levothyroxine increases the effects of warfarin, resulting in an increased risk of bleeding.

Lab Tests: Unknown

Herbal/Food: Soybean flour (infant formula), cottonseed meal, walnuts, and dietary fiber may bind and decrease the absorption of levothyroxine sodium from the GI tract. Calcium or iron supplements should be taken at least 4 hours after taking levothyroxine to prevent interference with drug absorption.

Treatment of Overdose: Overdose can cause serious thyrotoxicosis, which may not present until several days after the overdose. Treatment is symptomatic, usually targeted at preventing cardiac toxicity with beta-adrenergic antagonists such as propranolol.

Refer to MyNursingKit for a Nursing Process Focus specific to this drug.

Very high levels of circulating thyroid hormone may cause **thyroid storm,** a rare, life-threatening form of hyperthroidism. If untreated, it is associated with mortality rates of 80% to 90%, even with treatment. Symptoms include high fever, cardiovascular effects (tachycardia, heart failure, angina, MI), and CNS effects (agitation, restlessness, delirium, progressing to coma). Thyroid storm is treated with supportive measures, efforts to reduce body temperature while trying to avoid causing shivering, fluid, glucose and electrolyte replacement, and beta-adrenergic blockers. Antithyroid drugs may be used to decrease thyroid hormone production.

The two primary drugs for hyperthyroidism are propylthiouracil (PTU) and methimazole (Tapazole). These medications act by inhibiting the incorporation of iodine atoms into T_3 and T_4. Methimazole has a much longer half-life that offers the advantage of less-frequent dosing, although adverse effects can be more severe. Both drugs are pregnancy category D agents, but methimazole crosses the placenta more readily than propylthiouracil and is contraindicated in pregnant patients.

A third antithyroid drug, sodium iodide-131 (Iodotope) is a radioactive isotope that destroys overactive thyroid glands with ionizing radiation. Shortly after oral administration, I-131 accumulates in the thyroid gland, where it destroys follicular cells. The goal of pharmacotherapy with I-131 is to destroy just enough of the thyroid gland so that levels of thyroid function return to normal. Full benefits may take several months. Although most patients require only a single dose, others need multiple treatments. Small diagnostic doses of I-131 are used in nuclear medicine to determine the degree of iodide uptake in the thyroid gland.

Nonradioactive iodine is also available to treat other thyroid conditions. Lugol's solution is a mixture of 5% elemental iodine and 10% potassium iodide that is used to suppress thyroid function 10 to 15 days prior to thyroidectomy. Sodium iodide may be administered IV (along with

NURSING PROCESS FOCUS	PATIENTS RECEIVING PHARMACOTHERAPY WITH HYPOTHALAMIC AND PITUITARY HORMONES

Assessment	Potential Nursing Diagnoses
Baseline assessment prior to administration: ■ Understand the reason the drug has been prescribed in order to assess for therapeutic effects (e.g., treatment of specific disease condition such as diabetes insipidus, off-label use for nonendocrine-related conditions such as nocturnal enuresis). ■ Obtain a complete health history including cardiovascular, gastrointestinal, hepatic, or renal disease; pregnancy; or breast-feeding. Obtain a drug history including allergies, current prescription and OTC drugs, herbal preparations, alcohol use, or smoking. Be alert to possible drug interactions. ■ Evaluate appropriate laboratory findings (e.g., urine and serum osmolality, urine specific gravity, serum protein, CBC, electrolytes, glucose, hepatic and renal function studies). ■ Obtain baseline height, weight, and vital signs. Obtain an ECG on patients taking growth hormone antagonists.	■ Deficient Fluid Volume ■ Diarrhea ■ Delayed Growth and Development ■ Situational Low Self-Esteem (related to height, stature) ■ Impaired Urinary Elimination (nocturnal enuresis) ■ Deficient Knowledge (drug therapy)
Assessment throughout administration: ■ Assess for desired therapeutic effects dependent on the reason the drug is being given (e.g., measurable increase in height, slowed diuresis, return to normal urine output and serum osmolality, return to normal bowel activity). ■ Continue periodic monitoring of urine and serum osmolality, urine specific gravity, CBC, electrolytes, glucose, and hepatic and renal function studies. ■ Continue monitoring vital signs, height, and weight. Monitor the ECG for patients taking growth hormone antagonists. ■ Assess for adverse effects: nausea, vomiting, diarrhea, and headache. Hypo- or hypertension, tachycardia, dysrhythmias, or angina should be reported immediately.	

Planning: Patient Goals and Expected Outcomes

The patient will:
■ Experience therapeutic effects (e.g., height increase measurable over time, diuresis slows with urine and serum osmolality within normal limits, return to normal bowel function, nocturnal enuresis has stopped).
■ Be free from, or experience minimal, adverse effects.
■ Verbalize an understanding of the drug's use, adverse effects, and required precautions.
■ Demonstrate proper self-administration of the medication (e.g., dose, timing, when to notify provider).

Implementation

Interventions and (Rationales)	Patient and Family Education
Ensuring therapeutic effects: ■ *Patients taking growth hormone:* Monitor height and weight at each clinical visit. Report lack of growth to the health care provider. (Lack of growth after a period of consistent growth may indicate the development of antibodies against GH.) ■ *Patients taking growth hormone antagonists:* Monitor levels of serum GH. Monitor bowel sounds and for a decrease in diarrhea. (GH antagonists are given for acromegaly, severe diarrhea unresponsive to other drug therapy, and the treatment of portal hypertension. Monitoring levels of serum GH and bowel activity will evaluate therapeutic changes.) ■ *Patients taking antidiuretic hormones:* For patients with diabetes insipidus, monitor urine output, urine and serum osmolality, and urine specific gravity for return to normal limits. If given for nocturnal enuresis, have the patient, family, or caregiver keep a diary of sleep patterns, noting any bed-wetting. (Urine output, osmolality, and specific gravity should return to normal limits. Bed-wetting has slowed or stopped.)	■ Teach the patient, family, or caregiver to measure and record height and weight weekly and bring the record to each clinical visit. ■ Instruct the patient on the need to return periodically for lab work. ■ Instruct the patient to monitor output, provide measuring equipment as needed, and to keep a record of daily weight and output and bring the record to each provider visit. ■ Teach the patient, family, or caregiver to keep a diary of night-time sleep habits and any bedwetting. Limit oral fluids within 4 hours of bedtime. ■ Advise the patient of the drug's cost before beginning therapy. Explore the ability to maintain drug therapy for the duration of the treatment prescribed. Assess financial concerns and provide appropriate social service referral as needed.

(Continued)

NURSING PROCESS FOCUS   PATIENTS RECEIVING PHARMACOTHERAPY WITH HYPOTHALAMIC AND PITUITARY HORMONES (Continued)

Implementation

Interventions and (Rationales)	Patient and Family Education
Minimizing adverse effects: ▪ Monitor for any complaints of muscle, joint, or bone pain, particularly in the knee or hip, or any changes in gait. (Avascular necrosis is an adverse drug effect of growth hormone. Increasing or severe pain in joints or changes in gait should be reported promptly for follow-up evaluation.)	▪ Instruct the patient, family, or caregiver to report any changes in walking, discomfort or pain in knee or hip joints, bone pain, or consistent muscle pain over joint areas to the health care provider.
▪ Monitor glucose levels, particularly in diabetic patients. Report consistent elevations to the health care provider. (GH and GH antagonists may cause increases in glucose level. Diabetics may need alterations in their normal medication routines if hyperglycemia occurs.)	▪ Instruct the patient on the need to return periodically for lab work. ▪ Teach the diabetic patient to monitor capillary glucose levels more frequently during therapy. Report any consistent elevations in blood glucose to the health care provider.
▪ Continue to monitor vital signs, especially pulse and blood pressure for patients with cardiac disease. ECGs may be ordered periodically for patients with a history of dysrhythmias. Monitor daily weight, output, lung sounds, and for peripheral edema. (Fluid retention secondary to ADH treatment may lead to increased intravascular volume and hypertension.)	▪ Instruct the patient to immediately report pounding headache, dizziness, palpitations, or syncope. ▪ Teach the patient, family, or caregiver how to monitor pulse and blood pressure as appropriate. Ensure the proper use and functioning of any home equipment obtained. ▪ Instruct the patient to monitor output, provide measuring equipment as needed, and to keep a record of daily weight and output and bring the record to each provider visit.
▪ Monitor for signs of peripheral ischemia or angina and report immediately. (Vasoconstriction caused by vasopressin may cause cardiac or peripheral ischemia, angina, or infarction.)	▪ Instruct the patient to immediately report any chest pain, pain or numbness in toes or fingers, or cramping when walking to the health care provider.
▪ For patients taking intranasal medications, monitor nasal passages. Report any excoriation or bleeding. (Long-term intranasal ADH therapy may cause nasal irritation and ulceration.)	▪ Teach the patient to report nasal congestion, irritation, increase in nasal discharge, or nasal bleeding to the health care provider.
▪ Continue to monitor nutritional and fluid intake. (Chronic, severe diarrhea requiring treatment with a growth-hormone antagonist may result in nutritional deficits and dehydration until the diarrhea is corrected. Dietary consultation may be required.)	▪ Encourage increased fluid intake, up to 2 L per day, taken in frequent small amounts. ▪ Encourage small, high-calorie, nutrient-dense meals rather than large, infrequent meals.
Patient understanding of drug therapy: ▪ Use opportunities during administration of medications and during assessments to discuss the rationale for drug therapy, desired therapeutic outcomes, most common adverse effects, parameters for when to call the health care provider, and any necessary monitoring or precautions. (Using time during nursing care helps to optimize and reinforce key teaching areas.)	▪ The patient should be able to state the reason for the drug, appropriate dose and scheduling, and what adverse effects to observe for and when to report them.

Patient self-administration of drug therapy:
▪ When administering the medication, instruct the patient, family, or caregiver in the proper self-administration of the drug, e.g., during evening meal. (Proper administration will increase the effectiveness of the drug.)
	▪ Teach the patient to take the drug according to appropriate guidelines, as follows:
	  ▪ Reconstitute the parenteral drug exactly per package directions and do not shake the vial but rotate gently to avoid breaking down drug.
	  ▪ Direct nasal sprays high into the nasal cavity rather than back to the nasopharynx. Do not shake the nasal spray before using but rotate gently.
	  ▪ Store any unused reconstituted solutions in refrigerator. Nasal sprays may be kept at room temperature but avoid excessive heat over 80°F. Discard any discolored solution or if particulate matter is present.
	  ▪ Administer GH drugs in the evening to mimic the body's natural rhythms.
	  ▪ Administer a subcutaneous injections in the abdomen, buttock, or thigh areas.

Evaluation of Outcome Criteria

Evaluate the effectiveness of drug therapy by confirming that patient goals and expected outcomes have been met (see "Planning").

See Tables 43.1 & 2, for a list of drugs to which these nursing actions apply.

propylthiouracil) to manage thyroid storm. Potassium iodide (Thyro-Block, ThyroSafe) is administered to protect the thyroid from radiation damage following a nuclear bioterrorist act, as discussed in chapter 3∞.

ADRENAL GLAND DISORDERS

Though small, the adrenal glands secrete hormones that affect every body tissue. Adrenal disorders include those resulting from either *excess* hormone secretion or *deficient* hormone secretion. The specific pharmacotherapy depends on which portion of the adrenal gland is responsible for the abnormal secretion.

43.8 Normal Function of the Adrenal Gland

Weighing only two-tenths of an ounce, each adrenal gland is divided into two major portions: an inner medulla, and an outer cortex. The adrenal medulla secretes 75% to 80% epinephrine, with the remainder of its secretion being norepinephrine. Adrenal release of epinephrine is triggered by activation of the sympathetic division of the autonomic nervous system. These hormones are described in chapter 13∞.

The adrenal cortex secretes three classes of steroid hormones: the glucocorticoids, mineralocorticoids, and gonadocorticoids. Collectively, the glucocorticoids and mineralocorticoids are called *corticosteroids* or *adrenocortical hormones*. The terms *corticosteroid* and *glucocorticoid* are often used interchangeably in clinical practice. However, it should be understood that the term *corticosteroid* implies that a drug has both glucocorticoid *and* mineralocorticoid activity.

GONADOCORTICOIDS

The gonadocorticoids secreted by the adrenal cortex are mostly androgens (male sex hormones), though small amounts of estrogens are also produced. The amounts of these adrenal sex hormones are far less than the levels secreted by the testes or ovaries. It is believed that the adrenal gonadocorticoids contribute to the onset of puberty. The adrenal glands also are the primary source of endogenous estrogen in postmenopausal women. Tumors of the adrenal cortex can cause hypersecretion of gonadocorticoids, resulting in hirsutism and masculinization, signs that are more noticeable in females than males. The physiologic effects of androgens are detailed in chapter 46∞.

Pr Prototype Drug | Propylthiouracil (PTU)

Therapeutic Class: Drug for hyperthyroidism   **Pharmacologic Class:** Antithyroid agent

ACTIONS AND USES

Propylthiouracil is administered to patients with hyperthyroidism. It acts by interfering with the synthesis of T_3 and T_4 in the thyroid gland. It also prevents the conversion of T_4 to T_3 in the target tissues. Its action may be delayed from several days to as long as 6–12 weeks. Effects include a return to normal thyroid function: weight gain, reduction in anxiety, less insomnia, and slower pulse rate. Because it has a short half-life, PTU is usually administered several times a day. Propylthiouracil is the preferred antithyroid drug for treating thyroid storm.

ADMINISTRATION ALERTS

- Administer with meals to reduce GI distress.
- Pregnancy category D

PHARMACOKINETICS

Onset: 30–40 min

Peak: 1–1.5 h

Half-life: 1–2 h

Duration: 2–4 h

ADVERSE EFFECTS

Overtreatment with propylthiouracil produces symptoms of hypothyroidism. Rash and transient leucopenia are the most frequent adverse effects. A small percentage of patients experience agranulocytosis, which is its most serious adverse effect. Periodic laboratory blood counts and TSH values are necessary to establish proper dosage.

Contraindications: Propylthiouracil should not be given during pregnancy or lactation or to patients with known or suspected hypothyroidism.

INTERACTIONS

Drug–Drug: Propylthiouracil increases the actions of anticoagulants, which carries an increased risk of bleeding. Iodine-containing agents (amiodarone, potassium iodide, sodium iodide) and thyroid hormones can antagonize the effectiveness of this drug. Cross-hypersensitivity occurs in about 50% of patients who have experienced a hypersensitivity reaction to methimazole, the other major antithyroid medication.

Lab Tests: Propylthiouracil may increase prothrombin time and increase serum levels of aspartate aminotransferase (AST), alanine aminotransferase (ALT), and alkaline phosphatase (ALP).

Herbal/Food: Unknown

Treatment of Overdose: Overdose will cause signs of hypothyroidism. Treatment includes a thyroid agent, atropine for bradycardia, and symptomatic treatment as necessary.

Refer to MyNursingKit for a Nursing Process Focus specific to this drug.

NURSING PROCESS FOCUS   PATIENTS RECEIVING PHARMACOTHERAPY FOR THYROID DISORDERS: THYROID REPLACEMENT AND ANTITHYROID DRUGS

Assessment	Potential Nursing Diagnoses
Baseline assessment prior to administration: ■ Understand the reason the drug has been prescribed in order to assess for therapeutic effects (e.g., treatment of hypothyroidism or hyperthyroidism). ■ Obtain a complete health history including cardiovascular, gastrointestinal, hepatic, or renal disease; pregnancy; or breast-feeding. Obtain a drug history including allergies, current prescription and OTC drugs, herbal preparations, alcohol use, or smoking. Be alert to possible drug interactions. ■ Evaluate appropriate laboratory findings (e.g., T_3, T_4, and TSH levels, CBC, platelets, electrolytes, glucose, and lipid levels). ■ Obtain baseline height, weight, and vital signs. Obtain an ECG as needed.	■ Activity Intolerance ■ Fatigue ■ Constipation ■ Deficient Knowledge (drug therapy) ■ Risk for Infection (related to adverse drug effects)
Assessment throughout administration: ■ Assess for desired therapeutic effects dependent on the reason the drug is being given (e.g., T_3, T_4, and TSH levels return to normal, associated symptoms of hypo- or hyperthyroidism ease). ■ Continue periodic monitoring of T_3, T_4, and TSH levels; CBC; platelets; and glucose. ■ Continue monitoring vital signs, height, and weight. Monitor the ECG as needed. ■ Assess for adverse effects: nausea, vomiting, diarrhea, epigastric distress, skin rash, itching, headache, tachycardia, palpitations, dysrhythmias, sweating, nervousness, paresthesias, tremors, insomnia, heat intolerance, and angina. Hypo- or hypertension, tachycardia, especially associated with angina, should be reported immediately.	

Planning: Patient Goals and Expected Outcomes

The patient will:
■ Experience therapeutic effects (e.g., decrease in symptoms, thyroid lab studies return to within normal limits).
■ Be free from, or experience minimal, adverse effects.
■ Verbalize an understanding of the drug's use, adverse effects, and required precautions.
■ Demonstrate proper self-administration of the medication (e.g., dose, timing, when to notify provider).

Implementation

Interventions and (Rationales)	Patient and Family Education
Ensuring therapeutic effects: ■ Monitor vital signs, appetite, weight, sensitivity to heat or cold, sleep patterns, and ADLs for return to normal limits. (The patient should return to more normal ADLs and feelings of wellness. Weight and pulse rate are measured to assess therapeutic response to drug therapy.)	■ Advise the patient that the drug will help to stabilize thyroid hormone levels quickly, but full effects may take a week or longer to occur. ■ Instruct the patient to maintain consistent dosing during this initial period to allow the drug to reach therapeutic levels. ■ Instruct the patient to weigh self two to three times per week and to record the pulse rate. Bring the record of weight and pulse to each provider visit.
■ Monitor diet for iodine-containing foods (e.g., iodized salt, soy sauce, tofu, yogurt, milk, strawberries, eggs). (Increasing or decreasing normal iodine intake may result in adverse drug effects.)	■ Provide dietary instruction on foods to avoid. Provide dietitian consultation as needed.
■ Monitor thyroid function tests. (Results help determine the effectiveness of the drug therapy and the need for dosage changes.)	■ Instruct the patient on the need to return periodically for lab work.
Minimizing adverse effects: ■ Monitor for return of original symptoms and report consistent occurrence. (Daily fluctuations in symptoms may occur. Significant increases in original symptoms may signal suboptimal results. Dramatic "opposite" effect and hypo- or hyperthyroid symptoms may signal drug toxicity.)	■ Teach the patient that small daily fluctuations may occur, especially during periods of stress or illness. Any significant or increasing changes in pulse rate, weight, nervousness or fatigue, intolerance to heat or cold, and diarrhea or constipation should be reported to the health care provider.

NURSING PROCESS FOCUS   **PATIENTS RECEIVING PHARMACOTHERAPY FOR THYROID DISORDERS: THYROID REPLACEMENT AND ANTITHYROID DRUGS** *(Continued)*

Implementation

Interventions and (Rationales)	Patient and Family Education
■ Monitor for signs of infection, CBC and platelet counts. (Antithyroid drugs may cause agranulocytosis.)	■ Instruct the patient to report fever, rashes, sore throat, chills, malaise, or weakness to the health care provider.
■ Monitor symptoms in older adults more frequently. (Older adults are more sensitive to thyroid replacement therapy. Minor changes in daily thyroid levels may cause a significant change in symptoms.)	■ Teach the patient and family or caregiver that the lowest dose will be started and gradually increased to find the optimum level. Any significant change in symptoms should be reported to the health care provider promptly.
■ Monitor serum glucose levels, especially in patients with diabetes. Diabetics should monitor capillary levels more frequently. (Thyroid and antithyroid drugs may cause changes in glucose levels.)	■ Teach the diabetic patient to monitor capillary glucose levels more frequently during therapy. Report any consistent elevations in blood glucose to the health care provider.
■ Ensure patient safety, especially in older adults. Observe for dizziness and monitor ambulation until the effects of the drug are known. (Dizziness may be secondary to changes in pulse or blood pressure. Effects of thyroid hormone on bone remodeling may place the patient at risk for fractures.)	■ Instruct the patient to call for assistance prior to getting out of bed or attempting to walk alone if dizziness occurs. ■ Assess the safety of the home environment and discuss modifications that may be needed with the family or caregiver.
■ Ensure patient and caregiver safety if radioactive iodine is used. (Radioactive iodine provides low-dose radiation but prolonged contact by health care providers or visitors should be avoided.)	■ Teach the patient to limit contact with family to 1 hour per day per person until the treatment period is over. Young children and pregnant women should avoid contact. ■ Advise the patient to increase fluid intake and to void frequently to avoid irradiation to gonads from radioactivity in the urine. ■ Instruct the patient not to expectorate and to cover the mouth when coughing. Any contaminated tissues should be disposed of per the protocol of the health care provider.
Patient understanding of drug therapy: ■ Use opportunities during administration of medications and during assessments to discuss the rationale for drug therapy, desired therapeutic outcomes, most common adverse effects, parameters for when to call the health care provider, and any necessary monitoring or precautions. (Using time during nursing care helps to optimize and reinforce key teaching areas.)	■ The patient should be able to state the reason for the drug, appropriate dose and scheduling, and what adverse effects to observe for and when to report them.

Patient self-administration of drug therapy:
■ When administering the medication, instruct the patient, family, or caregiver in the proper self-administration of the drug, e.g., take the drug in the morning at the same time each day. (Proper administration will increase the effectiveness of the drug.)
	■ Teach the patient to take the drug according to appropriate guidelines, as follows:
	   ■ Take the drug at the same time each morning to approximate normal body hormone levels.
	   ■ Take the drug with food or a meal.
	   ■ Avoid foods high in iodine unless approved by the health care provider.
	   ■ To ensure a therapeutic response, take the same brand of drug and request same manufacturer each time the drug is filled. Do not switch brand names without the approval of the health care provider.

Evaluation of Outcome Criteria

Evaluate the effectiveness of drug therapy by confirming that patient goals and expected outcomes have been met (see "Planning").

See Table 43.3 for a list of drugs to which these nursing actions apply.

MINERALOCORTICOIDS

Aldosterone accounts for more than 95% of the mineralocorticoids secreted by the adrenals. The primary function of aldosterone is to regulate plasma volume by promoting sodium reabsorption and potassium excretion by the renal tubules. When plasma volume falls, the kidney secretes renin, which results in the production of angiotensin II. Angiotensin II then causes aldosterone secretion, which promotes sodium and water retention. Attempts to modify this pathway led to the development of the angiotensin-converting enzyme (ACE) inhibitor class of medications, which are often preferred drugs for treating hypertension and heart failure (chapters 23 and 24 ∞). Certain adrenal tumors cause excessive secretion of aldosterone, a condition known as *hyperaldosteronism,* which is characterized by hypertension and hypokalemia.

GLUCOCORTICOIDS

More than 30 glucocorticoids are secreted from the adrenal cortex, including cortisol, corticosterone, and cortisone. Cortisol, also called *hydrocortisone,* is secreted in the highest amount, and is the most important pharmacologically. Glucocorticoids affect the metabolism of nearly every cell and prepare the body for long-term stress. The effects of glucocorticoids are diverse, and include the following:

- Increasing the level of blood glucose (hyperglycemic effect) by inhibiting insulin secretion and promoting gluconeogenesis, the synthesis of carbohydrates from lipid and protein sources
- Increasing the breakdown of proteins and lipids and promoting their utilization as energy sources
- Suppressing the inflammatory and immune responses (chapters 32 and 33 ∞)
- Increasing the sensitivity of vascular smooth muscle to norepinephrine and angiotensin II
- Increasing the breakdown of bony matrix, resulting in bone demineralization
- Promoting bronchodilation by making bronchial smooth muscle more responsive to sympathetic nervous system activation
- Influencing the CNS by affecting mood and maintaining normal brain excitability

43.9 Regulation of Glucocorticoid Secretion

Control of glucocorticoid levels in the blood begins with corticotropin-releasing factor (CRF), secreted by the hypothalamus. CRF travels to the pituitary where it causes the release of **adrenocorticotropic hormone (ACTH).** ACTH then travels through the blood to reach the adrenal cortex, causing it to release glucocorticoids. When the level of cortisol in the blood rises, it provides negative feedback to the hypothalamus and the pituitary to shut off further release of glucocorticoids. This negative feedback mechanism is shown in ➤ Figure 43.4.

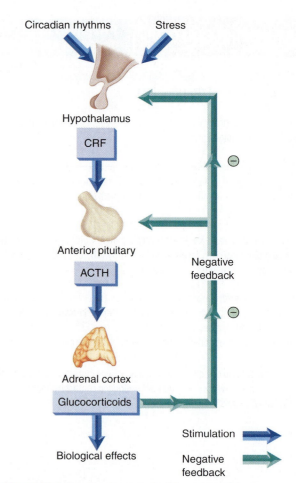

➤ **Figure 43.4** Feedback control of the adrenal cortex

Lack of adequate glucocorticoid production, known as **adrenocortical insufficiency,** may be caused by either hyposecretion of the adrenal cortex or inadequate secretion of ACTH from the pituitary. Cosyntropin (Cortrosyn) closely resembles ACTH and is used to diagnose the cause of the adrenocortical insufficiency. After administration of a small dose of cosyntropin, plasma levels of cortisol are measured to determine if the adrenal gland responded to the stimulation. A rise in plasma cortisol level indicates that the adrenal cortex is responsive to the ACTH challenge; the cause of the patient's adrenocortical insufficiency is likely at the level of the pituitary. Lack of cortisol increase suggests that the adrenal gland is unreceptive to the ACTH stimulation; the cause of the patient's adrenocortical insufficiency is likely at the level of the adrenal gland.

GLUCOCORTICOIDS

The glucocorticoids are used as replacement therapy for patients with adrenocortical insufficiency and to dampen inflammatory and immune responses. The glucocorticoids, listed in Table 43.4, are one of the most widely prescribed drug classes.

TABLE 43.4	Selected Glucocorticoids	
Drug	**Route and Adult Dose (max dose where indicated)**	**Adverse Effects**
SHORT ACTING		
cortisone	PO; 20–300 mg/day	*Sodium/fluid retention, nausea, acne, anxiety, insomnia, mood swings, increased appetite, weight gain, facial flushing*
⊕ hydrocortisone (Cortef, Hydrocortone, others)	PO; 10–320 mg/day in three to four divided doses	
	IV/IM; 15–800 mg/day in three to four divided doses (max: 2 g/day)	
INTERMEDIATE ACTING		Impaired wound healing, masking of infections, adrenal atrophy, hypokalemia, peptic ulcers, glaucoma, osteoporosis, muscle wasting/weakness, CHF, edema, worsening of psychoses
methylprednisolone (Dep-Medrol, Medrol, others)	PO; 2–60 mg one to four times/day	
prednisolone	PO; 5–60 mg one to four times/day	
prednisone (see page 471 for the Prototype Drug box ∞)	PO; 5–60 mg one to four times/day	
triamcinolone (Aristospan, Kenalog)	PO; 4–48 mg one to two times/day	
LONG ACTING		
betamethasone (Celestone, Betacort, others)	PO; 0.6–7.2 mg/day	
dexamethasone	IM; 0.5–9 mg/day	
	PO; 0.25–9 mg bid–qid	

Italics indicate common adverse effects; underlining indicates serious adverse effects.

43.10 Pharmacotherapy with Glucocorticoids

Symptoms of adrenocortical insufficiency include hypoglycemia, fatigue, hypotension, increased skin pigmentation, and GI disturbances such as anorexia, vomiting, and diarrhea. Low plasma cortisol, accompanied by high plasma ACTH levels, is diagnostic, because this indicates that the adrenal gland is not responding to ACTH stimulation. *Primary* adrenocortical insufficiency, known as **Addison's disease,** is quite rare and includes a deficiency of both glucocorticoids and mineralocorticoids. Autoimmune destruction of both adrenal glands is the most common cause of Addison's disease. *Secondary* adrenocortical insufficiency is more common than primary and can occur when corticosteroids are suddenly withdrawn during pharmacotherapy.

When glucocorticoids are taken as medications for prolonged periods, they provide negative feedback to the pituitary to stop secreting ACTH. Without stimulation by ACTH, the adrenal cortex shrinks and stops secreting *endogenous* glucocorticoids, a condition known as *adrenal atrophy.* If the glucocorticoid medication is abruptly discontinued, the shrunken adrenal glands will not be able to secrete sufficient glucocorticoids, and symptoms of acute adrenocortical insufficiency will appear. Symptoms include nausea, vomiting, lethargy, confusion, and coma. Immediate administration of IV therapy with hydrocortisone is essential, as shock may quickly result if symptoms remain untreated. Acute adrenocortical insufficiency can be prevented by discontinuing glucocorticoids gradually. Other possible causes of acute adrenocortical insufficiency include infection, trauma, and cancer. The development of adrenal atrophy following corticosteroid administration is shown in Pharmacotherapy Illustrated 43.1.

For chronic adrenocortical insufficiency, replacement therapy with glucocorticoids is indicated. The goal of replacement therapy is to achieve the same physiologic level of hormones in the blood that would be present if the adrenal glands were functioning properly. Patients requiring replacement therapy usually must take glucocorticoids their entire lifetime, and concurrent therapy with a mineralocorticoid such as fludrocortisone (Florinef) is necessary.

In addition to treating adrenal insufficiency, glucocorticoids are prescribed for a large number of "nonendocrine" disorders. Their ability to quickly and effectively suppress the inflammatory and immune responses gives them tremendous therapeutic utility to treat a diverse set of conditions. Indeed, no other drug class is used for so many different indications. Following are the indications for pharmacotherapy with glucocorticoids:

- Adrenal insufficiency
- Allergies, including allergic rhinitis (chapter 38 ∞)
- Asthma (chapter 39 ∞)
- Inflammatory bowel disease, including ulcerative colitis and Crohn's disease (chapter 41 ∞)
- Edema associated with hepatic, neurologic, and renal disorders
- Cancer, including Hodgkin's disease, leukemias, and lymphomas (chapter 37 ∞)
- Transplant rejection prophylaxis (chapter 32 ∞)
- Rheumatic disorders, including rheumatoid arthritis, ankylosing spondylitis, and bursitis (chapter 47 ∞)
- Shock (chapter 29 ∞)
- Skin disorders, including contact dermatitis and rashes (chapter 48 ∞)

PHARMACOTHERAPY ILLUSTRATED

43.1 Corticosteroids (Glucocorticoids) and Adrenal Atrophy

1. Normal adrenal glands

Corticosteroid Therapy

2. Adrenal gland atrophy following corticosteroid therapy

Gradual Discontinuation   Sudden Discontinuation

3. Gradual withdrawal of corticosteroids allows adrenal glands to resume normal function

4. Sudden withdraw of corticosteroids leads to acute
- adrenal insufficiency
- hypotension
- lethargy
- renal failure
- asthenia
- nausea/vomiting

More than 20 glucocorticoids are available as medications, and choice of a particular agent depends primarily on the pharmacokinetic properties of the drug. The duration of action, which is often used to classify these agents, ranges from short to long acting. Some, such as hydrocortisone, have mineralocorticoid activity that causes sodium and fluid retention; others, such as prednisone, have no such effect. Some glucocorticoids are available by only one route: for example, topical for dermal conditions or intranasal for allergic rhinitis.

Glucocorticoids interact with many drugs. Their hyperglycemic effects may decrease the effectiveness of antidiabetic agents. Combining glucocorticoids with other ulcerogenic drugs such as aspirin and other NSAIDs markedly increases the risk of peptic ulcer disease. Administration with non–potassium-sparing diuretics may lead to hypocalcemia and hypokalemia.

High doses of glucocorticoids taken for prolonged periods offers a significant risk for serious adverse effects. These adverse effects, shown in Table 43.5, can impact nearly any body system. The following strategies are used to limit the incidence of serious adverse effects from glucocorticoids:

- Keep doses to the lowest possible amount that will achieve a therapeutic effect.
- Administer glucocorticoids every other day (alternate-day dosing) to limit adrenal atrophy.
- For acute conditions, give patients large amounts for a few days and then gradually decrease the drug dose until it is discontinued.

Give the drugs locally by inhalation, intra-articular injections, or topical applications to the skin, eyes, or ears, when feasible, to diminish the possibility of systemic effects.

43.11 Pharmacotherapy of Cushing's Syndrome

Cushing's syndrome occurs when high levels of glucocorticoids are present in the body over a prolonged period. Although hypersecretion of these hormones can be due to pituitary

TABLE 43.5	Adverse Effects of Long-Term Glucocorticoid Therapy
Type of Adverse Event	**Description**
Immune response	Suppression of the immune and inflammatory responses increases patients' susceptibility to infections. Their anti-inflammatory actions may mask the signs of an existing infection.
Peptic ulcers	Development of peptic ulcers may occur, especially when combined with nonsteroidal anti-inflammatory drugs (NSAIDs).
Osteoporosis	Up to 50% of patients on long-term therapy will suffer a fracture due to osteoporosis.
Behavioral changes	Psychologic changes may be minor, such as nervousness or moodiness, or may involve hallucinations and increased suicidal tendencies.
Eye changes	Cataracts and open-angle glaucoma are associated with long-term therapy.
Metabolic changes	Their hyperglycemic effect raises serum glucose and can cause glucose intolerance. Mobilization of lipids may cause hyperlipidemia and abnormal fat deposits. Electrolyte changes include hypocalcemia, hypokalemia, and hypernatremia. Fluid retention, weight gain, hypertension, and edema are common.
Myopathy	Muscle wasting causes weakness and fatigue; may involve ocular or respiratory muscles.

Pr Prototype Drug | Hydrocortisone *(Cortef, Hydrocortone, others)*

Therapeutic Class: Adrenal hormone   **Pharmacologic Class:** Corticosteroid

ACTIONS AND USES

Structurally identical with the natural hormone cortisol, hydrocortisone is a synthetic corticosteroid that is the drug of choice for treating adrenocortical insufficiency. When used for replacement therapy, it is given at physiologic doses. Once proper dosing is achieved, its therapeutic effects should mimic those of endogenous corticosteroids. Hydrocortisone is also available for the treatment of inflammation, allergic disorders, and many other conditions. Intra-articular injections may be given to decrease severe inflammation in affected joints.

Hydrocortisone is available in six different formulations. Hydrocortisone base (Aeroseb-HC, Alphaderm, Cetacort, others) and hydrocortisone acetate (Anusol HC, Cortaid, Cortef Acetate) are available as oral preparations, creams, and ointments. Hydrocortisone cypionate (Cortef Fluid) is an oral suspension. Hydrocortisone sodium phosphate (Hydrocortone Phosphate) and hydrocortisone sodium succinate (A-Hydrocort, Solu-Cortef) are for parenteral use only. Hydrocortisone valerate (Westcort) is only for topical applications.

ADMINISTRATION ALERTS

- Administer exactly as prescribed and at the same time every day.
- Administer oral formulations with food.
- Pregnancy category C

PHARMACOKINETICS

Onset: 1–2 h PO; 20 min IM

Peak: 1 h PO; 4–8 h IM

Half-life: 1.5–2 h

Duration: 1–1.5 days PO or IM

ADVERSE EFFECTS

When used at low doses for replacement therapy, or by the topical or intranasal routes, adverse effects of hydrocortisone are rare. However, signs of Cushing's syndrome can develop with high doses or with prolonged use. If taken for longer than 2 weeks, hydrocortisone should be discontinued gradually. Hydrocortisone possesses some mineralocorticoid activity, so sodium and fluid retention may be noted. A wide range of CNS effects have been reported, including insomnia, anxiety, headache, vertigo, confusion, and depression. Cardiovascular effects may include hypertension and tachycardia. Long-term therapy may result in peptic ulcer disease.

Contraindications: Hydrocortisone is contraindicated in patients who are hypersensitive to the drug or who have known infections, unless the patient is being treated concurrently with anti-infectives. Patients with diabetes, osteoporosis, psychoses, liver disease, or hypothyroidism should be treated with caution.

INTERACTIONS

Drug–Drug: Barbiturates, phenytoin, and rifampin may increase hepatic metabolism, thus decreasing hydrocortisone levels. Estrogens potentiate the effects of hydrocortisone. Use with nonsteroidal anti-inflammatory drugs (NSAIDS) increases the risk of peptic ulcers. Cholestyramine and colestipol decrease hydrocortisone absorption. Diuretics and amphotericin B increase the risk of hypokalemia. Anticholinesterase agents may produce severe weakness. Hydrocortisone may cause a decrease in immune response to vaccines and toxoids.

Lab Tests: Hydrocortisone may increase serum values for glucose, cholesterol, sodium, uric acid, or calcium. It may decrease serum values of potassium and T_3/T_4.

Herbal/Food: Use of hydrocortisone with senna, cascara, or buckthorn may cause potassium deficiency with chronic use.

Treatment of Overdose: Hydrocortisone has no acute toxicity and deaths are rare. No specific therapy is available and patients are treated symptomatically.

Refer to MyNursingKit for a Nursing Process Focus specific to this drug.

Assessment	Potential Nursing Diagnoses
Baseline assessment prior to administration: ■ Understand the reason the drug has been prescribed in order to assess for therapeutic effects (e.g., replacement therapy, treatment of specific conditions such as autoimmune disorders or allergic responses). ■ Obtain a complete health history including cardiovascular, respiratory, neurologic, hepatic, or renal disease; pregnancy; or breast-feeding. Obtain a drug history including allergies, current prescription and OTC drugs, herbal preparations, caffeine, nicotine, and alcohol use. Be alert to possible drug interactions. ■ Obtain baseline vital signs and weight. ■ Evaluate appropriate laboratory findings (e.g., CBC, platelets, electrolytes, glucose, lipid profile, hepatic or renal function studies).	■ Deficient Knowledge (drug therapy) ■ Risk for Fluid Volume Excess (related to fluid retention properties of glucocorticoids) ■ Risk for Injury (related to adverse drug effects) ■ Risk for Infections (related to adverse drug effects) ■ Risk for Impaired Skin Integrity (related to adverse drug effects)
Assessment throughout administration: ■ Assess for desired therapeutic effects (e.g., signs and symptoms of inflammation such as redness or swelling are decreased). ■ Continue periodic monitoring of CBC, platelets, electrolytes, glucose, lipid profile, and hepatic or renal function studies. ■ Assess vital signs and weight periodically or if symptoms warrant. Obtain the weight daily and report any weight gain over 1 kg in a 24-hour period or more than 2 kg in 1 week. ■ Assess for and promptly report adverse effects: nausea, vomiting, symptoms of GI bleeding (dark or "tarry" stools, hematemesis or coffee-ground emesis, blood in the stool), abdominal pain, dizziness, confusion, agitation, euphoria or depression, palpitations, tachycardia, hypertension, increased respiratory rate and depth, pulmonary congestion, significant weight gain, edema, blurred vision, fever, and infections.	

Planning: Patient Goals and Expected Outcomes

The patient will:
■ Experience therapeutic effects (e.g., decreased signs and symptoms of inflammation or allergic response).
■ Be free from, or experience minimal, adverse effects.
■ Verbalize an understanding of the drug's use, adverse effects, and required precautions.
■ Demonstrate proper self-administration of the medication (e.g., dose, timing, when to notify provider).

Implementation

Interventions and (Rationales)	Patient and Family Education
Ensuring therapeutic effects: ■ Continue assessments as described earlier for therapeutic effects. (Diminished inflammation, allergic response, and increased feelings of wellness should begin after taking the first dose and continue to improve.)	■ Teach the patient to report any return of original symptoms or increase in inflammation, allergic response, or generalized malaise to the health care provider.
Minimizing adverse effects: ■ Continue to monitor vital signs, especially blood pressure and pulse. Immediately report tachycardia or BP over 140/90 mm Hg, or per parameters as ordered, to the health care provider. (Corticosteroids may cause increased blood pressure, hypertension, and tachycardia due to the increased retention of fluids.)	■ Teach the patient how to monitor the pulse and blood pressure. Ensure the proper use and functioning of any home equipment obtained. Immediately report tachycardia, palpitations, or increased BP to the health care provider.
■ Continue to monitor periodic lab work: CBC, electrolytes, glucose, lipid levels, and hepatic and renal function tests. (Corticosteroids affect the CBC, and may cause hyperglycemia, hypernatremia, hyperlipidemia, and hypokalemia. Diabetics may require a change in their antidiabetic medication if the blood glucose remains elevated.)	■ Instruct the patient on the need to return periodically for lab work. ■ Advise the patient taking corticosteroids long term to carry a wallet identification card or wear medical identification jewelry indicating corticosteroid therapy. ■ Teach the diabetic patient to test the blood glucose more frequently, notifying the health care provider if a consistent elevation is noted.
■ Monitor for abdominal pain, black or tarry stools, blood in the stool, hematemesis or coffee-ground emesis, dizziness, and hypotension, especially if associated with tachycardia. (GI bleeding is an adverse drug effect.)	■ Instruct the patient to immediately report any signs or symptoms of GI bleeding. ■ Teach the patient to take the drug with food or milk to decrease GI irritation. Alcohol use should be avoided or eliminated.

NURSING PROCESS FOCUS　　**PATIENTS RECEIVING SYSTEMIC GLUCOCORTICOID THERAPY** *(Continued)*

Implementation

Interventions and (Rationales)	Patient and Family Education
■ Monitor for signs and symptoms of infection. (Corticosteroids suppress the immune and inflammatory responses and may mask the signs of infection.)	■ Instruct the patient to immediately report any signs or symptoms of infections (e.g., increasing temperature or fever, sore throat, redness or swelling at site of injury, white patches in mouth, vesicular rash).
■ Monitor for osteoporosis [e.g., bone density testing] periodically in patients on long-term corticosteroids. Encourage adequate calcium intake, avoidance of carbonated sodas, and weight-bearing exercise. (Corticosteroids affect bone metabolism and may cause osteoporosis and fractures. Weight-bearing exercise stresses bone and encourages normal bone remodeling. Excessive or long-term consumption of carbonated sodas has been linked to an increased risk of osteoporosis.)	■ Teach the patient to maintain adequate calcium in the diet, avoid carbonated sodas, and to do weight-bearing exercises at least three to four times per week. ■ Teach the postmenopausal woman to consult with her provider about the need for additional drug therapy (e.g., bisphosphonates) for osteoporosis.
■ Monitor for unusual changes in mood or affect. (Corticosteroids may cause an increased or decreased mood, euphoria, depression, or severe mental instability.)	■ Teach the patient, family, or caregiver to promptly report excessive mood swings or unusual changes in mood.
■ Weigh the patient daily and report weight gain or increasing peripheral edema. Measure the intake and output in the hospitalized patient. (Daily weight is an accurate measure of fluid status and takes into account intake, output, and insensible losses.)	■ Instruct the patient to weigh self daily, ideally at the same time of day. The patient should report a weight gain of more than 1 kg (approximately 2 lb) in a 24-hour period or more than 2 kg (approximately 4–5 lb) per week, or increasing peripheral edema.
■ Monitor vision periodically in patients on corticosteroids. (Corticosteroids may cause increased intraocular pressure and an increased risk or glaucoma, and may cause cataracts.)	■ Teach the patient to maintain eye exams twice yearly or more frequently as instructed by the provider. Immediately report any eye pain, rainbow halos around lights, diminished vision, or blurring and inability to focus.
■ Do not stop the drug abruptly. The drug must be tapered off if used longer than 1 or 2 weeks. (Adrenal insufficiency and crisis may occur with profound hypotension, tachycardia, and other adverse effects if drug is stopped abruptly.)	■ Teach the patient to not stop corticosteroids abruptly and to notify the health care provider if unable to take the medication for more than 1 day due to illness.

Implementation

Interventions and (Rationales)	Patient and Family Education
Patient understanding of drug therapy: ■ Use opportunities during administration of medications and during assessments to discuss the rationale for drug therapy, desired therapeutic outcomes, most commonly observed adverse effects, parameters for when to call the health care provider, and any necessary monitoring or precautions. (Using time during nursing care helps to optimize and reinforce key teaching areas.)	■ The patient, family, or caregiver should be able to state the reason for the drug; appropriate dose and scheduling; what adverse effects to observe for and when to report them; and the anticipated length of medication therapy.
Patient self-administration of drug therapy: ■ When administering the medication, instruct the patient, family or caregiver in the proper self-administration of drug, e.g., with food or milk. (Proper administration will increase the effectiveness of the drug.)	■ The patient and family or caregiver are able to discuss appropriate dosing and administration needs, including: 　■ Take drug in the morning at the same time each day. 　■ Take drug with food, milk, or a meal to prevent GI upset. 　■ Household measuring devices such as teaspoons differ significantly in size and amount and should not be used for pediatric or liquid doses.

Evaluation of Outcome Criteria

Evaluate the effectiveness of drug therapy by confirming that patient goals and expected outcomes have been met (see "Planning").

See Table 43.4 for a list of drugs to which these nursing actions apply.

(due to excess ACTH) or adrenal tumors, the most common cause of Cushing's syndrome is long-term therapy with high doses of systemic glucocorticoids. Signs and symptoms include adrenal atrophy, osteoporosis, hypertension, increased risk of infections, delayed wound healing, acne, peptic ulcers, general obesity, and a redistribution of fat around the face (moon face), shoulders, and neck (buffalo hump). Mood and personality changes may occur, and the patient may become psychologically dependent on the drug. Some glucocorticoids, including hydrocortisone, also have mineralocorticoid activity and can cause retention of sodium and water. Because of their anti-inflammatory properties, glucocorticoids may mask signs of infection, and a resulting delay in antibiotic therapy may result.

Because Cushing's syndrome has a high mortality rate, the primary therapeutic goal is to identify and treat the cause of the excess glucocorticoid secretion. If the patient is receiving high doses of a glucocorticoid medication, gradual discontinuation of the agent is often sufficient to reverse the syndrome. When the cause of the hypersecretion is an adrenal tumor or perhaps an ectopic tumor secreting ACTH, surgical removal is indicated.

Metyrapone (Metopirone) is an antiadrenal drug used for diagnostic purposes. A single dose is administered orally at midnight, and blood samples are taken 8 hours later. Levels of ACTH and glucocorticoids are measured to determine if the adrenal glands responded to the inhibiting action of metyrapone. The drug may also be used off-label to treat Cushing's disease.

The antifungal drug ketoconazole (Nizoral) has become a preferred drug for patients with Cushing's disease who need long-term therapy. This drug rapidly blocks the synthesis of glucocorticoids, lowering serum levels. Unfortunately, patients often develop tolerance to the drug and glucocorticoids eventually return to abnormally high levels. Ketoconazole should not be used during pregnancy because it has been shown to be teratogenic in animals.

Mifepristone (Mifeprex) is a steroid that occupies glucocorticoid receptors; it does not block the synthesis of glucocorticoids or decrease their amounts. Although it has antiadrenal actions, its primary use is as an abortifacient: The drug is pregnancy category X and will induce abortion early in pregnancy.

None of the above drug therapies cure Cushing's disease. Their use is temporary until the tumor can be removed or otherwise treated with radiation or antineoplastics.

Chapter REVIEW

KEY CONCEPTS

The numbered key concepts provide a succinct summary of the important points from the corresponding numbered section within the chapter. If any of these points are not clear, refer to the numbered section within the chapter for review.

43.1 The endocrine system maintains homeostasis by using hormones as chemical messengers that are secreted in response to changes in the internal environment. Negative feedback prevents over-responses by the endocrine system.

43.2 The hypothalamus secretes releasing hormones, which direct the anterior pituitary gland to release specific hormones. The posterior pituitary releases its hormones in response to nerve signals from the hypothalamus.

43.3 Hormones are used in replacement therapy, as antineoplastics, and for their natural therapeutic effects, such as their suppression of body defenses. Hormone blockers are used to inhibit actions of certain hormones.

43.4 Only a few pituitary and hypothalamic hormones, including growth hormone and ACTH, have clinical applications as drugs. Growth hormone and ADH are examples of pituitary hormones used as drugs for replacement therapy.

43.5 The thyroid gland secretes thyroxine (T_4) and triiodothyronine (T_3), which control the basal metabolic rate and affect every cell in the body.

43.6 Hypothyroidism may be treated by administering thyroid hormone agents, especially levothyroxine (T_4).

43.7 Hyperthyroidism is treated by administering agents such as the thioamides that decrease the activity of the thyroid gland or by using radioactive iodide, which kills overactive thyroid cells.

43.8 The adrenal cortex secretes glucocorticoids, gonadocorticoids, and mineralocorticoids. The glucocorticoids mobilize the body for long-term stress and influence carbohydrate, lipid, and protein metabolism in most cells.

43.9 Glucocorticoid release is stimulated by ACTH secreted by the pituitary. ACTH and related agents are rarely used as medications.

43.10 Adrenocortical insufficiency may be acute or chronic. Glucocorticoids are prescribed for adrenocortical insufficiency, allergies, neoplasms, and a wide variety of other conditions.

43.11 Antiadrenal drugs may be used to treat severe Cushing's syndrome by inhibiting corticosteroid synthesis. They are not curative, and their use is usually limited to 3 months of therapy.

NCLEX-RN® REVIEW QUESTIONS

1 The nurse recognizes that drugs from which of the following classes cause increased risk for peptic ulcers, decreased wound healing, and increased capillary fragility?
1. Glucocorticoids
2. Antidiuretic hormones
3. Growth hormones
4. Antithyroid hormones

2 When administering hydrocortisone (Cortef, hydrocortone, others), the nurse recognizes it may mask which symptoms?
1. Signs and symptoms of infection
2. Signs and symptoms of heart failure
3. Hearing loss
4. Skin infections

3 When hydrocortisone use is discontinued abruptly, the nurse must assess for which side effect?
1. Development of myxedema
2. Circulatory collapse
3. Development of Cushing's syndrome
4. Development of diabetes insipidus

4 A patient who is taking levothyroxine (Synthroid) begins to develop weight loss, diarrhea, and stress intolerance. The nurse should be aware that this might be an indication of what hormonal condition?
1. Addison's disease
2. Hyperthyroidism
3. Cushing's syndrome
4. Development of acromegaly

5 What precautions should a patient who is receiving radioactive iodine be made aware of? (Select all that apply.)
1. Drink plenty of fluids, especially those high in calcium.
2. Avoid close contact with children or pregnant women for 1 week after administration of the drug.
3. Be aware of symptoms of tachycardia, increased metabolic rate, and anxiety.
4. Wear a mask if around children and pregnant women.
5. Signs and symptoms of hypothyroidism include general weakness, muscle cramps, and dry skin.

6 A patient with diabetes insipidus has stabilized but will be discharged home on desmopressin (DDAVP, Stimate) by nasal spray. When administering desmospressin intranasally, all of the following administration guidelines should be followed EXCEPT:
1. gently rotate the nasal spray bottle before spraying but do not shake.
2. store the bottle at room temperature but avoid excessive heat over 80° F.
3. spray the nasal spray high into nasal cavity, avoiding the back of the throat.
4. use the spray each morning at the same time of day.

CRITICAL THINKING QUESTIONS

1. A 5-year-old girl requires treatment for diabetes insipidus acquired following a case of meningitis. The child has suffered serious complications including blindness and mental retardation. Her diabetes insipidus is being treated with intranasal desmopressin, and the child's mother has been asked to help evaluate the drug's effectiveness using urine volumes and urine specific gravity. Discuss the changes that would indicate that the drug is effective.

2. A 17-year-old adolescent with a history of severe asthma is admitted to the intensive care unit. He is comatose, appears much younger than his listed age, and has short stature. The nurse notes that the asthma has been managed with prednisone for 15 days, until 3 days ago. The patient's father is extremely anxious and says that he was unable to refill his son's prescription for medicine until he got his paycheck. What is the nurse's role in this situation?

3. A 9-year-old boy has been diagnosed with growth hormone deficiency. His parents have decided to proceed with a prescribed regimen of somatotropin (Humatrope). Outline the basic information the parents need to know regarding this regimen, side effects, and evaluation of effectiveness.

See Appendix D for answers and rationales for all activities.

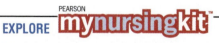

EXPLORE **mynursingkit™**

MyNursingKit is your one stop for online chapter review materials and resources. Prepare for success with additional NCLEX®-style practice questions, interactive assignments and activities, web links, animations and videos, and more!

Register your access code from the front of your book at
www.mynursingkit.com.

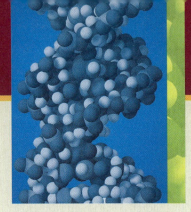

Chapter 44

Drugs for Diabetes Mellitus

DRUGS AT A GLANCE

INSULIN *page 680*
- **Pr** *human regular insulin (Humulin R, Novolin R)* *page 683*

ORAL HYPOGLYCEMICS *page 683*
- **Pr** *metformin (Fortamet, Glucophage, Glumetza, others)* *page 689*

LEARNING OUTCOMES

After reading this chapter, the student should be able to:

1. Describe the endocrine and exocrine functions of the pancreas.
2. Compare and contrast type 1 and type 2 diabetes mellitus.
3. Compare and contrast types of insulin.
4. Describe the signs and symptoms of insulin overdose and underdose.
5. Describe the nurse's role in the pharmacologic management of diabetes mellitus.
6. Identify drug classes used to treat type 2 diabetes mellitus.
7. For each of the drug classes listed in Drugs at a Glance, know representative drug examples, and explain the mechanisms of drug action, primary actions, and important adverse effects.
8. Use the nursing process to care for patients receiving drug therapy for diabetes mellitus.

KEY TERMS

Diabetes is one of the leading causes of death in the U.S. Mortality due to diabetes has been steadily increasing, causing some public health officials to refer to it as an epidemic. Diabetes can lead to serious acute and chronic complications, including heart disease, cerebrovascular accident (CVA), blindness, kidney failure, and amputations. Because nurses frequently care for patients with diabetes, it is imperative that the disorder, its treatment, and possible complications are well understood.

44.1 Regulation of Blood Glucose Levels

Located behind the stomach and between the duodenum and spleen, the pancreas is an organ essential to both the digestive and endocrine systems. It is responsible for the secretion of several enzymes into the duodenum that assist in the chemical digestion of nutrients (chapter 41∞). This is its exocrine function. Clusters of cells in the pancreas, called **islets of Langerhans,** are responsible for its endocrine function: the secretion of glucagon and insulin.

Glucose is one of the body's most essential molecules. The body prefers to use glucose as its primary energy source: The brain relies almost exclusively on glucose for its energy needs. Because of this need, blood levels of glucose must remain relatively constant throughout the day. Although many factors contribute to maintaining a stable serum glucose level, the two pancreatic hormones play major roles: **insulin** acts to *decrease* blood glucose levels, and **glucagon** acts to *increase* blood glucose levels (➤ Figure 44.1).

Following a meal, the pancreas recognizes the rising serum glucose level and releases insulin. Without insulin, glucose stays in the bloodstream and is not able to enter cells of the body. Cells may be virtually surrounded by glucose but they are unable to use it until insulin arrives. It may be helpful to visualize insulin as a transporter or "gatekeeper." When present, insulin swings open the gate, transporting glucose inside cells: no insulin, no entry. Thus, insulin is said to have a **hypoglycemic effect,** because its presence causes glucose to *leave* the blood and serum glucose to *fall*. The physiologic actions of insulin can be summarized as follows:

- Promotes the entry of glucose into cells
- Provides for the storage of glucose, as glycogen
- Inhibits the breakdown of fat and glycogen
- Increases protein synthesis and inhibits **gluconeogenesis;** the production of "new" glucose from noncarbohydrate molecules

The pancreas also secretes glucagon, which has actions *opposite* those of insulin. When levels of blood glucose fall, glucagon is secreted. Its primary function is to maintain adequate serum levels of glucose between meals. Thus, glucagon has a **hyperglycemic effect,** because its presence causes blood glucose to *rise*. ➤ Figure 44.2 illustrates the relationships among blood glucose, insulin, and glucagon.

Blood glucose levels are usually kept within a normal range by insulin and glucagon; however, other hormones and drugs can affect glucose metabolism. *Hyperglycemic* hormones include epinephrine, thyroid hormone, growth hormone, and glucocorticoids. Common drugs that can raise blood glucose levels include phenytoin, NSAIDs, and diuretics. Drugs with a *hypoglycemic* effect include alcohol, lithium, angiotensin-converting enzyme (ACE) inhibitors, and beta-adrenergic blockers. It is important that serum glucose be periodically monitored in patients receiving medications that exhibit hypoglycemia or hypoglycemic effects.

ALPHA CELL
Glucagon-secreting cell

BETA CELL
Insulin-secreting cell

Islet of Langerhans in pancreas

Glucagon—raises blood glucose level
Insulin—lowers blood glucose level

➤ *Figure 44.1* Glucagon- and insulin-secreting cells in the islets of Langerhans
Source: Pearson Education/PH College.

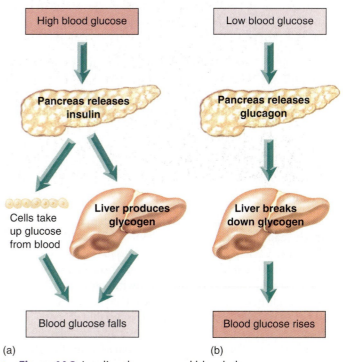

High blood glucose → Pancreas releases insulin → Cells take up glucose from blood / Liver produces glycogen → Blood glucose falls

Low blood glucose → Pancreas releases glucagon → Liver breaks down glycogen → Blood glucose rises

(a)   (b)

➤ *Figure 44.2* Insulin, glucagon, and blood glucose

DIABETES MELLITUS

Diabetes mellitus (DM) is a metabolic disease in which there is deficient insulin secretion or decreased sensitivity of insulin receptors on target cells, resulting in hyperglycemia. Worldwide, approximately 135 million people are believed to have DM; by 2025, this number is expected to have increased to 300 million. The etiology of DM includes a combination of genetic and environmental factors. The recent increase in the frequency of the disease is probably the result of trends toward more sedentary and stressful lifestyles, increasing consumption of highly caloric foods with resultant obesity, and increased longevity.

44.2 Etiology and Characteristics of Type 1 Diabetes Mellitus

Type 1 diabetes mellitus accounts for 5% to 10% of all cases of DM and is one of the most common diseases of childhood. Type 1 DM was previously called *juvenile-onset diabetes*, because it is often diagnosed between the ages of 11 and 13. Because approximately 25% of patients with type 1 DM develop the disease in adulthood, this is not the most accurate name for this disorder. This type of diabetes is also referred to as insulin-dependent diabetes mellitus.

Type 1 DM results from the autoimmune destruction of pancreatic beta cells, resulting in a lack of insulin secretion. The disease is thought to be an interaction of genetic, immunologic, and environmental factors. Because children and siblings of those with DM have a higher risk of acquiring the disorder, there is an obvious genetic component to the disease.

The signs and symptoms of type 1 DM are consistent from patient to patient, with the most diagnostic sign being sustained hyperglycemia. Following are the typical signs and symptoms:

- Hyperglycemia—fasting blood glucose greater than 126 mg/dL on at least two separate occasions
- Polyuria—excessive urination
- Polyphagia—increased hunger
- Polydipsia—increased thirst
- Glucosuria—high levels of glucose in the urine
- Weight loss
- Fatigue

Untreated DM produces long-term damage to arteries, which leads to heart disease, stroke, kidney disease, and blindness. Lack of adequate circulation to the feet may cause gangrene of the toes, requiring amputation. Nerve degeneration, or neuropathy, is common, with symptoms ranging from tingling in the fingers or toes to complete loss of sensation of a limb. Because glucose is unable to enter cells, lipids are utilized as an energy source and **ketoacids** are produced as waste products. These ketoacids can give the patient's breath an acetone-like, fruity odor. More important, high levels of ketoacids lower the pH of the blood, causing

diabetic ketoacidosis (DKA), which may progress to coma and possible death if untreated. DKA occurs primarily in patients with Type 1 DM.

Insulin

Insulin first became available as a medication in 1922. Prior to that time, type 1 diabetics were unable to adequately maintain normal blood glucose levels, experienced many complications, and usually died at a young age. Increased insulin availability and improvements in insulin products, personal blood glucose monitoring devices, and the insulin pump have made it possible for patients to maintain more exact control of their blood glucose levels.

44.3 Pharmacotherapy with Insulin

Patients with type 1 DM are severely deficient in insulin production; thus, insulin replacement therapy is required in normal physiologic amounts. Insulin is also required for those with type 2 diabetes who are unable to manage their blood glucose levels with diet, exercise, and oral antidiabetic agents. Among adults with diabetes in the United States, 16% take only insulin, 12% take insulin with oral agents, 57% take oral agents only, and 15% take neither insulin nor oral medication (CDC, 2005).

Because normal insulin secretion varies greatly in response to daily activities such as eating and exercise, insulin administration must be carefully planned in conjunction with proper meal planning and lifestyle habits. The desired outcome of insulin therapy is to prevent the long-term consequences of the disorder by strictly maintaining blood glucose levels within the normal range.

The fundamental principle to remember about insulin therapy is that the right amount of insulin must be available to cells when glucose is available in the blood. Administering insulin when glucose is *not* available can lead to serious hypoglycemia and coma. This situation occurs when a patient administers insulin correctly but skips a meal; the insulin is available to cells, but glucose is not. In another example, the patient participates in heavy exercise. The insulin may have been administered on schedule, and food eaten, but the active muscles quickly use up all the glucose in the blood, and the patient becomes hypoglycemic. Patients with diabetes who engage in competitive sports need to consume food or sports drinks just prior to or during the activity to maintain their blood sugar at normal levels.

Patients with diabetes who skip or forget their insulin dose face equally serious consequences. Again, remember the fundamental principle of insulin pharmacotherapy: The right amount of insulin must be available to cells when glucose is available in the blood. Without insulin present, glucose from a meal can build up to high levels in the blood, causing hyperglycemia and possible coma. Proper teaching and planning by the nurse is essential to successful outcomes and patient compliance with therapy.

Many types of insulin are available, differing in their source, time of onset and peak effect, and duration of action. Until the 1980s, the source of all insulin was beef or pork pancreas. Almost all insulin today, however, is human insulin obtained through recombinant DNA technology because it is more effective, causes fewer allergies, and has a lower incidence of resistance. Pharmacologists have modified human insulin to create certain pharmacokinetic advantages, such as a more rapid onset of action (Humalog) or a more prolonged duration of action (Lantus). These modified forms are called **insulin analogs**. The different types of insulin available are listed in Table 44.1.

Doses of insulin are highly individualized for the precise control of blood glucose levels in each patient. Some patients require two or more injections daily for proper diabetes management. For ease of administration, two different compatible types of insulin may be mixed, using a standard method, to obtain the desired therapeutic effects. Some of these combinations are marketed in cartridges containing premixed solutions. A long-acting insulin may be taken daily to provide a basal blood level, and supplemented with rapid-acting insulin given shortly before a meal. It is important for nurses and patients to know the time of peak action of any insulin, because that is when the risk for hypoglycemic adverse effects is greatest.

Because the GI tract destroys insulin, it must be given by injection. Some patients have an insulin pump (➤ Figure 44.3). This pump is usually abdominally anchored and is programmed to release small subcutaneous doses of insulin into the abdomen at predetermined intervals, with larger boluses administered manually at mealtime if necessary. Most pumps contain an alarm that sounds to remind patients to take their insulin. Figure 44.3 shows an insulin pump.

The primary adverse effect of insulin therapy is overtreatment; insulin may remove too much glucose from the blood, resulting in hypoglycemia. This occurs when a patient with type 1 DM has more insulin in the blood than is needed to balance the amount of circulating blood glucose. Hypoglycemia may occur when the insulin level peaks, during exercise, when the patient receives too much insulin due to a medication error, or if the patient skips a meal. Some of the symptoms of hypoglycemia are the same as those of diabetic ketoacidosis. Those that differ and help in determining that a patient is hypoglycemic include pale, cool, and moist skin, with blood glucose less than 50 mg/dL and a sudden onset of symptoms. Left untreated, severe hypoglycemia may result in death.

TABLE 44.1	Types of Insulin: Actions and Administration					
Drug	Action	Onset	Peak	Duration	Administration and Timing	Compatibility
insulin aspart (NovoLog)	Rapid	10–20 min	1–3 h	3–5 h	Subcutaneous; 5–10 min before a meal	Can give with NPH; draw aspart up first and give immediately
insulin lispro (Humalog)	Rapid	5–15 min	1–1.5 h	3–4 h	Subcutaneous; 5–10 min before a meal	Can give with NPH; draw lispro up first and give immediately
insulin glulisine (Apidra)	Rapid	15–30 min	1 h	3–4 h	Subcutaneous; 15 min before a meal	Can give with NPH; draw glulisine up first and give immediately
insulin regular (Humulin R, Novolin R)	Short	30–60 min	1–5 h	6–10 h	Subcutaneous; 30–60 min before a meal; IV	Can mix with NPH, sterile water, or normal saline; do not mix with glargine
isophane susp (NPH, Humulin N)	Intermediate	1–2 h	6–14 h	16–24 h	Subcutaneous; mix (cloudy)	Can mix with aspart, lispro, or regular; do not mix with glargine
insulin detemir (Levemir)	Long	Gradual	6–8 h	To 24 h	Subcutaneous; 1/day or 2/day	Do not mix with any other insulin
insulin glargine (Lantus)	Long	1.1 h	No peak	To 24 h	Subcutaneous; 1/day, same time each day	Do not mix with any other insulin

MyNursingKit Administering Subcutaneous Medications

MyNursingKit Administering Subcutaneous Medications (Abdomen)

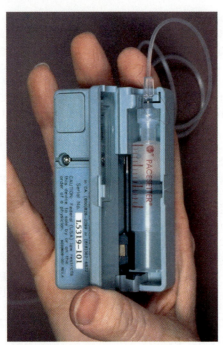

➤ *Figure 44.3* Insulin pump
Source: Pfizer Inc.

If the hypoglycemia is mild to moderate, symptoms can be reversed by giving food or drinks containing glucose. The quickest way to reverse serious hypoglycemia is to give IV glucose in a dextrose solution. The hormone glucagon is also used for the emergency treatment of severe hypoglycemia in patients unable to take IV glucose. Glucagon (1 mg) can be given IV, IM, or subcutaneously to reverse hypoglycemic symptoms in 20 minutes or less, depending on the route.

Other adverse effects of insulin include localized allergic reactions at the injection site, generalized urticaria, and swollen lymph glands. Some patients will experience **Somogyi phenomenon**, a rapid decrease in blood glucose, usually during the night, which stimulates the release of hormones that elevate blood glucose (epinephrine, cortisol, and glucagon) resulting in a high morning blood glucose level. Additional insulin above the patient's normal dose may produce a rapid rebound hypoglycemia.

44.4 Etiology and Characteristics of Type 2 Diabetes Mellitus

Type 2 diabetes mellitus is the more common form of DM, representing 90% to 95% of people with disorder. Because type 2 DM first appears in middle-aged adults, it has been referred to as *age-onset diabetes* or *maturity-onset diabetes*. These are inaccurate descriptions of this disorder, however, because increasing numbers of children are being diagnosed with type 2 DM. Patients with type 2 DM are often asymptomatic and may have the condition for years before their diagnosis.

The primary physiologic characteristic of type 2 DM is **insulin resistance**; target cells become unresponsive to insulin due to a defect in insulin receptor function. Essentially, the pancreas produces sufficient amounts of insulin but target cells do not recognize it.

As cells become more resistant to insulin, blood glucose levels rise and the pancreas responds by secreting even more insulin. Eventually, the hypersecretion of insulin causes beta cell exhaustion, and ultimately leads to beta cell death. As type 2 DM progresses, it becomes a disorder characterized by insufficient insulin levels as well as insulin resistance. The activity of insulin receptors can be increased by physical exercise and lowering the level of circulating insulin. In fact, adhering to a healthy diet and a regular exercise program has been shown to reverse insulin resistance, and delay or prevent the development of type 2 DM.

Many patients with type 2 DM are obese, have dyslipidemias, and will need a medically supervised plan to reduce weight gradually and exercise safely. This is an important lifestyle change for such patients; they will need to maintain these healthy lifestyle habits for their lifetime. Patients with poorly managed type 2 DM suffer from the same complications as patients with type 1 DM (e.g., retinopathy, neuropathy, and nephropathy).

Hyperosmolar hyperglycemic state (HHS) is a serious, acute condition with a mortality rate of 20% to 40% that occurs in persons with type 2 DM. This condition was formerly called hyperosmolar nonketotic coma (HNKC). HHS is caused by insufficient circulating insulin. The onset of HHS is gradual and is sometimes mistaken for a cerebrovascular accident. Seen most often in older adults, the skin appears flushed, dry, and warm. Blood glucose levels may be extreme and rise above 600 mg/dL. Treatment consists of fluid replacement, correction of electrolyte imbalances, and low-dose insulin given by slow IV infusion to lower glucose levels to 250 to 300 mg/dL. Although less common, HHS has a higher mortality rate than diabetic ketoacidosis.

Pr Prototype Drug | Human Regular Insulin *(Humulin R, Novolin R)*

Therapeutic Class: Antidiabetic agent; pancreatic hormone   **Pharmacologic Class:** Short-acting hypoglycemic agent

ACTIONS AND USES

Human regular insulin is used to help maintain blood glucose levels within normal limits. The primary effects of human regular insulin are: to promote cellular uptake of glucose, amino acids, and potassium; to promote protein synthesis, glycogen formation and storage, and fatty acid storage as triglycerides; and to conserve energy stores by promoting the utilization of glucose for energy needs, and inhibiting gluconeogenesis. Because regular insulin is short acting, it is most often used in combination with intermediate or long-acting insulin to achieve 24-hour glucose control. Indications for insulin include the following:

- As monotherapy to lower blood glucose levels in patients with type 1 diabetes
- In combination with oral antidiabetic agents in patients with type 2 diabetes
- For the emergency treatment of diabetic ketoacidosis
- For gestational diabetes

ADMINISTRATION ALERTS

- Ensure that the patient has sufficient food and is not hypoglycemic before administering regular insulin.
- Regular insulin is the only type of insulin that may be used for IV injection.
- Rotate injection sites. When the patient is hospitalized, use sites not normally used by the patient when at home.
- Administer approximately 30 minutes before meals so insulin will be absorbed and available when the patient begins to eat.
- Pregnancy category B

PHARMACOKINETICS

Onset: 30–60 min subcutaneous; 15 min IV

Peak: 2–4 h subcutaneous; 30–60 min IV

Half-life: Up to 13 h

Duration: 6–10 h subcutaneous; 30–60 min IV

ADVERSE EFFECTS

The most common adverse effect of insulin therapy is hypoglycemia. Hypoglycemia may result from taking too much insulin, not properly timing the insulin injection with food intake, or skipping a meal. Signs of hypoglycemia include tachycardia, confusion, sweating, and drowsiness. Irritation at injection sites may occur, including lipohypertrophy, the accumulation of fat in the area of injection. This effect is lessened with rotation of injection sites. Weight gain is a possible side effect.

Contraindications: Insulin is used with caution in pregnancy, renal impairment or failure, fever, thyroid disease, and among older adults, children, or infants. Insulin should not be administered to patients with hypoglycemia. Patients with hypokalemia should be monitored carefully because insulin may worsen this condition.

INTERACTIONS

Drug–Drug: The following substances may potentiate hypoglycemic effects: alcohol, salicylates, MAOIs, anabolic steroids, and guanethidine. The following substances may antagonize hypoglycemic effects: corticosteroids, thyroid hormone, and epinephrine. Serum glucose levels may be increased with furosemide or thiazide diuretics. Symptoms of hypoglycemic reaction may be masked with beta-adrenergic blockers.

Lab Tests: Insulin may increase urinary vanillylmandelic acid (VMA) and interfere with liver tests and thyroid function tests. It may decrease levels of serum potassium, calcium, and magnesium.

Herbal/Food: Garlic, bilberry, and ginseng may potentiate the hypoglycemic effects of insulin.

Treatment of Overdose: Overdose causes hypoglycemia. Mild cases are treated with oral glucose, and severe episodes are treated with parenteral glucagon or intravenous glucose.

See Refer to MyNursingKit for a Nursing Process Focus specific to this drug.

Oral Hypoglycemics

Type 2 DM is usually controlled with oral hypoglycemic agents, which are prescribed after diet and exercise have failed to reduce blood glucose to normal levels. As the disease progresses, insulin may become necessary for type 2 diabetics, or it may be required temporarily during times of stress such as illness or loss.

44.5 Pharmacotherapy with Oral Hypoglycemics

The six primary groups of oral antidiabetic drugs are classified by their chemical structures and their mechanisms of action. These include sulfonylureas, biguanides, meglitinides, thiazolidinediones (or glitazones), alpha-glucosidase inhibitors, and incretin therapies. Therapy with oral antidiabetic agents is not effective for persons with type 1 DM. All oral hypoglycemics have in common the action of lowering

RESEARCH SHOWS

The Question: Does lowering blood lipid levels help to improve the therapeutic outcomes of diabetic patients?

The Study: Researchers analyzed 12 studies that examined the benefits of lipid-lowering drugs in patients with diabetes. Each study lasted for 3 years and looked at the incidence of adverse cardiovascular events in diabetics versus nondiabetics. Although both groups benefited from lipid-lowering drugs (over 20% fewer cardiovascular adverse events), diabetic patients appeared to benefit more than nondiabetics.

Nursing Implications: Nurses should teach diabetic patients the importance of managing their blood lipid levels, as well as blood glucose levels.

Source: Costa, J., Borges, M., David, C. & Carneiro, A.V. (2006). Efficacy of lipid lowering drug treatment for diabetic and non-diabetic patients: meta-analysis of randomized controlled trials. British Medical Journal 332:1115–1124.

NURSING PROCESS FOCUS PATIENTS RECEIVING INSULIN THERAPY

Assessment	Potential Nursing Diagnoses
Baseline assessment prior to administration: ▪ Understand the reason the drug has been prescribed in order to assess for therapeutic effects and to plan for teaching needs (e.g., new onset of diabetes with hyperglycemia present, change in insulin type/amount, sliding scale coverage, treatment of hyperkalemia). ▪ Obtain a complete health history including endocrine, cardiovascular, hepatic, or renal disease; pregnancy; or breast-feeding. Obtain a drug history including allergies, current prescription and OTC drugs, herbal preparations, caffeine, nicotine, and alcohol use. Be alert to possible drug interactions. ▪ Obtain a history of current symptoms, duration and severity, and other related signs or symptoms (e.g., paresthesias of hands or feet). Assess feet and lower extremities for possible ulcerations. ▪ Obtain a dietary history including caloric intake if on an ADA diet, and the number of meals and snacks per day. Assess fluid intake and the type of fluids consumed. ▪ Obtain baseline vital signs, height, and weight. ▪ Evaluate appropriate laboratory findings (e.g., CBC, electrolytes, glucose, A1c level, lipid profile, osmolality, hepatic and renal function studies).	▪ Imbalanced Nutrition, Less Than Body Requirements (type I diabetes, related to lack of insulin availability for normal metabolism) ▪ Imbalanced Nutrition, More Than Body Requirements (type 2 diabetes, related to insulin resistance and intake more than body needs) ▪ Deficient Knowledge (drug therapy) ▪ Ineffective Therapeutic Regimen Management (related to deficient knowledge or altered compliance with prescribed treatment) ▪ Altered Compliance, Noncompliance (related to complexity of treatment plan, deficient knowledge) ▪ Risk for Deficient Fluid Volume (related to polyuria from hyperglycemia) ▪ Risk for Injury (related to adverse drug effects, lack of sensation in extremities from neuropathies) ▪ Risk for Infection (related to hyperglycemia, impaired circulation to extremities, neuropathies)
Assessment throughout administration: ▪ Assess for desired therapeutic effects dependent on the reason the drug is given (e.g., glucose levels, electrolytes and osmolality remain within normal limits, A1c levels demonstrate adequate control of glucose). ▪ Assess for and promptly report any adverse effects: signs of hypoglycemia (e.g., nausea, paleness, sweating, diaphoretic, tremors, irritability, headache, light-headedness, anxious, decreased level of consciousness) and hyperglycemia (e.g., flushed, dry skin, polyuria, polyphagia, polydipsia, drowsiness, glycosuria, ketonuria, acetone breath), lipodystrophy, and infection.	

Planning: Patient Goals and Expected Outcomes

The patient will:
▪ Experience therapeutic effects (e.g., blood sugar within normal limits).
▪ Be free from, or experience minimal, adverse effects.
▪ Verbalize an understanding of the drug's use, adverse effects, and required precautions.
▪ Demonstrate proper self-administration of the medication (e.g., dose, timing, when to notify provider).

Implementation

Interventions and (Rationales)	Patient and Family Education
Ensuring therapeutic effects: ▪ Continue assessments as described earlier for therapeutic effects. (Dependent on the severity of hyperglycemia, blood glucose levels should gradually return to normal.)	▪ Teach the patient to report any return of original symptoms. ▪ Teach the patient the symptoms of hyper- and hypoglycemia to observe for and instruct the patient to check the capillary glucose level (see "Minimizing adverse effects" later in this table) routinely and if symptoms are present. Promptly report any noticeable symptoms and concurrent capillary glucose level to the health care provider.
▪ Administer insulin correctly and per the schedule ordered [e.g., routine dosing with or without sliding-scale coverage], planning insulin administration and peak times around meal times. (See "Minimizing adverse effects" later in this table. Maintaining a steady level of insulin with meal times arranged to match peak insulin activity will assist in maintaining a stable blood glucose level.)	▪ Teach the patient, family, or caregiver appropriate administration techniques for all types of insulin used, followed by return-demonstration until the patient, family, or caregiver is comfortable with the technique and is able to perform it correctly. (See "Patient self-administration of drug therapy" later in this table.) ▪ Teach the patient, family, or caregiver the importance of peak insulin levels and the need to ensure that adequate food sources are consumed to avoid hypoglycemia. Provide written materials for future reference whenever possible.

NURSING PROCESS FOCUS   PATIENTS RECEIVING INSULIN THERAPY *(Continued)*

Implementation

Interventions and (Rationales)	Patient and Family Education
■ Ensure dietary needs are met based on the need to lose, gain, or maintain current weight and glucose levels. Consult with a dietitian as needed. Limit or eliminate alcohol use. (Adequate caloric amounts and protein, carbohydrates, and fats supports the insulin regimen for glucose control. Activity and lifestyle will also be factored into dietary management. Alcohol can raise and then precipitously lower blood glucose as alcohol is metabolized, raising the risk of hypoglycemia.)	■ Review current diet, lifestyle, and activity level with the patient. Arrange a dietitian consult based on the need to alter diet or food choices. Teach the patient to limit or eliminate alcohol use. If alcoholic beverages are consumed, limit to one per day and take along with a complete meal to ensure that intake balances alcohol metabolism.
Minimizing adverse effects:	
■ Continue to monitor capillary glucose levels. Hold insulin dose if the blood sugar level is less than 70 mg/dL or per parameters as ordered by the health care provider. (Daily glucose levels, especially before meals, will assist in maintaining stable blood glucose and will aid in assessing the appropriateness of the current insulin regimen.)	■ Instruct the patient on blood glucose monitoring appropriate techniques to obtain capillary blood glucose levels, followed by return-demonstration, and when to contact the health care provider (e.g., glucose less than 70 mg/dL). Monitor use and ensure the proper functioning of all equipment to be used at home.
■ Continue to monitor periodic lab work: CBC, electrolytes, glucose, A1c level, lipid profile, osmolality, and hepatic and renal function studies. (Periodic monitoring of lab work assists in determining glucose control, the need for any change in insulin needs, and assesses for complications. A1c levels provide a measure of glucose control over several months' time.)	■ Instruct the patient on the need to return periodically for lab work.
■ Assess for symptoms of hypoglycemia, especially around time of insulin peak activity. If symptoms of hypoglycemia are noted, provide a quick-acting carbohydrate source (e.g., juice or other simple sugar), and then check capillary glucose level. Report to the health care provider if the glucose level is less than 70 mg/dL or as ordered. If meal time is not immediate, provide a longer-acting protein source to ensure that hypoglycemia does not recur. (Hypoglycemia is especially likely to occur around peak insulin activity, especially if food sources are inadequate. Providing a quick-acting carbohydrate source and *then* checking the capillary glucose level will ensure that glucose does not decrease further while locating the glucose testing equipment. When in doubt, treating symptoms for suspected hypoglycemia is safer than allowing further decreases in glucose and possible loss of consciousness with adverse effects. Small additional amounts of carbohydrates will not dramatically increase blood sugar if testing shows a hyperglycemic episode.)	■ Teach the patient to always carry a quick-acting carbohydrate source in case symptoms of hypoglycemia occur. If unsure whether symptoms indicate hypo- or hyperglycemia, treat as hypoglycemia and then check capillary glucose. If symptoms are not relieved in 10 to 15 minutes, or if blood sugar is below 70 mg/dL (or parameters as ordered), notify the health care provider immediately.
■ Monitor blood glucose more frequently during periods of illness or stress. (Insulin needs may increase or decrease during periods of illness or stress. Frequent monitoring during these times helps to ensure adequate glucose control.)	■ Instruct the patient to check glucose levels more frequently when ill or under stress. Illness, especially associated with anorexia, nausea, or vomiting, may decrease insulin needs. Notify the health care provider if unable to eat normal meals during periods of illness or stress for a possible change in insulin dose.
■ Encourage increased physical activity but monitor blood glucose before and after exercise and begin any new or increased exercise routine gradually. Continue to monitor for hypoglycemia up to 48 hours after exercise. (Exercise assists muscles to use glucose more efficiently and increases insulin receptor sites in the tissues, lowering blood glucose. Benefits of exercise and lowered blood sugar may continue for up to 48 hours, increasing the risk of hypoglycemia during this time.)	■ Teach the patient the benefits of increased activity but to begin any new routine or increase in exercise gradually. Exercise should occur 1 hour after a meal or after a 10- or 15-g carbohydrate snack to prevent hypoglycemia. If exercise is prolonged, small, frequent carbohydrate snacks can be consumed every 30 minutes during exercise to maintain blood sugar. ■ Instruct the patient to check glucose levels more frequently, before and after exercise.

(Continued)

45.6 Pharmacotherapy with Progestins

Secreted by the corpus luteum, endogenous progesterone prepares the uterus for implantation of the embryo and pregnancy. If implantation does not occur, levels of progesterone fall dramatically and menses begins. If pregnancy occurs, the ovary continues to secrete progesterone to maintain a healthy endometrium until the placenta develops sufficiently to begin producing the hormone. Whereas the function of estrogen is to cause proliferation of the endometrium, progesterone limits and stabilizes endometrial growth.

Dysfunctional uterine bleeding can have a number of causes, including early abortion, pelvic neoplasms, thyroid disorders, pregnancy, and infection. Types of dysfunctional uterine bleeding include the following:

- Amenorrhea—absence of menstruation
- Endometriosis—abnormal location of endometrial tissues
- Oligomenorrhea—infrequent menstruation
- Menorrhagia—prolonged or excessive menstruation
- Breakthrough bleeding—hemorrhage between menstrual periods
- Premenstrual syndrome (PMS)—symptoms develop during the luteal phase
- Postmenopausal bleeding—hemorrhage following menopause
- Endometrial carcinoma—cancer of the endometrium

Dysfunctional uterine bleeding is often caused by a hormonal imbalance between estrogen and progesterone. Although estrogen increases the thickness of the endometrium, bleeding occurs sporadically unless balanced by an adequate amount of progesterone. Administration of a progestin in a pattern starting 5 days after the onset of menses and continuing for the next 20 days can sometimes reestablish a normal, monthly cyclic pattern. Oral contraceptives may also be prescribed for this disorder.

LIFESPAN CONSIDERATIONS

Estrogen Use and Psychosocial Issues

Because undesirable adverse effects may occur with estrogen use, the nurse should communicate these prior to implementing drug therapy. The nurse can explore the patient's reaction to these potential risks. An assessment of the patient's emotional support system should also be made before initiating drug therapy. Hirsutism, loss of hair, or a deepening of the voice can occur in the female patient. Men may develop secondary female characteristics such as a higher voice, lack of body hair, and increased breast size. Impotence may also develop and is typically viewed as a concern by most men.

Patients should be taught that these adverse effects are reversible and may subside with adjustment of dosage or discontinuation of estrogen therapy. This knowledge may allow both men and women patients to remain compliant when adverse effects occur. During therapy, patients may need emotional support to assist in dealing with these body image issues. The nurse can encourage this support, discuss these issues with family members, and refer patients for counseling. For the female patient, the nurse can refer to an aesthetician for hair removal or wig fitting. The male patient and his sexual partner may need a referral to deal with issues surrounding impotence and its effect on their relationship.

Pr Prototype Drug | Medroxyprogesterone Acetate (Provera)

Therapeutic Class: Hormone; agent for dysfunctional uterine bleeding

Pharmacologic Class: Progestin

ACTIONS AND USES

Medroxyprogesterone is a synthetic progestin with a prolonged duration of action. As with its natural counterpart, the primary target tissue for medroxyprogesterone is the endometrium of the uterus. It inhibits the effect of estrogen on the uterus, thus restoring normal hormonal balance. Applications include dysfunctional uterine bleeding, secondary amenorrhea, and contraception. Medroxyprogesterone may also be given IM for the palliation of metastatic uterine or renal carcinoma and as a sustained release form (Depo-Provera) for contraception.

ADMINISTRATION ALERTS

- Give PO with meals to avoid gastric distress.
- Observe IM sites for abscess: presence of lump and discoloration of tissue.
- Pregnancy category X

PHARMACOKINETICS (PO)
Onset: Unknown
Peak: 2–4 h
Half-life: 30 days
Duration: Unknown

ADVERSE EFFECTS

The most frequent adverse effects of medroxyprogesterone are breast tenderness, breakthrough bleeding, and other menstrual irregularities. Weight gain, depression, hypertension, nausea, vomiting, dysmenorrhea, and vaginal candidiasis may also occur. The most serious adverse effect is an increased risk for thromboembolic disease. The drug has a black box warning that use of the drug may cause a loss of bone mineral density.

Contraindications: Medroxyprogesterone is contraindicated during pregnancy and in women with known or suspected carcinoma of the breast. Caution should be used when treating patients with a history of thromboembolic disease, hepatic impairment, or undiagnosed vaginal bleeding. The drug should be used cautiously in patients with a history of psychic depression and the drug discontinued at the first sign of recurring depression.

INTERACTIONS

Drug–Drug: Serum levels of medroxyprogesterone are decreased by aminoglutethimide, barbiturates, primidone, rifampin, rifabutin, and topiramate.

Lab Tests: Medroxyprogesterone may increase values for alkaline phosphatase, glucose tolerance test (GTT), and HDL.

Herbal/Food: St. John's wort may decrease the effectiveness of medroxyprogesterone and cause abnormal menstrual bleeding.

Treatment of Overdose: There is no specific treatment for overdose.

Refer to MyNursingKit for a Nursing Process Focus specific to this drug.

In cases of heavy bleeding, high doses of conjugated estrogens may be administered for 3 weeks prior to adding medroxyprogesterone for the last 10 days of therapy. Treatment with nonsteroidal anti-inflammatory drugs (NSAIDs) sometimes helps to reduce bleeding and ease painful menstrual flow. In 2009, the FDA approved tranexamic acid (Lysteda) for the treatment of cyclic heavy menstrual bleeding. If aggressive hormonal therapy fails to stop the heavy bleeding, dilation and curettage (D & C) may be necessary.

Progestins are occasionally prescribed for the treatment of metastatic endometrial carcinoma. In these cases, they are used for palliation, usually in combination with other antineoplastics. Selected progestins and their dosages are listed in Table 45.5.

LABOR AND BREAST-FEEDING

Several agents are used to manage uterine contractions and to stimulate lactation. **Oxytocics** are agents that *stimulate* uterine contractions to promote the induction of labor. **Tocolytics**, are used to *inhibit* uterine contractions during premature labor. These agents are listed in Table 45.6.

TABLE 45.5	Selected Estrogens and Progestins	
Drug	Route and Adult Dose (max dose where indicated)	Adverse Effects
ESTROGENS		
estradiol (Climara, Estraderm, Estrace, Vivelle, others)	PO; 0.5–2 mg daily Transdermal patch; 1 patch either once weekly (Climara) or twice weekly (0.025–0.1 mg/day) Topical gel; Approximately 1.25 g/day Intravaginal cream; Insert 2–4 g/day for 2 wk, then reduce to ½ the initial dose for 2 wk, then use 1 g one to three times/week	*Breakthrough bleeding, spotting, breast tenderness, libido changes* <u>Hypertension, gallbladder disease, thromboembolic disorders, increased cancer risk</u>
estradiol cypionate	IM; 1–5 mg every 3–4 wk	
estradiol valerate (Delestrogen, Duragen-10, Valergen)	IM; 10–20 mg every 4 wk	
estrogen, conjugated (Cenestin, Enjuvia, Premarin)	PO; 0.3–1.25 mg/day for 21 days each month	
estropipate (Ogen)	PO; 0.75–6 mg/day for 21 days each month	
PROGESTINS		
● medroxyprogesterone (Depo Provera, depo-subQ-Provera, Provera, Cycrin)	PO; 5–10 mg daily on days 1–12 of menstrual cycle IM (Depo-Provera); 150 mg daily for 3 months. Give the first dose during the first 5 days of the menstrual period or within the first 5 days postpartum if not breast-feeding Subcutaneous (depo-subQ-Provera); 104 mg daily for 3 months. Give the first dose during the first 5 days of the menstrual period or at the 6th week postpartum if not breast-feeding	*Breakthrough bleeding, spotting, breast tenderness, weight gain* <u>Amenorrhea, dysmenorrhea, depression, thromboembolic disorders</u>
norethindrone (Micronor, Nor-Q.D.)	PO; 0.35 mg/day beginning on day 1 of menstrual cycle	
progesterone (Crinone, Endometrin, Prochieve, Prometrium)	Amenorrhea or functional uterine bleeding: IM; 5–10 mg/day Assisted reproductive technology: Intravaginal; 90 mg gel once daily or 100-mg tablets two to three times/day	
ESTROGEN–PROGESTIN COMBINATIONS		
● conjugated estrogens (equine)/medroxyprogesterone (Premphase, Prempro)	PO; Premphase: estrogen 0.625 mg/daily on days 1–28; add 5 mg medroxyprogesterone daily on days 15–28 PO; Prempro: estrogen 0.3 mg and medroxyprogesterone 1.5 mg daily Intravaginal cream: insert ½ to 2 g daily for 3–6 months.	See above for adverse effects of estrogens and progestins
estradiol/norgestimate (Prefest)	PO; 1 tablet of 1 mg estradiol for 3 days, followed by 1 tablet of 1 mg estradiol combined with 0.09 mg norgestimate for 3 days. Regimen is repeated continuously without interruption.	
ethinyl estradiol/norethindrone acetate (Activella)	PO; 1 tablet daily, which contains 0.5–0.1 mg of estradiol and 0.5–1 mg norethindrone Transdermal patch; 1 patch, twice weekly	

Italics indicate common adverse effects; <u>underlining</u> indicates serious adverse effects.

TABLE 45.6	Uterine Stimulants and Relaxants	
Drug	**Route and Adult Dose (max dose where indicated)**	**Adverse Effects**
OXYTOCICS		
oxytocin (Pitocin)	To control postpartum bleeding: 10–40 units per infusion pump in 1,000 mL of IV fluid To induce labor: IV 0.5–2 milliunits/min, gradually increasing the dose no greater than 1–2 milliunits/min at 30–60 minute intervals until contraction pattern is established	*Nausea, vomiting, maternal dysrhythmias* Fetal bradycardia, uterine rupture, fetal intracranial hemorrhage, water intoxication, fetal brain hemorrhage
ERGOT ALKALOIDS		
ergonovine maleate (Ergotrate)	PO; 1 tablet (0.2 mg) tid–qid after childbirth for a maximum of 1 wk	*Nausea, vomiting, uterine cramping*
methylergonovine maleate (Methergine)	PO; 0.2–0.4 mg bid–qid	Shock, severe hypertension, dysrhythmias
PROSTAGLANDINS		
carboprost (Hemabate)	IM; initial: 250 mcg (1 mL) repeated at 1 1/2–3 1/2-h intervals if indicated by uterine response	*Nausea, vomiting, diarrhea, headache, chills, uterine cramping*
dinoprostone (Cervidil, Prepidil, Prostin E₂)	Intravaginal; 10 mg	Uterine lacerations or perforation due to intense contractions
misoprostol (Cytotec)	Intravaginal: 25 mcg (1/4 of 100 mcg tablet); may repeat every 3–6 h	
TOCOLYTICS		
magnesium sulfate	IV; 1–4 g in 5% dextrose by slow infusion (initial max dose = 10–14 g/day, then no more than 30–40 g/day at a max rate of 1–2 g/h)	*Flushing, sweating, muscle weakness* Complete heart block, circulatory collapse, respiratory paralysis
nifedipine (Adalat, Procardia)	PO; Initial dosage of 20 mg, followed by 20 mg orally after 30 min If contractions persist, therapy can be continued with 20 mg orally every 3–8 h for 48–72 h with a maximum dose of 160 mg/day After 72 hours, if maintenance is still required, long-acting nifedipine 30–60 mg daily can be used	*Flushing, sweating, muscle weakness* Complete heart block, circulatory collapse, respiratory paralysis
terbutaline sulfate (Brethine)	IV; 2.5–10 mcg/min; increase every 10-20 minutes; duration of infusion = 12 h (max: 17.5–30 mcg/min) PO; maintenance dose: 2.5–10 mg every 4–6 h	*Nervousness, tremor, drowsiness* Bronchoconstriction, dysrhythmias, altered maternal and fetal heart rate

Italics indicate common adverse effects; underlining indicates serious adverse effects.

45.7 Pharmacologic Management of Uterine Contractions

The most widely used oxytocic is the natural hormone oxytocin, which is secreted by the posterior portion of the pituitary gland. The target organs for oxytocin are the uterus and the breast. As the growing fetus distends the uterus, oxytocin is secreted in increasingly larger amounts. The rising blood levels of oxytocin provide a steadily increasing stimulus to the uterus to contract, thus promoting labor and the delivery of the baby and the placenta. As pregnancy progresses, the number of oxytocin receptors in the uterus increases, making it even more sensitive to the effects of the hormone. When used as a drug, oxytocin rapidly causes uterine contractions and induces labor.

In postpartum women, oxytocin is released in response to suckling, which causes milk to be *ejected* (let down) from the mammary glands. Oxytocin does not increase the *volume* of milk production. This function is provided by the pituitary hormone prolactin, which increases the synthesis of milk. The actions of oxytocin during breast-feeding are illustrated in ➤ Figure 45.4.

Several prostaglandins are also used as uterine stimulants. Unlike most hormones, which travel through the blood to affect distant tissues, **prostaglandins** are local hormones that act directly at the site where they are secreted. Although the body makes dozens of different prostaglandins, only a few have clinical utility. In the uterus, prostaglandins cause intense smooth muscle contractions. Carboprost (Hemabate) is often used to control postpartum hemorrhage. Dinoprostone (Prepidil, Cervidil) and misoprostol (Cytotec) are prostaglandins used to promote cervical ripening, a softening and dilation of the cervix that must occur prior to vaginal delivery. The prostaglandins may also be used to induce pharmacologic abortion.

It is important to note that oxytocin and other uterine stimulants are only indicated when there are demonstrated risks to the mother or fetus in continuing the pregnancy. Because of potential adverse effects, they should never be used for elective induction of labor.

Some women enter labor before the baby has reached a normal stage of development. Premature birth is a leading cause of infant death. Tocolytics are uterine relaxants prescribed to suppress preterm labor contractions. Suppressing labor allows additional time, usually 24–72 hours, for the fetus to develop and may permit the pregnancy to reach normal term. Typically, the mother is given a monitor with a sensor that records uterine contractions, and this information is used to determine the doses and timing of tocolytic medications.

Only a few drugs are available as tocolytics. For over 30 years, magnesium sulfate has been the traditional drug of choice for suppressing preterm labor, but evidence suggests it may be ineffective and poses undue risks to the fetus and mother. The only drug that is FDA-approved for this indication is ritodrine (Yutopar) but it is no longer being manufactured for use in the United States. Calcium channel blockers such as nifedipine (Adalat, Procardia) and beta-adrenergic agonists such as terbutaline (Brethine) appear to be effective but are not approved for this indication.

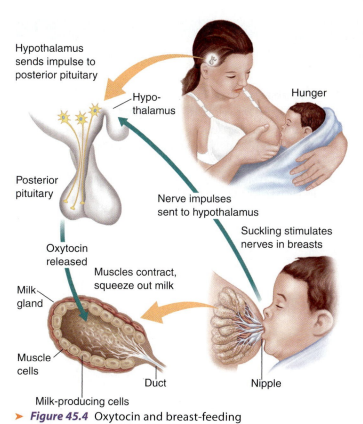

➤ *Figure 45.4* Oxytocin and breast-feeding

Pr Prototype Drug | Ocytocin *(Pitocin)*

Therapeutic Class: Drug to induce labor; uterine stimulant

Pharmacologic Class: Hormone; oxytocic

ACTIONS AND USES

Oxytocin is a natural hormone secreted by the posterior pituitary that is a drug of choice for inducing labor. Oxytocin is given by several different routes depending on its intended action. Given antepartum by IV infusion, oxytocin induces labor by increasing the frequency and force of uterine contractions. It is timed to the final stage of pregnancy, after the cervix has dilated, membranes have ruptured, and presentation of the fetus has occurred. Doses in an IV infusion are increased gradually, every 15–60 minutes, until a normal labor pattern is established.

Oxytocin may also be administered postpartum to reduce hemorrhage after expulsion of the placenta, and to aid in returning normal muscular tone to the uterus. Intranasal forms once used to promote milk letdown are no longer available in the United States.

ADMINISTRATION ALERTS
- Dilute 10 units oxytocin in 1,000 mL IV fluid prior to administration. For postpartum administration, may add up to 40 units in 1,000 mL IV fluid.
- Incidence of allergic reactions is higher when given IM or by IV injection, rather than IV infusion.
- Pregnancy category X

PHARMACOKINETICS
Onset: Immediate
Peak: Unknown
Half-life: 3–5 min
Duration: 1 h

ADVERSE EFFECTS

The most common adverse effects of oxytocin are rapid, painful uterine contractions and fetal tachycardia. When given IV, vital signs of the fetus and mother are monitored continuously to avoid complications in the fetus, such as dysrhythmias or intracranial hemorrhage. Serious complications in the mother may include uterine rupture, seizures, or coma. Risk of uterine rupture increases in women who have delivered five or more children. Though experience has shown the use of oxytocin to be quite safe, labor should be induced by this drug only when there are demonstrated risks to the mother or fetus in continuing the pregnancy.

Contraindications: Antepartum use is contraindicated in the following: significant cephalopelvic disproportion; unfavorable fetal positions that are undeliverable without conversion before delivery; obstetrical emergencies in which the benefit-to-risk ratio for the fetus or mother favors surgical intervention; fetal distress when delivery is not imminent; when adequate uterine activity fails to achieve satisfactory progress; when the uterus is already hyperactive or hypertonic; when vaginal delivery is contraindicated, such as invasive cervical carcinoma, active genital herpes, total placenta previa, vasa previa, and cord presentation or prolapse of the cord.

INTERACTIONS
Drug–Drug: Vasoconstrictors used concurrently with oxytocin may cause severe hypertension.

Lab Tests: Unknown

Herbal/Food: None known

Treatment of Overdose: Overdose causes strong uterine contractions, which may lead to uterine lacerations or rupture. Immediate discontinuation of the drug is necessary, along with symptomatic treatment.

Refer to MyNursingKit for a Nursing Process Focus specific to this drug.

NURSING PROCESS FOCUS   PATIENTS RECEIVING OXYTOCIN

Assessment	Potential Nursing Diagnoses
Baseline assessment prior to administration: - Understand the reason the drug has been prescribed in order to assess for therapeutic effects (e.g., labor induction, control of postpartum bleeding). - Obtain a complete health history including current length of pregnancy duration; presence of pre-eclampsia or eclampsia; recent labor; type of delivery; history of labors or caesarean sections; cardiovascular, neurologic, hepatic, or renal disease; diabetes; and breast-feeding. - Obtain a drug history including allergies, current prescription and OTC drugs, herbal preparations, alcohol use, and smoking. Be alert to possible drug interactions. - Evaluate appropriate laboratory findings (e.g., CBC, platelets, coagulation studies, electrolytes, glucose, magnesium level, hepatic and renal function studies). - Obtain baseline height, weight, and vital signs. - Obtain fetal heart rate and intrauterine positioning. - Check for the presence of cervical dilation and effacement. Monitor quality and duration of any existing contractions. Monitor fetal response to contractions, noting any sign of fetal distress. - Check for postpartum bleeding and note the number of pads saturated.	- Pain (acute, related to strong uterine contractions) - Ineffective Breastfeeding, Potential for Effective Breast-Feeding - Deficient Knowledge (drug therapy) - Risk of Injury (patient or fetus), related to adverse drug effects, strong uterine contractions - Risk for Imbalanced Fluid Volume (excess, related to water intoxication from the drug's antidiuretic hormone effects)
Assessment throughout administration: - Assess for desired therapeutic effects dependent on the reason the drug is given (e.g., strong, regular contractions supportive of labor). - Continuously monitor timing, quality, and duration of contractions. Immediately report sustained uterine contractions to the health care provider. - Continuously monitor the fetal heart rate and response to contractions. Immediately report signs of fetal distress to the health care provider. - Continue periodic monitoring of CBC, platelets, electrolytes, glucose, and magnesium level. - Monitor vital signs frequently and immediately report any BP above 140/90 mmHg or less than 90/60 mmHg especially if accompanied by tachycardia, or per parameters, to the health care provider. - Continue to monitor postpartum bleeding and pad count. Notify the health care provider if more than two full-size pads are saturated in 2 hours' time. - Assess for adverse effects: nausea, vomiting, and headache. Tachycardia, palpitations, and hypertension, especially associated with angina, severe headache, or dyspnea should be reported immediately. Immediately report any severe abdominal pain, sustained uterine contraction, diminished urine output, dizziness, drowsiness, confusion, changes in level of consciousness, or seizures.	

Planning: Patient Goals and Expected Outcomes

The patient will:

- Experience therapeutic effects (e.g., strong labor contractions supportive of labor, adequate milk letdown supportive of breast-feeding, postpartum bleeding is diminished).
- Be free from, or experience minimal, adverse effects.
- Verbalize an understanding of the drug's use, adverse effects, and required precautions.
- Demonstrate proper self-administration of the medication (e.g., dose, timing, when to notify provider).

NURSING PROCESS FOCUS   PATIENTS RECEIVING OXYTOCIN *(Continued)*

Implementation

Interventions and (Rationales)	Patient and Family Education
Ensuring therapeutic effects: ▪ Monitor appropriate medication administration for optimum results. Intravenous oxytocin must be given via an infusion pump to allow for precise dosing. (Infusion pumps allow for rapid dosage adjustments to maintain uterine contractions supportive of labor and cervical dilation has reached approximately 5 to 6 cm.)	▪ Instruct the patient about the rationale for all IV and monitoring equipment and the need for frequent monitoring, to allay anxiety. ▪ Teach the patient that labor contractions will gradually increase and that the drug will be decreased or stopped once contractions reach an optimum level. ▪ Encourage the patient in labor to use pain-control measures (e.g., therapeutic breathing) or use pain control drugs as needed and ordered.
Minimizing adverse effects: ▪ Monitor the timing, quality, and duration of contractions continuously. Immediately report any sustained uterine contractions to the health care provider. Stop the infusion, infusing normal saline or solution as ordered, and place the patient on her side until follow-up orders are obtained if contractions continue sustained. (Oxytocin may cause sustained uterine muscle contraction with potential uterine rupture. Uterine contractions must be continuously monitored.)	▪ Teach the patient that labor contractions will increase in strength and duration and will be monitored throughout. Instruct the patient to immediately report any sustained contraction or any severe abdominal pain.
▪ Continuously monitor fetal heart rate and response to contractions. Immediately report signs of fetal distress to the health care provider. (Uterine contractions can affect the amount of blood flow through the placenta with diminished oxygenation to the fetus. Changes in fetal heart rate may signal fetal distress and the patient should be placed on her side, oxygen administered, the infusion stopped, and the health care provider notified.)	▪ Teach the patient that the fetal heart rate will also be monitored along with uterine contractions. Explain the purpose for all monitoring equipment to allay anxiety.
▪ Monitor vital signs and urine output frequently and report any BP above 140/90 mmHg or less than 90/60 mmHg, especially if accompanied by tachycardia, or diminished urine output, to the health care provider immediately. (Oxytocin has vasoconstrictive properties and water-retention properties. BP or pulse rate exceeding parameters, increasing disorientation or confusion, and diminished urine output may signify adverse drug effects or possible complications.)	▪ Instruct the patient to immediately report any headache, dizziness, disorientation or confusion, palpitations, or chest pressure or pain.
▪ Monitor fundal firmness and location, and postpartum bleeding and pad count. (Oxytocin may be given to control postpartum bleeding. Lochia that increases, or if two or more pads are saturated over a 2-hour period, should be reported to the health care provider immediately.)	▪ Instruct the patient to report any sudden increase in lochia, dizziness or light-headedness, or if more than two pads are saturated after 2 hours.
Patient understanding of drug therapy: ▪ Use opportunities during administration of medications and during assessments to discuss the rationale for drug therapy, desired therapeutic outcomes, most commonly observed adverse effects, parameters for when to call the health care provider, and any necessary monitoring or precautions. (Using time during nursing care helps to optimize and reinforce key teaching areas.)	▪ The patient should be able to state the reason for the drug, appropriate dose and scheduling, monitoring needs, and what adverse effects to observe for and when to report them.

Evaluation of Outcome Criteria

Evaluate the effectiveness of drug therapy by confirming that patient goals and expected outcomes have been met (see "Planning").

See Tables 45.3 & 45.6 for a list of drugs to which these nursing actions apply.

FEMALE INFERTILITY

Infertility is the inability to become pregnant after at least 1 year of frequent unprotected intercourse. Infertility is a common disorder, with as many as 25% of couples experiencing difficulty in conceiving children at some point during their reproductive lifetimes. It is estimated that females contribute to approximately 60% of the infertility disorders. Agents used to treat infertility are listed in Table 45.7.

45.8 Pharmacotherapy of Female Fertility

The three primary causes of female infertility are pelvic infections, physical obstruction of the uterine tubes, and lack of ovulation. Extensive testing is often necessary to determine the exact cause and it is not uncommon to find multiple etiologies for the infertility. For women whose infertility has been determined to have an endocrine etiology, pharmacotherapy may be of value. Endocrine disruption of reproductive function can occur at the level of the hypothalamus, pituitary, or ovary, and pharmacotherapy is targeted to the specific cause of the dysfunction.

Ovulation (and thus pregnancy) cannot occur unless the ovarian follicles receive a hormonal signal to mature each month. This signal is normally supplied by LH and FSH during the first few weeks of the menstrual cycle. Lack of regular ovulation is a cause of infertility that can be successfully treated with drug therapy. Clomiphene (Clomid, Milophene, Serophene) is a preferred drug for female infer-

tility because it stimulates the release of LH, resulting in the maturation of more ovarian follicles than would normally occur. The rise in LH level is sufficient to induce ovulation in about 90% of treated women. The pregnancy rate of patients taking clomiphene is high, and twins occur in about 5% of treated patients. If ovulation is not induced by clomiphene, human chorionic gonadotropin (HCG) may be added to the regimen. Made by the placenta during pregnancy, HCG is similar to LH and can mimic the LH surge that normally causes ovulation.

If the infertility is a result of disruption at the pituitary level, therapy with human menopausal gonadotropin (HMG) or gonadotropin-releasing hormone (GnRH) may be indicated. These therapies are generally indicated only after clomiphene has failed to induce ovulation. Also known as menotropins (Pergonal, Humegon), HMG acts on the ovaries to increase follicle maturation, and results in a 25% incidence of multiple pregnancies. Newer formulations use recombinant DNA technology to synthesize gonadotropins containing nearly pure FSH. Other medications used to stimulate ovulation are gonadorelin (Factrel), bromocriptine (Parlodel), and HCG.

Premature ovulation, the expulsion of an oocyte from the ovary before it has fully matured, is another cause of infertility. GnRH antagonists such as ganirelix (Orgalutran) and cetrorelix (Cetrotide) suppress LH surges, thus preventing ovulation until the follicles are mature.

Endometriosis, a common cause of infertility, is characterized by the presence of endometrial tissue that has implanted outside the uterus, in locations such as the surface of pelvic organs or the ovaries. Being responsive to hor-

TABLE 45.7	Agents for Female Infertility
Drug	**Mechanism**
bromocriptine (Parlodel)	Reduction of high prolactin levels
clomiphene (Clomid, Milophene, Serophene)	Promotion of follicle maturation and ovulation
danazol (Danocrine)	Anabolic steroid; suppression of FSH control of endometriosis
FSH AND LH ENHANCING DRUGS	
chorionic gonadotropin-HCG (Novarel, Ovidrel, Pregnyl)	Promotion of follicle maturation and ovulation
menotropins (Humegon, Repronex)	
follitropin alfa (Gonal-F)	
follitropin beta (Follistim)	
urofollitropin (Bravelle))	
GnRH ANTAGONISTS	
cetrorelix acetate (Cetrotide)	Prevention of premature ovulation or control of endometriosis
ganirelix acetate (Orgalutran)	
GnRH ANALOGS/AGONISTS	
goserelin acetate (Zoladex)	Suppression of FSH and control of endometriosis
leuprolide (Lupron, Lupron Depot)	
nafarelin (Synarel)	

monal stimuli, this abnormal tissue can cause pain, dysfunctional bleeding, and dysmenorrhea.

Leuprolide (Lupron) and nafarelin (Synarel) are GnRH agonists that produce an initial release of LH and FSH, followed by suppression due to the negative feedback effect on the pituitary. Many women experience relief from the symptoms of endometriosis after 3 to 6 months of therapy.

As an alternative choice, danazol (Danocrine) is an anabolic steroid that suppresses FSH production, which in turn shuts down both ectopic and normal endometrial activity. While leuprolide is given only by the parenteral route, danazol is given orally. Estrogen–progestin oral contraceptives are also useful in treating endometriosis.

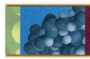

Chapter REVIEW

KEY CONCEPTS

The numbered key concepts provide a succinct summary of the important points from the corresponding numbered section within the chapter. If any of these points are not clear, refer to the numbered section within the chapter for review.

45.1 Female reproductive function is controlled by the secretion of GnRH from the hypothalamus, and FSH and LH from the pituitary.

45.2 Estrogens are secreted by ovarian follicles and are responsible for maturation of the sex organs and the secondary sex characteristics of the female. Progestins are secreted by the corpus luteum and prepare the endometrium for implantation.

45.3 Low doses of estrogens and progestins prevent conception by blocking ovulation. Long-term formulations are available that offer greater convenience.

45.4 Drugs for emergency contraception may be administered within 72 hours after unprotected sex to prevent implantation of the fertilized egg. Other agents may be given to

stimulate uterine contractions to expel the implanted embryo.

45.5 Estrogen–progestin combinations are used for hormone replacement therapy during and after menopause; however, their long-term use may have serious adverse effects.

45.6 Progestins are prescribed for dysfunctional uterine bleeding. High doses of progestins are also used as antineoplastics.

45.7 Oxytocics are drugs that stimulate uterine contractions and induce labor. Tocolytics slow uterine contractions to delay labor.

45.8 Medications may be administered to stimulate ovulation, to increase female fertility.

NCLEX-RN® REVIEW QUESTIONS

1 The patient is admitted with pain in the calf, shortness of breath, and severe chest pain. A medical history reveals that the patient is taking oral contraceptives. Based on this assessment, the patient may be experiencing a:
1. cerebrovascular accident.
2. hypertensive crisis.
3. hyperglycemic reaction.
4. thromboembolism.

2 The nurse includes which of the following discharge instructions to the patient receiving HRT?
1. Avoid foods that contain caffeine.
2. Take medication 30 minutes before meals.
3. Discontinue medication if uterine bleeding begins.
4. Monitor for a sudden increase in LDL cholesterol.

3 The nurse's assessment of the patient receiving an IV infusion of oxytocin notes that uterine contractions are 4 minutes apart and 60 seconds in duration. Which of the following nursing interventions is most important based on this assessment?

1. Administer oxygen via face mask.
2. Monitor the patient for water intoxication.
3. Position the patient on her left side.
4. Discontinue the infusion immediately.

4 The patient has made the decision to use Ortho-Novum 1/35 for contraception. The nurse includes which of the following instructions to the patient about this medication? (Select all that apply.)
1. Take the first pill of the pack on the fifth day of the menstrual cycle.
2. The placebo must be taken to decrease estrogen-related adverse effects.
3. Possible side effects include intolerance to contact lenses, abdominal cramps, dysmenorrhea, and breast fullness.
4. Barrier contraceptives are needed if a daily dose is missed.
5. Breakthrough bleeding indicates that ovulation has occurred.

5 The patient questions the nurses about how she could have become pregnant while she was taking oral contraceptives. Which of the following statements best describes the primary reason a patient would become pregnant while on oral contraceptives?
1. Antibiotics were taken in conjunction with the oral contraceptive.
2. Two or more doses of the oral contraceptive were skipped.
3. The dosage of the estrogen in the oral contraceptive was too low.
4. The oral contraceptive was taken in combination with an anticonvulsant.

6 A patient has started taking clomiphene (Clomid, Serophene) after an infertility workup and asks the nurse why she is not having in-vitro fertilization. Which of the following nursing statements would be most helpful in explaining the use of clomiphene to the patient?
1. Her diagnostic workup suggested that infrequent ovulation may be the cause for her infertility and clomiphene increases ovulation.
2. In-vitro fertilization is expensive and since clomiphene is less expensive, it is always tried first.
3. There is less risk of multiple births with clomiphene.
4. Her past history of oral contraceptive use has prevented her from ovulating. Clomiphene is given to stimulate ovulation again in these conditions.

CRITICAL THINKING QUESTIONS

1. A 28-year-old woman has a 3-year history of pelvic pain, dyspareunia, and infertility. She has been diagnosed with endometriosis and is prescribed leuprolide (Lupron) once a month per intramuscular injection. Discuss the mechanism of action of leuprolide in managing the patient's endometriosis. What information should be included in a teaching plan for a patient receiving this drug?

2. A labor and delivery nurse places one fourth of a tablet (crushed) of misoprostol (Cytotec) on the cervix of a patient who is being induced because she is 2 weeks past her due date. After several hours, the patient begins to have contractions, and the nurse notes late decelerations on the monitor. The nurse flushes the drug out of the patient's vagina with saline per hospital protocol. What is the use and action of misoprostol?

3. A nurse is assessing a 32-year-old postpartum patient and notes 2+ pitting edema of the ankles and pretibial area. The patient denies having "swelling" prior to delivery. The nurse reviews the patient's chart and notes that she was induced with oxytocin (Pitocin) over a 23-hour period. What is the relationship between this drug regimen and the patient's current presentation? What additional assessments should be made?

See Appendix D for answers and rationales for all activities.

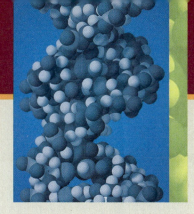

Chapter 46

Drugs for Disorders and Conditions of the Male Reproductive System

LEARNING OUTCOMES

After reading this chapter, the student should be able to:

1. Describe the roles of the hypothalamus, pituitary, and testes in regulating male reproductive function.
2. Identify indications for pharmacotherapy with androgens.
3. Describe the misuse and dangers associated with the use of anabolic steroids to enhance athletic performance.
4. Explain the role of medications in the treatment of male infertility.
5. Describe the etiology, pathogenesis, and pharmacotherapy of erectile dysfunction.
6. Describe the pathogenesis and pharmacotherapy of benign prostatic hyperplasia.
7. Describe the nurse's role in the pharmacologic management of disorders and conditions of the male reproductive system.
8. For each of the drugs/classes listed in Drugs at a Glance, know representative drugs, and explain the mechanism of drug action, primary actions, and important adverse effects.
9. Use the nursing process to care for patients who are receiving drug therapy for disorders and conditions of the male reproductive system.

KEY TERMS

As in women, reproductive function in men is regulated by a small number of hormones from the hypothalamus, pituitary, and gonads. Because hormonal secretion in men is relatively constant throughout the adult life span, the pharmacologic treatment of reproductive disorders in men is less complex, and more limited, than in women. This chapter examines drugs used to treat disorders and conditions of the male reproductive system.

46.1 Hypothalamic and Pituitary Regulation of Male Reproductive Function

The same pituitary hormones that control reproductive function in women also affect men. Although the name **follicle-stimulating hormone (FSH)** applies to its target in the female ovary, this hormone also regulates sperm production in men. **Leuteinizing hormone (LH),** more accurately called *interstitial cell–stimulating hormone* (ICSH) in the male reproductive system, regulates the production of testosterone.

Although they are also secreted in small amounts by the adrenal glands in women, **androgens** are considered male sex hormones. The testes secrete **testosterone,** the primary androgen responsible for maturation of the male sex organs and the secondary sex characteristics of men. Unlike the 28-day cyclic secretion of estrogen and progesterone in women, testosterone secretion is relatively constant in adult men. Beginning in puberty, testosterone production increases rapidly and continues to be maintained at a high level until late adulthood, after which it slowly declines. If the level of testosterone in the blood rises above normal, negative feedback to the pituitary shuts off the secretion of LH and FSH. The relationship between the hypothalamus, pituitary, and the male reproductive hormones is illustrated in ➤ Figure 46.1.

Testosterone has profound metabolic effects in tissues outside the reproductive system. Of particular note is its ability to build muscle mass, which contributes to differences in muscle strength and body composition between men and women.

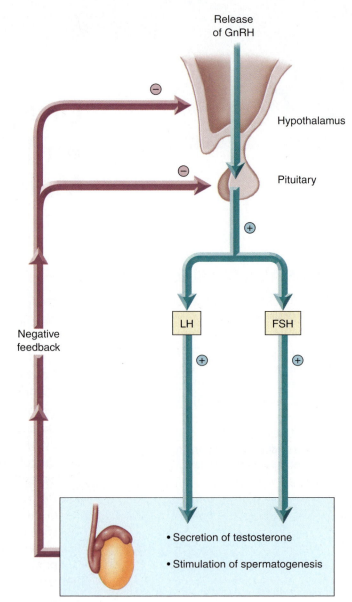

➤ **Figure 46.1** Hormonal control of the male reproductive hormones

ANDROGENS

Androgens include testosterone and related hormones that support male reproductive function. Other important androgens include androstenedione and dehydroepiandrosterone (DHEA). Therapeutically androgens are used to treat hypogonadism and certain cancers. These agents are in Table 46.1.

46.2 Pharmacotherapy with Androgens

Lack of sufficient testosterone secretion by the testes can result in male **hypogonadism.** Hypogonadism may be congenital or acquired later in life. When the condition is caused by a testicular disorder, it is called *primary* hypogonadism. Examples of disease states that may cause primary testicular

TABLE 46.1	Selected Androgens	
Drug	Route and Adult Dose (max dose where indicated)	Adverse Effects
danazol (Danocrine)	PO; 200–400 mg bid for 3–6 mo	*Acne, gynecomastia, hirsutism and male sex characteristics (in women), sodium and water retention, hypercholesterolemia* <u>Anaphylaxis, testicular atrophy and oligospermia at high doses</u>
fluoxymesterone (Halotestin)	PO; 5 mg one to four times/day	
methyltestosterone capsules (Android, Testred, Virilon); methyltestosterone tablets (Methitest)	PO; 10–50 mg/day Buccal: 5–25 mg/day	
nandrolone	IM; 50–200 mg/wk	
oxandrolone (Oxandrin)	PO; 2.5–20 mg/day divided two to four times/day for 2–4 wks	
oxymetholone (Androl-50)	PO; 1–5 mg/kg/day	
⊕ testosterone (Striant)	Buccal; 30 mg every 12 h	
(Testoderm TTS, Androderm, others)	Transdermal; Testoderm TTS patch: apply 1 daily; Androderm patch: apply 2.5–7.5 mg patch daily	
(AndroGel, Testim)	Gel; apply 5 grams daily (max 10 grams)	
testosterone cypionate (Depotest, Andro-Cyp, Depo-Testosterone)	IM; 50–400 mg every 2–4 wk	
testosterone enanthate (Andro L.A., Delatest, Delatestryl)	IM; 50–400 mg every 2–4 wk	

Italics indicate common adverse effects; <u>underlining</u> indicates serious adverse effects.

failure include mumps, testicular trauma or inflammation, and certain autoimmune disorders.

Without sufficient FSH and LH secretion by the pituitary, the testes will lack their stimulus to produce testosterone. This condition is known as *secondary* hypogonadism. Lack of FSH and LH secretion may have a number of causes, including Cushing's syndrome, thyroid disorders, estrogen-secreting tumors, and therapy with GnRH agonists such as leuprolide (Lupron).

Symptoms of male hypogonadism include a diminished appearance of the secondary sex characteristics of men: sparse axillary, facial, and pubic hair; increased subcutaneous fat; and small testicular size. In adult men, lack of testosterone can lead to erectile dysfunction, low sperm counts, and decreased **libido,** or interest in intercourse. Nonspecific complaints may include fatigue, depression, and reduced muscle mass. In young men, lack of sufficient testosterone secretion may lead to delayed puberty.

Pharmacotherapy of hypogonadism includes replacement therapy with testosterone or other androgens. Within days or weeks of initiating therapy, androgens improve libido and correct erectile dysfunction caused by low testosterone levels. Male sex characteristics reappear, a condition called *masculinization* or **virilization.** Depression resolves, and muscle strength rapidly improves. Therapy with androgens is targeted to return serum testosterone to normal levels. Above-normal levels serve no therapeutic purpose and increase the risk of adverse effects. Testosterone is available in a variety of different formulations, as listed in Table 46.2, to better meet the individual patient preferences and lifestyles.

Androgens have important physiologic effects outside the reproductive system. Testosterone promotes the synthesis of erythropoietin, which explains why men usually have a slightly higher hematocrit than women. Testosterone has a profound anabolic effect on skeletal muscle, which is the rationale for giving this drug to debilitated patients who have muscle-wasting disease.

Anabolic steroids are testosterone-like compounds with hormonal activity that are taken inappropriately by athletes who hope to build muscle mass and strength, thereby obtaining a competitive edge. Use of steroids is high among teens, who sometimes take these drugs because they believe it improves their appearance. When taken in large doses for prolonged periods, anabolic steroids can produce significant adverse effects, some of which may persist for months after discontinuing the drugs. These agents tend to raise cholesterol levels and may cause low sperm counts and impotence in men. In female athletes, menstrual irregularities are likely, with an obvious increase in masculine appearance. Oral androgens are hepatotoxic, and permanent liver damage may result with prolonged use. Behavioral changes include aggression and psychologic dependence. The use of anabolic steroids to improve athletic performance is illegal and strongly discouraged by health care providers and athletic associations. Most androgens are classified as Schedule III drugs because of their abuse potential.

High doses of androgens are occasionally used as a palliative measure to treat certain types of breast cancer, in combination with other antineoplastics. At the high doses required for breast cancer treatment, some virilization will occur in most patients. Because the growth of most prostate carcinomas is testosterone dependent, androgens should not be prescribed for older men unless the possibility of prostate cancer has been ruled out. Patients with prostate carcinoma are sometimes given a GnRH agonist such as leuprolide (Lupron) to reduce circulating testosterone levels.

TABLE 46.2	Androgen Formulations		
Route	Drug	Advantages	Disadvantages
Implantable pellets (subcutaneous)	Testopel: 1–6 pellets are implanted on the anterior abdominal wall depending upon the dose required.	Doses last 3–4 mo	Inflammation or infection may occur around insertion site.
Intramuscular (IM)	testosterone cypionate (Depo-Testosterone) and testosterone enanthate (Delatestryl)	Doses last 2–4 wk	Serum testosterone levels will vary widely after administration, causing the patient to experience fluctuations in their libido and energy, and experience mood swings. Patients tend to complain of soreness at the site of injection.
Testosterone buccal tablet	Striant tablet is applied to the gum area just above the incisor, holding it in place for 30 seconds.	Produces a continuous supply of testosterone in the blood.	Some men require twice-daily dosing. Local irritation to the buccal mucosa may occur.
Transdermal testosterone gel	AndroGel and Testim are applied once daily to the upper arms, shoulders, or abdomen.	The drug is absorbed into the skin in about 30 minutes and released slowly to the blood. Causes less skin irritation than patches.	Gel can be transferred to another person by skin-to-skin contact causing virilization of female contacts and fetal harm.
Transdermal testosterone patch	Androderm patch is applied daily to the upper arm, thigh, back or abdomen, rotating application sites.	Easy to use	Rash may occur at the site of patch application.

LIFESPAN CONSIDERATIONS

Human Chorionic Gonadotropin (hCG) Abuse by Athletes

Most health care providers are familiar with the serious problem of anabolic steroid use by athletes and teens. Fewer, however, are familiar with abuse of the placental hormone hCG in this population. hCG is not an anabolic steroid. Why would an athlete take a placental hormone? There are several reasons.

Men taking anabolic steroids experience a natural negative feedback phenomenon. The high levels of anabolic steroids provide feedback to the hypothalamus and pituitary to shut down production of testosterone by the testes. When the athlete stops taking the steroids the testes need several weeks to recover, and the man may suffer from loss of muscle strength, testicular atrophy, loss of libido, and impotence. Taking injectable hCG during this time immediately raises the man's testosterone level because hCG resembles leutenizing hormone, the natural stimulus for testosterone production. Thus, hCG is used to transition to regular (i.e., nonsteroid) training. hCG also masks steroid use by changing the types of steroids, and the amounts, that show up on laboratory tests conducted by athletic organizations.

The nurse needs to teach patients taking these illegal substances that hCG and anabolic steroids both have major adverse effects. These effects are those of excessive testosterone levels: testicular atrophy, feminization (excess testosterone is metabolized to estrogen), stunting of growth (it closes epiphyses in young teens), liver damage, and serious psychiatric disorders.

MALE INFERTILITY

It is estimated that 30% to 40% of infertility among couples is caused by difficulties with the male reproductive system. Male infertility may have a psychologic etiology, which must be ruled out before pharmacotherapy is considered.

46.3 Pharmacotherapy of Male Infertility

Like female infertility, male infertility may have a number of complex causes. The most obvious etiology is lack of sufficient sperm production. **Oligospermia**, the presence of less than 20 million sperm/mL of ejaculate, is considered abnormal and can lower reproductive success. **Azoospermia**, the complete absence of sperm in an ejaculate, may indicate an obstruction of the vas deferens or ejaculatory duct that can be corrected surgically. Infections such as mumps, chronic tuberculosis, and sexually transmitted diseases can contribute to infertility. The possibility of erectile dysfunction must be considered and treated, as discussed in Section 46.4. Infertility may occur with or without signs of hypogonadism.

The goal of endocrine pharmacotherapy of male infertility is to increase sperm production. Therapy often begins with IM injections of human chorionic gonadotropin (hCG), three times per week over 1 year. Although hCG is secreted by the placenta, its effects in men are identical to those of LH: increased testosterone secretion and spermatogenesis. Sperm counts are conducted periodically to assess therapeutic progress. If hCG is unsuccessful, therapy with menotropins (Pergonal) may be attempted. Menotropin consists of a mixture of purified FSH and LH. For infertile patients exhibiting signs of hypogonadism, testosterone therapy also may be indicated.

Other pharmacologic approaches to treating male infertility have been attempted. Antiestrogens such as tamoxifen (Nolvadex) and clomiphene (Clomid) have been used to block the negative feedback of estrogen (from the adrenal

Pr Prototype Drug | Testosterone

Therapeutic Class: Male sex hormone   **Pharmacologic Class:** Androgen; anabolic steroid; antineoplastic

ACTIONS AND USES

The primary therapeutic uses of testosterone are for the treatment of delayed puberty and hypogonadism in males. The drug promotes virilization, including enlargement of the sexual organs, growth of facial hair, and a deepening of the voice. In adult males, testosterone administration will increase libido and restore masculine characteristics that may be deficient. Testosterone is approved to treat erectile dysfunction that is caused by low androgen levels. The drug is also FDA approved for the palliative treatment of inoperable breast cancer in women.

Testosterone acts by stimulating RNA synthesis and protein metabolism. High doses may suppress spermatogenesis. Testosterone base is administered by the IM route, although other salts are available for the transdermal, implantable pellet, and buccal routes.

ADMINISTRATION ALERTS

- If using a patch, place on hair-free, dry skin of the abdomen, back, thigh, upper arm, or as directed.
- Alternate patch site daily, rotating sites every 7 days.
- Give IM injection into gluteal muscles.
- Pregnancy category X

PHARMACOKINETICS

Onset: Unknown

Peak: Unknown

Half-life: Unknown

Duration: 1–3 days (2–4 weeks for IM and pellet forms)

ADVERSE EFFECTS

An obvious adverse effect of testosterone therapy is virilization, which is usually only of concern when the drug is taken by female patients. Increased libido may occur. Salt and water are often retained, causing edema, and a diuretic may be indicated. Liver damage is rare, although it is a potentially serious adverse effect with some of the orally administered androgens. Acne and skin irritation is common during therapy. Females may experience suppression of ovulation or menstruation. Extreme doses in men (anabolic steroid abuse) may cause feminization rather than virilization because excess testosterone is metabolized to estrogen.

Contraindications: Testosterone is contraindicated in men with known or suspected breast or prostatic carcinomas and in women who are or may become pregnant (category X). The drug should be used with caution in patients with pre-existing renal or hepatic disease.

INTERACTIONS

Drug–Drug: Testosterone may potentiate the effects of oral anticoagulants and increase the risk of severe bleeding. Concurrent use of testosterone with corticosteroids may cause additive edema, which can be a serious concern for those with heart failure. Hepatotoxic drugs should be avoided because use with testosterone can cause additive liver damage.

Lab Tests: Values of the following may be decreased: T4, thyroxine-binding globulin, serum calcium, and clotting factors II, V, VII, and X. Creatinine may be increased, and cholesterol may be either increased or decreased.

Herbal/Food: The risk of hepatotoxicity may increase when testosterone is used with echinacea.

Treatment of Overdose: There is no specific treatment for overdose.

Refer to MyNursingKit for a Nursing Process Focus specific to this drug.

---

glands) to the pituitary and hypothalamus, thus increasing the levels of FSH and LH. Testolactone (Teslac), an aromatase inhibitor, has been administered to block the metabolic conversion of testosterone to estrogen. Various nutritional supplements have been tested, such as zinc to improve sperm production, L-arginine to improve sperm motility, and vitamins C and E as antioxidants to reduce reactive intermediates. Unfortunately, these and other therapies have not conclusively been shown to have any positive effect on male infertility.

Drug therapy of male infertility is not as successful as fertility pharmacotherapy in women, because only about 5% of infertile males have an endocrine etiology for their disorder. Many years of therapy may be required. Because of the expense of pharmacotherapy and the large number of injections needed, other means of conception may be explored, such as in vitro fertilization or intrauterine insemination.

ERECTILE DYSFUNCTION

Erectile dysfunction, or **impotence,** is a common disorder in men. The defining characteristic of this condition is the consistent inability to either obtain an erection or to sustain an erection long enough to achieve successful intercourse.

46.4 Pharmacotherapy of Erectile Dysfunction

The incidence of erectile dysfunction increases with age, although it may occur in a adult male of any age. Certain diseases, most notably atherosclerosis, diabetes, kidney disease, stroke, and hypertension, are associated with a higher incidence of the condition. Smoking increases the risk of erectile dysfunction by 30% to 60%, in a dose-dependent manner. Psychogenic causes may include depression, fatigue, guilt, or fear of sexual failure. A number of common drugs cause impotence as an adverse effect, including thiazide diuretics, phenothiazines, selective serotonin reuptake inhibitors (SSRIs), tricyclic antidepressants (TCAs), beta- and alpha-adrenergic blockers, and angiotensin converting enzyme (ACE) inhibitors. Low testosterone secretion can cause an inability to develop an erection, due to a loss of libido.

Penile erection has both neuromuscular and vascular components. Autonomic nerves dilate arterioles leading to the major erectile tissues of the penis, called the **corpora cavernosa.** The corpora have vascular spaces that fill with blood to cause rigidity. In addition, constriction of veins draining

MyNursingKit Erectile Dysfunction Resources

NURSING PROCESS FOCUS — PATIENTS RECEIVING ANDROGEN THERAPY

Assessment	Potential Nursing Diagnoses
Baseline assessment prior to administration: ■ Understand the reason the drug has been prescribed in order to assess for therapeutic effects (e.g., adult testicular failure, delayed puberty in boys over 15, hypogonadism). ■ Obtain a complete health history including cardiovascular, peripheral vascular, thyroid, hepatic, or renal disease; diabetes; prostatic hypertrophy; or prostatic or breast cancer. ■ Obtain a drug history including allergies, current prescription and OTC drugs, herbal preparations, alcohol use, and smoking. Be alert to possible drug interactions. ■ Evaluate appropriate laboratory findings (e.g., CBC, electrolytes, glucose, lipid levels, PSA). ■ Obtain baseline height, weight, and vital signs.	■ Disturbed Body Image (related to drug effects, aging process) ■ Sexual Dysfunction (related to drug effects) ■ Fluid Volume Excess (related to adverse drug effects) ■ Deficient Knowledge (drug therapy)
Assessment throughout administration: ■ Assess for desired therapeutic effects dependent on the reason the drug is given (e.g., hormone levels normalize, normal signs of masculinization are present). ■ Continue periodic monitoring of CBC, electrolytes, glucose, lipid levels, hepatic and renal function labs, and PSA levels. ■ Monitor vital signs, height, and weight at each health care visit. ■ Assess for adverse effects: nausea, vomiting, headache, weight gain, fluid retention, edema, increased blood pressure, changes in mood, irritability, and agitation. Also assess for tachycardia, palpitations, or hypertension, especially associated with angina or dyspnea; abdominal pain; or signs of hepatotoxicity.	

Planning: Patient Goals and Expected Outcomes

The patient will:
■ Experience therapeutic effects (e.g., normal virilization and development of secondary sex characteristics continues).
■ Be free from, or experience minimal, adverse effects.
■ Verbalize an understanding of the drug's use, adverse effects, and required precautions.
■ Demonstrate proper self-administration of the medication (e.g., dose, timing, when to notify provider).

Implementation

Interventions and (Rationales)	Patient and Family Education
Ensuring therapeutic effects: ■ Monitor appropriate medication administration. (Appropriate administration, especially of gels or transdermal forms, will optimize drug absorption and therapeutic effects.)	■ Teach the patient appropriate administration techniques (see "Patient self-administration of drug therapy" later in this table).
Minimizing adverse effects: ■ Monitor blood pressure at each clinical visit. Check body weight and for the presence of edema. (Androgens cause sodium and water retention with resulting increases in weight, blood pressure, and possible edema. Report promptly any BP over 140/90 mmHg, peripheral edema, or significant weight gain over a short amount of time.)	■ Teach the patient to monitor blood pressure on a weekly basis, ensuring proper functioning of any equipment used at home. Report any BP over 140/90 mmHg or as directed by the health care provider. Report any weight gain over 2 lb in 24 hours or 5 lb in 1 week. Report any peripheral edema.
■ Continue to monitor electrolytes, lipid levels, and hepatic function labs periodically. (Androgens may increase cholesterol and calcium levels. Hepatotoxicity and hepatic neoplasms are rare but potential adverse effects.)	■ Instruct the patient to return periodically for lab tests. ■ Teach the patient to immediately report any symptoms of abdominal or right upper quadrant discomfort or pain, yellowing of the skin or sclera, fatigue, anorexia, darkened urine or clay-colored stools, weakness, lethargy, nausea, or vomiting.

NURSING PROCESS FOCUS   PATIENTS RECEIVING ANDROGEN THERAPY (Continued)

Implementation

Interventions and (Rationales)	Patient and Family Education
▪ Monitor blood glucose levels in diabetic patients frequently. (Androgens may affect carbohydrate metabolism, leading to increased glucose levels. Men with diabetes should monitor their capillary blood glucose more frequently.)	▪ Teach men with diabetes to monitor capillary blood glucose more frequently while on drug and report consistent elevations to the health care provider.
▪ Monitor height and growth in children and adolescents. (Androgen administration may cause premature closure of epiphyses, and loss of normal growth patterns.)	▪ Teach the patient, family, or caregiver to measure height once per month or as directed. Return for clinical assessments as needed approximately every 6 months to monitor bone growth.
▪ Monitor use closely in adolescent patients. (Abuse of androgens and anabolic steroids may occur, along with resulting adverse effects.)	▪ Teach the adolescent patient to maintain daily dosing as instructed and not to increase dosage unless instructed to do so by the health care provider. The drug should never be shared with others.
Patient understanding of drug therapy: ▪ Use opportunities during administration of medications and during assessments to discuss the rationale for drug therapy, desired therapeutic outcomes, most commonly observed adverse effects, parameters for when to call the health care provider, and any necessary monitoring or precautions. (Using time during nursing care helps to optimize and reinforce key teaching areas.)	▪ The patient should be able to state the reason for the drug, appropriate dose and scheduling, and what adverse effects to observe for and when to report them.

Patient self-administration of drug therapy:
▪ When administering the medication, instruct the patient, family, or caregiver in the proper self-administration of drug, e.g., consistently at the same time each day to help remember the dose. (Proper administration will increase the effectiveness of the drug.)
	▪ Teach the patient to take the drug following appropriate guidelines:
	  ▪ Oral drugs should be taken at the same time each day to maintain consistent drug levels.
	  ▪ Transdermal patches should be applied to the scrotal area after dry shaving; do not use depilatories. Change patch and rotate sites daily and report any skin irritation.
	  ▪ Buccal tablets should be placed between the cheek and upper gum and held in place for 30 seconds. Rotate from side to side, avoiding areas of irritation.
	  ▪ Gels and creams should be applied to the upper torso, extremities, or abdomen. Swimming and showering should be avoided for several hours following administration. Do not allow women or children to come in contact with drug or application sites as the drug may rub off and cause adverse effects.
	  ▪ Transdermal pellets are implanted in the abdominal wall every 3 to 6 months.
	  ▪ Injections should be given into deep gluteal muscle. If the patient is to administer own injections, teach the appropriate technique, followed by return-demonstration until the patient is comfortable and demonstrates proper technique.

Evaluation of Outcome Criteria

Evaluate the effectiveness of drug therapy by confirming that patient goals and expected outcomes have been met (see "Planning").

See Table 46.1 for a list of drugs to which these nursing actions apply.

blood from the corpora allows the penis to remain rigid long enough for successful penetration. After ejaculation, the veins dilate, blood leaves the corpora, and the penis quickly loses its rigidity. Organic causes of erectile dysfunction may include damage to the nerves or blood vessels involved in the erection reflex.

The development of sildenafil (Viagra), an inhibitor of the enzyme phosphodiesterase-5 (PDE-5), revolutionized the medical therapy of erectile dysfunction. When sildenafil was approved as the first pharmacologic treatment for erectile dysfunction in 1998, it set a record for pharmaceutical sales for any new drug in U.S. history. Prior to the discovery of sildenafil, rigid or inflatable penile prostheses were implanted into the corpora. As an alternative to prostheses, drugs such as alprostadil (Caverject) or the combination of papaverine plus phentolamine were injected directly into

TABLE 46.3 Drugs for Erectile Dysfunction

Drug	Route and Adult Dose (max dose where indicated)	Adverse Effects
sildenafil (Viagra)	PO; 50 mg approximately 30–60 min before intercourse (max: 100 mg once/day)	*Nasal congestion, headache, facial flushing, dizziness, vision abnormalities, myalgia*
tadalafil (Cialis)	PO; 10 mg approximately 30 min before intercourse (max: 20 mg once/day)	
	Once-daily dosing: 2.5–5 mg daily	<u>Hypotension when taken with nitrates, priapism, hearing loss, nonarteritic anterior ischemic optic neuropathy</u>
vardenafil (Levitra)	PO; 10 mg approximately 1 h before intercourse (max: 20 mg once/day)	

Italics indicate common adverse effects; <u>underlining</u> indicates serious adverse effects.

the corpora cavernosa just prior to intercourse. Penile injections cause pain and reduce the spontaneity associated with pleasurable intercourse. These alternative therapies are rare today, though they may be used for patients in whom phosphodiesterase-5 inhibitors are contraindicated.

The PDE-5 inhibitors do not *cause* an erection; they merely *enhance* the erection resulting from physical contact or other sexual stimuli by maintaining relaxation of the smooth muscle in the penis and increasing blood flow. These drugs are not as effective in promoting erections in men who do not have ED. Despite considerable research interest, PDE-5 inhibitors have no effects on female sexual function, and these drugs are not approved for use by women.

Two other phosphodiesterase-5 inhibitors have been approved by the FDA. Vardenafil (Levitra), acts by the same mechanism as sildenafil but has a faster onset and slightly longer duration of action. Tadalafil (Cialis) acts within 30 minutes and has a prolonged duration lasting from 24 to 36 hours. Drugs for erectile dysfunction are listed in Table 46.3.

The three phosphodiesterase-5 inhibitors are equally effective at promoting erections in 60% to 80% of male patients, and adverse effects are similar. The most common adverse effects are nasal congestion, headache, facial flushing, and dizziness. These drugs produce a 5- to 10-mm fall in blood pressure, but this drop is usually not clinically important. In patients who are taking nitrates or multiple antihypertensive medications, however, this blood pressure change may produce symptoms of hypotension. Phosphodiesterase-5 inhibitors are contraindicated in patients taking nitrates. Tadalafil produces less blood pressure decrease than the other drugs in this class.

Pr Prototype Drug | Sildenafil (Viagra)

Therapeutic Class: Drug for treating impotence **Pharmacologic Class:** Phosphodiesterase (PDE)-5 inhibitor

ACTIONS AND USES
Sildenafil acts by relaxing smooth muscles in the corpora cavernosa, thus allowing increased blood flow into the penis. The increased blood flow results in a firmer and longer lasting erection in about 70% of men taking the drug. The onset of action is relatively rapid, less than 1 hour, and its effects last up to 4 hours. Sildenafil blocks the enzyme phosphodiesterase-5.

Sildenafil is also used for the treatment of pulmonary arterial hypertension. Blocking phosphodiesterase-5 in pulmonary vascular smooth muscle causes vasodilation and reduction in arterial hypertension. The drug improves exercise capacity in these patients.

ADMINISTRATION ALERTS
- Avoid administration of sildenafil with meals, especially high-fat meals, because absorption is decreased.
- Avoid grapefruit juice when administering sildenafil.

PHARMACOKINETICS
Onset: 20–60 min
Peak: 30–120 min
Half-life: 4 h
Duration: 24 h

ADVERSE EFFECTS
Sildenafil is well tolerated and adverse effects are usually transient and mild. Common adverse effects include headache, dizziness, flushing, rash, and nasal congestion. The most serious adverse effect, hypotension, occurs in patients concurrently taking organic nitrates for angina and can result in MI and sudden cardiac death. Sildenafil can produce blurred vision, increased sensitivity to light, or changes in color perception. Priapism, a sustained erection lasting longer than 6 hours, has been reported with sildenafil use and this may lead to permanent damage to penile tissues.

Contraindications: Sildenafil is contraindicated in patients taking nitrates and in those with hypersensitivity to the drug. These agents are contraindicated in patients with severe cardiovascular disease, recent MI, stroke, heart failure, dysrhythmias, and in the presence of anatomical deformities of the penis.

INTERACTIONS
Drug–Drug: Cimetidine, erythromycin, and ketoconazole will increase serum levels of sildenafil and necessitate lower drug doses. Use with nitrates will result in hypotension. Protease inhibitors (ritonavir, amprenavir, others) will cause increased sildenafil levels, which may lead to toxicity. Rifampin may decrease sildenafil levels, leading to decreased effectiveness.

Lab Tests: Unknown

Herbal/Food: Grapefruit juice increases the plasma concentrations of sildenafil and may cause adverse effects.

Treatment of Overdose: There is no specific treatment for overdose.

Refer to MyNursingKit for a Nursing Process Focus specific to this drug.

NURSING PROCESS FOCUS   PATIENTS RECEIVING TREATMENT FOR ERECTILE DYSFUNCTION

Assessment	Potential Nursing Diagnoses
Baseline assessment prior to administration: ■ Understand the reason the drug has been prescribed in order to assess for therapeutic effects (e.g., inability to obtain or sustain an erection). ■ Obtain a complete health history including cardiovascular, peripheral vascular, thyroid, hepatic, or renal disease; diabetes; and prostatic hypertrophy. ■ Obtain a drug history including allergies, current prescription and OTC drugs, herbal preparations, alcohol use, and smoking. Be alert to use of any antihypertensives and any possible drug interactions. ■ Evaluate appropriate laboratory findings (e.g., CBC, electrolytes, glucose, lipid levels, PSA). ■ Obtain baseline vital signs, especially blood pressure.	■ Sexual Dysfunction ■ Disturbed Body Image ■ Deficient Knowledge (drug therapy) ■ Risk for Injury (related to adverse drug effects)
Assessment throughout administration: ■ Assess for desired therapeutic effects dependent on the reason the drug is given (e.g., report of ability to achieve or maintain an erection). ■ Monitor vital signs, especially blood pressure. Report any blood pressure below 90/60 mmHg, or per parameters, to the health care provider. ■ Assess for adverse effects: nausea, vomiting, decreased blood pressure, or dizziness. Tachycardia, palpitations, or hypotension, especially associated with angina or dyspnea, should be reported immediately.	

Planning: Patient Goals and Expected Outcomes

The patient will:
■ Experience therapeutic effects (e.g., ability to achieve and maintain an erection).
■ Be free from, or experience minimal, adverse effects.
■ Verbalize an understanding of the drug's use, adverse effects, and required precautions.
■ Demonstrate proper self-administration of the medication (e.g., dose, timing, when to notify provider).

Implementation

Interventions and (Rationales)	Patient and Family Education
Ensuring therapeutic effects: ■ Monitor appropriate medication administration for optimum results. (Appropriate administration will optimize drug absorption and therapeutic effects.)	■ Teach the patient appropriate administration techniques (see "Patient self-administration of drug therapy" later in this table).
Minimizing adverse effects: ■ Monitor blood pressure at each clinical visit. Report any BP below 90/60 mmHg, especially if accompanied by tachycardia, dizziness, or chest pain, to the health care provider. Assess for concurrent use of nitrates or antihypertensives and review any new prescription. (Phosphodiesterase inhibitors cause vasodilation and may result in significant hypotension.)	■ Teach the patient to monitor blood pressure on a weekly basis, ensuring proper functioning of any equipment used at home. Report any BP below 90/60 mmHg. ■ Instruct the patient to not take the drug if currently taking nitrates for chest pain, even if only on a prn basis, and consult with the health care provider before starting any new prescription, especially for hypertension.
■ Monitor for changes in vision, including blurred vision, changes in the ability to view colors and for any sudden eye pain or lights or flashes in eyes. (Phosphodiesterase inhibitors may affect the ability to see colors, especially blue and green, and may cause blurred vision. Optic neuritis is a rare but serious adverse effect and significant visual changes or eye pain should be reported immediately.)	■ Caution the patient to exercise caution when driving or with activities involving visual acuity until effects of the drug are known. Patients who pilot aircraft should check with their employer or FAA regulations about the use of the drug before flying. ■ Instruct the patient to immediately report any significant changes in visual acuity, eye pain, lights, or flashes in the eyes to the health care provider.
■ Monitor for the development of priapism. (Any erection lasting longer than 4 hours should be reported to the health care provider for prompt treatment as tissue necrosis may occur.)	■ Instruct the patient to report any sustained erection lasting over 4 hours, or an erection with significant pain, to the health care provider and seek prompt medical treatment.

(Continued)

NURSING PROCESS FOCUS   PATIENTS RECEIVING PHARMACOTHERAPY FOR OSTEOPOROSIS AND OTHER BONE DISORDERS

Assessment	Potential Nursing Diagnoses
Baseline assessment prior to administration: ■ Understand the reason the drug has been prescribed in order to assess for therapeutic effects (e.g., replacement therapy for deficiencies or disease, preventative health maintenance). ■ Obtain a complete health history including musculoskeletal, gastrointestinal, cardiovascular, neurologic, endocrine, hepatic, or renal disease. Obtain a drug history including allergies, current prescription and OTC drugs, herbal preparations, alcohol use, or smoking. Be alert to possible drug interactions. ■ Obtain a history of any current symptoms and effect on ADLs. Assess muscle strength, gait, and note any pain or discomfort on movement or at rest. Obtain bone density studies as ordered. ■ Obtain a dietary history noting adequacy of essential vitamins, minerals, and nutrients obtained through food sources, particularly Ca, vitamin D, and Mg. Note the amount of soda intake daily. ■ Note sunscreen use and the amount of sun exposure. ■ Obtain baseline height, weight, and vital signs. ■ Evaluate appropriate laboratory findings (e.g., CBC; electrolytes; calcium, phosphorus, and magnesium levels; hepatic and renal function studies).	■ Acute or Chronic Pain (bone or joints) (related to disease condition) ■ Deficient Knowledge (drug therapy) ■ Risk for Injury, Risk for Falls (related to disease condition, adverse drug effects)
Assessment throughout administration: ■ Assess for desired therapeutic effects (e.g., calcium, phosphate, and magnesium levels are within normal limits; bone density studies show improvement). ■ Continue monitoring lab values as appropriate, especially Ca, phosphorus, and Mg. ■ Assess for and promptly report adverse effects: nausea, vomiting, abdominal pain, esophageal irritation, constipation or diarrhea, and electrolyte imbalances. Severe GI irritation or pain should be reported immediately.	

Planning: Patient Goals and Expected Outcomes

Patient will:
■ Experience therapeutic effects (e.g., maintenance of adequate bone density, lessened fracture risk).
■ Be free from, or experience minimal, adverse effects.
■ Verbalize an understanding of the drug's use, adverse effects, and required precautions.
■ Demonstrate proper self-administration of the medication (e.g., dose, timing, when to notify provider).

Implementation

Interventions and (Rationales)	Patient and Family Education
Ensuring therapeutic effects: ■ Review the dietary history with the patient and discuss food source options for correcting any calcium or vitamin D deficiencies. Encourage the patient to adopt a healthy lifestyle of increased physical activity, adequate sun exposure, limited caffeine and soda intake, and limited or eliminated alcohol consumption. (Adequate amounts of Ca, vitamin D, and Mg are needed for bone health. Any deficiencies should be corrected before bisphosphonates are started. Adequate sun exposure may assist in vitamin D formation. Excessive soda or caffeine intake may increase the risk of osteoporosis.)	■ Encourage adequate amounts of Ca, vitamin D, and Mg from food sources. Provide educational pamphlets or web-based references to reputable sources. Provide dietitian referral as needed. ■ Encourage limited amounts of sun exposure daily without sunscreens, approximately 15 to 20 minutes. Discourage prolonged sun exposure. ■ Teach the patient that excessive soda intake may take the place of beverages with milk or dairy. Excessive caffeine consumption may diminish the absorption of dietary calcium. ■ Encourage adequate activity, especially weight-bearing exercise, three to five times per week.

NURSING PROCESS FOCUS	PATIENTS RECEIVING PHARMACOTHERAPY FOR OSTEOPOROSIS AND OTHER BONE DISORDERS *(Continued)*

Implementation

Interventions and (Rationales)	Patient and Family Education
▪ Follow administration guidelines for optimum results. (Ca supplements and vitamin D should be taken with meals or within 1 hour after meals. Bisphosphonates should be taken on an empty stomach with a full glass of water and the patient should remain upright for 30 minutes to 1 hour. Bisphosphonates and calcium preparations should be taken 2 hours apart.)	▪ Teach the patient appropriate administration guidelines. Ensure that the patient is able to remain upright after administration if bisphosphonates are used.
Minimizing adverse effects: ▪ Monitor for GI irritation or abdominal pain. (Bisphosphonates may cause esophageal irritation and erosion. Increasing nausea and gastric or abdominal pain should be reported immediately.)	▪ Instruct the patient to immediately report any new onset of nausea or any increasing or severe chest or abdominal discomfort or pain.
▪ Continue to monitor periodic lab work, especially Ca, Mg, phosphorus levels, and creatinine as needed. Assess for signs or symptoms of hypo- or hypercalcemia. (Ca, Mg, and phosphorus levels should return to, and remain within, normal limits. Increased creatinine levels may required discontinuation of medications.)	▪ Instruct the patient on the need to return periodically for lab work. ▪ Instruct the patient to immediately report symptoms of hypocalcemia (muscle spasms, facial grimacing, irritability, hyper-reflexes) or hypercalcemia (increased bone pain, anorexia, nausea, vomiting, constipation, thirst, lethargy, fatigue).
▪ Increase fluid intake, avoiding caffeine or soda. (Increased fluid intake decreases the risk of renal calculi formation.)	▪ Encourage the patient to increase fluid intake to 2 L of fluid per day, divided throughout the day, but avoid highly caffeinated beverages and excessive soda intake.
▪ Monitor adherence to recommended regimen. (Bone remodeling occurs over several months' time. The patient may discontinue drug because of perceived lack of response.)	▪ Teach the patient to continue taking the drug therapy regularly to ensure full effects. Therapeutic response may take 1 to 3 months and effects continue after the drug has been discontinued.
Patient understanding of drug therapy: ▪ Use opportunities during administration of medications and during assessments to discuss the rationale for drug therapy, desired therapeutic outcomes, most commonly observed adverse effects, parameters for when to call the health care provider, and any necessary monitoring or precautions. (Using time during nursing care helps to optimize and reinforce key teaching areas.)	▪ The patient should be able to state the reason for the drug; appropriate dose and scheduling; what adverse effects to observe for and when to report; and the anticipated length of medication therapy.
Patient self-administration of drug therapy: ▪ When administering the medication, instruct the patient, family, or caregiver in the proper self-administration of the drug, e.g., taken with additional fluids. (Proper administration increases the effectiveness of the drugs.)	▪ The patient is able to discuss appropriate dosing and administration needs.

Evaluation of Outcome Criteria

Evaluate the effectiveness of drug therapy by confirming that patient goals and expected outcomes have been met (see "Planning").

See Tables 47.1 & 47.2 for a list of drugs to which these nursing actions apply.

addition to treating osteoporosis, calcitonin is indicated for Paget's disease and hypercalcemia. For osteoporosis, calcitonin is less effective than other therapies and is considered a second-line treatment.

OTHER DRUGS FOR MBD

Cinacalcet (Sensipar) is a calcium modifier approved to treat hypercalcemia caused by parathyroid gland cancer or for hyperparathyroidism due to chronic kidney disease. Cinacalcet is a calcium mimic; the drug is recognized as calcium by the parathyroid glands. When the drug is present, the parathyroid glands shut down the production of PTH, serum calcium falls, and bone resorption diminishes. Cinacalcet is an oral drug. Nausea, vomiting, and diarrhea are common during therapy.

Teriparatide (Forteo) is a form of human PTH, produced by recombinant DNA technology. The actions of teriparatide are identical to those of endogenous PTH. It is the only drug available that will increase bone formation. The only approved indication for teriparatide is for the treatment of osteoporosis in men and postmenopausal women. The drug is usually reserved for patients with a high risk of bone fractures.

A disadvantage of the drug is that it must be given daily by the subcutaneous route. The drug is well tolerated with dizziness and leg cramps being the most frequent adverse effects.

TREATING THE DIVERSE PATIENT

The Impact of Ethnicity and Lifestyle on Osteoporosis

Women of Caucasian and Asian American descent have a higher incidence of osteoporosis than those of African American descent, although postmenopausal women are at the highest risk in all ethnic groups. It is important to remember that men also can develop this disease.

Even though medications are available to halt bone deterioration, prevention by establishing and maintaining a healthy lifestyle is the key to conquering osteoporosis. During childhood and adolescence, the focus should be on building bone mass. Children should be encouraged to eat foods high in calcium and vitamin D, exercise regularly, and avoid smoking and excessive use of alcohol. During adulthood, the focus should be on maintaining bone mass and continuing healthy dietary and exercise habits. Vitamin supplements may be taken on the advice of the health care provider. Postmenopausal women should focus on preventing bone loss. In addition to maintaining a healthy lifestyle, patients should have bone density tests and should discuss the possibility of taking medication to prevent or treat osteoporosis with their health care provider.

JOINT DISORDERS

Joint conditions such as osteoarthritis, rheumatoid arthritis, and gout are frequent indications for pharmacotherapy. Because joint pain is common to all three disorders, analgesics and anti-inflammatory drugs are important components of pharmacotherapy. A few additional drugs are specific to the particular joint pathology.

AVOIDING MEDICATION ERRORS

The evening nurse on duty administers medications at 10:15 p.m. When a nurse enters Ms. Brown's room, Ms. Brown is already in bed and falling asleep. The nurse gently shakes her and says, "I have your 10 p.m. medications, Ms. Brown." Although the patient awakens, she is not fully awake. The nurse hands her the medication and a glass of water. Ms. Brown takes the medication and quickly returns to sleeping. In leaving, the nurse notices the room number and realizes that medication was just given to Ms. Crown, who is in a room down the hall from Ms. Brown. What should the nurse have done differently?

See Appendix D for the suggested answer.

Pr Prototype Drug | Raloxifene *(Evista)*

Therapeutic Class: Drug for osteoporosis prevention   **Pharmacologic Class:** Selective estrogen receptor modulator

ACTIONS AND USES

Raloxifene is a selective estrogen receptor modulator (SERM). It decreases bone resorption and increases bone mass and density by acting through the estrogen receptor. Raloxifene is primarily used for the prevention of osteoporosis in postmenopausal women. Although the drug reduces vertebral fractures caused by osteoporosis of the spine, it does not appear to reduce the incidence of fractures at nonvertebral sites. This drug also reduces serum total cholesterol and LDL (low-density lipoprotein) without lowering HDL (high-density lipoprotein) or triglycerides.

In 2007, raloxifene was approved for invasive breast cancer prophylaxis in postmenopausal women at high risk for breast cancer. It is important for nurses and patients to understand that this drug is for the prevention, not treatment, of breast carcinoma.

ADMINISTRATION ALERTS

- Give with or without food.
- Pregnancy category X

PHARMACOKINETICS

Onset: 8 weeks

Peak: Unknown

Half-life: 27–33 h

Duration: Unknown

ADVERSE EFFECTS

The most common adverse effects of raloxifene therapy are hot flashes, leg cramps, and weight gain. Less common effects include fever, arthralgia, depression, insomnia, chest pain, peripheral edema, decreased serum cholesterol, nausea, vomiting, flatulence, cystitis, migraine headache, flulike symptoms, endometrial disorder, breast pain, and vaginal bleeding. Raloxifene has two black box warnings. First it may increase the risk for deep vein thrombosis or pulmonary embolism. Second, use of raloxifene may increase the risk of death due to stroke in women with coronary heart disease.

Contraindications: This drug is contraindicated during lactation and pregnancy, and in women who may become pregnant. Patients with a history of venous thromboembolism and those hypersensitive to raloxifene should not take this drug.

INTERACTIONS

Drug–Drug: Concurrent use with warfarin may decrease prothrombin time. Decreased raloxifene absorption will result from concurrent use with ampicillin or cholestyramine. Use of raloxifene with other highly protein-bound drugs (ibuprofen, indomethacin, diazepam, etc.) may interfere with binding sites. Patients should not take cholesterol-lowering drugs or estrogen replacement therapy concurrently with this medication.

Lab Tests: Raloxifene increases values of apolipoprotein A_1, corticosteroid-binding globulin, and thyroxine-binding globulin. It may decrease values of cholesterol, fibrinogen, apolipoprotein B, and lipoprotein (a), calcium, phosphate, total protein, and albumin.

Herbal/Food: Black cohosh has estrogenic effects and may interfere with the actions of raloxifene.

Treatment of Overdose: There is no specific treatment for overdose.

Refer to MyNursingKit for a Nursing Process Focus specific to this drug.

Arthritis

- Between 20 and 40 million people in the United States are affected by osteoarthritis.

- After age 40, more than 90% of the population have symptoms of osteoarthritis in major weight-bearing joints. After 70 years of age, almost all patients have symptoms of osteoarthritis.

- Of the world's population, 1% have rheumatoid arthritis, which most often affects patients between 30 and 50 years of age. Women are three to five times more likely to develop rheumatoid arthritis than men.

- Between 1% and 3% of the U.S. population are affected by gout. Most of the patients are men between the ages of 30 and 60. Most women are affected after menopause.

47.5 Pharmacotherapy of Osteoarthritis and Rheumatoid Arthritis

Arthritis is a general term meaning inflammation of a joint. There are several types of arthritis, each having somewhat different characteristics based on the etiology. Gouty arthritis is presented in Section 47.7.

Nonpharmacologic therapies are sometimes effective at relieving arthritis pain. The use of nonimpact and passive range-of-motion (ROM) exercises to maintain flexibility along with adequate rest is encouraged. Splinting may help keep joints positioned correctly and relieve pain. Other therapies commonly used to relieve pain and discomfort include thermal therapies, meditation, visualization, distraction techniques, and massage. Knowledge of proper body mechanics and posture may offer some benefit. Surgical procedures such as joint replacement and reconstructive surgery may become necessary when other methods are ineffective.

OSTEOARTHRITIS

Osteoarthritis (OA) is a progressive, degenerative joint disease caused by the breakdown of articular cartilage. It is the most common type of arthritis. Weight-bearing joints such as the knee, spine, and hip are most frequently affected. Symptoms include localized pain and stiffness, joint and bone enlargement, and limitations in movement. OA is not accompanied by the severe degree of inflammation associated with other forms of arthritis. Many consider this condition to be a normal part of the aging process. A patient with OA is shown in ➤ Figure 47.4.

The goals of pharmacotherapy for OA include reduction of pain and inflammation. The initial treatment of choice is acetaminophen because it is inexpensive and relatively safe. For patients whose pain is unrelieved by acetaminophen, nonsteroidal anti-inflammatory drugs (NSAIDs), including naproxen and ibuprofen-like drugs, are usually given. Because high doses of NSAIDs can cause GI bleeding and affect platelet aggregation, patients must be carefully monitored. Aspirin is no longer recommended because the high doses needed to produce pain relief in OA patients may cause GI bleeding. Tramadol (Ultram) has become a popular drug for

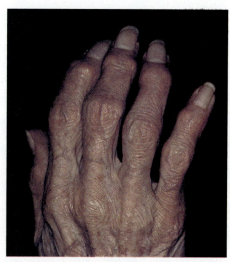

➤ *Figure 47.4* Patient with osteoarthritis

the treatment of moderate to severe pain. Although classified as an opioid, tramadol does not have abuse potential and is not a scheduled drug. Opioids such as codeine may be combined with acetaminophen for severe pain. The student should refer to chapter 18 for a complete discussion of the actions and side effects of analgesics∞. In acute cases, intra-articular glucocorticoids may be used on a temporary basis. Note that all these therapies are symptomatic; none of these drugs modify the progressive course of OA.

Many patients with osteoarthritis use OTC topical creams, gels, sprays, patches, or ointments that include salicylates (Aspercreme and Sportscreme), capsaicin (Capzasin), and counterirritants (Ben-Gay and Icy Hot). These therapies are well tolerated and produce few adverse effects.

A newer approach to treating patients with moderate OA who do not respond adequately to analgesics includes sodium hyaluronate (Hyalgan), a chemical normally found in high amounts within synovial fluid. Administered by injection directly into the knee joint, this drug replaces or supplements the body's natural hyaluronic acid that deteriorated because of the inflammation of osteoarthritis. Treatment consists of one injection per week for three to five injections. By coating the articulating cartilage surface, Hyalgan helps provide a barrier that prevents friction and further inflammation of the joint.

RHEUMATOID ARTHRITIS

Rheumatoid arthritis (RA) is a chronic, progressive disease that is characterized by disfigurement and inflammation of multiple joints. RA occurs at an earlier age than osteoarthritis and has an autoimmune etiology. In RA, **autoantibodies** called *rheumatoid factors* attack the person's tissues, activating complement and drawing leukocytes into the area, where they attack the cells of the synovial membranes and blood. This results in persistent injury and the formation of inflammatory fluid within the joints. Joint capsules, tendons, ligaments, and skeletal muscles may also be affected. Unlike OA, which causes local pain in affected joints, RA may produce systemic manifestations that include infections, pulmonary disease, pericarditis, abnormal numbers of blood cells, and symptoms of metabolic dysfunction such as fatigue, anorexia, and weakness. A patient with RA is shown in ➤ Figure 47.5.

The primary goals of RA pharmacotherapy are to control inflammation, reduce pain, and minimize physical disability. Pharmacotherapy for the relief of pain associated with RA is begun with NSAIDs, because these agents relieve both pain and inflammation. NSAIDs for RA patients are usually given in higher doses than those for patients with osteoarthritis. Aspirin is not recommended for long-term therapy due to its adverse effects on the GI system and platelet aggregation. Acetaminophen is effective at relieving pain and fever, but has no anti-inflammatory actions. Although these analgesics relieve symptomatic pain, they have little effect on disease progression. Because of their potent anti-inflammatory action, glucocorticoids may be used for RA flare-ups but are not used for long-term therapy because of their adverse effects.

Unlike OA, the progression of RA can be modified with drug therapy. These **disease-modifying antirheumatic drugs (DMARDs)** belong to several drug classes and have been found to reduce mortality due to RA. DMARDs are administered after pain and anti-inflammatory medications have failed to achieve the desired treatment outcomes. Many physicians begin therapy with a DMARD within the first few months after a confirmed diagnosis of RA. It would not be unusual for a patient to be taking several DMARDs and analgesics concurrently. Maximum therapeutic effects may take several months to achieve. Because many of these drugs can be toxic, patients must be closely monitored. These agents and their adverse effects are listed in Table 47.3.

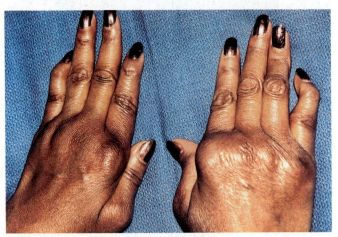

➤ **Figure 47.5** Patient with rheumatoid arthritis
Source: Courtesy of Dr. Jason L. Smith.

TABLE 47.3	Selected Disease-Modifying Antirheumatic Drugs (DMARDs)	
Drug	**Route and Adult Dose (max dose where indicated)**	**Adverse Effects**
abatacept (Orencia)	IV; 500–1,000 mg given on 0, 2, and 4 wks, then every 4 wks thereafter	*Local reactions at injection site (pain, erythema, myalgia), headache, nasopharyngitis*
adalimumab (Humira)	Subcutaneous; 40 mg every other week	
anakinra (Kineret)	Subcutaneous; 100 mg/day	<u>Opportunistic infections (including TB, sepsis, hepatitis B reactivation, and invasive fungal infections), lupus-like syndrome, tumor lysis syndrome (rituximab), worsening of heart failure (certolizumab, infliximab), Stevens–Johnson syndrome, hepatotoxicity (leflunomide, infliximab), malignancies (especially lymphomas)</u>
certolizumab pegol (Cimza)	Subcutaneous; 400 mg initially and at weeks 2 and 4, followed by 200 mg every other wk	
etanercept (Enbrel)	Subcutaneous; 25 mg twice weekly; or 0.08 mg/kg or 50 mg once weekly	
golimumab (Simponi)	Subcutaneous; 50 mg once monthly	
infliximab (Remicade)	IV; 3mg/kg at weeks 0, 2, and 6, then every 8 wk	
leflunomide (Arava)	PO; 100 mg loading dose for 3 days, then 20 mg/day	
rituximab (Rituxan)	IV; 1,000 mg every 2 wk for a total of two doses	
azathioprine (Imuran, Azasan)	PO; 1 mg/kg/day once or in divided doses bid for 6–8 wk (max: 2.5 mg/kg/day); Maintenance dose is 1–2.5 mg/kg/day as a single dose or divided	*Chills, fever, malaise, myalgia* <u>Myelosuppression, hepatoxicity, lymphoproliferative disorders</u>
ⓟ hydroxychloroquine (Plaquenil)	PO; 400–600 mg/day for 4–12 wk, then 200–400 mg once daily Maintenance dose: 10–20 mg/day	*Anorexia, nausea, vomiting, headache, personality changes* <u>Retinopathy, agranulocytosis, aplastic anemia, seizures</u>
methotrexate (Rheumatrex, Trexall)	PO; 7.5 mg once/wk or 2.5 mg every 12 h for three doses once/wk (max: 20 mg/wk)	*Headache, glossitis, gingivitis, mild leukopenia, nausea* <u>Ulcerative stomatitis, myelosuppression, aplastic anemia, hepatic cirrhosis, nephrotoxicity, sudden death, pulmonary fibrosis, agranulocytosis, hemolytic anemia, aplastic anemia, renal failure, teratogenicity</u>
sulfasalazine (Azulfidine)	PO; 500–1,000 mg/day (max: 3 g/day)	*Headache, anorexia, nausea, vomiting* <u>Anaphylaxis, Stevens–Johnson syndrome, agranulocytosis, leukopenia, reversible oligospermia</u>
Italics indicate common adverse effects; <u>underlining</u> indicates serious adverse effects.		

Glucosamine and Chondroitin for Osteoarthritis

Glucosamine is a natural substance that is an important building block of cartilage. With aging, glucosamine is lost with the natural thinning of cartilage. As cartilage wears down, joints lose their normal cushioning ability, resulting in the pain and inflammation of osteoarthritis. Glucosamine sulfate is available as an OTC dietary supplement. Some studies have shown it to be more effective than a placebo in reducing mild arthritis and joint pain. It is purported to promote cartilage repair in the joints. A typical dose is 500 to 10,000 mg/day.

Chondroitin is another dietary supplement purported to promote cartilage repair. It is a natural substance that forms part of the matrix between cartilage cells. Chondroitin is safe and almost free of side effects. A typical dose is 400 to 1,500 mg/day for 1–2 months. Chondroitin is usually combined with glucosamine in specific arthritis formulas. Research shows that glucosamine and chondroitin may be effective only for moderate to severe osteoarthritis pain (Clegg et al., 2006).

The choice of specific DMARD depends upon the experiences of the health care provider and the response of the patient to therapy. Therapy often begins with hydroxychloroquine (Plaquenil), methotrexate (Rheumatrex, Trexall), or sulfasalazine (Azulfidine), because these drugs have the most research-based evidence for reducing mortality due to RA. Gold salts, D-penicillamine (Cuprimine), azathioprine (Imuran), cyclosporine (Neoral), and cyclophosphamide (Cytoxan) are used as second-line drugs because they are more toxic. Biologic therapies such as etanercept (Enbrel), anakinra (Kineret), and the recently approved certolizumab pegol (Cimza) are newer therapies that block steps in the inflammatory response. The biologic agents appear to be effective and relatively nontoxic, although they are more expensive than first-line therapies.

47.6 Pharmacotherapy of Gout

Gout is a form of acute arthritis caused by an accumulation of uric acid (urate) crystals in the joints and other body tissues, causing inflammation. These crystals are the result of increased metabolism of nucleic acids or the reduced excretion of uric acid by the kidneys. Uric acid is a waste product created by the metabolic breakdown of DNA and RNA. An important metabolic step in the pharmacotherapy of this disease is the conversion of hypoxanthine to uric acid by the enzyme xanthine oxidase.

In patients with gout, uric acid accumulates and **hyperuricemia**, an elevated blood level of uric acid, occurs. Patients with mild hyperuricemia may be asymptomatic. Once the level of uric acid rises to saturation levels in body fluids, urate crystals form and symptoms appear, usually with a sudden onset.

Gout may be classified as primary or secondary. *Primary gout* is caused by a hereditary defect in uric acid metabolism that causes uric acid to be produced faster than it can be excreted by the kidneys. *Secondary gout* is caused by diseases or drugs that increase the metabolic turnover of nucleic acids, or that interfere with uric acid excretion. Examples of drugs that may cause gout include thiazide diuretics,

---

Pr Prototype Drug | Hydroxychloroquine *(Plaquenil)*

Therapeutic Class: Antirheumatic drug; antimalarial **Pharmacologic Class:** Disease-modifying antirheumatic drug

ACTIONS AND USES
Hydroxychloroquine is an older drug that is prescribed for rheumatoid arthritis and lupus erythematosus in patients who have not responded well to other anti-inflammatory drugs. This drug is also used for prophylaxis and treatment of malaria, but chloroquine (Aralen) is the preferred agent for this parasitic infection (chapter 35 ∞). Hydroxychloroquine relieves the severe inflammation characteristic of these disorders, although its mechanism of action is not known. For full effectiveness, hydroxychloroquine is most often prescribed with salicylates and glucocorticoids.

ADMINISTRATION ALERTS
- Take at the same time every day.
- Administer with milk to decrease GI upset.
- Store drug in safe place, as it is very toxic to children.
- Pregnancy category C

PHARMACOKINETICS
Onset: 4–6 weeks for antirheumatic response
Peak: 1–2 h
Half-life: 32–52 days
Duration: Unknown

ADVERSE EFFECTS
Adverse effects include anorexia, GI disturbances, loss of hair, headache, and mood and mental changes. Possible ocular effects include blurred vision, photophobia, diminished ability to read, and blacked-out areas in the visual field. With high doses or prolonged therapy, these retinal changes may be irreversible in some patients.

Contraindications: Patients hypersensitive to the drug or who exhibit retinal or visual field changes associated with quinoline drugs should not receive hydroxychloroquine.

INTERACTIONS
Drug–Drug: Antacids containing aluminum or magnesium may prevent absorption of hydroxychloroquine. Hydroxychloroquine may increase the risk of liver toxicity when administered with hepatotoxic drugs; alcohol use should be eliminated during therapy. This drug also may lead to increased digoxin levels, and may interfere with the patient's response to rabies vaccine.

Lab Tests: Unknown

Herbal/Food: Unknown

Treatment of Overdose: Overdose may be life threatening, especially in children. Therapy with anticonvulsants, vasopressors, and antidysrhythmics may be necessary.

Refer to MyNursingKit for a Nursing Process Focus specific to this drug.

Pr Prototype Drug | Colchicine *(Colcrys)*

Therapeutic Class: Drug for gout   **Pharmacologic Class:** Uric acid inhibitor

ACTIONS AND USES

Colchicine is a natural product obtained from the autumn crocus that has been the traditional oral drug of choice for the treatment of acute gouty arthritis. It has been used for centuries, and was approved by the FDA in 1939. It is most effective if taken within 24 hours after the onset of symptoms. The drug reduces inflammation associated with acute gouty arthritis by inhibiting the synthesis of microtubules, subcellular structures responsible for helping white blood cells infiltrate an area. Although colchicine has no analgesic properties, patients experience pain relief due to the reduction in inflammation. It may be taken to prevent or treat acute gout, often in combination with other uric acid-inhibiting agents. In 2009, colchicine became the first drug approved by the FDA to treat familial Mediterranean fever (FMF), a hereditary disorder characterized by acute inflammation and arthritis.

ADMINISTRATION ALERTS

- Take on an empty stomach, when symptoms first appear.
- Pregnancy category C. Parenteral doses must not be given to pregnant women.

PHARMACOKINETICS
Onset: 12 h
Peak: 0.5–2 h
Half-life: 1.7–20 h
Duration: Unknown

ADVERSE EFFECTS

Adverse effects such as nausea, vomiting, diarrhea, anorexia, and abdominal pain are common at the beginning of therapy. The drug may cause bone marrow toxicity, and aplastic anemia, leucopenia, thrombocytopenia, or agranulocytosis may occur.

Contraindications: This drug is contraindicated in patients with a known hypersensitivity to colchicine, and in those with serious GI, renal, hepatic, or cardiac impairment. Patients with blood dyscrasias should not receive colchicine.

INTERACTIONS

Drug–Drug: Concurrent use with NSAIDs may increase the risk of GI symptoms. Colchicine may exhibit additive bone marrow toxicity with cyclosporine, phenylbutazone, and other drugs that adversely affect bone marrow. Erythromycin may increase serum colchicine levels. Loop diuretics may decrease colchicine effects. Alcohol or products that contain alcohol may cause skin rashes and result in additive liver damage. Colchicine may increase sensitivity to CNS depressants.

Lab Tests: Colchicine may interfere with urinary steroid determinations, and may give false-positive values for urinary erythrocytes and Hgb.

Herbal/Food: Colchicine may interfere with the absorption of vitamin B_{12}. Foods that are rich in purines, including alcohol, salmon, sardines, and organ meats should be avoided. Foods that cause the urine to become more alkaline may increase the risk of kidney stones, including milk, fruits, carbonated drinks, most vegetables, molasses, and baking soda.

Treatment of Overdose: Overdoses (including accidental ingestion of autumn crocus) may cause severe GI distress, shock, paralysis, delirium, respiratory failure, and death. Treatment is symptomatic and may include gastric lavage and hemodialysis.

Refer to MyNursingKit for a Nursing Process Focus specific to this drug.

---

aspirin, cyclosporine, and alcohol, when ingested on a chronic basis. Conditions that can cause secondary gout include diabetic ketoacidosis, kidney failure, and diseases associated with a rapid cell turnover such as leukemia, hemolytic anemia, and polycythemia.

Acute gouty arthritis occurs when needle-shaped uric acid crystals accumulate in joints, resulting in extremely painful, red, and inflamed tissue. Attacks have a sudden onset, often occur at night, and may be triggered by ingestion of alcohol, dehydration, stress, injury to the joint, or fever. Gouty arthritis most often occurs in the big toes, heels, ankles, wrists, fingers, knees, or elbows. Of patients with gout, 90% are men. Kidney stones occur in 10% to 25% of patients with gout and are more likely to occur in patients with low fluid intake and when the urine is acidic.

The goals of gout pharmacotherapy are twofold: termination of acute attacks and prevention of future episodes. NSAIDs are the drugs of choice for treating the pain and inflammation of acute attacks. Indomethacin (Indocin) and naproxen (Naprosyn) are NSAIDs that have been widely used for acute gout. Glucocorticoids may be used to treat exacerbations of acute gout, particularly when the symptoms are in a single joint, and the medication can be delivered intra-articularly.

Prophylactic therapy of gout includes drugs that lower serum uric acid. Prophylactic therapy is used for patients who suffer frequent and acute gout attacks. Combination therapy using uric acid inhibitors such as colchicine and antigout medications such as probenecid (Benemid) and allopurinol (Zyloprim) are the mainstay of gout prophylaxis. Colchicine reduces the accumulation of uric acid in the blood or uric acid crystals within the joints. Probenecid increases the excretion of uric acid by blocking its reabsorption in the kidney. Allopurinol blocks xanthine oxidase, thus inhibiting the formation of uric acid. When uric acid accumulation is blocked, symptoms associated with gout diminish. In 2009, the first new antigout drug in over 40 years was approved by the FDA. Febuxostat (Uloric) acts by the same mechanism as allopurinol but is safer for patients with renal impairment because it is not excreted by the kidneys. Drugs for gout are listed in Table 47.4.

A plan for gout management should include dietary changes and avoidance of drugs that worsen the condition in addition to treatment with antigout medications. Patients should avoid high-purine foods such as meat, legumes, alcoholic beverages, mushrooms, and oatmeal, because nucleic acids will be formed when they are metabolized.

TABLE 47.4	**Drugs for Gout**	
Drug	Route and Adult Dose (max dose where indicated)	Adverse Effects
allopurinol (Lopurin, Zyloprim, others)	PO (primary); 100 mg/day; may increase by 100 mg/wk (max: 800 mg/day) PO (secondary); 200–800 mg/day for 2–3 days or longer	*Drowsiness, skin rash, diarrhea* <u>Severe skin reactions, bone marrow depression, hepatotoxicity, renal failure</u>
ⓟ colchicine (Colcrys)	PO; 0.5–1.2 mg, followed by 0.5–0.6 mg every 1–2 h until pain is relieved (max: 1.2 mg/day)	*Nausea, vomiting, diarrhea, GI upset* <u>Bone marrow depression, aplastic anemia, leukopenia, thrombocytopenia and agranulocytosis, severe diarrhea, nephrotoxicity</u>
febuxostat (Uloric)	PO; 40-80 mg once daily	*Nausea, rash* <u>Liver function abnormalities</u>
probenecid (Benemid, Probalan)	PO; 250 mg bid for 1 wk, then 500 mg bid (max: 3 g/day)	*Nausea, vomiting, headache, anorexia, flushed face* <u>Anaphylaxis, severe skin reactions, hepatotoxicity</u>
sulfinpyrazone (Anturane)	PO; 100–200 mg bid for 1 wk, then increase to 200–400 mg bid	*GI distress, rash* <u>Blood dyscrasias, nephrolithiasis</u>

Italics indicate common adverse effects; <u>underlining</u> indicates serious adverse effects.

NURSING PROCESS FOCUS   PATIENTS RECEIVING ANTIGOUT THERAPY

Assessment	Potential Nursing Diagnoses
Baseline assessment prior to administration: ■ Understand the reason the drug has been prescribed in order to assess for therapeutic effects (e.g., decreasing acute inflammatory stage, preventing recurrence). ■ Obtain a complete health history including musculoskeletal, gastrointestinal, cardiovascular, neurologic, endocrine, hepatic, or renal disease. Obtain a drug history including allergies, current prescription and OTC drugs, herbal preparations, alcohol use, or smoking. Be alert to possible drug interactions. ■ Obtain a history of any current symptoms and affect on ADLs. Assess for inflammation, location, and note any pain or discomfort on movement or at rest. ■ Obtain a dietary history, noting correlations between food intake and increase in symptoms. Assess fluid intake. ■ Obtain baseline weight and vital signs. ■ Evaluate appropriate laboratory findings (e.g., uric acid level, CBC, hepatic and renal function studies, urinalysis).	■ Acute Pain (related to acute stage of disease) ■ Activity Intolerance (related to joint pain) ■ Disturbed Body Image (related to joint inflammation and swelling) ■ Deficient Knowledge (drug therapy) ■ Risk for Injury (related to acute inflammatory condition)
Assessment throughout administration: ■ Assess for desired therapeutic effects dependent on the reason for the drug (e.g., symptoms of acute inflammation are diminished or absent, no return of symptoms). ■ Continue monitoring of vital signs and urine output. ■ Continue to monitor uric acid level, CBC, and hepatic and renal studies. ■ Assess for and promptly report adverse effects: nausea, vomiting, abdominal pain, skin rash, pruritus, paresthesias, diminished urine output, fever, and infections.	

Planning: Patient Goals and Expected Outcomes

The patient will:

■ Experience therapeutic effects (e.g., diminished inflammation, decreased or absent joint pain, increased ability to continue ADLs).

■ Be free from, or experience minimal, adverse effects.

■ Verbalize an understanding of the drug's use, adverse effects, and required precautions.

■ Demonstrate proper self-administration of the medication (e.g., dose, timing, when to notify provider).

(Continued)

NURSING PROCESS FOCUS   **PATIENTS RECEIVING ANTIGOUT THERAPY** *(Continued)*

Implementation

Interventions and (Rationales)	Patient and Family Education
Ensuring therapeutic effects: ■ Review the dietary history, noting any correlation between diet and symptoms, especially after ingestion of purine-containing foods. Avoid large doses of vitamin C. (Gout may occur due to overproduction or underexcretion of uric acid or a combination of both. Correlating symptoms to intake of high-purine foods assists in determining the most effective drug therapy. Large doses of vitamin C may acidify the urine leading to formation of uric acid stones.)	■ Encourage the patient to keep a food diary, noting any occurrence or increasing of symptoms related to food or beverage intake. ■ Teach the patient to limit intake of high-purine foods [e.g., salmon, sardines, organ meats, alcohol, mushrooms, legumes, oatmeal] and to limit or eliminate alcohol consumption.
■ Increase fluid intake to 2 to 4 L per day. Monitor urine output and obtain periodic urinalysis. (Increased fluid intake increases uric acid excretion and prevents urinary uric acid crystal formation or renal calculi.)	■ Teach the patient to increase fluid intake to 2 to 4 L per day, taken throughout the day.
■ Continue to monitor serum and urinary uric acid levels and note improvement in symptoms of acute inflammation, gouty tophi, and improved movement with less pain of affected joints. (As uric acid levels decrease, inflammation due to uric acid crystals should improve.)	■ Encourage the patient to maintain consistent drug dosing to ensure uric acid levels are diminishing. ■ Instruct the patient on the need to return for periodic lab testing and urinalysis.
Minimizing adverse effects: ■ Monitor serum and urinary uric acid levels and symptoms associated with acute inflammatory period. (Continued or increasing inflammation may indicate the need for additional medication.)	■ Instruct the patient to report any continued inflammation, pain, increased joint involvement, or general worsening of symptoms promptly.
■ Monitor daily weight and urinary output. (Uric acid excretion may cause urate crystal formation in the kidneys with resulting renal impairment. Daily weight is an accurate measure of overall body fluid volume.)	■ Instruct the patient to report any diminished urine output, changes in urine appearance, or flank pain, and to return periodically for urinalysis. ■ Have the patient weigh self daily at the same time each day and report any weight gain of over 2 lb (1 kg) in a 24-hour period to the health care provider.
■ Decrease the intake of purine-containing foods. Avoid large doses of vitamin C. (Intake of high-purine foods and alcohol may increase production of uric acid. Large doses of vitamin C may increase the formation of uric acid stones.)	■ Teach the patient to avoid foods with a high purine content, decrease or eliminate alcohol consumption, and avoid increased vitamin C intake or supplementation. Provide a dietitian consult as needed.
■ Observe for skin rashes, fever, stomatitis, flulike symptoms, or general malaise. (Bone marrow suppression may occur with antigout drugs and result in leukopenia and an increased risk of infection. Severe dermatologic reactions are possible and any skin rashes, especially with the appearance of blisters and discoloration, should be reported immediately.)	■ Teach the patient to immediately report any flulike symptoms, fever, mouth irritation or soreness, or skin rashes.
Patient understanding of drug therapy: ■ Use opportunities during administration of medications and during assessments to discuss the rationale for drug therapy, desired therapeutic outcomes, most common adverse effects, parameters for when to call the health care provider, and any necessary monitoring or precautions. (Using time during nursing care helps to optimize and reinforce key teaching areas.)	■ The patient should be able to state the reason for the drug; appropriate dose and scheduling; what adverse effects to observe for and when to report; and the anticipated length of medication therapy.
Patient self-administration of drug therapy: ■ When administering the medication, instruct the patient, family, or caregiver in the proper self-administration of the drug, e.g., taken on an empty stomach or with meals, with additional fluids. (Proper administration increases the effectiveness of the drugs.)	■ The patient is able to discuss appropriate dosing and administration needs including taking medications at the first sign of gout attack. ■ Colchicine should be taken on an empty stomach. Other antigout medications should be taken with food or meals.

Evaluation of Outcome Criteria

Evaluate the effectiveness of drug therapy by confirming that patient goals and expected outcomes have been met (see "Planning").

See Table 47.4 for a list of drugs to which these nursing actions apply.

Chapter REVIEW

KEY CONCEPTS

The numbered key concepts provide a succinct summary of the important points from the corresponding numbered section within the chapter. If any of points these are not clear, refer to the numbered section within the chapter for review.

47.1 Adequate levels of calcium in the body are necessary to properly transmit nerve impulses, prevent muscle spasms, and provide stability and movement. Adequate levels of vitamin D, parathyroid hormone, and calcitonin are also necessary for these functions.

47.2 Hypocalcemia is a serious condition that requires immediate therapy with calcium supplements, often concurrently with vitamin D.

47.3 Pharmacotherapy of osteomalacia includes calcium and vitamin D supplements.

47.4 Pharmacotherapy of osteoporosis includes bisphosphonates, estrogen modulator drugs, and calcitonin.

47.5 For osteoarthritis, the main drug therapy is pain medication that includes aspirin, acetaminophen, NSAIDs, or stronger analgesics. Drug therapy for rheumatoid arthritis includes analgesics, anti-inflammatory drugs, glucocorticoids, and disease-modifying antirheumatic drugs.

47.6 Gout is characterized by a buildup of uric acid in either the blood or the joint cavities. Drug therapy includes agents that inhibit uric acid buildup or enhance its excretion.

NCLEX-RN® REVIEW QUESTIONS

1 The nurse completing a physical exam on a child diagnosed with osteomalacia would expect to find:
1. bowlegs and a pigeon breast.
2. deformities of the fingers and toes.
3. shortness of breath.
4. the use of crutches for walking.

2 The patient's calcium level is reported as 5.6 mg/dL. The nurse should assess the patient for:
1. headache.
2. anorexia.
3. muscles spasms.
4. drowsiness.

3 The patient receiving allopurinol (Lopurin) for treatment of gout asks why he should avoid consumption of alcohol. The nurse's response is based on the knowledge that alcohol:
1. causes liver damage.
2. interferes with the absorption of antigout medications.
3. raises uric acid levels.
4. causes the urine to become more alkaline.

4 The patient is admitted with a diagnosis of hypercalcemia. The nurse would assess for which of the following? (Select all that apply.)

1. Cardiac dysrhythmias
2. Fatigue
3. Bone fractures
4. Increased muscle strength
5. Hunger

5 Sodium hyaluronate (Hyalgan) is prescribed for a patient with osteoarthritis. The nurse explains this drug will be administered by which method?
1. Intramuscularly
2. Directly into the joint
3. Intravenously
4. Subcutaneously

6 A patient has received a prescription for alendronate (Fosamax) for treatment of osteoporosis. The nurse would be concerned about this order if the patient reported: (Select all that apply.)
1. she enjoys milk, yogurt, and other dairy products and tries to consume some with each meal.
2. she is unable to sit upright for prolonged periods because of severe back pain.
3. she is lactose intolerant and rarely consumes dairy products.
4. she has had trouble swallowing and has been told she has "problems with her esophagus."

CRITICAL THINKING QUESTIONS

1. A young woman calls the triage nurse in her health care provider's office with questions concerning her mother's medication. The mother, age 76, has been taking alendronate (Fosamax) after a bone-density study revealed a decrease in bone mass. The daughter is worried that her mother may not be taking the drug correctly and asks for information to minimize the potential for drug adverse effects. What information should the triage nurse incorporate in a teaching plan regarding the oral administration of alendronate?

2. A community health nurse has decided to discuss the benefits of oral calcium supplements with an 82-year-old female patient. The patient had a stroke 6 years ago and requires help with most activities of daily living. Since her husband's death 18 months ago, she rarely leaves home. She has lost 25 lb because she "just can't get interested" in her meals. She refuses to drink milk. What considerations must the nurse make before recommending calcium supplementation?

3. A 36-year-old man comes to the emergency department complaining of severe pain in the first joint of his right big toe. The triage nurse inspects the toe and notes that the joint is red, swollen, and extremely tender. Recognizing this as a typical presentation for acute gouty arthritis, what historical data should the nurse obtain relevant to this disease process?

See Appendix D for answers and rationales for all activities.

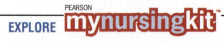

EXPLORE

MyNursingKit is your one stop for online chapter review materials and resources. Prepare for success with additional NCLEX®-style practice questions, interactive assignments and activities, web links, animations and videos, and more!

Register your access code from the front of your book at
www.mynursingkit.com.

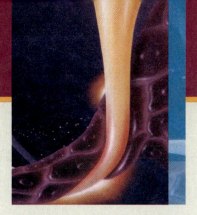

Chapter 48

Drugs for Skin Disorders

DRUGS AT A GLANCE

LEARNING OUTCOMES

After reading this chapter, the student should be able to:

1. Identify the structure and functions of the skin layers and associated structures.
2. Explain the process by which superficial skin cells are replaced.
3. Describe drug therapies for skin infections, mite and lice infestations, acne vulgaris, rosacea, dermatitis, and psoriasis.
4. Describe the prevention and management of minor burns.
5. Describe the nurse's role in the pharmacologic management of skin disorders.
6. For each of the classes listed in Drugs at a Glance, know representative drugs, and explain the mechanisms of drug action, primary actions, and important adverse effects.
7. Use the nursing process to care for patients who are receiving drug therapy for skin disorders.

KEY TERMS

The integumentary system consists of the skin, hair, nails, sweat glands, and oil glands. The largest and most visible of all organs, skin provides an effective barrier between the outside environment and the body's internal organs. At times, however, external conditions become too extreme, or conditions within the body change, resulting in unhealthy skin. When this occurs, pharmacotherapy may be utilized to improve the skin's condition. The purpose of this chapter is to examine the broad scope of skin disorders and the drugs used for skin pharmacotherapy.

48.1 Structure and Function of the Skin

To understand the actions of dermatologic drugs, it is necessary to have a thorough knowledge of skin structure. The skin comprises three primary layers: the epidermis, dermis, and subcutaneous layer. Each layer of skin is distinct in form and function and provides the basis for how drugs are injected or topically applied.

EPIDERMIS   The epidermis is the visible, outermost layer that constitutes about 5% of the skin depth. The epidermis has either four or five sublayers depending on its thickness. The five layers from the innermost to outermost are *stratum basale* (also referred to as the *stratum germinativum*), *stratum spinosum*, *stratum granulosum*, *stratum lucidum*, and the strongest layer, the *stratum corneum*. The stratum corneum contains an abundance of the protein keratin, which forms an effective barrier that repels bacteria and foreign matter: Most substances cannot penetrate this barrier.

The deepest epidermal sublayer, the stratum basale, supplies the epidermis with new cells after older superficial cells have been damaged or lost through normal wear. Over time, these newly created cells migrate from the stratum basale to the outermost layers of the skin. As these cells are pushed to the surface they are flattened and covered with a water-insoluble material, forming a protective seal. On average, it takes a cell about 3 weeks to move from the stratum basale to the body surface. Specialized cells within the deeper layers of the epidermis, called *melanocytes,* secrete the dark pigment *melanin,* which offers a degree of protection from the sun's ultraviolet rays. The number and type of melanocytes determine the overall pigment of the skin. The more melanin, the darker the skin color.

DERMIS   The middle layer of the skin is the dermis, which accounts for about 95% of the entire skin thickness. The dermis provides a foundation for the epidermis and accessory structures such as hair and nails. Most sensory nerves that transmit the sensations of touch, pressure, temperature, pain, and itch are located within the dermis, as well as the oil glands and sweat glands.

SUBCUTANEOUS TISSUE   Beneath the dermis is the subcutaneous layer, or *hypodermis,* consisting mainly of adipose tissue, which cushions, insulates, and provides a source of energy for the body. The amount of subcutaneous tissue varies in an individual, and is determined by nutritional status and heredity. Some sources consider the subcutaneous layer as being separate from the skin, and not one of its layers.

48.2 Causes of Skin Disorders

Of the many types of skin disorders, some have vague, generalized signs and symptoms, and others have specific and easily identifiable causes. **Urticaria** is a hypersensitivity response characterized by hives, often accompanied by pruritus, or itching. Allergies to foods often manifest as urticaria. **Pruritus** is a general condition associated with dry, scaly skin, or a parasite infestation. Pruritus may also be a sign of *systemic* pathology, such as serious hepatic or renal impairment. A substantial number of drugs have urticaria or pruritus listed as potential adverse effects. **Erythema** or redness of the skin accompanies inflammation and many other skin disorders. Inflammation is a characteristic of burns and trauma to the skin.

One simple method of classifying skin disorders is to group them as infectious, inflammatory, or neoplastic. Skin disorders, however, are diverse and difficult to classify because they frequently have overlapping symptoms and causes. For example, lesions characteristic of acne may be inflamed and become infected. Characteristics of these three classes of skin disorders are summarized in Table 48.1.

Dermatologic signs and symptoms often result from disease processes occurring in other body systems. Skin abnormalities such as changes in skin turgor and in the color,

TABLE 48.1	Classification of Skin Disorders
Type	Examples
Infectious	Bacterial infections: boils, impetigo, and infected hair follicles
	Fungal infections: ringworm, athlete's foot, jock itch, and nail infection
	Parasitic infections: ticks, mites, and lice
	Viral infections: cold sores, fever blisters (herpes simplex), chicken pox, warts, shingles (herpes zoster), measles (rubeola), and German measles (rubella)
Inflammatory	Injury and exposure to the sun
	Combination of overactive glands, increased hormone production, and/or infection such as acne and rosacea
	Disorders with itching, cracking, and discomfort such as atopic dermatitis, contact dermatitis, seborrheic dermatitis, stasis dermatitis, and psoriasis
Neoplastic	Skin cancers: squamous cell carcinoma, basal cell carcinoma, and malignant melanoma
	Benign neoplasms include keratosis and keratoacanthoma

size, types, and character of surface lesions may have systemic causes such as liver or renal impairment, cardiovascular insufficiency, metastatic tumors, recent injury, and poor nutritional status. The relationship between the integumentary system and other body systems is illustrated in ➤ Figure 48.1.

The pharmacotherapy of skin disorders may be conducted with oral or topical drugs. In general, topical drugs are preferred because this route delivers the medication directly to the site of pathology and systemic adverse effects are rare. If the skin condition involves deeper skin layers or is extensive, oral or parenteral drug therapy may be indicated. Some conditions such as lice infestation or sunburn with minor irritation warrant only short-term pharmacotherapy. Prolonged and extensive therapy is sometimes required of eczema, dermatitis, and psoriasis.

PharmFacts

Skin Disorders

- An estimated 3 million people with new cases of lice infestation are treated each year in the United States.
- Nearly 17 million people in the United States have acne, making it the most common skin disease.
- More than 15 million people in the United States have symptoms of dermatitis.
- Of infants and young children, 10% experience symptoms of dermatitis; roughly 60% of these infants continue to have symptoms into adulthood.
- Psoriasis affects 1% to 2% of the U.S. population. This disorder occurs in all age groups—adults mainly—affecting about the same number of men as women.

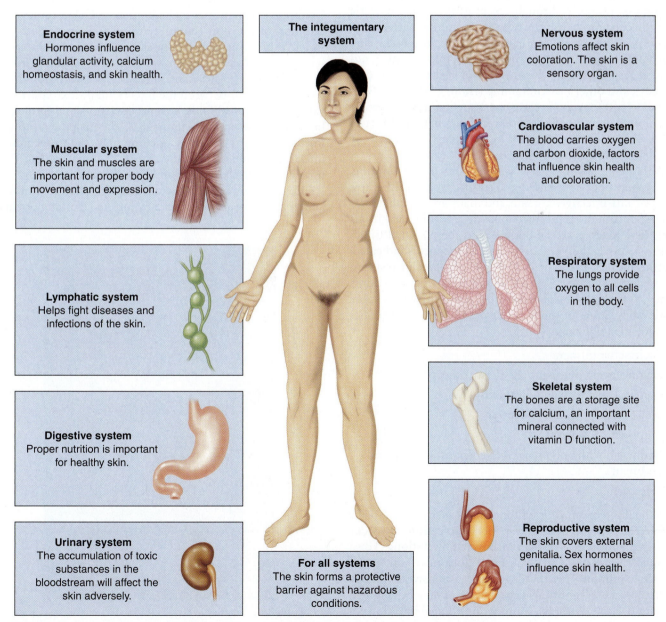

Endocrine system
Hormones influence glandular activity, calcium homeostasis, and skin health.

Muscular system
The skin and muscles are important for proper body movement and expression.

Lymphatic system
Helps fight diseases and infections of the skin.

Digestive system
Proper nutrition is important for healthy skin.

Urinary system
The accumulation of toxic substances in the bloodstream will affect the skin adversely.

The integumentary system

For all systems
The skin forms a protective barrier against hazardous conditions.

Nervous system
Emotions affect skin coloration. The skin is a sensory organ.

Cardiovascular system
The blood carries oxygen and carbon dioxide, factors that influence skin health and coloration.

Respiratory system
The lungs provide oxygen to all cells in the body.

Skeletal system
The bones are a storage site for calcium, an important mineral connected with vitamin D function.

Reproductive system
The skin covers external genitalia. Sex hormones influence skin health.

➤ *Figure 48.1* Interrelationships of the integumentary system with other body systems

SKIN INFECTIONS

The skin is normally populated with microorganisms or flora that include a diverse collection of viruses, fungi, and bacteria. As long as the skin remains healthy and intact, it provides an effective barrier against infection from these organisms. The skin is very dry, and keratin is a poor energy source for microbes. Although perspiration often provides a wet environment, its high salt content discourages microbial growth. Furthermore, the outer layer is continually being sloughed off, and the microorganisms leave with the dead skin.

48.3 Pharmacotherapy of Bacterial, Fungal, and Viral Skin Infections

Bacterial skin infections can occur when the skin is punctured or cut, or when the outer layer is abraded through trauma or removed through severe burns. Some bacteria also infect hair follicles. The two most common bacterial infections of the skin are caused by *Staphylococcus* and *Streptococcus*, which are also normal skin inhabitants. *S. aureus* is responsible for furuncles (boils), carbuncles (abscesses), and other pus-containing lesions of the skin. Both *S. aureus* and *S. pyogenes* can cause impetigo, a skin disorder commonly occurring in school-age children. Cellulitis is an acute skin and subcutaneous tissue infection caused by *Staphylococcus* and *Streptococcus*.

Although many skin bacterial infections are self-limiting, others may be serious enough to require pharmacotherapy. Topical anti-infectives are safe, and many are available OTC for self-treatment. If the infection is deep within the skin, affects large regions of the body, or has the potential to become systemic, then oral or parenteral therapy is indicated. Furthermore, the incidence of methicillin-resistant *Staphylococcus aureus* (MRSA) skin infections is increasing, which often requires pharmacotherapy with two or more antibiotics. Some of the more common topical antibiotics include the following:

- Bacitracin ointment
- Erythromycin ointment (Eryderm, others)
- Gentamicin cream and ointment
- Metronidazole cream and lotion
- Mupirocin (Bactroban)
- Neomycin with polymyxin B (Neosporin), cream and ointment
- Tetracycline

Fungal infections of the skin or nails such as tinea pedis (athlete's foot) and tinea cruris (jock itch) commonly occur in warm, moist areas of the skin covered by clothing. Tinea capitis (ringworm of the scalp) and tinea unguium (nails) are also common. These pathogens are responsive to therapy with topical OTC antifungal agents such as undecylenic acid (Cruex, Desenex, others). More serious fungal infections of the skin and mucous membranes, such as *Candida albicans*

infections that occur in immunocompromised patients, require systemic antifungals (chapter 35∞). Clotrimazole (Mycelex, Lotrimin, others) and miconazole (Monistat, others) are common antifungals available as creams or ointments that are used for a variety of dermatologic mycoses.

Certain viral infections can manifest with skin lesions, including varicella (chicken pox), rubeola (measles), and rubella (German measles). Usually, these infections are self-limiting and nonspecific, so treatment is directed at controlling the extent of skin lesions. Viral infections of the skin in adults include herpes zoster (shingles) and herpes simplex (cold sores and genital lesions). Pharmacotherapy of severe or persistent viral skin lesions may include topical or oral antiviral therapy with acyclovir (Zovirax), as discussed in chapter 36∞.

SKIN PARASITES

Common skin parasites include mites and lice. Scabies is an eruption of the skin caused by the female mite, *Sarcoptes scabiei*, which burrows into the skin to lay eggs that hatch after about 5 days. Scabies mites are barely visible without magnification and are smaller than lice. Scabies lesions most commonly occur between the fingers, on the extremities, in axillary and gluteal folds, around the trunk, and in the pubic area, as shown in ➤ Figure 48.2. The major symptom is intense itching; vigorous scratching may lead to secondary infections. Scabies is readily spread through contact with upholstery and shared bed and bath linens.

Lice are larger than mites, measuring from 1 to 4 mm in length. They are readily spread by infected clothing or close

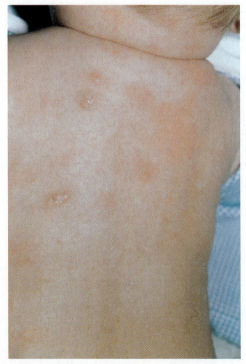

➤ *Figure 48.2* Scabies
Source: Courtesy of Dr. Jason L. Smith.

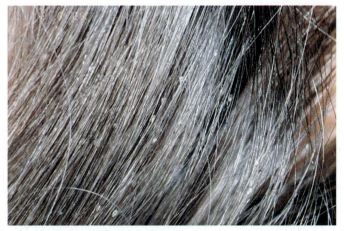

➤ **Figure 48.3** Pediculus capitis
Source: Courtesy of Dr. Jason L. Smith.

personal contact. These parasites require human blood for survival and die within 24 hours without the blood of a human host. Lice (singular: louse) often infest the pubic area or the scalp and lay eggs, referred to as **nits,** which attach to body hairs. Head lice are referred to as *Pediculus capitis* (➤ Figure 48.3), body lice as *P. corpus,* and pubic lice as *Phthirus pubis.* The pubic louse is referred to as a *crab louse,* because it looks like a tiny crab when viewed under the microscope. Individuals with pubic lice will sometimes say that they have "crabs." Pubic lice may produce sky-blue macules on the inner thighs or lower abdomen. The bite of the louse and the release of saliva into the wound lead to intense itch-

ing followed by vigorous scratching. Secondary infections can result from scratching.

48.4 Pharmacotherapy with Scabicides and Pediculicides

Scabicides are drugs that kill mites, and **pediculicides** are drugs that kill lice. Some drugs are effective against both types of parasites. The choice of drug depends on where the infestation is located, as well as factors such as age, pregnancy, or breast-feeding.

The preferred drug for lice infestation is permethrin, a chemical derived from chrysanthemum flowers and formulated as a 1% liquid (Nix). This drug is considered the safest agent, especially for infants and children. Pyrethrin (RID, others) is a related product also obtained from the chrysanthemum plant. Permethrin and pyrethrins, which are also widely used as insecticides on crops and livestock, kill lice and their eggs on contact. These agents are effective in about 90% to 99% of patients, although a repeat application may be needed. Side effects are generally minor and include stinging, itching, or tingling. Malathion (Ovide) is an alternative for resistant organisms.

Permethrin is also a preferred drug for scabies. The 5% permethrin cream (Elimite) is applied to the entire skin surface and allowed to remain for 8 to 14 hours before bathing. A single application cures 95% of the patients, although itching may continue for several weeks as the dead mites are removed from the skin. Crotamiton (Eurax) is an alternative scabicide available by prescription as a 10% cream.

Pr Prototype Drug | **Permethrin** *(Acticin, Elimite, Nix)*

Therapeutic Class: Antiparasitic   **Pharmacologic Class:** Scabicide; pediculicide

ACTIONS AND USES
Nix is marketed as a cream, lotion, or shampoo to kill head and crab lice and mites, and to eradicate their ova. A 1% lotion is approved for lice and a 5% lotion for mites. The medication should be allowed to remain on the hair and scalp 10 minutes before removal. Patients should be aware that penetration of the skin with mites causes itching, which lasts up to 2 or 3 weeks even after the parasites have been killed.

Successful elimination of parasite infections should include removal of nits with a nit comb, washing bedding, and cleaning or removal of objects that have been in contact with the head or hair.

ADMINISTRATION ALERTS
- Do not use on premature infants and children younger than 2 years.
- Do not use on areas of skin that have abrasions, rash, or inflammation.
- Pregnancy category B

PHARMACOKINETICS
Onset: 10 min
Peak: Unknown
Half-life: Unknown
Duration: 3 h

ADVERSE EFFECTS
Permethrin causes few systemic effects. Local reactions may occur and include pruritus, rash, transient tingling, burning, stinging, erythema, and edema of the affected area.

Contraindications: Contraindications include hypersensitivity to pyrethrins, chrysanthemums, sulfites, or other preservatives. Permethrin should be used cautiously over inflamed skin, in those with asthma, or in lactating women.

INTERACTIONS
Drug–Drug: No clinically significant interactions have been documented.

Lab Tests: Unknown

Herbal/Food: Unknown

Treatment of Overdose: No specific treatment for overdose is available.

Refer to MyNursingKit for a Nursing Process Focus specific to this drug.

NURSING PROCESS FOCUS   PATIENTS RECEIVING THERAPY WITH SCABICIDES AND PEDICULICIDES

Assessment	Potential Nursing Diagnoses
Baseline assessment prior to administration: ■ Understand the reason the drug has been prescribed in order to assess for therapeutic effects (e.g., specific type of infestation such as lice). ■ Obtain a complete health history including dermatologic and social history of recent exposure. ■ Obtain a drug history including allergies, current prescription and OTC drugs, herbal preparations, alcohol use, and smoking. Be alert to possible drug interactions. ■ Assess skin areas to be treated for signs of infestation (e.g., lice or nits in hair, reddened track areas between webs of fingers, around belt or elastic lines), irritation, excoriation, or drainage. ■ Obtain baseline height, weight, and vital signs.	■ Disturbed Body Image ■ Impaired Skin Integrity (related to pruritus and possible skin lesions) ■ Deficient Knowledge (drug therapy) ■ Risk for Poisoning (related to incorrect use of the drug, adverse drug effects)
Assessment throughout administration: ■ Assess for desired therapeutic effects dependent on the reason the drug is given (e.g., visible infestation is gone, nits are removed, skin healing is visible). ■ Assess for adverse effects: localized tingling, pruritus, stinging, or burning. Severe skin reactions or edema should be reported promptly.	

Planning: Patient Goals and Expected Outcomes

The patient will:
■ Experience therapeutic effects (e.g., infestation has cleared).
■ Be free from, or experience minimal, adverse effects.
■ Verbalize an understanding of the drug's use, adverse effects, and required precautions.
■ Demonstrate proper self-administration of the medication (e.g., dose, timing, when to notify provider).

Implementation

Interventions and (Rationales)	Patient and Family Teaching
Ensuring therapeutic effects: ■ Monitor appropriate medication administration for optimum results. Monitor the affected area after treatment over the following 1 to 2 weeks to ensure the infestation has been eliminated. (Appropriate administration will optimize therapeutic effects and limit need for retreatment.)	■ Teach the patient appropriate administration techniques (see "Patient self-administration of drug therapy" later in this table).
Minimizing adverse effects: ■ Monitor the area of infestation over the next 1 to 2 weeks. Reinfestations may appear within 1 week and need to be retreated at that time. (Most treatments are highly effective when administered correctly. Retreatment may be needed dependent on the type of infestation.)	■ Instruct the patient, family, or caregiver to continue to assess the area daily for 1 to 2 weeks and contact the health care provider for a second prescription if reinfestation is noted.
■ Monitor family members, those in close care of patient, or sexual contacts for infestation. Bedding and personal objects should be cleansed before reuse. (Reinfestation may recur if those in close contact with the patient are infested. Close contacts should be treated at the same time as the patient.)	■ Instruct the patient, family, or caregiver to wash bedding, clothing used currently, and combs and brushes in soapy water and dry thoroughly. Vacuum furniture or fabric that cannot be cleaned to remove any errant vermin. Dry clean hats or caps that cannot be washed. Seal children's toys in plastic bags for 2 weeks if they cannot be washed.
■ Monitor skin in areas that have been treated. Promptly report any irritation, broken skin, erythema, rashes, or edema. (Skin reactions are relatively uncommon but may occur. Allergic reactions should be reported promptly.)	■ Teach the patient, family, or caregiver to report any redness, swelling, itching, or excoriation, or if complaints of burning occur, to the health care provider.
Patient understanding of drug therapy: ■ Use opportunities during administration of medications and during assessments to discuss the rationale for drug therapy, desired therapeutic outcomes, common adverse effects, parameters for when to call the health care provider, and any necessary monitoring or precautions. (Using time during nursing care helps to optimize and reinforce key teaching areas.)	■ The patient should be able to state the reason for the drug, appropriate dose and scheduling, and what adverse effects to observe for and when to report them.

Implementation

Interventions and (Rationales)	Patient and Family Teaching
Patient self-administration of drug therapy: ■ When administering the medication, instruct the patient, family, or caregiver in the proper self-administration of the drug, e.g., use exactly as directed or per package directions. (Proper administration increases the effectiveness of the drugs.)	■ Teach the patient to take the drug following appropriate guidelines: ■ Apply the drug per package directions and allow to remain in the hair or on the skin the prescribed length of time (usually approximately 10 minutes). Most packages contain enough drug for one treatment although a second package may be required if the hair is long. ■ Dry thoroughly after showering or shampooing the drug out of the hair or skin. ■ Comb through hair with the small-toothed comb provided to remove any remaining dead lice, nits, or nit casings. ■ If eyelashes are infested, apply a thin coat of petroleum jelly to eyelashes once a day for 1 week. Comb through using a small-gauge comb. ■ Check hair, webbings of fingers and toes, and belt or elastic lines for signs of reinfestation over the next week. If needed, a second application of the drug can be used after 1 week.

Evaluation of Outcome Criteria

Evaluate the effectiveness of drug therapy by confirming that patient goals and expected outcomes have been met (see "Planning").

The traditional drug of choice for many decades for both mites and lice was lindane (Kwell). Because lindane has the potential to cause serious nervous system toxicity, it is now prescribed only after other less toxic drugs have failed to produce a therapeutic response.

All scabicides and pediculicides must be used strictly as directed, because excessive use has the potential to cause serious systemic effects and skin irritation. Drugs for the treatment of lice or mites must not be applied to the mouth, open skin lesions, or eyes, because this will cause severe irritation.

ACNE AND ROSACEA

Acne vulgaris and rosacea are two disorders that produce similar-appearing lesions on the face. Although the two conditions have some visual similarities and share a few common treatments, the pharmacotherapy of the disorders is very different.

48.5 Pharmacotherapy of Acne and Rosacea

Medications used for acne and related disorders are available OTC and by prescription. Because of their increased toxicity, prescription agents are reserved for more severe, persistent cases. These drugs are listed in Table 48.2.

ACNE VULGARIS **Acne vulgaris** is a common disorder of the hair and sebaceous glands that affects up to 80% of adolescents. Although acne occurs most often in teenagers, it is not unusual to find patients with acne who are older than 30 years, a condition referred to as *mature acne* or *acne tardive*. Acne vulgaris is more common in men but tends to persist longer in women.

Although the precise cause of acne is unknown, several factors associated with acne vulgaris include abnormal formation of keratin that blocks oil glands and **seborrhea**, the overproduction of sebum by oil glands. The bacterium *Propionibacterium acnes* grows within oil gland openings and changes sebum to an acidic and irritating substance.

HOME & COMMUNITY CONSIDERATIONS

Psychosocial and Community Impact of Scabies and Pediculosis

Children and parents, particularly those in relatively affluent areas, may express feeling unclean or that their self-esteem has been lowered when they are diagnosed with scabies or pediculosis. Some patients think that only homeless persons or people of low income get these disorders. Educate the patient and family members about the ways in which people contract scabies or pediculosis and the ways in which these infestations may be prevented. Help those affected to maintain their self-esteem and adopt a healthy attitude. Persons with scabies or pediculosis may tend to isolate socially, but this is unnecessary if precautions are taken to not share clothing, combs, or other hygiene supplies or have bodily contact with others.

Scabies or lice can rapidly spread in a school, nursing home, residential treatment center, or hospital and become a community health problem. School nurses must assess the potential for students or patients contacting scabies or lice and take preventive measures. This may include frequent assessments of the hair, scalp, and exposed skin, and elimination of coat and hat racks and opportunities to share or swap clothing and/or towels. School children and their families need education on prevention and treatment. Patients and their families reporting scabies or pediculosis to the nurse should be treated in an accepting, professional, helpful manner.

TABLE 48.2	Drugs for Acne
Drug	**Remarks**
adapalene (Differin)	Retinoid-like compound used to treat acne formation
azelaic acid (Azelex, Finacea, others)	For mild to moderate inflammatory acne
benzoyl peroxide (Benzalin, Fostex, others)	Keratolytic available OTC: sometimes combined with erythromycin (Benzamycin) or clindamycin (BenzaClin) for acne caused by *P. acnes*
clindamycin and tretinoin (Ziana)	Combination product with an antibiotic and a retinoid in a gel base; for mild to moderate acne
ethinyl estradiol (Estinyl)	Oral contraceptives are sometimes used for acne; example: ethinyl estradiol plus norgestimate (Ortho Tri-Cyclen-28)
isotretinoin (Accutane)	For severe acne with cysts or acne formed in small, rounded masses; pregnancy category X
sulfacetamide (Cetamide, Klaron, others)	For sensitive skin; sometimes combined with sulfur to promote peeling, as in the condition rosacea; also used for conjunctivitis
tazarotene (Tazorac)	A retinoid drug that may also be used for plaque psoriasis; has antiproliferative and anti-inflammatory effects
tetracyclines	Antibiotics; refer to chapter 34 ∞
⊕ tretinoin (Retin-A, others)	To prevent clogging of pore follicles; also used for the treatment of acute promyelocytic leukemia and wrinkles

As a result, small inflamed bumps appear on the surface of the skin. Other factors associated with acne include androgens, which stimulate the sebaceous glands to produce more sebum. This is clearly evident in teenage boys and in patients who are administered testosterone.

Acne lesions include open and closed comedones. Blackheads, or open **comedones,** occur when sebum has plugged the oil gland, causing it to become black because of the presence of melanin granules. Whiteheads, or closed comedones, develop just beneath the surface of the skin and appear white rather than black. Some closed comedones may rupture, resulting in papules, inflammatory pustules, and cysts. Mild papules and cysts drain on their own without treatment. Deeper lesions can cause scarring of the skin. Acne is graded as mild, moderate, or severe, depending on the number and type of lesions present.

The goal of acne therapy is to treat existing lesions and to prevent or lessen the severity of future recurrences. The regimen used depends on the extent and severity of the acne. Mechanisms of action of antiacne medications include the following:

- Inhibit sebaceous gland overactivity
- Reduce bacterial colonization
- Prevent follicles from becoming plugged with keratin
- Reduce inflammation of lesions

Benzoyl peroxide (Benzalin, Triaz, others) is the most common topical OTC medication for acne. Benzoyl peroxide has a **keratolytic** effect, which helps dry out and shed the outer layer of epidermis. In addition, this drug suppresses sebum production and exhibits antibacterial effects against *P. acnes*. Benzoyl peroxide is available as a topical lotion, cream, or gel in various percent concentrations. Typically, the patient applies benzoyl peroxide once daily and in many instances, this is the only treatment needed. The drug is very safe, with local redness, irritation, and drying being the most common side effects. Other kera-

tolytic agents used for severe acne include resorcinol, salicylic acid, and sulfur.

Retinoids are a class of drug closely related to vitamin A that are used in the treatment of inflammatory skin conditions, dermatologic malignancies, and acne. The topical formulations are often drugs of choice for patients with mild to moderate acne, particularly those with the presence of inflammatory cysts. Tretinoin (Retin-A) is an older drug with an irritant action that decreases comedone formation and increases extrusion of comedones from the skin. Tretinoin also has the ability to improve photodamaged skin and is used for wrinkle removal. Other retinoids include isotretinoin (Accutane), an oral vitamin A metabolite medication that aids in reducing the size of sebaceous glands, thereby decreasing oil production and the occurrence of clogged pores. Although extremely effective, isotretinoin is rarely used due to the potential for birth defects (pregnancy category X) and the fact it has been associated with a risk of suicidal ideation. Therapy with retinoids may require 8 to 12 weeks to achieve maximum effectiveness. Common reactions to retinoids include burning, stinging, and sensitivity to sunlight. Adapalene (Differin) is a third-generation retinoid that causes less imitation than the older agents. Additional retinoid-like agents and related compounds used to treat acne are listed in Table 48.2.

Antibiotics are sometimes used in combination with acne medications to lessen the severe redness and inflammation associated with the disorder, especially when the acne is inflammatory and results in cysts and pustules. Doxycycline (Vibramycin, others), minocycline, and tetracycline, administered in small doses over a long period, have been the traditional antibiotics used in acne therapy. Erythromycin and clindamycin are frequently used topically and have a low incidence of adverse effects.

Oral contraceptives containing ethinyl estradiol and norgestimate may be used to help clear the skin of acne. The agents are reserved for women who are unable to take oral antibiotics or when antibiotic therapy has

Pr Prototype Drug | Tretinoin *(Avita, Retin-A, Trentin-X, others)*

Therapeutic Class: Antiacne agent   **Pharmacologic Class:** Retinoid

ACTIONS AND USES

Tretinoin is a natural derivative of vitamin A that is indicated for the early treatment and control of mild to moderate acne vulgaris. Renova is a topical form of tretinoin approved to treat fine facial wrinkles and hyperpigmentation associated with photodamaged skin. Tretinoin has antineoplastic actions; an oral form (Vesanoid) is approved to treat acute promyelocytic leukemia and may be prescribed off-label for skin malignancies.

Symptoms take 4–8 weeks to improve, and maximum therapeutic benefit may take 5–6 months. Because of potentially serious adverse effects, this drug is most often reserved for cystic acne or severe keratinization disorders.

ADMINISTRATION ALERTS

- Avoid administering OTC acne medications and using skin products that cause excessive drying of the skin during therapy.
- Avoid direct exposure to sunlight or UV lamps.
- Do not administer to patients who are allergic to fish (the product contains fish proteins).
- Pregnancy category C

> **PHARMACOKINETICS**
> **Onset:** Unknown
> **Peak:** 1–2 h
> **Half-life:** 0.2–2 h
> **Duration:** Unknown

ADVERSE EFFECTS

Nearly all patients using topical tretinoin will experience redness, scaling, erythema, crusting, and peeling of the skin. Skin irritation can be severe and cause discontinuation of therapy; a lower strength solution may be necessary. Dermatologic adverse effects resolve once therapy is discontinued. Oral therapy can also cause skin adverse effects.

Very high oral doses can result in serious adverse effects, including bone pain, fever, headache, nausea, vomiting, rash, stomatitis, pruritus, sweating, and ocular disorders. The oral drug has several black box warnings, including the potential for rapid development of leukocytosis and the possibility of severe reactions in patients with promyelocytic leukemia.

Contraindications: Contraindications for topical administration include eczema, exposure to sunlight or UV rays, sunburn, hypersensitivity to the drug or vitamin A preparation, and children less than 12 years of age. This drug is contraindicated during lactation or pregnancy. Oral tretinoin is contraindicated in patients who have hepatic disease, leukopenia or neutropenia, or who are hypersensitive to the drug.

INTERACTIONS

Drug–Drug: Topical acne keratinolytics (sulfur, resorcinol, benzoyl peroxide, and salicylic acid) may increase inflammation and peeling; topical products containing alcohol or menthol may cause stinging. Additive phototoxicity can occur if tretinoin is used concurrently with other phototoxic drugs such as tetracyclines, fluoroquinolones, or sulfonamides.

Lab Tests: None known

Herbal/Food: Excessive amounts of vitamin A or St. John's wort may result in photosensitivity.

Treatment of Overdose: Overuse of the topical drug will lead to excessive skin drying and peeling. Symptoms of oral overdose are nonspecific and resolve with symptomatic treatment.

Refer to MyNursingKit for a Nursing Process Focus specific to this drug.

---

proved ineffective. For the actions and contraindications of oral contraceptives, see chapter 45 ∞.

ROSACEA   Rosacea is an inflammatory skin disorder of unknown etiology with lesions affecting mainly the face. Unlike acne, which most commonly affects teenagers, rosacea is a progressive disorder with an onset between 30 and 50 years of age. Rosacea is characterized by small papules or inflammatory bumps without pus that swell, thicken, and become painful, as shown in ➤ Figure 48.4. The face takes on a reddened or flushed appearance, particularly around the nose and cheek area. With time, the redness becomes more permanent, and lesions resembling acne appear. The soft tissues of the nose may thicken, giving the nose a reddened, bullous, irregular swelling called **rhinophyma**.

Rosacea is exacerbated by factors such as sunlight, stress, increased temperature, and agents that dilate facial blood vessels including alcohol, spicy foods, skin care products, and warm beverages. It affects more women than men, although men more often develop rhinophyma.

The two most effective treatments for rosacea are topical metronidazole (MetroGel, MetroCream) and azelaic acid

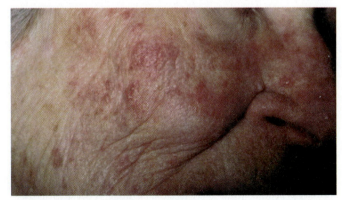

➤ **Figure 48.4** Rosacea
Source: Courtesy of Dr. Jason L. Smith.

(Finacea). Benzoyl peroxide may be applied as needed. Alternative medications include topical clindamycin (Cleocin-T, ClindaMax) and sulfacetamide. Tetracycline antibiotics are of benefit to rosacea patients with multiple pustules or with ocular involvement. Severe, resistant cases may respond to isotretinoin (Accutane).

NURSING PROCESS FOCUS   PATIENTS RECEIVING ANTIACNE MEDICATIONS

Assessment	Potential Nursing Diagnoses
Baseline assessment prior to administration: ■ Understand the reason the drug has been prescribed in order to assess for therapeutic effects (e.g., treatment of acne, signs of aging, component of cancer treatment). ■ Obtain a complete health history including dermatologic, hepatic, or renal disease; psychiatric disorders; pregnancy; or breast-feeding. ■ Obtain a drug history including allergies, current prescription and OTC drugs, herbal preparations, alcohol use, and smoking. Be alert to possible drug interactions. ■ Evaluate appropriate laboratory findings (e.g., CBC, lipid profiles, hepatic or renal function labs). ■ Obtain baseline vital signs.	■ Disturbed Body Image ■ Impaired Skin Integrity (related to skin condition or adverse drug effects) ■ Deficient Knowledge (drug therapy) ■ Risk for Injury (related to adverse drug effects)
Assessment throughout administration: ■ Assess for desired therapeutic effects (e.g., skin is clearing of acne lesions). ■ Continue periodic monitoring of CBC, lipid profile, glucose, and hepatic funtion tests if on oral drug. ■ Monitor vital signs at each health care visit. ■ Monitor eye health periodically with eye examinations every 6 months while on oral drug therapy. ■ Assess for adverse effects: localized skin irritation, erythema, pruritus, or dry or peeling skin, dry mouth, eyes, or nose may occur. Changes in mood, especially depression or suicidal thoughts, should be reported immediately in patients on oral isotretinoin.	

Planning: Patient Goals and Expected Outcomes

The patient will:
■ Experience therapeutic effects (e.g., acne lesions are clearing, appearance of wrinkles or skin damage is improving).
■ Be free from, or experience minimal, adverse effects.
■ Verbalize an understanding of the drug's use, adverse effects, and required precautions.
■ Demonstrate proper self-administration of the medication (e.g., dose, timing, when to notify provider).

Implementation

Interventions and (Rationales)	Patient and Family Education
Ensuring therapeutic effects: ■ Monitor appropriate medication administration for optimum results. (Topical treatment areas should show signs of improvement within 2–4 weeks. Oral treatment is usually successful within one course and a second course may be delayed for several weeks to monitor continuing improvement.)	■ Teach the patient appropriate administration techniques (see "Patient self-administration of drug therapy" later in this table).
Minimizing adverse effects: ■ Monitor area under topical treatment for excessive dryness and irritation. (Over-cleansing or over-drying of the skin may make the condition worse.)	■ Teach the patient to gently cleanse the skin using a nonoily soap and avoiding vigorous scrubbing. If excessive dryness occurs, use a nonoily lotion to areas of dryness.
■ Monitor patients on isotretinoin for emotional health or changes in mood. (Depression, including with suicidal ideation, has been noted as an adverse effect.)	■ Instruct the patient, family, or caregiver to immediately report any signs of decreased mood, affect, depression, or expressed suicidal thoughts to the health care provider.
■ Monitor CBC, lipid levels, and hepatic function labs periodically for patients on oral medication. (Lipid levels may increase in up to 70% of patients on oral acne therapy. Hepatotoxicity is an adverse effect of oral drugs.)	■ Instruct the patient to return periodically for lab tests. ■ Teach patient to report any symptoms of abdominal or right upper quadrant discomfort or pain, yellowing of the skin or sclera, fatigue, anorexia, darkened urine or clay-colored stools immediately.
■ Monitor for vision changes. (Corneal opacities or cataracts are an adverse effect of oral antiacne medications. Dryness of eyes during treatment is common. Night vision may be diminished during treatment.)	■ Instruct the patient to maintain regular eye exams and to report any changes in visual acuity, especially with night driving. ■ Teach the patient that artificial tear solutions may assist in relieving eye dryness.

NURSING PROCESS FOCUS **PATIENTS RECEIVING ANTIACNE MEDICATIONS** *(Continued)*	
Implementation	
Interventions and (Rationales)	**Patient and Family Education**
▪ Monitor the patient's exposure to the sun and UV light. (Drying, skin sensitivity, and peeling skin are possible adverse effects, especially for patients on tretinoin. Protection from sun exposure is essential.)	▪ Teach the patient to use sunscreens of SPF 15 or higher and to wear protective clothing to avoid sun exposure to areas under treatment. ▪ Teach the patient that UV light therapy from a health care provider is monitored and tanning beds are not a substitute and should be avoided.

▪ Monitor compliance with "iPledge" requirements for patients on isotretinoin. (iPledge is required of all patients on isotretinoin before receiving a prescription or refills of the drug. It requires the patient to ensure that all requirements to prevent teratogenic effects have been met.)	▪ Instruct the patient on isotretinoin of the requirements of the iPledge mandatory program to ensure continued prescriptions including:
	  ▪ Females of child-bearing age must use two methods of birth control while on the drug.
	  ▪ Females of child-bearing age must have two negative pregnancy tests one month before, during, and after drug therapy, conducted at certified labs.
	  ▪ Male patients must verify that they will use a barrier method of birth control and not donate blood while on the drug.

Patient understanding of drug therapy: ▪ Use opportunities during administration of medications and during assessments to discuss the rationale for drug therapy, desired therapeutic outcomes, most common adverse effects, parameters for when to call the health care provider, and any necessary monitoring or precautions. (Using time during nursing care helps to optimize and reinforce key teaching areas.)	▪ The patient should be able to state the reason for the drug, appropriate dose and scheduling, and what adverse effects to observe for and when to report them.

Patient self-administration of drug therapy:
▪ When administering the medication, instruct the patient, family, or caregiver in the proper self-administration of the drug, e.g., topical drug is used appropriately, iPledge program is followed. (Proper administration will increase the effectiveness of the drug.)
	▪ Teach the patient to take the drug following appropriate guidelines:
	  ▪ Gently cleanse the affected skin twice daily with nonoily soap, avoiding excessive or vigorous scrubbing.
	  ▪ Apply a thin layer of topical drug after cleansing skin. Allow to dry and avoid contact with clothing, towels, or bedding to avoid staining or bleaching.
	  ▪ For oral medications, take in the morning and if twice-a-day dosing is ordered, take the second dose approximately 8 hours after the first.

Evaluation of Outcome Criteria	
Evaluate the effectiveness of drug therapy by confirming that patient goals and expected outcomes have been met (see "Planning").	

DERMATITIS

Dermatitis is general term that refers to superficial inflammatory disorders of the skin. General symptoms include local redness, pain, and pruritus. Intense scratching may lead to **excoriation**, scratches that break the skin surface and fill with blood or serous fluid to form crusty scales.

48.6 Pharmacotherapy of Dermatitis

A large number of factors can cause dermatitis, and symptoms may differ depending on the causative agent. The three most common types that respond to topical pharmacotherapy are atopic, contact, and seborrheic.

Atopic dermatitis, or **eczema**, is a chronic, inflammatory skin disorder with a genetic predisposition. Patients presenting with eczema often have a family history of asthma and hay fever as well as allergies to a variety of irritants such as cosmetics, lotions, soaps, pollens, food, pet dander, and dust. About 75% of patients with atopic dermatitis have had an initial onset before 1 year of age. In those babies predisposed to eczema, breast-feeding seems to offer protection, as it is rare for a breast-fed child to develop eczema before the introduction of other foods. In infants and small children, lesions usually begin on the face and scalp, and then progress to other parts of the body. A frequent and prominent symptom in infants is the appearance of red cheeks.

Contact dermatitis can be caused by a hypersensitivity response, resulting from exposure to specific natural or synthetic allergens such as plants, chemicals, latex, drugs, metals, or foreign proteins. Accompanying the allergic reaction may be various degrees of cracking, bleeding, or small blisters.

Seborrheic dermatitis is a form of eczema that can affect patients at any age. The exact cause of seborrheic dermatitis is unknown, but hormone levels, coexisting fungal infections, nutritional deficiencies, and immunodeficiency states are associated with the disease. Seborrheic dermatitis presents as greasy, not dry, scales that affect the scalp, central face, and anterior chest, often presenting as scalp scaling, or dandruff. Other symptoms may include redness of the nasolabial fold, particularly during times of stress, blepharitis, otitis externa, and acne vulgaris.

Pharmacotherapy of dermatitis is symptomatic and involves lotions and ointments to control itching and skin flaking. Antihistamines may be used to control inflammation and reduce itching, and analgesics or topical anesthetics may be prescribed for pain relief. Atopic dermatitis can be controlled, but not cured, by medications. Part of the management plan must include the identification and elimination of allergic triggers that cause flare-ups.

Topical corticosteroids are the most effective treatment for controlling the inflammation and itching of dermatitis. Creams, lotions, solutions, gels, and pads containing these drugs are specially formulated to penetrate deep into the skin layers. Topical corticosteroids are classified by potency, as listed in Table 48.3. The high-potency agents are used to treat acute flare-ups and are limited to 2 to 3 weeks of therapy. The moderate-potency formulations are for more prolonged therapy of chronic dermatitis. The low-potency glucocorticoids are prescribed for children.

Long-term corticosteroid use may cause irritation, redness, hypopigmentation, and thinning of the skin. High-potency formulations are not advised for the head or neck regions because of potential adverse effects. If absorption occurs, topical corticosteroids may produce undesirable systemic effects including adrenal insufficiency, mood changes, serum imbalances, and loss of bone mass, as discussed in chapter 43∞. To avoid serious adverse effects, careful attention must be given to the amount of glucocorticoid applied, the frequency of application, and how long it has been used.

Several alternatives to corticosteroids are available. Patients with persistent atopic dermatitis not responsive to corticosteroids may benefit from oral immunosuppressive agents, such as cyclosporine. This drug is generally used for the short-term treatment of severe disease. The topical calcineurin inhibitors pimecrolimus 1% (Elidel) and tacrolimus 0.03%, 0.1% (Protopic) are available for patients older than 2 years of age. These medications may be used over all skin surfaces (including face and neck) because they have fewer adverse effects than the topical corticosteroids. Adverse effects include burning and stinging on broken skin.

TABLE 48.3	Topical Corticosteroids
Generic Name	Trade Names
VERY HIGH POTENCY	
betamethasone dipropionate, augmented, cream	Diprolene
clobetasol propionate	Temovate
diflorasone diacetate	Maxiflor
HIGH POTENCY	
amcinonide	Cyclocort
fluocinonide	Lidex
halcinonide	Halog
MEDIUM POTENCY	
betamethasone benzoate	Uticort
betamethasone valerate	Valisone
clocortolone	Cloderm
desoximetasone, cream	Topicort
fluocinolone acetonide	Synalar
flurandrenolide, cream	Cordran
fluticasone propionate, cream	Cutivate
hydrocortisone valerate	Westcort
mometasone furoate	Elocon
triamcinolone acetonide	Aristocort, Kenalog
LOWEST LEVEL OF POTENCY	
alclometasone dipropionate	Aclovate
desonide	Desonate, DesOwen, Verdeso
dexamethasone	Decaspray
hydrocortisone	Cortizone, Hycort

PSORIASIS

Psoriasis is a chronic, noninfectious, inflammatory skin disorder that affects 1% to 2% of the population and appears with greater frequency in people of European ancestry. The onset of psoriasis is generally established by 20 years of age, although it may occur throughout the life span.

48.7 Pharmacotherapy of Psoriasis

Psoriasis is characterized by red, raised patches of skin covered with flaky, thick, silver scales called *plaques,* as shown in ▶ Figure 48.5. These plaques shed the scales, which are sometimes grayish. The reason for the appearance of plaques is an extremely fast skin turnover rate, with skin cells reaching the surface in 4 to 7 days instead of the usual 14 days. Plaques are ultimately shed from the surface, while the underlying skin becomes inflamed and irritated. Lesion size varies, and the shape tends to be round. Lesions are usually discovered on the scalp, elbows, knees, and extensor surfaces of the arms and legs, sacrum, and occasionally around the nails. The various forms of psoriasis are described in Table 48.4.

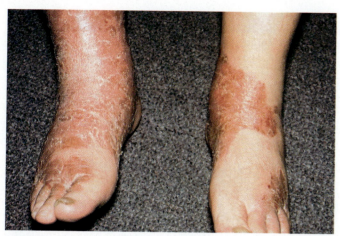

➤ **Figure 48.5** Psoriasis
Source: Courtesy of Dr. Jason L. Smith.

Although the etiology of psoriasis is incompletely understood, it appears to have both genetic and autoimmune components. About 50% of the cases have a genetic basis, with a close family member also having the disorder. One theory of causation is that psoriasis is an autoimmune condition, because overactive immune cells release cytokines that increase the production of skin cells. There is also a strong environmental component to the disease: factors such as stress, smoking, alcohol, climate changes, and infections can trigger flare-ups. In addition, certain drugs act as triggers, including angiotensin-converting enzyme (ACE) inhibitors, beta-adrenergic blockers, tetracyclines, and nonsteroidal anti-inflammatory drugs (NSAIDs).

The goal of psoriasis pharmacotherapy is to reduce skin reddening, plaques, and scales to improve the cosmetic appearance of the patient, leading to more normal lifestyle activities. This is accomplished by reducing epidermal cell turnover and promoting healing of the psoriatic lesions. Choice of therapy depends on the type and extent of the disease, and the history of response to previous psoriasis treatment. A number of prescription and OTC drugs are available for the treatment of psoriasis and are listed in Table 48.5. Therapy is often conducted in a stepwise manner. Psoriasis is lifelong, and there is no pharmacologic cure.

TOPICAL THERAPIES

Topical corticosteroids are the primary, initial treatment for psoriasis. These drugs are effective, inexpensive, and relatively safe. Examples include betamethasone (Diprosone) ointment, lotion, or cream and hydrocortisone acetate (Cortaid, Caldecort, others) cream or ointment. Topical corticosteroids reduce the inflammation associated with fast skin turnover. Initial therapy may begin with a high potency agent for 2 to 3 weeks, to obtain rapid clearing of lesions or to treat acute flare-ups. The high potency formulations are best applied to areas thickest with plaque, such as hands or feet, and should not used on the face and genital areas. For chronic, maintenance therapy, the patient is switched to moderate- and low-potency corticosteroids because they have a lower potential for adverse effects.

Topical immunomodulators (TIMS) are another class of agents that suppress the immune system. One example is the calcineurin inhibitor tacrolimus (Protopic) ointment. Other agents applied topically are retinoid-like compounds such as calcipotriene (Dovonex), a synthetic vitamin D ointment, cream, or scalp solution; and tazarotene (Tazorac), a vitamin A derivative gel or cream. These drugs provide the same benefits as topical corticosteroids but exhibit a lower incidence of adverse effects. Calcipotriene may produce hypercalcemia if applied over large areas of the body or used in higher doses than recommended. This drug is usually not used on an extended basis.

Other skin therapy techniques may be used with or without additional psoriasis medications. These include various forms of tar treatment (coal tar) and anthralin, which are applied to the skin's surface. Tar and anthralin inhibit DNA synthesis and arrest abnormal cell growth. These are considered second-line therapies.

TABLE 48.4	Types of Psoriasis		
Form of Psoriasis	Description	Most Common Location of Lesions	Comments
Guttate (droplike) or eruptive psoriasis	Lesions smaller than those of psoriasis vulgaris	Upper trunk and extremities	More common in early-onset psoriasis; can appear and resolve spontaneously a few weeks following a streptococcal respiratory infection
Psoriasis vulgaris	Lesions are papules that form into erythematous plaques with thick, silver, or gray plaques that bleed when removed; plaques in dark-skinned individuals often appear purple	Skin over scalp, elbows, and knees; lesions possible anywhere on the body	Most common form; requires long-term specialized management
Psoriatic arthritis	Resembles rheumatoid arthritis	Fingers and toes at distal interphalangeal joints; can affect skin and nails	About 20% of patients with psoriasis also have arthritis
Psoriatic erythroderma or exfoliative dermatitis	Generalized scaling; erythema without lesions	All body surfaces	Least common form
Pustular psoriasis	Eruption of pustules; presence of fever	Trunk and extremities; can appear on palms, soles, and nail beds	Average age of onset is 50 years

TABLE 48.5	Selected Drugs for Psoriasis and Related Disorders	
Drug	**Route and Adult Dose (max dose where indicated)**	**Adverse Effects**
TOPICAL MEDICATIONS*		
calcipotriene (Dovonex)	Topical: Apply thin layer to lesions one to two times/day	*Burning, stinging, folliculitis, itching* No serious adverse effects
coal tar (Balnetar, Cutar, others)	Topical: Apply to affected areas once qid	*Folliculitis, irritation, photosensitivity* No serious adverse effects
salicylic acid (Salax, Neutrogena, others)	Topical: Apply to affected areas tid–qid in concentrations ranging from 2–10%	*Erythema, pruritus, stinging of the skin* No serious adverse effects
tazarotene (Tazorac)	Acne: Apply thin film to clean, dry area daily Plaque psoriasis: Apply thin film daily in the evening	*Pruritus, burning, stinging, skin irritation, transient worsening of psoriasis* No serious adverse effects
SYSTEMIC MEDICATIONS		
acitretin (Soriatane)	PO; 25–50 mg/day with the main meal	*Dry mouth, alopecia, cheilitis, dry skin, dry mucous membranes* Increased triglycerides and cholesterol, paresthesia, rigors, arthralgia, skin peeling, pseudotumor cerebri, depression, elevated liver function tests, teratogenicity
adalimumab (Humira)	Subcutaneous; 40–80 mg every other week	*Upper respiratory infection, injection site reactions, headache, rash* Malignancies, serious infections
alefacept (Amevive)	IM; 15 mg once weekly for 12 weeks	*Pharyngitis, dizziness, cough, nausea, pruritus, myalgia, chills, injection site reactions* Malignancies, serious infections, hepatotoxicity, lymphopenia
cyclosporine (Sandimmune, Neoral) (see page 459 for the Prototype Drug box ∞)	PO; 1.25 mg/kg bid (max: 4 mg/kg/day)	*Hirsutism, tremor, vomiting, headache, pruritus, nausea, vomiting, diarrhea* Hypertension, MI, nephrotoxicity, hyperkalemia, gingival enlargement, paresthesias, hepatotoxicity, infection
etanercept (Enbrel)	Subcutaneous; 25 mg twice/wk or 0.08 mg/kg or 50 mg once/wk	*Local reactions at injection site (pain, erythema, myalgia), abdominal pain, vomiting, headache* Infections, pancytopenia, MI, heart failure
infliximab (Remicade)	IV; 5 mg/kg with additional doses 2 and 6 wk after the initial infusion, then every 8 wk thereafter	*Rash, minor infections* Infusion-related reactions, serious infections, malignancies, worsening of heart failure, hepatotoxicity
methotrexate (Rheumatrex , Trexall) (see page 558 for the Prototype Drug box ∞)	PO; 2.5–5 mg bid for three doses each week (max: 25–30 mg/wk) IM/IV; 10–25 mg/wk	*Headache, glossitis, gingivitis, mild leukopenia, nausea* Ulcerative stomatitis, myelosuppression, aplastic anemia, hepatic cirrhosis, nephrotoxicity, sudden death, pulmonary fibrosis
ustekinumab (Stelara)	Subcutaneous; 45–90 mg initially and 4 weeks later, followed by 45–90 mg every 12 weeks	*Nasopharyngitis, upper respiratory tract infection, headache, fatigue* Serious infections, malignancies

*See Table 48.3 for topical corticosteroids for psoriasis.

Italics indicate common adverse effects; underlining indicates serious adverse effects.

SYSTEMIC THERAPIES

Some patients have severe psoriasis that is resistant to topical therapy. Because these drugs have the potential to cause more serious adverse effects, they are generally only used when topical drugs and phototherapy fail to produce an adequate response. In some cases, systemic drugs may be used for a few weeks to produce a rapid improvement in symptoms before beginning topical therapy.

The most often prescribed systemic drug for severe psoriasis is methotrexate. Methotrexate (Rheumatrex, Trexall) is used for a variety of disorders, including carcinomas and rheumatoid arthritis, in addition to being used for the treatment of psoriasis. Methotrexate is presented as a prototype drug in chapter 37∞.

Other systemic drugs for psoriasis include acitretin (Soriatane), which is taken orally to inhibit excessive skin cell growth. Cyclosporine (Sandimmune, Neoral), an immunosuppressive agent, may be used for severe conditions. The newest psoriasis therapies include biologic agents such as alefacept (Amevive), adalimumab (Humira), ustekinumab (Stelara), etanercept (Enbrel), and infliximab (Remicade). These drugs act by suppressing specific aspects of the inflammatory and immune responses. Several of these are also used to treat rheumatoid arthritis (chapter 47∞). A major disadvantage of these biologic drugs is that they are very expensive and not available in oral formulations.

NONPHARMACOLOGIC THERAPIES

Phototherapy with ultraviolet-A (UVA) and ultraviolet-B (UVB) light is used in cases of severe debilitating psoriasis. Phototherapy with UVA is combined with methoxsalen, a drug from a chemical family known as the **psoralens**. The concurrent use of UVA and the drug is called PUVA therapy. Psoralens are oral or topical agents that produce a photosensitive reaction when exposed to UV light. This reaction reduces the number of lesions, but unpleasant side effects such as headache, nausea, and skin sensitivity still occur, limiting the effectiveness of this therapy.

UVB therapy is less hazardous than UVA therapy. The wavelength of UVB is similar to sunlight, and it reduces lesions covering a large area of body that normally resist topical treatments. With close supervision, this type of phototherapy can be administered at home. Keratolytic pastes are often applied between treatments.

SUNBURN AND MINOR BURNS

Burns are a unique type of stress that may affect all layers of the skin. Minor, first-degree burns affect only the outer layers of the epidermis, are characterized by redness, and are analogous to sunburn. Sunburn results from overexposure of the skin to UV light, and is associated with light skin complexions, prolonged exposure to the sun during the more hazardous hours of the day (10 a.m. until 3 p.m.), and lack of protective clothing when outdoors. Chronic sun exposure can result in serious conditions, including eye injury, cataracts, and skin cancer.

48.8 Pharmacotherapy of Sunburn and Minor Skin Irritation

In addition to producing local skin damage, sun overexposure releases toxins that may produce systemic effects. The signs and symptoms of sunburn include erythema, intense pain, nausea, vomiting, chills, edema, and headache. These symptoms usually resolve within a matter of hours or days, depending on the severity of the exposure. Once sunburn has occurred, medications can only alleviate the symptoms; they do not speed recovery time.

The best treatment for sunburn is *prevention*. Sunscreens are liquids or lotions applied for chemical or physical protection. *Chemical* sunscreens absorb the spectrum of UV light that is responsible for most sunburns. Chemical sunscreens include those that contain benzophenone for protection against UVA rays; those that work against UVB rays include cinnamates, p-aminobenzoic acid (PABA), and salicylates. *Physical* sunscreens such as zinc oxide, talc, and titanium dioxide reflect or scatter light to prevent the penetration of both UVA and UVB rays. Parsol is another sunscreen product that is being used more frequently as a key ingredient in lip balm.

Treatment for sunburn consists of addressing symptoms with soothing lotions, rest, prevention of dehydration, and topical anesthetic agents, if needed. Treatment is usually done on an outpatient basis. Topical anesthetics for minor burns include benzocaine (Solarcaine), dibucaine (Nupercainal), lidocaine (Xylocaine), and tetracaine HCl (Pontocaine). Aloe vera is a popular natural therapy for minor skin irritations and burns. These same agents may also provide relief from minor pain due to insect bites and pruritus. In more severe cases, oral analgesics such as aspirin or ibuprofen may be indicated.

Chapter REVIEW

KEY CONCEPTS

The numbered key concepts provide a succinct summary of the important points from the corresponding numbered section within the chapter. If any of these points are not clear, refer to the numbered section within the chapter for review.

48.1 Three layers of skin, epidermis, dermis, and subcutaneous layer, provide effective barrier defenses for the body.

48.2 Skin disorders that may benefit from pharmacotherapy are acne, sunburns, infections, dermatitis, and psoriasis.

48.3 When the skin integrity is compromised, bacteria, viruses, and fungi can gain entrance and cause infections. Anti-infective therapy may be indicated.

48.4 Scabicides and pediculicides are used to treat parasitic mite and lice infestations, respectively. Permethrin is an agent of choice for these infections.

48.5 The pharmacotherapy of acne includes treatment with benzoyl peroxide, retinoids, and antibiotics. Therapies for rosacea include retinoids and metronidazole.

48.6 The most effective treatment for dermatitis is topical glucocorticoids, which are classified by their potency.

48.7 Both topical and systemic drugs, including corticosteroids, immunomodulators, and methotrexate, are used to treat psoriasis.

48.8 The pharmacotherapy of sunburn includes the symptomatic relief of pain using soothing lotions, topical anesthetics, and analgesics.

NCLEX-RN® REVIEW QUESTIONS

1 The patient is treated for head lice with permethrin (Acticin, Elimite, Nix). Following treatment, the nurse reinforces instructions to:
1. remain isolated for 48 hours.
2. inspect the hair shaft, checking for nits daily for 1 week following treatment.
3. shampoo with permethrin three times per day.
4. wash linens with cold water and bleach.

2 Careful attention to directions for application of permethrine (Acticin, Elimite, Nix) is emphasized by the nurse. Signs of inappropriate over-application include: (Select all that apply.)
1. nausea and vomiting.
2. headache.
3. eye irritation.
4. diaphoresis.
5. restlessness.

3 The nurse evaluates the patient's understanding of the procedure for application of triamcinolone (Kenalog, Aristocort) cream for acute contact dermatitis of the neck, secondary to a reaction to perfume. The patient asks why she "can't just use up some fluocinonide (Lidex) cream she has left over from a poison ivy dermatitis last month." The nurse's response will be based on the knowledge that:

1. high-potency corticosteroid creams should be avoided in the neck or face because of the possibility of additional adverse effects.
2. all creams should be discarded after the initial condition has resolved.
3. fluocinonide cream is too low-potency to use for contact dermatitis.
4. contact dermatitis from perfume is harder to treat than poison ivy dermatitis.

4 The teaching plan for a 24-year-old female receiving tretinoin (Avita, Retin-A, Trentin-X) for treatment of acne should include instructions to: (Select all that apply.)
1. obtain 20 to 30 minutes of sun exposure per day to help dry the skin and prevent breakouts.
2. wash face with a mild soap, avoiding scrubbing, twice a day.
3. use oil-free sunscreens, sun hats, and protective clothing to avoid sun exposure.
4. expect some dryness, redness, and peeling while on the drug but report severe skin irritation.

5 A 15-year-old patient started using topical benzoyl peroxide (Benzalin, Fostex) 1 week ago for treatment of acne
and is discouraged that her acne is still visible. The nurse's
best response will be:
1. "The cream should've started working by now. Check
with your provider about switching to a different type."
2. "Some improvement will be noticed quickly but full
effects may take several weeks to a month or longer."
3. "Acne is very difficult to treat. It may be several months
before you notice any effects."
4. "If your acne is not gone by now, you may need an
antibiotic too. Ask your provider."

6 After trying many other treatments, a 28-year-old female
is started on isotretinoin (Accutane) for treatment of severe acne. While she is on this medication, she must follow explicit instructions to: (Select all that apply.)
1. use two forms of birth control and have pregnancy tests
before beginning, during, and after she is on the therapy.
2. have vision checks performed every 6 months.
3. increase intake of vitamin A–rich foods.
4. return every 2 to 3 months for lab tests.

CRITICAL THINKING QUESTIONS

1. A senior nursing student is participating in well-baby
screenings at a public health clinic. While examining a 4-
month-old infant, the student notes an extensive, conflu-
ent diaper rash. The baby's mother is upset and asks the
student nurse about the use of OTC corticosteroid ointment and wonders how she should apply the cream. How
should the student nurse respond?

2. A 14-year-old girl has been placed on oral doxycycline
(Doxy-Caps) for acne vulgaris because she has not responded to topical antibiotic therapy. After 3 weeks of
therapy, the patient returns to the dermatologist's office
complaining about episodes of nausea and epigastric pain.
The nurse learns that the patient is "so busy with school
activities" that she often forgets a morning dose and "doubles up" on the drug before bedtime. Devise a teaching
plan relevant to drug therapy that takes into consideration
the major side effects of this drug and the cognitive abilities of this patient.

3. A 37-year-old woman is referred to a dermatologist for increasing redness and painful "acne" lesions. The patient is
frustrated with her attempts to camouflage her "teenage
face" with makeup. She relates to the nurse that she had
acne as a teen but had no further problem until the last 11
months. After consultation, the dermatologist suggests a
3-month trial of isotretinoin (Accutane). What are the
specific reproductive considerations for this patient? What
information should this patient be provided in relation to
reproductive concerns?

See Appendix D for answers and rationales for all activities.

EXPLORE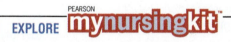

PEARSON

MyNursingKit is your one stop for online chapter review materials and
resources. Prepare for success with additional NCLEX®-style practice
questions, interactive assignments and activities, web links, animations
and videos, and more!

Register your access code from the front of your book at
www.mynursingkit.com.

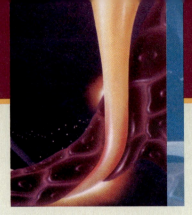

Chapter 49

Drugs for Eye and Ear Disorders

LEARNING OUTCOMES

After reading this chapter, the student should be able to:

1. Identify the basic anatomic structures of the eye.
2. Describe the major risk factors associated with glaucoma.
3. Compare and contrast open-angle and closed-angle glaucoma.
4. Explain the two primary mechanisms by which drugs reduce intraocular pressure.
5. Describe the nurse's role in the pharmacologic management of eye and ear disorders.
6. Identify drugs for treating glaucoma and explain their basic actions and adverse effects.
7. Identify drugs that dilate or constrict pupils, relax ciliary muscles, constrict ocular blood vessels, or moisten eye membranes.
8. Identify drugs for treating ear conditions.
9. Use the nursing process to care for patients who are receiving drug therapy for eye and ear disorders.

The senses of vision and hearing provide the primary means for us to communicate with the world around us. Disorders affecting the eye and ear can result in problems with self-care, mobility, safety, and communication. The eye is vulnerable to a variety of conditions, many of which can be prevented, controlled, or reversed with proper pharmacotherapy. The first part of this chapter covers drugs used for the treatment of glaucoma and those used routinely by ophthalmic health care providers. The remaining part of the chapter presents drugs used for treatment of common ear disorders, including infections, inflammation, and the buildup of ear wax.

49.1 Anatomy of the Eye

A firm knowledge of basic ocular anatomy is required to understand eye disorders and their pharmacotherapy. Important structures of the eye are shown in ➤ Figures 49.1 and 49.2.

A fluid called **aqueous humor** is found in the anterior cavity of the eye, which has two divisions. The *anterior* chamber extends from the cornea to the anterior iris; the *posterior* chamber lies between the posterior iris and the lens. The aqueous humor is formed by the *ciliary body*, a muscular structure in the posterior chamber.

Aqueous humor helps retain the shape of the eye and circulates to bring nutrients to the area and remove wastes. From its origin in the ciliary body, aqueous humor flows from the posterior chamber through the pupil and into the anterior chamber. Within the anterior chamber and around the periphery is a network of spongy connective tissue, or *trabecular meshwork*, that contains an opening called the canal of Schlemm. The aqueous humor drains into the canal of Schlemm and out of the anterior chamber into the venous system, thus completing its circulation. Under normal circumstances, the rate of aqueous humor production (inflow) is equal to its outflow, which helps to maintain intraocular pressure (IOP) within a normal range. Interference with either the inflow or outflow of aqueous humor, however, can lead to an increase in IOP.

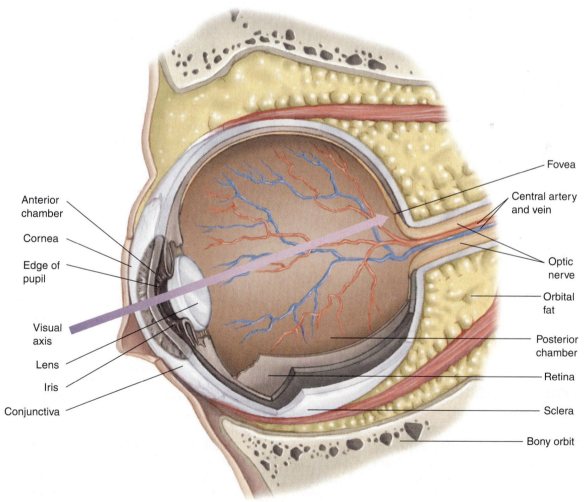

➤ *Figure 49.1* Internal structures of the eye
Source: Pearson Education/PH College.

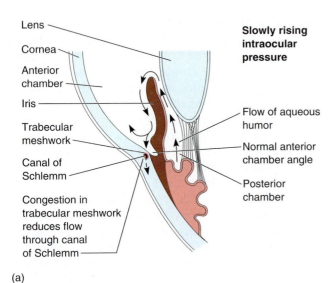

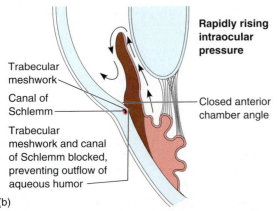

> **Figure 49.2** Forms of primary adult glaucoma: (a) in chronic open-angle glaucoma, the anterior chamber angle remains open, but drainage of aqueous humor through the canal of Schlemm is impaired; (b) in acute closed-angle glaucoma, the angle of the iris and anterior chamber narrows, obstructing the outflow of aqueous humor

GLAUCOMA

Glaucoma is an eye disease caused by damage to the optic nerve that results in a gradual loss of vision, possibly advancing to blindness. This disorder is usually accompanied by increased intraocular pressure (IOP). Glaucoma may occur so gradually that patients do not seek medical intervention until late in the disease process.

49.2 Types of Glaucoma

Glaucoma occurs when the IOP becomes so high that it causes damage to the optic nerve. Although the median IOP in the population is 15 to 16 mmHg, normal pressure varies greatly with age, daily activities, and even time of day. As a rule, IOPs consistently above 21 mmHg are considered abnormal and at risk for glaucoma. Many patients, however, tolerate IOPs in the mid to high 20s without damage to the optic nerve. IOPs above 30 mmHg require treatment because they are associated with permanent vision changes.

Some patients of Asian descent may experience glaucoma at "normal" IOP values, below 21 mmHg. In addition, patients who have had Lasik surgery, which removes corneal tissue to correct myopia, may appear to have normal IOPs yet have glaucoma.

Glaucoma usually occurs as a *primary* condition without an identifiable cause and is most frequently found in persons older than 60 years. In some cases, glaucoma is associated with genetic factors; it can be congenital and occur in young children. Glaucoma can also be *secondary* to eye trauma, infection, diabetes, inflammation, hemorrhage, tumor, or cataracts. Some medications may contribute to the development or progression of glaucoma, including the long-term use of topical corticosteroids, some antihypertensives, antihistamines, and antidepressants. Other major risk factors associated with glaucoma include high blood pressure, migraine headaches, high degrees of nearsightedness or farsightedness, and normal aging. Glaucoma is the leading cause of *preventable* blindness.

The two principal types of primary glaucoma are closed-angle glaucoma and open-angle glaucoma, as illustrated in Figure 49.2. Both disorders result from the same problem: a buildup of aqueous humor in the anterior cavity. This buildup is caused either by *excessive production* of aqueous humor or by a *blockage of its outflow*. In either case, IOP increases, leading to progressive damage to the optic nerve. As degeneration of the optic nerve occurs, the patient will first notice a loss of visual field, then a loss of central visual acuity, and finally total blindness. Major differences between closed-angle glaucoma and open-angle glaucoma include how quickly the IOP develops and whether there is narrowing of the anterior chamber angle between the iris and cornea.

Closed-angle glaucoma, also called *narrow-angle* glaucoma accounts for only 5% of all primary glaucoma. The incidence is higher in older adults and in persons of Asian descent. This type of glaucoma is usually unilateral and may be caused by stress, impact injury, or medications. It is typically caused by the normal thickening of the lens and may develop progressively over several years. Pressure inside the anterior chamber increases suddenly because the iris is being pushed over the area where the aqueous humor normally drains. The displacement of the iris is due in part to the dilation of the pupil or accommodation of the lens, causing the angle between the posterior cornea and the anterior iris to narrow or close. Signs and symptoms, caused by acute obstruction of the outflow of aqueous humor from the eye, include dull to severe eye pain, headaches, bloodshot eyes, foggy vision with halos around bright lights, and a bulging iris. Ocular pain may be so severe that it causes vomiting. Once the outflow is totally closed, closed-angle glaucoma constitutes an emergency. Laser or conventional surgery is indicated for this condition. Options include iridectomy, laser trabeculoplasty, trabeculectomy, and drainage implants.

Open-angle glaucoma is the most common type, accounting for more than 90% of the cases. Its cause is not known and many patients are asymptomatic. It is usually bilateral, with intraocular pressure developing over years. It is called "open angle" because the iris does not cover the trabecular meshwork;

PharmFacts

Glaucoma

- Worldwide, more than 5 million people have lost their vision due to glaucoma. More than 50,000 of these people are in the United States.
- Only 50% of the people with glaucoma are aware that they have the disease.
- The incidence of glaucoma in people of African heritage is three to five times higher than in any other ethnic group.
- Glaucoma is most common in patients older than 60 years.
- Acute glaucoma is often caused by head trauma, cataracts, tumors, or hemorrhage.
- Chronic simple glaucoma accounts for 90% of all glaucoma cases.

it remains open. If discovered early, most patients with open-angle glaucoma can be successfully treated with medications.

49.3 General Principles of Glaucoma Pharmacotherapy

Some health care providers initiate glaucoma pharmacotherapy in all patients with an IOP greater than 21 mmHg. Because of the expense of pharmacotherapy and the potential for adverse drug effects, other health care providers will instead carefully monitor the patient through regular follow-up exams and wait until the IOP rises to 28 to 30 mmHg before initiating drug therapy. If signs of optic nerve damage or visual field changes are evident, the patient is treated regardless of the IOP.

When beginning glaucoma pharmacotherapy, a target IOP is established. During therapy, revaluation of the IOP and the extent of visual field changes is performed after 2 to 4 months to check for therapeutic effectiveness. Some of the antiglaucoma drugs take 6 to 8 weeks to reach peak effect. If the therapeutic goals are not achieved with a single medication, it is common to add a second drug from a different class to the regimen to produce an additive decrease in IOP. Some of the drugs may continue to have effects on the eye for 2 to 4 weeks after they are discontinued.

Drugs for glaucoma work by one of two mechanisms: increasing the outflow of aqueous humor at the canal of Schlemm or decreasing the formation of aqueous humor at the ciliary body. Many agents for glaucoma act by affecting the autonomic nervous system (chapter 13).

49.4 Antiglaucoma Drugs

There are many drugs available to treat glaucoma. Although topical drugs are most frequently prescribed, oral medications are available for severe disease. Drugs for glaucoma, listed in Table 49.1, include the following classes:

- Prostaglandins
- Autonomic agents, including beta-adrenergic blockers, nonselective sympathomimetics, alpha$_2$-adrenergic agonists, and cholinergic agonists
- Carbonic anhydrase inhibitors
- Osmotic diuretics

PROSTAGLANDINS

Prostaglandin analogs are a more recent therapy for glaucoma, and one of the most effective. They are often drugs of choice for glaucoma because they have long durations of action and produce fewer adverse effects than drugs from other classes. They may be used as monotherapy or combined with beta-adrenergic blockers to produce an additive reduction in IOP in patients with resistant glaucoma.

Prostaglandin analogs decrease IOP by enhancing the outflow of aqueous humor. Latanoprost (Xalatan), available as an eye drop solution, is one of the most frequently prescribed prostaglandin analogs and is a prototype drug in this chapter. Several other ocular prostaglandins have been approved, including bimatoprost (Lumigan), travaprost (Travatan), and unoprostone (Rescula). An occasional adverse effect of these medications is heightened pigmentation, which turns a blue iris to a more brown color. This change may be irreversible. Many patients experience thicker and longer eyelashes. These drugs cause local irritation, stinging of the eyes, and redness during the first month of therapy. Because of these effects, prostaglandins are normally administered just before bedtime.

Autonomic Drugs

Several structures within the eye receive signals from the sympathetic and parasympathetic divisions of the autonomic nervous system. As such, a significant number of autonomic agents have been used to treat glaucoma and to aid in ophthalmic examinations of the eye.

BETA-ADRENERGIC BLOCKERS Before the discovery of the prostaglandin analogs, beta-adrenergic blockers were drugs of choice for open-angle glaucoma. These drugs act by decreasing the production of aqueous humor by the ciliary body, and can lower IOP by 20% to 30%. Beta-adrenergic blockers generally produce fewer ocular adverse effects than other autonomic drugs. In most patients, the topical administration of beta blockers does not result in significant systemic absorption. Should absorption occur, however, systemic adverse effects may include bronchoconstriction, dysrhythmias, and hypotension. Because of the potential for systemic effects, these drugs should be used with caution in patients with asthma or heart failure.

ALPHA$_2$-ADRENERGIC AGONISTS Alpha$_2$-adrenergic agonists act by decreasing the production of aqueous humor. Only two alpha$_2$-adrenergic agonists are currently approved for open-angle glaucoma, and neither of them is frequently prescribed. Apraclonidine (Iopidine) is indicated for the reduction in IOP during or following eye surgery and brimonidine (Alphagan) is used as an adjunct in combination with other antiglaucoma agents. The most significant adverse effects are allergic reactions, headache, drowsiness, dry mucosal membranes, blurred vision, and irritated eyelids.

CHOLINERGIC AGONISTS Cholinergic agonists are autonomic drugs that activate cholinergic receptors in the eye

TABLE 49.1	**Selected Drugs for Glaucoma**	
Drug	Route and Adult Dose (max dose where indicated)	Adverse Effects
PROSTAGLANDIN ANALOGS		
bimatoprost (Lumigan)	1 drop of 0.03% solution daily in the evening	*Increased length and thickness of eyelashes, darkening of iris, sensation of foreign body in the eye*
latanoprost (Xalatan)	1 drop of 0.005% solution daily in the evening	
travoprost (Travatan)	1 drop of 0.004% solution daily in the evening	Serious adverse effects that may occur with systemic absorption: respiratory infection/flu, angina, muscle or joint pain
BETA-ADRENERGIC BLOCKERS		
betaxolol (Betoptic)	1 drop of 0.5% solution bid	*Local burning and stinging, blurred vision, headache*
levobunolol (Betagan)	1–2 drops of 0.25–0.5% solution one to two times/day	
metipranolol (OptiPranolol)	1 drop of 0.3% solution bid	Serious adverse effects that may occur with systemic absorption: angina, anxiety, bronchoconstriction, hypertension, dysrhythmias
timolol (Betimol, Istalol, Timoptic)	1–2 drops of 0.25–0.5% solution one to two times/day	
	Gel (salve): apply daily	
ALPHA$_2$-ADRENERGIC AGONISTS		
apraclonidine (Lopidine)	1 drop of 0.5% solution bid	*Local itching and burning, blurred vision, dry mouth*
brimonidine (Alphagan)	1 drop of 0.2% solution tid	Allergic conjunctivitis, conjunctival hyperemia, hypertension
CARBONIC ANHYDRASE INHIBITORS		
acetazolamide (Diamox)	PO; 250 mg one to four times/day	*For topical agents: blurred vision, bitter taste, dry eye, blepharitis, local itching, sensation of foreign body in the eye, headache*
brinzolamide (Azopt)	1 drop of 1% solution tid	
dorzolamide (Trusopt)	1 drop of 2% solution in affected eye(s) tid	For oral route: diuresis, electrolyte imbalances, blood dyscrasias, flaccid paralysis, hepatic impairment
methazolamide (Neptazane)	PO; 50–100 mg bid–tid	
CHOLINERGIC AGONISTS		
carbachol (Miostat)	1–2 drops of 0.75–3% solution in lower conjunctival sac every 4 h tid	*Induced myopia, reduced visual acuity in low light, eye redness, headache*
echothiophate iodide (Phospholine Iodide)	1 drop of 0.03–0.25% solution one to two times/day	Serious adverse effects that may occur with systemic absorption: salivation, tachycardia, hypertension, bronchospasm, sweating, nausea, vomiting
pilocarpine (Isopto Carpine, Pilopine)	Acute glaucoma: 1 drop of 1–2% solution every 5–10 min for 3–6 doses	
	Chronic glaucoma: 1 drop of 0.5–4% solution every 4–12 h	
NONSELECTIVE SYMPATHOMIMETICS		
dipivefrin HCl (Propine)	1 drop of 0.1% solution bid	*Local burning and stinging, blurred vision, headache, photosensitivity*
		Tachycardia, hypertension
OSMOTIC DIURETICS		
isosorbide (Ismotic)	PO; 1–3 g/kg one to two times/day	*Orthostatic hypotension, facial flushing, headache, palpitations, anxiety, nausea*
mannitol (Osmitrol)	IV; 1.5–2 mg/kg as a 15–25% solution over 30–60 min	Severe headache, electrolyte imbalances, edema

Italics indicate common adverse effects; underlining indicates serious adverse effects.

and produce **miosis,** constriction of the pupil, and contraction of the ciliary muscle. These actions physically pull open the trabecular meshwork to allow greater outflow of aqueous humor and a lowering of IOP. The cholinergic agonists are applied topically to the eye. Pilocarpine (Isopto-Carpine, Pilopine) is the most commonly prescribed cholinergic agonist. Adverse effects include headache, induced myopia, and decreased vision in low light. Because of their greater toxicity and more frequent dosing requirements, cholinergic agonists are normally used only in patients with open-angle glaucoma who do not respond to other agents.

NONSELECTIVE SYMPATHOMIMETICS *Nonselective sympathomimetics* activate the sympathetic nervous system to produce **mydriasis** (pupil dilation), which increases the outflow of

Pr Prototype Drug | Latanoprost (Xalatan)

Therapeutic Class: Antiglaucoma drug   **Pharmacologic Class:** Prostaglandin analog

ACTIONS AND USES
Latanoprost is a prostaglandin analog that reduces IOP by increasing the outflow of aqueous humor. It is used to treat open-angle glaucoma. The recommended dose is one drop in the affected eye(s) in the evening. It is metabolized to its active form in the cornea, reaching its peak effect in about 12 hours.

ADMINISTRATION ALERTS
- Remove contact lens before instilling eye drops. Do not reinsert contact for 15 minutes.
- Avoid touching the eye or eyelashes with any part of the eyedropper to avoid cross-contamination.
- Wait 5 minutes before/after instillation of a different eye prescription to administer eye drop(s).
- Pregnancy category C

PHARMACOKINETICS
Onset: 3–4 h
Peak: 8–12 h
Half-life: 17 min
Duration: Unknown

ADVERSE EFFECTS
Adverse effects include ocular symptoms such as conjunctival edema, tearing, dryness, burning, pain, irritation, itching, sensation of foreign body in eye, photophobia, and/or visual disturbances. The eyelashes on the treated eye may grow thicker, and darker. Changes may occur in pigmentation of the iris of the treated eye and in the periocular skin.

Contraindications: Contraindications include hypersensitivity to the drug or another component in the solution, pregnancy, lactation, intraocular infection, or conjunctivitis. It should not be administered to patients with closed-angle glaucoma.

INTERACTIONS
Drug–Drug: Latanoprost interacts with the preservative thimerosal: If used concurrently with other eye drops containing thimerosal, precipitation may occur.

Lab Tests: Unknown

Herbal/Food: Unknown

Treatment of Overdose: Overdose with ophthalmic solution is unlikely.

Refer to MyNursingKit for a Nursing Process Focus specific to this drug.

Pr Prototype Drug | Timolol (Betimol, Istalol, Timoptic)

Therapeutic Class: Drug for glaucoma   **Pharmacologic Class:** Miotic; beta-adrenergic antagonist

ACTIONS AND USES
Timolol is a nonselective beta-adrenergic blocker available in several ophthalmic formulations. Betimol and Timoptic are 0.25% or 0.5% ophthalmic solutions taken twice daily. Timoptic XE and Istalol are long-acting solutions that allow for once daily dosing. Timolol lowers IOP in chronic open-angle glaucoma by reducing the formation of aqueous humor. The drug has no significant effects on visual acuity, pupil size, or accommodation. Treatment may require 2 to 4 weeks for maximum therapeutic effect. As an oral medication, timolol is prescribed to treat mild hypertension, stable angina, prophylaxis of myocardial infarction, and migraines.

ADMINISTRATION ALERTS
- Proper administration lessens the danger that the drug will be absorbed systemically. Systemic absorption can mask symptoms of hypoglycemia.
- Pregnancy category C

PHARMACOKINETICS
Onset: 30 min
Peak: 1–2 h
Half-life: Unknown
Duration: 12–24 h

ADVERSE EFFECTS
The most common adverse effects are local burning and stinging on instillation. Vision may become temporarily blurred. In most patients there is not enough absorption to cause systemic adverse effects as long as timolol is applied correctly. If absorption occurs, hypotension or dysrhythmias are possible.

Contraindications: Timolol is contraindicated in patients with asthma, severe chronic obstructive pulmonary disease, sinus bradycardia, second- or third-degree atrioventricular block, heart failure, cardiogenic shock, or hypersensitivity to the drug.

INTERACTIONS
Drug–Drug: Drug interactions may result if significant systemic absorption occurs. Timolol should be used with caution in patients taking other beta blockers due to additive cardiac effects. Concurrent use with anticholinergics, nitrates, reserpine, methyldopa, or verapamil could lead to hypotension and bradycardia. Epinephrine use could lead to hypertension followed by severe bradycardia.

Lab Tests: Unknown

Herbal/Food: Unknown

Treatment of Overdose: Overdose with ophthalmic solution is unlikely.

See Refer to MyNursingKit for a Nursing Process Focus specific to this drug.

NURSING PROCESS FOCUS   PATIENTS RECEIVING OPHTHALMIC SOLUTIONS FOR GLAUCOMA

Assessment	Potential Nursing Diagnoses
Baseline assessment prior to administration: ■ Understand the reason the drug has been prescribed in order to assess for therapeutic effects (e.g., open angle or closed angle, secondary to eye trauma). ■ Obtain a complete health history including ophthalmologic, respiratory, cardiovascular, and endocrine disease. ■ Assess visual acuity and visual fields. Assess for the presence of eye pain, visual disturbances such as halos around lights, diminished "foggy" vision, or loss of peripheral vision. ■ Assess for history of recent eye trauma or infection. ■ Obtain a drug history including allergies, current prescription and OTC drugs, herbal preparations, alcohol use, and smoking. Be alert to possible drug interactions. ■ Obtain baseline vital signs.	■ Disturbed Sensory Perception (Visual) ■ Anxiety (related to concerns of loss of vision, eye pain) ■ Pain (disease condition, treatment adverse effects) ■ Deficient Knowledge (drug therapy) ■ Risk for Injury (related to visual acuity deficits) ■ Deficient Self-Care Ability (related to impaired vision)
Assessment throughout administration: ■ Assess for desired therapeutic effects dependent on the reason the drug is given (e.g., intraocular pressure remains below 20 mmHg or at target value, improvement in visual acuity or fields). ■ Assess for adverse effects: conjunctival edema, tearing, dryness, burning, pain, irritation, itching, sensation of foreign body in eye, or photophobia. Severe visual disturbances or eye pain should be promptly reported to the health care provider.	

Planning: Patient Goals and Expected Outcomes

The patient will:
■ Experience therapeutic effects (e.g., eye pressure has normalized, visual acuity and visual fields remain stable).
■ Be free from, or experience minimal, adverse effects.
■ Verbalize an understanding of the drug's use, adverse effects, and required precautions.
■ Demonstrate proper self-administration of the medication (e.g., dose, timing, when to notify provider).

Implementation

Interventions and (Rationales)	Patient and Family Education
Ensuring therapeutic effects: ■ Monitor visual acuity, vision fields, and intraocular eye pressure. (Eye pressure should remain less than 20 mmHg or per parameters set by health care provider. Visual acuity and fields remain intact.)	■ Instruct the patient to immediately report changes in vision, eye pain, light-sensitivity, halos around lights, or headache to the health care provider.
Minimizing adverse effects: ■ Monitor appropriate administration of drug to avoid extraocular effects. (Eye drops should be instilled into the conjunctival sac and the lacrimal duct area held with gentle pressure for 1 full minute to prevent drug leakage into the nasopharynx with possible systemic effects.)	■ Teach the patient proper administration techniques for eye drops. Oral medications should be taken as regularly throughout the day as possible and with consistent dosing.
■ Monitor intraocular pressure periodically. (Consistent readings above the target value may indicate worsening disease or improper use of drug therapy.)	■ Instruct the patient of the importance to return for and maintain regular eye exams.
■ Monitor for increasing eye redness, pain, light sensitivity, or changes in visual acuity. (Eye changes or pain may indicate worsening disease, infection, or adverse drug effects.)	■ Instruct the patient to avoid touching the eye drop tip to the conjunctival sac when instilling eye drops. Immediately report any increasing redness, eye pain, eye drainage, or changes in vision.
■ Remove contact lenses before administering ophthalmic solutions. (Contact lenses may hinder the eye solution from fully reaching all eye surfaces or may absorb solution, resulting in higher than expected amounts in eye over time.)	■ Instruct the patient to remove contact lenses prior to administering eye drops and wait at least 15 minutes before reinserting them.

NURSING PROCESS FOCUS   PATIENTS RECEIVING OPHTHALMIC SOLUTIONS FOR GLAUCOMA *(Continued)*

Implementation

Interventions and (Rationales)	Patient and Family Education
■ Monitor vital signs periodically for signs of systemic absorption of topical preparations. (Ophthalmic drugs such as beta blockers or cholinergic drugs may result in hypotension or bradycardia if the drug is absorbed systemically. Ensure the patient is administering drops appropriately if changes in blood pressure are noted.)	■ Teach the patient to return to the health care provider periodically for monitoring. Assess blood pressure once per week and report any values less than 90/60 mmHg or per parameters. Immediately report any dizziness, headache, palpitations, or syncope.
■ Provide for eye comfort such as adequately lighted room. (Ophthalmic drugs such as beta blockers used in the treatment of glaucoma can cause miosis and difficulty seeing in low light levels.)	■ Caution the patient about driving or other activities in low-light conditions or at night until the effects of the drug are known.
■ Monitor adherence to the treatment regimen. (Nonadherence may result in the total loss of vision.)	■ Teach the patient of the importance in adhering to the medication schedule as prescribed. ■ Address any concerns the patient may have about cost and discomfort related to drug therapy and provide appropriate referrals (e.g., social service agency) as needed.
Patient understanding of drug therapy: ■ Use opportunities during administration of medications and during assessments to discuss the rationale for drug therapy, desired therapeutic outcomes, most common adverse effects, parameters for when to call the health care provider, and any necessary monitoring or precautions. (Using time during nursing care helps to optimize and reinforce key teaching areas.)	■ The patient should be able to state the reason for the drug, appropriate dose and scheduling, and what adverse effects to observe for and when to report them.
Patient self-administration of drug therapy: ■ When administering the medication, instruct the patient, family, or caregiver in the proper self-administration of the drug, e.g., appropriate instillation of eye drops. (Proper administration increases the effectiveness of the drug.)	■ Teach the patient to take the drug following the guidelines provided by the health care provider.

Evaluation of Outcome Criteria

Evaluate the effectiveness of drug therapy by confirming that patient goals and expected outcomes have been met (see "Planning").

See Table 49.1 for a list of drugs to which these nursing actions apply.

aqueous humor, resulting in a lower IOP. They are not as effective as the beta-adrenergic blockers or the prostaglandin analogs in treating open-angle glaucoma. Epinephrine is no longer available for glaucoma. Dipivefrin is converted to epinephrine in the eye; thus, its effects are identical to those of epinephrine. If epinephrine reaches the systemic circulation, it increases blood pressure and heart rate. Because of the potential for systemic adverse effects, these are rarely prescribed for glaucoma.

Carbonic Anhydrase Inhibitors

Carbonic anhydrase inhibitors (CAIs) may be administered topically or systemically to reduce IOP in patients with open-angle glaucoma. They act by decreasing the production of aqueous humor.

CAIs are grouped into topical or oral formulations. Dorzolamide (Trusopt) is used topically to treat open-angle glaucoma, either as monotherapy or in combination with other agents. Dorzolamide and other topical CAIs are well tolerated and produce few significant adverse effects other than photosensitivity. Oral formulations such as acetazolamide (Diamox) are very effective at lowering IOP, but are rarely used because they produce more systemic adverse effects than drugs from other classes. Systemic effects include lethargy, nausea, vomiting, depression, paresthesias, and drowsiness. Patients must be cautioned when taking these medications because they contain sulfur and may cause an allergic reaction. Because the oral formulations are diuretics and can reduce IOP quickly, serum electrolytes should be monitored during treatment.

Osmotic Diuretics

Osmotic diuretics are occasionally used preoperatively and postoperatively with ocular surgery or as emergency treatment for acute closed-angle glaucoma attacks. Examples include isosorbide (Ismotic), urea, and mannitol (Osmitrol). Because they have the ability to quickly reduce plasma volume (chapter 30 ∞), these drugs are effective in reducing the formation of aqueous humor. Adverse effects include headache, tremors, dizziness, dry mouth, fluid and electrolyte imbalances, and thrombophlebitis or venous clot formation near the site of IV administration.

49.5 Pharmacotherapy for Eye Exams and Minor Eye Conditions

Various drugs are used to enhance diagnostic eye examinations. **Mydriatic drugs** dilate the pupil to allow better assessment of retinal structures. **Cycloplegic drugs** not only dilate the pupil but also paralyze the ciliary muscle and prevent the lens from moving during assessment. Agents used for eye examinations include anticholinergics such as atropine (Isopto Atropine) and tropicamide (Mydriacyl), and sympathomimetics such as phenylephrine (Mydfrin).

Mydriatics cause intense photophobia and pain in response to bright light. Mydriatics can worsen glaucoma by impairing aqueous humor outflow and thereby increasing IOP. Cycloplegics cause severe blurred vision and loss of near vision. The response to mydriatics and cycloplegics can last 3 hours up to several days. The patient needs to be taught to wear sunglasses and that the ability to drive, read, and perform visual tasks will be affected during treatment.

Drugs for minor irritation and dryness come from a broad range of classes. Some agents lubricate only the eye's surface, whereas others are designed to penetrate and affect a specific area of the eye. Vasoconstrictors are commonly used to treat minor eye irritation. Common vasoconstrictors include phenylephrine (Neo-Synephrine), naphazoline (ClearEyes), and tetrahydrozoline (Altazine, Murine Tears Plus, Visine). Adverse effects of the vasoconstrictors are usually minor and include blurred vision, tearing, headache, and rebound vasodilation with redness. Examples of cycloplegic, mydriatic, and lubricant drugs are listed in Table 49.2.

Conjunctivitis is an inflammation or infection of the lining of the eyelids. Topical corticosteroids and nonsteroidal anti-inflammatory agents (NSAIDs), such as ketorolac (Acular), can be used to treat conjunctivitis and other inflammatory conditions. Several medications, including antihistamines and mast cell stabilizers, are used to decrease the redness and itching associated with allergic conjunctivitis. Topical mast cell stabilizers, with or without an antihistamine, are the preferred treatment for allergic conjunctivitis because they do not cause excessive drying of the eyes. Two more recent drugs, olopatadine (Patanol) and pemirolast (Alamast), provide for daily dosed treatments for allergic conjunctivitis. Azelastine (Optivar) and epinastine (Elestat) are combination antihistamine–mast cell stabilizers, indicated for twice-daily dosing. Bepotastine (Bepreve) is an antihistamine approved in 2009 for itching associated with allergic conjunctivitis.

EAR CONDITIONS

The ear has two major sensory functions: hearing and maintenance of equilibrium and balance. As shown in ▶ Figure 49.3,

TABLE 49.2	Drugs for Mydriasis, Cycloplegia, and Lubrication of the Eye	
Drug	**Route and Adult Dose (max dose where indicated)**	**Adverse Effects**
MYDRIATICS: SYMPATHOMIMETICS		
phenylephrine (Mydfrin, Neo-Synephrine) (see page 133 for the Prototype Drug box ∞)	1 drop 2.5% or 10% solution before eye exam	*Eye pain, photosensitivity, eye irritation, headache* Hypertension, tremor, dysrhythmias
CYCLOPLEGICS: ANTICHOLINERGICS		
atropine (Isopto Atropine, others) (see page 144 for the Prototype Drug box ∞)	1 drop of 0.5% solution each day	*Eye irritation and redness, dry mouth, local burning or stinging, headache, blurred vision, photosensitivity, eczematoid dermatitis (scopolamine and tropicamide)*
cyclopentolate (Cyclogyl, Pentolair)	1 drop of 0.5–2% solution 40–50 min before eye exam	
homatropine (Isopto Homatropine, others)	1–2 drops of 2% or 5% solution before eye exam	Somnolence, tachycardia, convulsions, mental changes, keratitis, increased intraocular pressure (homatropine)
scopolamine hydrobromide (Isopto Hyoscine)	1–2 drops of 0.25% solution 1 h before eye exam	
tropicamide (Mydriacyl, Tropicacyl)	1–2 drops of 0.5–1% solution before eye exam	
LUBRICANTS AND VASOCONSTRICTORS		
lanolin alcohol (Lacril-lube)	Apply a thin film to the inside of the eyelid	*Temporary burning or stinging, eye itching or redness, headache*
methylcellulose (Methulose, Visculose, others)	1–2 drops prn	
naphazoline (Albalon, Allerest, ClearEyes, others)	1–3 drops of 0.1% solution every 3–4 h prn	No serious adverse effects
oxymetazoline (OcuClear, Visine LR)	1–2 drops of 0.025% solution qid	
polyvinyl alcohol (Liquifilm, others)	1–2 drops prn	
tetrahydrozoline (Collyrium, Murine Plus, Visine, others)	1–2 drops of 0.05% solution bid–tid	

Italics indicate common adverse effects; underlining indicates serious adverse effects.

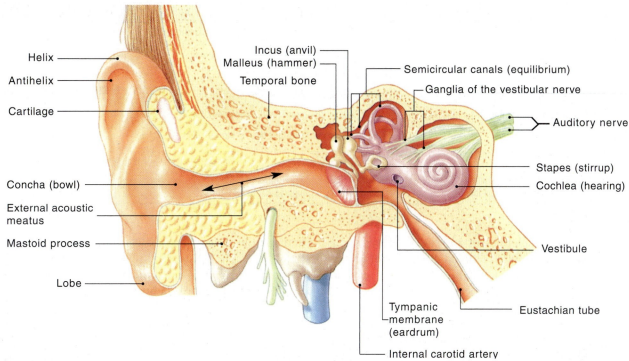

> **Figure 49.3** Structures of the external ear, middle ear, and inner ear
> *Source: Pearson Education/PH College.*

---

three structural areas, the outer ear, middle ear, and inner ear, carry out these functions. The basic treatment for ear conditions is topical preparations in the form of ear drops.

49.6 Pharmacotherapy with Otic Preparations

Otitis, or inflammation of the ear, is a common indication for pharmacotherapy. **External otitis**, commonly called *swimmer's ear*, is inflammation of the outer ear that is most often associated with water exposure. **Otitis media**, inflammation of the middle ear, is most often associated with upper

MyNursingKit | National Library of Medicine

TABLE 49.3	**Otic Preparations**	
Drug	Route and Adult Dose (max dose where indicated)	Adverse Effects
acetic acid and hydrocortisone (VoSoL HC)	3–5 drops every 4 h qid for 24 h, then 5 drops tid–qid	*Ear irritation, local stinging or burning, dizziness*
benzocaine and antipyrine (Auralgan)	Fill ear canal with solution tid for 2–3 days	
carbamide peroxide (Debrox)	1–5 drops 6.5% solution bid for 4 days	<u>Allergic reactions (antibiotics)</u>
ciprofloxacin and dexamethasone (CiproDex)	Children to adult: 4 drops in affected ears bid for 7 days	
ciprofloxacin and hydrocortisone (Cipro)	3 drops of the suspension instilled into ear bid for 7 days	
polymyxin B, neomycin, and hydrocortisone (Cortisporin)	4 drops in ear tid–qid	

Italics indicate common adverse effects; <u>underlining</u> indicates serious adverse effects.
Refer also to chapter 3 "Principles of Drug Administration," for proper administration technique for ear drops ∞.

MyNursingKit | Administering Ear Drops

respiratory infections, allergies, or auditory tube irritation. Of all ear infections, the most difficult ones to treat are inner ear infections. **Mastoiditis,** or inflammation of the mastoid sinus, can be a serious problem because if left untreated, it can result in hearing loss.

Chloramphenicol (Chloromycetin, Pentamycetin) and ciprofloxacin (Cipro otic) are commonly used topical otic antibiotics. Otitis media is treated with a course of systemic rather than topical antibiotics. Amoxicillin, at a dose of 80 to 90 mg/kg/day, is prescribed for most children.

In cases of otitis media, drugs for pain, edema, and itching may also be necessary. Topical corticosteroids are often combined with antibiotics or other drugs when inflammation is present. Examples of these drugs are listed in Table 49.3. Acetaminophen or NSAIDs such as ibuprofen are used to relieve pain and reduce fever.

Mastoiditis is frequently the result of chronic or recurring bacterial otitis media. The infection moves into the bone and surrounding structures of the middle ear. The treatment of acute mastoiditis involves aggressive antibiotic therapy. Intravenous gentamicin or ticarcillin may be used initially; therapy may be adjusted once culture and sensitivity results are obtained. Therapy is continued for at least 14 days. If the antibiotics are not effective and symptoms persist, surgery such as mastoidectomy or meatoplasty may be indicated.

Cerumen (ear wax) softeners are also used for proper ear health. When cerumen accumulates, it narrows the ear canal and may interfere with hearing. This procedure usually involves instillation of an earwax softener and then a gentle lavage of the wax-impacted ear with tepid water using an asepto syringe to gently insert the water. An instrument called an *ear loop* may be used to help remove earwax, but should be used only by health care providers who are skilled in using it. Examples of earwax softeners include carbamide peroxide (Debrox) and triethanolamine.

Chapter REVIEW

KEY CONCEPTS

The numbered key concepts provide a succinct summary of the important points from the corresponding numbered section within the chapter. If any of these points are not clear, refer to the numbered section within the chapter for review.

49.1 Knowledge of basic eye anatomy is fundamental to understanding eye disorders and pharmacotherapy.

49.2 Glaucoma develops because the flow of aqueous humor in the anterior eye cavity becomes disrupted, leading to increased intraocular pressure. The two principal types of glaucoma are closed-angle glaucoma and open-angle glaucoma. Therapy of acute glaucoma may require laser surgery to correct the underlying pathology.

49.3 The goal of glaucoma pharmacotherapy is to prevent damage to the optic nerve by lowering IOP. Combination therapy may be necessary to achieve this goal.

49.4 Drugs used for glaucoma decrease IOP by increasing the outflow of aqueous humor or by decreasing the formation of aqueous humor. Drug classes include prostaglandins, beta-adrenergic blockers, alpha$_2$-adrenergic agonists, carbonic anhydrase inhibitors, nonselective sympathomimetics, cholinergic agonists, and osmotic diuretics.

49.5 Drugs routinely used for eye examinations include mydriatics, which dilate the pupil, and cycloplegics, which cause both dilation and paralysis of the ciliary muscle.

49.6 Otic preparations treat infections, inflammation, and earwax buildup.

NCLEX-RN® REVIEW QUESTIONS

1 A patient with a history of glaucoma who has been taking latanoprost (Xalatan) eye drops complains of severe pain in the eye, severe headache, and blurred vision. The appropriate nursing action is to:
1. document the occurrence; this symptom is expected.
2. medicate the patient with a narcotic analgesic.
3. notify the health care provider immediately.
4. place the patient in a quiet darkened environment.

2 The patient should be aware of potential side effects of prostaglandins used in the treatment of glaucoma. The nurse should include which of the following in the teaching plan?
1. Hypertension
2. Loss of lashes
3. Dilation of pupils
4. Brown pigmentation of treated eye

3 Beta-adrenergic agents may be used to treat glaucoma. The nurse should teach the patients and family to:
1. monitor urine output.
2. monitor blood glucose.
3. monitor pulse and blood pressure.
4. monitor respiratory rate.

4 The nurse emphasizes to the patient with glaucoma the importance of notifying the health care provider performing an eye examination of a glaucoma diagnosis because of potential adverse reactions to which drugs?
1. Antibiotic drops
2. Cycloplegic drops
3. Anti-inflammatory drops
4. Anticholinergic mydriatic drops

5 The patient is prescribed timolol (Timoptic) for treatment of glaucoma. The nurse assesses for which of the following medical disorders during the history and physical, which may be a contraindication to the use of this drug? (Select all that apply.)
1. Heart block
2. Congestive heart failure
3. Liver disease
4. COPD
5. Renal disease

6 Appropriate administration is key for patients taking eye drops for the treatment of glaucoma to optimize therapeutic effects and reduce adverse effects. The nurse would be concerned if the patient reports administering the drops:
1. into the conjunctival sac.
2. holding slight pressure on the tear duct (lacrimal duct) for 1 minute after using the eye drops.
3. avoiding direct contact with the eye dropper tip and the eye.
4. leaving contact lenses in to be sure the eye drop is maintained in the eye.

CRITICAL THINKING QUESTIONS

1. A 3-year-old girl is playing nurse with her dolls. She picks up her mother's flexible metal necklace and places the tips of the necklace in her ears for her "stethoscope." A few hours later, she cries to her mother that her "ears hurt." The child's mother takes her to see the health care provider at an after-hours clinic. An examination reveals abrasions in the outer ear canal and some dried blood. The health care provider prescribes corticosporin otic drops. What does the nurse need to teach the mother about instillation of this medication?

2. A 64-year-old man has been diagnosed with primary open-angle glaucoma. He has COPD following a 40-year history of smoking. Is he a candidate for treatment with timolol (Timoptic)? Why or why not? Is there a preferred agent?

3. To determine a patient's ability to administer glaucoma medications, the nurse asks the 82-year-old woman to instill her own medications prior to discharge. The nurse notes that the patient is happy to cooperate and watches as the patient quickly drops her head back, opens her eyes, and drops the medication directly onto her cornea. The patient blinks several times, smiles at the nurse, and says, "There, it is no problem at all!" What correction should the nurse make in the patient's technique?

See Appendix D for answers and rationales for all activities.

ISMP'S LIST OF HIGH-ALERT MEDICATIONS

High-alert medications are drugs that bear a heightened risk of causing significant patient harm when they are used in error. Although mistakes may or may not be more common with these drugs, the consequences of an error are clearly more devastating to patients. The nurse should use this list to determine which medications require special safeguards to reduce the risk of errors. This may include strategies like improving access to information about these drugs; limiting access to high-alert medications; using auxiliary labels and automated alerts; standardizing the ordering, storage, preparation, and administration of these products; and employing redundancies such as automated or independent double-checks when necessary. (Note: manual independent double-checks are not always the optimal error-reduction strategy and may not be practical for all of the medications on the list.)

Classes/Categories of Medications

adrenergic agonists: IV (e.g., epinephrine, phenylephrine, norepinephrine)

adrenergic antagonists: IV (e.g., propranolol, metoprolol, labetalol)

anesthetic agents: general, inhaled, and IV (e.g., propofol, ketamine)

antiarrhythmics: IV (e.g., lidocaine, amiodarone)

antithrombotic agents (anticoagulants), including warfarin, low-molecular-weight heparin: IV unfractionated heparin, Factor Xa inhibitors (fondaparinux), direct thrombin inhibitors (e.g., argatroban, lepirudin, bivalirudin), thrombolytics (e.g., alteplase, reteplase, tenecteplase), and glycoprotein IIb/IIIa inhibitors (e.g., eptifibatide)

cardioplegic solutions

chemotherapeutic agents: parenteral and oral

dextrose, hypertonic, 20% or greater

dialysis solutions: peritoneal and hemodialysis

epidural or intrathecal medications

hypoglycemics: oral

inotropic medications: IV (e.g., digoxin, milrinone)

liposomal forms of drugs (e.g., liposomal amphotericin B)

moderate sedation agents: IV (e.g., midazolam)

moderate sedation agents: oral, for children (e.g., chloral hydrate)

narcotics/opiates: IV, transdermal, and oral (including liquid concentrates, immediate and sustained-release formulations)

neuromuscular blocking agents (e.g., succinylcholine, rocuronium, vecuronium)

radiocontrast agents: IV

total parenteral nutrition solutions

Specific Medications

epoprostenol (Flolan): IV

insulin: subcutaneous and IV

magnesium sulfate injection

methotrexate: oral, nononcologic use

opium tincture

oxytocin: IV

nitroprusside sodium for injection

potassium chloride for injection concentrate

potassium phosphates injection

promethazine: IV

sodium chloride for injection, hypertonic (greater than 0.9% concentration)

sterile water for injection, inhalation, and irrigation (excluding pour bottles) in containers of 100 mL or more

Background

Based on error reports submitted to the USP-ISMP Medication Errors Reporting Program, reports of harmful errors in the literature, and input from practitioners and safety experts, ISMP created and periodically updates a list of potential high-alert medications. During February–April 2007, 770 practitioners responded to an ISMP survey designed to identify which medications were most frequently considered high-alert drugs by individuals and organizations. Further, to assure relevance and completeness, the clinical staff at ISMP, members of our advisory board, and safety experts throughout the United States were asked to review the potential list. This list of drugs and drug categories reflects the collective thinking of all who provided input.

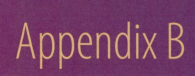

Appendix B

TOP 100 DRUGS RANKED BY NUMBER OF PRESCRIPTIONS

Rank	Top 100 Generic Drugs	Rank	Top 100 Generic Drugs	Rank	Top 100 Brand Name Drugs	Rank	Top 100 Brand Name Drugs
1.	hydrocodone w/APAP	51.	doxycycline	1.	Lipitor	51.	Detrol LA
2.	lisinopril	52.	carisoprodol	2.	Nexium	52.	Chantix
3.	simvastatin	53.	allopurinol	3.	Lexapro	53.	Avapro
4.	levothyroxine	54.	methylprednisolone tabs	4.	Singulair	54.	Proventil HFA
5.	amoxicillin	55.	meloxicam	5.	Plavix	55.	Abilify
6.	azithromycin	56.	amlodipine/benazepril	6.	Synthroid	56.	Yasmin 28
7.	hydrochlorothiazide	57.	potassium chloride	7.	Prevacid	57.	Budeprion XL
8.	alprazolam	58.	clonidine	8.	Advair Diskus	58.	Niaspan
9.	atenolol	59.	promethazine tabs	9.	Effexor XR	59.	Combivent
10.	metformin	60.	isosorbide mononitrate	10.	Diovan	60.	Januvia
11.	metoprolol succinate	61.	folic acid	11.	Crestor	61.	Boniva
12.	furosemide oral	62.	spironolactone	12.	Vytorin	62.	TriNessa
13.	metoprolol tartrate	63.	glimepiride	13.	Cymbalta	63.	NuvaRing
14.	sertraline	64.	pantoprazole	14.	Pro-Air HFA	64.	Risperdal
15.	omeprazole	65.	glyburide	15.	Klor-Con	65.	Polymagma Plain
16.	zolpidem tartrate	66.	verapamil SR	16.	Diovan HCT	66.	Flovent HFA
17.	oxycodone w/APAP	67.	albuterol nebulizer solution	17.	Levaquin	67.	Imitrex oral
18.	ibuprofen	68.	cefdidnir	18.	Actos	68.	Evista
19.	prednisone oral	69.	temazepam	19.	Flomax	69.	Avelox
20.	fluoxetine	70.	triamcinolone acetonide topical	20.	Seroquel	70.	Depakote ER
21.	warfarin	71.	penicillin VK	21.	Zetia	71.	Protonix
22.	cephalexin	72.	oxycodone	22.	Tricor	72.	Avalide
23.	lorazepam	73.	metformin HCl ER	23.	Celebrex	73.	Lioderm
24.	clonazepam	74.	benazepril	24.	Nasonex	74.	Zyprexa
25.	citalopram	75.	glipizide	25.	Premarin-Tabs	75.	Namenda
26.	tramadol	76.	clindamycin systemic	26.	Lantus	76.	Tussionex
27.	gabapentin	77.	ramipril	27.	Viagra	77.	Thyroid, Armour
28.	ciprofloxacin	78.	metronidazole tabs	28.	Yaz	78.	Humalog
29.	propoxyphene w/APAP	79.	digoxin	29.	Lyrica	79.	Vigamox
30.	lisinopril/HCTZ	80.	metoclopramide	30.	Adderall XR	80.	Tamiflu
31.	triamterene/HCTZ	81.	estradiol oral	31.	Valtrex	81.	Budeprion SR
32.	amoxicillin/clavulanate	82.	hydroxyzine	32.	Cozaar	82.	Suboxone
33.	cyclobenzaprine	83.	amphetamine salt combination	33.	Topamax	83.	Lanoxin
34.	trazodone	84.	diclofenac	34.	Concerta	84.	Loestrin 24 Fe
35.	fexofenadine	85.	gemfibrozil	35.	Levoxyl	85.	Avodart
36.	fluticasone nasal	86.	propranolol HCl	36.	Actonel	86.	Coumadin tabs
37.	paroxetine	87.	vitamin D	37.	Ambien CR	87.	Wellbutrin XL
38.	lovastatin	88.	quinapril	38.	Spiriva	88.	Endocet
39.	trimethoprim/sulfa	89.	promethazine/codeine	39.	Benicar	89.	Skelaxin
40.	albuterol aerosol	90.	doxazosin	40.	Xalatan	90.	Nasacort AQ
41.	diazepam	91.	mirtazapine	41.	Benicar HCT	91.	Keppra
42.	pravastatin	92.	glipizide ER	42.	Aricept	92.	Allegra D 12 hr
43.	acetaminophen/codeine	93.	phentermine	43.	Ortho Tri-Cyclen Lo	93.	Strattera
44.	alendronate	94.	acyclovir	44.	Hyzaar	94.	Lovaza
45.	amitriptyline	95.	meclizine	45.	Tri-Sprintec	95.	Avandia
46.	naproxen	96.	potassium chloride	46.	Cialis	96.	Ocella
47.	fluconazole	97.	nitrofurantoin	47.	OxyContin	97.	Vyvanse
48.	enalapril	98.	sulfamethoxazole/trimethoprim	48.	AcipHex	98.	Toprol XL
49.	carvedilol	99.	fentanyl transdermal	49.	Lunesta	99.	Levitra
50.	ranitidine	100.	buspirone	50.	Lamictal	100.	Astelin

Source: Data from http://drugtopics.modernmedicine.com/drugtopics/data/articlestandard//drugtopics/222009/599844/article.pdf and http://drugtopics.modernmedicine.com/drugtopics/data/articlestandard//drugtopics/222009/599845/article.pdf, accessed September 24, 2009.

BIBLIOGRAPHY AND REFERENCES

General References

Audesirk, T., Audesirk, G., & Beyers, B. E. (2008). *Biology: Life on earth* (8th ed.). San Francisco, CA: Benjamin Cummings.

Beers, M. H., & Berkow, R. (Eds.). (2006). *Merck manual: Diagnosis and therapy* (18th ed.). Whitehouse Station, NJ: Merck & Co.

Holland, N., & Adams, M. (2007). *Core concepts in pharmacology* (2nd ed.). Upper Saddle River, NJ: Prentice Hall.

Krogh, D. (2009). *Biology: A guide to the natural world* (4th ed.). Upper Saddle River, NJ: Prentice Hall.

LeMone, P., & Burke, K. M. (2008). *Medical-surgical nursing: Critical thinking in client care* (4th ed.). Upper Saddle River, NJ: Prentice Hall.

Martini, F. H. (2004). *Fundamentals of human anatomy and physiology* (6th ed.). San Francisco, CA: Benjamin Cummings.

Medical Economics (Ed.). (2004). *Physician's desk reference for herbal medicines* (3rd ed.). Montvale, NJ: Author.

Medical Economics (Ed.). (2001). *Physician's desk reference for nutritional supplements.* Montvale, NJ: Author.

Medical Economics (Ed.). (2006). *Physician's desk reference* (60th ed.). Montvale, NJ: Author.

Mulvihill, M. L., Zelman, P., Holdaway, P., Tompary, E., & Turchany, J. (2010). *Human diseases: A systemic approach* (7th ed.). Upper Saddle River, NJ: Prentice Hall.

Rice, J. (2005). *Medical terminology with human anatomy* (5th ed.). San Francisco, CA: Benjamin Cummings.

Silverthorn, D. U. (2010). *Human physiology: An integrated approach* (5th ed.). San Francisco, CA: Benjamin Cummings.

Wilson, B. A., Shannon, M. T., & Shields, K. L. (2010). *Nurse's drug guide 2010.* Upper Saddle River, NJ: Prentice Hall.

Chapter 1

Moore, T. J., Cohen, M. R., Furberg, C. D. QuarterWatch 2008 quarter 2. Retrieved from Institute for Safe Medication Practices website: http://www.ismp.org/QuarterWatch/200901.pdf

Newton, G. D., Pray, W. S., & Popovich, N. G. (2001). New OTC drugs and devices 2000: A selective review. *Journal of the American Pharmaceutical Association, 41*(2), 273–282.

Ng, R. (2004). *Drugs: From discovery to approval.* Hoboken, NJ: Wiley.

Oates, J. A. (2006). The science of drug therapy. In L. L. Brunton, J. S. Lazo, & K. L. Parker (Eds.), *Goodman & Gilman's The pharmacological basis of therapeutics* (11th ed., pp. 117–136). New York, NY: McGraw-Hill.

Olsen, D. P. (2000). The patient's responsibility for optimum healthcare. *Disease Management & Health Outcomes, 7*(2), 57–65.

Chapter 2

Bond, C. A., Raehl, C. L., & Franke, T. (2001). Medication errors in United States hospitals. *Pharmacotherapy, 21*(9), 1023–1036.

Brass, E. P. (2001). Drug therapy: Changing the status of drugs from prescription to over-the-counter availability. *New England Journal of Medicine, 345,* 810–816.

Brown, S. D., & Landry, F. J. (2001). Recognizing, reporting, and reducing adverse drug reactions. *Southern Medical Journal, 94*(4), 370–373.

Force, M. V., Deering, L., Hubbe, J., Andersen, M., Hagemann, B., Cooper-Hahn, M., & Peters, W. (2006). Effective strategies to increase reporting of medication errors in hospitals. *Journal of Nursing Administration, 36*(1) 34–41.

Gaither, C. A., Kirking, D. M., Ascione, F. J., & Welage, L. S. (2001). Consumers' views on generic medications. *Journal of the American Pharmaceutical Association, 41*(5), 729–736.

Phillips, K. A., Veenstra, D. L., Oren, E., Lee, J. K., & Sardee, W. (2001). Potential role of pharmacogenomics in reducing adverse drug reactions: A systematic review. *Journal of the American Medical Association, 286,* 2270–2279.

Chapter 3

Armitage, G., & Knapman, H. (2003). Adverse events in drug administration: A literature review. *Journal of Nursing Management, 11*(2), 130–140.

Berman, A. J., Snyder, S., Kozier, B., & Erb, G. (2008). *Kozier & Erb's Fundamentals of Nursing Concepts, Process, and Practice* (8th ed.). Upper Saddle River, NJ: Prentice Hall.

Blais, K. K., Hayes, J., Kozier, B., & Erb, G. (2002). *Professional nursing practice: Concepts and perspectives* (4th ed.). Upper Saddle River, NJ: Prentice Hall.

Deedwania, P. C. (2002). The changing face of hypertension: Is systolic blood pressure the final answer? *Archives of Internal Medicine, 162*(5), 506–508.

Hallgren, J., Tengvall–Linder, M., Persson, M., & Wahlgren, C. F. (2003). Stevens–Johnson syndrome associated with ciprofloxacin: A review of adverse cutaneous events reported in Sweden as associated with this drug. *Journal of the American Academy of Dermatology, 49* (5 Suppl), S267–S269.

Koo, M. M., Krass, I., & Aslani, P. (2003). Factors influencing consumer use of written drug information. *Annals of Pharmacotherapy, 37*(2), 259–267.

Kozma, C. M. (2002). Why aren't we doing more to enhance medication compliance? *Managed Care Interface, 15*(1), 59–60.

Madlon, K., Diane, J., & Mosch, F. S. (2000). Liquid medication dosing errors. *Journal of Family Practice, 49*(1), 741–744.

Olsen, J. L., Giangrasso, A. P., & Shrimpton, D. M. (2004). *Medical dosage calculations* (8th ed.). Upper Saddle River, NJ: Prentice Hall.

Seal. R. (2000). How to promote drug compliance in the elderly. *Community Nurse, 6*(1), 41–42.

Smith, D. I. (2001). Taking control of your medicines. Newsletter 1(1). *Consumer Health Information Corporation.* Retrieved from www.consumer-health.com

Smith, S., Duell, D., & Martin, B. (2000). *Clinical nursing skills: Basic to advanced skills* (5th ed.). Upper Saddle River, NJ: Prentice Hall Health.

Wooten, J. (2001). Toxic epidermal necrolysis. *Nursing 2001 64*(10), 35–38.

Chapter 4

Bateman, D. N. (2001). Introduction to pharmacokinetics and pharmacodynamics. *Journal of Toxicology: Clinical Toxicology, 39*(3), 207.

Bhattaram, V. B., Graefe, U., Kohlert, C., Veit, M., & Derendorf, H. (2002). Pharmacokinetics and bioavailability of herbal medicinal products. *Phytomedicine, 9,* 1–33.

Brunton, L. L., Lazo, J. S., & Parker, K. L. (Eds.). (2006). *Goodman & Gilman's The pharmacological basis of therapeutics* (11th ed.). New York, NY: McGraw-Hill.

Buxton, I. L. O. (2006). Pharmacokinetics and pharmacodynamics: The dynamics of drug absorption, distribution, action, and elimination. In L. L. Brunton, J. S. Lazo, & K. L. Parker (Eds.), *Goodman & Gilman's The pharmacological basis of therapeutics* (11th ed., pp. 1–40). New York, NY: McGraw-Hill.

Doucet, J., Jego, D., Noel, D., Geffroy, C. E., Capet, C., Coquard, A., . . . & Bercoff, E. (2002). Preventable and nonpreventable risk factors for adverse drug events related to hospital admission in the elderly. *Clinical Drug Investigation, 22*(6), 385–392.

Kanneh, K. (2002a). Paediatric pharmacological principles: An update part 2, Pharmacokinetics: Absorption and distribution. *Paediatric Nursing, 14*(9), 39–44.

Kanneh, K. (2002b). Paediatric pharmacological principles: An update part 3, Pharmacokinetics: Metabolism and excretion. *Paediatric Nursing, 14*(10), 39–43.

Lampela, P., Hartikainen, S., Sulkava, R., & Huupponen, R. (2007). Adverse drug effects in elderly people – A disparity between clinical examination and adverse effects self-reported by the patient. *European Journal of Clinical Pharmacology, 63*, 979–980.

Levy, R. H., Thummel, K. E., Trager, W. F., Hansten, P. D., & Eichelbaum, M. (Eds.). (2000). *Metabolic drug interactions.* Philadelphia, PA: Lippincott, Williams, & Wilkins.

Rollins, D. E. (2000). Clinical pharmacokinetics. In A. R. Gennaro (Ed.), *Remington: The science and practice of pharmacy* (pp. 1145–1155). Philadelphia, PA: Lippincott, Williams, & Wilkins.

Scott, G. N., & Elmer, G. W. (2002). Update on natural product–drug interactions. *American Journal of Health-System Pharmacy, 59*(4), 339–347.

Suggs, D. M. (2000). Pharmacokinetics in children: History, considerations, and applications. *Journal of the American Academy of Nurse Practitioners, 12*(6), 236–240.

White, R. J., & Park, G. (2001). Safe drug prescribing in the critically ill. In G. Park & M. Shelly (Eds.), *Pharmacology of the critically ill.* London, England: BMI Books.

Chapter 5

Berg, M. J. (2002, August 31–September 5). *Does sex matter?* Paper presented at the Congress of the 62nd International Pharmaceutical Federation. Nice, France. *Medscape Pharmacists, 3*(2).

Bottles, K. (2001). A revolution in genetics: Changing medicine, changing lives. *Physician Executive, 27*, 58–63.

Buxton, I. L. O. (2006). Pharmacokinetics and pharmacodynamics: The dynamics of drug absorption, distribution, action, and elimination. In L. L. Brunton, J. S. Lazo, & K. L. Parker (Eds.), *Goodman & Gilman's The pharmacological basis of therapeutics* (11th ed., pp. 1–40). New York, NY: McGraw-Hill.

du Souich, P. (2001). In human therapy, is the drug–drug interaction or the adverse drug reaction the issue? *Canadian Journal of Clinical Pharmacology, 8*, 153–161.

Ginsburg, G. S., & McCarthy, J. J. (2001). Personalized medicine: Revolutionizing drug discovery and patient care. *Trends in Biotechnology, 19*, 491–496.

Hughes, R. (2001). *A manual of pharmacodynamics.* New Delhi, India: B. Jain.

Kramer, T. (2003). Side effects and therapeutic effects. *Medscape General Medicine, 5*(1).

Kuo, G. M. (2003). Pharmacodynamic basis of herbal medicine. *Annals of Pharmacotherapy, 37*(2), 308.

Ma, M. K., Woo, M. A., & McLeod, H. L. (2002). Genetic basis of drug metabolism. *American Journal of Health-System Pharmacy, 59*(21), 2061–2069.

Nightingale, C. H., Murakawa, T., & Ambrose, P. G. (Eds.). (2002). *Antimicrobial pharmacodynamics in theory and clinical practice.* New York, NY: Marcel Dekker.

Oates, J. A. (2006). The science of drug therapy. In L. L. Brunton, J. S. Lazo, & K. L. Parker (Eds.), *Goodman & Gilman's The pharmacological basis of therapeutics* (11th ed., pp. 117–136). New York, NY: McGraw-Hill.

Relling, M. V., & Dervieux, T. (2001). Pharmacogenetics and cancer therapy. *Nature Reviews Cancer, 1*, 99–108.

Roses, A. D. (2001). Pharmacogenetics. *Human Molecular Genetics, 10*, 2261–2267.

Ross, J. S., & Ginsburg, G. S. (2003). The integration of molecular diagnostics with therapeutics. *American Journal of Clinical Pathology, 119*(1), 26–36.

Steimer, W., & Potter, J. M. (2001). Pharmacogenetic screening and therapeutic drugs. *Clinica Chimica Acta, 315*, 137–155.

Wortman, M. (2001, January/February). Medicine gets personal. *Technology Review,* 72–78.

Chapter 6

Berman, A. J., Snyder, S., Kozier, B., & Erb, G. (2008). *Kozier & Erb's Fundamentals of Nursing Concepts, Process, and Practice* (8th ed.). Upper Saddle River, NJ: Prentice Hall.

D'Amica, D., & Barbarito, C. (2007). Health and physical assessment in nursing. Upper Saddle River, NJ: Prentice Hall.

Gardner, P. (2003). *Nursing process in action.* New York, NY: Thompson Delmar Learning.

Hogan, M. A., Bowles, D., & White, J. E. (2003). *Nursing fundamentals: Reviews & rationales.* Upper Saddle River, NJ: Prentice Hall.

Jahraus, D., Sokolosky, S., Thurston, N., & Guo, D. (2002). Evaluation of an education program for patients with breast cancer receiving radiation therapy. *Cancer Nursing, 24*(4), 266–275.

North American Nursing Diagnosis Association. (2003). *Nursing diagnoses: Definitions and classification 2003–2004.* Philadelphia, PA: Author.

Smith, S. F., Duell, D. J., & Martin, B. C. (2004). *Clinical nursing skills* (6th ed.). Upper Saddle River, NJ: Prentice Hall.

Wilkinson, J. M. (2005). *Nursing diagnosis handbook: NIC interventions and NOC outcomes* (8th ed.). Upper Saddle River, NJ: Prentice Hall.

Wilkinson, J. M. (2007). *Nursing process and critical thinking* (4th ed.). Upper Saddle River, NJ: Prentice Hall.

Chapter 7

American Academy of Pediatrics, Committee on Drugs. (2001). The transfer of drugs and other chemicals into human breast milk. *Pediatrics, 3*, 776–782.

Andrade, S. E., Gurwitz, J. H., Davis, R. L., Chan, K. A., Finkelstein, J. A., Fortman, K., et al. (2004). Prescription drug use in pregnancy. *American Journal of Obstetrics and Gynecology, 191*(2), 398–407.

Anwar, A. (2007). Prescribing in pregnancy and lactation: Factors to consider. *Nurse Prescribing, 5*(6), 245–249.

Ball, J. W., & Bindler, R. C. (2003). *Pediatric nursing: Caring for children.* Upper Saddle River, NJ: Prentice Hall.

Beers, M. H., & Berkow, R. (Eds.). (2000). *The Merck manual of geriatrics* (3rd ed.). Whitehouse Station, NJ: Merck & Company, Inc.

Bressler, R., & Katz, M. (2003). *Geriatric pharmacology* (2nd ed.). New York, NY: McGraw-Hill Professional.

Briggs, G. G. (2002). Drug effects on the fetus and breast-fed infant. *Clinical Obstetrics and Gynecology, 45*(1), 6–21, 170–171.

Hale, T. W. (2004). Maternal medications during breastfeeding. *Clinical Obstetrics and Gynecology, 47*(3), 696–711.

Leipzig, R. M. (Ed.). (2003). *Drug prescribing for older adults: An evidence-based approach.* Philadelphia, PA: American College of Physicians.

Olsen, C. G., Tindall, W. N., & Clasen, M. E. (2007). *Geriatric pharmacotherapy: A guide for the helping professional.* Washington, DC: American Pharmacists Association.

Spencer, J. P., Gonzalez, L. S., III, & Barnhart, D. J. (2001). Medications in the breast-feeding mother. *American Family Physician, 64*, 19–126.

U.S. Food and Drug Administration, Department of Health and Human Services. (2005). *Regulations requiring manufacturers to* assess the safety and effectiveness of new drugs and biological products in pediatric patients. Retrieved May 1, 2008, from http://www.fda.gov/cder/guidance/pedrule.htm

Chapter 8

Andrus, M. R., & Roth, M. T. (2002). Health literacy: A review. *Pharmacotherapy, 22*(3), 282–302.

Chen, J. (2002, October 20–23). *The role of ethnicity in medication use.* Paper presented at the American College of Clinical Pharmacy 2002 Annual Meeting, Albuquerque, NM.

Davidhizar, R. (2002). Strategies for providing culturally appropriate pharmaceutical care to the Hispanic patient. *Hospital Pharmacy, 37*(5), 505–510.

Franconi, F., Brunelleschi, S., Steardo, L., & Cuomo, V. (2007). Gender differences in drug responses. *Pharmacological Research, 55*(2), 81–85.

Gallagher, R. M. (2002). *The pain–depression conundrum: Bridging the body and mind.* Medscape clinical update based on session presented at the 21st Scientific Meeting of the American Pain Society. Retrieved from http://www.medscape.com/viewprogram/2030

Humma, L. M., & Terra, S. G. (2002). Pharmacogenetics and cardiovascular disease: Impact on drug response and applications to disease management. *American Journal of Health-System Pharmacy, 59*(13), 1241–1252.

Kudzma, E. C. (2001). Cultural competence: Cardiovascular medications. *Progress in Cardiovascular Nursing, 16*(4), 152–160, 169.

Martin, L., Miracle, A. W., & Bonder, B. R. (2001). *Culture in clinical care.* Thorofare, NJ: Slack.

Richardson, L. G. (2003). Psychosocial issues in patients with congestive heart failure. *Progressive Cardiovascular Nursing, 18*(1), 19–27.

Salimbene, S. (2005). *What language does your patient hurt in? A practical guide to culturally competent patient care* (2nd ed.). Amherst, MA: Diversity Resources.

Simpson, R. J. (2006). Challenges for improving medication adherence. *Journal of the American Medical Association, 296*(21), 2614–2616.

Sleath, B., & Wallace, J. (2002). Providing pharmaceutical care to Spanish-speaking patients. *Journal of the American Pharmaceutical Association, 42,* 799–801.

Spector, R. E. (2004). *Cultural diversity in health and illness* (6th ed.). Upper Saddle River, NJ: Prentice Hall.

Chapter 9

Bates, D. W., Clapp, M., Federico, F., Goldmann, D., Kaushal, R., Landrigan, C., & McKenna, K. J. (2001). Medication errors and adverse drug events in pediatric inpatients. *Journal of the American Medical Association, 285*(16), 2114–2120.

Berman, A. J., Snyder, S., Kozier, B., & Erb, G. (2008). *Kozier & Erb's Fundamentals of Nursing Concepts, Process and Practice* (8th ed.). Upper Saddle River, NJ: Prentice Hall.

Burns, J. P., Mitchell, C., Griffith, J. L., & Truog, R. D. (2001). End-of-life care in the pediatric intensive care: Attitudes and practices of pediatric critical care physicians and nurses. *Critical Care Medicine, 29*(3), 658–664.

Committee on Drugs and Committee on Hospital Care. (2003). Prevention of medication errors in the pediatric inpatient setting. *Pediatrics, 112,* 431–436.

Federal Drug Administration. (2001, October 1). Med error reports to FDA show a mixed bag. Drug Topics. Retrieved from www.drugtopics.com

Ghaleb, M. A., Barber, N., Franklin, B. D., Yeung, V., Khaki, Z. F., & Wong, I. (2006). Systematic review of medication errors in pediatric patients: Suggestions to prevent medication errors in children. *The Annals of Pharmacotherapy, 40*(10), 1766–1776.

Goldman, E. (2006, May 1). PDA-based drug dose calculator slashes NICU med errors. *Family Practice News,* 55.

Guido, G. W. (2001). *Legal and ethical issues in nursing* (3rd ed.). Upper Saddle River, NJ: Prentice Hall.

Institute for Safe Medication Practices. (2005). *ISMP medication safety alert! Acute care edition, January 1996–September 2004.* Author.

Joanna Briggs Institute. (2006). Strategies to reduce medication errors with reference to older adults. *Nursing Standard, 20,* 53–57.

Kane-Gill, S., & Weber, R. J. (2006). Principles and practices of medication safety in the ICU. *Critical Care Clinics, 22,* 273–290.

Koczmara, C., Jelincic, V., & Perri, D. (2006). Communication of medication orders by telephone—"writing it right." *Dynamics, 17,* 20–24.

Meadows, M. (2003) Strategies to reduce medication errors. How the FDA is working to improve medication safety and what you can do to help. *FDA Consumer, 37*(3), 20–27.

Mitchell, A. (2001). Challenges in pediatric pharmacotherapy: Minimizing medication errors. *Medscape Pharmacists, 2*(1), 1–8.

National Coordinating Council for Medication Error and Reporting (NCC MERP). *Recommendations to enhance accuracy in prescription writing.* Adopted September 4, 1996. Revised June 2, 2005. Retrieved from http://www.nccmerp.org/council/council1996-09-04.html

O'Dell K. (2006). Allergy documentation: Strategies for patient safety. *Oklahoma Nurse, 51,* 16.

Page, K., & McKinney, A. A. (2006, July 11). Addressing medication errors: The role of undergraduate nurse education. *Nurse Education Today,* (epub).

Phillips, J., Beam, S., Brinker, A., Holquist, C., Honig, P., Lee, L. Y., & Palmer, C. (2001). Retrospective analysis of mortalities associated with medication errors. *American Journal of Health-System Pharmacy, 58,* 1835–1841.

Santell J. P., & Cousins, D. (2004). Preventing medication errors that occur in the home. *U.S. Pharmacist, 29*(9), 64–68.

Shuttleworth, A. (2006). How to keep up to date with practice. *Nursing Times, 102,* 54–55.

USP. (2003). Pediatric population can benefit from USP recommendations. *Quality Review,* 7.

Chapter 10

Blumenthal, M. (Ed.). (2000). *Herbal medicine: Expanded commission E monographs.* Austin, TX: American Botanical Council.

Ebadi, M. (2002). *Pharmacodynamic basis of herbal medicine.* Boca Raton, FL: CRC Press.

Fontaine, K. L. (2009). *Complementary and alternative therapies for nursing practice* (3rd ed.). Upper Saddle River, NJ: Prentice Hall.

Foster, S., & Hobbs, C. (2002). *A field guide to Western medicinal plants and herbs.* Boston, MA and New York, NY: Houghton Mifflin.

Goldman, P. (2001). Herbal medicines today and the roots of modern pharmacology. *Annals of Internal Medicine, 135*(8), 594–597.

Marcus, D. M., & Snodgrass, W. R. (2005). Do no harm: Avoidance of herbal medicines during pregnancy. *Obstetrics & Gynecology, 105,* 1119–1122.

Medical Economics Staff (Ed.). (2007). *PDR for herbal medicines* (4th ed.). Montvale, NJ: Thomson Healthcare.

The review of natural products: 2005 (4th ed.). Missouri, MO: Facts and Comparisons®, Publisher.

Scott, G. N., & Elmer, G. W. (2002). Update on natural product–drug interactions. *American Journal of Health-System Pharmacy, 59*(4), 339–347.

Sierpina, V. S., Wollschlaeger, B., & Blumenthal, M. (2003). Ginkgo biloba. *American Family Physician, 68*(5), 923–926.

White House commission on complementary and alternative medicine policy, final report. (2002, March). Retrieved May 8, 2008, at http://govinfo.library.unt.edu/whccamp/

Chapter 11

Barangan, C. J., & Alderman, E. M. (2002). Management of substance abuse. *Pediatrics in Review, 23*(4), 123–131.

Chychula, N. M., & Sciamanna, C. (2002). Help substance abusers attain and sustain abstinence. *Nurse Practitioner, 27*(11), 30–47.

Fraschini, F., Demartini, G., & Esposti, D. (2002). Pharmacology of silymarin. *Clinical Drug Investigation, 22*(1), 51–65.

Freese, T. E., Miotto, K., & Reback, C. J. (2002). The effects and consequences of selected club drugs. *Journal of Substance Abuse Treatment, 23*(2), 151–156.

Gable, R. (2006). The toxicity of recreational drugs. *American Scientist, 94*(3), 206.

Hardie, T. L. (2002). The genetics of substance abuse. *American Association of Critical Care Nursing Clinical Issues, 13*(4), 511–522.

Haseltine, E. (2001). The unsatisfied mind: Are reward centers in your brain wired for substance abuse? *Discover, 22*(11), 88.

Jason, L. A., Davis, M. I., Ferrari, J. R., & Bishop, P. D. (2001). A review of research and implications for substance abuse recovery and community research. *Journal of Drug Education, 31*(1), 1–28.

Kandel, D. B. (2003). Does marijuana use cause the use of other drugs? *Journal of the American Medical Association, 289*(4), 482–483.

Manoguerra, A. S. (2001). Methamphetamine abuse. *Journal of Toxicology: Clinical Toxicology, 38*(2), 187.

Naegle, M. A., & D'Avanzo, C. E. (2001). *Addictions and substance abuse: Strategies for advanced practice nursing.* Upper Saddle River, NJ: Prentice Hall.

Sindelar, J. L., & Fiellin, D. A. (2001). Innovations in treatment for drug abuse: Solutions to a public health problem. *Annual Review of Public Health, 22*, 249.

Song, Z., Deaciuc, I., Song, M., Lee, D. Y., Liu, Y., Ji, X., & McClain, C. (2006). Silymarin protects against acute ethanol-induced hepatotoxicity in mice. *Alcoholism, Clinical and Experimental Research, 30*(3), 407–413.

Tuttle, J., Melnyk, B. M., & Loveland-Cherry, C. (2002). Adolescent drug and alcohol use. Strategies for assessment, intervention, and prevention. *Nursing Clinics of North America, 37*(3), ix, 443–460.

Wasilow-Mueller, S., & Erickson, C. K. (2001). Drug abuse and dependency: Understanding gender differences in etiology and management. *Journal of the American Pharmaceutical Association, 41*(1), 78–90.

Chapter 12

Bartlett, J. G., Sifton, D. W., & Kelly, G. L. (Eds.). (2002). *PDR guide to biological and chemical warfare response.* Montvale, NJ: Medical Economics.

Blendon, R. J., Des Roches, C. M., Benson, J. M., Herrmann, M. J., Taylor-Clark, K., & Weldon, K. J. (2003). The public and the smallpox threat. *New England Journal of Medicine, 348*(5), 426–432.

Bozeman, W. P., Dilbero, D., & Schauben, J. L. (2002). Biologic and chemical weapons of mass destruction. *Emergency Medical Clinics of North America, 20*(4), xii, 975–993.

Cangemi, C. W. (2002). Occupational response to terrorism. *American Association of Occupational Health Nurses Journal, 50*(4), 190–196.

Chyba, C. F. (2001). Biological security in a changed world. *Science, 293*(5539), 2349.

Crupi, R. S., Asnis, D. S., Lee, C. C., Santucci, T., Marino, M. J., & Flanz, B. J. (2003). Meeting the challenge of bioterrorism: Lessons learned from West Nile virus and anthrax. *American Journal of Emergency Medicine, 21*(1), 77–79.

Donnellan, C. (2002). New law funds nursing's role in bioterrorism response: The ANA establishes the National Nurses Response Team. *American Journal of Nursing, 102*(8), 23.

Fidler, D. P. (2001). The malevolent use of microbes and the rule of law: Legal challenges presented by bioterrorism. *Clinical Infectious Diseases, 33*(5), 686–689.

Henderson, D. A., Inglesby, T. V., & O'Toole, T. (2002). *Bioterrorism: Guidelines for medical and public health management.* Chicago, IL: American Medical Association.

Hughes, J. M. (2001). Emerging infectious diseases: A CDC perspective. *Emerging Infectious Diseases, 7*(3, Suppl.), 494–496.

Khan, A. S., Swerdlow, D. L., & Juranek, D. D. (2001). Precautions against biological and chemical terrorism directed at food and water supplies. *Public Health Reports, 116*(1), 3–14.

Kimmel, S. R., Mahoney, M. C., & Zimmerman, R. K. (2003). Vaccines and bioterrorism: Smallpox and anthrax. *Journal of Family Practice, 52*(1), S56–S61.

McLaughlin, S. (2001). Thinking about the unthinkable. Where to start planning for terrorism incidents. *Health Facilities Management, 14*(7), 26–30, 32.

Morse, A. (2002). Bioterrorism preparedness for local health departments. *Journal of Community Health Nursing, 19*(4), 203–211.

Mortimer, P. P. (2003). Can postexposure vaccination against smallpox succeed? *Clinical Infectious Diseases, 36*(5), 622–629.

O'Connell, K. P., Menuey, B. C., & Foster, D. (2002). Issues in preparedness for biologic terrorism: A perspective for critical care nursing. *American Association of Critical-Care Nurses Clinical Issues, 13*(3), 452–469.

O'Toole, T. (2001). Emerging illness and bioterrorism: Implications for public health. *Journal of Urban Health, 78*(2), 396–402.

Rose, M. A., & Larrimore, K. L. (2002). Knowledge and awareness concerning chemical and biological terrorism: Continuing education implications. *Journal of Continuing Education in Nursing, 33*(6), 253–258.

Salazar, M. K., & Kelman, B. (2002). Planning for biological disasters. Occupational health nurses as "first responders." *American Association of Occupational Health Nurses Journal, 50*(4), 174–181.

Spencer, R. C., & Lightfoot, N. F. (2001). Preparedness and response to bioterrorism. *Journal of Infection, 43*(2), 104–110.

Stephenson, J. (2003). Smallpox vaccine program launched amid concerns raised by expert panel, unions. *Journal of the American Medical Association, 289*(6), 685–686.

Stillsmoking, K. (2002). Bioterrorism—Are you ready for the silent killer? *Association of PeriOperative Registered Nurses Journal, 76*(3), 434, 437–442, 444–446.

Tasota, F. J., Henker, R. A., & Hoffman, L. A. (2002). Anthrax as a biological weapon: An old disease that poses a new threat. *Critical Care Nurse, 22*(5), 21–32, 34.

Chapter 13

Bouchard, R., Weber, A. R., & Geiger, J. D. (2002). Informed decision-making on sympathomimetic use in sports and health. *Clinical Journal of Sports Medicine, 12*(4), 209–224.

Chapple, C. R., Yamanishi, T., & Chess-Williams, R. (2002). Muscarinic receptor subtypes and management of the overactive bladder. *Urology, 60* (5 Suppl. 1), 82–88; discussion 88–89.

Cilliers, L., & Retief, F. P. (2003). *Poisons, poisoning, and the drug trade in ancient Rome.* Retrieved from www.sun.ac.za

Defilippi, J., & Crismon, M. L. (2003). Drug interactions with cholinesterase inhibitors. *Drugs and Aging, 20*(6), 437–444.

Herbison, P., Hay-Smith, J., Ellis, G., & Moore, K. (2003). Effectiveness of anticholinergic drugs compared with placebo in the treatment of overactive bladder: Systematic review. *British Medical Journal, 326*, 841–844.

Kolpuru, S. (2003). Doctor corner: Approach to a case of Down syndrome. *Pediatric OnCall™.* Retrieved from www.pediatriconcall.com

Lemstra, A. W., Eikelenboom, P., & van Gool, W. A. (2003). The cholinergic deficiency syndrome and its therapeutic implications. *Gerontology, 49*(1), 55–60.

McCrory, D. C., & Brown, C. D. (2002). Anticholinergic bronchodilators versus beta$_2$-sympathomimetic agents for acute exacerbations of chronic obstructive pulmonary disease. *Cochrane Database of Systematic Reviews, 2003*(1), CD003900.

Medical Economics (Ed.). (2000). *PDR for herbal medicines*. Montvale, NJ: Author.

Miller, C. A. (2002). Anticholinergics: The good and the bad. *Geriatric Nursing, 23*(5), 286–287.

MSN Health. (2003). *Drugs & herbs: Phenylephrine ophthalmic*. Retrieved from http://health.msn.com

National Parkinson Foundation. (2004). *What you should know about acetylcholine, anticholinergic drugs, the autonomic nervous system, and Botox*. Retrieved from http://www.parkinson.org

National Toxicology Program, National Institutes of Health. (2001). *NTP chemical repository: Phenylephrine*. Retrieved from http://www.ntp-server.niehs.nih.gov

Rodrigo, G. J., & Rodrigo, C. (2002). The role of anticholinergics in acute asthma treatment: An evidence-based evaluation. *Chest, 121*(6), 1977–1987.

Roe, C. M., Anderson, M. J., & Spivack, B. (2002). Use of anticholinergic medications by older adults with dementia. *Journal of the American Geriatrics Society, 50*, 836–842.

ThinkQuest On-line Library. (2003). *Poisonous plants and animals. Atropa belladonna, deadly nightshade*. Retrieved from http://www.thinkquest.org/pls/html/think.library

Wang, H. E. (2002). Street drug toxicity resulting from opiates combined with anticholinergics. *Prehospital Emergency Care, 6*(3), 351–354.

Westfall, T. C., & Westfall, D. P. (2005). Neurotransmission: The autonomic and somatic motor nervous systems. In L. L. Brunton, J. S. Lazo, & K. L. Parker (Eds.), *Goodman & Gilman's The pharmacological basis of therapeutics* (11th ed., pp. 137–182). New York, NY: McGraw-Hill.

Chapter 14

Andai-Otlong, D. (2006). Patient education guide: Anxiety disorders. *Nursing 2006, 36*(3), 48–49.

Baldessarini, R. J. (2005). Drug therapy of depression and anxiety disorders. In L. L. Brunton, J. S. Lazo, & K. L. Parker (Eds.), *Goodman & Gilman's The pharmacological basis of therapeutics* (11th ed., pp. 429–460). New York, NY: McGraw-Hill.

Charney, D. S., Mihic, J., & Harris, A. (2006). Hypnotics and sedatives. In L. L. Brunton, J. S. Lazo, & K. L. Parker (Eds.), *Goodman & Gilman's The pharmacological basis of therapeutics* (11th ed., pp. 401–428). New York, NY: McGraw-Hill.

Ernst, E. (2006). Herbal remedies for anxiety—a systematic review of controlled clinical trials. *Phytomedicine, 13*(3), 205–208.

Gorman, J. N. (2001). Generalized anxiety disorder. *Clinical Cornerstone, 3*(3), 37–46.

Health A to Z. (2003). *Benzodiazepines*. Retrieved from http://www.healthatoz.com

Kennedy, D. O., Little, W., Haskell, C. F., & Schoey, A. B. (2006). Anxiolytic effects of a combination of *Melissa officinalis* and *Valerian officinalis* during laboratory induced stress. *Phytotherapy Research, 20*(2), 96–102.

Lippmann, S., Mazour, I., & Shahab, H. (2001). Insomnia: Therapeutic approach. *Southern Medical Journal, 94*(9), 866–873.

Medical Economics (Ed.). (2001). *PDR for nutritional supplements*. Montvale, NJ: Author.

Miyasaka, L. S., Atallah, A. N., & Soares, B. G. O. (2006). Valerian for anxiety disorders. *Cochrane Database of Systematic Reviews, 2006*(4). doi:10.1002/14651858.CD004515.pub2

National Institute for Drug Abuse (NIDA). (2006). *Prescription medications*. Retrieved from http://www.nida.nih.gov/drugpages/prescription.html

Smock, T. K. (2001). *Physiological psychology: A neuroscience approach*. Upper Saddle River, NJ: Prentice Hall.

The Nurse Practitioner: The American Journal of Primary Health Care (2005). *Medication update; FDA: Antidepressants a risk for kids*. Retrieved from http://www.tnpj.com

United States Drug Enforcement Agency (DEA). (2003). *Benzodiazepines*. Retrieved from http://www.usdoj.gov/dea

United States Drug Enforcement Agency (DEA). (2003). *Depressants*. Retrieved from http://www.usdoj.gov/dea

Vitiello, M. V. (2000). Effective treatment of sleep disturbances in older adults. *Clinical Corner, 2*(5), 16–27.

Chapter 15

Burstein, A. H., Horton, R. L., Dunn, T., Alfaro, R. H., Piscitelli, S. C., & Theodore, W. (2000). Lack of effect of St. John's wort on carbamazepine pharmacokinetics in healthy volunteers. *Clinical Pharmacology and Therapeutics, 68*, 6.

Cross, J. H. (2009). The ketogenic diet. *Advances in Clinical Neurosciences & Rehabilitation, 8*(6), 8–10.

Johnson, K. (2002). Epilepsy and pregnancy. *Medscape Ob/Gyn & Women's Health, 7*(2).

Levy, R. G., & Cooper, P. P. (2003). Ketogenic diet for epilepsy. *Cochrane Database of Systematic Reviews, 2003*(3). doi:10.1002/14651858.CD001903

Murphy, P. A., & Blaylock, R. L. (2001). *Treating epilepsy naturally: A guide to alternative and adjunct therapies*. New York, NY: McGraw-Hill Contemporary Books.

Pack, A. M., & Morrell, M. J. (2003). Treatment of women with epilepsy. *Seminars in Neurology, 22*(3), 289–298.

Patel, P., & Mageda, M. (2002, April). *Vitamin K deficiency*. E-Medicine: Instant access to the minds of medicine. Retrieved from http://www.emedicine.com

Snelson, C., & Dieckman, B. (2000, June). Recognizing and managing purple glove syndrome. *Critical Care Nurse, 20*(3), 54–61.

Tierney, L. M., McPhee, S. J., & Papadakis, M. A. (Eds.). (2002). The nervous system. In M. J. Minoff (Ed.), *Current medical diagnosis and treatment*. New York, NY: Lange Medical Books/McGraw-Hill Medical.

Trimble, M., & Schmitz, B. (Eds.). (2002). *The neuropsychiatry of epilepsy*. New York, NY: Cambridge University Press.

United States National Library, National Institutes of Health. (2003). *Neural tube defects*. Retrieved from http://www.nlm.nih.gov/medlineplus

University of Illinois at Chicago, College of Pharmacy Drug Information Center. (2003). *Is there an interaction between phenytoin and enteral feedings?* Retrieved from http://www.uic.edu

Wyllie, E. (2001). *The treatment of epilepsy: Principles and practice* (3rd ed.). Philadelphia, PA: Lippincott, Williams, & Wilkins.

Chapter 16

American Academy of Pediatrics. (2000). Diagnosis and evaluation of the child with attention deficit–hyperactivity disorder. *Pediatrics, 105*(5), 1158–1170.

Aschenbrenner, D. S. (2005). Drug watch. *American Journal of Nursing, 105*(11), 87–89.

Baldessarini, R. J. (2006). Drug therapy of depression and anxiety disorders. In L. L. Brunton, J. S. Lazo, & K. L. Parker (Eds.), *Goodman & Gilman's The pharmacological basis of therapeutics* (11th ed., pp. 429–460). New York, NY: McGraw-Hill.

Bodkin, J. A., & Amsterdam, J. D. (2002). Transdermal selegiline in major depression: A double-blind, placebo-controlled study in outpatients. *Journal of Psychiatry, 159*(11), 1869–1875.

Desai, H. D., & Jann, M. W. (2000). Major depression in women: A review of the literature. *Journal of the American Pharmaceutical Association, 40*(4), 525–537.

Eli Lilly & Company. (2003). *Strattera: Safety information for health care professionals*. Indianapolis, IN: Author. Retrieved from http://www.strattera.com

Fugh-Berman, A. (2000). Herb-drug interactions. *Lancet, 355*(9198), 134–138.

Gastpar, M., Singer, A., & Zeller, K. (2006). Comparative efficacy and safety of a once-daily dosage of hypericum extract STW3-VI and citalopram in patients with moderate depression: A double-blind, randomised, multicentre, placebo-controlled study. *Pharmacopsychiatry, 39*(2), 66–75.

Janicak, P. (2002). *TMS vs. ECT in depressed patients.* (Research report). Chicago, IL: University of Illinois.

Lin, K. M. (1982). Cultural aspects in mental health for Asian Americans. In A. Gaw (Ed.), *Cross cultural psychiatry* (pp. 69–73). Boston, MA: John Wright.

Linde, K., Berner, M. M., & Kriston, L. (2008). St John's wort for major depression. *Cochrane Database of Systematic Reviews, 2008*(4). doi:10.1002/14651858.CD000448.pub3

Medical Economics (Ed.). (2000). *PDR for herbal medicines.* Montvale, NJ: Author.

Moses, S. (2003). *Family practice notebook: Imipramine.* Lino Lakes, MN: Family Practice Notebook, LLC. Retrieved from http://www.fpnotebook.com

National Association of State Boards of Education. (2003). The use and abuse of Ritalin. *Policy Update, 7*(18).

Spector, R. E. (2000). *Cultural diversity in health and illness.* Upper Saddle River, NJ: Prentice Hall.

The Nurse Practitioner: The American Journal of Primary Health Care. (2004). *Medication update: Antidepressant treats neuropathy in diabetes.* Retrieved from http://www.tnpj.com

Chapter 17

Bailey, K. (2003). Aripiprazole: The newest antipsychotic agent for the treatment of schizophrenia. *Psychosocial Nursing and Mental Health Services, 41*(2), 14–18.

Baldessarini, R. J., & Tarazi, F. I. (2006). Pharmacotherapy of psychosis and mania. In L. L. Brunton, J. S. Lazo, & K. L. Parker (Eds.), *Goodman & Gilman's The pharmacological basis of therapeutics* (11th ed., pp. 461–500). New York, NY: McGraw-Hill.

Barclay, L. (2002, July 1). Quetiapine well-tolerated, effective in refractory schizophrenia. *Medscape Medical News.* Retrieved from http://www.medscape.com

Barthel, R. (2002, October 27). Early interventions in psychosis. *Medscape Medical News.* Retrieved from http://www.medscape.com

Brown University Child and Adolescent Psychopharmacology Update. (2002, July 19). *Drugs in the pipeline: New drugs and indications for children and adolescents.* Retrieved from http://www.medscape.com

Brown University Geriatric Psychopharmacology Update. (2002, December 9). *Treating bipolar disorder in older adults: Gaps in knowledge remain.* Retrieved from http://www.medscape.com

Burns, M. J. (2001). The pharmacology and toxicology of atypical antipsychotic agents. *Journal of Toxicology: Clinical Toxicology, 39*(1), 1.

Cada, D., Levien, T., & Baker, D. (2003). Aripiprazole. *Hospital Pharmacy, 38*(3), 247–254.

Kneisl, C. R., Wilson, H. S., & Trigoboff, E. (2004). *Contemporary psychiatric–mental health nursing.* Upper Saddle River, NJ: Prentice Hall.

Medical Economics (Ed.). (2000). *PDR for herbal medicines.* Montvale, NJ: Author.

Medscape Medical News. (2003, February 13). *Dispensing errors reported for serzone and seroquel.* Retrieved from http://www.medscape.com

Vitiello, B. (2001). Psychopharmacology for young children: Clinical needs and research opportunities. *Pediatrics, 108*(4), 983.

Wahlbeck, K., Cheine, M., & Essali, M. A. (2002, April 1). Clozapine versus typical neuroleptic medication for schizophrenia. *Cochrane Review Abstracts.* Retrieved from http://www.medscape.com

Chapter 18

Barkin, R. L., & Barkin, D. (2001). Pharmacologic management of acute and chronic pain: Focus on drug interactions and patient-specific pharmacotherapeutic selection. *Southern Medical Journal, 94*(8), 756–812.

Bayer ASA side effects and ASA drug interactions. (2003). Retrieved from http://www.rxlist.com/cgi/generic/asa_ad.htm

Bell, J., Kimber, J., Mattick, R., Ali, R., Lintzers, N., Monhert, B., . . . & White, J. (2003). *Interim clinical guidelines: Use of naltrexone in relapse prevention for opioid dependence* (abbreviated version).

Washington, DC: Office of Disease Prevention and Health Promotion, United States Department of Health and Human Services. Retrieved from http://www.health.gov

Broadbent, C. (2000). The pharmacology of acute pain. Part 3. *Nursing Times, 96*(26), 39.

Clinical aspects of G6PD deficiency (2003). Retrieved from http://www.rialto.com

Diamond, M. (2003). *Emergency treatment of headache.* Chicago, IL: Internal Medicine Department, Columbus Hospital. Retrieved from http://www.usdoctor.com

Dog, L. T (2005). Menopause: A review of botanical dietary supplements. *American Journal of Medicine. 118*(Suppl 12B), 98–108.

Evans, R. W., & Taylor, F. R. (2006). "Natural" or alternative medications for migraine prevention. *Headache: The Journal of Head and Face Pain, 46*(6), 1012–1018.

Glajchen, M. (2001). Chronic pain. Treatment barriers and strategies for clinical practice. *Journal of the American Board of Family Practice, 14*(3), 178–183.

Guay, D. R. P. (2001). Adjunctive agents in the management of chronic pain. *Pharmacotherapy, 21*(9), 1070–1081.

Gunsteuin, H., & Akil, H. (2006). Opioid analgesics. In L. L. Brunton, J. S. Lazo, & K. L. Parker (Eds.), *Goodman & Gilman's The pharmacological basis of therapeutics* (11th ed., pp. 569–620). New York, NY: McGraw-Hill.

Khouzam, H. R. (2000). Chronic pain and its management in primary care. *Southern Medical Journal, 93*(10), 946–952.

Little, C. V., & Parsons, T. (2000). Herbal therapy for treating rheumatoid arthritis. *Cochrane Database of Systematic Reviews, 2000*(4). doi:10.1002/14651858.CD002948

Moses, S. (Ed.). (2002). Subarachnoid hemorrhage. *Family Practice Notebook.* Retrieved from http://www.fpnotebook.com/NEU33.htm

National Reye's Syndrome Foundation, Inc. (2000). *Aspirin or salicylate-containing medications.* Retrieved from http://www.reyessyndrome.org/aspirin.htm

Office of Disease Prevention and Health Promotion, United States Department of Health and Human Services. (2003). *Section 11: Gastrointestinal system.* Retrieved from http://www.health.gov

Tepper, S. J., & Rapoport, A. M. (1999). The triptans: A summary. *CNS Drugs, 12*(5), 403–417.

Tfelt-Hansen, P., DeVries, P., & Sexena, P. R. (2000). Triptans in migraine: A comparative review of pharmacology, pharmacokinetics, and efficacy. *Drugs, 60*(6), 1259–1287.

Chapter 19

Alqareer, A., Alyahya, A., & Andersson, L. (2006). The effect of clove and benzocaine versus placebo as topical anesthetics. *Journal of Dentistry, 34*(10), 747–750.

Catterall, W. A., & Mackie, K. (2006). Local anesthetics. In L. L. Brunton, J. S. Lazo, & K. L. Parker (Eds.), *Goodman & Gilman's The pharmacological basis of therapeutics* (11th ed., pp. 367–384). New York, NY: McGraw-Hill.

Colbert, B. J., & Mason, B. J. (2006). *Integrated cardiopulmonary pharmacology.* Upper Saddle River, NJ: Prentice Hall.

Evers, A., & Crowder, C. M. (2006). General anesthetics. In L. L. Brunton, J. S. Lazo, & K. L. Parker (Eds.), *Goodman & Gilman's The pharmacological basis of therapeutics* (11th ed., pp. 337–366). New York, NY: McGraw-Hill.

KidsHealth for Parents. (2003). *Your child's anesthesia.* The Nemours Foundation. Retrieved from http://www.kidshealth.org

Nagelhout, J. J., Nagelhout, K., & Zaglaniczny, V. H. (2001). *Handbook of nurse anesthesia* (2nd ed.). Philadelphia, PA: W. B. Saunders.

National Institutes of Health. (2003). *General anesthesia.* Retrieved from http://www.nlm.nih.gov/medlineplus/

Chapter 20

About Alzheimer's. Retrieved from http://www.alzfdn.org

Alzheimer's disease; Unraveling the mystery: The search for new treatments. (2003, April 11). Retrieved from http://www.alzheimers.org

Birks, J., Grimley-Evans, J., & Van Dongen, M. (2003). Ginkgo biloba for cognitive impairment and dementia. *Medscape.* Retrieved from http://www.medscape.com

Birks, J., Grimley, E., and VanDongen, M. (2002). Ginkgo biloba for cognitive impairment and dementia. *Cochrane Database of Systematic Reviews,* (4), CD003120. Retrieved from http://www.cochrane.org

Borek, C. (2006). Garlic reduces dementia and heart-disease risk. *Journal of Nutrition, 136*(3 Suppl), 810S–812S.

Capozza, K. (2003, April 2). Drug slows progression of Alzheimer's. *Medline Plus.* Retrieved from http://www.nlm.nih.gov/medlineplus

DeKosky, S. T., Williamson, J. D., Fitzpatrick, A. L., Kronmal, R. A., Ives, D. G., Saxton, J. A., . . . & Furberg, C. D. (2008). Ginkgo biloba for prevention of dementia: A randomized controlled trial. *Journal of the American Medical Association, 300*(19), 2253–2262.

Dooley, M., & Lamb, H. M. (2000). Donepezil: A review of its use in Alzheimer's disease. *Drugs and Aging, 16*(3), 199–226.

Gruetzner, H. (2001). *Alzheimer's: A caregiver's guide and sourcebook* (3rd ed.). Indianapolis, IN: Wiley.

Hristove, A. H., & Koller, W. C. (2000). Early Parkinson's disease: What is the best approach in treatment? *Drugs and Aging, 17*(3), 165–181.

Kahle, P., & Haass, C. (Eds.). (2003). *Molecular mechanisms in Parkinson's disease.* Georgetown, TX: Landes Bioscience/Eurekah.com

Lambert, D., & Waters, C. H. (2000). Comparative tolerability of the new generation antiparkinson agents. *Drugs and Aging, 16*(1), 55–65.

Richter, R. (Ed.). (2003). *Alzheimer's disease: The physician's guide to practical management.* Totowa, NJ: Human Press.

Sierpina, V. S., Wollschlaeger, B., & Blumenthal M. (2003). Ginkgo biloba. *American Family Physician, 68*(5), 923–926.

Standaert, D. G., & Young, A. B. (2006). Treatment of central nervous system degenerative disorders. In L. L. Brunton, J. S. Lazo, & K. L. Parker (Eds.), *Goodman & Gilman's The pharmacological basis of therapeutics* (11th ed., pp. 527–546). New York, NY: McGraw-Hill.

Chapter 21

American Society for Aesthetic Plastic Surgery. (2003). *Your image.* Retrieved from http://surgery.org/EFFECTIVE_METHODS.HTML

Dystonia Medical Research Foundation. (2003a). *Botulism toxin injections.* Retrieved from http://www.dystonia-foundation.org/pages/botulinum_toxin_injections/124.php

Dystonia Medical Research Foundation. (2003b). *Complementary therapy.* Retrieved from http://www.dystonia-foundation.org/pages/complementary_therapy/156.php

Dystonia Medical Research Foundation. (2003c). *Dystonia defined.* Retrieved from http://www.dystonia-foundation.org/defined/

National Institutes of Health. (2003). *Spasticity.* Retrieved from http://www.nlm.nih.gov/medlineplus/ency/article/003297.htm

National Institutes of Health, National Institute of Neurological Disorders and Stroke. (2003). *NINDS spasticity information page.* Retrieved from http://nindsupdate.ninds.nih.gov/health_and_medical/disorders/spasticity_doc.htm

Nelson, A. J., Ragan, B. G., Bell, G. W., Ichiyama, R. M., & Iwamoto, G. A. (2004). Capsaicin-based analgesic balm decreases pressor responses evoked by muscle afferents. *Medicine & Science in Sports & Exercise, 36*(3), 444–450.

Chapter 22

Ballantyne, C. M., O'Keefe, J. H., Jr., & Gotto, A. M., Jr. (2005). *Dyslipidemia essentials.* Royal Oak, MI: Physician's Press.

Citkowitz, E. (2007). Hypercholesterolemia, familial. *emedicine.* Retrieved July 3, 2008, from http://www.emedicine.com/med/TOPIC1072.HTM

Law, M., & Rudnicka, A. (2006). Statin safety: A systematic review. *American Journal of Cardiology, 97*(8), S52–S60.

Levy, H. B., & Kohlhaas, H. K. (2006). Considerations for supplementing with coenzyme Q10 during statin therapy. *Annals of Pharmacotherapy, 40*(2), 290–294.

Littarru, G. P., & Tiano, L. (2005). Clinical aspects of coenzyme Q10: An update. *Current Opinion in Clinical Nutrition and Metabolic Care, 8*(6), 641–646.

Mahley, R. W., & Bersot, T. P. (2006). Drug therapy for hypercholesterolemia and dyslipidemia. In L. L. Brunton, J. S. Lazo, & K. L. Parker (Eds.), *Goodman & Gilman's The pharmacological basis of therapeutics* (11th ed., pp. 933–964). New York, NY: McGraw-Hill.

McLoughlin, C. (2004). Statins. *Professional Nurse, 19*(11), 51–52.

Nichols, N. (2004). Clinical practice guidelines for the management of dyslipidemia. *Canadian Journal of Cardiovascular Nursing, 14*(2), 7–10.

O'Riordan, M. (2005). Coenzyme Q10 improves myopathic pain in statin-treated patients. Medscape Medical News. Retrieved from http://www.medscape.com/viewarticle/538168

Robinson, A. W., Sloan, H. L., & Arnold, G. (2001). Use of niacin in the prevention and management of hyperlipidemia. *Progress in Cardiovascular Nursing, 16*(1), 14–20.

U.S. Food and Drug Administration Center for Food Safety and Applied Nutrition, Office of Nutritional Products, Labeling, and Dietary Supplements. (2001, February). *New dietary ingredients in dietary supplements* (updated September 10, 2001). Washington, DC: Author.

Xydakis, A. M., & Ballantyne, C. M. (2004). Management of metabolic syndrome: Statins. *Endocrinology and Metabolism Clinics of North America, 33*(3), 509–523.

Chapter 23

Biujsee, B., Feskens, E. J., Kok, F. J., & Kromhout, D. (2006). Cocoa intake, blood pressure, and cardiovascular mortality. *Archives of Internal Medicine, 166,* 411–417.

Chang, W. T., Shao, Z. H., Vanden Hoek, T. L., McEntee, E., Mehendale, S. R., Li, J., . . . & Yuan, C. S. (2006). Cardioprotective effects of grape seed proanthocyanidins, baicalin, and wogonin. *American Journal of Chinese Medicine, 34*(2), 363–365.

Chaudhry, S. I., Krumholz, H. M., & Foody, J. M. (2004). Systolic hypertension in older persons. *Journal of the American Medical Association, 292*(9), 1074–1080.

Colbert, B. J., & Mason, B. J. (2008). *Integrated cardiopulmonary pharmacology.* (2nd ed.). Upper Saddle River, NJ: Prentice Hall.

Ding, E. L., Hutfless, S. M., Ding, X., & Girotra, S. (2006). Chocolate and prevention of cardiovascular disease: A systematic review. *Nutrition and Metabolism, 3,* 2.

Grassi, D., Lippi, C., Necozione, S., Desideri, G., & Ferri, C. (2005). Short-term administration of dark chocolate is followed by a significant increase in insulin sensitivity and a decrease in blood pressure in healthy persons. *American Journal of Clinical Nutrition, 81*(3), 611–614.

Hoffman, B. B. (2006). Therapy of hypertension. In L. L. Brunton, J. S. Lazo, & K. L. Parker. (Eds.), *Goodman & Gilman's The pharmacological basis of therapeutics* (11th ed., pp. 845–868). New York, NY: McGraw-Hill.

Israili, Z. H., Hernandez-Hernandez, R., & Valasco, M. (2007). The future of antihypertensive treatment. *American Journal of Therapeutics, 14*(2), 121–134.

Klag, M. J., Wang, N. Y., Meoni, L. A., Brancati, F. L., Cooper, L. A., Liang, K. Y., . . . & Ford, D. E. (2002). Coffee: Intake and risk of hypertension. The Johns Hopkins Precursors Study. *Archives of Internal Medicine, 162,* 657–662.

Manach, C., Mazur, A. & Scalbert, A. (2005). Grape seed extract. *Drug Digest.* Retrieved from http://www.drugdigest.org/wps/portal/ddigest

National Center for Complementary and Alternative Medicine (NCCAM). (2008). *Grape seed extract.* Retrieved from http://nccam.nih.gov/health/grapeseed/

National High Blood Pressure Education Program. National Heart, Lung & Blood Institute. (2003). *JNC-7 Express: The Seventh Report of the Joint National Committee on Prevention, Detection, Evaluation, and Treatment of High Blood Pressure*. Bethesda, MD: Author.

National High Blood Pressure Education Program Working Group on High Blood Pressure in Children and Adolescents. (2004). The fourth report on the diagnosis, evaluation, and treatment of high blood pressure in children and adolescents. *Pediatrics, 114*(Suppl. 2), 555–576.

National Institutes of Health. (2003). NHLBI issues new high blood pressure clinical practice guidelines. *NIH NEWS*. Retrieved from http://www.nhlbi.nih.gov

Oates, J. A., & Brown, N. J. (2006). Antihypertensive agents and the drug therapy of hypertension. In L. L. Brunton, J. S. Lazo, & K. L. Parker (Eds.), *Goodman & Gilman's The pharmacological basis of therapeutics* (11th ed., pp. 871–900). New York, NY: McGraw-Hill.

Ong, K. L., Cheung, B. M. Y., Man, Y. B., Lau, C. P., & Lam, K. S. L. (2007). Prevalence, awareness, treatment, and control of hypertension among United States adults 1999–2004. *Hypertension, 49*(12), 69–75.

Poudre Valley Health System. (2003). *Herbal medicines and dietary supplements: Information for people with heart disease*. Retrieved from http://www.pvhs.org

Simpson, C. (2003). *Autonomic nervous system agents: Adrenergics and adrenergic blocking agents*. Retrieved from http://www.cotc.edu/Pages/index.aspx

Thadhani, R., Camargo, C. A., Jr., Stampfer, M. J., Curhan, G. C., Willett, W. C., & Rimm, E. B. (2002). Prospective study of moderate alcohol consumption and risk of hypertension in young women. *Archives of Internal Medicine, 162*, 569–574.

Vlachopoulos, C., Aznaouridis, K., Alexopoulos, N., Economou, E., Andreadou, I., & Stefanadis, C. (2005). Effect of dark chocolate on arterial function in healthy individuals. *American Journal of Hypertension, 18*(6), 785–791.

Chapter 24

Albert, N. M. (2006). Evidence-based nursing care for patients with heart failure. *AACN Advanced Critical Care, 17*(2), 170–185.

Albrant, D. H. (2001). Drug treatment protocol: Management of chronic systolic heart failure. *Journal of the American Pharmaceutical Association, 41*(5), 672–681.

Chang, W. T., Dao, J., & Shao, Z. H. (2005). Hawthorn: Potential roles in cardiovascular disease. *American Journal of Chinese Medicine, 33*(1), 1–10.

Ferrari R., Merli, E., Cicchitelli, G., Mele, D., Fucili, A., & Ceconi, C. (2004). Therapeutic effects of l-carnitine and propionyl-l-carnitine on cardiovascular diseases: A review. *Annals of New York Academy of Science, 1033*(12), 79–91.

Gomberg-Maitland, M., Baran, D. A., & Fuster, V. (2001). Treatment of congestive heart failure: Guidelines for the primary care health care provider and the heart failure specialist. *Archives of Internal Medicine, 161*, 342–352.

Hudson, S., & Tabet, N. (2003). Acetyl-L-carnitine for dementia. *Cochrane Database of Systematic Reviews*, (2). doi: 10.1002/14651858.CD003158

Jamali, A. H., Tang, A. H. W., Khot, U. N., & Fowler, M. B. (2001). The role of angiotensin receptor blockers in the management of chronic heart failure. *Archives of Internal Medicine, 161*, 667–672.

Kendler, B. S. (2006). Supplemental conditionally essential nutrients in cardiovascular disease therapy. *Journal of Cardiovascular Nursing, 21*(1), 9–16.

Kennedy, E. B., & Ignatavicius, D. D. (2006). Interventions for clients with cardiac problems. In D. D. Ignatavicius & L. H. Workman (Eds.), *Medical–surgical nursing: Critical thinking for collaborative care* (5th ed., pp. 749–776). St. Louis, MO: W.B. Saunders.

McCarthy, P. M., & Young, J. B. (Eds.). (2007). *Heart failure: A combined medical and surgical approach*. Malden, MA: Blackwell.

Paul, S. (2002). Balancing diuretic therapy in heart failure: Loop diuretics, thiazides, and antagonists. *Congestive Heart Failure, 8*(6), 307–312.

Pittler, M. H., Schmidt, K., & Ernst, E. (2003). Hawthorn extract for treating chronic heart failure: Meta-analysis of randomized trials. *American Journal of Medicine, 114*(8), 665–674.

Richardson, L. G. (2003). Psychosocial issues in patients with congestive heart failure. *Progress in Cardiovascular Nursing, 18*(1), 19–27.

Rocco, T. P., & Fang, J. C. (2006). Pharmacotherapy of congestive heart failure. In L. L. Brunton, J. S. Lazo, & K. L. Parker (Eds.), *Goodman & Gilman's The pharmacological basis of therapeutics* (11th ed., pp. 869–898). New York, NY: McGraw-Hill.

Tankanow, R., Tamer, H. R., Streetman, D. S., Smith, S. G., Welton, J. L., Annesley, T., . . . & Bleske, B. E. (2003). Interaction study between digoxin and a preparation of hawthorn (*Crataegus oxyacantha*). *Journal of Clinical Pharmacology, 43*(6), 637–642.

Wagner, J. A. (2006). Top ten challenges in heart failure management. *Journal for Nurse Practitioners, 2*(8), 528–532.

Chapter 25

Aronow, W. S., Frishman, W. H., & Cheng-Lai, A. (2007). Cardiovascular drug therapy in the elderly. *Cardiology in Review, 15*(4), 195–215.

Danchin, N., & Durand, E. (2003). Acute myocardial infarction. *Clinical Evidence, 10*, 37–63.

Freestone, B., Lip, G. Y. H., Scott, P. A., & Pancioli, A. M. (2003). Stroke prevention. *Clinical Evidence, 11*, 257–283.

Kurth, T., Glynn, R. J., Walker, A. M., Chan, K. A., Buring, J. E., Hennekens, C. H., & Gaziano, J. M. (2003). Inhibition of clinical benefits of aspirin on first myocardial infarction by nonsteroidal antiinflammatory drugs. *Circulation, 108*(10), 1191–1195.

Levine, G. N., Ali, M. N., & Schafer, A. I. (2001). Antithrombotic therapy in patients with acute coronary syndromes. *Archives of Internal Medicine, 161*, 937–948.

Michel, T. (2006). Treatment of myocardial ischemia. In L. L. Brunton, J. S. Lazo, & K. L. Parker (Eds.), *Goodman & Gilman's The pharmacological basis of therapeutics* (11th ed., pp. 823–844). New York, NY: McGraw-Hill.

Parchure, N., & Brecker, S. J. (2002). Management of acute coronary syndromes. *Current Opinions in Critical Care, 8*(3), 230–235.

Rasmussen, J. N., Chong, A., & Alter, D. A. (2007). Relationship between adherence to evidence-based pharmacotherapy and long-term mortality after acute myocardial infarction. *Journal of the American Medical Association, 297*(2), 177–186.

Staniforth, A. D. (2001). Contemporary management of chronic stable angina. *Drugs and Aging, 18*(2), 109–121.

Tong, G. M., & Rude, R. K. (2005). Magnesium deficiency in critical illness. *Journal of Intensive Care Medicine, 20*(1), 3–17.

Ueshima, K. (2005). Magnesium and ischemic heart disease: A review of epidemiological, experimental, and clinical evidences. *Magnesium Research, 18*(4), 275–284.

Chapter 26

American College of Cardiology, American Heart Association Task Force, European Society of Cardiology. (2006). ACC/AHA/ESC 2006 guidelines for management of patients with ventricular arrhythmias and the prevention of sudden cardiac death—Executive Summary. *Journal of the American College of Cardiology, 48*, 1064–1108. Retrieved July 15, 2008, from http://content.onlinejacc.org/cgi/content/full/48/5/1064

Beattie, W. S., & Elliot, R. F. (2005). Magnesium supplementation reduces the risk of arrhythmia after cardiac surgery. *Evidence-based Cardiovascular Medicine, 9*(1), 82–85.

Berry, C., Rankin, A. C., & Brady, A. (2004). Bradycardia and tachycardia occurring in older people: An introduction. *British Journal of Cardiology, 11*(1), 61–64.

Dayer, M., & Hardman, S. (2002). Special problems with antiarrhythmic drugs in the elderly: Safety, tolerability, and efficacy. *American Journal of Geriatric Cardiology, 11*(6), 370–375.

Ellison, K. E., Stevenson, W. G., Sweeney, M. O., Epstein, L. M., & Maisel, W. H. (2003). Management of arrhythmias in heart failure. *Congestive Heart Failure, 9*(2), 91–99.

Haugh, K. H. (2002). Antidysrhythmic agents at the turn of the twenty-first century: A current review. *Critical Care Nursing Clinics of North America, 14*(1), 53–69.

Huikuri, H. V., Castellanos, A., & Myerburg, R. J. (2001). Medical progress: Sudden death due to cardiac arrhythmias. *New England Journal of Medicine, 345,* 1473–1482.

Kern, L. S. (2004). Postoperative atrial fibrillation: New directions in prevention and treatment. *Journal of Cardiovascular Nursing, 19*(2), 103–115.

Piotrowski, A. A., & Kalus, J. S. (2004). Magnesium for the treatment and prevention of atrial tachyarrhythmias. *Pharmacotherapy, 24*(7), 879–895.

Roden, D. M. (2006). Antiarrhythmic drugs. In L. L. Brunton, J. S. Lazo, & K. L. Parker (Eds.), *Goodman & Gilman's The pharmacological basis of therapeutics* (11th ed., pp. 899–932). New York, NY: McGraw-Hill.

Somberg, J. C., Cao, W., Cvetanovic, I., Ranade, V. V., & Molnar, J. (2005). The effect of magnesium sulfate on action potential duration and cardiac arrhythmias. *American Journal of Therapeutics, 12*(3), 218–222.

Tong, G. M., & Rude, R. K. (2005). Magnesium deficiency in critical illness. *Journal of Intensive Care Medicine, 20*(1), 3–17.

Ueshima, K. (2005). Magnesium and ischemic heart disease: A review of epidemiological, experimental, and clinical evidences. *Magnesium Research, 18*(4), 275–284.

Chapter 27

Allison, G. L., Lowe, G. M., & Rahman, K. (2006). Aged garlic extract and its constituents inhibit platelet aggregation through multiple mechanisms. *Journal of Nutrition, 136*(Suppl. 3), 782S–788S.

Cooney, M. F. (2006). Heparin-induced thrombocytopenia: Advances in diagnosis and treatment. *Critical Care Nurse, 26*(6), 30–36.

Coumadin: Prescription drug reference. (2003). Retrieved from http://www.healthsquare.com

Hiatt, W. R. (2001). Drug therapy: Medical treatment of peripheral arterial disease and claudication. *New England Journal of Medicine, 344,* 1608–1621.

Hirsh, J., Guyatt, G., Albers, G. W., Harrington, R., & Shünemann, H. J. (2008). Antithrombotic and thrombolytic therapy: American College of Chest Physicians Guidelines (8th ed.). *Chest, 133,* 110S–112S. Retrieved July 17, 2008, from http://www.chestjournal.org/content/vol133/6_suppl/

Rahman, K., & Lowe, G. M. (2006). Garlic and cardiovascular disease: A critical review. *Journal of Nutrition, 136*(3), 736S–740S.

Segal, J. B., Streiff, M. B., Hofmann, L. V., Thornton, K., & Bass, E. B. (2007). Management of venous thromboembolism: A systematic review for a practice guideline. *Annals of Internal Medicine, 146*(3), 211–222.

Shamseer, L., Charrois, T. L., & Vohra, S. (2006). Complementary, holistic, and integrative medicine: Garlic. *Pediatrics in Review, 27*(12), e77–e80.

Chapter 28

Bailey, L. B., Rampersaud, G. C., & Kauwell, G. P. (2003). Folic acid supplements and fortification affect the risk for neural tube defects, vascular disease, and cancer: Evolving science. *Journal of Nutrition, 133*(6), 1961S–1968S.

Dharmarajan, T. S., Adiga, G. U., & Norkus, E. P. (2003). Vitamin B$_{12}$ deficiency. Recognizing subtle symptoms in older adults. *Geriatrics, 58*(3), 30–34, 37–38.

Eden, A. N. (2003). Preventing iron deficiency in toddlers: A major public health problem. *Contemporary Pediatrics, 20*(2), 57–67.

Gozzard, D. I. (2006). Diagnosing and treating iron deficiency. *Nursing in Practice: The Journal for Today's Primary Care Nurse, 29,* 57–58, 61.

Kaushansky, K., & Kipps, T. J. (2006). Hematopoietic agents: Growth factors, minerals, & vitamins. In L. L. Brunton, J. S. Lazo, & K. L. Parker (Eds.), *Goodman & Gilman's The pharmacological basis of therapeutics* (11th ed., pp. 1433–1466). New York, NY: McGraw-Hill.

Oh, R., & Brown, D. L. (2003). Vitamin B$_{12}$ deficiency. *American Family Health Care Provider, 67*(5), 979–986.

Rampersaud, G. C., Kauwell, G. P., & Bailey, L. B. (2003). Folate: A key to optimizing health and reducing disease risk in the elderly. *Journal of the American College of Nutrition, 22*(1), 1–8.

Somer, E. (2003). Ironing out anemia. *WebMDHealth.* Retrieved from http://my.webmd.com

Wolff, T., Takacs-Witkop, K., Miller, M., & Syed, S. (2009). Folic acid supplementation for the prevention of neural tube defects: An update of the evidence for the U.S. Preventive Services Task Force. *Annals of Internal Medicine, 150,* 632–639.

Chapter 29

Brown, S. G. (2005). Cardiovascular aspects of anaphylaxis: Implications for treatment and diagnosis. *Current Opinion in Allergy and Clinical Immunology, 5*(4), 359–364.

Dellinger, R. P. (2003). Cardiovascular management of septic shock. *Critical Care Medicine, 31*(3), 946–955.

Hasdai, D., Berger, P. B., Battler, A., & Holmes, D. R. (2002). *Cardiogenic shock: Diagnosis and treatment.* Totowa, NJ: Humana Press.

Kolecki, P., & Menckhoff, C. R. (2001, December 11). Hypovolemic shock. *eMedicine Journal, 2*(12).

Leone, M., & Martin, C. (2008). Vasopressor use in septic shock: An update. *Current Opinion in Anaesthesiology, 21*(2), 141–147.

Menon, V., & Fincke, R. (2003). Cardiogenic shock: A summary of the randomized SHOCK trial. *Congestive Heart Failure, 9*(1), 35–39.

Murray, J. J. (2005). Cardiovascular risks associated with beta-agonist therapy. *Chest, 127*(6), 2283–2285.

Pittler, M. H., & Ernst, E. Horse chestnut seed extract for chronic venous insufficiency. *Cochrane Database of Systematic Reviews, 2006*(1). doi:10.1002/14651858.CD003230.pub3

Von Rosenstiel, N., von Rosenstiel, I., & Adam, D. (2001). Management of sepsis and septic shock in infants and children. *Paediatric Drugs, 3*(1), 9–27.

Chapter 30

Charlesworth, J. A., Gracey, D. M., & Pussell, B. A. (2008). Adult nephrotic syndrome: Non-specific strategies for treatment. *Nephrology, 13*(1), 45–50.

Costello-Boerrigter, L. C., Boerrigter, G., & Burnett, J. C. (2003). Revisiting salt and water retention: New diuretics, aquaretics, and natriuretics. *Medical Clinics of North America, 87*(2), 475–491.

Howell, A. B., Reed, J. D., Krueger, C. G., Winterbottom, R., Cunningham, D. G., & Leahy, M. (2005). A-type cranberry proanthocyanidins and uropathogenic bacterial anti-adhesion activity. *Phytochemistry, 66*(18), 2281–2291.

Jackson, E. K. (2006). Diuretics. In L. L. Brunton, J. S. Lazo, & K. L. Parker (Eds.), *Goodman & Gilman's The pharmacological basis of therapeutics* (11th ed., pp. 737–770). New York, NY: McGraw-Hill.

Jepson, R. G., Mihaljevic, L., & Craig, J. (2006). Cranberries for preventing urinary tract infections. *Cochrane Database of Systematic Reviews, 2004*(1), CD001321.

National Center for Complementary and Alternative Medicine (NCCAM). (2008). Retrieved from http://nccam.nih.gov/health/cranberry/

National Kidney Foundation. (2008). *End stage renal disease in the United States.* Retrieved July 8, 2008, from http://www.kidney.org/news/newsroom/fsitem.cfm?id=38

Sica, D., Gehr, T., & Frishman, W. (2006). Use of diuretics in the treatment of heart failure in the elderly. *Heart Failure Clinics, 3*(4), 455–464.

Chapter 31

Ayers, P., & Warrington, L. (2008). Diagnosis and treatment of simple acid–base disorders. *Nutrition in Clinical Practice, 23*(2), 122–127.

Bunn, F.,Trivedi, D., & Ashraf, S. (2007). Colloid solutions for fluid resuscitation. *Cochrane Database of Systematic Reviews, 4.* (Art. No.: CD001319, DOI:10.1002/14651858.CD001319.pub2).

Joy, M. S., & Hladik, G. A. (2005). Disorders of sodium, water, calcium, and phosphorous homeostasis. In J. T. DiPiro, R. L. Talbert, C. Y. Yee, G. R. Matzke, B. G. Wells, & L. M. Posey (Eds.), *Pharmacotherapy: A pathophysiologic approach* (6th ed., pp. 937–966). New York: McGraw-Hill.

Matzke, G. R., & Palevsky, P. M. (2005). Acidbase disorders. In J. T. DiPiro, R. L.Talbert, C. Y. Yee, G. R. Matzke, B. G.Wells, & L. M. Posey (Eds.), *Pharmacotherapy: A pathophysiologic approach* (6th ed., pp. 51–73). New York: McGraw-Hill.

Mitch, W. E. (2006). Metabolic and clinical consequences of metabolic acidosis. *Journal of Nephrology, 19*(Suppl. 9) S70–S75..

Chapter 32

Advisory Committee on Immunization Practices, Centers for Disease Control. Prevention of varicella: Recommendations of the Advisory Committee on Immunization Practices. (2007). *Morbidity and Mortality Weekly Report, 56*(RR-4), 1–40.

Agnew, L. L., Guffogg, S. P., Matthias, A., Lehmann, R. P., Bone, K. M., & Watson, K. (2005). Echinacea intake induces an immune response through altered expression of leucocyte hsp70, increased white cell counts, and improved erythrocyte antioxidant defences. *Journal of Clinical Pharmacy and Therapeutics, 30*(4), 363–369.

Centers for Disease Control and Prevention (CDC). (2003). *National Vaccine Program Office: Immunization laws.* Retrieved from http://www.cdc.gov/od/nvpo/law.htm

Children's Defense Fund. (2003). *Every child deserves a healthy start.* Retrieved from http://www.childrensdefense.org

Goel, V., Lovlin, R., Chang, C., Slama, J. V., Barton, R., Gahler, R., . . . & Basu, T. K. (2005). A proprietary extract from the echinacea plant (*Echinacea purpurea*) enhances systemic immune response during a common cold. *Phytotherapy Research, 19*(8), 689–694.

Karam, U. S., & Reddy, K. R. (2003). Pegylated interferons. *Clinical Liver Disease, 7*(1), 139–148.

Krensky, A. M., Strom, T. B., & Bluestone, J. A. (2006). Immunomodulators: Immunosuppressive agents, toleragens, and immunostimulants. In L. L. Brunton, J. S. Lazo, & K. L. Parker (Eds.), *Goodman & Gilman's The pharmacological basis of therapeutics* (11th ed., pp. 1463–1484). New York, NY: McGraw-Hill.

Santamaria, P. (2003). *Cytokines and autoimmune disease.* New York, NY: Kluwer Academic/Plenum.

Schoop, R., Klein, P., Suter, A., & Johnston, S. L. (2006). Echinacea in the prevention of induced rhinovirus colds: A meta-analysis. *Clinical Therapeutics, 28*(2), 174–183.

Sharma, M., Arnason, J. T., Burt, A., & Hudson, J. B. (2006). Echinacea extracts modulate the pattern of chemokine and cytokine secretion in rhinovirus-infected and uninfected epithelial cells. *Phytotherapy Research, 20*(2), 147–152.

Sur, D. K., Wallis, D. H., & O'Connell, T. X. (2003). Vaccinations in pregnancy. *American Family Physician, 68,* E299–E309.

Thomson, A. W., & Lotze, M. T. (2003). *The cytokine handbook* (4th ed., vols. 1–2). Burlington, MA: Elsevier Science & Technology Books.

Chapter 33

Burke, A., Smythe, E. M., & Fitzgerald, G. A. (2006). Analgesic-antipyretic agents: Pharmacotherapy of gout. In L. L. Brunton, J. S. Lazo, & K. L. Parker (Eds.), *The pharmacological basis of therapeutics* (11th ed., pp. 671–716). New York: McGraw-Hill.

Carson, S. (2003). Alternating acetaminophen and ibuprofen in the febrile child: Examination of the evidence regarding efficacy and safety. *Pediatric Nursing, 18,* 428–432.

Galley, H. F. (2002). *Critical care focus: Vol. 10. Inflammation and immunity.* London, England: BMJ Books.

Oh, R. (2005). Practical applications of fish oil (omega-3 fatty acids) in primary care. *Journal of the American Board of Family Practice, 18*(1), 28–36.

Rostom, A., Muir, K., Dube, C., Jolicoeur, E., Boucher, M., Joyce, J., et al. (2007). Gastrointestinal safety of cyclooxygenase-2 inhibitors: A Cochrane collaboration systematic review. *Clinical Gastroenterology and Hepatology, 5*(7), 18–28.

Stillman, M. J., & Stillman, M. T. (2007). Choosing nonselective NSAIDs and selective COX-2 inhibitors in the elderly. A clinical use pathway. *Geriatrics, 62*(2), 26–34.

Chapter 34

Bradbury, B. J., & Pucci, M. J. (2008). Recent advances in bacterial topoisomerase inhibitors. *Current Opinion in Pharmacology, 8*(3), 132–145.

Chambers, H. F. (2006). General considerations of antimicrobial therapy. In L. L. Brunton, J. S. Lazo, & K. L. Parker (Eds.), *Goodman & Gilman's The pharmacological basis of therapeutics* (11th ed., pp. 1095–1110). New York, NY: McGraw-Hill.

Cisneros-Farrar, F., & Parsons, L. (2007). Antimicrobials: Classifications and uses in critical care. *Critical Care Nursing Clinics of North America, 19*(1), 43–51.

McFarland, L., Beneda, H., Clarridge, J., & Raugi, G. (2007). Implications of the changing face of *Clostridium difficile* disease for health care practitioners. *American Journal of Infection Control, 35*(4), 237–253.

Moran, G. J., & Mount, J. (2003). Update on emerging infections: News from the Centers for Disease Control and Prevention. *Annals of Emergency Medicine, 41*(1), 148–151.

Nicolau, D. P. (2008). Carbapenems: A potent class of antibiotics. *Expert Opinion on Pharmacotherapy, 9*(1), 23–27.

Parsons, L., & Krau, S. (2007). Bacterial infections: Management by acute and critical care nurses. *Critical Care Nursing Clinics of North America, 19*(1), 17–26.

Petri, W. A. (2006a). Sulfonamides, trimethoprim-sulfamethoxazole, quinolones, and agents for urinary tract infections. In L. L. Brunton, J. S. Lazo, & K. L. Parker (Eds.), *Goodman & Gilman's The pharmacological basis of therapeutics* (11th ed., pp. 1111–1126). New York, NY: McGraw-Hill.

Petri, W. A. (2006b). Penicillins, cephalosporins, and other beta-lactam antibiotics. In L. L. Brunton, J. S. Lazo, & K. L. Parker (Eds.), *Goodman & Gilman's The pharmacological basis of therapeutics* (11th ed., pp. 1127–1154). New York, NY: McGraw-Hill.

Petri, W. A. (2006c). Chemotherapy of tuberculosis, *Mycobacterium avium* complex disease, and leprosy. In L. L. Brunton, J. S. Lazo, & K. L. Parker (Eds.), *Goodman & Gilman's The pharmacological basis of therapeutics* (11th ed., pp. 1203–1224). New York, NY: McGraw-Hill.

Tillotson, G. S., Blondeau, J. M., & Carroll, J. (2007). Hospital-based strategies to reduce antibiotic resistance: Are they valid in the community setting? *Expert Review of Anti-Infective Therapy, 5*(1), 53–59.

Wooten, J., & Sakind, A. (2003). Superbugs: Unmasking the threat. *RN, 66*(3), 37–43.

Chapter 35

Bennet, J. E. (2006). Antifungal agents. In L. L. Brunton, J. S. Lazo, & K. L. Parker (Eds.), *Goodman & Gilman's The pharmacological basis of therapeutics* (11th ed., pp. 1225–1242). New York, NY: McGraw-Hill.

Dickson, R., Awasthi, S., Demellweek, C., & Williamson, P. (2003). Anthelmintic drugs for treating worms in children: Effects on growth and cognitive performance. *Cochrane Database of Systematic Reviews, 2005*(2), CD000371. Retrieved from http://www.medscape.com

Kontoyiannis, D. P., Mantadakis, E., & Samonis, G. (2003). Systemic mycoses in the immunocompromised host: An update in antifungal therapy. *Journal of Hospital Infection, 53*(4), 243–258.

Martin, K. W., & Ernst, E. (2004). Herbal medicines for treatment of fungal infections: A systematic review of controlled clinical trials. *Mycoses, 47*(3–4), 87–92.

Pasqualotto, A. C., & Denning, D. W. (2008). New and emerging treatments for fungal infections. *Journal of Antimicrobial Chemotherapy, 61*(Supplement 1), i19–i30.

Perlroth, J., Choi, B., & Spellberg, B. (2007). Nosocomial fungal infections: Epidemiology, diagnosis, and treatment. *Medical Mycology, 45*(4), 321–346.

Pray, W. S. (2001). Treatment of vaginal fungal infections. *U.S. Pharmacist, 26*(9), 15–27.

Shapiro, T. A., & Goldberg, D. E. (2006). Chemotherapy of protozoal infections: Malaria. In L. L. Brunton, J. S. Lazo, & K. L. Parker (Eds.), *Goodman & Gilman's The pharmacological basis of therapeutics* (11th ed., pp. 869–898). New York, NY: McGraw–Hill.

Steile, R. W. (2002). Focus on infection, prevention, detection, and treatment. *Medscape Medical News.* Retrieved from http://www .medscape.com

Re, V. L., & Gluckman, S. J. (2003). Prevention of malaria in travelers. *American Family Physician, 68,* 509–514, 515–516.

Smith, C. M., & Kagan, S. H. (2005). Prevention of systemic mycoses by reducing exposure to fungal pathogens in hospitalized and ambulatory neutropenic patients. *Oncology Nursing Forum, 32*(3), 565–579.

Wilson, C. (2005). Recurrent vulvovaginitis candidiasis: An overview of traditional and alternative therapies. *Advance for Nurse Practitioners, 13*(5), 24–29.

Chapter 36

Almuente, V. (2002). Herbal therapy in patients with HIV. *Medscape Pharmacists, 3*(2), 1–4.

Centers for Disease Control and Prevention (CDC). (2008). Prevention and control of influenza: Recommendations of the Advisory Committee on Immunization Practices (ACIP), *Morbidity and Mortality Weekly Report, 57*(Early Release), 1–60.

Idemyor, V. (2003). Twenty years since human immunodeficiency virus discovery: Considerations for the next decade. *Pharmacotherapy, 23,* 384–387.

Kirkbride, H. A., & Watson, J. (2003). Review of the use of neuraminidase inhibitors for prophylaxis of influenza. *Communicable Disease and Public Health, 6*(2), 123–127.

Kuritzkes, D. R., Boyle, B. A., Gallant, J. E., Squires, K. E., & Zolopa, A. (2003). Current management challenges in HIV: Antiretroviral resistance. *AIDS Reader, 13*(3), 133–135, 138–142.

Lesho, E. P., & Gey, D. C. (2003). Managing issues related to antiretroviral therapy. *American Family Physician, 68,* 675–686, 689–690.

Maltezou, H. C. (2008). Nosocomial influenza: New concepts and practice. *Current Opinion in Infectious Diseases, 21*(4), 337–343.

Mills, E., Montori, V., Perri, D., Phillips, E., & Koren, G. (2005). Natural health product–HIV drug interactions: A systematic review. *International Journal of STDs and AIDS, 16*(3), 181–186.

Morbidity and Mortality Weekly Report, Centers for Disease Control and Prevention. (2005). *Antiretroviral postexposure prophylaxis after sexual, injection-drug use, or other nonoccupational exposure to HIV in the United States.* Recommendations from the U.S. Department of Health and Human Services, 54(R07), 1–20. Retrieved August 20, 2008, from http://www.cdc.gov/mmwr/ preview/mmwrhtml/rr5402a1.htm

National Institutes of Health (NIH), the Centers for Disease Control and Prevention (CDC), and the HIV Medicine Association of the Infectious Diseases Society of America (HIVMA/IDSA). (2008, June 18). *Guidelines for prevention and treatment of opportunistic infections in HIV-infected adults and adolescents.* Retrieved August 20, 2008, from http://aidsinfo.nih.gov/ contentfiles/Adult_OI.pdf

Ofotokun, I., & Pomeroy, C. (2003). Sex differences in adverse reactions to antiretroviral drugs. *Topics in HIV Medicine, 11*(2), 55–59.

Panel on Antiretroviral Guidelines for Adults and Adolescents, Department of Health and Human Services. (2008, January 29). *Guidelines for the use of antiretroviral agents in HIV-1-infected adults and adolescents.* Retrieved August 20, 2008, from http:// www.aidsinfo.nih.gov/ContentFiles/AdultandAdolescentGL.pdf

Public Health Service Task Force, Perinatal HIV Guidelines Working Group. (2008, July 8). *Recommendations for use of antiretroviral drugs in pregnant HIV-infected women for maternal health and interventions to reduce perinatal HIV-1 transmission in the United States.* Retrieved August 2, 2008, from http://aidsinfo .nih.gov/contentfiles/PerinatalGL.pdf

Sandhu, R. S., Prescilla, R. P., Simonelli, T. M., & Edwards, D. J. (2003). Influence of goldenseal root on the pharmacokinetics of indinavir. *Journal of Clinical Pharmacology, 43*(11), 1283–1288.

Wilson, T. R. (2005). The ABCs of hepatitis. *Nurse Practitioner, 30*(6), 12–21.

Chapter 37

American Cancer Society. (2008). *Making treatment decisions: Staging.* Retrieved August 5, 2008, from http://www.cancer.org/ docroot/ETO/content/ETO_1_2X_Staging.asp

Birner, A. (2003). Safe administration of oral chemotherapy. *Clinical Journal of Oncology Nursing, 2,* 158–162.

Breed, C. D. (2003). Diagnosis, treatment, and nursing care of patients with chronic leukemia. *Seminars in Oncology Nursing, 19*(2), 109–117.

Chabner, B. A., Amrein, P. C., Druker, B., Michaelson, M. D., Mitsiades, C. S., Goss, P. E., et al. (2006). Chemotherapy of neoplastic diseases. In L. L. Brunton, J. S. Lazo, & K. L. Parker (Eds.), *The pharmacological basis of therapeutics* (11th ed., pp. 1315–1403). New York: McGraw-Hill.

Hood, L. E. (2003). Chemotherapy in the elderly: Supportive measures for chemotherapy-induced myelotoxicity. *Clinical Journal of Oncology Nursing, 7*(2), 185–190.

Lee, S. O., Yeon Chun, J., Nadiminty, N., Trump, D. L., Ip, C., Dong, Y., & Gao, A.C. (2006). Monomethylated selenium inhibits growth of LNCaP human prostate cancer xenograft accompanied by a decrease in the expression of androgen receptor and prostate-specific antigen (PSA). *The Prostate, 66*(10), 1070–1075.

Peters, U., Chatterjee, N., Church, T. R., Mayo, C., Sturup, S., Foster, C. B., . . . & Hayes, R. B. (2006). High serum selenium and reduced risk of advanced colorectal adenoma in a colorectal cancer early detection program. *Cancer Epidemiology, Biomarkers, and Prevention, 15*(2), 315–320.

Reid, M. E., Duffield-Lillico, A. J., Sunga, A., Fakih, M., Alberts, D. S., & Marshall, J. R. (2006). Selenium supplementation and colorectal adenomas: An analysis of the nutritional prevention of cancer trial. *International Journal of Cancer, 118*(7), 1777–1781.

Smith, B., Waltzman, R., & Rugo, H. (2002, December 10). *Living longer with cancer: Preserving quality of life.* Retrieved from http:// healthology.com

Szetala, A., & Gibson, D. (2007). How the new oral antineoplastics affect nursing practice. *American Journal of Nursing, 107*(12), 40–49.

U.S. Preventive Services Task Force. (2003). Chemoprevention of breast cancer: Recommendations and rationale. *American Family Physician, 67*(6), 1309–1314.

Chapter 38

Berger, W. E. (2003). Overview of allergic rhinitis. *Annals of Allergy, Asthma, and Immunology, 90*(6, Suppl. 3), 7–12.

Braunstahl, G., & Hellings, P. W. (2003). Allergic rhinitis and asthma: The link further unraveled. *Current Opinion in Pulmonary Medicine, 9*(1), 46–51.

Chang, A. B., & Glomb, W. B. (2006). Guidelines for evaluating chronic cough in pediatrics: ACCP evidence-based clinical practice guidelines. *Chest, 129*(1 Suppl.), 260S–283S.

Hayden, M., & Womack, C. (2007). Caring for patients with allergic rhinitis. *Journal of the American Academy of Nurse Practitioners, 19*(6), 290–298.

Nathan, R. A. (2003). Pharmacotherapy for allergic rhinitis: A critical review of leukotriene receptor antagonists compared with other treatments. *Annals of Allergy, Asthma, and Immunology, 90*(2), 182–190.

Ratner, P. H., Stoloff, S., Metzer, E.O., & Hadley, J. A. (2007). Intranasal corticosteroids in the treatment of allergic rhinitis. *Allergy and Asthma Proceedings, 28*(Suppl. 1), s25–s32.

Rogers, D. F. (2003). Airway hypersecretion in allergic rhinitis and asthma: New pharmacotherapy. *Current Allergy and Asthma Reports, 3*(3), 238–248.

Rosenwasser, L. J. (2002). Treatment of allergic rhinitis. *American Journal of Medicine, 16*(113, Suppl. 9A), 17S–24S.

Smith, S. M., Schroeder, K., & Fahey, T. (2008). Over-the-counter medications for acute cough in children and adults in ambulatory settings. *Cochrane Database of Systematic Reviews 2007, 3.* Art. No.: CD001831. DOI: 10.1002/14651858.CD001831.pub3.

Chapter 39

Altman, E. E. (2004). Update on COPD. Today's strategies improve quality of life. *Advance for Nurse Practitioners, 12*(3), 49–54.

Banasiak, N. (2007). Childhood asthma part one: Initial assessment, diagnosis, and education. *Journal of Pediatric Health Care, 21*(1), 44–48.

Celli, B. (2003). *Pharmacotherapy in chronic obstructive pulmonary disease.* New York, NY: Marcel Dekker.

Joint Task Force on Practice Parameters Representing the American Academy of Allergy, Asthma, and Immunology, the American College of Allergy, Asthma, and Immunology, and the Joint Council of Allergy, Asthma, and Immunology. (2005). Obtaining optimal asthma control: A practice parameter. *Journal of Allergy and Clinical Immunology.* Retrieved September 4, 2008, from http://www.jaconline.org/webfiles/images/journals/YMAI/5412.pdf

Luggen, A. S. (2004). Pharmacology tips: Medications that complicate asthma control in older people. *Geriatric Nursing, 25*(3), 184.

Matsuyama, W., Mitsuyama, H., Watanabe, M., Oonakahara, K., Higashimoto, I., Osame, M., & Arimura, K. (2005). Effects of omega-3 polyunsaturated fatty acids on inflammatory markers in COPD. *Chest, 128*(6), 3817–3827.

National Asthma Education and Prevention Program Coordinating Committee. (2007). *Expert panel report 3 (EPR3): Guidelines for the diagnosis and management of asthma.* Coordinated by the National Heart, Lung, and Blood Institute of the National Institutes of Health. Retrieved September 5, 2008, from http://www.nhlbi.nih.gov/guidelines/asthma/asthgdln.htm

Rogers, D. F. (2003). Airway hypersecretion in allergic rhinitis and asthma: New pharmacotherapy. *Current Allergy Asthma Reports, 3*(3), 238–248.

Roy, S. R. (2003). Asthma. *Southern Medical Journal, 96*(11), 1061–1067.

Stevens, N. (2003). Inhaler devices for asthma and COPD: Choice and technique. *Professional Nurse, 18*(11), 641–645.

Undem, B. J. (2006). Pharmacotherapy of asthma. In L. L. Brunton, J. S. Lazo, and K. L. Parker (Eds.), *Goodman & Gilman's The pharmacological basis of therapeutics* (11th ed., pp. 717–735). New York, NY: McGraw-Hill.

Vega, C. (2005). Budesonide/formoterol may be effective for maintenance and acute relief of asthma. *American Journal of Respiratory Critical Care Medicine, 171,* 129–136.

Weir, P. (2004). Quick asthma assessment: A stepwise approach to treatment. *Advance for Nurse Practitioners, 12*(1), 53–56.

Chapter 40

Chaiyakunapruk, N., Nathisuwan, S., Leeprakobboon, K., & Leelasettagool, C. (2006). The efficacy of ginger for the prevention of postoperative nausea and vomiting: A meta-analysis. *American Journal of Obstetrics and Gynecology, 194,* 95–99.

Feldman, M., & Le, M. (2007). *Gastroenterology II: Peptic ulcer diseases, May 2007 update.* Philadelphia: APCMedicine.

Gold, B., Scheiman, J., Sabesin, S., & Vitat, P. (2007). Updates on the management of upper gastrointestinal disorders in the primary care setting: NSAID-related gastropathies and pediatric reflux disease. *Journal of Family Practice, 56*(3), S1–S12.

Hoogerwerf, W. A., & Pasricha, P. J. (2006). Pharmacotherapy of gastric acidity, peptic ulcers, and gastroesophageal reflux disease. In L. L. Brunton, J. S. Lazo, and K. L. Parker (Eds.), *Goodman & Gilman's The pharmacological basis of therapeutics* (11th ed., pp. 967–982). New York, NY: McGraw-Hill.

Huggins, R. M., Scates, A. C., & Latour, J. K. (2003). Intravenous proton-pump inhibitors versus H_2-antagonists for treatment of GI bleeding. *Annals of Pharmacotherapy, 37*(3), 433–437.

Petersen, A. M. (2003). *Helicobacter pylori:* An invading microorganism? A review. *FEMS Immunology and Medical Microbiology, 36*(3), 117–126.

Sharma, P., & Vakil, N. (2003). Review article: *Helicobacter pylori* and reflux disease. A*limentary Pharmacology and Therapeutics, 17*(3), 297–305.

Stanghellini, V. (2003). Management of gastroesophageal reflux disease. *Drugs Today, 39*(Suppl A), 15–20.

Vanderhoff, B. T., & Tahboub, R. M. (2002). Proton pump inhibitors: An update. *American Family Physician, 66,* 273–280.

Chapter 41

Barclay, L. (2007). New guidelines for treatment of irritable bowel syndrome in adults. *Medscape Medical News.* Retrieved August 15, 2008, from http://www.medscape.com/viewarticle/556356

Feagan, B. G., Dieckgraefe, B. K., & Hanauer, S. B. (2006). *Advances in the treatment of Crohn's disease: From research to clinical practice.* Retrieved from http://www.medscape.com/viewprogram/5211

Franz, J., VanWormer, A., Crain, J., Boucher, T., Histon, W., Caplan, J., . . . & Pronk, N. P. (2007). Weight-loss outcomes: A systematic review and meta-analysis of weight-loss clinical trials with a minimum 1-year follow-up. *Journal of the American Dietetic Association, 107*(10), 1755–1767.

Glazer, G. (2001). Long-term pharmacotherapy of obesity: A review of efficacy and safety. *Archives of Internal Medicine, 161,* 1814–1824.

Guglietta, A. (2003). *Pharmacotherapy of gastrointestinal inflammation.* Basel, Switzerland: Birkhauser Verlag.

Herrstedt, J. (2008). Antiemetics: An update and the MASCC guidelines applied to clinical practice. *Nature Clinical Practice Oncology, 5*(1), 32–43.

Knutson, D., Greenberg, G., & Cronau, H. (2003). Management of Crohn's disease: A practical approach. *American Family Physician, 68,* 707–714, 717–718.

Metcalf, C. (2007). Chronic diarrhea: Investigation, treatment, and nursing care. *Nursing Standard, 21*(21), 48–56.

Pasricha, P. J. (2006). Treatment of disorders of bowel motility and water flux; antiemetics; agents used in biliary and pancreatic disease. In L. L. Brunton, J. S. Lazo, and K. L. Parker (Eds.), *Goodman & Gilman's The pharmacological basis of therapeutics* (11th ed., pp. 983–1008). New York, NY: McGraw-Hill.

Pray, W. S., and Pray, J. J. (2005). Diarrhea: Sweeping changes in the OTC market. *U.S. Pharmacist, 30*(1), 17–27.

Scorza, K., Williams, A., Phillips, J. D., & Shaw, J. (2007). Evaluation of nausea and vomiting. *American Family Physician, 76*(1), 76–84.

Sellin, J. H., and Pasricha, P. J. (2006). Pharmacotherapy of inflammatory bowel disease. In L. L. Brunton, J. S. Lazo, and K. L. Parker (Eds.), *Goodman & Gilman's The pharmacological basis of therapeutics* (11th ed., pp. 1009–1020). New York, NY: McGraw-Hill.

Spanier, J. A., Howden, C. W., & Jones, M. P. (2003). A systematic review of alternative therapies in the irritable bowel syndrome. *Archives of Internal Medicine, 163*(3), 265–274.

Spiller, R. (2008). Review article: Probiotics and prebiotics in irritable bowel syndrome. *Alimentary Pharmacology and Therapeutics, 28*(4), 385–396.

Weigle, D. S. (2003). Pharmacological therapy of obesity: Past, present, and future. *Journal of Clinical Endocrinology and Metabolism, 88*(6), 2462–2469.

Chapter 42

Bailey, L. B., Rampersaud, G. C., & Kauwell, G. P. (2003). Folic acid supplements and fortification affect the risk for neural tube defects, vascular disease, and cancer: Evolving science. *Journal of Nutrition, 133*(6), 1961S–1968S.

Dharmarajan, T. S., Adiga, G. U., & Norkus, E. P. (2003). Vitamin B_{12} deficiency. Recognizing subtle symptoms in older adults. *Geriatrics, 58*(3), 30–34, 37–38.

Douglas, R. M., Hemilä, H., Chalker, E., & Treacy, B. Vitamin C for preventing and treating the common cold. *Cochrane Database of Systematic Reviews, 2004*(4), CD000980.

Eden, A. N. (2003). Preventing iron deficiency in toddlers: A major public health problem. *Contemporary Pediatrics, 20*(2), 57–67.

Huisman-deWaal, G., Schoonhoven, L., Jansen, J., Wanten, G., & vanAchterberg, T. (2007). The impact of home parenteral nutrition on daily life. *Clinical Nutrition, 26*(3), 275–288.

Jean-Marie, S. (2007). Vitamin supplements: Ensuring a healthy start in life. *Nursing in Practice: The Journal for Today's Primary Care Nurse, 18*(33), 43–44, 46.

Joque, L., & Jatoi, A. (2005). Total parenteral nutrition in cancer patients: Why and when? *Nutrition in Clinical Care, 8*(2), 89–92.

Kaushansky, K., & Kipps, T. J. (2006). Hematopoietic agents: Growth factors, minerals, and vitamins. In L. L. Brunton, J. S. Lazo, and K. L. Parker (Eds.), *Goodman & Gilman's The pharmacological basis of therapeutics* (11th ed., pp. 1433–1466). New York, NY: McGraw-Hill.

More, J. (2007). Who needs vitamin supplements? *Journal of Family Health Care, 17*(2), 57–60.

Morin, K. (2005). Infant nutrition: Water-soluble vitamins. *American Journal of Maternal/Child Nursing, 30*(4), 271.

Oh, R. C., & Brown, D. L. (2003). Vitamin B_{12} deficiency. *American Family Physician, 67*, 979–986, 993–994.

Padayatty, S. J., Katz, A., Wang, Y., Eck, P., Kwon, O., Lee, J. H., . . . & Levine, M. (2003). Vitamin C as an antioxidant: Evaluation of its role in disease prevention. *Journal of the American College of Nutrition, 22*(1), 18–35.

Ragione, F. (2003). Vitamin A and infancy. Biochemical, functional, and clinical aspects. *Vitamins and Hormones, 66*, 457–591.

Rampersaud, G. C., Kauwell, G. P., & Bailey, L. B. (2003). Folate: A key to optimizing health and reducing disease risk in the elderly. *Journal of the American College of Nutrition, 22*(1), 1–8.

Risser, N., & Murphy, M. (2004). Literature review: Enteral nutrition. *Nurse Practitioner: American Journal of Primary Health Care, 29*(3), 49–59.

Tharp, R. (2007). *Complications of enteral nutrition.* Retrieved August 21, 2008, from http://www.rxkinetics.com/tpntutorial/ 2_1.html

Chapter 43

Andrioli, M., Giraldi, F. P., De Martin, M., & Cavagnini, F. (2007). Therapies for adrenal insufficiency. *Expert Opinion on Therapeutic Patents, 17*(11), 1323–1329.

Dahlgren, J., & Wikland, K. A. (2005). Final height in short children born small for gestational age treated with growth hormone. *Pediatric Research, 57*(2), 216–222.

Farwell, A. P., & Braverman, L. E. (2006). Thyroid and antithyroid drugs. In L. L. Brunton, J. S. Lazo, and K. L. Parker (Eds.), *Goodman & Gilman's The pharmacological basis of therapeutics* (11th ed., pp. 1511–1540). New York, NY: McGraw-Hill.

Griffiths, H., & Jordan, S. (2002). Corticosteroids: Implications for nursing practice. *Nursing Standard, 17*(12), 43–53.

Holcomb, S. S. (2002). Thyroid diseases: A primer for the critical care nurse. *Dimensions of Critical Care Nursing, 21*(4), 127–133.

Parker, K. L., & Schimmer, B. P. (2006). Pituitary hormones and their hypothalamic releasing factors. In L. L. Brunton, J. S. Lazo, and K. L. Parker (Eds.), *Goodman & Gilman's The pharmacological basis of therapeutics* (11th ed., pp. 1489–1510). New York, NY: McGraw-Hill.

Schori-Ahmed, D. (2003). Defenses gone awry: Thyroid disease. *RN, 66*(6), 38–43.

Chapter 44

American Diabetes Association. (2007). *From insulin to incretins: A report from the 67th Scientific Session of the American Diabetes Association.* Chicago: Author.

Bates, N. (2002). Overdose of insulin and other diabetic medication. *Emergency Nurse, 10*(7), 22–26.

Bohannon, N. J. V. (2002). Treating dual defects in diabetes: Insulin resistance and insulin secretion. *American Journal of Health-System Pharmacists, 59*(Suppl. 9), S9–S13.

Costa, J., Borges, M., David, C., & Carneiro, A.V. (2006). Efficacy of lipid lowering drug treatment for diabetic and non-diabetic patients: Meta-analysis of randomised controlled trials. *British Medical Journal, 332*, 1115–1124.

Davis, S. N. (2006). Insulin, oral hypoglycemic agents, and the pharmacology of the endocrine pancreas. In L. L. Brunton, J. S. Lazo, and K. L. Parker (Eds.), *Goodman & Gilman's The pharmacological basis of therapeutics* (11th ed., pp. 1613–1646). New York, NY: McGraw-Hill.

Feig, D. S., Briggs, G. G., & Koren, G. (2007). Oral antidiabetic agents in pregnancy and lactation: A paradigm shift? *Annals in Pharmacotherapy, 41*(7), 1174–1180.

Gregersen, S., Jeppesen, P. B., Holst, J. J., & Hermansen, K. (2004). Antihyperglycemic effects of stevioside in type 2 diabetic subjects. *Metabolism, 53*(1), 73–76.

Hjelm, K., Mufunda, E., Nambozi, G., & Kemp, J. (2003). Preparing nurses to face the pandemic of diabetes mellitus: A literature review. *Journal of Advanced Nursing, 41*, 424–435.

Hovens, M. M., Tamsma, J. T., Beishuizen, E. D., & Huisman, M. V. (2005). Pharmacological strategies to reduce cardiovascular risk in type 2 diabetes mellitus: An update. *Drugs, 65*(4), 433–445.

McKnight-Menci, H., Sababu, S., & Kelly, S. D. (2005). The care of children and adolescents with type 2 diabetes. *Journal of Pediatric Nursing, 20*(2), 96–106.

Mokdad, A. H., Bowman, B. A., & Ford, E. S. (2001). The continuing epidemics of obesity and diabetes in the United States. *Journal of the American Medical Association, 286*, 1195–1200.

VandeLaar, F. A., Akkermans, R. P., & van Binsbergen, J. J. (2007). Limited evidence for effects of diet for type 2 diabetes from systematic reviews. *European Journal of Clinical Nutrition, 61*(8), 929–937.

Chapter 45

Davidson, M. R., London, M. L., & Ladewig, P. L. (2008). *Maternal newborn nursing and women's health across the lifespan* (8th ed.).Upper Saddle River, NJ: Prentice Hall.

David, P. S., Boatwright, E. A., Tozer, B. S., Verma, D. P., Blair, J. E., Mayer, A. P., et al. (2006). Hormonal contraception update. *Mayo Clinic Proceedings, 81*(7), 949–955.

Erkkola, R. (2007). Recent advances in hormonal contraception. *Current Opinion in Obstetrics & Gynecology, 19*(6), 547–553.

Hansen, L. B., & Portman, D. (2006). Hormone therapy update: Current recommendations for menopausal symptoms. *US Pharmacist, 31*(9), 89–96.

Leeman, L., Fontaine, P., King, V., Klein, M. C., & Ratcliffe, S. (2003). The nature and management of labor pain: Part II. Pharmacologic pain relief. *American Family Physician, 68*, 1115–1120, 1121–1122.

Loose, D. S., & Stancel, G. M. (2006). Estrogens. In L. L. Brunton, J. S. Lazo, and K. L. Parker (Eds.), *Goodman & Gilman's The pharmacological basis of therapeutics* (11th ed., pp. 1541–1572). New York, NY: McGraw-Hill.

Ludwig, M., Westergaard, L. G., Diedrich, K., & Andersen, C. Y. (2003). Developments in drugs for ovarian stimulation. *Best Practice and Research. Clinical Obstetrics and Gynecology, 17*(2), 231–247.

Olds, S. B., London, M. L., Ladewig, P. A., & Davidson, M. R. (2008). *Maternal–newborn nursing and women's health care* (8th ed.). Upper Saddle River, NJ: Prentice Hall Health.

Osmers, R., Friede, M., Liske, E., Schnitker, J., Freudenstein, J., & Henneicke-von Zepelin, H. H. (2005). Efficacy and safety of isopropanolic black cohosh extract for climacteric symptoms. *Obstetrics and Gynecology, 105*(5 pt 1), 1074–1083.

Prine, L. (2007). Emergency contraception: Myths and facts. *Obstetrics and Gynecology Clinics of North America, 34*(1), 127–136.

Stearns, V. (2007). Clinical update: New treatments for hot flashes. *The Lancet, 369*(9579), 2062–2064.

Chapter 46

Bent, S., Kane, C., Shinohara, K., Neuhaus, J., Hudes, E. S., Goldberg, H., & Avins, A. L. (2006). Saw palmetto for benign prostatic hyperplasia. *New England Journal of Medicine, 354*(6), 557–566.

Bullock, T. L., & Andriole, G. L. (2006). Emerging drug therapies for benign prostatic hyperplasia. *Expert Opinion on Emergency Drugs, 11*(1), 111–123.

Carrier, S. (2003). Pharmacology of phosphodiesterase 5 inhibitors. *Canadian Journal of Urology, 10*(Suppl. 1), 12–16.

Ficorelli, C. (2007). Untangling the complexities of male infertility. *Nursing, 2007, 37*(1), 24–26.

Gordon, A. E., & Shaughnessy, A. F. (2003). Saw palmetto for prostate disorders. *American Family Physician, 67*(6), 1281–1283.

Kassabian, V. S. (2003). Sexual function in patients treated for benign prostatic hyperplasia. *Lancet, 361*(9351), 60–62.

Khastgir, J., Arya, M., Shergill, I. S., Kalsi, J. S., Minhas, S., & Mundy, A. R. (2002). Current concepts in the pharmacotherapy of benign prostatic hyperplasia. *Expert Opinion on Pharmacotherapy, 3*(12), 1727–1737.

Mcleod, D. G. (2003). Hormonal therapy: Historical perspective to future directions. *Urology, 61*(2, Suppl. 1), 3–7.

Snyder, P. J. (2006). Androgens. In L. L. Brunton, J. S. Lazo, and K. L. Parker (Eds.), *Goodman & Gilman's The pharmacological basis of therapeutics* (11th ed., pp. 1573–1586). New York, NY: McGraw-Hill.

Spencer, M. (2007, March 30). Management of erectile dysfunction in primary care. *GP: General Practitioner,* 36–37.

Steiner, B. S. (2002). Hypogonadism in men. A review of diagnosis and treatment. *Advance for Nurse Practitioners, 10*(4), 22–27, 29.

Chapter 47

Burke, A., Smyth, E. M., & Fitzgerald, G. A. (2006). Analgesic–antipyretic agents; Pharmacotherapy of gout. In L. L. Brunton, J. S. Lazo, and K. L. Parker (Eds.). *Goodman & Gilman's The pharmacological basis of therapeutics* (11th ed., pp. 671–716). New York, NY: McGraw-Hill.

Clegg, D. O., Reda, D. J., Harris, C. L., Klein, M. A., O'Dell, J. R., Hooper, M. M., . . . & Williams, H. J. (2006). Glucosamine, chondroitin sulfate, and the two in combination for painful knee osteoarthritis. *New England Journal of Medicine, 354*(8), 795–808.

Curry, L. C., & Hogstel, M. O. (2002). Osteoporosis. *American Journal of Nursing, 102,* 26–32.

Friedman, P. A. (2006). Agents affecting mineral ion homeostasis and bone turnover. In L. L. Brunton, J. S. Lazo, and K. L. Parker (Eds.), *Goodman & Gilman's The pharmacological basis of therapeutics* (11th ed., pp. 1647–1677). New York, NY: McGraw-Hill.

Kuehn, B. (2007). Knee therapies probed. *Journal of the American Medical Association, 298*(20), 2361.

Love, C. (2003). Dietary needs for bone health and the prevention of osteoporosis. *British Journal of Nursing, 12*(1), 12–21.

Olsen, N. J., & Stein, C. M. (2004). New drugs for rheumatoid arthritis. *New England Journal of Medicine, 350*(21), 2167–2179.

Qaseem, A., Snow, V., Shekelle, P., Hopkins Jr., R., Forciea, M. A., & Owens, D. K. (2008). Screening for osteoporosis in men: A clinical practice guideline from the American College of Physicians. *Annals of Internal Medicine, 148*(9), 680–684.

Secrist, J. (2003). Osteoporosis. Part IV. Rapid review of drug therapies (A to Z) for preventing male osteoporosis/fractures. *Urology Nursing, 23*(2), 168–174.

Watts, N. B. (2003). Bisphosphonate treatment of osteoporosis. *Clinical Geriatric Medicine,19*(2), 395–414.

Chapter 48

Bayliffe, A. I., Brigandi, R. A., Wilkins, H. J., & Levick, M. P. (2004). Emerging therapeutic targets in psoriasis. *Current Opinions in Pharmacology, 4*(3), 306–310.

Fox, L. P., Merk, H. F., & Bickers, D. R. (2006). Dermatological pharmacology. In L. L. Brunton, J. S. Lazo, and K. L. Parker (Eds.), *Goodman & Gilman's The pharmacological basis of therapeutics* (11th ed., pp. 1679–1706). New York, NY: McGraw-Hill.

Jesitus, J. (2007). Rosacea requires multifaceted approach. *Dermatology Times, 28*(1), 50–63.

Lebwohl, M. (2003). Psoriasis. *Lancet, 361,* 1197–1206.

Leung, D. Y., & Boguniewicz, M. (2003). Advances in allergic skin diseases. *Journal of Allergy and Clinical Immunology, 111*(Suppl. 3), S805–S812.

Murphy, K. D., Lee, J. O., & Herndon, D. N. (2003). Current pharmacotherapy for the treatment of severe burns. *Expert Opinion on Pharmacotherapy, 4*(3), 369–384.

Nash, K. (2007). Options still limited for age-old problem. *Dermatology Times, 28*(6), 40–41.

Schwartz, R. A., Janusz, C. A., & Janniger, C. K. (2006). Seborrheic dermatitis. *American Family Physician, 74*(1), 125–130.

Smith, G. (2003). Cutaneous expression of cytochrome P-450 CYP25: Individuality in regulation by therapeutic agents for psoriasis and other skin diseases. *Lancet, 361,* 1336–1344.

Smolinski, K. N., & Yan, A. C. (2004). Acne update: 2004. *Current Opinion in Pediatrics, 16*(4), 385–391.

Snow, M. (2007). The truth about scabies. *Nursing, 37*(2), 28–30.

Chapter 49

American Academy of Family Physicians and American Academy of Pediatrics. (2004). *Diagnosis and management of acute otitis media.* Retrieved September 8, 2008, from http://www.aafp.org/online/en/home/clinical/clinicalrecs/aom.html

Beers, S. L., & Abramo, T. J. (2004). Otitis externa review. *Pediatric Emergency Care, 20*(4), 250–256.

Fingeret, M. (2007). Understanding glaucoma medications. *Review of Optometry, 144,* 13–15.

Friedman, D. (2007). Primary angle closure glaucoma. *Review of Optometry, 144,* 26–27.

Henderer, J. D., & Rapuano, C. J. (2006). Ocular pharmacology. In L. L. Brunton, J. S. Lazo, and K. L. Parker (Eds.), *Goodman & Gilman's The pharmacological basis of therapeutics* (11th ed., pp. 1707–1737). New York, NY: McGraw-Hill.

McCarter, D., Courtney, A., & Porter, S. (2007). Cerumen impaction. *American Family Physician, 75*(10), 1523–1528.

Osguthorpe, J. D., & Nielsen, D. R. (2006). Otitis externa: Review and clinical update. *American Family Physician, 74*(9), 1510–1516.

Schwartz, K. A., & Budenz, D. B. (2004). Current management of glaucoma. *Current Opinion in Ophthalmology, 15*(2), 119–126.

Tripathi, R. C., Tripathi, B. J., & Haggerty, C. (2003). Drug-induced glaucomas: Mechanism and management. *Drug Safety, 26*(11), 749–767.

Wright, J. (2005). Common ear problems in the primary care setting. *Journal of Community Nursing, 19*(9), 43–46.

ANSWERS

Chapter 1

Answers to Critical Thinking Questions

1 The patient may choose OTC drugs rather than more effective prescription medications for a variety of reasons. OTC drugs do not require the patient to see a health care provider to write a prescription for the drug. By not seeing a health care provider, the patient saves time and money. OTC drugs are obtained much more easily than prescription drugs. Patients often think they can effectively treat themselves and that OTC drugs do not have as many side effects as prescription drugs.

2 The FDA is the agency responsible for determining whether prescription and OTC drugs may be used for therapy. By reviewing the availability of safe, effective drugs, the FDA is responsible for keeping unsafe and ineffective drugs off the market. Another of the agency's goals is to improve the health of Americans and ensure that drug information is clear and easily understandable. Over the years, the scope of the FDA has been broadened to include information on biologics, which include serums, vaccines, and blood products. The FDA also has the authority to recommend civil penalties if the guidelines are not followed and to remove dietary supplements that cause a significant risk to the public.

3 The FDA takes part in the postmarketing surveillance stage of the drug approval process. In this phase, the drug is monitored for harmful effects in the larger population. The FDA holds public meetings to receive feedback from patients and organizations regarding the safety and effectiveness of new drug therapies.

4 Nurses are responsible for the safe administration of medications, monitoring for therapeutic and adverse effects of those drugs, and for providing education for their patients who are taking drugs. Learning pharmacology, the proper administration of medications, and patient education are all nursing responsibilities. During the drug approval process, some nurses may administer medications to patients participating in phase II and III clinical trials, but all nurses participate in phase IV postmarketing surveillance by reporting adverse drug reactions.

Chapter 2

Answers to Critical Thinking Questions

1 The therapeutic classification is a method of organizing drugs based on their therapeutic usefulness in treating particular diseases. The pharmacologic classification refers to how an agent works at the molecular, tissue, and body system levels. A beta-adrenergic blocker is pharma-cologic; an oral contraceptive is therapeutic; a laxative is therapeutic; a folic acid antagonist is pharmacologic; an antianginal agent is therapeutic.

2 Prototype drugs exhibit typical or essential features of the drugs within a specific class.

3 Generic advantages include cost savings to the patient and the fact that only one name is assigned for the drug; therefore, the name is less complicated and easier to remember. However, because generic drug formularies may be different, the inert ingredients may be somewhat different and, consequently, may affect the ability of the drug to reach the target cells and produce an effect.

4 Schedules refer to the potential for abuse. These schedules help the nurse identify the potential for abuse and require the nurse to maintain complete records for all quantities. The higher the abuse potential, the more restrictions are placed on the health care provider and the filling of refills.

5 This Schedule III drug is a controlled substance restricted by the Controlled Substance Act of 1970 and is regulated by the DEA. A Schedule III drug has a moderate potential for abuse and physical dependency and a high potential for psychologic dependence.

Chapter 3

Answers to NCLEX-RN® Review Questions

1 *Answer: 1*
Rationale: The primary responsibility of the nurse is to ensure patient safety when administering prescribed medications. Patient compliance includes much more than watching the patient take medications. Accurate health care provider orders are a part of ensuring safe medication administration. ***Cognitive Level:*** Comprehension. ***Nursing Process:*** Implementation. ***Patient Need:*** Health Promotion and Maintenance.

2 *Answer: 3*
Rationale: The enteral route involves the process of swallowing by definition. ***Cognitive Level:*** Comprehension. ***Nursing Process:*** Assessment. ***Patient Need:*** Health Promotion and Maintenance.

3 *Answer: 3*
Rationale: This question asks for the highest priority; therefore, all the answers are correct, but one should stand out as the first action the nurse should take. Think about patient safety. In this example, the drug has been newly prescribed; therefore, notifying the health care provider of the patient's reaction takes priority so that new medication orders can be received to address the allergic reaction and to discontinue the present order. ***Cognitive Level:*** Analysis. ***Nursing Process:*** Implementation. ***Patient Need:*** Physiological Integrity.

4 *Answer: 2*

Rationale: STAT means immediately. *ASAP* orders should be administered within 30 minutes. ***Cognitive Level:*** Application. ***Nursing Process:*** Implementation. ***Patient Need:*** Physiological Integrity.

5 *Answers: 2, 3, 5*

Rationale: Enteric-coated tablets are designed to dissolve in the alkaline environment of the small intestine. Sustained-release medications dissolve very slowly over an extended period for a longer duration. IV medications are designed to enter directly into the bloodstream. Liquid forms or finely crushed tablets are the preferred forms. ***Cognitive Level:*** Application. ***Nursing Process:*** Implementation. ***Patient Need:*** Physiological Integrity.

6 *Answer: 4*

While a patient who is NPO for surgery is not usually allowed anything to eat or drink, crucial medications such as drugs to control blood sugar may be allowed or a different form (e.g., insulin by injection) may be given. The nurse should contact the health care provider and check if any additional orders are needed. ***Cognitive Level:*** Analysis. ***Nursing Process:*** Implementation. ***Patient Need:*** Physiological Integrity.

Answers to Critical Thinking Questions

1 Although the nurse is responsible for safe medication administration, errors continue because many disciplines are responsible for safe and accurate drug administration. Many steps are involved in the safe administration of medications, and there are multiple points where errors can occur.

2 To help ensure drug compliance, the nurse and patient should formulate an individualized plan of care using the nursing process. Including the patient in this process enables the patient to participate fully, which encourages compliance with the treatment plan.

3 The IV route has the fastest onset because medications are administered directly into the bloodstream. IV medications also bypass the digestive system and the first-pass effect. When administering parental medications (IV, intradermal, subcutaneous, and IM routes), the nurse must ensure that aseptic techniques are strictly used.

4 The metric system is much more accurate than the household or apothecary system. Using the metric system helps ensure that the safest, most accurate doses are prepared and administered.

Chapter 4

Answers to NCLEX-RN® Review Questions

1 *Answer: 1*

Rationale: Some medications can be affected by foods, beverages, or other drugs. The effect of calcium, iron, and magnesium on a tetracycline antibiotic is an example of a food–drug interaction that occurs in the absorption process.

2 *Answer: 1*

Rationale: The blood–brain barrier may cause difficulty in treating tumors. Most antitumor medications do not cross the blood–brain barrier. ***Cognitive Level:*** Analysis. ***Nursing Process:*** Assessment. ***Patient Need:*** Physiological Integrity.

3 *Answer: 1*

Rationale: The liver is the primary site of drug metabolism. Patients with severe liver damage, such as that caused by cirrhosis, will require reductions in drug dosage because of the decreased metabolic activity. ***Cognitive Level:*** Analysis. ***Nursing Process:*** Implementation. ***Patient Need:*** Physiological Integrity.

4 *Answer: 4*

Rationale: Some oral drugs are rendered inactive by hepatic metabolic reactions, during the process known as the first-pass effect. An alternative route may need to be assessed. ***Cognitive Level:*** Application. ***Nursing Process:*** Implementation. ***Patient Need:*** Physiological Integrity.

5 *Answer: 3*

Rationale: The kidneys are the primary site of excretion. Renal failure increases the duration of the drug's action because of decreased excretion. The patient must be assessed for drug toxicity. ***Cognitive Level:*** Analysis. ***Nursing Process:*** Assessment. ***Patient Need:*** Physiological Integrity.

6 *Answers: 1, 2, 3*

Rationale: Glandular activity is an elimination mechanism in which water-soluble drugs are excreted into saliva, sweat, and breast milk. Secretion of drugs in the bile is known as *biliary excretion*. ***Cognitive Level:*** Application. ***Nursing Process:*** Implementation. ***Patient Need:*** Physiological Integrity.

Answers to Critical Thinking Questions

1 For most medications, the greatest barrier is crossing the many membranes that separate the drug from its target cells. A drug taken by mouth must cross the plasma membranes of the mucosal cells of the gastrointestinal tract and the capillary endothelial cells to enter the bloodstream. To leave the bloodstream, it must again cross capillary cells, travel through interstitial fluid, and enter target cells by passing through their plasma membranes. Depending on the mechanism of action, the drug may also need to enter cellular organelles, such as the nucleus, which are surrounded by additional membranes. While seeking their target cells and attempting to pass through the various membranes, drugs are subjected to numerous physiologic substances such as stomach acids and digestive enzymes.

2 The plasma half-life is the time required for the concentration of the medication in the plasma to decrease to half its initial value after administration. This value is important to nurses because the longer the half-life, the longer it takes the medication to be excreted. The medication will then produce a longer effect in the body. The half-life

determines how often a medication will be administered. Renal and hepatic diseases will prolong the half-life of drugs, increasing the potential for toxicity.

3 The degree of ionization of a drug affects its absorption. The pH of the local environment directly influences drug absorption through its ability to ionize the drug. The relationship between pH and drug excretion can be used in critical situations to either increase or decrease excretion of the drug.

4 Many oral drugs are rendered inactive by hepatic metabolic reactions. Alternative routes of delivery that bypass the first-pass effect (sublingual, rectal, or parenteral routes) may need to be considered for these drugs.

Chapter 5

Answers to NCLEX-RN® Review Questions

1 *Answer: 2*

Rationale: Unpredictable and unexplained drug reactions are labeled *idiosyncratic*. **Cognitive Level:** Analysis. **Nursing Process:** Implementation. **Patient Need:** Physiological Integrity.

2 *Answer: 1*

Rationale: An antagonist occupies a receptor site and prevents endogenous chemicals from acting. An agonist produces the same type of response as the endogenous substance. A partial agonist is a medication that produces a weaker response than an agonist. **Cognitive Level:** Application. **Nursing Process:** Implementation. **Patient Need:** Physiological Integrity.

3 *Answer: 2*

Rationale: The most important property is efficacy. *Efficacy* is the magnitude of the maximal response that can be produced from a drug. **Cognitive Level:** Application. **Nursing Process:** Implementation. **Patient Need:** Physiological Integrity.

4 *Answer: 1*

Rationale: The term *efficacious* refers to the response that can be produced from a particular drug. **Cognitive Level:** Application. **Nursing Process:** Implementation. **Patient Need:** Physiological Integrity.

5 *Answer: 4*

Rationale: A drug that is more *efficacious* produces a higher maximal response. If other drugs for pain were not effective in relieving the pain, morphine would be considered to have a greater efficacy in relieving this type of pain. **Cognitive Level:** Application. **Nursing Process:** Implementation. **Patient Need:** Physiological Integrity.

6 *Answer: 2*

A narrow therapeutic index indicates that there is only a small amount of difference between the dosage needed to be effective (ED_{50}) and the dosage that will be toxic (LD_{50}). Extra caution should be taken with drugs with a narrow therapeutic index to avoid giving an excessive dose and to ensure

patient safety. **Cognitive Level**: Application. **Nursing Process**: Implementation. **Patient Need**: Physiological Integrity.

Answers to Critical Thinking Questions

1 The other 50% of the patients did not experience the desired effect from the dose.

2 An agonist binds to the receptor and produces the same or a greater response than the endogenous chemical. An antagonist occupies a receptor site and prevents the endogenous substance from acting. Antagonists compete with agonists for binding sites. An antihistamine would most likely be an antagonist.

Chapter 6

Answers to NCLEX-RN® Review Questions

1 *Answer: 1*

Rationale: NANDA classifies a nursing diagnosis as a clinical judgment about individual, family, or community responses to actual or potential health/life processes. Per NANDA, nursing diagnoses provide the basis for the selection of nursing interventions to achieve outcomes for which the nurse is accountable. **Cognitive Level:** Analysis. **Nursing Process:** Assessment. **Patient Need:** Health Promotion and Maintenance.

2 *Answer: 2*

Rationale: Goals focus on what a patient should be able to achieve and outcomes provide the specific, measurable criteria that will be used to measure goal attainment. "*The patient will demonstrate self-injection of insulin* (what should be achieved) *using a preloaded syringe, into the subcutaneous tissue of the thigh prior to discharge*" (specific, measurable criteria used to measure goal attainment). **Cognitive Level:** Application. **Nursing Process:** Evaluation. **Patient Need:** Physiological Integrity.

3 *Answer: 1*

Rationale: NANDA defines Deficient Knowledge as lacking the specific knowledge necessary to make informed choices. *Noncompliance* is incorrect because it assumes the patient has made an *educated* decision about the treatment plan. By stating that she "did not want to gain weight and is afraid of needle marks," this patient has identified a lack of knowledge related to the effects of insulin (effect on weight) and administration techniques (needle marks). The nurse plays a key role in educating the patient about the effects of insulin and appropriate administration techniques. **Cognitive Level:** Application. **Nursing Process:** Intervention. **Patient Need:** Psychological Integrity.

4 *Answer: 4*

Rationale: Evidence of therapeutic benefit (i.e., efficacy) is the most important factor to assess when evaluating the effectiveness of any medication. **Cognitive Level:** Application. **Nursing Process:** Evaluation. **Patient Need:** Physiological Integrity.

5 *Answer: 4*

Rationale: The purpose of evaluation in the nursing process is to determine whether the goals and outcomes have been adequately met by the patient. *Cognitive Level:* Application. *Nursing Process:* Assessment. *Patient Need:* Health Promotion and Maintenance.

6 *Answer: 3*

Rationale: By monitoring the patient for both therapeutic and adverse effects, the nurse carries out the evaluation phase of the nursing process. *Cognitive Level:* Analysis. *Nursing Process:* Evaluation. *Patient Need:* Physiological Integrity.

Answers to Critical Thinking Questions

1 The nurse would need to determine whether the patient and her mother have had sufficient information about the patient's type 1 diabetes in order to make appropriate choices regarding the patient's eating habits, weight, and diabetes management. A dietary history should be assessed including frequency of meals and snacks, types of foods consumed, overall number of calories per day, and the availability of healthy food choices at home, at school, and during athletic activities. An assessment of the type(s) and amount of insulin taken as well as an assessment for adverse effects should also be gathered. Cost issues related to insulin administration or equipment for monitoring should also be discussed with the patient and mother. If indicated, a physical exam should be recommended because weight loss is a symptom of uncontrolled type 1 diabetes. The nurse would also explore the patient's and her mother's understanding of the diagnosis, their expectations about the treatment plan, and any previous teaching given, correcting any misunderstandings or misinformation. *Noncompliance* assumes the patient has made an *educated* decision about the treatment plan. If insufficient knowledge about the condition, treatment plan, or care needs is the reason behind the health-seeking behavior in this case example, noncompliance would be an inappropriate nursing diagnosis.

2 Since an insulin pump will be a new component of the patient's treatment plan, the following nursing diagnoses would be appropriate for this patient:

- Deficient Knowledge (related to new or changed treatment routine)

- Ineffective Therapeutic Regimen Management (related to deficient knowledge or altered compliance with prescribed treatment)

- Risk for Infection (related to implanted subcutaneous catheter used for delivering insulin via pump)

- Risk for Injury (related to adverse drug effects, hypoglycemia or hyperglycemia related to insulin dosage)

3 State Nurse Practice Acts and accrediting organizations such as JCAHO consider patient education as a primary role for nurses. In order to ensure the safe and effective use of medications, patient education concerning medications should include the therapeutic uses and expected effects, monitoring for side and adverse effects and how to handle them, how to correctly administer the medication, and any other special requirements needed to ensure therapeutic effect. Each time a medication is administered presents an opportunity for patient education and small portions of information given over time are often better than large amounts of information presented all at once. It also provides the patient with an opportunity to ask questions about the medications or the treatment plan.

Chapter 7

Answers to NCLEX-RN® Review Questions

1 *Answer: 3*

Rationale: Isotretinoin (Accutane) is FDA pregnancy category X and is contraindicated during pregnancy. It should not be used at all during pregnancy. *Cognitive Level:* Application. *Nursing Process:* Implementation. *Patient Need:* Physiological Integrity.

2 *Answer: 4*

Rationale: Administration immediately after breast-feeding allows as much time as possible for the medication to be excreted from the mother's body prior to the next feeding. The other options do not provide enough time for the medication to be excreted. *Cognitive Level:* Analysis. *Nursing Process:* Implementation. *Patient Need:* Physiological Integrity.

3 *Answer: 3*

Rationale: Medications should be stored in child-resistant containers and out of reach of children. Patients with arthritic hands may request special easy-to-open medication containers to make self-administration easier. These two situations may be in conflict if elders and children are present in the same home. Toddlers are at risk for poisoning. If the patient cares for a young child, explore options for keeping the medication away from the child such as using a locked box or other safe storage options. This would allow the patient to continue to visit with or care for young children if desired. *Cognitive Level:* Analysis. *Nursing Process:* Evaluation. *Patient Need:* Physiological Integrity.

4 *Answer: 4*

Rationale: Toddlers may resist taking medications. Short explanations followed by immediate (kind but firm) drug administration are best. Children should not be told that medicine is candy for safety reasons. A toddler is not able to make a decision regarding medication administration. When medication is mixed with liquids or other food products, a small amount should be used; 8 oz is too much liquid to use for mixing. *Cognitive Level:* Analysis. *Nursing Process:* Implementation. *Patient Need:* Physiological Integrity.

5 *Answer: vastus lateralis*

Rationale: The middle third of the vastus lateralis muscle is the preferred site for intramuscular injection in the newborn. The middle third of the rectus femoris is an alternate site, but its proximity to major vessels and the sciatic nerve requires caution in using this site for injection. ***Cognitive Level:*** Comprehension. ***Nursing Process:*** Implementation. ***Patient Need:*** Physiological Integrity.

6 *Answer: 3*

Rationale: With each visit, the nurse should take a medication history of all OTC and prescription medications, noting any new medications not previously mentioned. A "pharmacy history" will draw attention to the possibility that the patient is obtaining medications from more than one pharmacy, a potential problem in polypharmacy. ***Cognitive Level:*** Analysis. ***Nursing Process:*** Implementation. ***Patient Need:*** Physiological Integrity.

Answers to Critical Thinking Questions

1 Pyelonephritis is frequently associated with preterm labor in pregnancy. Before initiating antibiotic therapy, the nurse should first determine the fetal gestational age. The potential for a drug to be teratogenic is highest during the first trimester. The nurse should also look up the pregnancy classification of the antibiotic. Selected agents, such as tetracyclines, should not be used during pregnancy. The nurse should address any concerns regarding the drug category with the health care provider.

2 Prior to considering a sedative agent, the nurse should assess the patient for other physical causes of confusion. For example, in the frail elderly, alterations in electrolytes, drug side effects, and rapid environmental changes can contribute to confusion. Attempts at reorientation should be made. The nurse should determine how diazepam (Valium) is distributed and metabolized. Valium is a fat-soluble drug; thus, because elderly patients have increased total body fat, the drug has a much longer half-life. In addition, numerous drugs decrease the metabolism of diazepam and may contribute to an increased half-life and enhanced CNS depression. If sedation is deemed necessary, other drugs should be considered.

3 The nurse should consult with the provider or pharmacist regarding the need to repeat the dose. Many oral elixirs are absorbed, to some degree, in the mucous membranes of the oral cavity. Therefore, the nurse may not need to repeat the dose. Acetaminophen can also be toxic to the liver in doses only slightly higher than normal and extra caution should be used for all drugs containing acetaminophen. The nurse should consider using an oral syringe to accurately measure and administer medications to infants. The syringe tip should be placed in the side of the mouth, not forced over the tongue. Conditions affecting the GI tract, such as gastroenteritis, can affect drug absorption because of their effect on peristalsis.

Chapter 8

Answers to NCLEX-RN® Review Questions

1 *Answer: 2*

Rationale: Many cultural groups believe in using herbs and other alternative therapies either along with or in place of traditional medicines. The nurse should examine how these herbal and alternative therapies will affect the desired pharmacotherapeutic outcomes of the prescribed medications. The physician or prescriber should be notified if the patient refuses to take the prescribed medications and for any questions the nurse may have concerning the safety of the herbal and prescribed medication interactions. ***Cognitive Level:*** Assessment. ***Nursing Process:*** Application. ***Patient Need:*** Physiological Integrity.

2 *Answers: 1, 2, 3*

Rationale: Written materials allow the patient and family to review information on additional occasions at home, but up to 48% of English-speaking patients do not have the basic ability to read, understand, and act on health information. This rate is even higher among non-English-speaking individuals and older patients. The nurse must be aware of the patient's literacy level and take appropriate action to ensure that information is understood. An assessment of visual impairment should also be made and large-print materials provided when necessary. ***Cognitive Level:*** Assessment. ***Nursing Process:*** Analysis. ***Patient Need:*** Health Promotion and Maintenance.

3 *Answer: 2*

Rationale: Women seek health care earlier than men. Men and women are both affected by Alzheimer's disease; however, women are one and a half to three times more likely to develop the disease. ***Cognitive Level:*** Analysis. ***Nursing Process:*** Diagnosis. ***Patient Need:*** Health Promotion and Maintenance.

4 *Answer: 2*

Rationale: When patients have strong spiritual or religious beliefs, these may greatly influence their perceptions of illness and their preferred modes of treatment. Ill health and spiritual issues can have an impact on wellness, nursing care, and pharmacotherapy. ***Cognitive Level:*** Analysis. ***Nursing Process:*** Assessment. ***Patient Need:*** Psychosocial Integrity.

5 *Answer: 1*

Rationale: Slow acetylators experience a delay in drug metabolism in the liver. This can cause the drug to build to toxic levels and result in drug toxicity. ***Cognitive Level:*** Application. ***Nursing Process:*** Evaluation. ***Patient Need:*** Psychological Integrity.

6 *Answer: 4*

Rationale: To treat a patient holistically, the nurse seeks to understand the multiple factors that may contribute or help solve a specific patient problem. By asking for the patient's own evaluation of the problem, the nurse can determine the severity of the problem and the impact it has on normal activities. These determinations help to develop a plan of care specifically tailored to individual patient needs. ***Cognitive Level:*** Application. ***Nursing Process:*** Assessment. ***Patient Need:*** Safe, Effective Care Environment.

Answers to Critical Thinking Questions

1 The primary concern for this patient would be the potential for drug–food interactions. Warfarin (Coumadin) achieves

its anticoagulant effect by interfering with the synthesis of vitamin K-dependent clotting factors. The anticoagulant effect of Coumadin can be decreased by a diet high in vitamin K. Fresh greens and tomatoes from the garden are excellent sources of vitamin K. The nurse must include questions related to the dietary intake of these foods. It is common for rural people to "eat out of their gardens" during the growing season. The nurse must also determine whether other medications have been added to the patient's regimen that could interfere with the action of Coumadin.

2 As women age, they experience a 10% decrease in total body water. In general, body weight also decreases in this aging population. The nurse should carefully assess the patient's current weight and compare it with the previously documented weight. In addition, because this patient's body weight has decreased, she may also have decreased serum protein. The dose of furosemide is dependent on the degree of protein binding; therefore, less serum protein could make the drug more pharmacologically active. The patient may need to have the dosage adjusted.

3 Per assessment in the clinic, it was noted that the patient is possibly a migrant farm worker, has limited English proficiency, and has a condition which has developed over time (abscessed teeth). This may indicate a potential lack of health care, a knowledge or a therapeutic management deficit, or other related concerns. Cost issues, fear related to potential immigration status, lack of available health care, misunderstandings related to limited English proficiency, or lack of time available to leave work and take care of his health care needs could all be factors leading to his condition. Further holistic assessment of the patient will help the nurse determine probable reasons for his present condition.

Chapter 9

Answers to NCLEX-RN® Review Questions

1 *Answer: 4*
Rationale: Nurse practice acts encompass all aspects of nursing, including the definition of professional nursing, medication administration, and definition of standards of care. *Cognitive Level:* Analysis. *Nursing Process:* Implementation. *Patient Need:* Safe, Effective Care Environment.

2 *Answer: 3*
Rationale: The nurse is responsible for documenting medication errors and completing an incident report for review by the facility's quality assurance personnel. *Cognitive Level:* Analysis. *Nursing Process:* Implementation. *Patient Need:* Safe, Effective Care Environment.

3 *Answer: 1*
Rationale: Prior to administering medications, the nurse should assess renal and liver function and impairments of other body systems that may affect pharmacotherapy. This is especially important when administering medications to elderly and severely debilitated patients. *Cognitive Level:*

Analysis. *Nursing Process:* Assessment. *Patient Need:* Physiological Integrity.

4 *Answer: 4*
Rationale: The Food and Drug Administration (FDA) and the National Coordinating Council for Medication Error Reporting and Prevention (NCC MERP) encourage nurses and other health care professionals to report medication errors. This aids in examining interdisciplinary causes of medication errors and developing methods to prevent them, thereby promoting medication safety. *Cognitive Level:* Analysis. *Nursing Process:* Implementation. *Patient Need:* Safe, Effective Care Environment.

5 *Answers: 1, 4, 5*
Rationale: After a medication error involving a medication given to the wrong patient, the nurse must notify the physicians for the patient who received the incorrect medication as well as the patient for whom the medication was intended if the medication was omitted. The medication as given should be charted on the MAR for the patient receiving the medication. A facility report of the error, sometimes referred to as an "Incident Report" or other related terms, documents the error and related corrective actions taken. Most facilities do not require notation of the error in the nursing notes. Vital signs should be assessed dependent on the medication given. *Cognitive Level:* Analysis. *Nursing Process:* Implementation. *Patient Need:* Safe, Effective Care Environment.

6 *Answer: 2*
Rationale: This approach best ensures a collaboration between the nurse and patient, allows the nurse to ensure the medication is taken, and provides an opportunity for the nurse to teach the patient about the medication. *Cognitive Level:* Application. *Nursing Process:* Implementation. *Patient Need:* Safe, Effective Care Environment.

Answers to Critical Thinking Questions

1 The nurse should be well organized in preparing for drug administration. The MAR must be assessed at the beginning of the shift, and the nurse should develop a system that will serve as a reminder of when drugs are due to be administered. In most institutions, regularly scheduled drugs may be administered 30 minutes before and 30 minutes after the assigned time. If administered within this time frame, the drugs are considered to have been given "on time." Institutional policies vary and should be consulted.

2 This order as written does not contain an indication for "right dose." Tylenol 3 could represent a combination drug of acetaminophen and codeine (i.e., "Tylenol #3"), or three plain Tylenol tablets, given orally. A potential error is to assume that the healthcare provider meant for the patient to have one "Tylenol #3" tablet by mouth. Prior to administering the dose, the nurse should consult with the healthcare provider to clarify the intent of the order.

3 There are numerous members of the health care team who may have contributed to the medication error for this pa-

tient. The prescriber could have assured that the appropriate dosage for the weight of the patient was ordered. The nurse may have checked the "Five Rights" of drug administration but did not note that the dose as written was not in the acceptable range given the patient variables of age and weight. The pharmacist is also responsible for checking the drug against patient-specific variables. In order to practice safe and effective drug administration, all members of the health care team must work together to ensure every drug and administration meets the five Rights. When new to a unit, particularly when administering unfamiliar drugs or drugs ordered in different dosages than the nurse has administered before, it is always safer to check the drug and dose along with patient variables such as weight before giving the medication. The nurse is the last link in the chain of administration and is often key to preventing medication errors.

Chapter 10

Answers to NCLEX-RN® Review Questions

1 *Answer: 4*

Rationale: Some herbal products contain ingredients that may serve as agonists or antagonists to prescription drugs. Herbal supplements should not be taken without discussing their use with the health care provider. Herbal supplements are considered less potent than prescription medications, but when similar drugs are taken together, there is the potential for adverse reactions. *Cognitive Level:* Analysis. *Nursing Process:* Implementation. *Patient Need:* Physiological Integrity.

2 *Answer: 1*

Rationale: Natural products contain many active ingredients, many of which have not been tested or identified. Patients with known allergies to food products or medicines should seek medical advice before using herbal supplements. Dietary supplements must state that the product is not intended to diagnose, treat, cure, or prevent any disease. *Cognitive Level:* Analysis. *Nursing Process:* Implementation. *Patient Need:* Physiological Integrity.

3 *Answer: 2*

Rationale: Saw palmetto is used to relieve urinary problems related to prostate enlargement. Cranberry juice (or the berries) is used to prevent urinary tract infections. Soy, evening primrose, and black cohosh are used for menopausal symptoms. *Cognitive Level:* Analysis. *Nursing Process:* Implementation. *Patient Need:* Physiological Integrity.

4 *Answer: 4*

Rationale: Feverfew may interact with aspirin, heparin, NSAIDs, and warfarin to cause increased bleeding. *Cognitive Level:* Analysis. *Nursing Process:* Assessment. *Patient Need:* Physiological Integrity.

5 *Answers: 1, 2, 3, 5*

Rationale: Serotonin syndrome is a rare but potentially life-threatening medical condition that may occur when pa-

tients are taking two or more drugs, one of which is a selective serotonergic medication. Symptoms include agitation, dizziness, sweating, and headache. Patients should discontinue use of the medication and seek medical care immediately. *Cognitive Level:* Analysis. *Nursing Process:* Assessment. *Patient Need:* Physiological Integrity.

6 *Answer: 3*

Rationale: Specialty supplements are nonherbal dietary products used to enhance a wide variety of body functions. In general, specialty supplements have a legitimate rationale for their use. But the link between most specialty supplements and their claimed benefits is unclear and the body may already have sufficient quantities of the substance. Taking additional amounts may be of no benefit and large amounts of some supplements may be harmful. Specialty supplements may give patients false hopes of an easy cure. *Cognitive Level:* Comprehension. *Nursing Process:* Implementation. *Patient Need:* Physiological Integrity.

Answers to Critical Thinking Questions

1 Tamoxifen is a selective estrogen receptor modulator (SERM) that acts by preventing estrogen from binding to the estrogen receptor in breast cells. Therefore, breast cell proliferation is inhibited. Many women assume that because they are taking a SERM, estrogen replacement is indicated. In fact, tamoxifen's effect in tissues other than the breast is similar to that of estrogen. Tamoxifen does not cause menopause and does not prevent pregnancy. If the patient takes a "natural" soy product, it may interfere with the desired action of tamoxifen. Her concern should be acknowledged, but she should be warned not to consume any herbal product without first consulting her health care provider.

2 Both garlic and ginseng have a potential drug interaction with the anticoagulant warfarin (Coumadin). It is known that ginseng is capable of inhibiting platelet activity. When taken in combination with an anticoagulant, these herbal products are capable of producing increased bleeding potential.

3 St. John's wort interacts with multiple drugs. It is important that the patient stop taking St. John's wort at least 3 weeks prior to the surgery, because it can potentiate sedation when combined with CNS depressants and opiate analgesics. St. John's wort can also decrease the effects of anticoagulants.

Chapter 11

Answers to NCLEX-RN® Review Questions

1 *Answer: 2*

Rationale: Some patients and health care professionals believe that therapeutic use of scheduled drugs creates large numbers of addicted patients. Prescription drugs rarely cause addiction when used according to accepted medical protocols. The risk of addiction for prescription medications is primarily a function of the dose and the length of therapy. **Cognitive Level:** Application. **Nursing Process:** Implementation. **Patient Need:** Physiological Integrity.

2 Answer: 2

Rationale: Tolerance is a biologic condition that occurs when the body adapts to a substance after repeated administration. Over time, higher doses of the drug are required to produce the same initial effect. **Cognitive Level:** Application. **Nursing Process:** Assessment. **Patient Need:** Physiological Integrity.

3 Answer: 4

Rationale: Use of marijuana slows motor activity, decreases coordination, and causes disconnected thoughts, feelings of paranoia, and euphoria. It increases thirst and craving for food, especially chocolate and other candies. Heroin produces a brief, intense rush of euphoria sought by addicts. Individuals experience a range of CNS effects from extreme pleasure to slowed body activities and profound sedation. Signs include constricted pupils, an increase in the pain threshold, and respiratory depression. Crack cocaine produces feelings of intense euphoria, a decrease in hunger, analgesia, illusions of physical strength, and increased sensory perception. Larger doses magnify these effects and also cause rapid heartbeat, sweating, dilation of the pupils, and an elevated body temperature. Large doses of barbiturates drugs suppress the respiratory centers in the brain. The user may stop breathing or lapse into a coma. **Cognitive Level:** Analysis. **Nursing Process:** Assessment. **Patient Need:** Physiological Integrity.

4 Answer: 3

Rationale: Patients experiencing alcohol withdrawal typically experience tremors, fatigue, anxiety, abdominal cramping, hallucinations, confusion, seizures, and delirium. **Cognitive Level:** Analysis. **Nursing Process:** Assessment. **Patient Need:** Physiological Integrity.

5 Answers: 1, 2, 4

Rationale: Symptoms of nicotine withdrawal include irritability, anxiety, restlessness, headaches, increased appetite, insomnia, inability to concentrate, and a decrease in heart rate and blood pressure. **Cognitive Level:** Application. **Nursing Process:** Implementation. **Patient Need:** Physiological Integrity.

6 Answer: 1

Rationale: Physical dependence and psychological dependence may occur together and result in drug-seeking behavior. But physical dependence occurs as the body adapts to the substance such that withdrawal symptoms will occur if the substance is stopped. Physical withdrawal symptoms do not occur with psychological dependence although an intense craving for the substance may be felt. **Cognitive Level:** Comprehension. **Nursing Process:** Assessment. **Patient Need:** Physiological Integrity.

Answers to Critical Thinking Questions

1 The National Institute on Drug Abuse offers a link titled InfoFacts, which provides a great deal of information about MDMA (www.drugabuse.gov). This drug is a neurotoxic agent. When taken in high doses it can produce malignant hyperthermia, which can lead to muscle damage and renal and cardiovascular system failure. Physical symptoms of MDMA use include muscle tension, nausea, rapid eye movement, faintness, chills, sweating, increased heart rate and blood pressure, and involuntary teeth clenching.

2 The NIDA InfoFacts sheet on steroids (www .drugabuse.gov) points out that aggression is a common psychiatric side effect of anabolic steroid abuse. Research indicates that users may experience paranoid jealousy, extreme irritability, delusions, and impaired judgment. Other symptoms are extreme mood changes and manic-like symptoms, even when the user reports feeling "good."

3 The principal danger associated with prolonged use of barbiturates is tolerance and physical addiction. Barbiturates generally lose their effectiveness as hypnotics within 2 weeks of continued use. This patient is demonstrating signs of developing tolerance. He needs to discontinue the drug gradually to decrease the risk of complications associated with sudden withdrawal. These symptoms include severe anxiety, tremors, marked excitement, delirium, and rebound rapid eye movement (REM) sleep. Today, nonbarbiturates are usually prescribed as first-line hypnotics.

Chapter 12

Answers to NCLEX-RN® Review Questions

1 Answers: 3, 5

Rationale: Anthrax affects the respiratory system. Fever, persistent cough, and dyspnea are all initial symptoms of inhaled anthrax. **Cognitive Level:** Analysis. **Nursing Process:** Assessment. **Patient Need:** Physiological Integrity.

2 Answer: 2

Rationale: The potassium iodine protects only the thyroid gland from I-131. No other body organs are protected by this medication. **Cognitive Level:** Analysis. **Nursing Process:** Implementation. **Patient Need:** Physiological Integrity.

3 Answer: 1

Rationale: Overstimulation of the neurotransmitter acetylcholine causes convulsions and loss of consciousness within seconds. **Cognitive Level:** Analysis. **Nursing Process:** Assessment. **Patient Need:** Physiological Integrity.

4 Answer: 3

Rationale: The antibiotic ciprofloxacin (Cipro) has been used for both prophylaxis and treatment of anthrax. **Cognitive Level:** Analysis. **Nursing Process:** Planning. **Patient Need:** Physiological Integrity.

5 Answer: 2

Rationale: The CDC has categorized biologic threats based on their potential impact on public health. The goal of biologic terrorism is to cause widespread casualties. **Cognitive Level:** Analysis. **Nursing Process:** Assessment. **Patient Need:** Safe, Effective Care Environment.

6 *Answers: 1, 2, 4, 5*

Rationale: Nurses and other health care providers may be consulted by neighbors, friends, and family in the event of a potential bioterrorism attack or for how to prepare. Participating in planning for any type of disaster, recognizing and reporting key signs or symptoms that may be related to an attack, having a list of agency resources available, and keeping up-to-date with emergency management protocols are all ways a nurse may benefit the community. Specific medications, antidotes, vaccines, and supplies are kept in strategic locations by the federal government and are available quickly for emergency use. They are not part of an individual's disaster preparedness strategy. *Cognitive Level:* Comprehension. *Nursing Process:* Implementation. *Patient Need:* Health Promotion and Maintenance.

Answers to Critical Thinking Questions

1 Mass vaccination of the general public for anthrax and smallpox should be avoided at this time because there is ongoing controversy regarding the safety and effectiveness of these vaccines.

2 KI tablets, if taken prior to or immediately after radiation exposure, can prevent up to 100% of radioactive iodine from entering the thyroid gland and damaging the thyroid tissues. Iodine is an integral component of thyroid hormone (T_3 and T_4) and as such, KI will concentrate predominately in the thyroid gland.

3 The SNS is designed to ensure immediate deployment of essential medical supplies to a community in the event of a large-scale chemical or biologic attack. Push packages of preassembled medical supplies and pharmaceuticals are designed to meet the needs of an unknown biologic or chemical attack. They are strategically located around the United States, can be deployed rapidly, and reach any affected community within 12 hours of an attack. VMI packages are shipped if necessary and require identification of the type of chemical or biologic attack. They contain supplies more specific to the type of attack and can reach an affected community within 24 to 36 hours.

4 Nurses play a key role in preparing for an emergency of any kind, natural or human-made, by educating patients and their communities, serving as volunteers for emergency medical corps, maintaining current knowledge of resources, and in the early detection of possible emergency conditions. Through educating their patients, families, and communities, they are also a primary source of information in the prevention of poisonings or for early treatment.

Chapter 13

Answers to NCLEX-RN® Review Questions

1 *Answer: 1*

Rationale: Adrenergic agonists stimulate the sympathetic nervous system and produce symptoms of the fight-or-flight response. Nausea, vomiting, nervousness, bronchial dilation, and hypertension are potential adverse reactions related to the use of adrenergic agonists. Hypotension is a potential adverse reaction related to the use of adrenergic antagonists. *Cognitive Level:* Assessment. *Nursing Process:* Application. *Patient Need:* Physiological Integrity.

2 *Answers: 1, 2, 4*

Rationale: Anticholinergics are used in the treatment of peptic ulcer disease, irritable bowel syndrome, and bradycardia because they suppress the effects of acetylcholine and stimulate the sympathetic nervous system. Anticholinergics may cause decreased sexual function because the parasympathetic impulses are blocked. Urine retention is a potential side effect of anticholinergics. *Cognitive Level:* Analysis. *Nursing Process:* Diagnosis. *Patient Need:* Physiological Integrity.

3 *Answer: 1*

Rationale: Potential adverse reactions associated with the use of adrenergic antagonists include tachycardia, edema, and heart failure. Bronchodilation is associated with the use of adrenergic agonists. *Cognitive Level:* Analysis. *Nursing Process:* Assessment. *Patient Need:* Physiological Integrity.

4 *Answer: 3*

Rationale: The nurse should monitor elderly patients for episodes of dizziness caused by CNS stimulation from the parasympathomimetic. Diaphoresis and dizziness are potential side effects related to the use of bethanechol. Bethanechol is used to treat nonobstructive urinary retention. *Cognitive Level:* Application. *Nursing Process:* Implementation. *Patient Need:* Physiological Integrity.

5 *Answer: 2*

Rationale: Anticholinergic medications slow intestinal motility; therefore, constipation is a potential side effect. Heartburn and hypothermia are not associated with the use of benztropine. *Cognitive Level:* Application. *Nursing Process:* Assessment. *Patient Need:* Physiological Integrity.

6 *Answer: 1*

Rationale: Overdosage of parasympathomimetics (cholinesterase inhibitors) may produce excessive sweating, drooling, dyspnea, or excessive fatigue. These symptoms should be promptly reported. *Cognitive Level:* Analysis. *Nursing Process:* Assessment. *Patient Need:* Physiological Integrity.

Answers to Critical Thinking Questions

1 Terbutaline (Brethine) is a sympathomimetic that was originally prescribed for the treatment of asthma. Terbutaline promotes bronchodilation and therefore reduces bronchospasm by inducing smooth-muscle relaxation. Today, terbutaline has found widespread use as a tocolytic because it also produces smooth-muscle relaxation in the uterus. Because terbutaline is a sympathomimetic, the nurse should prepare the patient for potential adverse reactions such as nervousness, tremor, and tachycardia. The nurse should also teach the patient to take the medication exactly as directed and on schedule, and instruct on the signs and symptoms of preterm labor in case they occur again.

2 Bethanechol is a direct-acting cholinergic agent that works by stimulating the parasympathetic nervous system. The desired effect, in this case, is an increase in smooth-muscle tone in the bladder. Any side effects would be related to an overstimulation of the parasympathetic nervous system. Following are suggested nursing diagnoses:

- Risk for Injury (related to side effects of cholinergic agents: hypotension, bradycardia, and syncope)

- Alteration in Comfort (related to adverse drug effects: abdominal cramping, nausea, and vomiting)

- Risk for Ineffective Individual Therapeutic Management (related to side effects and precautions of using cholinergic agents)

3 Benztropine (Cogentin) is an anticholinergic. Blocking the parasympathetic nerves allows the sympathetic nervous system to dominate. The drug is given as an adjunct in Parkinson's disease to reduce muscular tremor and rigidity. Anticholinergics affect many body systems and produce a wide variety of side effects. The nurse should monitor for decreased heart rate, dilated pupils, decreased peristalsis, and decreased salivation in addition to decreased muscular tremor and rigidity. Many of the side effects of anticholinergics are dose dependent. Adverse effects include typical signs of sympathetic nervous system stimulation.

Chapter 14

Answers to NCLEX-RN® Review Questions

1 **Answer: 3**

Rationale: CNS side effects for lorazepam (Ativan) include amnesia, weakness, disorientation, ataxia, blurred vision, diplopia, nausea, and vomiting. *Cognitive Level:* Analysis. *Nursing Process:* Assessment. *Patient Need:* Physiological Integrity.

2 **Answer: 4**

Rationale: The nurse should recognize that this medication is ordered for insomnia. Therefore, the patient should be experiencing relief from insomnia and reporting feeling rested when awakening. *Cognitive Level:* Analysis. *Nursing Process:* Evaluation. *Patient Need:* Physiological Integrity.

3 **Answer: 3**

Rationale: Flumazenil (Romazicon) is a benzodiazepine-receptor blocker which may be used to reverse CNS depressant effects. Naloxone (Narcan) is an opioid antagonist. *Cognitive Level:* Analysis. *Nursing Process:* Evaluation. *Patient Need:* Physiological Integrity.

4 **Answer: 3**

Rationale: Benzodiazepines should not be stopped abruptly. The health care provider should decide when and how to discontinue the medication. *Cognitive Level:* Analysis. *Nursing Process:* Evaluation. *Patient Need:* Physiological Integrity.

5 **Answer: 2**

Rationale: The statement by the patient needs to show clearly that the expected benefit of the medication therapy has been experienced by the patient. *Cognitive Level:* Analysis. *Nursing Process:* Evaluation. *Patient Need:* Physiological Integrity.

6 **Answer: 4**

Counseling or behavioral techniques such as stress reduction will assist in addressing the underlying problem and help ensure the drug is not taken longer than necessary. Benzodizepines are not stopped abruptly or rebound anxiety or cardiovascular effects may occur. *Cognitive Level*: Analysis. *Nursing Process*: Evaluation. *Patient Need*: Physiological Integrity.

Answers to Critical Thinking Questions

1 Pain is emphasized as being the fifth vital sign. The assessment and appropriate management of pain is a nursing function. A nurse might be tempted to give this patient a sleeping medication alone, fearing the side effects that might occur if given in combination with an opioid narcotic. Secobarbital is a short-acting barbiturate. Barbiturates are not effective analgesics and generally do not produce significant hypnosis in patients with severe pain. The barbiturate may intensify the patient's reaction to painful stimuli. Administering a barbiturate with a potent analgesic appears to reduce analgesic requirements by about 50%. The nurse may need to consult with the health care provider regarding lowering the dose of narcotic.

2 Lorazepam (Ativan) is used as an antianxiety agent but it also has an off-label use as an antiemetic. For a patient with severe nausea and vomiting, lorazepam may offer an additive effect when combined with the odanesetron for enhanced therapeutic effects.

3 A thorough assessment of the patient's sleep patterns should be conducted. In addition, nonpharmacological interventions such as a cool room, quieting activities before bedtime, and avoidance of heavy meals, alcohol, and caffeine before bedtime should also be considered. In older adults, the total amount of sleep does not change; however, the quality of sleep deteriorates. Time spent in REM sleep and stages 3 and 4 NREM sleep shortens. Older adults awaken more often during the night. This sleep disturbance can be compounded by the presence of a chronic illness. The alteration in sleep patterns may also be due to changes in the CNS that affect the regulation of sleep. After a thorough assessment, the nurse should discuss age-related issues, health concerns, and environmental factors that may be affecting the quality of sleep.

Chapter 15

Answers to NCLEX-RN® Review Questions

1 **Answer: 3**

Rationale: Seizures may be caused by inflammation, head injuries, or low blood sugar levels. Rapid-growing, space-occupying lesions in the brain, which increase intracranial pressure, may cause seizures, but not tumors, within the muscles. **Cognitive Level:** Analysis. **Nursing Process:** Evaluation. **Patient Need:** Physiological Integrity.

2   *Answer: 3*

Rationale: The influx of sodium into a neuron enhances neuronal activity. The delay of an influx suppresses neurotransmitter frequency. **Cognitive Level:** Analysis. **Nursing Process:** Assessment. **Patient Need:** Physiological Integrity.

3   *Answer: 2*

Rationale: GABA drugs mimic GABA by stimulating the influx of chloride ions into the neuron, leading to the suppression of neuron firing. **Cognitive Level:** Analysis. **Nursing Process:** Assessment. **Patient Need:** Physiological Integrity.

4   *Answer: 3*

Rationale: Valproic acid may produce an idiosyncratic response in children, including restlessness and psychomotor agitation. **Cognitive Level:** Analysis. **Nursing Process:** Assessment. **Patient Need:** Physiological Integrity.

5   *Answer: 3*

Rationale: Carbamazepine affects vitamin K metabolism and may lead to blood dyscrasias and bleeding. **Cognitive Level:** Application. **Nursing Process:** Implementation. **Patient Need:** Physiological Integrity.

6   *Answers: 1, 2, 4*

Rationale: The phenytoin-like drugs are used to treat partial seizures. Diazepam (Valium) is a benzodiazepine that is used to treat tonic–clonic seizures and status epilepticus. **Cognitive Level:** Analysis. **Nursing Process:** Implementation. **Patient Need:** Physiological Integrity.

Answers to Critical Thinking Questions

1   Carbamazepine (Tegretol) is the second most widely prescribed antiepileptic drug in the United States. Common side effects are drowsiness, dizziness, nausea, ataxia, and blurred vision. Serious and sometimes fatal blood dyscrasias secondary to bone marrow suppression have occurred with carbamazepine. The patient's hematocrit suggests anemia, and the petechiae and bruising suggest thrombocytopenia. The nurse should evaluate the patient for complaints of fever and sore throat that would suggest leukopenia. This patient needs immediate evaluation by the health care provider responsible for monitoring the seizure disorder.

2   This question requires that the student consult a laboratory reference manual. The therapeutic drug level of phenytoin (Dilantin) is 5 to 20 mg/dL. Patients may become drug toxic and demonstrate signs of CNS depression. Exaggerated effects of phenytoin can be seen if the drug has been combined with alcohol or other agents. Phenytoin also demonstrates dose-dependent metabolism. When hepatic enzymes necessary for metabolism are saturated, any increase in drug concentration results in a disproportionate increase in plasma concentration level.

3   Long-term phenytoin therapy can produce an androgenic stimulus. Reported skin manifestations include acne, hirsutism, and an increase in subcutaneous facial tissue—changes that have been characterized as "Dilantin facies." These changes, coupled with the risk for gingival hypertrophy, may be difficult for the adolescent to cope with. In addition, the adolescent with a seizure disorder may be prohibited from operating a motor vehicle at the very age when driving becomes key to achieving young-adult status. The thoughtful nurse will consider the range of possible support groups for this patient once she is discharged and will encourage the patient to discuss her concerns about the drug regimen with her health care provider.

Chapter 16

Answers to NCLEX-RN® Review Questions

1   *Answer: 4*

Anticholinergic effects such as blurred vision, dry mouth, and constipation may occur during the first weeks of therapy. Tolerance to anticholinergic effects tends to develop after several weeks of regular use. They can be managed symptomatically by increasing fluid intake, being cautious with activities that require visual acuity (e.g., driving), and increasing fiber in the diet. Psychomotor symptoms, tachycardia, hypertension, increase in respiratory rate, and tardive dyskinesias are potential adverse effects of TCA antidepressants but are not related to anticholinergic effects. **Cognitive Level**: Application. **Nursing Process**: Assessment. **Patient Need**: Physiological Integrity.

2   *Answer: 3*

Rationale: Methylphenidate (Ritalin) is a Schedule II drug with potential to cause drug dependence when used over an extended period. The drug holiday is to decrease the risk of dependence and to evaluate behavior. **Cognitive Level:** Application. **Nursing Process:** Implementation. **Patient Need:** Physiological Integrity.

3   *Answers: 1, 2, 5*

Rationale: Diarrhea, ataxia, hypotension, edema, slurred speech, and muscle weakness are signs of lithium toxicity. Dehydration can lead to lithium toxicity. **Cognitive Level:** Analysis. **Nursing Process:** Assessment. **Patient Need:** Physiological Integrity.

4   *Answer: 2*

Rationale: Taking St. John's wort with an MAOI could result in hypertensive crisis; patients should always consult with their health care provider before taking any medications or OTC drugs/herbal remedies. **Cognitive Level:** Application. **Nursing Process:** Implementation. **Patient Need:** Physiological Integrity.

5   *Answer: 3*

Rationale: Nardil is an MAOI. This class of drugs has many drug and food interactions that may cause a hypertensive crisis. **Cognitive Level:** Analysis. **Nursing Process:** Planning. **Patient Need:** Physiological Integrity.

6 *Answer: 3*

Antidepressant drugs such as the SSRIs may not have full effects for a month or longer but some improvement in mood and depression should be noticeable after beginning therapy. Anything less than a month is too early for *full* effects although some improvement may be noticed. *Cognitive Level*: Application. *Nursing Process*: Assessment. *Patient Need*: Physiological Integrity.

Answers to Critical Thinking Questions

1 Methylphenidate (Ritalin) therapy is usually administered twice a day, with one dose before breakfast and one dose before lunch. A child in school would be required to visit a school nurse to receive a dose of Ritalin before lunch. Amphetamine (Adderall) requires once-a-day dosing and may be better accepted by the child and his or her family because treatment can be privately managed at home. Although many children cope effectively with treatment for ADHD, a 12-year-old girl might be concerned about being "singled out" for therapy. She is old enough to realize her problems in performance. The self-esteem of children in this age group is tied to success in school, a characteristic of Erikson's developmental stage of industry versus inferiority. Children who have difficulty in school perceive themselves as being inferior to peers. Helping the child with ADHD pharmacologically may require the health care provider to be sensitive to social factors such as dosage regimens.

2 The nurse should teach the patient that it might take 2 to 4 weeks before she begins to notice therapeutic benefit. The nurse should help the patient identify a support person or network to help assist as she works through her grief. The nurse also needs to instruct the patient that both caffeine and nicotine are CNS stimulants and decrease the effectiveness of the medication.

3 The use of any drug during pregnancy must be carefully evaluated. Sertraline (Zoloft) is a pregnancy category B drug, which means that studies indicate no risk to animal fetuses, although safety in humans has not been established. The health care provider must weigh risks and benefits of any medication during pregnancy. The nurse should recognize this patient's risk for ineffective coping, as evidenced by her history of depression, and help the patient identify support groups in the community. She may be functioning in some degree of isolation from family or other parenting women, which is typical of women who suffer postpartum depression. Identifying community resources for the patient is one intervention designed to provide more holistic care.

Answer to Avoiding Medication Errors

Unless there is a health care provider's order, it is never permissible to leave medications at the bedside of a patient. It is possible that the patient will deliberately discard them, save them for a later overdose, or forget to take them. It is also possible that the medications could be inadvertently removed with the food tray or taken by another patient. Always supervise all medication administration and be certain that the drug is swallowed. Never leave medications unattended in a patient's room. If there are concerns that the patient may not have swallowed the medications, ask the patient to open his or her mouth. The risk that a depressed patient will take an intentional overdose increases as the medication begins to work and gives the patient more energy to carry out a suicide plan.

Chapter 17

Answers to NCLEX-RN® Review Questions

1 *Answer: 4*

Rationale: Symptoms of psychosis are likely to return and manifest as agitation, distrust, and frustration. *Cognitive Level:* Analysis. *Nursing Process:* Implementation. *Patient Need:* Physiological Integrity.

2 *Answer: 2*

Rationale: Acute dystonias occur early in the course of therapy. These are severe muscle spasms, particularly of the back, neck, tongue, and face. *Cognitive Level:* Analysis. *Nursing Process:* Planning. *Patient Need:* Physiological Integrity.

3 *Answer: 2*

Rationale: Antipsychotic drugs such as risperiodne (Risperdal) treat the positive and negative effects of the underlying mental disorder. A decrease in delusional thinking, lessened hallucinations, and overall improvement in mental thought processes should be noted. Improvement in sleep patterns, anxiety, and nutrition may be noted as secondary effects of treatment of the underlying thought disorder. Orthostatic hypotension, reflex tachycardia, or sedation are potential *adverse* effects. *Cognitive Level*: Application. *Nursing Process*: Assessment. *Patient Need*: Physiological Integrity.

4 *Answers: 1, 2, 4*

Rationale: Aluminum- and magnesium-based antacids decrease absorption of haloperidol (Haldol). Haldol also has a high incidence of EPS. Haldol must be taken as ordered for therapeutic results to occur. It is contraindicated in Parkinson's disease, seizure disorders, alcoholism, and severe mental depression. The sustained-release forms must not be opened or crushed. *Cognitive Level:* Analysis. *Nursing Process:* Implementation. *Patient Need:* Physiological Integrity.

5 *Answer: 3*

Rationale: Fluphenazine (Prolixin) is a phenothiazine drug. Use is contraindicated in patients with CNS depression, bone marrow depression, and alcohol withdrawal. *Cognitive Level:* Analysis. *Nursing Process:* Assessment. *Patient Need:* Physiological Integrity.

6 *Answer: 3*

Rationale: Acute dystonias are characterized by acute spasms of the face, tongue, neck, or back. Dry mouth, constipation, and blurred vision are adverse effects related to anticholinergic activity. Pacing and squirming are signs of akathisia, and bradykinesia and tremors are symptoms of pseudoparkinsonism. Involuntary lip-puckering and wormlike movements of the tongue are symptomatic of tardive dyskinesias. *Cognitive Level*: Application. *Nursing Process*: Assessment. *Patient Need*: Physiological Integrity.

Answers to Critical Thinking Questions

1 The patient is exhibiting signs of EPS. Initially, the nurse would assess the patient to ensure he had sustained no recent neck injury or trauma, but if the neck spasms started spontaneously, the nurse would then assess for the possibility of EPS. The patient probably needs to be on a medication such as benztropine (Cogentin) to decrease the EPS effects. The patient should be taught to recognize the symptoms of EPS and to seek medical evaluation when the symptoms occur.

2 The patient is elderly; thus, safety is a priority when administering this medication. Postural hypotension and dizziness are common; therefore, the patient needs to move and change position slowly. Constipation is also a concern for a patient on this medication, especially elderly patients.

3 The nurse should initially assess whether the patient has been taking the medication as ordered or has altered the dose in any way. It is not uncommon for a young person to "cheek" the medication or attempt to cut back on the dose because of the lack of desire to take the medication on a continual basis—especially when the patient begins to feel better. It is important that the patient understand the necessity of being on this medication for a lifetime, and that the dose is not to be adjusted without consulting a health care provider.

Chapter 18

Answers to NCLEX-RN® Review Questions

1 *Answer: 2*

Rationale: When used concurrently with medication, non-pharmacologic techniques may allow for lower doses and possibly fewer drug-related adverse effects. Relaxation techniques and imagery may also be used in the acute care setting. *Cognitive Level:* Analysis. *Nursing Process:* Implementation. *Patient Need:* Physiological Integrity.

2 *Answer: 3*

Rationale: Some opioid agonists, such as morphine, activate both mu and kappa receptors. *Cognitive Level:* Analysis. *Nursing Process:* Implementation. *Patient Need:* Physiological Integrity.

3 *Answer: 3*

Rationale: Vicodin is a combination drug of hydrocodone and acetaminophen. Acetaminophen can be hepatotoxic, and this patient has hepatitis B, a chronic liver disorder. *Cognitive Level:* Application. *Nursing Process:* Implementation. *Patient Need:* Physiological Integrity.

4 *Answers: 4, 5*

Rationale: Opioids activate mu and kappa receptors that may cause profound respiratory depression. The patient's respiratory rate should remain above 12 breaths per minute. Although the patient may also become drowsy, he or she should not become unresponsive after administration of morphine sulfate. *Cognitive Level:* Analysis. *Nursing Process:* Implementation. *Patient Need:* Physiological Integrity.

5 *Answer: 2*

Rationale: Opioids suppress intestinal contractility, increase anal sphincter tone, and inhibit fluids into the intestines, which can lead to constipation. *Cognitive Level:* Application. *Nursing Process:* Implementation. *Patient Need:* Physiological Integrity.

6 *Answer: 3*

Opioid pain relievers should be given as consistently as possible, and before the onset of acute pain, in the immediate postoperative period unless the patient's condition does not allow the consistent dosing (e.g., vital signs do not support regular doses). Giving the drug only when the family members report that the patient is complaining of pain, every time the patient complains of acute pain, or only when the nurse observes signs and symptoms of pain. These methods of drug administration would potentially allow pain to become severe before being adequately treated. Patients or family members may not always report pain or may downplay the severity. Cultural norms may also influence the patient's way of exhibiting pain. *Cognitive Level*: Analysis. *Nursing Process*: Implementation. *Patient Need*: Physiological Integrity.

Answers to Critical Thinking Questions

1 The nurse should initially manage the patient's airway, breathing, and circulation (ABCs) by opening the airway and providing oxygen support, and then stop the PCA pump. Although the nurse's first reaction may be to go directly to the PCA to stop the medication, it is important initially to manage the patient's airway before stopping the PCA because it is unknown how long the patient has been hypoxic. The nurse then needs to administer IV naloxone (Narcan), which is a narcotic antagonist. After these initial steps have been completed and the patient is stabilized, the nurse must inform the health care provider of this adverse effect of the morphine.

2 Sumatriptan (Imitrex) is not recommended for patients with CAD, diabetes, or hypertension because of the drug's vasoconstrictive properties. The nurse should refer the patient to the health care provider for review of medications and possible adverse reactions related to sumatriptan.

3 The patient should be taught not to take any medication, including OTC medications, without the approval of the health care provider. This patient is taking an anticoagulant, and aspirin increases bleeding time. The patient needs to be taught how to recognize the signs and symptoms of bleeding related to the anticoagulant therapy. The patient should review with the health care provider all her

medications. Possibly, her anti-inflammatory medication can be changed from aspirin to another drug for treatment of arthritis.

Chapter 19

Answers to NCLEX-RN® Review Questions

1 *Answer: 1*
Rationale: The throat is anesthetized during a gastroscopy. Monitor the patient for return of the gag reflex before the patient drinks or eats. Ensuring an airway is the priority when caring for these patients. Abdominal pain, ability to stand, and ability to urinate are not priorities. *Cognitive Level:* Application. *Nursing Process:* Assessment. *Patient Need:* Physiological Integrity.

2 *Answer: 4*
Rationale: Solutions of lidocaine containing preservatives or epinephrine are intended for local anesthesia only and must never be given IV for dysrhythmias. *Cognitive Level:* Analysis. *Nursing Process:* Implementation. *Patient Need:* Physiological Integrity.

3 *Answer: 3*
Rationale: The first step of the nursing process is assessment. Assessment of prior knowledge provides the basis for the development of a teaching plan. The other options take place after a thorough assessment. *Cognitive Level:* Application. *Nursing Process:* Assessment. *Patient Need:* Physiological Integrity.

4 *Answer: 3*
Rationale: Nitrous oxide suppresses the pain mechanisms within the CNS, thereby causing analgesia. It does not produce complete loss of consciousness or profound relaxation of skeletal muscles. Nitrous oxide does not induce stage 3 analgesia or cause a loss of consciousness. *Cognitive Level:* Analysis. *Nursing Process:* Implementation. *Patient Need:* Physiological Integrity.

5 *Answers: 1, 4*
Rationale: Succinylcholine (Anectine) can cause complete paralysis of the diaphragm and intercostal muscles. Bradycardia and respiratory depression are expected. Mechanical ventilation should be available. *Cognitive Level:* Analysis. *Nursing Process:* Assessment. *Patient Need:* Physiological Integrity.

6 *Answer: 4*
Rationale: Neuroleptanalgesia drugs such as ketamine do not result in full loss of consciousness but cause disconnection from events occurring. Confusion, anxiety, fear, or panic may occur in the immediate postprocedure period if sensory stimulation is misinterpreted. Sensory stimulation should be kept to a minimum during this period for this reason. Frequent assessments above those required for patient safety increase sensory stimulation and may result in extreme patient reactions. *Cognitive Level:* Analysis. *Nursing Process:* Implementation. *Patient Need:* Physiological Integrity.

Answers to Critical Thinking Questions

1 The nurse should question the health care provider regarding this order. Lidocaine is an appropriate choice for a local anesthesia but not if it includes epinephrine. Epinephrine has alpha-adrenergic properties, is a potent vasoconstrictor, and may cause cardiac dysrhythmias in this elderly patient. Epinephrine is traditionally not used in the areas of "fingers, nose, penis, and toes," because these areas may suffer adverse effects from the vasoconstrictive properties of the drug.

2 The nurse understands that this drug is a depolarizing medication and therefore has the potential to increase potassium release. The nurse is aware that this patient is on digoxin (Lanoxin) and has renal failure, and therefore is not a good candidate for this drug because of the potential hyperkalemia that may result in life-threatening cardiac dysrhythmias.

3 The priority postoperative drug is St. John's wort because it may prolong the effects of anesthesia and opioids in the patient's system, causing depression of the CNS and respiratory system. The patient should also be monitored for postoperative bleeding related to the use of ibuprofen. The digoxin concentration should be at a therapeutic level prior to surgery to decrease possible adverse effects of the cardiovascular system postoperatively.

Chapter 20

Answers to NCLEX-RN® Review Questions

1 *Answer: 2*
Rationale: Extrapyramidal symptoms may be life threatening without intervention. The patient should be immediately transported to the emergency department. Diphenhydramine must be given parenterally for effective treatment. The drug dosage should not be increased, because symptoms may become worse. *Cognitive Level:* Analysis. *Nursing Process:* Implementation. *Patient Need:* Physiological Integrity.

2 *Answer: 2*
Rationale: Pharmacotherapy does not cure or stop the disease process but does improve the patient's ability to perform normal activities such as eating, bathing, and walking. Depending on the drug therapy, EPS may be an adverse effect. *Cognitive Level:* Analysis. *Nursing Process:* Implementation. *Patient Need:* Physiological Integrity.

3 *Answer: 4*
Rationale: A decrease in kidney and liver function may slow the metabolism and excretion of the drug, leading to overdose and toxicity. Levodopa does not cause the urine to turn orange. It is not reasonable for a patient to monitor his or her blood pressure every 2 hours during the first 2 weeks of therapy. *Cognitive Level:* Analysis. *Nursing Process:* Implementation. *Patient Need:* Physiological Integrity.

4 *Answer: 1*
Rationale: The cause is unknown; however, structural damage consisting of amyloid plaques and neurofibrillary tan-

gles has been found within the brain at autopsy. Alzheimer's disease has not been associated with intracranial bleeding, loss of circulation to the brain, or loss of dopamine receptors. **Cognitive Level:** Application. **Nursing Process:** Implementation. **Patient Need:** Physiological Integrity.

5 **Answers: 1, 3**

Rationale: Symptoms of overdose include severe nausea and vomiting, sweating, salivation, hypotension, bradycardia, convulsions, and increased muscle weakness, including respiratory muscles. Tachycardia, hypertension, emotional withdrawal, tachypnea, and increased muscle strength are not associated with overdose of these drugs. **Cognitive Level:** Analysis. **Nursing Process:** Assessment. **Patient Need:** Physiological Integrity.

6 **Answer: 3**

Rationale: Blepharospam (spasmodic eye winking) and muscle twitching are early signs of potential overdose or toxicity. Orthostatic hypotension, drooling, nausea, vomiting, and diarrhea are potential adverse effects unrelated to toxicity or overdosage. **Cognitive Level**: Analysis. **Nursing Process**: Implementation. **Patient Need**: Physiological Integrity.

Answers to Critical Thinking Questions

1 The patient should reassess with a health care provider the need for regular Mylanta. This drug contains magnesium, which may cause increased absorption and toxicity. The patient needs teaching on decreasing foods that contain vitamin B_6 (for example, bananas, wheat germ, and green vegetables) because vitamin B_6 may also cause an increase in the absorption of the medication. Teaching should include information about a potential loss of glycemic control (because this patient is diabetic) and safety issues related to postural hypotension.

2 A patient on benztropin (Cogentin) has a decreased ability to tolerate heat. Arizona in July is hot, so the patient should be taught to avoid hot climates, if at all possible, or to increase rest periods, avoid exertion, and observe for signs of heat intolerance. When symptoms occur, the patient must immediately get out of the heat and rest.

3 The nurse should refer the patient and his wife to a health care provider regarding the appropriateness of this medication (this is not a nursing function). The couple should be educated regarding safety issues such as postural hypotension and bradycardia that may occur with this medication. Anorexia is also a potential problem; this patient has diabetes and thus may have glycemic issues.

Chapter 21

Answers to NCLEX-RN® Review Questions

1 **Answers: 1, 2, 5**

Rationale: Adverse reactions to cyclobenzaprine include drowsiness, dizziness, dry mouth, rash, and tachycardia. Because medication can cause drowsiness and dizziness, ensuring patient safety must be a priority. Usually, patients experiencing back pain have orders for limited ambulation

until muscle spasms have subsided. **Cognitive Level:** Analysis. **Nursing Process:** Implementation. **Patient Need:** Physiological Integrity.

2 **Answer: 4**

Rationale: An adverse effect of botulinum is pain. The drug is injected directly into the muscle. Pain associated with injections is usually blocked by a local anesthetic. Treatment with botulinum helps improve muscle strength, but therapeutic effects are usually delayed by a few days. **Cognitive Level:** Analysis. **Nursing Process:** Implementation. **Patient Need:** Physiological Integrity.

3 **Answer: 1**

Rationale: Elevated serum liver enzymes should be reported to the health care provider. Cyclobenzaprine may cause serious liver damage. The medication should be held until the health care provider has been notified. **Cognitive Level:** Analysis. **Nursing Process:** Implementation. **Patient Need:** Physiological Integrity.

4 **Answer: 3**

Rationale: Muscle relaxers such as cyclobenzaprine may cause hypotension. Given concurrently with antihypertensives such as propranolol may increase the risk of hypotension. Cyclobenzaprine may have CNS effects such as drowsiness, dizziness, or fatigue but should not result in neurologic changes. Giving the drugs concurrently greatly increases the risk of hypotension. While renal functioning labs may be monitored periodically, propranolol will not have direct effects on that lab test result. **Cognitive Level**: Analysis. **Nursing Process**: Assessment. **Patient Need**: Physiological Integrity.

5 **Answer: 4**

Rationale: Patients should be instructed to report side effects such as muscle weakness, drowsiness, dry mouth, dizziness, nausea, diarrhea, tachycardia, erratic blood pressure, photosensitivity, and urine retention. Until effects are known, the patient should not drive. It may take a few hours for the drug to become effective. **Cognitive Level:** Analysis. **Nursing Process:** Evaluation. **Patient Need:** Physiological Integrity.

6 **Answer: 1**

Rationale: Muscle relaxers such as baclofen work best when taken consistently and not prn. Noting consistently of dosing helps to determine the appropriateness of dose, frequency, and drug effects. Consumption of alcohol or increasing the dose of muscle relaxers will increase the risk of sedation and drowsiness. The patient's log of symptoms and drug dose and frequency may assist the provider in determining the therapeutic outcome of the medication. The patient's report of pain or continued spasms should be considered an accurate account. **Cognitive Level**: Analysis. **Nursing Process**: Assessment. **Patient Need**: Physiological Integrity.

Answers to Critical Thinking Questions

1 The nurse would anticipate a decrease in the patient's spasticity after 1 week of therapy. If there has been no

improvement in 45 days, the medication regimen is usually discontinued. In this case, the nurse should evaluate the patient's muscle firmness, pain experience, range of motion, and ability to maintain posture and alignment when in a wheelchair. When spasticity is used to maintain posture, dantrolene should not be used. In this case, the patient's spasticity involved only the lower extremities.

2 Leg and foot cramps have been anecdotally associated with tamoxifen, an antiestrogenic drug. Tamoxifen, which has been shown to reduce the recurrence of some breast cancers, has been demonstrated to preserve bone density. Tamoxifen has several side effects that affect lifestyle, including the potential for weight gain and leg cramps. The nurse should assess the following factors before responding to this patient's concerns:

- What is the patient's activity level? Muscle cramps are associated with muscle fatigue.

- Does she take exogenous calcium?

- Can she tolerate dietary sources of calcium?

Interventions for leg cramps include the following:

- Stretching exercises before sleep

- Daily calcium and magnesium supplements

- Increasing dietary calcium intake

- Drinking a glass of tonic water (containing quinine) at bedtime

This patient needs to relate her concerns to the oncologist. A health care provider may consider starting the patient on quinine 200 to 300 mg at bedtime. This is an off-label use and requires careful patient evaluation.

3 Cyclobenzaprine (Flexeril) has been demonstrated to produce significant anticholinergic activity. Students should recall that anticholinergics block the action of the neurotransmitter acetylcholine at the muscarinic receptors in the parasympathetic nervous system. This allows the activities of the sympathetic nervous system to dominate. In this case, the result has been a decrease in oral secretions and relaxation of the smooth muscle of the GI tract. Decreased peristalsis and motility can result in constipation. The anticholinergic effect is also responsible for urine retention because of increased constriction of the internal sphincter.

Chapter 22

Answers to NCLEX-RN® Review Questions

1 *Answer: 2*
Rationale: HMG-CoA reductase inhibitors may cause rhabdomyolysis, a rare but serious adverse effect. Constipation and hemorrhoids may result from bile acid sequestrants. Flushing or hot flash–type effects may result from nicotinic acid. *Cognitive Level*: Analysis. *Nursing Process*: Assessment. *Patient Need*: Physiological Integrity.

2 *Answer: 3*
Rationale: The goal of lipid-lowering therapy is to decrease total cholesterol and LDL, while raising HDL levels. The other choices do not decrease the levels of harmful lipid levels. *Cognitive Level*: Analysis. *Nursing Process*: Evaluation. *Patient Need*: Physiological Integrity.

3 *Answer: 4*
Rationale: One adult-strength aspirin taken 30 minutes before the nicotinic acid may reduce the adverse effects of flushing and feelings of hot flashes. Taking the drug one hour before meals with plenty of water, mixing the drug thoroughly in water before taking, and taking other medications 1 hour before or 4 hours after the drug are guidelines recommended for bile acid sequestrant drugs. *Cognitive Level*: Application. *Nursing Process*: Implementation. *Patient Need*: Physiological Integrity.

4 *Answer: 3*
Rationale: The nurse teaches the patient with a diagnosis of hyperlipidemia about lipids in the body. The nurse informs the patient that the major storage form of fat in the body is triglycerides. *Cognitive Level:* Analysis. *Nursing Process:* Implementation. *Patient Need:* Health Promotion and Maintenance.

5 *Answers: 1, 2*
Rationale: Long-term use of lipid-lowering therapy may cause depletion or decreased absorption of folic acid and the fat-soluble vitamins. Decrease in potassium, iodine, chloride, and protein is not a direct-effect of lipid-lowering therapy. *Cognitive Level*: Application. *Nursing Process*: Implementation. *Patient Need*: Physiological Integrity.

6 *Answers: 1, 2, 4*
Rationale: Vegetables such as broccoli and carrots, most nuts, and fish such as salmon and sardines provide soluble fiber and are good sources of omega-3 fatty acids and coenzyme Q10. Grapefruit and grapefruit juice may inhibit the metabolism of the statins and lead to potentially toxic levels. *Cognitive Level*: Application. *Nursing Process*: Implementation. *Patient Need*: Physiological Integrity.

Answers to Critical Thinking Questions

1 Photosensitivity is a major problem with atorvastatin (Lipitor), so the patient must take precautions such as using sunscreen, wearing sunglasses and protective clothing, and staying out of the direct sun as much as possible. This will probably be a lifestyle change for this patient, and education with reinforcement is necessary.

2 This medication has the possibility of causing esophageal irritation, so taking the proper fluids or food with this medication is important. Pulpy fruit such as applesauce could be used for dual purposes with this drug, because the applesauce works for the esophageal irritation, and it also may help prevent the constipation caused by the drug.

3 The nurse should advise this patient to seek medical advice before self-medicating—especially because this patient has diabetes, and many drugs affect hyperglycemic

medications and blood glucose levels. Niacin can cause hyperglycemia in this patient, so serum glucose levels should be evaluated. The flushing and hot flashes are normal side effects of this medication.

Answer to Avoiding Medication Errors

The nurse should have administered cholestyramine at least 4 hours before or 2 hours after digoxin and tetracycline because there is decreased absorption if they are administered together.

Chapter 23

Answers to NCLEX-RN® Review Questions

1 *Answer: 3*

Rationale: Furosemide was prescribed as an adjunct treatment for hypertension. Blood pressure within normal limits indicates that treatment has been effective. Absence of edema, weight loss, and frequency of voiding is related to fluid status. *Cognitive Level:* Analysis. *Nursing Process:* Evaluation. *Patient Need:* Physiological Integrity.

2 *Answer: 1*

Rationale: HCTZ is a thiazide diuretic. It acts on the kidney tubules to decrease the reabsorption of sodium. When reabsorption is blocked, more sodium is sent into the urine. The most common side effect of HCTZ is electrolyte sodium and potassium depletion. The patient's potassium level is decreased at 2.8 mEq/ml. Administering HCTZ could further deplete the patient's potassium level. *Cognitive Level:* Analysis. *Nursing Process:* Diagnosis. *Patient Need:* Physiological Integrity.

3 *Answer: 2*

Rationale: The advantage of using two drugs is that lower doses of each may be used, resulting in fewer side effects. Compliance will increase due to fewer uncomfortable side effects. *Cognitive Level:* Application. *Nursing Process:* Planning. *Patient Need:* Physiological Integrity.

4 *Answer: 3*

Rationale: ACE inhibitors block the effects of angiotensin II, decreasing blood pressure through two mechanisms: lowering peripheral resistance and decreasing blood volume. *Cognitive Level:* Application. *Nursing Process:* Assessment. *Patient Need:* Physiological Integrity.

5 *Answers: 2, 3, 4, 5*

Side effects of ACE inhibitors include persistent cough and postural hypotension. Hyperkalemia may occur and can be a major concern for those with diabetes or renal impairment and in patients taking potassium-sparing diuretics. Though rare, the most serious adverse effect of ACE inhibitors is the development of angioedema. *Cognitive Level:* Analysis. *Nursing Process:* Assessment. *Patient Need:* Physiological Integrity.

6 *Answer: 2*

Rationale: Propranolol and other beta-blocking drugs are used to prevent reflex tachycardia that may occur as a result of treatment with direct-acting vasodilators. Giving two antihypertensive drugs together may also lower blood pressure further but the beta-blocking drugs also lower the heart rate and are given in this case to reduce the chance for reflex tachycardia. Propranolol has not been demonstrated to have effects in preventing lupus and is not a diuretic, although judicious diuretic therapy may be necessary if excessive fluid gain is an adverse effect of direct-acting vasodilator therapy. *Cognitive Level:* Analysis. *Nursing Process:* Implementation. *Patient Need:* Physiological Integrity.

Answers to Critical Thinking Questions

1 Traditionally, if the patient has a systolic blood pressure of less than 110 mmHg, the dose should be held unless verified with the health care provider that the dose should be given. The patient is on a low-sodium, low-protein diet, which may contribute to hypotension. Because the patient has mild renal failure, the excretion of the drug may be prolonged and also contribute to the hypotensive effects. If the health care provider wants the patient to receive the benazepril (Lotensin), then the blood pressure should be rechecked at 30 minutes and 60 minutes after the medication is given. The patient should be cautioned about postural hypotension.

2 Atenolol (Tenormin) is a beta$_1$-adrenergic blocker that works directly on the heart. The nurse and the patient need to be aware that the patient's heart rate will rarely go above 80 beats per minute because of the action of the medication. Tachycardia is one of the adrenergic signs of hypoglycemia that would not be evident with this patient. Both the nurse and patient need to be aware of the more subtle signs of hypoglycemia (or any other condition that may be recognized by tachycardia) that would not be evident with a patient on beta-blocking medications.

3 The nurse must be careful that the patient's blood pressure is not lowered too dramatically, or hypotension may occur. This is an example of a case in which 120/80 mmHg is not necessarily an ideal blood pressure reading. Typically, the blood pressure is not lowered below 160 mmHg systolic. The patient is reevaluated and then (often many hours later) the blood pressure is brought down further. This drip is light sensitive and must remain covered with foil during infusion. Once prepared, the drip is stable for only 24 hours. Nitroprusside is a cyanide by-product; therefore, any patient on this drug must be monitored for cyanide toxicity.

Chapter 24

Answers to NCLEX-RN® Review Questions

1 *Answers: 3, 4*

Rationale: Digoxin helps increase the contractility of the heart thus increasing cardiac output. The heart rate will decrease with the use of digoxin. *Cognitive Level:* Analysis. *Nursing Process:* Evaluation. *Patient Need:* Physiological Integrity.

2 Answer: 2

Rationale: Normal serum potassium level is 3.5 to 5.0 mEq/L. Hypokalemia may predispose the patient to digitalis toxicity. *Cognitive Level:* Analysis. *Nursing Process:* Implementation. *Patient Need:* Physiological Integrity.

3 Answer: 3

Rationale: ACE inhibitors can cause severe hypotension with initial doses. The nurse should monitor the patient closely for several hours. *Cognitive Level:* Analysis. *Nursing Process:* Implementation. *Patient Need:* Physiological Integrity.

4 Answer: 2

Rationale: Potassium levels should be closely monitored. Encouraging the eating of foods rich in potassium could help maintain potassium levels. *Cognitive Level:* Application. *Nursing Process:* Planning. *Patient Need:* Physiological Integrity.

5 Answers: 1, 3, 4, 5

Rationale: Side effects of this medication may include cough, headache, dizziness, change in sensation of taste, vomiting and diarrhea, and hypotension. Hyperkalemia may occur, especially when the drug is taken concurrently with potassium-sparing diuretics. *Cognitive Level:* Analysis. *Nursing Process:* Assessment. *Patient Need:* Physiological Integrity.

6 Answer: 3

Rationale: Digoxin and other positive inotropic drugs increase myocardial contractility, allowing the ventricles to eject blood more forcefully and maintaining organ perfusion. In heart failure, blood pressure may be lower than normal or hypotensive due to decreased cardiac output and urinary output declines as renal perfusion decreases. Therapeutic effects include normalized blood pressure and urine output. Positive inotropes exert effects on heart rate through increases in cardiac output. In addition, digoxin slows heart rate do to effects on the conduction system. Positive inotropes do not have diuretic effects. Increased urine output is secondary to increased renal perfusion. While digoxin exerts effects on the cardiac conduction system, not all positive inotropes affect the conduction system. *Cognitive Level:* Analysis. *Nursing Process:* Implementation. *Patient Need:* Physiological Integrity.

Answers to Critical Thinking Questions

1 The nurse should first note improved signs of perfusion if this medication is effective. The nurse would evaluate the patient's skin signs, blood pressure, heart rate, and urine output. If the medication is effective, all these will be within normal limits, or at least improved from the patient's baseline. The ECG may show improvement with a normal sinus rhythm once the digoxin (Lanoxin) has reached a therapeutic level.

2 The nurse understands that there is a cross sensitivity between sulfa and furosemide (Lasix) and therefore would inform the health care provider of the patient's allergy status so a different diuretic might be utilized. Morphine is an appropriate medication for this patient, not only for its analgesic and sedative effects but also for the increased venous capacitance that it causes.

3 This diabetic patient needs to be educated about the importance of regular glucose checks, because this medication may cause the blood sugar to vary sporadically. Typically, hypoglycemia is more of a problem, so the patient needs to be especially aware of the symptoms and treatment of hypoglycemia. Safety should be emphasized, especially regarding postural hypotension.

Chapter 25

Answers to NCLEX-RN® Review Questions

1 Answer: 2

Rationale: At the initial onset of chest pain, sublingual nitroglycerin is administered to assist in the diagnosis, and three doses may be taken 5 minutes apart. Pain that persists 5 to 10 minutes after the initial dose may indicate a myocardial infarction, and the patient should seek medical assistance. *Cognitive Level:* Application. *Nursing Process:* Implementation. *Patient Need:* Physiological Integrity.

2 Answer: 4

Rationale: Antianginal drugs act by decreasing myocardial oxygen demand. This is accomplished by decreasing heart rate, preload, contractility, and afterload. *Cognitive Level:* Application. *Nursing Process:* Implementation. *Patient Need:* Physiological Integrity.

3 Answer: 1

Rationale: Beta blockers decrease the workload of the heart by slowing heart rate and reducing contractility. Calcium channel blockers decrease peripheral resistance. Nitrates relax arterial and venous smooth muscles. *Cognitive Level:* Application. *Nursing Process:* Assessment. *Patient Need:* Physiological Integrity.

4 Answer: 4

Rationale: Patients are often instructed to remove the transdermal patch for 6 to 12 hours each day or withhold the night-time dose of the oral medications to delay the development of tolerance. Because the oxygen demands of the heart during sleep are diminished, the patient with stable angina experiences few anginal episodes during this drug-free interval. *Cognitive Level:* Application. *Nursing Process:* Implementation. *Patient Need:* Physiological Integrity.

5 Answers: 3, 2, 1, 4

Rationale: Prior to administering nitrates for chest pain, the nurse must first assess location, quality, and intensity of pain. Nitrates should not be administered if the patient is hypotensive or if the heart rate is below 60 beats per minute. Once nitrates are administered, blood pressure must be monitored, because hypotension may occur. Documentation of interventions and outcomes is essential to the patient's health history.

Cognitive Level: Application. *Nursing Process:* Implementation. *Patient Need:* Physiological Integrity.

6 Answer: 2

Rationale: Erectile dysfunction drugs such as sildenafil (Viagra), vardenafil (Levitra), and tadalafil (Cialis) decrease blood pressure. When combined with nitrates, severe and prolonged hypotension may result. Erectile dysfunction drugs do not contain nitrates. These drugs are not recognized as useful for the treatment of anginal pain. These drugs do not contain nitrates and do not lead to nitrate tolerance. *Cognitive Level*: Analysis. *Nursing Process*: Implementation. *Patient Need*: Physiological Integrity.

Answers to Critical Thinking Questions

1 The nurse needs to verify blood pressure. A major adverse effect of nitroglycerin is hypotension. If the systolic blood pressure remains below 100 mmHg, the nurse needs to notify the health care provider of the patient's chest pain and blood pressure.

2 Beta blockers slow the heart rate to a desired 50 to 65 beats per minute (beats/min). Many patients suffer from postural hypotension if the heart rate drops below 60 beats/min; therefore, the nurse needs to educate the patient about the necessity of changing positions slowly. The nurse must be aware that a cardinal sign of decreasing cardiac output is tachycardia—a heart rate greater than 100 beats/min for the patient not on beta blockers. If the patient is on beta-blocking medication, the heart rate may not go above 80 to 85 beats/min and is considered tachycardia for this type of patient.

3 Diltiazem (Cardizem) has been given to lower the heart rate and to decrease the myocardial oxygen consumption for this patient with chest pain. The nurse must monitor closely for hypotension, because this medication lowers the heart rate but also lowers the blood pressure, and this patient already has a borderline low blood pressure of 100/60 mmHg. The patient should be on a cardiac monitor with frequent monitoring of blood pressure.

Chapter 26

Answers to NCLEX-RN® Review Questions

1 Answer: 4

Rationale: Beta blockers decrease the body's adrenergic "fight-or-flight" response and may block the symptoms and signals of hypoglycemia that a diabetic normally perceives as the blood sugar drops. Beta blockers may inhibit glycogenolysis, resulting in *hypo*glycemia and have no effect on the development of insulin resistance. *Cognitive Level*: Analysis. *Nursing Process*: Implementation. *Patient Need*: Physiological Integrity.

2 Answer: 1

Rationale: In the absence of ECG monitoring, the nurse would assess the pulse for rate, regularity, quality, and volume, noting any changes. The nurse should also teach the patient to monitor the pulse for rate and regularity, before sending the patient home. The nurse is monitoring for the therapeutic effects of antidysrhythmic therapy. While blood pressure and drug level may also be monitored, they do not evaluate the therapeutic effects of the drug. Urine output may change related to the type of drug given and any effects on cardiac output, but frequent output monitoring is not indicated in routine antidysrhythmic therapy and will not assess for therapeutic drug effects. *Cognitive Level*: Analysis. *Nursing Process*: Assessment. *Patient Need*: Physiological Integrity.

3 Answer: 3

Rationale: Calcium channel blockers such as verapamil (Calan) are used cautiously or are contraindicated in patients with heart failure because of the negative inotropic effects on cardiac muscle which may precipitate or worsen heart failure. Verapamil and calcium channel blockers are often prescribed to treat these conditions. *Cognitive Level*: Analysis. *Nursing Process*: Assessment. *Patient Need*: Physiological Integrity.

4 Answers: 1, 3, 4

Rationale: Because antidysrhythmics can slow the heart rate, the patient may experience hypotension, dizziness, or weakness. *Cognitive Level:* Analysis. *Nursing Process:* Assessment. *Patient Need:* Physiological Integrity.

5 Answer: 2

Rationale: Beta blockers such as propranolol should never be stopped abruptly because of the possible rebound hypertension and increased dysrhythmias that may occur. The nurse may teach the patient to take the medication on an empty stomach and to be cautious with drowsiness while taking beta blockers. However, these are not as significant as the hypertension or dysrhythmias that may occur from abrupt cessation. Therefore, these are secondary teaching points. Hearing loss is not a common side effect of beta blockers. *Cognitive Level*: Analysis. *Nursing Process*: Implementation. *Patient Need*: Physiological Integrity.

6 Answer: 4

Rationale: Potassium channel blockers such as amiodarone, like other antidysrhythmics, may cause significant bradycardia and hypotension. The light-headedness and dizziness may be associated with a drop in cardiac output due to bradycardia and hypotension. The significant finding of dizziness would first be assessed in relation to the known adverse effects of the drug. If pulse and blood pressure are within normal limits, the nurse could consider sleep deprivation, allergies, and drug blood level as a cause of these symptoms. *Cognitive Level*: Analysis. *Nursing Process*: Assessment. *Patient Need*: Physiological Integrity.

Answers to Critical Thinking Questions

1 Propranolol (Inderal) is a nonselective beta-adrenergic blocker, which means it acts on both the intended system (heart) and the lungs. This may cause the patient to have untoward lung problems such as shortness of breath; therefore, this patient should not be taking propranolol.

2 The patient should be monitored closely for hypotension, especially in the first few weeks of treatment, and should be taught about postural hypotension. Pulmonary toxicity is a major complication of this drug, so the patient should be monitored for cough or shortness of breath. Because both digoxin (Lanoxin) and amiodarone (Cordarone) slow the heart rate, the patient must be monitored closely for bradycardia. Safety and pulmonary symptoms are priorities of care for this patient. Amiodarone often increases the effects of digoxin and warfarin (Coumadin) and thus must be closely monitored.

3 Bradycardia is a potential problem for a patient taking verapamil (Isoptin) and digoxin. The patient may exhibit signs of decreased cardiac output, such as pale skin, chest pain, dyspnea, hypotension, and altered level of consciousness. The patient needs to be taught how to recognize the signs of decreasing cardiac output as well as how to assess heart rate.

Answer to Avoiding Medication Errors

The nurse should not administer the medication. Research the correct dosage and administration. The correct dose of lidocaine is 1 to 1.5 mg/kg IV every 3 to 5 minutes up to a maximum dose of 3 mg/kg. It should be given over a 2-minute period, and the nurse should obtain an apical heart rate. The instructions regarding the continuous infusion are unclear. Lidocaine is generally administered 1 to 4 mg/min after a bolus dose. Nurses should never proceed with drug administration until they are confident of the correct parameters for the particular medication.

Chapter 27

Answers to NCLEX-RN® Review Questions

1 *Answer: 4*

Rationale: Prothrombinase converts prothrombin to thrombin. Thrombin then converts fibrinogen to long strands of fibrin, which provide a framework for the clot. Thrombin and fibrin are formed only after the injury occurs. Fibrin strands form an insoluble web over the injured area to stop blood loss. *Cognitive Level:* Analysis. *Nursing Process:* Implementation. *Patient Need:* Physiological Integrity.

2 *Answer: 2*

Rationale: Anticoagulants do not change the viscosity of the blood. Instead, anticoagulants exert a negative charge on the surface of the platelets, so that clumping or aggregation of cells is inhibited. *Cognitive Level:* Analysis. *Nursing Process:* Implementation. *Patient Need:* Physiological Integrity.

3 *Answers: 1, 2, 3, 4*

Rationale: Enoxaparin is a low-molecular-weight heparin (LMWH). This class of drugs has fewer side effects, including being less likely to cause thrombocytopenia. Patients and family can be taught to give subcutaneous injections at home. Teaching should include not taking any other medications without first consulting the health care provider and recognizing the signs and symptoms of bleeding.

Enoxaparin is given to prevent development of DVT. Patients should be taught signs and symptoms of DVT to observe for and should contact their health care provider immediately if these develop. *Cognitive Level:* Analysis. *Nursing Process:* Implementation. *Patient Need:* Physiological Integrity.

4 *Answer: 4*

Rationale: aPT is the coagulation study that monitors oral anticoagulant use, such as warfarin. A result of one and a half to two and a half times the control value indicates adequate anticoagulation. aPTT is the coagulation study that monitors heparin use. An aPT level of one would indicate a less-than-therapeutic level of anticoagulation. *Cognitive Level*: Analysis. *Nursing Process*: Assessment. *Patient Need*: Physiological Integrity.

5 *Answer: 3*

Rationale: Thrombolytic agents dissolve existing clots rapidly and continue to have effects for 2 to 4 days. All forms of bleeding must be monitored and reported immediately. Skin rash with urticaria, wheezing with labored respirations, and temperature elevation of 100.8°F are not symptoms of adverse effects directly attributed to thrombolytic therapy. *Cognitive Level*: Analysis. *Nursing Process*: Assessment. *Patient Need*: Physiological Integrity.

6 *Answer: 2*

Rationale: Antiplatelet drugs such as clopidogrel are given to inhibit platelet aggregation and thus reduce the risk of thrombus formation. Antiplatelet drugs do not exert anti-inflammatory, antipyretic, or analgesic effects. The antiplatelet and anticoagulant drugs do not prevent emboli formation. Thrombolytics dissolve existing blood clots. *Cognitive Level*: Analysis. *Nursing Process*: Implementation. *Patient Need*: Physiological Integrity.

Answers to Critical Thinking Questions

1 The nurse should question the health care provider about this order. No patient who appears to be having a CVA (brain attack) should have heparin until a CT scan of the brain has been done. Approximately 20% of CVAs are hemorrhagic; these types of CVAs must be ruled out before an anticoagulant is given.

2 The major adverse effect of a fibrinolytic drug is bleeding. All tubes (nasogastric, Foley catheter, or endotracheal) must be inserted, blood needs to be drawn, and IVs need to be inserted before the medication is given. Otherwise, the drugs may potentiate bleeding in this patient.

3 Whether the nurse gives this drug or is teaching the patient to self-administer the medication, proper placement of the needle in the abdomen is vital. The injection must be given at least 1 to 2 inches away from the umbilicus. Major blood vessels run close to the umbilicus, and if the LMWH is given near one of these vessels, there is an increased chance of bleeding into the abdomen or formation of a large (and often initially occult) hematoma in the abdomen.

Answer to Avoiding Medication Errors

Most health care providers recommend that mothers not breast-feed while taking warfarin (Coumadin). Heparin is considered safe for breast-feeding mothers. Warfarin is pregnancy category X. Heparin is not excreted into the breast milk.

Chapter 28

Answers to NCLEX-RN® Review Questions

1 *Answers: 1, 2, 3*

Rationale: Iron preparations should be taken on an empty stomach, diluted, and taken through a straw if liquid preparations are used. In addition, extra fluid and fiber will help prevent constipation. Sustained-release medications are specially formulated to absorb slowly and should never be crushed or dissolved. ***Cognitive Level***: Application. ***Nursing Process***: Implementation. ***Patient Need***: Physiological Integrity.

2 *Answer: 3*

Rationale: Secreted by the kidney, erythropoietin travels to the bone marrow, where it interacts with receptors on hematopoietic stem cells with the message to increase erythrocyte production. The primary signal for the increased secretion of erythropoietin is a reduction in oxygen reaching the kidney. ***Cognitive Level:*** Analysis. ***Nursing Process:*** Assessment. ***Patient Need:*** Physiological Integrity.

3 *Answer: 2*

Rationale: This medication does not cure the primary disease condition; however, it helps reduce the anemia that dramatically affects the patient's ability to function. The hematocrit and hemoglobin levels will provide reference for evaluating the drug's effectiveness. ***Cognitive Level:*** Analysis. ***Nursing Process:*** Evaluation. ***Patient Need:*** Physiological Integrity.

4 *Answer: 1*

Rationale: This drug increases the risk of thromboembolic disease. The patient should be monitored for early signs of CVA or MI. ***Cognitive Level:*** Analysis. ***Nursing Process:*** Assessment. ***Patient Need:*** Safe, Effective Care Environment.

5 *Answer: 2*

Rationale: Filgrastim stimulates granulocytes (WBCs). Filgrastim does not stimulate RBC production or enhance/replace electrolytes. ***Cognitive Level***: Application. ***Nursing Process***: Implementation. ***Patient Need***: Physiological Integrity.

6 *Answer: 1*

Filgrastim stimulates granulocytes (WBCs) and is used in the treatment of conditions such as cancer and in HIV. The patient remains at risk for infections until WBC counts increase. Routine monitoring of vital signs is followed and ECG or intake and output levels may be monitored based on patient condition but are not required specific to filgrastim. ***Cognitive Level***: Application. ***Nursing Process***: Implementation. ***Patient Need***: Physiological Integrity.

Answers to Critical Thinking Questions

1 Patients with chronic renal failure often have decreased secretion of endogenous erythropoietin and therefore require a medication such as epoetin alfa (Epogen) to stimulate RBC production and reduce the potential of becoming anemic (or to decrease the effects of anemia). Teaching points should include the importance of monitoring blood pressure for hypertension. Side effects such as nausea, vomiting, constipation, redness/pain at the injection site, confusion, numbness, chest pain, and difficulty breathing should be reported to the health care provider. The patient should also be instructed to maintain a healthy diet and follow any dietary restrictions necessary because of renal failure.

2 Patients who are receiving filgrastim (Neupogen) should have their vital signs assessed every 4 hours (especially pulse and temperature) to monitor for signs of infection related to a low WBC count. Other nursing interventions include assessing for signs and symptoms of myocardial infarction, dysrhythmias, and hepatic dysfunction during treatment.

3 Patients taking this drug need to be educated about the GI distress that may occur while on iron supplements. This medication may be taken with food to reduce the potential for GI upset. Constipation is a common complaint of patients on this medication, so preventive measures need to be taken. The patient needs to ensure that this medication has a child-resistant cap and is safely secured, because overdose of iron supplements is a common toxicology emergency for children.

Chapter 29

Answers to NCLEX-RN® Review Questions

1 *Answers: 1, 2, 4*

Rationale: Crystalloid solutions such as lactated Ringer's closely approximate the electrolytes and concentration of blood plasma. They help increase vascular volume by replacing fluid and promoting adequate urine output, and help maintain normal intracellular volume. Crystalloid solutions are given to maintain osmolarity and intracellular volume within normal limits. ***Cognitive Level***: Analysis. ***Nursing Process***: Implementation. ***Patient Need***: Physiological Integrity.

2 *Answers: 1, 2*

Rationale: With increased cardiac output, renal function should improve, and there should be an increase in urine output. BUN and creatinine levels should be normal. Blood pressure should increase. ***Cognitive Level***: Analysis. ***Nursing Process:*** Evaluation. ***Patient Need:*** Physiological Integrity.

3 *Answer: 2*

Rationale: Dobutamine is beneficial when shock is caused by heart failure. The drug increases contractility and has the potential to cause dysrhythmias. ***Cognitive Level:*** Analysis. ***Nursing Process:*** Assessment. ***Patient Need:*** Physiological Integrity.

4 *Answer: 3*

Rationale: Anaphylactic reactions may occur with the use of plasma protein fraction (Plasmanate). Symptoms include periorbital edema, urticaria, wheezing, and respiratory difficulties. *Cognitive Level:* Analysis. *Nursing Process:* Assessment. *Patient Need:* Physiological Integrity.

5 *Answer: 1*

Rationale: Albumin is a colloid solution. Colloids pull fluid into the vascular space. Circulatory overload may occur. The nurse should assess the patient for symptoms of heart failure. *Cognitive Level:* Analysis. *Nursing Process:* Assessment. *Patient Need:* Physiological Integrity.

6 *Answers: 1, 3, 4*

Rationale: As fluid volume increases beyond the ability of the heart to adequately pump the volume, pulmonary congestion may occur; changes in level of consciousness may indicate increasing intracranial pressure due to increased cerebral volume; and an increase in daily weight may indicate fluid retention. Crystalloid solutions may affect electrolyte levels but these are not accurate indicators of fluid volume excess. aPTT, aPT, or INR levels are monitored when patients are given colloid solutions. *Cognitive Level*: Application. *Nursing Process*: Assessment. *Patient Need*: Physiological Integrity.

Answers to Critical Thinking Questions

1 A major action of this vasopressor medication is its positive inotropic effect on damaged myocardium that is having difficulty maintaining a good cardiac output (and, therefore, blood pressure). Nursing assessments include constant monitoring blood pressure, heart rate and rhythm, fluid volume status, and urine output. The drip must be slowly tapered to a point at which the blood pressure is well maintained, normally a systolic blood pressure of greater than 100 mmHg. The nurse must never consider a blood pressure reading as okay and shut off the vasopressor drip—the patient may immediately become acutely hypotensive.

2 This isotonic solution is appropriate for this patient. Based on history and assessment, the patient is demonstrating signs of being hypovolemic (heart rate of 122 beats per minute) and requires a solution that will meet the intracellular need. The patient must be monitored for hypernatremia and hyperchloremia if more than 3 L of normal saline is given. As the patient responds to the fluid, the nurse will note a corresponding decrease in the heart rate.

3 This is not an appropriate IV solution for a patient with a head injury. Once this IV solution is infused into the patient, it is considered to be a hypotonic solution that moves fluids into the cells. A patient with an increased ICP cannot tolerate an increase of fluid at the cellular level because this may cause the brain to herniate and lead to death.

Chapter 30

Answers to NCLEX-RN® Review Questions

1 *Answer: 1*

Rationale: Because the kidneys excrete most drugs, patients with renal failure will need a significantly lower dosage of medications that may damage the kidneys, to avoid fatal consequences. *Cognitive Level:* Analysis. *Nursing Process:* Implementation. *Patient Need:* Physiological Integrity.

2 *Answer: 1*

Rationale: Potassium is a serious side effect of loop diuretics, and this is a serious concern for patients being treated with digoxin (Lanoxin). *Cognitive Level:* Analysis. *Nursing Process:* Evaluation. *Patient Need:* Physiological Integrity.

3 *Answer: 3*

Rationale: Rapid excretion of large amounts of fluid predisposes the patient to potassium deficits and is manifested by hypotension, dizziness, cardiac dysrhythmias, and fainting. Polydipsia is not associated with hypokalemia, but with diabetes. Hypertension is an indication for the use of diuretics. Diarrhea can be associated with hyperkalemia. *Cognitive Level:* Analysis. *Nursing Process:* Assessment. *Patient Need:* Physiological Integrity.

4 *Answer: 2*

Mannitol increases osmolarity of glomerular filtrate, which raises osmotic pressure in renal tubules and decreases absorption of water and electrolytes. Although mannitol increases urine output, it does not draw excess fluid from tissue spaces and should be used with caution in patients with CHF. Acetazolamide (Diamox) is used to decrease intraocular fluid pressure patients with open-angle glaucoma. Bumetanide (Bumex) and ethacrynic acid (Edecrin) are loop diuretics. *Cognitive Level:* Analysis. *Nursing Process:* Assessment. *Patient Need:* Physiological Integrity.

5 *Answers: 2, 4*

Rationale: Type 2 diabetes is the most common cause of chronic renal failure; hypertension is the second leading cause. *Cognitive Level:* Application. *Nursing Process:* Assessment. *Patient Need:* Physiological Integrity.

6 *Answer: 4*

Rationale: ACE inhibitors or ARBs taken concurrently with potassium-sparing diuretics increase the risk of hyperkalemia. NSAIDs are used cautiously with all diuretics because they are excreted through the kidney. Corticosteroids and loop diuretics may cause *hypo*kalemia and may be paired with a potassium-sparing diuretic to reduce the risk of hypokalemia developing if a diuretic is needed. *Cognitive Level*: Application. *Nursing Process*: Implementation. *Patient Need*: Physiological Integrity.

Answers to Critical Thinking Questions

1 Losartan (Cozaar) is an angiotensin II receptor antagonist commonly prescribed for hypertension. Because

some patients do not respond adequately to monotherapy, a drug that offers combined therapy, Hyzaar, is added. Hyzaar combines losartan with hydrochlorothiazide, a diuretic. This combination decreases blood pressure initially by reducing blood volume and arterial resistance. Over time, the diuretic is effective in maintaining the desired change in sodium balance with a resultant decrease in the sensitivity of vessels to norepinephrine. Angiotensin II–receptor antagonists appear to prevent the hypokalemia associated with thiazide therapy.

2 The nurse should carefully monitor fluid status. Because the primary concern is cardiopulmonary, the nurse should assess and document lung sounds, vital signs, and urine output. Depending on the patient's condition, a Foley catheter may be inserted to permit the measurement of hourly outputs. Daily weights should be obtained. Edema should be evaluated and documented, as well as status of mucous membranes and skin turgor. Because furosemide (Lasix) is a loop diuretic, the nurse would anticipate rapid and profound diuresis. Therefore, the nurse should also observe for signs of dehydration and potassium depletion over the course of therapy.

3 Cerebral edema occurs as a result of the body's response to an initial head trauma. In this case, the patient sustained a skull fracture and underwent the trauma of required surgery. The nurse should explain to the mother that mannitol (Osmitrol) helps reduce swelling or cerebral edema at the site of her son's injury. The nurse might explain that the drug helps "pull" water from the site of injury and carry it to the kidneys, where it is eliminated. The patient's mother should understand that the goal of decreasing swelling is to promote tissue recovery. Nurses must be sensitive to the fact that family members may have severe emotional reactions to a patient's injury and need help to focus on short-term goals for recovery when the long-term prognosis is not known. For additional information on the action or administration of mannitol, students should consult a drug handbook.

Chapter 31

Answers to NCLEX-RN® Review Questions

1 *Answer: 1*

Rationale: Thirst is the most important regulator of fluid intake. **Cognitive Level:** Analysis. **Nursing Process:** Assessment. **Patient Need:** Physiological Integrity.

2 *Answer: 2*

Rationale: Dextran 40, a plasma volume expander, causes fluid to move rapidly from the tissues to vascular spaces, which places the patient at risk for fluid overload. **Cognitive Level:** Analysis. **Nursing Process:** Implementation. **Patient Need:** Physiological Integrity.

3 *Answers: 1, 4*

Rationale: Hypernatremia is defined as serum sodium levels higher than 148 mEq/L. A slight increase in sodium can be managed by diet. The health care provider should be noti-

fied of any elevated lab values. **Cognitive Level:** Analysis. **Nursing Process:** Implementation. **Patient Need:** Physiological Integrity.

4 *Answer: 4*

Rationale: Hyperkalemia, a serum potassium level greater than 5 mEq/L, predisposes the patient to cardiac and muscle irregularities such as cramping in the calves, paresthesia of the toes, and palpitations. **Cognitive Level:** Analysis. **Nursing Process:** Diagnosis. **Patient Need:** Physiological Integrity.

5 *Answer: 3*

Rationale: Bananas, strawberries, tomatoes, dried beans, and fresh meats are natural sources of potassium. The other food items have low levels of potassium but may be part of a healthy diet. **Cognitive Level:** Application. **Nursing Process:** Implementation. **Patient Need:** Physiological Integrity.

6 *Answer: 2*

Rationale: A weight gain of 1 kg (approximately 2 lb) or more may indicate fluid retention. Signs of fluid retention include hypertension and edema. A complete nursing assessment is needed to determine other signs or symptoms that may be present. Checking dietary history may be considered after the nursing assessment is completed. Changing diet or medications is part of the collaborative treatment plan with the health care provider. **Cognitive Level:** Analysis. **Nursing Process:** Assessment. **Patient Need:** Physiological Integrity.

Answers to Critical Thinking Questions

1 Aggressive treatment with loop diuretics is a common cause of hypokalemia. As in this example, hypokalemia can produce a myriad of sequelae including dysrhythmias. KCl is indicated for patients with low potassium levels and is preferred over other potassium salts because chloride is simultaneously replaced. The nurse administering KCl must keep in mind several critical concerns to safeguard the patient. The primary concern is the risk of potassium intoxication. High plasma concentrations of potassium may cause death through cardiac depression, arrhythmias, or arrest. The signs and symptoms of potassium overdose include mental confusion, weakness, listlessness, hypotension, and ECG abnormalities. In a patient with heart disease, cardiac monitoring may be indicated during potassium infusion. Students should consult their drug handbooks and look up the maximum rates for infusing KCl in adults and children.

To prevent potassium intoxication, the nurse should carefully regulate the infusion of IV fluids. Most institutions require that any solution containing KCl be administered using an infusion pump. Prior to beginning and throughout the infusion, the nurse should assess the patient's renal function (BUN and creatinine levels). A patient with diminished renal function is more likely to develop hyperkalemia.

2 The patient may be considered dehydrated despite her appearance as indicated by her elevated hematocrit and hemoglobin ("hemoconcentration"). Most pregnant women present with normal or slightly decreased hemoglobin and hematocrit levels related to the increase in intravascular volume during pregnancy. The midwife recognizes the need to increase the intravascular fluid compartment to promote renal and uterine perfusion. Careful monitoring of the patient's blood pressure, pulse, and weight should be maintained.

3 Excessive renal fluid loss due to diuretic therapy, such as with furosemide (Lasix), can contribute to fluid volume deficits in patients taking these medications. Because pharmacotherapy with thiazide or loop diuretics such as furosemide is the most common cause of potassium loss, patients taking these diuretics are usually instructed to take oral potassium supplements to prevent hypokalemia.

Answer to Avoiding Medication Errors

Student nurses are held to the same standard as nurses holding a license. Like the student nurse, the nursing instructor and the primary nurse are responsible if they checked the medication dosage prior to administration and did not question the order. The health care provider is responsible because the order was incorrect, but the errors should have been identified prior to reaching the patient. The nurse manager retains accountability for the unit.

Chapter 32

Answers to NCLEX-RN® Review Questions

1 *Answer: 4*
Rationale: Due to immune system suppression by the medication, infections are common. *Cognitive Level:* Application. *Nursing Process:* Diagnosis. *Patient Need:* Physiological Integrity.

2 *Answer: 4*
Rationale: Grapefruit juice increases cyclosporine levels 50% to 200%, resulting in drug toxicity. Hand washing is important to prevent infection. Renal toxicity and hypertension are adverse effects of cyclosporine therapy. *Cognitive Level:* Analysis. *Nursing Process:* Assessment. *Patient Need:* Physiological Integrity.

3 *Answer: 2*
Rationale: Seventy-five percent of patients on cyclosporine experience decreased renal output because of physiological changes in the kidneys, such as microcalcification and interstitial fibrosis. The serum creatinine test is a good indicator of renal function. *Cognitive Level:* Analysis. *Nursing Process:* Assessment. *Patient Need:* Physiological Integrity.

4 *Answers: 1, 2, 4, 5*
Rationale: Pregnancy, renal or liver disease, and metastatic cancer are contraindications to the use of immunostimulant drugs. Infection, immunodeficiency disease, and cancer are indications for use of these drugs. *Cognitive Level:* Analysis. *Nursing Process:* Assessment. *Patient Need:* Physiological Integrity.

5 *Answer: 1*
Rationale: Active immunity occurs when the patient has received the vaccine. Passive immunity is achieved by directly administering antibodies to a patient. A titer is a measurement of the amount of antibody produced after a vaccine. *Cognitive Level:* Application. *Nursing Process:* Assessment. *Patient Need:* Physiological Integrity.

6 *Answer: 4*
Rationale: Live vaccines may be contraindicated when patients present an exposure risk of the infectious agent to immunocompromised patients such as those on chemotherapy or immunosuppressant therapy. The patient's cousin having the flu is not a potential contraindication, assuming the cousin has a normal and active immune system. The mother would not be at risk and since she has received recent vaccinations, assessment of her immune system would have been completed at that time. Soreness of the injected arm is a potential (mild) adverse effect of immunizations and can be managed symptomatically. *Cognitive Level:* Application. *Nursing Process:* Assessment. *Patient Need:* Physiological Integrity.

Answers to Critical Thinking Questions

1 Sirolimus (Rapamune) is an immunosuppressant. The nurse should assess for any signs and symptoms of bleeding or jaundice and infection. The nurse should question the patient regarding activities that may cause bleeding. The nurse should also assess for signs and symptoms of liver impairment. The nurse should notify the health care provider of the laboratory findings and educate the patient to report any bleeding to the provider. The patient should also report signs and symptoms of infection.

2 The patient needs the protection of this passive form of immunity after an exposure to such an illness. The gamma globulin will act as a protective mechanism for 3 weeks while the patient is in the window of opportunity for developing hepatitis A. This drug does not stimulate the patient's immune system but will help protect the patient from developing the disease. The nurse should inform the patient that the shot is far less debilitating than the disease.

3 Cyclosporine is a toxic medication with many serious adverse effects. The nurse must understand that this drug cannot be given with grapefruit juice; patients who take this medication need their kidney function assessed regularly (not because of the kidney transplant but because cyclosporine reduces urine output). The nurse also must assess whether this patient is taking steroids, which are often given concurrently with cyclosporine, as the serum glucose needs to be monitored regularly.

Answer to Avoiding Medication Errors

Methotrexate is given for rheumatoid arthritis in smaller doses than when used in cancer chemotherapy. It is thought to block metabolism of folic acid. For rheumatoid arthritis, patients take 10 to 12 mg once a week. It may modify the disease manifestations, or it may just improve symptoms and quality of life.

Chapter 33

Answers to NCLEX-RN® Review Questions

1 *Answer: 3*

Rationale: Acetaminophen has analgesic and antipyretic properties, but no anti-inflammatory actions. *Cognitive Level:* Analysis. *Nursing Process:* Implementation. *Patient Need:* Physiological Integrity.

2 *Answer: 3*

Rationale: High doses of aspirin can produce side effects of tinnitus, dizziness, headache, and sweating. *Cognitive Level:* Analysis. *Nursing Process:* Implementation. *Patient Need:* Physiological Integrity.

3 *Answer: 4*

Rationale: Side effects that need to be reported immediately include difficulty breathing; heartburn; chest, abdomen, or joint or bone pain; nosebleed; blood in sputum when coughing; blood in vomitus, urine, or stools; fever; chills or signs of infection; increased thirst or urination; fruity breath odor; falls; or mood swings. *Cognitive Level:* Analysis. *Nursing Process:* Implementation. *Nursing Process:* Physiological Integrity.

4 *Answer: 4*

Rationale: Monitor for development of Cushing's syndrome (adrenocortical excess) with signs and symptoms of bruising and a characteristic pattern of fat deposits in the cheeks (moon face), shoulders (buffalo hump), and abdomen. *Cognitive Level:* Analysis. *Nursing Process:* Diagnosis. *Patient Need:* Physiological Integrity.

5 *Answer: 1*

Rationale: Excessive doses of acetaminophen or regular consumption of alcohol may increase the risk of hepatic toxicity when acetaminophen is used. Renal damage, thrombotic effects, and pulmonary damage are not adverse effects associated specifically with acetaminophen. *Cognitive Level:* Application. *Nursing Process:* Assessment. *Patient Need:* Physiological Integrity.

6 *Answer: 4*

Rationale: Aspirin and salicylates are associated with an increased risk of Reye's syndrome in children under 18, especially in the presence of viral infections. Acetaminophen is not quantifiably different than aspirin or salicylates for the treatment of fever. Use of aspirin or salicylates should not increase fever although may cause nausea or vomiting related to GI irritation but is not contraindicated in children specifically for this reason. *Cognitive Level:* Application. *Nursing Process:* Implementation. *Patient Need:* Physiological Integrity.

Answers to Critical Thinking Questions

1 This patient has many potential problems related to the use of prednisone over a sustained period. The primary current concern is the hyperglycemia—an adverse effect of the prednisone that can become serious when the patient is diabetic. Blood pressure must be monitored for potential hypertension, which is related to sodium retention and, therefore, increased water retention caused by the prednisone. The patient is also at high risk for infection while on prednisone because of suppression of the immune system, also related to the diabetes.

2 The nurse should give the patient celecoxib (Celebrex) for the elbow inflammation and pain. This medication should provide adequate relief of the symptoms for this patient. Ensure that the patient is not allergic to sulfa prior to giving this medication. The patient should not take acetaminophen (Tylenol) because of related potential liver compromise secondary to alcohol abuse. The patient should not take ibuprofen (Motrin) because of the potential for gastric bleeding. The patient's stomach is already at risk because of alcohol abuse, and the chance for bleeding is elevated because of potential liver problems secondary to alcohol abuse.

3 The nurse should educate the mother that aspirin and aspirin-containing products should not be given to children younger than age 18. These drugs have been implicated in the development of Reye's syndrome. Acetaminophen is the antipyretic of choice for treating most fevers. The nurse should also further question the mother regarding the length and severity of symptoms.

Chapter 34

Answers to NCLEX-RN® Review Questions

1 *Answer: 4*

When normal host flora are decreased or killed by antibacterial therapy, opportunistic organisms such as viral and fungal infections may occur. The other options are not definitions of superinfections although they may be adverse drug effects of antibacterial therapy. *Cognitive Level:* Application. *Nursing Process:* Assessment. *Patient Need:* Physiological Integrity.

2 *Answer: 2*

Rationale: Many people will discontinue medication after improvement is noted. All antibiotic regimens must be completed to prevent recurrence of infection. Some penicillins (amoxicillin) should be taken with meals, whereas all others should be taken 1 hour before or 2 hours after meals. Penicillins should be used with caution during breastfeeding. *Cognitive Level:* Analysis. *Nursing Process:* Implementation. *Patient Need:* Physiological Integrity.

3 *Answer: 4*

Rationale: This drug has the ability to cause permanent mottling and discoloration of teeth, and therefore is not appropriate for children younger than 8 years of age. Tetracyclines have one of the broadest spectrums of the antibiotics and are contraindicated in pregnancy. *Cognitive Level:* Analysis. *Nursing Process:* Implementation. *Patient Need:* Physiological Integrity.

4 *Answer: 4*

Rationale: This anti-infective is noted for its toxic effects on kidneys and vestibular apparatus. Patients should be monitored for ototoxicity and nephrotoxicity during and after therapy. Aminoglycosides do not cause discoloration of the teeth. Fluid intake should be increased with aminoglycosides. Aminoglycosides are poorly absorbed from the GI tract and are administered parentally for systemic bacterial infections. *Cognitive Level:* Analysis. *Nursing Process:* Implementation. *Patient Need:* Physiological Integrity.

5 *Answers: 1, 2, 3*

Rationale: For the medication to reach the microorganism, it is critical that the medicine be taken for 6 to 12 months, and possibly as long as 24 months. Antitubercular drugs are also used for prevention and treatment. Multiple drug therapy is necessary because the mycobacteria grow slowly, and resistance is common. Using multiple drugs in different combinations during the long treatment period lowers the potential for resistance and increases the chances for successful therapy. *Cognitive Level:* Analysis. *Nursing Process:* Implementation. *Patient Need:* Physiological Integrity.

6 *Answer: 2*

Penicillin antibiotics may significantly decrease the effectiveness of oral contraceptives and another method of birth control should be suggested during the time the drug is taken. The other options are not adverse drug effects associated directly with penicillin antibiotics. Given the age of this patient, concern for possible pregnancy prevention would be a high priority. *Cognitive Level*: Application. *Nursing Process*: Assessment. *Patient Need*: Physiological Integrity.

Answers to Critical Thinking Questions

1 This patient should not be on tetracycline (Achromycin) while pregnant because tetracycline is a category D drug that has teratogenic effects on the fetus. Counseling should be provided for alternative sources of care for her acne as well as for use of drugs when pregnant.

2 The nurse should not give the erythromycin. This patient has a history of hepatitis B, and this medication is metabolized by the liver. An alternative type of antibiotic should be utilized.

3 This medication is typically reserved for more serious infections because of its higher potential for toxicity. Renal function is a priority assessment for this patient. The nurse should monitor urine output, urine protein, and serum BUN and creatinine on a regular basis. A secondary priority is hearing assessment, because ototoxicity is common for patients on gentamicin.

Answer to Avoiding Medication Errors

The nurse should have questioned the health care provider regarding Bactrim, which contains sulfamethoxazole. Because the patient has an allergy to sulfa drugs, he would be allergic to Bactrim as well. Some individuals experience nausea, a side effect of sulfa drugs. True allergies involve histamine-mediated responses and result in symptoms such as a rash or hives. In severe cases, bronchospasm and cardiovascular compromise are possible. Because the drug is a large tablet, it is permissible to break the tablet in half and provide a large glass of water.

Chapter 35

Answers to NCLEX-RN® Review Questions

1 *Answer: 3*

Rationale: Systemic antifungal drugs have little or no antibacterial activity. Fluid intake should be increased with this medication because it can affect renal function. The full course of therapy should be completed. All intramuscular sites have the potential to bruise. *Cognitive Level:* Analysis. *Nursing Process:* Implementation. *Patient Need:* Physiological Integrity.

2 *Answer: 2*

Rationale: The patient needs to be assessed for pre-existing cardiovascular disease, and an ECG should be done. Quinine therapy does not require a consent to be signed, but education is needed. All medication should be continued unless otherwise specified. *Cognitive Level:* Analysis. *Nursing Process:* Implementation. *Patient Need:* Physiological Integrity.

3 *Answer: 4*

Rationale: Chloroquine (Aralen) is the classic antimalarial for treating the acute stage. Proguanil (Paludrine) is the prototype antimalarial for prophylaxis. Rizatriptan (Maxalt) is used in the treatment of migraines. *Cognitive Level:* Analysis. *Nursing Process:* Implementation. *Patient Need:* Physiological Integrity.

4 *Answers: 1, 2, 3, 4*

Rationale: Play habits and hygiene of children can contribute to the transmission and reinfestation of pinworms and roundworms. It is important that all family members understand the importance of hand washing to prevent the transmission of worms. Correct hand washing should be taught, and children should not be allowed to play in sandboxes that are left uncovered. Children should also wear shoes when outside playing to prevent skin invasion. *Cognitive Level:* Analysis. *Nursing Process:* Implementation. *Patient Need:* Safe, Effective Care Environment.

5 *Answer: 4*

Rationale: Concurrent use of alcohol during metronidazole treatment may cause a disulfiram-like reaction with excessive nausea, vomiting, and possible hypotension. The other options may have slight GI effects (e.g., mild nausea) but would not be a cause for concern if taken with the metronidazole. *Cognitive Level*: Application. *Nursing Process*: Implementation. *Patient Need*: Physiological Integrity.

6 *Answers: 1, 2, 4, 5*

Rationale: Metronidazole may cause a metallic drug taste during therapy and may cause urine to darken. Taking the drug with food or milk may help reduce GI effects. Current sexual partners do not usually require treatment for *Giardia* infections unless they are also experiencing symptoms. The entire course of metronidazole therapy should be completed, even if symptoms are diminished or absent, to ensure adequate treatment. **Cognitive Level**: Application. **Nursing Process**: Implementation. **Patient Need**: Physiological Integrity.

Answers to Critical Thinking Questions

1 As always, the ABCs are a priority for any patient and must be considered. The nurse must monitor the patient's airway for evidence of bronchospasm or decreased gas exchange, such as coughing, poor color, and decreased oxygen saturation. The nurse must understand that leukopenia is a problem for these patients (related to the amphotericin B and the patient's own depressed immune status); therefore, prevention of infection is always a priority. The patient's renal status (urine output, serum BUN, and creatinine) also must be closely monitored because approximately 30% of patients on this medication suffer renal damage.

2 This patient has vaginal candidiasis, so it must be stressed that her partner be treated concurrently or reinfection may result. Alcohol must be avoided while on this medication to prevent profound vomiting. It is important to stress that alcohol is found not only in alcoholic drinks but also in products such as cough medicine, vanilla extract, and even in perfume that is absorbed via the skin.

3 This drug can have profound adverse effects, and the patient must be carefully screened and educated about this drug prior to taking it. The patient must have a baseline physical assessment, including an ECG and blood pressure assessment, liver and renal function tests, and a hearing and visual assessment screening. Because the patient may suffer permanent organ damage while taking this medication, baseline information is crucial.

Chapter 36

Answers to NCLEX-RN® Review Questions

1 *Answer: 2*

Rationale: Drug therapy has not produced a cure but has resulted in a number of therapeutic successes. There is no vaccine for HIV. **Cognitive Level:** Application. **Nursing Process:** Implementation. **Patient Need:** Physiological Integrity.

2 *Answers: 3, 4*

Rationale: Two laboratory tests used to guide pharmacotherapy are an absolute CD4 count and an HIV RNA measurement. Clotting factors and a CBC do not provide information for guiding HIV-AIDS therapy. **Cognitive Level:** Analysis. **Nursing Process:** Implementation. **Patient Need:** Physiological Integrity.

3 *Answer: 1*

Rationale: The medication should be taken on an empty stomach for maximum absorption. **Cognitive Level:** Analy-

sis. **Nursing Process:** Implementation. **Patient Need:** Physiological Integrity.

4 *Answer: 2*

Rationale: Oseltamivir (Tamiflu) and zanamivir (Relenza) are available and may prevent the flu or if taken within 48 hours of symptoms, may limit the length of the disease. Immunity begins approximately 2 weeks after immunization. Vaccination is recommended for high-risk populations and for healthy adults over 65. Flu may be highly contagious and at-risk patients should not wait until symptoms begin to seek vaccination or treatment. **Cognitive Level**: Application. **Nursing Process**: Implementation. **Patient Need**: Physiological Integrity.

5 *Answer: 3*

Rationale: Neurologic adverse effects may occur but dizziness, sleep disorders, nightmares, and difficulty thinking clearly tend to improve after 3 to 4 weeks. Neurotoxicity may occur and increasing confusion, delusions, or seizures should be reported immediately. Drugs for HIV-AIDS help limit the viral load and maintain a longer symptom-free period. All drugs used for HIV-AIDS have significant adverse effects. Taking efavirenz (Sutiva) with a high-fat meal may increase its absorption by as much as 50%, leading to toxicity. **Cognitive Level**: Application. **Nursing Process**: Implementation. **Patient Need**: Physiological Integrity.

6 *Answers: 1, 2*

Rationale: Acyclovir can be renal toxic and fluids should be increased throughout therapy. Neurotoxicity may occur and increasing dizziness, tremors, or any confusion should be reported immediately. Fluid intake should be increased, not decreased, and the drug must be taken consistently throughout the entire course of therapy. Suppressive therapy may also be ordered. **Cognitive Level**: Application. **Nursing Process**: Implementation. **Patient Need**: Physiological Integrity.

Answers to Critical Thinking Questions

1 The best approach to influenza infection is *prevention* through annual vaccination. Those who benefit greatly from vaccinations include residents of long-term care facilities. The drug amantadine (Symmetrel) is used to prevent and treat influenza. The nurse should work with the health care provider to obtain an order and make arrangements to administer the medication.

2 This medication may cause bone marrow suppression. This patient is already immunocompromised, and the potential for leukopenia is high. The patient should be taught to watch for any evidence of infection, monitor temperature, and have regular lab tests. The patient also needs instruction about the importance of good hand washing and safeguarding against potential sources of infection.

3 The nurse should inform the health care provider that the medication needs to be administered over a minimum of 1 hour, and that the nurse is unable to give the medication as a bolus or IV piggyback for less than 1 hour. The IV site

must be monitored closely for potential infiltration while the medication is infusing. If this occurs, the IV must be stopped immediately.

Chapter 37

Answers to NCLEX-RN® Review Questions

1 *Answer: 2*

Rationale: Effectiveness of chemotherapy is increased by use of multiple drugs from different classes that attack cancer cells at different points in the cell cycle. Thus, lower doses of each individual agent can be used to reduce side effects. A third benefit of combination chemotherapy is reduced incidence of drug resistance. *Cognitive Level:* Application. *Nursing Process:* Implementation. *Patient Need:* Physiological Integrity.

2 *Answer: 3*

Rationale: For maximum effect, patients starting therapy with agents with high emetic potential should be given an antiemetic prior to the start of treatment. *Cognitive Level:* Application. *Nursing Process:* Implementation. *Patient Need:* Physiological Integrity.

3 *Answers: 4, 5*

Rationale: Patient and family members should avoid receiving live virus vaccinations or becoming exposed to chicken pox. The patient could have an exacerbation or a more pronounced episode of chicken pox. The patient should also avoid crowds. *Cognitive Level:* Analysis. *Nursing Process:* Implementation. *Patient Need:* Physiological Integrity.

4 *Answer: 3*

Rationale: The nurse should monitor for blood dyscrasias resulting from bone marrow suppression by monitoring the CBC with differential and platelet count. *Cognitive Level:* Analysis. *Nursing Process:* Evaluation. *Patient Need:* Physiological Integrity.

5 *Answer: 2*

Rationale: The most serious side effect of vincristine is nervous system toxicity. Paralytic ileus is likely in young children. *Cognitive Level:* Analysis. *Nursing Process:* Implementation. *Patient Need:* Physiological Integrity.

6 *Answer: 2*

Rationale: The nadir is the point of greatest bone marrow suppression, as measured by the lowest neutrophil count. Nadir does not refer to chemotherapy dose, level, or patient symptoms. *Cognitive Level:* Application. *Nursing Process:* Assessment. *Patient Need:* Physiological Integrity.

Answers to Critical Thinking Questions

1 The patient needs to be taught strategies for coping with the side effects of the chemotherapy regimen. Nutrition is a major focus. The patient should always take antiemetics 1 hour prior to chemotherapy, eat small frequent meals, drink high-calorie liquids if unable to eat solid food, and increase fluids if diarrhea occurs.

2 The patient and family should be taught about the potential for infection related to immunosuppression. The nurse should stress frequent hand washing, avoiding large crowds, self-assessing temperature accurately at home, and knowing when to call the health care provider. Nurses take these basics for granted even though patients often have misconceptions about them.

3 The nurse should remain with the solution and call for someone to bring the chemo spill kit immediately. While waiting for the spill kit, the nurse may cover the contaminated fluid with paper towels (the nurse must not touch the solution without wearing protective equipment). The nurse should clean up the spill and dispose of the waste per hospital protocols. At no time should the chemotherapy spill be left unattended.

Chapter 38

Answers to NCLEX-RN® Review Questions

1 *Answer: 1*

Rationale: Prolonged use of oxymetazoline causes hypersecretion of mucus and worsening nasal congestion, resulting in increased daily use. This medication should not be used for longer than 3 days and should be used only as directed. *Cognitive Level:* Application. *Nursing Process:* Implementation. *Patient Need:* Physiological Integrity.

2 *Answers: 2, 3*

Rationale: The device delivers a metered spray that regulates the dosage and keeps it consistent. Use of intranasal glucocorticoids may require 2 to 4 weeks. Side effects include drying and bleeding of the nasal cavity. Saline nasal sprays may be used to alleviate drying. The medication should be used as prescribed. *Cognitive Level:* Application. *Nursing Process:* Implementation. *Patient Need:* Physiological Integrity.

3 *Answer: 1*

Rationale: First-generation H_1-receptor antagonists are contraindicated in patients with a history of dysrhythmias and heart failure. These medications can cause vasodilation of vessels due to H_1 stimulation. These medications have no relationship to weight gain or peptic ulcer disease. *Cognitive Level:* Analysis. *Nursing Process:* Assessment. *Patient Need:* Physiological Integrity.

4 *Answers: 1, 2, 5*

Rationale: The device must be primed prior to initial use. The nose should be cleared prior to administration, not afterward, so that medication remains in the nasal cavity. Any excess that drains into the mouth must not be swallowed but should be spit out. *Cognitive Level:* Application. *Nursing Process:* Implementation. *Patient Need:* Physiological Integrity.

5 *Answer: 1*

Rationale: A major side effect of antihistamines relates to their anticholinergic effects. Anticholinergic effects can also cause urinary hesitancy and should not be used in patients with a history of prostatic hypertrophy. *Cognitive Level:* Analysis. *Nursing Process:* Assessment. *Patient Need:* Physiological Integrity.

6 *Answer: 3*

Rationale: Single-symptom OTC preparations are preferred over multiuse preparations to avoid additional drugs that are not needed for symptom relief and to decrease risk of additional adverse effects. Dosing of any OTC preparation is carefully calculated to provide precise dosing for age and symptoms. Antibiotics may be required for serious infections but for common symptoms, OTC remedies are recognized as safe and effective but should not be used indefinitely without consultation with a health care provider. *Cognitive Level*: Application. *Nursing Process*: Implementation. *Patient Need*: Physiological Integrity.

Answers to Critical Thinking Questions

1 The nurse needs to ensure that the patient understands the potential side effects related to the anticholinergic effects of this medication. The patient (based on age) is at higher risk for urine retention, glaucoma (or other visual changes), and constipation.

2 Although codeine is a more powerful antitussive, it can cause dependence and constipation. Dextromethorphan is a more appropriate choice for this patient initially, with codeine syrup as a potential later choice for more severe cough symptoms.

3 Intranasal glucocorticoids, such as Flonase, may take as long as 2 to 4 weeks to work. The medication should not be discontinued prematurely. If a decongestant spray is being used along with the Flonase, the decongestant should always be administered first to clear the nasal passages, which will facilitate adequate application of the glucocorticoid mist.

Answer to Avoiding Medication Errors

Benzonatate is chemically related to the local anesthetic tetracaine (Pontocaine) and suppresses the cough reflex by anesthetizing stretch receptors in the lungs. The perles (capsules) must be swallowed whole and not be chewed or punctured so the liquid may be swallowed. The drug inside the perle can cause numbing of the mouth, pharynx, and epiglottis, leading to aspiration, respiratory distress, or arrest. If the patient cannot swallow the medication whole, the health care provider should be contacted for a possible change in orders.

Chapter 39

Answers to NCLEX-RN® Review Questions

1 *Answer: 2*

Rationale: An aerosol is a suspension of minute liquid droplets or fine solid particles in a gas. Aerosol therapy can give immediate relief for bronchospasm or can loosen thick mucus. The major advantage of aerosol therapy is that it delivers medications to the immediate sites of action, thus re-

ducing systemic side effects. The main disadvantage is that the precise dose received by the patient is difficult to measure because it depends on the patient's breathing pattern and the correct use of the aerosol device. *Cognitive Level:* Application. *Nursing Process:* Implementation. *Patient Need:* Physiological Integrity.

2 *Answer: 2*

Rationale: Beta-adrenergic agonists (sympathomimetics) act by relaxing bronchial smooth muscle, resulting in bronchodilation that lowers airway resistance and makes breathing easier for the patient. Beta-adrenergic agonists do not liquefy or reduce mucus production. *Cognitive Level:* Analysis. *Nursing Process:* Implementation. *Patient Need:* Physiological Integrity.

3 *Answer: 4*

Rationale: Tolerance may develop to the therapeutic effects of the beta-adrenergic agonists; therefore, the patient must be instructed to seek medical attention if the drugs become less effective with continued use. Increased heart rate is a side effect of beta-adrenergic agonists. The patient should not change the medication dosage without first consulting the health care provider. *Cognitive Level:* Analysis. *Nursing Process:* Implementation. *Patient Need:* Physiological Integrity.

4 *Answer: 3*

Rationale: Anticholinergic bronchodilators should be used cautiously in elderly men with benign prostatic hyperplasia and in patients with glaucoma. An enlarged liver and diarrhea have no relationship to the use of ipratropium. *Cognitive Level:* Analysis. *Nursing Process:* Implementation. *Patient Need:* Physiological Integrity.

5 *Answers: 3, 4*

Rationale: If taken for longer than 10 days, oral glucocorticoids can produce significant adverse effects, including adrenal gland atrophy, peptic ulcers, and hyperglycemia. Long-term oral glucocorticoids can cause osteoporosis. Changes in level of consciousness may be related to oxygenation levels and need to be reported to the health care provider. *Cognitive Level:* Analysis. *Nursing Process:* Assessment. *Patient Need:* Physiological Integrity.

6 *Answer: 3*

Rationale: Beta-adrenergic drugs such as albuterol (Proventil, Ventolin) are most often used for rapid bronchodilation. Glucocorticoids such as beclomethasone, leukotriene modifiers such as zileuton, and long-acting beta agonists such as salmeterol may be used for maintenance therapy to prevent or control asthma attacks but do not act quickly enough for acute attacks. *Cognitive Level*: Application. *Nursing Process*: Implementation. *Patient Need*: Physiological Integrity.

Answers to Critical Thinking Questions

1 The nurse needs to ensure that the patient understands the potential side effects related to anticholinergic effects of this medication. The patient (based on age) is at higher

risk for urine retention, glaucoma (or other visual changes), and constipation. These are also common problems for patients who are taking this medication.

2 Once the patient's condition begins to improve, the nurse should assess the patient's understanding of the asthma regimen. The patient should receive instruction on the side effects of glucocorticoid therapy. Glucocorticoids can suppress the hypothalamic–pituitary axis. Abruptly discontinuing a glucocorticoid after long-term therapy (greater than 10 days) can produce cardiovascular collapse. The patient needs to be instructed on the dosage regimen for prednisone, which may include an incremental decrease in the drug dosage when discontinuing the drug. The patient should be monitored for hyperglycemia, peptic ulcer disease, signs and symptoms of GI bleeding, poor wound healing, infections, and mood changes.

3 Key patient education points of emphasis regarding administering medications via an inhaler include the following:

1. Shake the canister well immediately before each use.

2. Exhale completely to the end of a normal breath.

3. With the inhaler in the upright position, place the mouthpiece just inside the mouth and use the lips to form a tight seal.

4. While pressing down on the inhaler, take a slow, deep breath and hold for approximately 10 seconds.

5. Wait approximately 2 minutes before taking a second inhalation of the drug.

6. Rinse the mouth with water after each use (especially after using steroid inhalers, because the drug may cause fungal infections of the mouth and throat).

Chapter 40

Answers to NCLEX-RN® Review Questions

1 *Answer: 3*

Rationale: Antacids are generally combinations of aluminum hydroxide and magnesium hydroxide. Hypermagnesemia can develop with use of OTC antacids while on renal dialysis because the kidneys are unable to excrete excess magnesium. Hyperkalemia is a complication of renal failure. Hypernatremia can occur with use of antacids. *Cognitive Level:* Analysis. *Nursing Process:* Implementation. *Patient Need:* Physiological Integrity.

2 *Answer: 1*

Rationale: Two or more antibiotics are used to lower the potential for bacterial resistance and increase the effectiveness of therapy. Bacterial infections can recur, requiring future treatment. *Cognitive Level:* Analysis. *Nursing Process:* Implementation. *Patient Need:* Physiological Integrity.

3 *Answer: 1*

Rationale: Simethicone is used along with other GI drugs or alone to decrease the amount of gas bubbles that accumulate with GI disorders or indigestion. Simethicone will not affect the acid-fighting ability of medications, or prevent constipation or diarrhea from developing. *Cognitive Level:* Application. *Nursing Process:* Implementation. *Patient Need:* Physiological Integrity.

4 *Answers: 2, 3*

Rationale: Bismuth compounds may be added to the regimen treatment of *Helicobacter pylori.* These products inhibit bacterial growth and prevent *H. pylori* from adhering to the gastric mucosa H_2-receptor blockers are also used to help eradicate *H. pylori.* None of the other options is used in the treatment of *H. pylori.* *Cognitive Level:* Analysis. *Nursing Process:* Implementation. *Patient Need:* Physiological Integrity.

5 *Answers: 1, 2, 3, 5*

Rationale: Risk factors associated with peptic ulcer disease include a family history of peptic ulcer disease; blood group O; smoking tobacco; caffeine, aspirin, glucocorticoid, and NSAID use; excessive stress; and *H. pylori.* Type 2 diabetes mellitus has not been associated with peptic ulcer disease. *Cognitive Level:* Analysis. *Nursing Process:* Assessment. *Patient Need:* Physiological Integrity.

6 *Answer: 4*

Rationale: Proton-pump inhibitors such as omeprazole are recommended for short-term therapy and are associated with a possible increased risk of gastric cancer when taken long term. If symptoms of epigastric pain and discomfort continue, other therapies and screening for *H. pylori* may be indicated. Switching to another proton pump inhibitor still exceeds the recommended time of use for this category of drugs. H_2-receptor blockers may be indicated but their use should be evaluated by a health care provider because more definitive treatment (e.g., for *H. pylori*) may be required. Proton pump inhibitors should be taken 30 minutes *before* meals. *Cognitive Level:* Application. *Nursing Process:* Implementation. *Patient Need:* Physiological Integrity.

Answers to Critical Thinking Questions

1 Regular use of aluminum hydroxide (Amphojel) may cause hypercalcemia because calcium and phosphorus have a reciprocal relationship; that is, if the calcium goes up, the phosphorus goes down. A patient with low serum phosphorus often exhibits signs of increasing weakness. The treatment is to replace the aluminum hydroxide with a different antacid and take oral phosphorus supplements until serum phosphorus returns to a normal level.

2 The stomach is empty during the sleep cycle, the time when the protective protein peptide TFF2 is most effective at repairing the mucoprotective lining of the stomach. For the TFF2 protein to reach its maximum effectiveness, the person needs a minimum of 6 hours of

uninterrupted sleep, which is uncommon in people who sleep during the daytime.

3 This patient has a history of PUD; therefore, alcohol and smoking are contraindicated because they will exacerbate the condition. This patient is on ranitidine (Zantac), and smoking decreases the effectiveness of the medication. Alcohol is a depressant and can cause increased drowsiness in combination with ranitidine. This patient should be advised to stop smoking and drinking alcohol if PUD is to be resolved.

Chapter 41

Answers to NCLEX-RN® Review Questions

1 *Answer: 1*

Rationale: When contents lost from the stomach are strongly acidic, vomiting may change the pH of the blood, resulting in metabolic acidosis. With severe loss, acid–base disturbances can lead to vascular collapse. Patients' respirations may increase with prolonged vomiting. Esophageal tears with prolonged vomiting occur rarely. *Cognitive Level:* Analysis. *Nursing Process:* Assessment. *Patient Need:* Physiological Integrity.

2 *Answer: 1*

Rationale: Dramamine is most effective when taken at least 20 to 60 minutes before the intended use. The other options are not within the range of optimal effectiveness. *Cognitive Level:* Application. *Nursing Process:* Implementation. *Patient Need:* Physiological Integrity.

3 *Answer: 1*

Rationale: Stress is one of the major factors in developing IBS. *Helicobacter pylori* is associated with development of peptic ulcers. GERD is associated with esophageal disorders. *Cognitive Level:* Analysis. *Nursing Process:* Assessment. *Patient Need:* Physiological Integrity.

4 *Answers: 2, 5*

Rationale: Prochlorperazine (Compazine) and promethazine hydrochloride (Phenergan) can cause the anticholinergic side effects of dry mouth, constipation, urine retention, and a rapid heart rate. Peppermint induces a calming effect. Loperamide (Imodium, Kaopectate) and dipheroxylate (Lamotil) are antidiarrheals. *Cognitive Level:* Analysis. *Nursing Process:* Implementation. *Patient Need:* Physiological Integrity.

5 *Answers: 1, 2, 3, 4*

Rationale: Sibutramine (Meridia) is a CNS agent that is contraindicated in patients with a history of hypertension, CAD, and renal and hepatic impairments. The patient should be assessed for abdominal pain after medication has been initiated. *Cognitive Level:* Analysis. *Nursing Process:* Assessment. *Patient Need:* Physiological Integrity.

6 *Answer: 2*

Rationale: Prochlorperazine may cause decreased blood pressure or hypotension as an adverse effect. The blood pressure

should be taken before administering and the drug held if the blood pressure is below 90/60 mmHg or below parameters as ordered by the provider. The pulse will be taken along with the blood pressure but may increase in relationship to hypotension (i.e., reflex tachycardia). Prochlorperazine does not directly affect lung sounds or temperature. *Cognitive Level*: Application. *Nursing Process*: Implementation. *Patient Need*: Physiological Integrity.

Answers to Critical Thinking Questions

1 A priority for the nurse is to assess the potential for dehydration. The nurse should assess the patient for possible hypotension and tachycardia. The cause of this ongoing diarrhea needs to be investigated by the health care provider.

2 The patient needs to be informed that prochlorperazine (Compazine) is administered in its own syringe and must not be mixed with any other drug. The nurse could notify the health care provider that the patient wants a change of antiemetic to one that can be combined with an analgesic and given in the same syringe.

3 This patient needs to take a contact laxative to stimulate the nerve endings and facilitate a bowel movement. A bulk-forming laxative promotes bowel regularity. The liquid stool may be a result of fecal impaction, in which only liquid seeps out. If this patient has ongoing bowel irregularity problems, the bulk-forming laxative may be helpful later. The nurse should assess the abdomen for bowel sounds and educate the patient to drink plenty of fluids when taking bulk-forming laxatives.

Chapter 42

Answers to NCLEX-RN® Review Questions

1 *Answer: 4*

Pernicious anemia results in the inability to absorb vitamin B_{12} due to the lack of intrinsic factor in the gut. Replacement therapy must be administered via intramuscular injection because oral supplementation will not be absorbed. Pernicious anemia affects vitamin B_{12} absorption. *Cognitive Level*: Application. *Nursing Process*: Implementation. *Patient Need*: Physiological Integrity.

2 *Answers: 2, 3, 4*

Rationale: Circulatory collapse, complete heart block, and respiratory failure are all known to occur in patients receiving magnesium sulfate intravenously. The therapy should be used cautiously in patients with renal impairment. *Cognitive Level:* Analysis. *Nursing Process:* Assessment. *Patient Need:* Physiological Integrity.

3 *Answer: 3*

Rationale: Hypomagnesemia should be assessed. Patients experiencing hypomagnesemia may experience general weakness, dysrhythmias, hypertension, loss of deep tendon reflexes, and respiratory depression. *Cognitive Level:* Analysis. *Nursing Process*: Assessment. *Patient Need:* Physiological Integrity.

4 Answer: 4

Rationale: Alcohol is known for its ability to inhibit the absorption of thiamine and folic acid. Alcohol abuse is the most common cause of thiamine deficiency. **Cognitive Level:** Analysis. **Nursing Process:** Implementation. **Patient Need:** Physiological Integrity.

5 Answer: 3

Rationale: Vitamin K should be given to the patient to improve clotting. Without vitamin K, abnormal prothrombin is produced and blood clotting is affected. **Cognitive Level:** Analysis. **Nursing Process:** Implementation. **Patient Need:** Physiological Integrity.

6 Answer: 3

Rationale: TPN access sites, tubing, and parenteral nutrition bag are all areas at risk for contamination and for bacteria to enter the patient. The nurse should assess the IV access site for redness, streaking, swelling, or drainage and all tubing and bag for signs of cracks, cloudiness, or precipitate. Glucose levels and TPN orders will be assessed periodically but do not directly contribute to the development of infection. Periodic chest x-ray monitoring may be ordered and should be obtained if adventitious breath sounds are noted. **Cognitive Level:** Application. **Nursing Process:** Implementation. **Patient Need:** Physiological Integrity.

Answers to Critical Thinking Questions

1 The patient is experiencing a normal reaction to the niacin but should be instructed to follow up with the health care provider for guidance on the appropriate dose of niacin to take.

2 This patient should be instructed to see a health care provider regarding the appropriate doses of vitamins. Vitamin A can cause increased intracranial pressure, which could be the cause of the headaches. Patients need to be instructed about the appropriate amounts of vitamins and potential adverse effects—especially when taking megadoses of vitamins.

3 This patient needs to be assessed for possible renal calculi. The patient is taking 500 mg of vitamin C daily to prevent an upper respiratory infection, but vitamin C is contraindicated in patients with a history of renal calculi because the vitamin may exacerbate the problem.

Chapter 43

Answers to NCLEX-RN® Review Questions

1 Answer: 1

Rationale: Glucocorticoids can increase the risk of peptic ulcers, decrease wound healing, and increase capillary fragility. Glucocorticoids place the patient at increased risk for infection. The other options do not cause increased risk for peptic ulcers, delayed wound healing, or infection. **Cognitive Level:** Analysis. **Nursing Process:** Implementation. **Patient Need:** Physiological Integrity.

2 Answer: 1

Rationale: This drug may mask the signs and symptoms of infection. Hydrocortisone is contraindicated in patients with known infections or hypersensitivity to the drug. Skin infections, heart failure, and hearing loss are not associated with the use of hydrocortisone. **Cognitive Level:** Analysis. **Nursing Process:** Implementation. **Patient Need:** Physiological Integrity.

3 Answer: 2

Rationale: Circulatory collapse can occur if hydrocortisone use is discontinued abruptly. The patient may experience nausea, vomiting, lethargy, and confusion, progressing to coma and death. Diabetes insipidus is caused by ADH deficiency. Myxedema is related to hypothyroidism. Cushing's syndrome is caused by excess glucocorticoids. **Cognitive Level:** Analysis. **Nursing Process:** Assessment. **Patient Need:** Physiological Integrity.

4 Answer: 2

Rationale: The patient may have the hormonal condition hyperthyroidism. Symptoms of hyperthyroidism include diarrhea, stress intolerance, and weight loss. The other disease processes are not related to the thyroid gland. **Cognitive Level:** Analysis. **Nursing Process:** Implementation. **Patient Need:** Physiological Integrity.

5 Answers: 2, 5

Rationale: Because small doses of radiation will be emitted for up to 1 week, patients should avoid close contact with children or pregnant women after drug administration. Radioactive iodine is used to permanently decrease thyroid function. Patients may experience hypothyroidism, including signs and symptoms such as general weakness, muscle cramps, and dry skin. Fluids do not affect radiation levels. **Cognitive Level:** Application. **Nursing Process:** Implementation. **Patient Need:** Physiological Integrity.

6 Answer: 4

Rationale: Desmopressin nasal spray should be used in the evening to mimic the body's own natural rhythms. Gently rotating the bottle rather than shaking, storing the bottle in room temperature conditions unless excessive heat is present, and spraying the drug high into the nasal cavity are all appropriate administration techniques. **Cognitive Level:** Application. **Nursing Process:** Implementation. **Patient Need:** Physiological Integrity.

Answers to Critical Thinking Questions

1 To answer this question the student should refer to a medical–surgical text or a laboratory manual. A child with diabetes insipidus produces large amounts of pale or colorless urine with a low specific gravity of 1.001 to 1.005. Daily urine volume may be 4 to 10 L or more and result in excessive thirst and rapid dehydration. Desmopressin is a synthetic analog of ADH. It may be administered intranasally and therefore may be better tolerated by a child. With pharmacotherapy, there should be an imme-

diate decrease in urine production and an increase in urine concentration. The child's mother or caregiver should be taught to use a urine dipstick to check specific gravity during the initiation of therapy. A normal specific gravity would range from 1.005 to 1.030 and would indicate that the kidneys are concentrating urine. The caregiver also should be taught to monitor urine volume, color, and odor until a dosing regimen is established.

2 The nurse must be empathetic with the patient's father and allow him to express his concerns. He may feel guilty about contributing to his son's current health crisis. Once the patient's condition begins to improve, the nurse should assess the father's understanding of the asthma regimen. The father and the patient should receive instruction about the side effects of glucocorticoid therapy. Glucocorticoids used for anti-inflammatory purposes can suppress the hypothalamic–pituitary axis. Abruptly discontinuing a glucocorticoid after long-term therapy (more than 10 days) can produce cardiovascular collapse. The father needs to be instructed about the dosage regimen for prednisone, which may include an incremental decrease in the drug dosage when discontinuing the drug. The nurse might also be concerned about the family's economic needs. Referrals to a resource providing financial support for medication is appropriate.

3 The instruction needed by the parents should include the following points:

a. Drug action: The drug stimulates growth of most body tissues, especially epiphyseal plates; it also increases cellular size.

b. Instructions for reconstituting the medication, site selection, and technique for IM or subcutaneous injection.

c. Dosing schedule: Somatropin injections are usually scheduled 48 hours apart.

d. Pain and swelling at the injection site.

e. Importance of regular follow-up with the health care provider, including checks on height, weight, and bone age.

f. A discussion of the cost of the medication and an opportunity for the parents to raise any concerns they may have for appropriate referral to the prescriber or social services department.

Answer to Avoiding Medication Errors

No. The infant's weight of 2000 g is equivalent to 2 kg. Therefore, 25 mg/kg/day would be 50 mg. When given in two equally divided doses, the correct dose is 25 mg.

Chapter 44

Answers to NCLEX-RN® Review Questions

1 *Answer: 1600*

Rationale: The onset of NPH is between 1 and 4 hours, and it peaks between 8 and 12 hours. **Cognitive Level:** Application. **Nursing Process:** Assessment. **Patient Need:** Physiological Integrity.

2 *Answer: 1*

Rationale: Humalog is a rapid-acting insulin that is administered for elevated glucose levels and should be given 0 to 15 minutes before breakfast. Hypoglycemic reactions may occur rapidly if Humalog insulin is not supported by sufficient food intake. The medication can be mixed in one syringe. **Cognitive Level:** Application. **Nursing Process:** Implementation. **Patient Need:** Physiological Integrity.

3 *Answer: 3*

Rationale: Additional teaching is needed. The clear solution (regular insulin) should be drawn into the syringe first followed by the cloudy solution (NPH). The other options demonstrate an understanding of discharge instructions. **Cognitive Level:** Analysis. **Nursing Process:** Evaluation. **Patient Need:** Physiological Integrity.

4 *Answers: 1, 2, 3, 4*

Rationale: The patient needs to understand that exercise may increase insulin needs. Blood glucose levels should be monitored prior to starting and after ending exercise, and addressed appropriately. A complex carbohydrate should be consumed prior to strenuous exercise. **Cognitive Level:** Analysis. **Nursing Process:** Implementation. **Patient Need:** Physiological Integrity.

5 *Answer: 4*

Rationale: The health care provider should be contacted for further orders. The need for oral hypoglycemic medication may have been overlooked or other measures, such as insulin, to treat glucose needs during the surgery may be planned. Contacting the provider ensures that the provider is aware that the patient is a diabetic and is aware that no medications for diabetes were ordered. Holding all medications as ordered will not address the patient's glucose needs during surgery. Intravenous fluids during this time may contain glucose solutions, resulting in a hyperglycemic condition. It is not within the nurse's scope of practice to independently change a medication dosage order or to give medications when an NPO order has been written. The provider should be contacted before these decisions are carried out. **Cognitive Level:** Application. **Nursing Process:** Implementation. **Patient Need:** Physiological Integrity.

6 *Answer: 1*

Rationale: The stress of hospitalization and infection may cause the release of glucose as a response to this stress. Blood glucose levels will continue to be monitored and control may improve as the infection clears and the patient is discharged. The pathogenesis of type I and type II diabetes is different. Type II diabetics may eventually need insulin but for reasons other than the pathogenesis of type I. Immediate changes in response to an oral hypoglycemic drug are not known and diabetics may continue to take all-oral medications while in the hospital. **Cognitive Level:** Application. **Nursing Process:** Implementation. **Patient Need:** Physiological Integrity.

Answers to Critical Thinking Questions

1 The nurse should first explain that management of type 1 diabetes is initiated with diet, exercise, and home blood glucose monitoring. Compliance with prescribed regimens may reduce the patient's fasting and postprandial blood glucose values to acceptable levels. Mothers with type 1 diabetes must keep their blood glucose level within a very narrow range to prevent the numerous complications that can occur because of elevated blood glucose during pregnancy. These complications can range from fetal deformity to fetal macrosomia and its subsequent sequelae. Some authorities recommend that the fasting blood glucose levels be maintained at or below 100 mg/dL and the postprandial glucose below 120 mg/dL. The nurse should prepare the patient for insulin therapy in case diet and exercise fail to maintain control. Oral hypoglycemic agents cross placental membranes and have been implicated as teratogenic agents. Their use is not recommended during pregnancy.

2 Beta-blocking drugs such as propranolol have the potential to affect type II diabetics on oral hypoglycemics by altering the way hypoglycemia is perceived. In recent studies, hypoglycemia was perceived differently in patients taking concurrent beta-blocker therapy than patients who were not. Diaphoresis was a common symptom when blood sugar decreased among those patients on beta blockers along with their oral hypoglycemic drug. The nurse should teach the patient to be aware that should his blood sugar begin to decrease, symptoms normally felt (e.g., nervousness, tremors, agitation) may be perceived differently and that should diaphoresis occur, he should check his blood sugar immediately.

3 Insulin glargine (Lantus) is a newer agent that is a recombinant human insulin analog. It must not be mixed in the syringe with any other insulin and must be administered subcutaneously. Insulin glargine appears to have a constant long-duration hypoglycemic effect with no defined peak effect. It is prescribed once daily, at bedtime. The nurse should question the order for Lantus to be administered every morning.

Chapter 45

Answers to NCLEX-RN® Review Questions

1 Answer 4

Rationale: Use of oral contraceptives puts a patient at risk for thromboembolism, which is manifested by calf pain, shortness of breath, and chest pain. *Cognitive Level:* Analysis. *Nursing Process:* Assessment. *Patient Need:* Physiological Integrity.

2 Answer: 1

Rationale: Caffeine and estrogen may lead to increased CNS stimulation. *Cognitive Level:* Analysis. *Nursing Process:* Implementation. *Patient Need:* Physiological Integrity.

3 Answer: 2

Rationale: The assessment of the patient is within normal parameters for a patient in labor. Antidiuretic hormone can cause water intoxication in patients with prolonged IV infusion of oxytocin. *Cognitive Level:* Analysis. *Nursing Process:* Assessment. *Patient Need:* Physiological Integrity.

4 Answers: 1, 2

Rationale: Barrier contraception is needed only when two or more doses are missed. Placebos are usually iron, which has no effect on estrogen-related adverse effects. Side effects include intolerance to contact lenses, abdominal cramps, dysmenorrhea, breast fullness, headache, acne, skin rash, hypertension, and thromboembolic disorders. *Cognitive Level:* Analysis. *Nursing Process:* Implementation. *Patient Need:* Physiological Integrity.

5 Answer: 2

Rationale: Although some antibiotics and anticonvulsants can reduce the efficacy of oral contraceptives, the most common cause of pregnancy in patients using oral contraceptives is skipping two or more doses. *Cognitive Level:* Analysis. *Nursing Process:* Implementation. *Patient Need:* Physiological Integrity.

6 Answer: 1

Rationale: Infertility may result from physical obstruction, pelvic infections, or endocrine-related reasons resulting in lack of ovulation. If a fertility workup suggests that infrequent or anovulation is a primary cause, clomiphene may be tried to increase ovulation and is approximately 90% effective for patients with ovulatory-related infertility. Clomiphene will not be therapeutic if the causes of infertility are other than lack of ovulation. The risk of multiple births is higher with ovulatory stimulants with approximately 25% resulting in multiple births. Contraceptives do not continue to suppress ovulation after they have been discontinued. *Cognitive Level:* Application. *Nursing Process:* Implementation. *Patient Need:* Physiological Integrity.

Answers to Critical Thinking Questions

1 The student should be able to use this example to help illustrate neuroendocrine control of the female reproductive system. Leuprolide acetate is a synthetic GnRH agonist that acts by stimulating the anterior pituitary to secrete FSH and LH. The pituitary receptors become desensitized, which causes a decrease in FSH and LH secretion. Consequently, estrogen production, which is dependent on ovarian stimulation, is diminished and the patient's menstrual cycle is suppressed. The goal of suppressing the menstrual cycle is to decrease hormonal stimuli to abnormal endometrial tissue. It is expected that amenorrhea will result and that endometriosis lesions will decrease. A decrease in lesions will likely enhance the patient's fertility or improve her level of comfort during menstruation. The patient will remain on this drug therapy for approximately 6 months. Menstrual periods usually resume 2 months after the completion of therapy.

2 Misoprostol (Cytotec) is a prostaglandin that may be prescribed as an antiulcer agent. The drug also has two off-label uses, which include cervical ripening prior to

induction of labor, or termination of pregnancy when used with mifepristone. It is known that prostaglandins have a role in the initiation of labor, as has been demonstrated with the vaginal application of prostaglandin E. Misoprostol is a prostaglandin E analog that has clearly been demonstrated to produce uterine contractions. In this example, the fetus was not tolerating the uterine contractions and the nurse used correct judgment in quickly acting to remove the drug.

3 Oxytocin exerts an antidiuretic effect when administered in doses of 20 milliunits/min or greater. Urine output decreases, and fluid retention increases. Most patients begin a postpartum diuresis and are able to balance fluid volumes relatively quickly. However, the nurse should evaluate the patient for signs of water intoxication, which include drowsiness, listlessness, headache, and oliguria.

Chapter 46

Answers to NCLEX-RN® Review Questions

1 *Answers: 2, 3*

Rationale: A side effect of testosterone therapy is fluid retention. Testosterone is also used to increase muscle mass and strength. The hematocrit usually increases with the use of testosterone, because it promotes the synthesis of erythropoietin. *Cognitive Level:* Analysis. *Nursing Process:* Assessment. *Patient Need:* Physiological Integrity.

2 *Answer: 1*

Rationale: The primary use of testosterone is to treat hypogonadism in men with delayed puberty. Testosterone therapy promotes normal gonadal development and often restores reproductive function. Secondary sex characteristics or virilization also occur. *Cognitive Level:* Analysis. *Nursing Process:* Assessment. *Patient Need:* Physiological Integrity.

3 *Answer: 3*

Rationale: In men, some medications such as phenothiazides, thiazide diuretics, SSRIs, TCAs, propranolol, and diazepam cause impotence because of low testosterone secretion. *Cognitive Level:* Analysis. *Nursing Process:* Assessment. *Patient Need:* Physiological Integrity.

4 *Answer: 1*

Rationale: Life-threatening hypotension is an adverse effect in patients who are taking sildenafil (Viagra) and organic nitrates. *Cognitive Level:* Analysis. *Nursing Process:* Assessment. *Patient Needs:* Physiological Integrity.

5 *Answer: 4*

Rationale: Finasteride promotes shrinking of enlarged prostates and helps restore urinary function. Tadalafil and sildenafil are used in patients experiencing erectile dysfunction. Testosterone is used in the treatment of hypogonadism. *Cognitive Level:* Analysis. *Nursing Process:* Implementation. *Patient Need:* Physiological Integrity.

6 *Answers: 1, 3, 4*

Rationale: Enlarged prostatic tissue will decrease over a period of 3 to 6 months. The drug is teratogenic and should not be handled by pregnant women. Blood donation should not occur while taking finasteride because it may be given to a woman. Finasteride in lower doses is given under the trade name "Propecia" for treatment of baldness. *Cognitive Level:* Application. *Nursing Process:* Implementation. *Patient Need:* Physiological Integrity.

Answers to Critical Thinking Questions

1 This patient's age puts him at risk for a variety of health problems. Conditions such as renal or hepatic dysfunction may alter the manner in which the drug is metabolized or excreted. The potential impact on patients with coronary artery disease who are using nitrates has been well documented. Because the patient is requesting a prescription for sildenafil (Viagra), the nurse should ensure that the history includes the following data: sexual dysfunction, cardiovascular disease and use of organic nitrates, severe hypotension, and renal or hepatic impairment—which requires a decrease in the prescribed dose. Nurses can be effective in initiating conversations about sexuality. Studies have shown that patients are often forthcoming with concerns about sexual performance when an interviewer is open and professional.

2 According to Erikson's theory of psychosocial development, this young man is in the stage of identity versus isolation. The family has been replaced in its influence largely by the adolescent's peer group. This young man's desire to be accepted as an athlete and a team member may produce a willingness to do what it takes to fit in. In addition, the young man may have aspirations of a career in sports and recognize the need to be in optimum physical condition. This patient may not realize that the use of testosterone in immature men has not been associated with significant increases in muscle mass. Such an increase has been documented only in mature men. In addition, testosterone can produce premature epiphyseal closure, potentially affecting this young man's adult height.

3 Finasteride (Proscar), an androgen inhibitor, is used to shrink the prostate and relieve symptoms associated with BPH. Finasteride inhibits 5-alpha-reductase, an enzyme that converts testosterone to the potent androgen 5-alpha-dihydrotestosterone (DHT). The prostate gland depends on this androgen for its development, but excessive levels can cause prostate cells to increase in size and divide. A regimen of 6 to 12 months may be necessary to determine patient response. Saw palmetto is an herbal preparation derived from a shrublike palm tree that is native to the southeastern United States. This phytomedicine compares pharmacologically with finasteride in that it is an antiandrogen. The mechanism of action is virtually the same in these two agents. Authorities note no significant adverse effects of saw palmetto extract and no known drug–drug interactions. Just as with finasteride, long-term use is required.

Chapter 47

Answers to NCLEX-RN® Review Questions

1 *Answer: 1*

Rationale: Osteomalacia, referred to as *rickets* in children, is a disorder characterized by softening of bones without alteration in basic bone structure. Classic signs of rickets in children include bowlegs and a pigeon breast. Shortness of breath, crutch walking, and finger and toe deformities are not associated with osteomalacia. *Cognitive Level:* Analysis. *Nursing Process:* Assessment. *Patient Need:* Physiological Integrity.

2 *Answer: 3*

Rationale: A normal serum calcium level is 8.5 to 11.5 mg/dL. Signs of hypocalcemia include seizures, muscle spasms, facial twitching, and paresthesias. Anorexia, headache, and drowsiness may be associated with hypercalcemia. *Cognitive Level:* Analysis. *Nursing Process:* Assessment. *Patient Need:* Physiological Integrity.

3 *Answer: 3*

Rationale: Gout is a metabolic disorder characterized by the accumulation of uric acid in the bloodstream or joint cavities. Alcohol increases uric acid levels. Although long-term alcohol use may affect the liver, it is not related to uric acid. Alcohol does not affect the absorption of antigout medications. Alcohol increases urine acidity. *Cognitive Level:* Analysis. *Nursing Process:* Assessment. *Patient Need:* Physiological Integrity.

4 *Answers: 1, 2, 3*

Rationale: Signs and symptoms of hypercalcemia include anorexia, vomiting, excessive thirst, fatigue, and confusion. Kidney stones may occur, and bones may fracture easily. Cardiac dysrhythmias may occur, because calcium ions influence the excitability of all neurons. Whenever calcium concentrations are too high, sodium permeability decreases across cell membranes. This is a dangerous state, because nerve conduction depends on the proper influx of sodium into cells. *Cognitive Level:* Analysis. *Nursing Process:* Assessment. *Patient Need:* Physiological Integrity.

5 *Answer: 2*

Rationale: Sodium hyaluronate (Hyalgan) is administered by injection directly into the knee joint. This medication replaces or supplements the body's natural hyaluronic acid that deteriorated because of the inflammation of osteoarthritis. All other routes are incorrect. *Cognitive Level:* Analysis. *Nursing Process:* Implementation. *Patient Need:* Physiological Integrity.

6 *Answers: 2, 3, 4*

Rationale: Bisphosphonates such as alendronate require the patient to take the drug on an empty stomach and remain upright for 30 minutes to 1 hour. Adequate serum calcium levels should be confirmed before starting bisphosphonates and adequate calcium and vitamin D intake should be encouraged while on drug therapy. Any narrowing of the esophagus may place the patient at risk of increased adverse esophageal effects from the drug. Adequate calcium intake is advised while on bisphosphonates to maintain normal serum calcium levels. *Cognitive Level*: Application. *Nursing Process*: Assessment. *Patient Need*: Physiological Integrity.

Answers to Critical Thinking Questions

1 Alendronate (Fosamax) is poorly absorbed after oral administration and can produce significant GI irritation. It is important that the patient be educated regarding several elements of drug administration. To promote absorption, the drug should be taken first thing in the morning with 8 oz of water before food or beverages are ingested or any other medications are taken. It has been shown that certain beverages, such as orange juice and coffee, interfere with drug absorption. By delaying eating for 30 minutes or more, the patient is promoting absorption of the drug. Additionally, the patient should be taught to sit upright after taking the drug to reduce the risk of esophageal irritation. Alendronate must be used carefully in patients with esophagitis or gastric ulcer. If the patient misses a dose, she should be told to skip it and not to double the next dose. Alendronate has a long half-life, and missing an occasional dose will do little to interfere with the therapeutic effect of the drug.

2 Frail elderly patients may be susceptible to hypocalcemia caused by dietary deficiencies of calcium and vitamin D or decreased physical activity and lack of exposure to sunshine. This patient has all these risk factors. She is uninterested in eating, has physical limitations, and is not able to get out of the house into the sunshine without assistance. Orally administered calcium requires vitamin D for absorption to take place. Because this patient does not consume milk, the most recognizable source of vitamin D, she needs to be encouraged to increase her intake of other dietary sources of this vitamin. Foods rich in vitamin D include canned salmon, cereals, lean meats, beans, and potatoes. To promote the effectiveness of calcium supplementation, the nurse must remember the importance of drug–nutrient interactions.

3 The triage nurse should obtain information about the onset of symptoms, degree of discomfort, and frequency of attacks. A familial history of gout can be predictive, because primary gout is inherited as an X-linked trait. A past medical history of renal calculi may also be predictive of acute gouty arthritis. The nurse should ask the patient questions about his diet and fluid intake. An attack of gout can be precipitated by alcohol intake (particularly beer and wine), starvation diets, and insufficient fluid intake. In addition, the nurse should obtain information about prescribed drugs and the use of OTC drugs containing salicylates. Thiazide diuretics and salicylates can precipitate an attack. The nurse should also ask about recent lifestyle events. Stress, illness, trauma, or strenuous exercise can precipitate an attack of gouty arthritis.

Answer to Avoiding Medication Errors

This error occurred because the nurse administered the medication to the wrong patient. Patients must be correctly identified by checking the identification band or by another identifying method and not by relying on patients to respond to calling them by name. When there are two patients with similar names, it is particularly important to double-check the room number and identification band. Perhaps Ms. Brown was responding to being awoken. Best practice requires that proper patient identification occur prior to any medication administration. The nurse must adhere to the five rights of medication administration:

1. Right patient
2. Right drug
3. Right dose
4. Right route
5. Right time

Chapter 48

Answers to NCLEX-RN® Review Questions

1 Answer: 2

Rationale: To ensure the effectiveness of drug therapy, patients should inspect hair shafts after treatment, checking for nits by combing with a fine-toothed comb after the hair is dry. This procedure must be conducted daily for at least 1 week after treatment. The patient does not require isolation. Linens should be washed with hot water; bleach is not required. *Cognitive Level:* Analysis. *Nursing Process:* Implementation. *Patient Need:* Physiological Integrity.

2 Answers: 1, 2, 5

Rationale: The directions for scabicides and pediculicides must be followed carefully. If these doses are overapplied, wrongly applied, or accidentally ingested, the patient may experience headaches; nausea or vomiting; irritation of the nose, ears, or throat; dizziness; tremors; restlessness; or convulsions. Eye irritation does not occur with overapplication. *Cognitive Level:* Analysis. *Nursing Process:* Implementation. *Patient Need:* Physiological Integrity.

3 Answer: 1

Rationale: High-potency corticosteroid creams such as fluocinonide should be avoided in the highly vascular neck and facial regions because of the possibility of adverse effects. Topical corticosteroid creams may be kept at room temperature until the expiration date unless there are signs of discoloration of the cream, unless otherwise stated on the label or as instructed by the health care provider. Fluocinonide is one of the higher potency creams available for topical use. Contact dermatitis is a skin reaction to contact with antigenic material and the body's reaction depends on the antigen–antibody response, not necessarily to the antigen itself. *Cognitive Level:* Application. *Nursing Process:* Implementation. *Patient Need:* Physiological Integrity.

4 Answers: 2, 3, 4

Rationale: Washing the face gently with a mild soap and using sunscreens and protection from sun exposure are part of the care required for patients taking tretinoin. Mild dryness, redness, and peeling skin are all possible adverse effects that are expected but any severe skin irritation or pain should be reported. Sun exposure should be avoided unless specifically instructed to do so by the health care provider. *Cognitive Level*: Application. *Nursing Process*: Implementation. *Patient Need*: Physiological Integrity.

5 Answer: 2

Rationale: Initial drying of the skin caused by benzoyl peroxide will help to clear acne lesions in the early stages of treatment but it may take several weeks before full effects are visible. One week of keratolytic therapy for acne should demonstrate the beginning of therapeutic effects. Most acne is responsive to keratolytic therapy but may need an antibiotic included as part of the treatment plan after a full course of the keratolytic has been tried. Only in severe cases is oral drug therapy usually considered, after other treatment options have not been successful. *Cognitive Level*: Application. *Nursing Process*: Implementation. *Patient Need*: Physiological Integrity.

6 Answers: 1, 2, 4

Rationale: Isotretinoin is teratogenic and pregnancy must be avoided while on this medication. To be eligible for treatment, female patients must agree to frequent pregnancy tests and commit to using two forms of birth control while on the drug. Because of adverse visual, hepatic, and lipid effects, periodic vision screening and lab work must be monitored. Isotretinoin is a retinoid closely related to vitamin A. Vitamin A may be toxic when taken in large doses and normal daily intake is usually sufficient to meet the body's needs without supplementation. *Cognitive Level*: Application. *Nursing Process*: Implementation. *Patient Need*: Physiological Integrity.

Answers to Critical Thinking Questions

1 To establish a rapport with the baby's mother, the nurse should first respond to the mother's anxiety. She should validate that the baby's condition is cause for concern and commend the mother for seeking medical guidance. The nursing student should recognize that the availability of OTC preparations can be a temptation to a young mother who only wants to see her infant more comfortable and relieved of symptoms.

However, the student nurse must also recognize that topical use of corticosteroid ointments can be potentially harmful, especially for young children. Corticosteroids, when absorbed by the skin in large enough quantities over a long period can result in adrenal suppression and skin atrophy. Children have an increased risk of toxicity from topically applied drugs because of their greater ratio of skin surface area to weight compared with that of adults. The student nurse should ensure that the health care provider at the public health clinic sees this patient. Once a drug treatment modality is prescribed, the student nurse should make sure that the baby's mother understands the correct method for drug administration.

2 According to Piaget, this 14-year-old patient is capable of formal operations, the highest level of cognitive development. A young person in this age group is able to think logically and make decisions regarding health care problems and take control of a treatment regimen. To safely self-medicate, the teenager needs information about the medication, its administration, and side effects. Teenagers need clear instructions and often respond to a caregiver outside the family as a resource for information.

The nurse should recognize that this patient is experiencing GI side effects that are common in doxycycline and all tetracycline treatment. Recent studies have demonstrated cases of esophagitis in teenage patients. To develop an effective teaching plan, the nurse will need to assess the patient's dosing regimen and current dietary patterns. A teaching plan would include the following:

- Encouraging oral fluids to maintain hydration even if nausea occurs

- Drinking a full glass of water with the medication to reduce gastric irritation

- Sitting up for 30 minutes after the night-time dose to reduce gastric irritation and reflux

- Consuming small frequent meals to ensure adequate nutrition

- Taking the drug 1 hour before or 2 hours after meals to promote its absorption and effectiveness (if nausea persists, however, the patient should be encouraged to take the doxycycline with food)

- Taking doxycycline with milk products or antacids decreases the absorption of the drug; therefore, other remedies for GI irritation will need to be discussed with the health care provider

3 This patient's presentation is typical of rosacea. To prevent long-term changes in the skin, therapy should be aggressive despite the fact that this patient is also of child-bearing age. Isotretinoin (Accutane) is a pregnancy category X drug and has a picture of a fetus overlaid by the "No" symbol on the package. Reported teratogenic effects include severe CNS abnormalities such as hydrocephalus, microcephalus, cranial nerve deficits, and compromised intelligence scores.

This patient needs to understand that she must use contraception while receiving drug therapy and for up to 6 months after therapy is discontinued. She should not begin therapy unless she first demonstrates a negative pregnancy test. In addition, she should be taught to begin therapy on the second or third day of her normal menstrual cycle. Teenagers who are on isotretinoin should anticipate monthly pregnancy tests.

Chapter 49

Answers to NCLEX-RN® Review Questions

1 *Answer: 3*

Rationale: Closed-angle glaucoma is an acute type of glaucoma that is caused by stress, impact injury, or medications. Pressure inside the anterior chamber increases suddenly because the iris is pushed over the area where the aqueous fluid normally drains. Signs and symptoms include intense headaches, difficulty concentrating, bloodshot eyes, blurred vision, and a bulging iris. Closed-angle glaucoma constitutes an emergency. All other options are inappropriate in this emergency. *Cognitive Level:* Application. *Nursing Process:* Implementation. *Patient Need:* Physiological Integrity.

2 *Answer: 4*

Rationale: Side effects include eye irritation, conjunctival edema, burning, stinging, redness, blurred vision, pain, itching, the sensation of a foreign body in the eye, photophobia, and visual disturbances. The patient may experience the phenomenon of increasing amounts of brown pigmentation in the treated eye only and thickening of the eyelashes and hair adjacent to the treated eye. General body symptoms such as flulike symptoms, rash, or headache may occur. Loss of lashes, hypertension, and dilation of the pupils do not occur with the use of prostaglandins. *Cognitive Level:* Analysis. *Nursing Process:* Implementation. *Patient Need:* Physiological Integrity.

3 *Answer: 3*

Rationale: Beta-adrenergic drugs may reduce resting heart rate and blood pressure. The patient and family should be taught how to check the pulse and blood pressure before administration and to notify the health care provider if extremes occur. Beta-adrenergic drugs do not affect urine output, respiratory rate, or glucose levels. *Cognitive Level:* Analysis. *Nursing Process:* Implementation. *Patient Need:* Physiological Integrity.

4 *Answer: 4*

Rationale: Some drugs are specifically designed for examining the eyes of patients. These include cycloplegic drugs to relax ciliary muscles and mydriatic drugs to dilate the pupils. One has to be especially careful with anticholinergic mydriatics, because these drugs can worsen glaucoma by impairing aqueous humor outflow and thereby increasing intraocular pressure. *Cognitive Level:* Analysis. *Nursing Process:* Implementation. *Patient Need:* Physiological Integrity.

5 *Answers: 1, 2, 4*

Rationale: The nurse needs to notify the health care provider if the patient has second- or third-degree heart block, bradycardia, cardiac failure, CHF, or COPD because timolol may be contraindicated for patients with these conditions. If the drug is absorbed systemically, it will worsen these conditions. Proper administration lessens the danger that the drug will be absorbed systemically. The renal and hepatic systems are not affected by timolol. *Cognitive Level:* Analysis. *Nursing Process:* Assessment. *Patient Need:* Physiological Integrity.

6 *Answer: 4*

Rationale: Contact lenses should be removed before instilling eye drops and remain out for a minimum of 15 minutes after instilling eye drops. Administering eye drops into the conjunctival sac, applying slight pressure to the lacrimal duct for 1 full minute, and avoiding direct contact with the dropper tip and the eye are all appropriate techniques to use when administering eye drops. *Cognitive Level*: Application. *Nursing Process*: Implementation. *Patient Need*: Physiological Integrity.

Answers to Critical Thinking Questions

1 Cortisporin Otic is a combination of neomycin, polymyxin B, and 1% hydrocortisone. The technique for instilling this drug applies to most eardrops. The nurse needs to instruct the mother to position her daughter in a side-lying position with the affected ear facing up. The mother needs to inspect the ear for the presence of drainage or cerumen and, if present, gently remove it with a cotton-tipped applicator. Any unusual odor or drainage could indicate a ruptured tympanic membrane and should be reported to the health care provider. Next, the mother should be taught to straighten the child's external ear canal by pulling down and back on the auricle to promote distribution of the medication to deeper external ear structures. After the drops are instilled, the mother can further promote medication distribution by gently pressing on the tragus of the ear. The mother should be taught to keep her daughter in a side-lying position for 3 to 5 minutes after the drops are instilled. If a cotton ball has been prescribed, the cotton ball should be placed in the ear without applying pressure. The cotton ball can be removed in 15 minutes.

2 Timoptic, a beta-adrenergic blocking agent, is contraindicated in individuals with COPD. This agent has been known to produce bronchospasm by blocking the stimulation of beta$_2$-adrenergic receptors. When beta$_2$ receptors are stimulated, relaxation of bronchial smooth muscles is facilitated. Timolol is contraindicated in COPD, an air-trapping disorder, and may be contraindicated in chronic asthma. In both cases, the beta-adrenergic blocking effect of timolol could be potentially life threatening. Betaxolol (Betoptic) is also a beta-adrenergic blocking agent but is considered safer for use in patients with COPD who require treatment for glaucoma.

3 All ophthalmic agents should be administered in the conjunctival sac. The cornea is highly innervated, and direct application of medication to the cornea can result in excessive burning and stinging. The conjunctival sac normally holds one or two drops of solution. The patient should be reminded to place pressure on the inner canthus of the eye following administration of the medication to prevent the medication from flowing into the nasolacrimal duct. This maneuver helps prevent systemic absorption of medication and decreases the risk of side effects commonly associated with antiglaucoma agents.

Appendix E

CALCULATING DOSAGES

I. CALCULATING DOSAGE USING RATIOS AND PROPORTIONS

A. A *ratio* is used to express a relationship between two or more quantities. Ratios may be written using the following notations.

1:10 means 1 part of drug A to 10 parts of solution/solvent

In drug calculations, ratios are usually expressed as a fraction:

$$\frac{1 \text{ part drug A}}{10 \text{ parts solution}} = \frac{1}{10}$$

A *proportion* shows the relationship between two ratios. It is a simple and effective means for calculating certain types of doses.

$$\frac{\text{Dose on hand}}{\text{Quantity on hand}} = \frac{\text{Desired dose}}{\text{Quantity desired } (X)}$$

Using cross multiplication, we can write the same formula as follows:

$$\text{Quantity desired } (X) =$$
$$\frac{\text{Desired dose}}{\text{Dose on hand} \times \text{quantity on hand}}$$

Example 1: The health care provider orders erythromycin 500 mg. It is supplied in a liquid form containing 250 mg in 5 mL. How much drug should the nurse administer?

To calculate the dosage, use the formula:

$$\frac{\text{Dose on hand (250 mg)}}{\text{Quantity on hand (5 mL)}} = \frac{\text{Desired dose (500 mg)}}{\text{Quantity desired } (X)}$$

Then, cross-multiply:

$$250 \text{ mg} \times X = 5 \text{ mL} \times 500 \text{ mg}$$

Therefore, the dose to be administered is 10 mL.

B. The same proportion method can be used to solve solid dosage calculations.

Example 2: The health care provider orders methotrexate 20 mg/day. The methotrexate is available in 2.5-mg tablets. How many tablets should the nurse administer each day?

$$\frac{\text{Dose on hand (2.5 mg)}}{1 \text{ tablet}} = \frac{\text{Desired dose (20 mg)}}{\text{Quantity desired } (X \text{ tablets})}$$

Cross-multiplication gives:

$$2.5 \text{ mg } X = 20 \text{ mg} \times 1 \text{ tablet}$$

Therefore the nurse should administer 8 tablets daily.

II. CALCULATING DOSAGE BY WEIGHT

Doses for pediatric patients are often calculated by using body weight. The nurse must use caution to convert between pounds and kilograms, as necessary (see Table 3.2 in Chapter 3, page 21). Use the formula:

$$\text{Body weight} \times \text{amount/kg} = X \text{ mg of drug}$$

Example 3: The health care provider orders 10 mg/kg of methsuximide for a client who weighs 90 kg. How much should be administered?

The patient should receive 900 mg of methsuximide.

Example 4: The health care provider orders 5 mg/kg/day of amiodarone. The patient weighs 110 pounds. How much of the drug should be administered daily?

Step 1: Convert pounds to kilograms.

$$110 \text{ lb} \times 1 \text{ kg/2.2 lb} = 50 \text{ kg}$$

Step 2: Perform the drug calculation.

$$50 \text{ kg (body weight)} \times 5 \text{ mg/kg} = 250 \text{ mg}$$

The patient should receive 250 mg of amiodarone per day.

III. CALCULATING DOSAGE BY BODY SURFACE AREA

Many antineoplastic drugs and most pediatric doses are calculated using body surface area (BSA).

The formula for BSA in metric units is:

$$\text{BSA} = \sqrt{\frac{\text{weight (kg)} \times \text{height (cm)}}{3600}}$$

The formula for BSA in household units is

$$\text{BSA} = \sqrt{\frac{\text{weight (lb)} \times \text{height (inches)}}{3131}}$$

Example 5: The health care provider orders 10 mg/m^2 of an antibiotic for a child who is 2 feet tall and weighs 30 lb. How many milligrams should be administered?

Step 1: Calculate the BSA of the child.

$$BSA = \sqrt{\frac{30 \times 24}{3131}}$$

$$BSA = \sqrt{\frac{720}{3131}}$$

$$BSA = \sqrt{0.230} = 0.48 \text{ m}^2$$

Step 2: Calculate the drug amount.

$$10 \text{ mg/m}^2 \times 0.48 \text{ m}^2$$

The nurse should administer 4.8 mg of the antibiotic to the child.

IV. CALCULATING IV INFUSION RATES

Intravenous fluids are administered over time in units of mL/min or gtt/min (gtt = drops). The basic equation for IV drug calculations is as follows:

$$\frac{\text{mL of solution} \times \text{gtt/mL}}{\text{h of administration} \times 60 \text{ min/h}} = \frac{\text{gtt}}{\text{min}}$$

Example 6: The health care provider orders 1,000 mL of 5% normal saline to infuse over 6 hours. What is the flow rate?

$$\frac{1,000 \text{ mL} \times 10 \text{ gtt/mL}}{6 \text{ h} \times 60 \text{ min/h}} = \frac{28 \text{ gtt}}{\text{min}}$$

Other IV conversion formulas you may use include the following:

$$\text{mcg/kg/h} \rightarrow \text{mL/h}$$

$$\text{kg} \times \frac{\text{mcg/kg}}{\text{h}} \times \frac{\text{mg}}{1,000 \text{ mcg}} \times \frac{\text{mL}}{\text{mg}} = \frac{\text{mL}}{\text{h}}$$

$$\text{mcg/m}^2/\text{h} \rightarrow \text{mL/h}$$

$$\text{m}^2 \times \frac{\text{mcg/m}^2}{\text{h}} \times \frac{\text{mg}}{1,000 \text{ mcg}} \times \frac{\text{mL}}{\text{mg}} = \frac{\text{mL}}{\text{h}}$$

$$\text{mcg/kg/min} \rightarrow \text{gtt/min}$$

$$\text{kg} \times \frac{\text{mcg/kg}}{\text{min}} \times \frac{\text{mg}}{1,000 \text{ mcg}} \times \frac{\text{mL}}{\text{mg}} \times \frac{10 \text{ gtt}}{\text{mL}} = \frac{\text{gtt}}{\text{min}}$$

Glossary

A-delta fibers nerves that transmit sensations of sharp pain

Absence seizure seizure with a loss or reduction of normal activity, including staring and transient loss of responsiveness

Absorption the process of moving a drug across body membranes

Acetylcholine primary neurotransmitter of the parasympathetic nervous system; also present at somatic neuromuscular junctions and at sympathetic preganglionic nerves

Acetylcholinesterase (AchE) enzyme that degrades acetylcholine within the synaptic cleft, enhancing effects of the neurotransmitter

Acidosis condition of having too much acid in the blood; plasma pH below 7.35

Acne vulgaris condition characterized by small inflamed bumps that appear on the surface of the skin

Acquired immunodeficiency syndrome (AIDS) infection caused by the human immunodeficiency virus (HIV)

Acquired resistance the capacity of a microbe to no longer be affected by a drug following anti-infective pharmacotherapy

Action potential electrical changes in the membrane of a muscle or nerve cell due to changes in membrane permeability

Activated partial thromboplastin time (PTT) blood test used to determine how long it takes clots to form to regulate heparin dosage

Active immunity resistance resulting from a previous exposure to an antigen

Acute gouty arthritis condition in which uric acid crystals accumulate in the joints of the big toes, ankles, wrists, fingers, knees, or elbows, resulting in red, swollen, or inflamed tissue

Acute radiation syndrome life-threatening symptoms resulting from acute exposure to ionizing radiation, including nausea, vomiting, severe leukopenia, thrombocytopenia, anemia, and alopecia

Addiction the continued use of a substance despite its negative health and social consequences

Addison's disease hyposecretion of glucocorticoids and aldosterone by the adrenal cortex

Adenohypophysis anterior portion of the pituitary gland

Adjuvant chemotherapy technique in which antineoplastics are administered *after* surgery or radiation to effect a cure

Adolescence period from 13 to 16 years of age

Adrenergic relating to nerves that release norepinephrine or epinephrine

Adrenergic antagonist drug that blocks the actions of the sympathetic nervous system

Adrenocorticotropic hormone (ACTH) hormone secreted by the anterior pituitary that stimulates the release of glucocorticoids by the adrenal cortex

Aerobic pertaining to an oxygen environment

Aerosol suspension of minute liquid droplets or fine solid particles in a gas

Affinity chemical attraction that impels certain molecules to unite with others to form complexes

Afterload pressure that must be overcome for the ventricles to eject blood from the heart

Agonist drug that is capable of binding with receptors to induce a cellular response

Akathisia inability to remain still; constantly moving

Aldosterone hormone secreted by the adrenal cortex that increases sodium reabsorption in the distal tubule of the kidney

Alkalosis condition of having too many basic substances in the blood; plasma pH above 7.45

Alkylation process by which certain chemicals attach to DNA and change its structure and function

Allergic reaction acquired hyperresponse of body defenses to a foreign substance (allergen)

Alopecia hair loss

Alpha receptor type of subreceptor found in the sympathetic nervous system

Alzheimer's disease most common dementia, characterized by loss of memory, delusions, hallucinations, confusion, and loss of judgment

Amenorrhea lack of normal menstrual periods

Amide type of chemical linkage found in some local anesthetics involving carbon, nitrogen, and oxygen (–NH–CO–)

Amyloid plaques abnormal protein fragments related to neuronal damage; a sign of Alzheimer's disease observed during autopsy

Anabolic steroids compounds resembling testosterone with hormonal activity commonly abused by athletes

Anaerobic pertaining to an environment without oxygen

Analgesic drug used to reduce or eliminate pain

Anaphylactic shock type of shock caused by an acute allergic reaction

Anaphylaxis acute allergic response to an antigen that results in severe hypotension and may lead to life-threatening shock if untreated

Anastomoses natural communication networks among the coronary arteries

Androgens steroid sex hormones that promote the appearance of masculine characteristics

Anemia lack of adequate numbers of red blood cells, or decreased oxygen-carrying capacity of the blood

Angina pectoris acute chest pain on physical or emotional exertion due to inadequate oxygen supply to the myocardium

Angiotensin II chemical released in response to falling blood pressure that causes vasoconstriction and release of aldosterone

Angiotensin-converting enzyme (ACE) enzyme responsible for converting angiotensin I to angiotensin II

Anions negatively charged ions

Anorexia loss of appetite

Anorexiant drug used to suppress appetite

Antacid drug that neutralizes stomach acid

Antagonist drug that blocks the response of another drug

Antepartum prior to the onset of labor

Anthrax microorganism that can cause severe disease and high mortality in humans

Antibiotic substance produced by a microorganism that inhibits or kills other microorganisms

Antibody protein produced by the body in response to an antigen; used interchangeably with the term *immunoglobulin*

Anticholinergic drug that blocks the actions of the parasympathetic nervous system

Anticoagulant agent that inhibits the formation of blood clots

Antidepressant drug that alters levels of two important neurotransmitters in the brain, norepinephrine and serotonin, to reduce depression and anxiety

Antiemetic drug that prevents vomiting

Antiflatulent agent that reduces gas bubbles in the stomach and intestines, thereby decreasing bloating and discomfort

Anti-infective general term for any medication that is effective against pathogens

Antipyretic drug that lowers body temperature

Antiretroviral drug that is effective against retroviruses

Antithrombin III protein that prevents abnormal clotting by inhibiting thrombin

Antitussive drug used to suppress cough

Anxiety state of apprehension and autonomic nervous system activation resulting from exposure to a nonspecific or unknown cause

Anxiolytics drugs that relieve anxiety

Apoprotein protein component of a lipoprotein

Apothecary system of measurement older system of measurement that uses drams; rarely used

Aqueous humor fluid that fills the anterior and posterior chambers of the eye

Aromatase inhibitor hormone inhibitor that blocks the enzyme aromatase, which normally converts adrenal androgen to estradiol

ASAP order (as soon as possible) order that should be available for administration to the patient within 30 minutes of the written order

Assessment appraisal of a patient's condition that involves gathering and interpreting data

Asthma chronic inflammatory disease of the lungs characterized by airway obstruction

Astringent effect drops or spray used to shrink swollen mucous membranes, or to loosen secretions and facilitate drainage

Atherosclerosis condition characterized by a buildup of fatty plaque and loss of elasticity of the walls of the arteries

Atonic seizure very-short-lasting seizure during which the patient may stumble and fall for no apparent reason

Atrioventricular (AV) node cardiac tissue that receives electrical impulses from the sinoatrial node and conveys them to the ventricles

Atrioventricular bundle cardiac tissue that receives electrical impulses from the AV node and sends them to the bundle branches; also known as the *bundle of His*

Attention-deficit disorder (ADD) inability to focus attention on a task for a sufficient length of time

Attention deficit/hyperactivity disorder (ADHD) disorder typically diagnosed in childhood and adolescence characterized by hyperactivity as well as attention, organization, and behavior control issues

Aura sensory cue such as bright lights, smells, or tastes that precedes a migraine

Autoantibodies proteins called *rheumatoid factors* released by B lymphocytes that tear down the body's own tissue

Automaticity ability of certain myocardial cells to spontaneously generate an action potential

Autonomic nervous system portion of the peripheral nervous system that governs involuntary actions of the smooth muscle, cardiac muscle, and glands

Azole term for the major class of drugs used to treat mycoses

Azoospermia complete absence of sperm in an ejaculate

Bacteriocidal substance that kills bacteria

Bacteriostatic substance that inhibits the growth of bacteria

Balanced anesthesia use of multiple medications to rapidly induce unconsciousness, cause muscle relaxation, and maintain deep anesthesia

Baroreceptors nerves located in the walls of the atria, aortic arch, vena cava, and carotid sinus that sense changes in blood pressure

Basal metabolic rate resting rate of metabolism in the body

Baseline data patient information that is gathered before pharmacotherapy is implemented

B cell lymphocyte responsible for humoral immunity

Beneficence ethical principle of doing good

Benign not life threatening or fatal

Benign prostatic hypertrophy/hyperplasia (BPH) nonmalignant enlargement of the prostate gland

Benzodiazepines major class of drugs used to treat anxiety disorders

Beriberi deficiency of thiamine

Beta-lactam ring chemical structure found in most penicillins and some cephalosporins

Beta-lactamase (penicillinase) enzyme present in certain bacteria that is able to inactivate many penicillins and some cephalosporins

Beta receptor type of subreceptor found in the sympathetic nervous system

Bile acid resin drug that binds bile acids, thus lowering cholesterol

Bioavailability ability of a drug to reach the bloodstream and its target tissues

Biologics substances that produce biologic responses within the body; they are synthesized by cells of the human body, animal cells, or microorganisms

Bioterrorism intentional use of infectious biologic agents, chemical substances, or radiation to cause widespread harm or illness

Bipolar disorder syndrome characterized by extreme and opposite moods, such as euphoria and depression

Bisphosphonates class of drugs that block bone resorption by inhibiting osteoclast activity

Blood–brain barrier anatomical structure that prevents certain substances from gaining access to the brain

Bone deposition opposite of bone resorption; the process of depositing mineral components into bone

Bone resorption process of bone demineralization or the breaking down of bone into mineral components

Botanical plant extract used to treat or prevent illness

Bradykinesia difficulty initiating movement and controlling fine muscle movements

Bradykinin chemical released by cells during inflammation that produces pain and side effects similar to those of histamine

Breakthrough bleeding hemorrhage at abnormal times during the menstrual cycle

Broad-spectrum antibiotic anti-infective that is effective against many different gram-positive and gram-negative organisms

Bronchospasm rapid constriction of the airways

Buccal route administration of a tablet or capsule by placing it in the oral cavity between the gum and the cheek

Buffer chemical that helps maintain normal body pH by neutralizing strong acids or bases

Bundle branch electrical conduction pathway in the heart leading from the AV bundle and through the wall between the ventricles

C fibers nerves that transmit dull, poorly localized pain

Calcifediol substance formed in the first step of vitamin D formation

Calcineurin intracellular messenger molecule to which immunosuppressants bind

Calcitonin hormone secreted by the thyroid gland that increases the deposition of calcium in bone

Calcitriol substance transformed in the kidneys during the second step of the conversion of vitamin D to its active form

Calcium channel blocker drug that blocks the flow of calcium ions into myocardial cells

Calcium ion channel pathway in a plasma membrane through which calcium ions enter and leave

Camptothecins class of antineoplastics that inhibit the enzyme topoisomerase

Cancer/carcinoma malignant disease characterized by rapidly growing, invasive cells that spread to other regions of the body and eventually kill the host

Capsid protein coat that surrounds a virus

Carbonic anhydrase enzyme that forms carbonic acid by combining carbon dioxide and water

Cardiac decompensation condition during heart failure in which the heart can no longer handle the workload, and symptoms such as dyspnea on exertion, fatigue, pulmonary congestion, and peripheral edema appear

Cardiac output amount of blood pumped by a ventricle in 1 minute

Cardiac remodeling change in the size, shape, and structure of the myocardial cells (myocytes) that occurs over time in heart failure

Cardiogenic shock type of shock caused by a diseased heart that cannot maintain circulation to the tissues

Cardioversion/defibrillation conversion of fibrillation to a normal heart rhythm

Carotene class of yellow-red pigments that are precursors to vitamin A

Catecholamines class of agents secreted in response to stress that include epinephrine, norepinephrine, and dopamine

Cathartic substance that causes complete evacuation of the bowel

Cations positively charged ions

CD4 receptor protein that accepts HIV and allows entry of the virus into the T4 lymphocyte

Central nervous system (CNS) division of the nervous system consisting of the brain and spinal cord

Chemical name strict chemical nomenclature used for naming drugs established by the International Union of Pure and Applied Chemistry (IUPAC)

Chemoreceptors nerves located in the aortic arch and carotid sinus that sense changes in oxygen content, pH, or carbon dioxide levels in the blood

Chemotherapy drug treatment of cancer

Chief cells cells located in the mucosa of the stomach that secrete pepsinogen, an inactive form of the enzyme pepsin that chemically breaks down proteins

Cholecalciferol vitamin D_3 formed in the skin by exposure to ultraviolet light

Cholinergic relating to nerves that release acetylcholine

Chronic bronchitis recurrent disease of the lungs characterized by excess mucus production, inflammation, and coughing

Chronic obstructive pulmonary disease (COPD) generic term used to describe several pulmonary conditions characterized by cough, mucus production, and impaired gas exchange

Chyme semifluid, partly digested food that is passed from the stomach to the duodenum

Clinical investigation second stage of drug testing that involves clinical phase trials

Clinical phase trials testing of a new drug in selected patients

Clonic spasm multiple, rapidly repeated muscular contractions

Closed-angle glaucoma acute glaucoma that is caused by decreased outflow of aqueous humor from the anterior chamber

Clotting factors substances contributing to the process of blood hemostasis

Coagulation process of blood clotting

Coagulation cascade complex series of steps by which blood flow stops

Colloid type of IV fluid consisting of large organic molecules that are unable to cross membranes

Colony-stimulating factors hormones that regulate the growth and maturation of specific WBC populations

Combination drug drug product with more than one active generic ingredient

Comedone type of acne lesion that develops just beneath the surface of the skin (whitehead) or as a result of a plugged oil gland (blackhead)

Complement a series of proteins involved in the nonspecific defense of the body that promote antigen destruction

Complementary and alternative medicine (CAM) treatments that consider the health of the whole person and promote disease prevention

Complementary and alternative therapies treatments considered outside the realm of conventional Western medicine

Compliance taking a medication in the manner prescribed by the health care provider, or, in the case of over-the-counter (OTC) drugs, following the instructions on the label

Conjugates side chains that, during metabolism, make drugs more water soluble and more easily excreted by the kidney

Constipation infrequent passage of abnormally hard and dry stools

Contractility the strength with which the myocardial fibers contract

Controlled substance in the United States, a drug whose use is restricted by the Comprehensive Drug Abuse Prevention and Control Act; in Canada, a drug subject to guidelines outlined in the Canadian Narcotic Control Act

Convulsion uncontrolled muscle contraction or spasm that occurs in the face, torso, arms, or legs

Coronary arterial bypass graft (CABG) surgical procedure performed to restore blood flow to the myocardium by using a section of the saphenous vein or internal mammary artery to go around the obstructed coronary artery

Coronary arteries vessels that bring oxygen and nutrients to the myocardium

Corpus cavernosum tissue in the penis that fills with blood during an erection

Corpus luteum ruptured follicle that remains in the ovary after ovulation and secretes progestins

Corpus striatum area of the brain responsible for unconscious muscle movement; a point of contact for neurons projecting from the substantia nigra

Crohn's disease chronic inflammatory bowel disease affecting the ileum and sometimes the colon

Cross-tolerance situation in which tolerance to one drug makes the patient tolerant to another drug

Crystalloid type of IV fluid resembling blood plasma minus proteins that is capable of crossing membranes

Culture set of beliefs, values, religious rituals, and customs shared by a group of people

Culture and sensitivity test laboratory exam used to identify bacteria and to determine which antibiotic is most effective

Cushing's syndrome condition of having an excessive concentration of corticosteroids in the blood; caused by excessive secretion by the adrenal glands or by overdosage with corticosteroid medication

Cyclooxygenase (COX-1 and COX-2) key enzyme in the prostaglandin metabolic pathway that is blocked by aspirin and other NSAIDs

Cycloplegic drugs drugs that relax or temporarily paralyze ciliary muscles and cause blurred vision

Cytokines chemicals produced by white blood cells, such as interleukins, leukotrienes, interferon, and tumor necrosis factor, that guide the immune response

Cytotoxic T cell lymphocyte responsible for cell-mediated immunity that kills target cells directly or by secreting cytokines

Defecation evacuation of the colon; bowel movement

Delusions false ideas and beliefs not founded in reality

Dementia degenerative disorder characterized by progressive memory loss, confusion, and the inability to think or communicate effectively

Dependence strong physiological or psychological need for a substance

Depolarization reversal of the plasma membrane charge such that the inside is made less negative

Depression disorder characterized by depressed mood, lack of energy, sleep disturbances, abnormal eating patterns, and feelings of despair, guilt, and misery

Dermatitis inflammatory condition of the skin characterized by itching and scaling

Dermatophytic relating to a superficial fungal infection

Designer drug substance produced in a laboratory and intended to mimic the effects of another psychoactive controlled substance

Diabetes insipidus disorder marked by excessive urination due to lack of secretion of antidiuretic hormone

Diabetes mellitus, type 1 metabolic disease characterized by hyperglycemia caused by a lack of secretion of insulin by the pancreas

Diabetes mellitus, type 2 chronic metabolic disease caused by insufficient secretion of insulin by the pancreas, and a lack of sensitivity of insulin receptors

Diabetic ketoacidosis a type of metabolic acidosis due to an excess of ketone bodies, most often occurring when diabetes mellitus is uncontrolled

Diarrhea abnormal frequency and liquidity of bowel movements

Diastolic pressure blood pressure during the relaxation phase of heart activity

Dietary fiber ingested substance that is neither digested nor absorbed that contributes to the fecal mass

Dietary supplement nondrug substance regulated by the Dietary Supplement Health and Education Act of 1994 (DSHEA)

Dietary Supplement Health and Education Act of 1994 (DSHEA) primary law in the United States regulating herb and dietary supplements

Digitalization procedure in which the dose of cardiac glycoside is gradually increased until tissues become saturated with the drug, and the symptoms of heart failure diminish

Disease-modifying antirheumatic drugs (DMARD) drugs from several classes that modify the progression of rheumatoid arthritis; include hydroxychloroquine (Plaquenil), methotrexate (Rheumatrex), and sulfasalazine (Azulfidine)

Distribution the process of transporting drugs through the body

Diuretic substance that increases urine output

Dopamine type-D_2 receptor receptor for dopamine in the basal nuclei of the brain that is associated with schizophrenia and antipsychotic drugs

Drug general term for any substance capable of producing biologic responses in the body

Drug–protein complex drug that has bound reversibly to a plasma protein, particularly albumin, that makes the drug unavailable for distribution to body tissues

Dry powder inhaler (DPI) device used to convert a solid drug to a fine powder for the purpose of inhalation

Dysentery severe diarrhea that may include bleeding

Dysfunctional uterine bleeding hemorrhage that occurs at abnormal times or in excessive quantity during the menstrual cycle

Dyslipidemia abnormal (excess or deficient) level of lipoproteins in the blood

Dysrhythmia abnormality in cardiac rhythm

Dystonia severe muscle spasms, particularly of the back, neck, tongue, and face; characterized by abnormal tension starting in one area of the body and progressing to other areas

Eclampsia pregnancy-induced hypertensive disorder

Ectopic focus, pacemaker cardiac tissue outside the normal cardiac conduction pathway that generates action potentials

Eczema also called *atopic dermatitis*; a skin disorder with unexplained symptoms of inflammation, itching, and scaling

Efficacy the ability of a drug to produce a desired response

Electrocardiogram (ECG) device that records the electrical activity of the heart

Electroconvulsive therapy (ECT) treatment used for serious and life-threatening mood disorders in patients who are unresponsive to pharmacotherapy

Electroencephalogram (EEG) diagnostic test that records brainwaves through electrodes attached to the scalp

Electrolytes charged substances in the blood such as sodium, potassium, calcium, chloride, and phosphate

Embolus blood clot carried in the bloodstream

Emesis vomiting

Emetic drug used to induce vomiting

Emetic potential usually applied to antineoplastic agents; degree to which an agent is likely to trigger the vomiting center in the medulla, resulting in nausea and vomiting

Emphysema terminal lung disease characterized by permanent dilation of the alveoli

Endogenous opioids chemicals produced naturally within the body that decrease or eliminate pain; they closely resemble the actions of morphine

Endometriosis presence of endometrial tissue in nonuterine locations such as the pelvis and ovaries; a common cause of infertility

Endothelium inner lining of a blood vessel

Enteral nutrition nutrients supplied orally or by feeding tube

Enteral route administration of drugs orally, and through nasogastric or gastrostomy tubes

Enteric coated referring to tablets that have a hard, waxy coating designed to dissolve in the alkaline environment of the small intestine

Enterohepatic recirculation recycling of drugs and other substances by the circulation of bile through the intestine and liver

Enzyme induction process in which a drug changes the function of the hepatic microsomal enzymes and increases metabolic activity in the liver

Epilepsy disorder of the CNS characterized by seizures and/or convulsions

Ergocalciferol activated form of vitamin D

Ergosterol lipid substance in fungal cell membranes

Erythema redness associated with skin irritation

Erythrocytic stage phase in malaria during which infected red blood cells rupture, releasing merozoites and causing fever and chills

Erythropoietin hormone secreted by the kidney that regulates the process of red blood cell formation, or erythropoiesis

Ester type of chemical linkage found in some local anesthetics involving carbon and oxygen (–CO–O–)

Estrogen class of steroid sex hormones secreted by the ovary

Ethnic referring to people having a common history and similar genetic heritage

Evaluation, systematic objective assessment of the effectiveness and impact of interventions

Excoriation scratch that breaks the skin surface and fills with blood or serous fluid to form a crusty scale

Excretion the process of removing substances from the body

Expectorant drug used to increase bronchial secretions

External otitis commonly called *swimmer's ear*, an inflammation of the outer ear

Extracellular fluid (ECF) compartment body fluid lying outside cells, which includes plasma and interstitial fluid

Extrapyramidal side effects symptoms of acute dystonia, akathisia, parkinsonism, and tardive dyskinesia often caused by antipsychotic drugs

Febrile seizure tonic–clonic motor activity lasting 1 to 2 minutes with rapid return of consciousness that occurs in conjunction with elevated body temperature

Ferritin one of two protein complexes that maintain iron stores inside cells (hemosiderin is the other)

Fetal–placental barrier special anatomical structure that inhibits entry of many chemicals and drugs to the fetus

Fibrillation type of dysrhythmia in which the chambers beat in a highly disorganized manner

Fibrin an insoluble protein formed from fibrinogen by the action of thrombin in the blood clotting process

Fibrinogen blood protein that is converted to fibrin by the action of thrombin in the blood coagulation process

Fibrinolysis removal of a blood clot

Fight-or-flight response characteristic set of signs and symptoms produced when the sympathetic nervous system is activated

Filtrate fluid in the nephron that is filtered at Bowman's capsule

First-pass effect mechanism whereby drugs are absorbed across the intestinal wall and enter into the hepatic portal circulation

Five rights of drug administration principles that offer simple and practical guidance for nurses to use during drug preparation, delivery, and administration

Folic acid/folate B vitamin that is a coenzyme in protein and nucleic acid metabolism

Follicle-stimulating hormone (FSH) hormone secreted by the anterior pituitary gland that regulates sperm or egg production

Follicular cells cells in the thyroid gland that secrete thyroid hormone

Food and Drug Administration (FDA) U.S. agency responsible for the evaluation and approval of new drugs

Formulary list of drugs and drug recipes commonly used by pharmacists

Frank–Starling law the greater the degree of stretch on the myocardial fibers, the greater will be the force by which they contract

Frequency response curve graphical representation that illustrates interpatient variability in responses to drugs

Fungi kingdom of organisms that includes mushrooms, yeasts, and molds

Gamma-aminobutyric acid (GABA) neurotransmitter in the CNS

Ganglion collection of neuron cell bodies located outside the CNS

Gastroesophageal reflux disease (GERD) regurgitation of stomach contents into the esophagus

General anesthesia medical procedure that produces unconsciousness and loss of sensation throughout the entire body

Generalized anxiety disorder (GAD) difficult-to-control, excessive anxiety that lasts 6 months or more, focuses on a variety of life events, and interferes with normal day-to-day functions

Generalized seizures seizures that travel throughout the entire brain

Generic name nonproprietary name of a drug assigned by the government

Genetic polymorphism changes in enzyme structure and function due to mutation of the encoding gene

Glucocorticoid class of hormones secreted by the adrenal cortex that help the body respond to stress

Glycoprotein IIb/IIIa enzyme that binds fibrinogen and von Willebrand's factor to begin platelet aggregation and blood coagulation

Goal any object or objective that the patient or nurse seeks to attain or achieve

Gonadotropin-releasing hormone hormone secreted by the hypothalamus that stimulates the secretion of follicle-stimulating hormone (FSH) and luteinizing hormone (LH)

Gout metabolic disorder characterized by the accumulation of uric acid in the bloodstream or joint cavities

Graded dose response relationship between and measurement of the patient's response obtained at different doses of a drug

Gram negative bacteria that do not retain a purple stain because they have an outer envelope

Gram positive bacteria that stain purple because they have no outer envelope

Graves' disease syndrome caused by hypersecretion of thyroid hormone

Growth fraction the ratio of the number of replicating cells to resting cells in a tumor

H^+, K^+-ATPase enzyme responsible for pumping acid onto the mucosal surface of the stomach

H_1 receptor site located on smooth muscle cells in the bronchial tree and blood vessels that is stimulated by histamine to produce bronchodilation and vasodilation

H_2 receptor site located on cells of the digestive system that is stimulated by histamine to produce gastric acid

H_2-receptor antagonist drug that inhibits the effects of histamine at its receptors in the GI tract

Hallucination seeing, hearing, or feeling something that is not real

Heart failure (HF) disease in which the heart muscle cannot contract with sufficient force to meet the body's metabolic needs

Helicobacter pylori bacterium associated with a large percentage of peptic ulcer disease

Helminth type of flat, round, or segmented worm

Helper T cell lymphocyte that coordinates both the humoral and cell-mediated immune responses and that is the target of the human immunodeficiency virus

Hematopoiesis process of erythrocyte production that begins with primitive stem cells that reside in bone marrow

Hemophilia hereditary lack of a specific blood clotting factor

Hemosiderin one of two protein complexes that maintain iron stores inside cells (ferritin is the other)

Hemostasis the slowing or stopping of blood flow

Hemostatic drug used to inhibit the normal removal of fibrin, used to speed clot formation, and keep the clot in place for a longer period

Hepatic microsomal enzyme system as it relates to pharmacotherapy, liver enzymes that inactivate drugs and accelerate their excretion; sometimes called the P-450 system

Hepatitis viral infection of the liver

Herb plant with a soft stem that is used for healing or as a seasoning

High-density lipoprotein (HDL) lipid-carrying particle in the blood that contains high amounts of protein and lower amounts of cholesterol; considered to be "good" cholesterol

Highly active antiretroviral therapy (HAART) drug therapy for HIV infection that includes high doses of multiple medications given concurrently

Hippocampus region of the brain responsible for learning and memory; a part of the limbic system

Histamine chemical released by mast cells in response to an antigen that causes dilation of blood vessels, bronchoconstriction, tissue swelling, and itching

HIV-AIDS acronym for human immunodeficiency virus–acquired immune deficiency syndrome; characterized by profound immunosuppression that leads to opportunistic infections and malignancies not commonly found in patients with functioning immune defenses

HMG-CoA reductase primary enzyme in the biochemical pathway for the synthesis of cholesterol

Holistic viewing a person as an integrated biologic, psychosocial, cultural, communicating whole, existing and functioning within the communal environment

Hormone chemical secreted by endocrine glands that acts as a chemical messenger to affect homeostasis

Hormone replacement therapy (HRT) drug therapy consisting of estrogen and progestin combinations; used to treat symptoms associated with menopause

Host flora normal microorganisms found in or on a patient

Household system of measurement older system of measurement that uses teaspoons, tablespoons, and cups

Humoral immunity branch of the immune system that produces antibodies

Hydrolysis breakdown of a substance into simpler compounds by the addition or taking up of water

Hypercholesterolemia high levels of cholesterol in the blood

Hyperemia increase in blood supply to a part or tissue space causing swelling, redness, and pain

Hyperglycemia high glucose level in the blood

Hyperlipidemia excess amount of lipids in the blood

Hypernatremia high sodium level in the blood

Hyperosmolar nonketotic coma life-threatening metabolic condition that occurs in people with type 2 diabetes

Hypertension high blood pressure

Hyperuricemia elevated blood level of uric acid, which causes gout

Hypervitaminosis excess intake of vitamins

Hypnotic drug that causes sleep

Hypoglycemia low glucose level in the blood

Hypogonadism below-normal secretion of the steroid sex hormones

Hyponatremia low sodium level in the blood

Hypovolemic shock type of shock caused by loss of fluids such as occurs during hemorrhage, extensive burns, or severe vomiting or diarrhea

Idiosyncratic response unpredictable and unexplained drug reaction

Ileum third portion of the small intestine extending from the jejunum to the ileocecal valve

Illusion distorted perception of actual sensory stimuli

Immune response specific reaction of the body to foreign agents involving B and/or T lymphocytes

Immunosuppressant any drug, chemical, or physical agent that lowers the immune defense mechanisms of the body

Impotence inability to obtain or sustain an erection; also called *erectile dysfunction*

Infant child younger than 1 year

Infertility inability to become pregnant after at least 1 year of frequent, unprotected intercourse

Inflammation nonspecific body defense that occurs in response to an injury or antigen

Influenza common viral infection; often called flu

Inotropic agent drug or chemical that changes the force of contraction of the heart

Inotropic effect change in the strength or contractility of the heart

Insomnia inability to fall asleep or stay asleep

Insulin analog modified human insulin with pharmacokinetic advantages, such as more rapid onset of action or prolonged duration of action

Insulin resistance occurs in type 2 diabetes mellitus; although insulin is secreted, insulin receptors in target tissues become *insensitive* to insulin, binding of insulin to these receptors decreases, less effect is achieved

Interferon type of cytokine secreted by T cells in response to antigens to protect uninfected cells

Interleukin class of cytokines synthesized by lymphocytes, monocytes, macrophages, and certain other cells that enhance the capabilities of the immune system

Intermittent claudication condition caused by insufficient blood flow to skeletal muscles in the lower limbs, resulting in ischemia of skeletal muscles and severe pain on walking, especially in calf muscles

Intervention action that produces an effect or that is intended to alter the course of a disease or condition

Intracellular fluid (ICF) compartment body fluid that is inside cells; accounts for about two thirds of the total body water

Intracellular parasite infectious microbe that lives inside host cells

Intradermal (ID) medication administered into the dermis layer of the skin

Intramuscular (IM) delivery of medication into specific muscles

Intravenous (IV) administration of medications and fluids directly into the bloodstream

Intrinsic factor chemical substance secreted by the parietal cells in the stomach that is essential for the absorption of vitamin B_{12}

Ionizing radiation radiation that is highly penetrating and can cause serious biologic effects

Irritable bowel syndrome (IBS) inflammatory disease of the small or large intestine characterized by intense abdominal cramping and diarrhea

Islets of Langerhans cell clusters in the pancreas responsible for the secretion of insulin and glucagon

Jejunum middle portion of the small intestine between the duodenum and the ileum

Kaposi's sarcoma vascular cancer that first appears on the skin and then invades internal organs; frequently occurs in AIDS patients

Kappa receptor type of opioid receptor

Keratolytic action that promotes shedding of old skin

Ketoacid acidic waste product of lipid metabolism that lowers the pH of the blood

Latent phase period of HIV infection during which there are no symptoms

Laxative drug that promotes defecation

Lecithin phospholipid that is an important component of cell membranes

Leukemia cancer of the blood characterized by overproduction of white blood cells

Leukotriene chemical mediator of inflammation stored and released by mast cells; effects are similar to those of histamine

Libido interest in sexual activity

Limbic system area in the brain responsible for emotion, learning, memory, motivation, and mood

Lipodystrophy atrophy increase or decrease of subcutaneous fat at an insulin injection site, resulting in an indenture or a raised area

Lipoprotein substance carrying lipids in the bloodstream that is composed of proteins bound to fat

Liposome small sac of lipids designed to carry drugs inside it

Loading dose comparatively large dose given at the beginning of treatment to rapidly obtain the therapeutic effect of a drug

Local anesthesia loss of sensation to a limited part of the body without loss of consciousness

Long-term insomnia inability to sleep for more than a few nights, often caused by depression, manic disorders, and chronic pain

Low-density lipoprotein (LDL) lipid-carrying particle that contains relatively low amounts of protein and high amounts of cholesterol; considered to be "bad" cholesterol

Low-molecular-weight heparins (LMWHs) drugs closely resembling heparin that inhibit blood clotting

Leutinizing hormone (LH) hormone secreted by the pituitary gland that triggers ovulation in the female and stimulates sperm production in the male

Lymphoma cancer of lymphatic tissue

Macromineral (major mineral) inorganic compound needed by the body in amounts of 100 mg or more daily

Maintenance dose dose that keeps the plasma drug concentration continuously in the therapeutic range

Malaria tropical disease characterized by severe fever and chills caused by the protozoan *Plasmodium*

Malignant life threatening or fatal

Mania condition characterized by an expressive, impulsive, excitable, and overreactive nature

Mast cell connective tissue cell located in tissue spaces that releases histamine following injury

Mastoiditis inflammation of the mastoid sinus

Mechanism of action the way in which a drug exerts its effects

Median effective dose (ED_{50}) dose required to produce a specific therapeutic response in 50% of a group of patients

Median lethal dose (LD_{50}) often determined in preclinical trials, the dose of drug that will be lethal in 50% of a group of animals

Median toxicity dose (TD_{50}) dose that will produce a given toxicity in 50% of a group of patients

Medication drug after it has been administered

Medication administration record (MAR) documentation of all pharmacotherapies received by the patient

Medication error any preventable event that may cause or lead to inappropriate medication use or patient harm while the medication is in the control of the health care provider, patient, or consumer

Medication error index categorization of medication errors according to the extent of the harm an error can cause

Menopause period of time during which females stop secreting estrogen and menstrual cycles cease

Menorrhagia prolonged or excessive menstruation

Metabolism total of all biochemical reactions in the body

Metastasis travel of cancer cells from their original site to a distant tissue

Metered dose inhaler (MDI) device used to deliver a precise amount of drug to the respiratory system

Methadone maintenance treatment of opioid dependence by using methadone

Methylxanthine chemical derivative of caffeine

Metric system of measurement most common system of drug measurement that uses grams and liters

Micromineral (trace mineral) inorganic compound needed by the body in amounts of 20 mg or less daily

Middle-age adulthood person from 40 to 65 years of age

Migraine severe headache preceded by auras that may include nausea and vomiting

Minimum effective concentration amount of drug required to produce a therapeutic effect

Miosis constriction of the pupil

Monoamine oxidase (MAO) enzyme that destroys norepinephrine in the nerve terminal

Monoamine oxidase inhibitor (MAOI) drug inhibiting monoamine oxidase, an enzyme that terminates the actions of neurotransmitters such as dopamine, norepinephrine, epinephrine, and serotonin

Mood disorder change in behavior such as clinical depression, emotional swings, or manic depression

Mood stabilizer drug that levels mood that is used to treat bipolar disorder and mania

Mu receptor type of opioid receptor

Mucolytic drug used to loosen thick mucus

Mucosa layer inner lining of the alimentary canal that provides a surface area for the various acids, bases, and enzymes to break down food

Mucositis inflammation of the epithelial lining of the digestive tract

Muscarinic type of cholinergic receptor found in smooth muscle, cardiac muscle, and glands

Muscle spasm involuntary contraction of a muscle or group of muscles, which become tightened, develop a fixed pattern of resistance, and result in a diminished level of functioning

Mutation permanent, inheritable change to DNA

Myasthenia gravis motor disorder caused by a destruction of nicotinic receptors on skeletal muscles and characterized by profound muscular fatigue

Mycoses diseases caused by fungi

Mydriatic drug agent that causes pupil dilation

Myocardial infarction blood clot blocking a portion of a coronary artery that causes necrosis of cardiac muscle

Myocardial ischemia lack of blood supply to the myocardium due to a constriction or obstruction of a blood vessel

Myoclonic seizure seizure characterized by brief, sudden contractions of a group of muscles

Myxedema condition caused by insufficient secretion of thyroid hormone

Narcotic natural or synthetic drug related to morphine; may be used as a broader legal term referring to hallucinogens, CNS stimulants, marijuana, and other illegal drugs

Narrow-spectrum antibiotic anti-infective that is effective against only one or a small number of organisms

Nausea uncomfortable wavelike sensation that precedes vomiting

NDA review third stage of new drug evaluation by the FDA

Nebulizer device used to convert liquid drugs into a fine mist for the purpose of inhalation

Negative feedback in homeostasis, the shutting off of the first hormone in a pathway by the last hormone or product in the pathway

Negative symptoms in schizophrenia, symptoms that subtract from normal behavior, including a lack of interest, motivation, responsiveness, or pleasure in daily activities

Neoplasm abnormal swelling or mass; same as *tumor*

Nephron structural and functional unit of the kidney

Nerve agent chemical used in warfare or by bioterrorists that can affect the central nervous system and cause death

Neurofibrillary tangles bundles of nerve fibers found in the brain of patients with Alzheimer's disease on autopsy

Neurogenic shock type of shock resulting from brain or spinal cord injury

Neurohypophysis posterior portion of the pituitary gland

Neurolepanalgesia type of general anesthesia that combines fentanyl with droperidol to produce a state in which patients are conscious though insensitive to pain and unconnected with surroundings

Neuroleptic malignant syndrome potentially fatal condition caused by certain antipsychotic medications characterized by an extremely high body temperature, drowsiness, changing blood pressure, irregular heartbeat, and muscle rigidity

Neuromuscular blocker drug used to cause total muscle relaxation

Neuropathic pain caused by injury to nerves and typically described as burning, shooting, or numb pain

Nicotinic type of cholinergic receptor found in ganglia of both the sympathetic and parasympathetic nervous systems

Nit egg of the louse parasite

Nociceptor receptor connected with nerves that receive and transmit pain signals to the spinal cord and brain

Nonmaleficence ethical obligation to not harm the patient

Nonspecific body defense defense such as inflammation that protects the body from invasion by general hazards

Nonspecific cellular response drug action that is independent of cellular receptors and is not associated with other mechanisms, such as changing the permeability of cellular membranes, depressing membrane excitability, or altering the activity of cellular pumps

Norepinephrine (NE) primary neurotransmitter in the sympathetic nervous system

Nosocomial infection infection acquired in a health care setting such as a hospital, physician's office, or nursing home

Nurse Practice Act legislation designed to protect the public by defining the legal scope of practice of nurses

Nursing diagnosis clinically based judgment about the patient and his or her response to health and illness

Nursing process five-part decision-making system that includes assessment, nursing diagnosis, planning, implementation, and evaluation

Objective data information gathered through physical assessment, laboratory tests, and other diagnostic sources

Obsessive-compulsive disorder recurrent, intrusive thoughts or repetitive behaviors that interfere with normal activities or relationships

Older adulthood person older than age 65

Oligomenorrhea infrequent menstruation

Oligospermia presence of less than 20 million sperm in an ejaculate

Oncogene gene responsible for the conversion of normal cells into cancer cells

Open-angle glaucoma chronic, simple glaucoma caused by hindered outflow of aqueous humor from the anterior chamber

Opiate substance closely related to morphine extracted from the poppy plant

Opioid substance obtained from the unripe seeds of the poppy plant; natural or synthetic morphine-like substance

Orthostatic hypotension fall in blood pressure that occurs when changing position from recumbent to upright

Osmolality number of dissolved particles, or solutes, in 1 kg (1 L) of water

Osmosis process by which water moves from areas of low solute concentration (low osmolality) to areas of high solute concentration (high osmolality)

Osteoarthritis disorder characterized by degeneration of joints; particularly the fingers, spine, hips, and knees

Osteomalacia rickets in children; caused by vitamin D deficiency; characterized by softening of the bones without alteration of basic bone structure

Osteoporosis condition in which bones lose mass and become brittle and susceptible to fracture

Otitis media inflammation of the middle ear

Ototoxicity having an adverse effect on the organs of hearing

Outcome objective measurement of goals

Ovulation release of an egg by the ovary

Oxytocin hormone secreted by the posterior pituitary gland that stimulates uterine contractions and milk ejection

Paget's disease disorder of bone formation and resorption characterized by weak, enlarged, and deformed bones

Palliation form of cancer chemotherapy intended to alleviate symptoms rather than cure the disease

Panic disorder anxiety disorder characterized by intense feelings of immediate apprehension, fearfulness, terror, or impending doom, accompanied by increased autonomic nervous system activity

Parafollicular cells cells in the thyroid gland that secrete calcitonin

Paranoia having an extreme suspicion and delusion that one is being followed and that others are trying to inflict harm

Parasympathetic nervous system portion of the autonomic nervous system that is active during periods of rest and that results in the rest-or-relaxation response

Parasympathomimetic drug that mimics the actions of the parasympathetic nervous system

Parenteral route dispensation of medications via a needle into the skin layers

Parietal cell cell in the stomach mucosa that secretes hydrochloric acid

Parkinson's disease degenerative disorder of the nervous system caused by a deficiency of the brain neurotransmitter dopamine that results in disturbances of muscle movement

Parkinsonism having tremor, muscle rigidity, stooped posture, and a shuffling gait

Partial (focal) seizure seizure that starts on one side of the brain and travels a short distance before stopping

Partial agonist medication that produces a weaker, or less efficacious, response than an agonist

Passive immunity immune defense that lasts 2 to 3 weeks; obtained by administering antibodies

Pathogen organism that is capable of causing disease

Pathogenicity ability of an organism to cause disease in humans

Pediculicides medications that kill lice

Pegylation process that attaches polyethylene glycol (PEG) to an interferon to extend its pharmacologic activity

Pellagra deficiency of niacin

Peptic ulcer erosion of the mucosa in the alimentary canal, most commonly in the stomach and duodenum

Percutaneous transluminal coronary angioplasty (PTCA) procedure by which a balloon-shaped catheter is used to compress fatty plaque against an arterial wall for the purpose of restoring normal blood flow

Perfusion blood flow through a tissue or organ

Peripheral nervous system division of the nervous system containing all nervous tissue outside the CNS, including the autonomic nervous system

Peripheral resistance amount of friction encountered by blood as it travels through the vessels

Peristalsis involuntary wavelike contraction of smooth muscle lining the alimentary canal

Pernicious (megaloblastic) anemia type of anemia usually caused by lack of secretion of intrinsic factor

pH measure of the acidity or alkalinity of a solution

Pharmacodynamics study of how the body responds to drugs

Pharmacogenetics area of pharmacology that examines the role of genetics in drug response

Pharmacokinetics study of how drugs are handled by the body

Pharmacologic classification method for organizing drugs on the basis of their mechanism of action

Pharmacology the study of medicines; the discipline pertaining to how drugs improve or maintain health

Pharmacopoeia medical reference indicating standards of drug purity, strength, and directions for synthesis

Pharmacotherapy treatment or prevention of disease by means of drugs

Phobia fearful feeling attached to situations or objects such as snakes, spiders, crowds, or heights

Phosphodiesterase enzyme in muscle cells that cleaves phosphodiester bonds; its inhibition increases myocardial contractility

Phospholipid type of lipid that contains two fatty acids, a phosphate group, and a chemical backbone of glycerol

Photosensitivity condition in which the skin is highly sensitive to sunlight

Physical dependence condition of experiencing unpleasant withdrawal symptoms when a substance is discontinued

Planning linkage of strategies or interventions to established goals and outcomes

Plaque fatty material that builds up in the lining of blood vessels and may lead to hypertension, stroke, myocardial infarction, or angina

Plasma cell cell derived from B lymphocytes that produces antibodies

Plasma half-life ($t_{1/2}$) the length of time required for the plasma concentration of a drug to decrease by half after administration

Plasmid small piece of circular DNA found in some bacteria that is able to transfer resistance from one bacterium to another

Plasmin enzyme formed from plasminogen that dissolves blood clots

Plasminogen protein that prevents fibrin clot formation; precursor of plasmin

Polarized condition in which the inside of a cell is more negatively charged than the outside of the cell

Polyene antifungal class containing amphotericin B and nystatin

Polypharmacy the taking of multiple drugs concurrently

Positive symptoms in schizophrenia, symptoms that add to normal behavior, including hallucinations, delusions, and a disorganized thought or speech pattern

Postmarketing surveillance evaluation of a new drug after it has been approved and used in large numbers of patients

Postpartum occurring after childbirth

Postsynaptic neuron in a synapse, the nerve that has receptors for the neurotransmitter

Post-traumatic stress disorder type of anxiety that develops in response to reexperiencing a previous life event that was psychologically traumatic

Potassium ion channel pathway in a plasma membrane through which potassium ions enter and leave

Potency the strength of a drug at a specified concentration or dose

Preclinical investigation procedure implemented after a drug has been licensed for public use, designed to provide information on use and on occurrence of side effects

Preload degree of stretch of the cardiac muscle fibers just before they contract

Prenatal preceding birth

Preschool child child from 3 to 5 years of age

Presynaptic neuron nerve that releases the neurotransmitter into the synaptic cleft when stimulated by an action potential

PRN order medication is administered as required by the patient's condition (Latin: *pro re nata*)

Prodrug drug that becomes more active after it is metabolized

Progesterone hormone secreted by the corpus luteum and placenta responsible for building up the uterine lining in the second half of the menstrual cycle and during pregnancy

Prolactin hormone secreted by the anterior pituitary gland that stimulates milk production in the mammary glands

Prostaglandins class of local hormones that promote local inflammation and pain when released by cells in the body

Protease viral enzyme that is responsible for the final assembly of the HIV virions

Prothrombin blood protein that is converted to thrombin in blood coagulation

Prothrombin activator enzyme in the coagulation cascade that converts prothrombin to thrombin; also called *prothrombinase*

Prothrombin time blood test used to determine the time needed for plasma to clot for the regulation of warfarin dosage

Proton pump inhibitor drug that inhibits the enzyme H^+, K^+-ATPase

Prototype drug well-understood model drug with which other drugs in a pharmacologic class may be compared

Protozoan single-celled animal

Provitamin inactive chemical that is converted to a vitamin in the body

Pruritus itching associated with dry, scaly skin

Psoralen drug used along with phototherapy for the treatment of psoriasis and other severe skin disorders

Psychedelic substance that alters perception and reality

Psychological dependence intense craving for a drug that drives people to continue drug abuse

Psychology science that deals with normal and abnormal mental processes and their impact on behavior

Purine building block of DNA and RNA, either adenine or guanine

Purkinje fibers electrical conduction pathway leading from the bundle branches to all portions of the ventricles

Pyrimidine building block of DNA and RNA, either thymine or cytosine in DNA, and cytosine and uracil in RNA

Rapid eye movement (REM) sleep stage of sleep characterized by quick, scanning movements of the eyes

Reabsorption movement of filtered substances from the kidney tubule back into the blood

Reasonable and prudent action defines the standard of care as the actions that a reasonable and prudent nurse with equivalent preparation would do under similar circumstances

Rebound insomnia increased sleeplessness that occurs when long-term antianxiety or hypnotic medication is discontinued

Receptor the structural component of a cell to which a drug binds in a dose-related manner, to produce a response

Recommended Dietary Allowance (RDA) amount of vitamin or mineral needed each day to avoid a deficiency in a healthy adult

Red-man syndrome rash on the upper body caused by certain anti-infectives

Reflex tachycardia temporary increase in heart rate that occurs when blood pressure falls

Refractory period time during which the myocardial cells rest and are not able to contract

Releasing hormone hormone secreted by the hypothalamus that affects secretions in the pituitary gland

Renin–angiotensin system series of enzymatic steps by which the body raises blood pressure

Respiration exchange of oxygen and carbon dioxide in the lungs; also, the process of deriving energy from metabolic reactions

Rest-and-digest response signs and symptoms produced when the parasympathetic nervous system is activated

Reticular activating system (RAS) responsible for sleeping and wakefulness and performs an alerting function for the cerebral cortex; includes the reticular formation, hypothalamus, and part of the thalamus

Reticular formation portion of the brain affecting awareness and wakefulness

Retinoid compound resembling vitamin A used in the treatment of severe acne and psoriasis

Reverse cholesterol transport the process by which cholesterol is transported away from body tissues to the liver

Reverse transcriptase viral enzyme that converts RNA to DNA

Reye's syndrome potentially fatal complication of infection associated with aspirin use in children

Rhabdomyolysis breakdown of muscle fibers usually due to muscle trauma or ischemia

Rheumatoid arthritis systemic autoimmune disorder characterized by inflammation of multiple joints

Rhinophyma reddened, bullous, irregular swelling of the nose

Risk management system of reducing medication errors by modifying policies and procedures within the institution

Rosacea chronic skin disorder characterized by clusters of papules on the face

Routine order order not written as STAT, ASAP, NOW, or PRN

Salicylism poisoning due to aspirin and aspirin-like drugs

Sarcoma cancer of connective tissue such as bone, muscle, or cartilage

Scabicide drug that kills scabies mites

Scabies skin disorder that results when the female mite burrows into the skin and lays eggs

Scheduled drug in the United States, a term describing a drug placed into one of five categories based on its potential for misuse or abuse

Schizoaffective disorder psychosis with symptoms of both schizophrenia and mood disorders

Schizophrenia psychosis characterized by abnormal thoughts and thought processes, withdrawal from other people and the outside environment, and apparent preoccupation with one's own mental state

School-age child child from 6 to 12 years of age

Scurvy deficiency of vitamin C

Seborrhea skin condition characterized by overactivity of oil glands

Second messenger cascade of biochemical events that initiates a drug's action by either stimulating or inhibiting a normal activity of the cell

Secretion in the kidney, movement of substances from the blood into the tubule after filtration has occurred

Sedative substance that depresses the CNS to cause drowsiness or sleep

Sedative–hypnotic drug with the ability to produce a calming effect at lower doses and to induce sleep at higher doses

Seizure symptom of epilepsy characterized by abnormal neuronal discharges within the brain

Selective estrogen receptor modulator (SERM) drug that produces an action similar to estrogen in body tissues; used for the treatment of osteoporosis in postmenopausal women

Selective serotonin reuptake inhibitor (SSRI) drug that selectively inhibits the reuptake of serotonin into nerve terminals; used mostly for depression

Septic shock type of shock caused by severe infection in the bloodstream

Serotonin syndrome set of signs and symptoms associated with overmedication with antidepressants that includes altered mental status, fever, sweating, and lack of muscular coordination

Shock condition in which there is inadequate blood flow to meet the body's metabolic needs

Short-term or behavioral insomnia inability to sleep that is often attributed to stress caused by a hectic lifestyle or the inability to resolve day-to-day conflicts within the home or workplace

Single order medication that is to be given only once, and at a specific time, such as a preoperative order

Sinoatrial (SA) node pacemaker of the heart located in the wall of the right atrium that controls the basic heart rate

Sinus rhythm number of beats per minute normally generated by the SA node

Situational anxiety anxiety experienced by people faced with a stressful environment

Sleep debt lack of sleep

Social anxiety fear of crowds

Sociology study of human behavior within the context of groups and societies

Sodium ion channel pathway in a plasma membrane through which sodium ions enter and leave

Somatic nervous system nerve division that provides voluntary control over skeletal muscle

Somatostatin synonym for growth hormone inhibiting factor from the hypothalamus

Somatotropin another name for growth hormone

Somogyi phenomenon rapid decrease in blood glucose level that stimulates the release of hormones (epinephrine, cortisol, glucagon) resulting in an elevated morning blood glucose

Spasticity inability of opposing muscle groups to move in a coordinated manner

Specialty supplement nonherbal dietary product used to enhance a wide variety of body functions

Spirituality the capacity to love, to convey compassion and empathy, to give and forgive, to enjoy life, and to find peace of mind and fulfillment in living

Stable angina type of angina that occurs in a predictable pattern, usually relieved by rest

Standards of care the skills and learning commonly possessed by members of a profession

Standing order order written in advance of a situation that is to be carried out under specific circumstances

STAT order any medication that is needed immediately and is to be given only once

Status epilepticus condition characterized by repeated seizures or one prolonged seizure attack that continues for at least 30 minutes

Stem cell cell that resides in the bone marrow and is capable of maturing into any type of blood cell

Steroid type of lipid consisting of four rings that is a structural component of certain hormones and drugs

Sterol nucleus ring structure common to all steroids

Strategic National Stockpile (SNS) program designed to ensure the immediate deployment of essential medical materials to a community in the event of a large-scale chemical or biologic attack

Stroke volume amount of blood pumped out by a ventricle in a single beat

Subcutaneous medication delivered beneath the skin

Subjective data information gathered regarding what a patient states or perceives

Sublingual route administration of medication by placing it under the tongue and allowing it to dissolve slowly

Substance abuse self-administration of a drug that does not conform to the medical or social norms within the patient's given culture or society

Substance P neurotransmitter within the spinal cord involved in the neural transmission of pain

Substantia nigra location in the brain where dopamine is synthesized that is responsible for regulation of unconscious muscle movement

Superficial mycosis fungal disease of the hair, skin, nails, and mucous membranes

Superinfection new infection caused by an organism different from the one causing the initial infection; usually a side effect of anti-infective therapy

Surgical anesthesia stage 3 of anesthesia, in which most major surgery occurs

Sustained release tablets or capsules designed to dissolve slowly over an extended time

Sympathetic nervous system portion of the autonomic system that is active during periods of stress and results in the fight-or-flight response

Sympathomimetic drug that stimulates or mimics the sympathetic nervous system

Synapse junction between two neurons consisting of a presynaptic nerve, a synaptic cleft, and a postsynaptic nerve

Synaptic transmission process by which a neurotransmitter reaches receptors to regenerate the action potential

Systemic mycosis fungal disease affecting internal organs

Systolic pressure blood pressure during the contraction phase of heart activity

Tardive dyskinesia unusual tongue and face movements such as lip smacking and wormlike motions of the tongue that occur during pharmacotherapy with certain antipsychotics

Taxanes alkaloids isolated from the bark of the Pacific yew and used for antineoplastic activity; current drugs include paclitaxel (Taxol) and docetaxel (Taxotere), but more than 19 others are being investigated

T cell type of lymphocyte that is essential for the cell-mediated immune response

Tension headache common type of head pain caused by stress and relieved by nonnarcotic analgesics

Teratogen drug or other agent that causes developmental birth defects

Testosterone primary androgen responsible for maturation of male sex organs and secondary sex characteristics of men; secreted by testes

Tetrahydrocannabinol (THC) the active chemical in marijuana

Therapeutic classification method for organizing drugs on the basis of their clinical usefulness

Therapeutic index the ratio of a drug's LD_{50} to its ED_{50}

Therapeutic range the dosage range or serum concentration that achieves the desired drug effects

Therapeutics the branch of medicine concerned with the treatment of disease and suffering

Three checks of drug administration in conjunction with the five rights, these ascertain patient safety and drug effectiveness

Thrombin enzyme that causes clotting by catalyzing the conversion of fibrinogen to fibrin

Thrombocytopenia reduction in the number of circulating platelets

Thromboembolic disorder condition in which the patient develops blood clots

Thrombolytic drug used to dissolve existing blood clots

Thrombopoietin hormone produced by the kidneys that controls megakaryocyte activity

Thrombus blood clot obstructing a vessel

Thyrotoxic crisis acute form of hyperthyroidism that is a medical emergency; also called *thyroid storm*

Tissue plasminogen activator (tPA) natural enzyme and a drug that dissolves blood clots

Titer measurement of the amount of a substance in the blood

Tocolytic drug used to inhibit uterine contractions

Tocopherol generic name for vitamin E

Toddlerhood term applied to children from 1 to 3 years of age

Tolerance process of adapting to a drug over a period of time and subsequently requiring higher doses to achieve the same effect

Tonic spasm single, prolonged muscular contraction

Tonic–clonic seizure seizure characterized by intense jerking motions and loss of consciousness

Tonicity the ability of a solution to cause a change in water movement across a membrane due to osmotic forces

Tonometry technique for measuring intraocular tension and pressure

Topoisomerase enzyme that assists in the repair of DNA damage

Total parenteral nutrition (TPN) nutrition provided through a peripheral or central vein

Toxic concentration level of drug that will result in serious adverse effects

Toxin chemical produced by a microorganism that is able to cause injury to its host

Toxoid substance that has been chemically modified to remove its harmful nature but is still able to elicit an immune response in the body

Trade name proprietary name of a drug assigned by the manufacturer; also called the brand name or product name

Tranquilizer older term sometimes used to describe a drug that produces a calm or tranquil feeling

Transferrin protein complex that transports iron to sites in the body where it is needed

Transplant rejection recognition by the immune system of a transplanted tissue as foreign and subsequent attack on the tissue

Tricyclic antidepressant (TCA) class of drugs used in the pharmacotherapy of depression

Triglyceride type of lipid that contains three fatty acids and a chemical backbone of glycerol

Tubercle cavity-like lesion in the lung characteristic of infection by *Mycobacterium tuberculosis*

Tumor abnormal swelling or mass

Tyramine form of the amino acid tyrosine that is found in foods such as cheese, beer, wine, and yeast products

Ulcerative colitis inflammatory bowel disease of the colon

Undernutrition lack of adequate nutrition to meet the metabolic demands of the body

Unstable angina severe angina that occurs frequently and that is not relieved by rest

Urinalysis diagnostic test that examines urine for the presence of blood cells, proteins, pH, specific gravity, ketones, glucose, and microorganisms

Vaccination immunization inoculation with a vaccine or toxoid to prevent disease

Vaccine biologic material that confers protection against infection; preparation of microorganism particles that is injected into a patient to stimulate the immune system, with the intention of preventing disease

Vasomotor center area of the medulla that controls baseline blood pressure

Vasospastic or Prinzmetal's angina type of angina in which the decreased myocardial blood flow is caused by *spasms* of the coronary arteries

Vendor Managed Inventory (VMI) supplies and pharmaceuticals that are shipped after a chemical or biologic threat has been identified

Ventilation process by which air is moved into and out of the lungs

Very-low-density lipoprotein (VLDL) lipid-carrying particle that is converted to LDL in the liver

Vesicant agent that can cause serious tissue injury if it escapes from an artery or vein during an infusion or injection (extravasation); many antineoplastics are vesicants

Vestibular apparatus portion of the inner ear responsible for the sense of position

Vinca alkaloid chemical obtained from the periwinkle plant that has antineoplastic activity

Virilization appearance of masculine secondary sex characteristics

Virion particle of a virus capable of causing an infection

Virulence the severity of disease that a pathogen is able to cause

Virus nonliving particle containing nucleic acid that is able to cause disease

Vitamin organic compound required by the body in small amounts

Vitiligo milk-white areas of depigmented skin

Vomiting center area in the medulla that controls the vomiting reflex

Von Willebrand's disease decrease in quantity or quality of von Willebrand factor (vWF), which acts as a carrier of factor VIII and has a role in platelet aggregation

Withdrawal physical signs of discomfort associated with the discontinuation of an abused substance

Withdrawal syndrome symptoms that result when a patient discontinues taking a substance on which he or she was dependent

Yeast type of fungus that is unicellular and divides by budding

Young adulthood term applied to persons from 18 to 40 years of age

Zollinger–Ellison syndrome disorder of excess acid secretion in the stomach resulting in peptic ulcer disease

Index

Page numbers followed by *f* indicate figures and those followed by *t* indicate tables, boxes, or special features. The titles of special features (e.g., Home and Community Considerations, PharmFacts, Treating the Diverse Patient) are also capitalized.

Prototype drugs appear in **boldface,** drug classifications are in SMALL CAPS, and trade names are capitalized and cross-referenced to their generic name. Disease, disorders, and conditions are in red type.

A

AAPMC (antibiotic-associated pseudomembranous colitis), 494
abacavir, 530*t*
abatacept, 742*t*
abbreviations:
    to avoid, 20*t*, 87*t*
    drug administration, 20*t*
abciximab, 349, 379*t*
Abel, John Jacob, 3
Abelcet. *See* **Amphotericin B**
Abilify. *See* Aripiprazole
abortion, pharmacological, drugs for:
    carboprost tromethamine, 703*t*, 704
    dinoprostone, 703*t*, 704
    methotrexate with misoprostol, 703*t*, 704
    mifepristone with misoprostol, 703*t*, 704
Abreva. *See* Docosanol
absence (petit mal) seizure, 168*t*, 169*t*, 172
absorption:
    definition, 37
    factors affecting, 38, 39*f*
    mechanisms, 37–38, 38*f*
    in older adults, 73
    in pregnancy, 64
acamprosate calcium, 108
acarbose, 687*t*, 688
Accolate. *See* **Zafirlukast**
Accretropin. *See* Somatotropin
Accupril. *See* Quinapril
Accuretic, 302*t*
Accutane. *See* Isotretinoin
ACE inhibitors. *See* ANGIOTENSIN-CONVERTING ENZYME (ACE) INHIBITORS
acebutolol:
    actions and uses, 136*t*
    for angina and myocardial infarction, 343*t*
    for dysrhythmias, 360*t*
    effects during breastfeeding, 67*t*
    for hypertension, 315*t*
Aceon. *See* Perindopril
acetaminophen, 472*t*
    actions and uses, 472*t*

administration alerts, 472*t*
adverse effects, 228*t*, 472*t*
alternation with ibuprofen in children, 472*t*
in cold/allergy combination drugs, 576*t*
ethnic/racial considerations, 473*t*
interactions, 472*t*
mechanisms of action, 229
overdose treatment, 472*t*
pharmacokinetics, 472*t*
route and adult dose, 228*t*
Acetazolam. *See* Acetazolamide
acetazolamide:
    for glaucoma, 770*t*, 773
    for pancreatitis, 635
    for renal failure, 424, 425*t*
acetic acid and hydrocortisone, 776*t*
acetylation, 81
acetylcholine (Ach):
    blockers. *See* NEUROMUSCULAR BLOCKERS
    physiology, 130, 139
    receptors. *See* Cholinergic receptors
acetylcholinesterase (AchE), 131, 264
acetylcholinesterase inhibitors. *See* CHOLINERGICS (PARASYMPATHOMIMETICS), INDIRECT ACTING
acetylcysteine, 123*t*, 472*t*, 583*t*
acetylsalicylic acid. *See* **Aspirin**
acetyltransferase, 81, 81*t*
Achromycin. *See* **Tetracycline**
acid–base imbalance, 440, 440*f*. See also Acidosis; Alkalosis
acidophilus, 100*t*, 623
acidosis:
    causes, 420*t*, 441*t*
    definition, 440, 440*f*
    pharmacotherapy, 440, 441*t*
AcipHex. *See* Rabeprazole
acitretin, 762*t*
Aclovate. *See* Alclometasone
acne tardive, 755
acne vulgaris:
    characteristics, 755
    Nursing Process Focus
        assessment, 758*t*
        evaluation of outcome criteria, 759*t*
        implementation
            interventions and rationales, 758–59*t*
            patient and family education, 758–59*t*
        planning: patient goals and expected outcomes, 758*t*
        potential nursing diagnoses, 758*t*
    pharmacotherapy
        adapalene, 756, 756*t*
        azelaic acid, 756*t*

benzoyl peroxide, 756, 756*t*
doxycycline. *See* Doxycycline
erythromycin, 756
ethinyl estradiol. *See* Ethinyl estradiol
isotretinoin, 756*t*
sulfacetamide, 756*t*
tazarotene, 756*t*
tetracycline. *See* **Tetracycline**
tretinoin. *See* **Tretinoin**
Acova. *See* Argatroban
acquired immune deficiency syndrome (AIDS), 528. *See also* HIV-AIDS
acquired resistance, 481–82, 482*f*
acromegaly, 659*t*, 660
Actaea racemosa. See Black cohosh
ACTH. *See* Adrenocorticotropic hormone; Corticotropin
ActHIB. *See* Haemophilus type B conjugate vaccine
Acticin. *See* **Permethrin**
Actifed. *See* Pseudoephedrine
Actifed Cold and Allergy, 576*t*
Actifed Cold and Allergy tablets, 576*t*
action potentials, 355
Actiq. *See* Fentanyl
Activase. *See* **Alteplase**
activated charcoal, 122
activated clotting time, 372*t*
activated partial thromboplastin time (aPTT), 371, 372*t*
active immunity, 449, 451*f*
active transport, 37
Activella. *See* Ethinyl estradiol/ norethindrone acetate
Actonel. *See* Risedronate
ACTOplus met. *See* Pioglitazone/ metformin
Actos. *See* Pioglitazone
Actron. *See* Ketoprofen
acute gouty arthritis, 744
acute pain, 219
acute radiation syndrome, 120
acyclovir, 539*t*
    actions and uses, 539*t*
    administration alerts, 539*t*
    adverse effects, 538*t*, 539*t*
    interactions, 539*t*
    pharmacokinetics, 539*t*
    route and adult dose, 538*t*
    for viral skin lesions, 752
Adalat. *See* **Nifedipine**
adalimumab, 625
Adamsite, 121*t*
adapalene, 756, 756*t*
Adapin. *See* Doxepin
ADD (attention-deficit disorder), 197
Adderall. *See* D- and L-amphetamine racemic mixture

Naprelan. *See* Naproxen
Naprosyn. *See* Naproxen
naproxen, 228*t*, 467*t*
naproxen sodium, 228*t*
naratriptan, 233*t*
Narcan. *See* **Naloxone hydrochloride**
narcotic, 220, 221
narcotic analgesics. *See* OPIOID (NARCOTIC) ANALGESICS
Nardil. *See* **Phenelzine**
Naropin. *See* Ropivacaine
narrow-spectrum antibiotics, 482. *See also* ANTIBACTERIALS
narrow-spectrum penicillins. *See* PENICILLINS
Nasacort AQ. *See* Triamcinolone
nasal drug administration, 25, 26*t*, 28*f*
Nasalide. *See* Flunisolide
Nasarel. *See* Flunisolide
Nascobal. *See* **Vitamin B₁₂ (cyanocobalamin)**
nasogastric (NG) tube, 23*t*, 24
Nasonex. *See* Mometasone
natalizumab, 625
nateglinide, 687*t*
National Cholesterol Education Program (NCEP), 285
National Coordinating Council for Medication Error Reporting and Prevention (NCC MERP), 86*f*, 87, 89*f*
National Formulary (NF), 5, 6*f*
Native Americans:
    mental illness treatment, 205*t*
Natrecor. *See* Nesiritide
Naturacil. *See* **Psyllium mucilloid**
Natural Health Products Directorate (NHPD), 9
natural penicillins, 484*t*
nausea, 625. *See also* Nausea and vomiting
nausea and vomiting:
    pathophysiology, 628–29
    pharmacotherapy. *See* ANTIEMETICS
Navane. *See* Thiothixene
NDA review, 7
NE. *See* **Norepinephrine**
Nebcin. *See* Tobramycin
nebulizer, 591, 591*f*
NebuPent. *See* Pentamidine
nedocromil sodium, 596*t*
nefazodone, 186*t*, 189
negative formulary list, 14
negative inotropic agents, 325
negative symptoms, 204
NegGram. *See* Nalidixic acid
Neisseria gonorrhoeae, 480*t*
Neisseria meningitidis, 480*t*
nelarabine, 555*t*
nelfinavir, 530*t*
Nembutal. *See* Pentobarbital sodium
Neoloid. *See* Castor oil
neomycin, 490, 490*t*

neomycin cream/ointment, 752
neomycin with polymyxin B cream/ointment, 752
neoplasm, 548
Neoral. *See* **Cyclosporine**
neostigmine, 123*t*, 139, 140*t*
Neo-Synephrine. *See* **Oxymetazoline; Phenylephrine**
nephron, 418, 419*f*
nephrotoxic drugs, 420*t*
Neptazane. *See* Methazolamide
nerve agents, 120, 121*t*
nerve block anesthesia, 240*f*, 241*t*
Nesacaine. *See* Chloroprocaine
nesiritide, 328*t*, 334
Nestrex. *See* Vitamin B₆
Neulasta. *See* Pegfilgrastim
Neumega. *See* Oprelvekin
Neupogen. *See* **Filgrastim**
neural tube defects, 644*t*
neurofibrillary tangles, 263, 265*f*
neurogenic shock, 407*t*
neurohypophysis, 657
NEUROKININ RECEPTOR ANTAGONIST:
    aprepitant, 629, 630*t*
neuroleptanalgesia, 248
neuroleptic malignant syndrome, 187*t*, 188*t*, 207*t*, 473
neuroleptics, 206. *See also* ANTIPSYCHOTICS
NEUROMUSCULAR BLOCKERS:
    depolarizing
        succinylcholine. *See* **Succinylcholine**
    as general anesthesia adjunct, 252
    nondepolarizing
        mivacurium, 252
        tubocurarine, 252, 252*t*
Neurontin. *See* Gabapentin
neuropathic pain, 219
Neutra-Phos. *See* Potassium and sodium phosphates
Neutra-Phos-K. *See* Potassium and sodium phosphates
Neutrogena. *See* Salicylic acid
nevirapine, 530*t*
    administration alerts, 533*t*
New Drug Application (NDA), 6*f*, 7
Nexavar. *See* Sorafenib
Nexium. *See* Esomeprazole
NF (*National Formulary*), 5, 6*f*
NHPD (Natural Health Products Directorate), 9
Niac. *See* Vitamin B₃
niacin. *See* Vitamin B₃
nicardipine, 307, 307*t*, 319
Nicobid. *See* Vitamin B₃
Nicolar. *See* Vitamin B₃
nicotine:
    characteristics, 111
    effects, 111
    toxicity signs, 106*t*
    withdrawal symptoms, 106*t*
nicotinic acid. *See* Vitamin B₃
nicotinic receptors, 131, 131*t*

nifedipine, 308*t*
    actions and uses, 307, 308*t*
    administration alerts, 308*t*
    adverse effects, 233*t*, 307*t*, 308*t*, 708*t*
    interactions, 308*t*
    mechanisms of action, 307
    overdose treatment, 308*t*
    pharmacokinetics, 308*t*
    for specific conditions
        angina and myocardial infarction, 343*t*
        hypertension, 307*t*
        migraine, 233*t*
        as tocolytic, 708*t*
nifurtimox, 521*t*
Nilandron. *See* Nilutamide
Nilstat. *See* **Nystatin**
nilutamide, 561*t*
Nimbex. *See* Cisatracurium
nimodipine, 233*t*
Nimotop. *See* Nimodipine
nisoldipine, 307*t*
Nitro-Bid. *See* **Nitroglycerin**
Nitro-Dur. *See* **Nitroglycerin**
nitrofurantoin, 495*t*
nitrogen mustard, 121*t*
NITROGEN MUSTARDS. *See also* ALKYLATING AGENTS
    bendamustine, 555*t*
    chlorambucil, 555*t*
    cyclophosphamide. *See* **Cyclophosphamide**
    estramustine, 555*t*
    ifosfamide, 555*t*
    mechlorethamine, 555*t*
    melphalan, 555*t*
nitroglycerin, 344*t*
    actions and uses, 344*t*
    administration alerts, 344*t*
    adverse effects, 343*t*, 344*t*
    interactions, 344*t*
    nursing process focus
        assessment, 344–45*t*
        evaluation of outcome criteria, 346*t*
        implementation
            interventions and rationales, 345–46*t*
            patient and family education, 345–46*t*
        planning: patient goals and expected outcomes, 345*t*
        potential nursing diagnoses, 344–45*t*
    overdose treatment, 344*t*
    pharmacokinetics, 344*t*
    route and adult dose, 343*t*
    in suspected myocardial infarction, 350
Nitropress. *See* Nitroprusside
nitroprusside, 318*t*, 319
NitroQuick. *See* **Nitroglycerin**
NITROSOUREAS. *See also* ALKYLATING AGENTS
    carmustine, 553, 555*t*
    lomustine, 555*t*
    streptozocin, 555*t*

Special Features

Avoiding Medication Errors

Home & Community Considerations

Complementary and Alternative Therapies

Treating the Diverse Patient

RESEARCH SHOWS

SPECIAL CONSIDERATIONS

NURSING PROCESS FOCUS

PROTOTYPE DRUG